Pharmacology and Physiology in Anesthetic Practice

Second Edition

Robert K. Stoelting, M.D.

Professor and Chairman
Department of Anesthesia
Indiana University School of Medicine
Indianapolis, Indiana

Pharmacology and Physiology in Anesthetic Practice

Second Edition

J.B. LIPPINCOTT COMPANY

Philadelphia   New York   London   Hagerstown

Acquisitions Editor: *Mary K. Smith*
Coordinating Editorial Assistant: *Anne Geyer*
Manuscript Editor: *Anne-Adele Wight*
Indexer: *Victoria Boyle*
Art Director: *Susan Hermansen*
Designer: *Doug Smock*
Production Manager: *Helen Ewan*
Production Coordinator: *Nannette Winski*
Compositor: *Graphic Sciences Corporation*
Printer/Binder: *R. R. Donnelley & Sons Company*

2nd Edition

6 5 4 3 2 1

Library of Congress Cataloging-in-Publication Data

Stoelting, Robert K.
    Pharmacology and physiology in anesthetic practice.
    Includes bibliographies and indexes.
    1. Anesthetics—Physiological effect. 2. Anesthesia.
3. Human physiology. 4. Pharmacology. I. Title.
[DNLM: 1. Anesthetics—pharmacodynamics. 2.
Physiology. QV 81 S872p]
RD81.S87   1987   615'.781   86-21017
ISBN 0-397-51129-9

The author and publisher have exerted every effort to
ensure that drug selection and dosage set forth in this
text are in accord with current recommendations and
practice at the time of publication. However, in view of
ongoing research, changes in government regulations,
and the constant flow of information relating to drug
therapy and drug reactions, the reader is urged to check
the package insert for each drug for any change in
indications and dosage and for added warnings and
precautions. This is particularly important when the
recommended agent is a new or infrequently employed
drug.

PREFACE

This second edition of *Pharmacology and Physiology in Anesthetic Practice* is intended to meet the same goals as the first edition—to provide students as well as practicing anesthesiologists with an in-depth but concise and current presentation of those aspects of pharmacology and physiology that are relevant either directly or indirectly to the perioperative anesthetic management of patients. Frequent revisions of a textbook related to pharmacology are necessary to keep pace with the continued evolution of understanding of drug actions, their benefits and risks. The *Pharmacology* section of this second edition provides the most current available information on the pharmacology of drugs relevant to the anesthesiologist's practice, as well as introducing several new drugs not discussed in the first edition. The *Physiology* section has been completely rewritten in the second edition to better describe those aspects of physiology uniquely relevant to anesthesiologists.

As with the first edition, special accolades for preparation of this second edition go to my secretary, Deanna Walker, for her skillful preparation of the many revisions. Again, Ellyn Traub receives my thanks for her skillful preparation of new art work. Nancy L. Mullins and Anne Geyer from J. B. Lippincott provided constant encouragement and direction in guiding the second edition to completion.

ROBERT K. STOELTING, M.D.

CONTENTS

Section 2
PHYSIOLOGY

Pharmacology and Physiology in Anesthetic Practice

Second Edition

Pharmacokinetics and Pharmacodynamics of Injected and Inhaled Drugs

INTRODUCTION

Pharmacokinetics is the quantitative study of the absorption, distribution, metabolism, and excretion of injected drugs and their metabolites. As such, pharmacokinetics may be viewed as *what the body does to a drug*. Combined with the dose of drug administered, pharmacokinetics determines the concentration of drug at its sites of action (receptors) and, thus, the intensity of the drug's effects with time. Pharmacokinetics may also determine variability in drug responses between patients, reflecting individual differences in absorption, distribution and elimination (Wood, 1989). Selection and adjustment of drug dosage schedules and interpretation of measured plasma concentrations of drugs are facilitated by an understanding of pharmacokinetic principles.

Pharmacodynamics is the study of the intrinsic sensitivity or responsiveness of receptors to a drug and the mechanisms by which these effects occur. As such, pharmacodynamics may be viewed as *what a drug does to the body*. Structure-activity relationships link the actions of drugs to their chemical structure and facilitate the design of drugs with more desirable pharmacologic properties. Intrinsic sensitivity of receptors is de-termined by measuring plasma concentrations of a drug required to evoke specific pharmacologic responses. Variability exists in the intrinsic sensitivity of receptors among patients. As a result, at similar plasma concentrations of drug, some patients show a therapeutic response, others show no response, and in others, toxicity develops.

Stereoisomers are nonsuperimposable mirror images of the same molecule. Such stereo-isomers are defined as enantiomers, and a 50:50 mixture of enantiomers is termed racemic. Drug enantiomers have identical physical properties, yet their affinities for receptors, tissues, and protein binding sites often differ. Likewise, distribution of drug in the body and metabolism often differ between enantiomers. As a result, pharmacologic effects of isomers of racemic mixtures of drugs (ketamine, epinephrine, atropine, propranolol) may be different.

DESCRIPTION OF DRUG RESPONSE

Hyperreactive is the term used for people in whom an unusually low dose of drug produces its expected pharmacologic effects. *Hypersensitive* is the term usually reserved for people who are allergic (sensitized) to a drug. *Hyporeactive* describes persons who require exceptionally large doses of drug to evoke expected pharmacologic effects. Hyporeactivity acquired from chronic exposure to a drug is better termed *tolerance*. Cross-tolerance frequently develops between drugs of different classes that produce similar pharmacologic effects (alcohol and inhaled anesthetics). Tolerance that develops acutely within only a few doses of a drug, such as thiopental, is termed *tachyphylaxis*. The most important factor in the development of tolerance to drugs such as opioids, barbiturates, and alcohol is neuronal adaptation, referred to as cellular tolerance. Other mechanisms of tolerance may include enzyme induction and depletion of neurotransmitters caused by sustained stimulation. Immunity is present when hyporeactivity is due to formation of antibodies. Idiosyncrasy is present when an unusual effect of a drug occurs in a small percentage of patients regardless of the dose of drug. More appropriately, unusual effects of drugs should be described precisely in terms of their documented or likely mechanisms, such as allergy or genetic differences.

An *additive* effect means that a second drug acting with the first drug will produce an effect equal to an algebraic summation. For example, the anesthetic effects of two different inhaled anesthetics are additive (see the section entitled "Minimum Alveolar Concentration"). Synergistic effect means that two drugs interact to produce an effect greater than an algebraic summation. Antagonism means that two drugs interact to produce an effect less than an algebraic summation.

A drug that activates a receptor by binding to the receptor is called an *agonist*. An *antagonist* is a drug that binds to the receptor without activating the receptor and at the same time prevents an agonist from stimulating the receptor. Competitive antagonism is present when increasing concentrations of the antagonist progressively inhibit the response to an unchanging concentration of agonist. Noncompetitive antagonism is present when, after administration of an antagonist, even high concentrations of agonist cannot completely overcome the antagonism.

Termination of drug effect is by metabolism, excretion, or redistribution. Redistribution is a factor in terminating drug effect primarily when a highly lipid-soluble drug is administered intravenously.

PHARMACOKINETICS OF INJECTED DRUGS

Pharmacokinetics of injected drugs usually is defined initially in healthy adults with a low fat-to-lean body ratio. Conversely, drugs are most likely to be administered to patients with chronic diseases (renal failure, cirrhosis of the liver, cardiac failure) at various extremes of age, hydration, and nutrition. General anesthesia and surgery may alter pharmacokinetics of injected drugs relative to the awake state because of alterations in renal blood flow, hepatic blood flow, and hepatic enzyme activity. Drug-induced changes in peripheral blood flow may further alter perioperative distribution of injected anesthetics. Commonly measured pharmacokinetic parameters of injected drugs are bioavailability, clearance, volume of distribution (Vd), and elimination half-time.

Compartmental Models

Pharmacokinetics of injected drugs has been simplified by considering the body to be composed of a number of compartments representing theoretical spaces with calculated volumes. A two-compartment model can be used to illustrate basic concepts of pharmacokinetics that also apply to more complex models (Fig. 1-1) (Stanski and Watkins, 1982). In the two-compartment model, drug is introduced by intravenous injection directly into the central compartment. Drug subse-

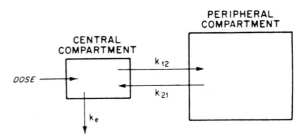

FIGURE 1–1. A two-compartment pharmacokinetic model as derived from a biexponential plasma decay curve (see Fig. 1–2). K_{12} and K_{21} are the rate constants that characterize intercompartmental transfer of drugs, and Ke is the rate constant for overall drug elimination from the body (From Stanski DR, Watkins WD. Drug disposition in anesthesia. New York, Grune and Stratton, 1982; with permission).

quently distributes to the peripheral compartment only to return eventually to the central compartment where clearance from the body occurs.

The central compartment includes intravascular fluid and highly perfused tissues (lungs, heart, brain, kidneys, liver) into which uptake of drug is rapid. In adults, these highly perfused tissues receive almost 75% of the cardiac output but represent about 10% of the body mass. This central compartment is defined only in terms of its apparent volume, which is calculated and does not necessarily correspond to actual anatomic volumes (see the section entitled "Volume of Distribution"). Likewise, the peripheral compartment (there may be more than one) is defined in terms of its calculated volume. A large calculated volume for the peripheral compartment suggests extensive uptake of drug by those tissues that constitute that peripheral compartment. The rate of drug transfer (rate constant, K) between compartments (intercompartmental clearance) may decrease with aging, resulting in greater plasma concentrations of drugs such as thiopental in elderly patients despite identical injected doses and similar Vd in young adults and elderly patients (see Fig. 4-5). (Avram et al, 1990; Stanski and Maitre, 1990). Any residual drug present in the peripheral compartment at the time of repeat intravenous injection will diminish the effect of distributive processes on the reduction of the plasma concentration and lead to exaggerated (cumulative) effects of the repeat dose. The degree of cumulative drug effect can be calculated knowing the drug's dosing interval and elimination half-time.

Plasma Concentration Curves

A graphic plot of the logarithm of the decrease in the plasma concentration of a drug vs time following a rapid (bolus) intravenous injection characterizes the distribution (alpha) and elimination phases (beta) of that drug (Fig. 1-2) (Stanski and Watkins, 1982). Logarithms provide a convenient means for plotting the large range in plasma concentrations present after intravenous injection of a drug. In addition, logarithms are appropriate for depiction of the first-order kinetics characteristic of the distribution and elimination of most drugs.

The distribution phase of the plasma concentration curve begins immediately after intravenous injection of a drug and reflects that drug's

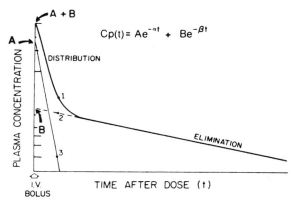

FIGURE 1–2. Schematic depiction of the decline in the plasma concentration of drug with time following rapid intravenous injection into the central compartment (see Fig. 1–1). Two distinct phases (biexponential) that characterize this curve are designated the distribution (alpha) and elimination (beta) phases (From Stanski DR, Watkins WD. Drug disposition in anesthesia. New York, Grune and Stratton, 1982; with permission.)

distribution from the circulation (central compartment) to peripheral tissues (peripheral compartments) (Figs. 1-1 and 1-2) (Stanski and Watkins, 1982). The elimination phase of the plasma concentration curve follows the initial distribution phase and is characterized by a more gradual decline in the drug's plasma concentration (Fig. 1-2) (Stanski and Watkins, 1982). This gradual decline reflects the drug's elimination from the circulation (central compartment) by renal and hepatic clearance mechanisms.

Elimination Half-Time

The rate of drug elimination is defined by the slope of the line representing the log plasma concentration of drug plotted against time during the elimination phase. *Elimination half-time* is the time necessary for the plasma concentration of drug to decline 50% during the elimination phase. Elimination half-time of a drug is directly proportional to its Vd and inversely proportional to its clearance. For this reason, renal or hepatic disease that alters Vd and/or clearance will alter the elimination half-time. Conversely, elimination half-time is independent of the dose of drug administered.

Elimination half-life, in contrast to elimination half-time, defines the time necessary to eliminate 50% of the drug from the body following its rapid intravenous injection. Elimination half-time and elimination half-life are not equal when the decrease in the drug's plasma concentration does not parallel its elimination from the body. The amount of drug remaining in the body is related to the number of elimination half-times that have elapsed (Table 1-1). For example, if 50% of a drug is eliminated in 10 minutes, another 10 minutes will be required for elimination of one-half of the remaining drug. About five elimination half-times are required for nearly total (96.9%) elimination of the drug from the body. For this reason, drug accumulation is predictable if dosing intervals are less than this period of time. Drug accumulation continues until the rate of its elimination equals the rate of its administration. As with drug elimination, the time necessary for a drug to achieve a steady-state plasma concentration (Cpss) with intermittent dosing is about five elimination half-times.

Route of Administration and Systemic Absorption of Drugs

The choice of route of administration for a drug should be based on an appreciation of factors that influence the systemic absorption of drugs. The systemic absorption rate of a drug determines its intensity and duration of action. Changes in the systemic absorption rate may necessitate an ad-

Table 1–1
Relationship of Half-Times to Amount of Drug Eliminated

Number of Half-Times	Fraction of Initial Amount Remaining	Percent of Initial Amount Eliminated
0	1	0
1	$1/2$	50
2	$1/4$	75
3	$1/8$	87.5
4	$1/16$	93.8
5	$1/32$	96.9
6	$1/64$	98.4

justment in the dose or time interval between repeated drug doses.

Systemic absorption, regardless of the route of drug administration, depends on the drug's solubility. Local conditions at the site of absorption alter solubility, particularly in the gastrointestinal tract. Blood flow to the site of absorption is also important in the rapidity of absorption. For example, increased blood flow evoked by rubbing or applying heat at the injection site enhances systemic absorption, whereas decreased blood flow owing to vasoconstriction impedes drug absorption. Finally, the area of the absorbing surface available for drug absorption is an important determinant of drug entry into the circulation.

Oral Administration

Oral administration of a drug is the most convenient and economic route of administration. Disadvantages of the oral route of administration include (1) emesis because of irritation of the gastrointestinal mucosa by the drug, (2) destruction of the drug by digestive enzymes or acidic gastric fluid, and (3) irregularities in absorption in the presence of food or other drugs. Furthermore, drugs may be metabolized by enzymes or bacteria in the gastrointestinal tract before systemic absorption can occur.

Following oral administration, the onset of drug effect is largely determined by the rate and extent of absorption from the gastrointestinal tract. The principal site of drug absorption after oral administration is the small intestine, reflecting the large surface area of this portion of the gastrointestinal tract. Changes in the pH of gastrointestinal fluid that favor the existence of a drug in its nonionized (lipid-soluble) fraction thus favor systemic absorption. Drugs (such as aspirin) that exist as weak acids become highly ionized in the alkaline environment of the small intestine, but absorption is still great because of the large surface area. Furthermore, absorption also occurs in the stomach, where the fluid is acidic.

FIRST-PASS EFFECT. Drugs absorbed from the gastrointestinal tract enter the portal venous blood and thus pass through the liver before entering the systemic circulation for delivery to tissue receptors (Fig. 1-3). This is known as the *first-pass*

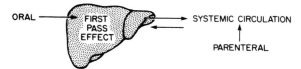

FIGURE 1–3. Drugs administered orally are absorbed from the gastrointestinal tract into the portal venous blood and pass through the liver (first-pass hepatic effect) before entering the systemic circulation for distribution to receptors. Conversely, intravenous administration of drugs allows rapid access to the systemic circulation without an initial impact of metabolism in the liver.

hepatic effect, and for drugs that undergo extensive hepatic extraction and metabolism (propranolol, lidocaine), this is the reason for large differences between effective oral and intravenous doses.

Oral Transmucosal Administration

The sublingual or buccal route of administration permits a rapid onset of drug effect, since it bypasses the liver and thus prevents the first-pass hepatic effect on the initial plasma concentration of drug. For example, venous drainage from the sublingual area is into the superior vena cava. Evidence of the value of bypassing the first-pass hepatic effect is the efficacy of sublingual nitroglycerin. Conversely, oral administration of nitroglycerin is ineffective because extensive first-pass hepatic metabolism prevents achievement of a therapeutic plasma concentration. Buccal administration is an alternative to sublingual placement of drug, being better tolerated and less likely to stimulate salivation. The nasal mucosa also provides an effective absorption surface for certain drugs.

Transdermal Administration

Transdermal administration of drugs provides sustained therapeutic plasma concentrations of the drug and decreases the likelihood of loss of therapeutic efficacy owing to peaks and valleys associated with conventional intermittent drug injections. This route of administration is devoid of the complexity of continuous intravenous infusion techniques, and the low incidence of side effects because of the small doses used contributes to high patient compliance. Characteristics of drugs that favor predictable transdermal absorption include (1) combined water and lipid solubility, (2) molecular weight less than 1000, (3) pH 5 to 9 in a saturated aqueous solution, (4) absence of histamine-releasing effects, and (5) dose requirements less than 10 mg·24 h^{-1}. Scopolamine, fentanyl, clonidine, and nitroglycerin are examples of drugs that are available in transdermal delivery systems (see Chapters 3, 10, 15, and 16). Unfortunately, sustained plasma concentrations provided by transdermal absorption of scopolamine and nitroglycerin may result in tolerance and loss of therapeutic effect.

It is likely that transdermal absorption of drugs initially occurs along sweat ducts and hair follicles that function as diffusion shunts. The rate-limiting step in transdermal absorption of drugs is diffusion across the stratum corneum of the epidermis. Differences in the thickness and chemistry of the stratum corneum are reflected in the skin's permeability. For example, skin may be 10 to 20 μm thick on the back and abdomen compared with 400 to 600 μm on the palmar surfaces on the hands. Likewise, skin permeation studies have shown substantial regional differences for systemic absorption of scopolamine. The postauricular zone, because of its thin epidermal layer and somewhat higher temperature, is the only area that is sufficiently permeable for predictable and sustained absorption of scopolamine. The stratum corneum sloughs and regenerates at a rate such that 7 days of adhesion appears to be the duration limit for one application of a transdermal system. Contact dermatitis at the site of transdermal patch application may occur in a significant number of patients.

Rectal Administration

Drugs injected into the proximal rectum are absorbed into the superior hemorrhoidal veins and thence transported via the portal system to the liver (first-pass hepatic effect), where they are exposed to metabolism before entering the systemic circulation. On the other hand, drugs absorbed from a low rectal injection site reach the general circulation without first passing through the liver. These factors, in a large part, explain the unpredictable responses that follow rectal administration of drugs. Furthermore, drugs may cause irritation of the rectal mucosa.

Parenteral Administration

Parenteral administration may be required to ensure absorption of the active form of the drug and is the only acceptable route of administration in an unconscious or otherwise uncooperative patient. Systemic absorption after subcutaneous or intramuscular injection is usually more rapid and predictable than after oral administration. Rate of systemic absorption is limited by the surface area of the absorbing capillary membranes and by solubility of the drug in interstitial fluid. Large aqueous channels in vascular endothelium account for the unimpeded diffusion of drug molecules, regardless of their lipid solubility.

The desired concentration of drug in the blood can be achieved more rapidly and precisely by the intravenous route of administration, which circumvents those factors that limit systemic absorption by other routes. Irritant drugs are administered more comfortably by the intravenous route because blood vessel walls are relatively insensitive and the injected drug is rapidly diluted, especially if the drug is injected into a large forearm vein.

Distribution of Drugs Following Systemic Absorption

Following systemic absorption of a drug, the highly perfused tissues (heart, brain, kidneys, liver) receive a disproportionately large amount of the total dose (Table 1-2). Subsequently, as the plasma concentration of drug decreases below that in highly perfused tissues, drug leaves these tissues to be redistributed to less well-perfused sites, such as skeletal muscles and fat (Table 1-2). For example, awakening after a single dose of

Table 1-2
Body Tissue Compartments

	Body Mass (percent of 70-kg adult)	Blood Flow (percent of cardiac output)
Vessel-rich group	10	75
Muscle group	50	19
Fat group	20	6
Vessel-poor group	20	<1

Table 1-3
Rate and Capacity of Tissue Uptake of Drugs

Determinants of Tissue Uptake of Drug
  Blood flow
  Concentration gradient
  Blood-brain barrier
  Physicochemical properties of drug
    Ionization
    Lipid solubility
    Protein binding

Determinants of Capacity of Tissue to Store Drug
  Solubility
  Tissue mass
  Binding to macromolecules
  pH

thiopental principally reflects redistribution of drug from the brain to less well-perfused tissues sites such as fat and skeletal muscles, where thiopental is considered to be pharmacologically inactive.

Uptake of a drug by tissues is principally determined by tissue blood flow if the drug in question can penetrate membranes rapidly. The concentration gradient for the diffusible fraction of drug (nonionized, lipid soluble, and unbound to protein) determines both the rate and direction of net transfer between plasma and the tissue. Initially, after administration of a drug, the concentration gradient favors drug passage from plasma into tissues. With continuing elimination of drug, the plasma concentration declines below that in tissues, and drug leaves tissues to reenter the circulation. Therefore, a tissue that accumulates drug preferentially may act as a reservoir to maintain the plasma concentration and thus prolong its duration of action. Similarly, repeated or large doses of drug may saturate inactive tissue sites, thus negating the role of these tissues in providing an inactive tissue site for redistribution. When this occurs, the duration of action of drugs such as thiopental and fentanyl is likely to be prolonged as waning of drug effect now depends on metabolism rather than redistribution.

Capacity of tissues to accept drug depends largely on the drug's solubility in the tissue and the mass of the tissue (Table 1-3). For example, a drug could exhibit limited solubility in skeletal muscles, but the large mass of this tissue (about 50% of the body weight) would exert a dominant role in distribution of the drug.

Uptake into the Lungs

The lungs have important functions in pharmacokinetics as reflected by uptake of injected drugs, especially basic lipophilic amines (pK greater than 8.0), into this tissue. For example, first-pass pulmonary uptake of the initial dose of lidocaine, propranolol, fentanyl, and meperidine is 65%, 75%, 75%, and 65%, respectively (Roerig et al, 1987). This degree of uptake into the lungs will influence the peak arterial concentrations of these drugs and serve as a reservoir to release drug back into the systemic circulation.

Central Nervous System Distribution

Distribution of ionized water-soluble drugs to the central nervous system from the circulation is restricted because of the limited permeability characteristics of brain capillaries known as the *blood-brain barrier.* Conversely, cerebral blood flow is the only limitation to permeation of the central nervous system by nonionized lipid-soluble drugs. It is important to recognize that the blood-brain barrier is subject to change and can be overcome by administration of large doses of drug. Furthermore, acute head injury and arterial hypoxemia may be associated with disruption of the blood-brain barrier.

Volume of Distribution

Volume of distribution (Vd) of a drug is a mathematical expression of the sum of the apparent volumes of the compartments that constitute the compartmental model (Fig. 1-1) (Stanski and Watkins, 1982). As such, this value depicts the distribution characteristics of a drug in the body. Volume of distribution is calculated as the dose of drug administered intravenously divided by the resulting plasma concentration of drug before elimination starts. As such, Vd is influenced by physicochemical characteristics of the drug, including (1) lipid solubility, (2) binding to plasma proteins, and (3) molecular size. Binding to plasma proteins and poor lipid solubility limit passage of drug to tissues, thus maintaining a high concentration in the plasma and a small calculated Vd. Examples of poorly lipid-soluble drugs with a Vd similar to extracellular fluid volume are the nondepolarizing neuromuscular blocking drugs. A lipid-soluble drug that is highly concentrated in tissues with a resulting low plasma concentration will have a calculated Vd that exceeds total body water. Examples of lipid-soluble drugs with a Vd that exceeds total body water are thiopental and diazepam.

Ionization

Most drugs are weak acids or bases that are present in solutions as both ionized and nonionized molecules. Solubility characteristics of the ionized and nonionized molecules determine the ease with which drugs may diffuse through lipid components of cell membranes. This diffusion is particularly important because drugs are often too large to pass through membrane channels.

Characteristics of Ionized and Nonionized Molecules

The nonionized drug molecule is usually lipid soluble and can diffuse across lipid cell membranes that constitute the blood-brain barrier, renal tubular epithelium, gastrointestinal epithelium, and hepatocytes (Table 1-4). As a result, this fraction of drug is pharmacologically active, undergoes reabsorption across renal tubules, is absorbed from the gastrointestinal tract, and is susceptible to hepatic metabolism. Conversely, the ionized fraction is poorly lipid soluble and cannot penetrate lipid cell membranes easily (Table 1-4). Ionization causes the drug to be repelled from portions of cells with similar charges. A high degree of ionization thus impairs absorption of drug from the gastrointestinal tract, limits access to drug-metabolizing enzymes in

Table 1-4
Characteristics of Nonionized and Ionized Drug Molecules

	Nonionized	*Ionized*
Pharmacologic effect	Active	Inactive
Solubility	Lipids	Water
Cross lipid barriers (gastrointestinal tract, blood-brain barrier, placenta)	Yes	No
Renal excretion	No	Yes
Hepatic metabolism	Yes	No

the hepatocytes, and facilitates renal excretion of unchanged drug, since reabsorption across the renal tubular epithelium is unlikely.

Determinants of Degree of Ionization

The degree of ionization of a drug is a function of its dissociation constant (pK) and the pH of the surrounding fluid. When the pK and pH are identical, 50% of the drug exists in the ionized form. Small changes in pH can result in large changes in the extent of ionization, especially if the pH and pK values are similar. Acidic drugs, such as barbiturates, tend to be highly ionized at an alkaline pH, whereas basic drugs, such as opioids and local anesthetics, are highly ionized at an acid pH.

Ion Trapping

A concentration difference of total drug can develop on two sides of a membrane that separates fluids with different pHs (Fig. 1-4) (Hug, 1978). As a result of this pH difference, the degree of ionization of a drug is also different on each side of the membrane. The nonionized lipid-soluble fraction of drug equilibrates across cell membranes, but the total concentration of drug is very different on each side of the membrane because

of the impact of pH on the fraction of drug that exists in the ionized form. This is an important consideration because one fraction of the drug may be more pharmacologically active than the other fraction.

Systemic administration of a weak base, such as an opioid, can result in accumulation of ionized drug (ion trapping) in the acid environment of the stomach. A similar phenomenon occurs in the transfer of basic drugs, such as local anesthetics, across the placenta from mother to fetus where the fetal pH is lower than maternal pH. The lipid-soluble nonionized fraction of local anesthetic crosses the placenta and is converted to the poorly lipid-soluble ionized fraction in the more acidic environment of the fetus. The ionized fraction in the fetus cannot easily cross the placenta to the maternal circulation and thus is effectively trapped in the fetus. At the same time, conversion of the nonionized to ionized fraction maintains a gradient for continued passage of local anesthetic into the fetus. The resulting accumulation of local anesthetic in the fetus is accentuated by the acidosis that accompanies fetal distress.

Protein Binding

A variable amount of most drugs is bound to plasma proteins that include albumin, alpha-1 acid glycoprotein, and lipoproteins (Wood, 1986). Most acidic drugs bind to albumin, whereas basic drugs select alpha-1 acid glycoprotein. Protein binding has an important effect on distribution of drugs because only the free or unbound fraction is readily available to cross cell membranes. Furthermore, Vd of a drug is inversely related to protein binding. For example, high protein binding limits passage of drug into tissues, thus resulting in high drug plasma concentrations and a small calculated Vd. Clearance of a drug is also influenced by protein binding because it is the unbound fraction in the plasma that has ready access to hepatic drug-metabolizing enzymes, and it is also this unbound fraction of drug that undergoes glomerular filtration.

The drug-protein complex is maintained by a weak bond (ionic, hydrogen, or van der Walls bond) and can dissociate when the plasma concentration of drug declines as a result of hepatic

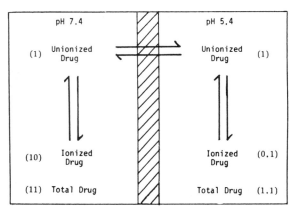

FIGURE 1–4. A concentration difference of total drug can develop on two sides of a membrane that separates fluids with different pHs. At steady state, the non-ionized (unionized) drug concentration on both sides of the membrane is similar, but the concentration of ionized drug differs (From Hug CC. Pharmacokinetics of drugs administered intravenously. Anesth Analg 1978; 57: 704–23; with permission.)

or renal clearance of the unbound drug fraction. In this regard, protein binding of drugs may actually facilitate elimination by acting as a transport mechanism to deliver drugs to sites of clearance.

Alterations in protein binding are usually important only for drugs that are highly protein bound, such as warfarin, propranolol, phenytoin, and diazepam. For example, for a drug that is 98% protein bound, a decrease in binding to 96% will double the plasma fraction of unbound drug, with potential associated increases in pharmacologic effects. Conversely, a decrease in protein binding from 70% to 68% results in only a 7% increase in the free fraction of drug in plasma.

Determinants of Protein Binding

The extent of protein binding parallels lipid solubility of the drug. For example, pentobarbital is less highly bound to protein than is its more lipid-soluble thioanalogue, thiopental. In addition to lipid solubility, the fraction of total drug in plasma that is protein bound is determined by the drug's plasma concentration and the number of available binding sites. Low plasma concentrations of drugs are likely to be more highly protein bound than are higher plasma concentrations of the same drug. Statements about the percent of protein binding of a drug are not meaningful unless the plasma concentration of drug and availability of binding sites (plasma concentration of albumin) are also known.

Binding of drugs to plasma albumin is often nonselective such that many drugs with similar physicochemical characteristics can compete with each other and with endogenous substances for the same protein binding sites. For example, sulfonamides can displace unconjugated bilirubin from binding sites on albumin, leading to the risk of bilirubin encephalopathy in the neonate. It is important to consider protein binding when comparing maternal to fetal ratios for drugs. For example, total body concentrations of drugs may be different, but the pharmacologic effects are similar because the free concentration of drug is similar.

Renal failure may decrease the fraction of drug bound to protein even in the absence of changes in plasma concentrations of albumin or other proteins. For example, the free fraction of phenytoin is increased in patients with renal failure such that toxic plasma concentrations are likely to occur if the total dose of drug is not decreased. This occurrence in the presence of normal plasma concentrations of albumin suggests that an alteration in protein structure or displacement of phenytoin from its protein binding sites by a metabolic factor that is normally excreted by the kidneys has occurred. Albumin concentrations tend to be lower in elderly patients, but the impact of this change is small compared with the effect of disease states that result in renal or hepatic dysfunction.

Increases in the plasma concentration of alpha-1 acid glycoprotein occur in response to surgery, chronic pain, and acute myocardial infarction (Wood, 1986). An increase of this protein fraction in patients with rheumatoid arthritis leads to increased protein binding of lidocaine and propranolol. The plasma concentrations of alpha-1 acid glycoprotein are reduced in neonates, resulting in decreased protein binding of several drugs, including d-tubocurarine, metocurine, diazepam, propranolol, sufentanil, and lidocaine (Wood and Wood, 1981).

Clearance of Drugs from the Systemic Circulation

Clearance is the volume of plasma cleared of drug by renal excretion and/or metabolism in the liver or other organs. Almost all drugs administered in the therapeutic dose ranges are cleared from the circulation at a rate proportional to the amount of drug present in the plasma (first-order kinetics). Even at therapeutic doses, however, a few drugs will exceed the metabolic or excretory capacity of the body to clear drugs by first-order kinetics. In this situation, a constant amount of drug is cleared per unit of time (zero-order kinetics).

Clearance is one of the most important pharmacokinetic variables to be considered when defining a constant drug infusion regimen. To maintain an unchanging plasma concentration of drug (steady state), the intravenous infusion rate must be equal to the rate of drug clearance by hepatic and renal mechanisms. Knowledge of the elimination half-time for a drug is crucial for achieving a constant plasma concentration of drug. Nevertheless, individual variations in Vd and clearance may alter the elimination half-time of a drug in an individual patient compared with values calculated from normal patients.

Hepatic Clearance

Hepatic clearance of a drug is the product of hepatic blood flow and the hepatic extraction ratio. If the hepatic extraction ratio is high (greater than 0.7), the clearance of drug will depend on hepatic blood flow, whereas changes in enzyme activity will have minimal influence (Fig. 1-5) (Wilkinson and Shand, 1975). Thus, a high hepatic extraction ratio results in *perfusion-dependent elimination.* If the hepatic extraction ratio is less than 0.3, only a small fraction of the drug delivered to the liver is removed per unit of time. As a result, an excess of drug is available for hepatic-elimination mechanisms, and changes in hepatic blood flow will not greatly influence hepatic clearance. A decrease in protein binding or an increase in enzyme activity, as associated with enzyme induction, will greatly increase hepatic clearance of a drug with a low hepatic extraction ratio. This type of hepatic elimination is termed *capacity-dependent elimination..*

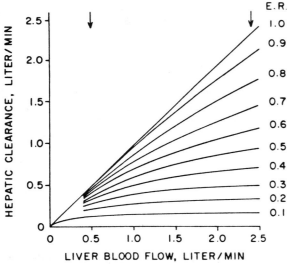

FIGURE 1–5. An increase in hepatic blood flow within the physiologic range denoted by the arrows produces minimal changes in hepatic clearance of drugs with a low extraction ratio (*ER*). Conversely, for drugs with a high ER, an increase in hepatic blood flow produces a nearly proportional increase in hepatic clearance (From Wilkinson GR, Shand DG. A physiologic approach to hepatic drug clearance. Clin Pharmacol Ther 1975; 18: 377–90; with permission.)

Biliary Excretion

Most of the metabolites of drugs produced in the liver are excreted in bile into the gastrointestinal tract. Often, these metabolites are reabsorbed from the gastrointestinal tract into the circulation for ultimate elimination in the urine. Organic anions, such as glucuronides, are transported actively into bile by carrier systems similar to those that transport these anions into renal tubules.

Renal Clearance

The kidneys are the most important organs for the elimination of unchanged drugs or their metabolites. Water-soluble compounds are excreted more efficiently by the kidneys than are compounds with high lipid solubility. This emphasizes the important role of metabolism in converting lipid-soluble drugs to water-soluble metabolites. Drug elimination by the kidneys is correlated with endogenous creatinine clearance or serum creatinine concentration. The magnitude of elevation of these indices provides an estimate of the necessary downward adjustment in drug dosage.

Renal excretion of drugs involves (1) glomerular filtration, (2) active tubular secretion, and (3) passive tubular reabsorption. The amount of drug that enters the renal tubular lumen depends on the fraction of drug bound to protein and the glomerular filtration rate. Renal tubular secretion involves active transport processes, which may be selective for certain drugs and metabolites, including protein-bound compounds. Reabsorption from renal tubules removes drug that has entered tubules by glomerular filtration and tubular secretion. This reabsorption is most prominent for lipid-soluble drugs that can easily cross cell membranes of renal tubular epithelial cells to enter pericapillary fluid. Indeed, a highly lipid-soluble drug, such as thiopental, is almost completely reabsorbed such that little or no unchanged drug is excreted in the urine. Conversely, production of less lipid-soluble metabolites limits renal tubule reabsorption and facilitates excretion in the urine.

The rate of reabsorption from renal tubules is influenced by factors such as pH and rate of renal tubular urine flow. Passive reabsorption of weak bases and acids is altered by urine pH, which influences the fraction of drug that exists in the ionized form. For example, weak acids are excreted more rapidly in an alkaline urine. This occurs because alkalinization of the urine results in more ionized drug that cannot easily cross renal tubular epithelial cells, resulting in less passive reabsorption.

Metabolism of Drugs

The role of metabolism (biotransformation) is to convert pharmacologically active, lipid-soluble drugs into water-soluble and often pharmacologically inactive metabolites. Increased water solubility reduces the Vd for a drug and enhances its renal excretion. A lipid-soluble parent drug is not likely to undergo extensive renal excretion because of the ease of reabsorption from the lumens of renal tubules into pericapillary fluid. In the absence of metabolism, a lipid-soluble drug, such as thiopental, would continue to undergo reabsorption from renal tubules and have an elimination half-time of about 100 years. Metabolism to water-soluble metabolites, however, reduces its reabsorption from renal tubules and, thus, facilitates elimination in the urine.

It is important to recognize that metabolism does not always lead to production of pharmacologically inactive metabolites. For example, diazepam and propranolol may be metabolized to active compounds. In some instances, an inactive parent compound (cyclophosphamide) is administered and subsequently undergoes metabolism to active metabolites. These examples emphasize that metabolism is not always synonymous with inactivation or even detoxification.

Rate of Metabolism

Rate of metabolism of most drugs is determined by the concentration of drug at the site of metabolism and by the intrinsic rate of the metabolism process. Hepatic blood flow often determines delivery and, thus, concentration of drug at the site of metabolism. The intrinsic rate of metabolism reflects factors that influence enzyme activity, such as genetics and enzyme induction.

FIRST-ORDER KINETICS. Most drug metabolism follows linear or first-order kinetics such that a constant fraction of available drug is metabolized in a given time period. First-order kinetics depends on the plasma concentration of drug in the sense that the absolute amount of drug eliminated per unit of time is greatest when its plasma concentration is greatest. However, the fraction of total drug that is eliminated during first-order kinetics is independent of the plasma concentration of drug.

ZERO-ORDER KINETICS. Zero-order kinetics occurs when the plasma concentration of drug exceeds the capacity of metabolizing enzymes. This reflects saturation of available enzymes and results in metabolism of a constant amount of drug per unit of time. This contrasts with the constant fraction of drug metabolized during first-order kinetics. As a result, the absolute amount of drug eliminated per unit of time during zero-order kinetics is the same, regardless of its plasma concentration. The intrinsic activity of enzymes determines the constant amount of drug metabolized per unit of time. Alcohol, aspirin, and phenytoin are drugs that exhibit zero-order kinetics at even therapeutic concentrations.

Pathways of Metabolism

The four basic pathways of metabolism are (1) oxidation, (2) reduction, (3) hydrolysis, and (4) conjugation. Phase I reactions include oxidation, reduction, and hydrolysis. Phase II reactions are when the parent drug, or a metabolite, reacts with an endogenous substrate, such as a carbohydrate or an amino acid, to form a water-soluble conjugate. Hepatic microsomal enzymes are responsible for the metabolism of most drugs. Other sites of drug metabolism include the plasma, lungs, kidneys, and gastrointestinal tract. The evolutionary development of drug-metabolizing enzymes is most likely related to ingestion of toxic alkaloids in plants. In this regard, drug metabolism has evolved as a means of protection against environmental toxins.

HEPATIC MICROSOMAL ENZYMES. Hepatic microsomal enzymes, which participate in the metabolism of many drugs, are located principally in hepatic smooth endoplasmic reticulum. These microsomal enzymes are also present in the kidneys, gastrointestinal tract, and adrenal cortex. The term *microsomal enzyme* is derived from the fact that centrifugation of homogenized cells (usually hepatocytes) concentrates fragments of the disrupted smooth endoplasmic reticulum in what is designated as the microsomal fraction.

The microsomal fraction also includes an iron-containing protein termed *cytochrome P-450*. The designation "cytochrome P-450" emphasizes this substance's absorption peak at 450 nm when it combines with carbon monoxide. The cytochrome P-450 system is also known as the mixed function oxidase system because it involves both oxidation and reduction steps. Cytochrome P-450 functions as the terminal oxidase in the electron transport scheme. Considering the large number of different drugs metabolized by the cytochrome P-450 system, it is likely that this system is actually a large number of different protein enzymes.

Microsomal enzymes catalyze most of the oxidation, reduction, and conjugation reactions that lead to metabolism of drugs. Lipid solubility of a drug favors passage across cell membranes and thus facilitates access by drugs to microsomal enzymes in hepatocytes and other cells. Hepatic microsomal enzyme activity is low in neonates, especially premature infants. Individual differences in microsomal enzyme activity are determined genetically. Indeed, rates of drug metabolism vary sixfold or more among individuals as a reflection of differences in microsomal enzyme activity.

ENZYME INDUCTION. A unique feature of hepatic microsomal enzymes is the ability of drugs or chemicals to stimulate activity of these enzymes. Increased enzyme activity produced by drugs or chemicals is known as *enzyme induction*. Enzyme induction also occurs to a limited extent in the lungs, kidneys, and gastrointestinal tract. Phenobarbital and polycyclic hydrocarbons are examples of substances that induce microsomal enzymes. The resulting increase in microsomal enzyme activity produced by phenobarbital is attributed to increased synthesis of cytochrome P-450 and cytochrome P-450 reductase.

NONMICROSOMAL ENZYMES. Nonmicrosomal enzymes catalyze reactions responsible for metabolism of drugs by conjugation, by hydrolysis, and, to a lesser extent, by oxidation and reduction. These nonmicrosomal enzymes are present principally in the liver but are also found in plasma and the gastrointestinal tract. All conjugation reactions except for conjugation to glucuronic acid

are catalyzed by nonmicrosomal enzymes. Nonspecific esterases in the liver, plasma, and gastrointestinal tract are examples of nonmicrosomal enzymes responsible for hydrolysis of drugs that contain ester bonds (succinylcholine, atracurium, esmolol, ester local anesthetics). Nonmicrosomal enzymes such as plasma cholinesterase and acetylating enzymes do not, however, undergo enzyme induction. The activity of these enzymes is determined genetically, as emphasized by patients with atypical cholinesterase enzyme and persons who are classified as being rapid or slow acetylators.

OXIDATIVE METABOLISM. Hepatic microsomal enzymes, including cytochrome P-450 enzymes, are crucial for the oxidation and resulting metabolism of many drugs. These enzymes require an electron donor in the form of reduced nicotinamide-adenine dinucleotide (NAD) and molecular oxygen for their activity. The molecule of oxygen is split, with one atom of oxygen oxidizing each molecule of drug and the other oxygen atom being incorporated into a molecule of water. A loss of electrons results in oxidation, whereas a gain of electrons results in reduction.

Examples of oxidative metabolism of drugs catalyzed by cytochrome P-450 enzymes include hydroxylation, deamination, desulfuration, dealkylation, and dehalogenation. Demethylation of morphine to normorphine is an example of oxidative dealkylation. Dehalogenation involves oxidation of a carbon-hydrogen bond to form an intermediate metabolite that is unstable and spontaneously loses a halogen atom. Halogenated volatile anesthetics are susceptible to dehalogenation, often leading to release of bromide, chloride, and fluoride ions. Aliphatic oxidation is oxidation of a side chain. For example, oxidation of the side chain of thiopental converts the highly lipid-soluble parent drug to the more water-soluble carboxylic acid derivative. Thiopental also undergoes desulfuration to pentobarbital by an oxidative step.

Epoxide intermediates in the oxidative metabolism of drugs are capable of covalent binding with macromolecules and may be responsible for drug-induced organ toxicity, such as hepatic dysfunction. Normally, these highly reactive intermediates have such a transient existence that they exert no biologic action. When enzyme induction occurs, however, large amounts of reactive intermediates may be produced, leading to organ damage. This is especially likely to occur if the antioxidant glutathione, which is in limited supply in the liver, is depleted by the reactive intermediates.

REDUCTIVE METABOLISM. Reductive pathways of metabolism, like oxidative pathways, involve cytochrome P-450 enzymes. Under conditions of low oxygen partial pressures, cytochrome P-450 enzymes transfer electrons directly to a substrate such as halothane rather than to oxygen. This electron gain imparted to the substrate occurs only when insufficient amounts of oxygen are present to compete for electrons.

HYDROLYSIS. Enzymes responsible for hydrolysis of drugs (often at an ester bond) do not involve the cytochrome P-450 system (see the section entitled "Nonmicrosomal Enzymes"). Hydrolysis of glucuronide conjugates secreted into the bile occurs in the gastrointestinal tract and is necessary for release of drug to become available for enterohepatic recirculation.

CONJUGATION. Conjugation with glucuronic acid involves cytochrome P-450 enzymes. Glucuronic acid is readily available from glucose. When conjugated to a lipid-soluble drug or metabolite, hydrophilic glucuronic acid renders the substance pharmacologically inactive and more water soluble. The resulting water-soluble glucuronide conjugates are unlikely to be reabsorbed into the systemic circulation and are then preferentially excreted in the bile and urine.

Reduced microsomal enzyme activity interferes with conjugation, leading to hyperbilirubinemia of the neonate and the risk of bilirubin encephalopathy. This decreased microsomal enzyme activity is responsible for increased toxicity in the neonate of drugs that are normally inactivated by conjugation with glucuronic acid. Conjugation with glucuronic acid is also reduced during pregnancy, presumably because of elevated levels of progesterone.

Dose-Response Curves

Dose-response curves depict the relationship between dose of drug administered and the resulting pharmacologic effect (Fig. 1-6). Logarithmic

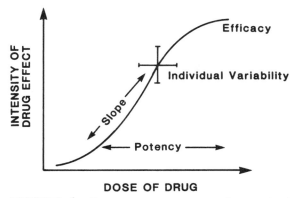

FIGURE 1–6. Dose-response curves are characterized by differences in potency, slope, efficacy, and individual responses.

transformation of dosage is frequently used, because it permits display of a wide range of doses. Dose-response curves are characterized by differences in (1) potency, (2) slope, (3) efficacy, and (4) individual responses.

Potency

Potency of a drug is depicted by its location along the dose axis of the dose-response curve. Factors that influence potency of a drug include (1) absorption, (2) distribution, (3) metabolism, (4) excretion, and (5) affinity for the receptor. For clinical purposes, the potency of a drug makes little difference as long as the effective dose of the drug can be administered conveniently. Doses required to produce a specified effect are designated as the *effective dose* (ED) necessary to produce that effect in a given percentage of patients (ED_{50}, ED_{90}). Increased affinity of a drug for its receptor moves the dose-response curve to the left.

Slope

The slope of the dose-response curve is influenced by the number of receptors that must be occupied before a drug effect occurs. For example, if a drug must occupy a majority of receptors before an effect occurs, the slope of the dose-response curve will be steep. A steep dose-response curve is characteristic of neuromuscular blocking drugs and inhaled anesthetics (MAC); it means that small increases in dose evoke intense increases in drug effect. For example, a 1-MAC concentration of volatile anesthetic prevents skeletal muscle movement in response to a surgical skin incision in 50% of patients, whereas a modest increase to about 1.3 MAC prevents movement in at least 95% of patients. Furthermore, when the dose-response curve is steep, the difference between a therapeutic and a toxic concentration may be small. This is true for volatile anesthetics that are characterized by small differences between the doses that produce desirable degrees of central nervous system depression and undesirable degrees of cardiac depression (see Chapter 2).

Efficacy

The maximal effect of a drug reflects its intrinsic activity or efficacy. This efficacy is depicted by the plateau in dose-response curves. It must be recognized that undesirable effects (side effects) of a drug may limit dosage to below the concentration associated with its maximal effect. Differences in efficacy are emphasized by pharmacologic effects of opioids versus aspirin in relieving pain. Opioids relieve pain of high intensity, whereas maximal doses of aspirin are effective only against mild discomfort. Efficacy and potency of a drug are not necessarily related.

Therapeutic index, or margin of safety, is the difference between the dose of drug that produces a desired effect and the dose that produces undesirable effects. In laboratory studies, the therapeutic index is often defined as the ratio between the median lethal dose and median effective dose (LD_{50}/ED_{50}). Drugs have multiple therapeutic indices, depending on the therapeutic response being considered and the dose of drug necessary to evoke that response. For example, the therapeutic index for aspirin to relieve headache is greatly different from the therapeutic index to relieve pain of rheumatoid arthritis.

Individual Responses

Individual responses to a drug may vary as reflections of differences in pharmacokinetics and/or pharmacodynamics among patients (Table 1-5) (Wood, 1989). This may even account for differences in pharmacologic effects of drugs in the

Table 1-5

Events Responsible for Variations in Drug Responses Between Individuals

Pharmacokinetics
  Bioavailability
  Renal function
  Liver function
  Cardiac function
  Patient age

Pharmacodynamics
  Enzyme activity
  Genetic differences

Drug Interactions

same patient at different times. The relative importance of the numerous factors that contribute to variations in individual responses to drugs depends, in part, on the drug itself and its usual route of excretion. Drugs that are excreted primarily unchanged by the kidneys tend to exhibit smaller differences in pharmacokinetics than do drugs that are metabolized. The most important determinant of metabolism rate is genetic. The dynamic state of receptor concentrations, as influenced by diseases and other drugs, also influences the variation in drug responses observed among patients (see the section entitled "Concentration of Receptors"). Finally, inhaled anesthetics, by altering circulatory, hepatic, and renal function, may influence the pharmacokinetics of injected drugs.

ELDERLY PATIENTS.   In elderly patients, variations in drug response most likely reflect (1) decreased cardiac output, (2) enlarged fat compartment, (3) reduced protein binding, and (4) a decline in renal function. Decreased cardiac output reduces hepatic blood flow and thus delivery of drug to the liver for metabolism. This decreased delivery, combined with the possibility of decreased hepatic enzyme activity, may prolong the duration of action of drugs such as lidocaine and fentanyl (Bentley et al, 1982). An enlarged fat compartment may increase the Vd and lead to the accumulation of lipid-soluble drugs such as diazepam and thiopental (Jung et al, 1982; Klotz et al, 1975). Increased total body fat content and decreased plasma protein binding of drugs accounts for the increased Vd that accompanies aging. A parallel decrease in total body water accompanies increased fat stores. The net effect of these changes is an increased vulnerability of elderly patients to cumulative drug effects. Aging does not seem to be accompanied by changes in receptor responsiveness.

ENZYME ACTIVITY. Alterations in enzyme activity as reflected by enzyme induction may be responsible for variations in drug responses among individuals. For example, cigarette smoke contains polycyclic hydrocarbons that induce mixed-function hepatic oxidases, leading to increased dose requirements for drugs such as theophylline and tricyclic antidepressants (Vestal and Wood, 1980). Acute alcohol ingestion can inhibit metabolism of drugs. Conversely, chronic alcohol use (greater than 200 g·day^{-1}) induces microsomal enzymes that metabolize drugs. Because of enzyme induction, this accelerated metabolism may manifest as tolerance to drugs such as barbiturates.

GENETIC DIFFERENCES. Variations in drug responses among individuals are due, in part, to genetic differences that may also affect receptor sensitivity. Genetic variations in metabolic pathways (rapid vs slow acetylators) may have important clinical implications for drugs such as isoniazid and hydralazine. Pharmacogenetics describes genetically determined disease states that are initially revealed by altered responses to specific drugs. Examples of diseases that are unmasked by drugs include (1) atypical cholinesterase enzyme revealed by prolonged neuromuscular blockade following administration of succinylcholine; (2) malignant hyperthermia triggered by succinylcholine or volatile anesthetics; (3) glucose-6-phosphate dehydrogenase deficiency, in which certain drugs cause hemolysis; and (4) intermittent porphyria, in which barbiturates may evoke an acute attack.

Drug Interactions

A drug interaction occurs when a drug alters the intensity of pharmacologic effects of another drug given concurrently. Drug interactions may reflect alterations in pharmacokinetics or pharmacodynamics. The net result of a drug interaction may be enhanced or diminished effects of one or both of the drugs, leading to desired or undesired effects.

An example of a beneficial drug interaction is the concurrent administration of propranolol with hydralazine so as to prevent compensatory increases in heart rate that would offset the blood pressure–lowering effects of hydralazine. Interactions between drugs are frequently used to counter the effects of agonist drugs, as reflected by the use of naloxone to antagonize opioids. Adverse drug interactions typically manifest as impaired therapeutic efficacy and/or enhanced toxicity. In this regard, one drug may interact with another to (1) impair absorption, (2) compete with the same plasma protein binding sites, (3) alter metabolism by enzyme induction or inhibition, or (4) change the rate of renal excretion.

PHARMACODYNAMICS OF INJECTED DRUGS

The most common mechanism by which drugs exert pharmacologic effects is by the interaction of the drug with a specific protein macromolecule in the lipid bilayer of cell membranes. This protein macromolecule in the cell membrane is referred to as a *receptor.* Receptors exist for endogenous regulatory substances such as hormones and neurotransmitters. A drug administered as an exogenous substance is an incidental "passenger" for these receptors. A drug-receptor interaction alters the function or conformation of a specific cellular component that initiates or prevents a series of changes that characterize pharmacologic effects of the drug.

Receptors

Receptors are identified and subsequently classified primarily by the effects of specific antagonists and by the relative potencies of known agonists. Such a classification serves as a practical basis for summarizing the pharmacologic effects of agonist drugs and the likely effects of antagonist drugs. Multiple subtypes of receptors (alpha-1 and alpha-2, beta-1 and beta-2, H-1 and H-2, mu-1 and mu-2) exist for many receptors. For example, there are differences in the ligand binding properties for acetylcholine at cholinergic nicotinic receptors present in ganglia of the automatic nervous system compared with those at the neuromuscular junction. This difference is emphasized by nondepolarizing neuromuscular blocking drugs that act at nicotinic receptors at the neuromuscular junction but exert minimal or no effect at nicotinic receptors in autonomic ganglia.

Concentration of Receptors

The concentration of receptors in the lipid portion of cell membranes is dynamic, either increasing (up-regulation) or decreasing (down-regulation) in response to specific stimuli. For example, an excess of endogenous ligand, as present in a patient with a pheochromocytoma, results in a decrease in the concentration of beta-adrenergic receptors in cell membranes in an attempt to reduce the intensity of stimulation. Likewise, prolonged treatment of asthma with a beta agonist may result in tachyphylaxis associated with a decrease in the concentration of receptors. Conversely, chronic interference with activity of receptors as produced by a beta antagonist may result in increased numbers of receptors in cell membranes such that an exaggerated response (hypersensitivity) occurs if the blockade is abruptly reversed as by the sudden discontinuation of propranolol in the perioperative period. Disease states may reflect the inappropriate regulation of the concentration of receptors in cell membranes. For example, antibodies against beta-adrenergic receptors may occur in patients with asthma, leading to a predominance of bronchoconstrictor activity. Patients with myasthenia gravis often manifest antibodies to receptors that respond to acetylcholine.

Changing concentrations of receptors in cell membranes emphasizes that receptors determine that pharmacologic responses to drugs are not static but rather are dynamic. This dynamic state is modulated by a variety of exogenous and endogenous factors that may influence the pharmacologic responses to drugs in different people or the same person at different times. If this concept is kept in mind, variable pharmacologic responses often evoked by drugs become more predictable (Wood, 1989).

Characteristics of Drug-Receptor Interaction

A drug or endogenous substance (ligand) is an agonist if the drug-receptor interaction elicits a pharmacologic effect by an alteration in the functional properties of receptors. A drug is an antagonist when it interacts with receptors but does not alter their functional properties and, at the same time, prevents their response to an agonist. If inhibition can be overcome by increasing the concentration of agonist, the antagonist drug is said to produce competitive blockade. This type of antagonism is produced by neuromuscular blocking drugs and beta-adrenergic antagonists that act reversibly at receptors. An agonist drug that binds only weakly to receptors may produce minimal pharmacologic effects even though a maximal concentration is present. Such a drug is known as a partial agonist. Examples of partial agonists are the opioid agonist-antagonist drugs.

RECEPTOR OCCUPANCY THEORY. It is traditionally assumed that the intensity of effect produced by binding of drugs to receptors is proportional to the fraction of receptors occupied by the drug. Conceptually, maximal drug effects occur when all the receptors are occupied. This receptor occupancy theory, however, does not explain differences in intrinsic activity between drugs that occupy the same number of receptors and produce responses ranging from full stimulation to antagonism.

STATE OF RECEPTOR ACTIVATION. A modification of the receptor occupancy theory that is consistent with differences in intrinsic activity of drugs is the concept of activated and nonactivated states for receptors. In this theory, when an agonist binds to receptors, it converts the receptors from a nonactivated to an activated state. Full agonists are able to convert most of the receptors they occupy to the activated state; partial agonists convert only a fraction of the receptors they occupy to the activated state; and antagonists do not activate any of the receptors they occupy to the activated state. Increasing doses of a partial agonist in the presence of a maximal effect produced by an agonist results in competitive antagonism of the effect of the agonist. Conversely, addition of a partial agonist in the presence of less than a maximal effect produced by the agonist will result in additional drug action to the maximal effect of the partial agonist. It is likely that opioid agonist-antagonists act in this way when administered in the presence of opioid agonists (see Chapter 3).

DRUG-RECEPTOR BOND.   The action of drugs on receptors requires binding to occur between drugs and receptors by a physicochemical force. It is likely that multiple types of bonds between drugs and receptors occur involving reactive groups on drugs and complimentary regions of receptors. A *covalent bond* is formed by sharing a pair of electrons between atoms, thus forming a strong bond that plays little role in reversible binding of drugs to receptors. Covalent bonding is involved in the inactivation of cholinesterase enzyme by organophosphates (insecticides) and alpha-adrenergic blockade as produced by phenoxybenzamine. *Ionic bonds* arise from electrostatic forces existing between groups of opposite charge. Acidic or basic drugs that are ionized at plasma pH can combine readily with charged groups on proteins. *Hydrogen bonds* occur between hydroxyl or amino groups and an electronegative carboxyl oxygen group. *Van der Walls* forces are weak bonds between two atoms or groups of atoms of different molecules. When the configuration between drug and receptor is sterically similar, these bonds can form readily.

Nonreceptor Drug Action

Drugs may act by mechanisms other than combination with receptors on cell membranes. For example, chelating drugs are capable of forming strong bonds with metallic cations that may be found normally or abnormally in the body. Antacids neutralize gastric acid by a direct action.

Plasma Drug Concentrations

Plasma drug concentrations are a reliable monitor of therapy only when interpreted in parallel with the clinical course of the patient. Furthermore, serial measurements of plasma drug concentrations at selected intervals are more informative than isolated determinations. It is misleading to measure the plasma concentrations of drugs during the rapidly changing distribution phase. Likewise, at a later time, when the gradient is reversed, drug concentrations at receptors are probably higher than that existing in plasma. In this regard, individual pharmacokinetic characteristics of each drug must be considered to determine an optimal time during the elimination phase for measurement of a steady-state plasma

concentration of drug. Finally, it is important to know whether the analytical technique used measures both free and protein-bound drug. Most often, the technique for determining the plasma concentration of a drug measures the total concentration of drug and does not discriminate between protein-bound or free drug. Nevertheless, pharmacologic effects usually reflect only the free fraction of drug in the plasma. Indeed, drug toxicity from phenytoin or diazepam is more frequent in patients with associated hypoalbuminemia, suggesting that measurement of the free fraction of these drugs would permit better prediction of drug toxicity.

Relationship of Plasma and Receptor Drug Concentration

In patients, the plasma concentration of drug is the most practical measurement for monitoring the receptor concentration. The plasma concentration should be proportional, if not equal to, the receptor concentration of drug. Typically, there is a direct relationship between the (1) dose of drug administered, (2) resulting plasma concentration, and (3) intensity of drug effect. Likewise, the onset and duration of drug effect are related to the increase and decrease of the drug concentration at responsive receptors as reflected by corresponding changes in the plasma concentration.

Initial and Maintenance Doses

An initial loading dose is necessary to establish promptly a therapeutic plasma concentration of drug. This initial dose will be larger than the subsequent maintenance dose. Changes in Vd will influence the size of the initial dose. For example, in the presence of an increased Vd, the drug is diluted in a large volume, and, thus, a larger initial dose is required to produce the same plasma concentration of drug that would be obtained with a smaller dose and a normal Vd. The maintenance dose of a drug must be adjusted downward in the presence of renal or hepatic dysfunction so as to prevent drug accumulation owing to a prolonged elimination half-time. This adjustment can be achieved by reducing the maintenance dose or increasing the time interval between doses.

Intermittent doses result in abrupt increases followed by decreases in the plasma concentration of drug such that a therapeutic plasma level is not sustained. A continuous variable-rate intravenous infusion of drug is more likely to maintain the plasma concentration in a therapeutic range without the wide oscillations characteristic of intermittent injections.

PHARMACOKINETICS OF INHALED ANESTHETICS

Pharmacokinetics of inhaled anesthetics describes their (1) absorption (uptake) from alveoli into pulmonary capillary blood, (2) distribution in the body, (3) metabolism, and (4) elimination, principally via the lungs. A series of partial pressure gradients beginning at the anesthetic machine serve to propel the inhaled anesthetic across various barriers (alveoli, capillaries, cell membranes) to their sites of action in the central nervous system. The principal objective of inhalation anesthesia is to achieve a constant and optimal brain partial pressure of the inhaled anesthetic.

The brain and all other tissues equilibrate with the partial pressures of inhaled anesthetics delivered to them by arterial blood (Pa) (Fig. 1-7). Likewise, arterial blood equilibrates with the alveolar partial pressures (PA) of anesthetics. This emphasizes that the PA of inhaled anesthetics mirrors the brain partial pressure (Pbr). This is the reason that PA is used as an index of (1) depth of anesthesia, (2) recovery from anesthesia, and (3) anesthetic equal potency (MAC). It is important to recognize that equilibration between two phases means the same partial pressure exists in both phases. Equilibration does not mean equality of concentrations in two phases. Understanding those factors that determine the PA and thus the Pbr permits control of the doses of inhaled anesthetics delivered to the brain so as to maintain a constant and optimal depth of anesthesia.

$$P_A \rightleftharpoons P_a \rightleftharpoons P_{br}$$

FIGURE 1-7. The alveolar partial pressure (*PA*) of an inhaled anesthetic is in equilibrium with the arterial blood (*Pa*) and brain (*Pbr*). As a result, the PA is an indirect measurement of anesthetic partial pressure at the brain.

Table 1-6
Factors Determining Partial Pressure Gradients Necessary for Establishment of Anesthesia

Transfer of Inhaled Anesthetic from Anesthetic Machine to Alveoli
  Inspired partial pressure
  Alveolar ventilation
  Characteristics of anesthetic breathing system

Transfer of Inhaled Anesthetic from Alveoli to Arterial Blood
  Blood:gas partition coefficient
  Cardiac output
  Alveolar-to-venous partial pressure difference

Transfer of Inhaled Anesthetic from Arterial Blood to Brain
  Brain:blood partition coefficient
  Cerebral blood flow
  Arterial-to-venous partial pressure difference

Determinants of the Alveolar Partial Pressure

The PA and ultimately the Pbr of inhaled anesthetics are determined by input (delivery) into alveoli minus uptake (loss) of the drug from alveoli into arterial blood (Table 1-6). Input of inhaled anesthetics depends on the (1) inhaled partial pressures (PI), (2) alveolar ventilation, and (3) characteristics of the anesthetic breathing system. Uptake of inhaled anesthetics from alveoli depends on (1) solubility of the anesthetic in body tissues, (2) cardiac output, and (3) alveolar to venous partial pressure differences (A-vD).

Inhaled Partial Pressure

A high PI delivered from the anesthetic machine is required during initial administration of the anesthetic. A high initial input offsets the impact of uptake, accelerating induction of anesthesia as reflected by the rate of rise in the PA and thus the Pbr. With time, as uptake into the blood decreases, the PI should be decreased to match the reduced anesthetic uptake and, therefore, maintain a constant and optimal Pbr. If the PI is maintained constant with time, the PA and the Pbr will increase progressively as uptake diminishes.

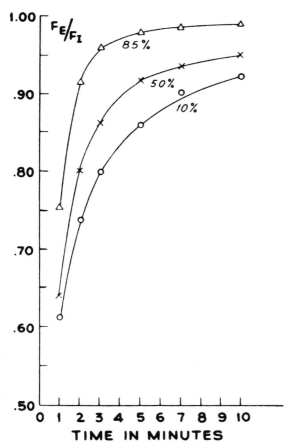

FIGURE 1–8. The impact of the inhaled concentration of an anesthetic on the rate at which the alveolar concentration approaches the inspired (F_E/F_I) is known as the concentration effect (From Eger EI. Effect of inspired anesthetic concentration on the rate of rise of alveolar concentration. Anesthesiology 1963; 24: 153–7; with permission.)

CONCENTRATION EFFECT. The impact of PI on the rate of rise of the PA of an inhaled anesthetic is known as the *concentration effect* (Fig. 1-8) (Eger, 1963.). The principle of the concentration effect states that the greater the PI, the more rapidly the PA approaches the PI. The greater PI provides input to offset uptake and thus speeds the rate at which the PA increases.

The concentration effect results from (1) a concentrating effect and (2) an augmentation of tracheal inflow (Stoelting and Eger, 1969a). The concentrating effect reflects concentration of the inhaled anesthetic in a smaller lung volume owing to uptake of all gases in the lung. At the same time, anesthetic input via tracheal inflow is increased to fill the space (void) produced by uptake of gases.

SECOND-GAS EFFECT. The second-gas effect reflects the ability of high-volume uptake of one gas (first gas) to accelerate the rate of rise of the PA of a concurrently administered companion gas (second gas) (Fig. 1-9) (Epstein et al, 1964). For example, the initial large-volume uptake of nitrous oxide accelerates the uptake of companion

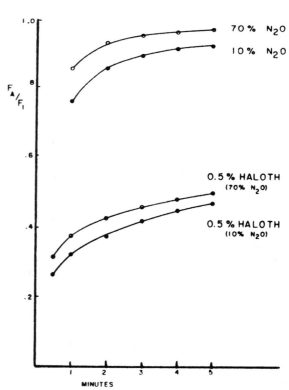

FIGURE 1–9. The second gas effect is the accelerated rise in the alveolar concentration of a second gas, halothane (*HALOTH*), toward the inspired (F_A/F_I) in the presence of a high inhaled concentration of the first gas (N_2O) (From Epstein RM, Rackow H, Salanitre E, Wolf G. Influence of the concentration effect on the uptake of anesthetic mixtures: The second gas effect. Anesthesiology 1964; 25: 364–71; with permission.)

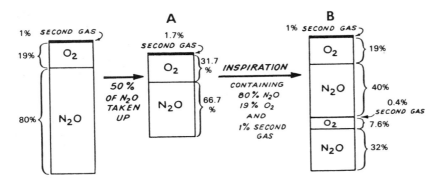

FIGURE 1–10. The second gas effect results from a concentrating effect (*A*) and an augmentation of tracheal inflow (*B*) (From Stoelting RK, Eger EI. An additional explanation for the second gas effect: A concentrating effect. Anesthesiology 1969; 30: 273–7; with permission.)

(second) gases such as oxygen and volatile anesthetics. This increased uptake of the second gas reflects increased tracheal inflow of all the inhaled gases (first and second gases) and concentration of the second gas or gases in a smaller lung volume (concentrating effect) owing to the high-volume uptake of the first gas (Fig. 1-10) (Stoelting and Eger, 1969a).

Alveolar Ventilation

Increased alveolar ventilation, like PI, promotes input of anesthetics to offset uptake. The net effect is a more rapid rate of rise in the PA and induction of anesthesia. In addition to increased input, the decreased $PaCO_2$ produced by hyperventilation of the lungs decreases cerebral blood flow. Conceivably, the impact of increased input on the rate of rise of the PA would be offset by decreased delivery of anesthetic to the brain. Decreased alveolar ventilation decreases input and thus slows the establishment of a PA and a Pbr necessary for the induction of anesthesia. Inhaled anesthetics influence their own uptake by virtue of dose-dependent depressant effects on alveolar ventilation. This, in effect, is a negative feedback mechanism that prevents establishment of an excessive depth of anesthesia when a high PI is administered during spontaneous breathing. This protective mechanism is lost when mechanical ventilation of the lungs replaces spontaneous breathing.

The impact of changes in alveolar ventilation on the rate of rise in the PA depends on the solubility of the anesthetic. For example, changes in alveolar ventilation influence the rate of rise of the PA of a soluble anesthetic more than a poorly soluble anesthetic. Indeed, the rate of rise in the PA of a poorly soluble anesthetic, such as nitrous oxide, is rapid regardless of the alveolar ventilation. This occurs because uptake of nitrous oxide is limited as a result of its poor solubility. Conversely, uptake of a soluble drug is large, and increasing alveolar ventilation provides more drug to offset loss by way of uptake. As a result, increases in alveolar ventilation greatly accelerate the rate at which the PA of a soluble anesthetic approaches the PI. This emphasizes that changing from spontaneous breathing to controlled ventilation of the lungs, which is likely also to be associated with increased alveolar ventilation, will probably increase the depth of anesthesia (PA) produced by a soluble anesthetic.

Anesthetic Breathing System

Characteristics of the anesthetic breathing system that influence the rate of rise of the PA are the (1) volume of the external breathing system, (2) the solubility of inhaled anesthetics in the rubber or plastic components of the breathing system, and (3) gas inflow from the anesthetic machine. The volume of the anesthetic breathing system acts as a buffer to slow achievement of the PA. High gas inflow rates (5 to 10 $L \cdot min^{-1}$) from the anesthetic machine negate this buffer effect. Solubility of inhaled anesthetics in the components of the anesthetic breathing system initially slows the rate at which the PA increases. At the conclusion of the administration of an anesthetic, however, reversal of the partial pressure gradient in the anesthetic breathing system results in elution of the anesthetic, which slows the rate at which the PA decreases.

Table 1-7
Comparative Solubilities of Inhaled Anesthetics

	Blood: Gas Partition Coefficient	Brain: Blood Partition Coefficient	Muscle: Blood Partition Coefficient	Fat: Blood Partition Coefficient	Oil: Gas Partition Coefficient
Soluble					
Methoxyflurane	12	2	1.3	48.8	970
Intermediate Solubility					
Halothane	2.4	1.9	3.4	51.1	224
Enflurane	1.9	1.5	1.7	36.2	98
Isoflurane	1.4	1.6	2.9	44.9	98
Poorly Soluble					
Nitrous oxide	0.46	1.1	1.2	2.3	1.4
Desflurane	0.42	1.3	2.0	27.2	18.7
Sevoflurane	0.59	1.7	3.1	47.5	55

Solubility

Solubility of inhaled anesthetics in blood and tissues is denoted by the partition coefficient (Table 1-7) (Yasuda et al, 1989). A partition coefficient is a distribution ratio describing how the inhaled anesthetic distributes itself between two phases at equilibrium (partial pressures equal in both phases). For example, a blood:gas partition coefficient of 2 means that the concentration of inhaled anesthetic is 2 in the blood and 1 in the alveolar gas when the partial pressures of that anesthetic in these two phases are identical (Fig. 1-11). The partition coefficient also may be thought of as reflecting the relative capacity of each phase to accept anesthetic. Partition coefficients are temperature dependent such that solubility of a gas in a liquid is increased when the temperature of the liquid decreases.

BLOOD:GAS PARTITION COEFFICIENTS. The rate of rise of the PA relative to a constant PI is related to the blood:gas partition coefficient of the inhaled anesthetic (Fig. 1-12) (Carpenter et al, 1986a). Based on their blood:gas partition coefficients, inhaled anesthetics are categorized traditionally as soluble, intermediately soluble, and poorly soluble (Table 1-7). Blood can be considered a pharmacologically inactive reservoir, the size of which is determined by the solubility of the anes-

thetic in blood. When the blood:gas partition coefficient is high, a large amount of anesthetic must be dissolved in the blood before the Pa equilibrates with the PA. For example, the high solubility of methoxyflurane in blood slows the rate at which the PA and Pa increase relative to the PI, and the induction of anesthesia is slow. The impact of high blood solubility on the rate of rise of the PA can be offset, to some extent, by increasing the PI. When blood solubility is low, as with nitrous oxide or desflurane, minimal amounts of the inhaled anesthetic must be dissolved before equilibrium is reached; therefore,

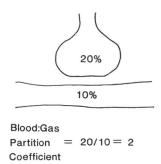

Blood:Gas
Partition   = 20/10 = 2
Coefficient

FIGURE 1-11. If at equilibrium, when the partial pressures are identical, the arterial concentration of an inhaled drug is 10% and the alveolar concentration is 20%, the blood:gas partition coefficient for this drug is 2.0.

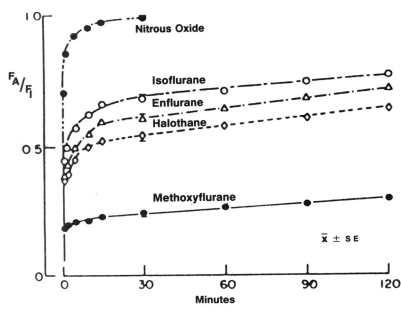

FIGURE 1–12. The rate of rise of the alveolar to the inspired concentration of inhaled anesthetics (F_A/F_I) with time parallels the blood:gas partition coefficients of these drugs (From Carpenter RL, Eger EI, Johnson BH, Unadkat JD, Sheiner LB. Pharmacokinetics of inhaled anesthetics in humans: Measurements during and after the simultaneous administration of enflurane, halothane, isoflurane, methoxyflurane, and nitrous oxide. Anesth Analg 1986; 65: 575–82; with permission.)

the rate of rise of PA and Pa, and thus the induction of anesthesia, are rapid. For example, the inhalation of nitrous oxide or desflurane for 10 minutes results in a PA that is greater than 80% of the PI. Associated with this rapid rise in the PA of nitrous oxide is the absorption of several liters (up to 10 L during the first 10 to 15 minutes) of this gas, reflecting its common administration at inhaled concentrations of 60% to 70%. This high-volume absorption of nitrous oxide is responsible for several unique effects of nitrous oxide when it is administered in the presence of volatile anesthetics or air-containing cavities (see the sections entitled "Concentration Effect", "Second Gas Effect", "Nitrous Oxide Transfer to Closed Gas Spaces"). Percutaneous loss of inhaled anesthetics occurs but is too small to influence the rate of rise in the PA (Stoelting and Eger, 1969b). With the possible exception of methoxyflurane, the magnitude of metabolism of inhaled anesthetics is too small to influence the rate of increase of the PA (Berman et al, 1973). This lack of effect reflects the large excess of anesthetic molecules administered and the saturation, by anesthetic concentrations of inhaled drugs, of enzymes responsible for anesthetic metabolism (Halsey et al, 1971; Sawyer et al, 1971).

Blood:gas partition coefficients are altered by individual variations in water, lipid, and protein content and by the hematocrit of whole blood (Laasberg and Hedley-White, 1970; Ellis and Stoelting, 1975). For example, blood:gas partition coefficients are about 20% less in blood with a hematocrit of 21% compared with blood with a hematocrit of 43%. Presumably, this decreased solubility reflects the reduction in lipid-dissolving sites normally presented by erythrocytes. Conceivably, reduced solubility of volatile anesthetics in anemic blood would manifest as an increased rate of rise in the PA and a more rapid induction of anesthesia. Ingestion of a fatty meal alters the composition of blood, resulting in an approximately 20% increase in the solubility of volatile anesthetics in blood (Munson et al, 1978).

TISSUE:BLOOD PARTITION COEFFICIENTS. Tissue:blood partition coefficients determine uptake of anesthetic into tissues and the time necessary for equilibration of tissues with the Pa. This time for equilibration can be estimated by calculating a time constant (amount of inhaled anesthetic that can be dissolved in the tissue divided by tissue blood flow) for each tissue. One time constant on an exponential curve represents 63% equilibration. Three time constants are equivalent to about 95% equilibration. For volatile anesthetics, equilibration between Pa and Pbr requires about 15 minutes (three time constants). Fat has an enormous capacity to hold anesthetic, and this combined with low blood flow to this tissue prolongs the time required to narrow anesthetic partial pressure differences between arterial blood and fat. For example, equilibration of fat with isoflurane (three time constants) based on this drug's fat:blood partition coefficient and an assumed fat blood flow of 2 to 3 ml·100 g⁻¹·min⁻¹ is estimated to be 25 to 46 hours. Fasting before elective operations results in transport of fat to the liver, which could increase anesthetic uptake by this tissue and modestly slow the rate of increase in the PA of a volatile anesthetic during induction of anesthesia (Fassoulaki and Eger, 1986).

OIL:GAS PARTITION COEFFICIENTS. Oil:gas partition coefficients parallel anesthetic requirements. For example, an estimated MAC can be calculated as 150 divided by the oil:gas partition coefficient. The constant, 150, is the average value of the product of oil:gas solubility and MAC for numerous inhaled drugs with widely divergent lipid solubilities. Using this constant, the calculated MAC for an anesthetic with an oil:gas partition coefficient of 100 would be 1.5%.

NITROUS OXIDE TRANSFER TO CLOSED GAS SPACES. The blood:gas partition coefficient of nitrous oxide (0.46) is about 34 times greater than nitrogen (0.014). This differential solubility means that nitrous oxide can leave the blood to enter an air-filled cavity 34 times more rapidly than nitrogen can leave the cavity to enter blood. As a result of this preferential transfer of nitrous oxide, the volume or pressure of an air-filled cavity increases. Passage of nitrous oxide into an air-filled cavity surrounded by a compliant wall (intestinal gas, pneumothorax, pulmonary blebs, air bubbles) causes the gas space to expand. Conversely, passage of nitrous oxide into an air-filled cavity surrounded by a noncompliant wall (middle ear, cerebral ventricles, supratentorial space) causes an increase in intracavitary pressure.

The magnitude of volume or pressure increase is influenced by the (1) partial pressure of nitrous oxide, (2) blood flow to the air-filled cavity, and (3) duration of nitrous oxide administration. In an animal model, the inhalation of 75%

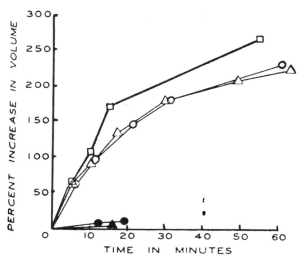

FIGURE 1–13. Inhalation of 75% nitrous oxide rapidly increases the volume of a pneumothorax (*open symbols*). Inhalation of oxygen (*solid symbols*) does not alter the volume of pneumothorax (From Eger EI, Saidman LJ. Hazards of nitrous oxide anesthesia in bowel obstruction and pneumothorax. Anesthesiology 1965; 26: 61–6; with permission.)

nitrous oxide doubles the volume of a pneumothorax in 10 minutes (Fig. 1-13) (Eger and Saidman, 1965). This finding emphasizes the high blood flow to this area. Likewise, air bubbles (emboli) expand rapidly when exposed to nitrous oxide (Fig. 1-14) (Munson and Merrick, 1966). In contrast to the rapid expansion of a pneumothorax, the increase in bowel gas volume produced by nitrous oxide is slow.

The middle ear is an air-filled cavity that vents passively by way of the eustachian tube when pressure reaches 20 to 30 cmH₂O. Nitrous oxide diffuses into the middle ear more rapidly than nitrogen leaves, and middle ear pressures may become elevated if eustachian tube patency is compromised by inflammation or edema. Indeed, tympanic membrane rupture has been attributed to this mechanism following administration of nitrous oxide. Negative middle ear pressures may develop after discontinuation of nitrous oxide, leading to serous otitis. Nausea and vomiting that follow anesthesia may be due to multiple mechanisms, but the possible role of altered middle ear pressures as a result of nitrous oxide should be considered.

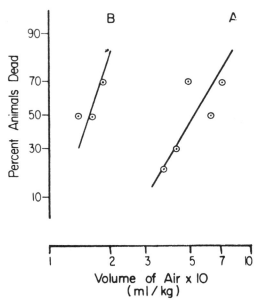

FIGURE 1–14. Nitrous oxide rapidly expands air bubbles as reflected by the volume of injected air necessary to produce 50% mortality in animals breathing nitrous oxide (0.16 ml·kg^{-1}) (*A*) compared with animals breathing oxygen (0.55 ml·kg^{-1}) (*B*) (From Munson ES, Merrick HC. Effect of nitrous oxide on venous air embolism. Anesthesiology 1966; 27: 783–7; with permission.)

Cardiac Output

Cardiac output (pulmonary blood flow) influences uptake and therefore PA by carrying away either more or less anesthetic from alveoli. An increased cardiac output results in more rapid uptake, so that the rate of rise in the PA and thus the induction of anesthesia are slowed. A decreased cardiac output speeds the rate of rise of the PA, because there is less uptake to oppose input.

The effect of cardiac output on the rate of increase in the PA may seem paradoxical. For example, the uptake of more drug by an increased cardiac output should speed the rate of rise of partial pressures in tissues and thus narrow the A-vD for anesthetics. Indeed, an increase in cardiac output does hasten equilibration of tissue anesthetic partial pressures with the Pa. Nevertheless, the Pa is lower than it would be if cardiac output were normal. Conceptually, a change in cardiac output is analogous to the effect of a change in solubility. For example, doubling cardiac output increases the capacity of blood to

hold anesthetic, just as solubility increases the capacity of the same volume of blood.

As with alveolar ventilation, changes in cardiac output most influence the rate of rise of the PA of a soluble anesthetic. Conversely, the rate of rise of the PA of a poorly soluble anesthetic, such as nitrous oxide, is rapid regardless of physiologic deviations of the cardiac output around its normal value. As a result, changes in cardiac output exert little influence on the rate of rise of the PA of nitrous oxide. In contrast, doubling the cardiac output will greatly increase the uptake of soluble anesthetic from alveoli, slowing the rate of rise of the PA. Conversely, a low cardiac output, as with shock, could produce an unexpectedly high PA of a soluble anesthetic.

Volatile anesthetics that depress cardiac output can exert a positive feedback response that contrasts with the negative feedback response on spontaneous breathing exerted by these drugs. For example, decreases in cardiac output owing to an excessive dose of volatile anesthetic results in an increase in the PA, which further increases anesthetic depth and thus cardiac depression. The administration of a volatile anesthetic that depresses cardiac output, plus controlled ventilation of the lungs, results in a situation characterized by unopposed input of anesthetic via alveolar ventilation combined with decreased uptake because of a reduced cardiac output. The net effect of this combination of events can be an unexpected, abrupt increase in the PA and an excessive depth of anesthesia.

Distribution of cardiac output will influence the rate of rise of the PA of an anesthetic. For example, increases in cardiac output are not necessarily accompanied by proportional increases in blood flow to all tissues. Preferential perfusion of vessel-rich–group tissues when the cardiac output increases results in a more rapid rise in the PA of anesthetic than would occur if the increased cardiac output was distributed equally to all tissues. Indeed, infants have a relatively greater perfusion of vessel-rich–group tissues than do adults and, consequently, show a faster rate of rise of the PA toward the PI (Salanitre and Rackow, 1969).

IMPACT OF A SHUNT. In the absence of an intracardiac or intrapulmonary right-to-left shunt, it is valid to assume that the PA and Pa of inhaled anesthetics are essentially identical. When a right-to-left shunt is present, the diluting effect of the shunted blood on the partial pressure of anesthetic in blood coming from ventilated alveoli results in a decrease in the Pa and a slowing in the rate of induction of anesthesia. A similar mechanism is responsible for the reduction in PaO_2 in the presence of a right-to-left shunt.

The relative impact of a right-to-left shunt on the rate of rise in the Pa depends on the solubility of the anesthetic. For example, a right-to-left shunt slows the rate of rise of the Pa of a poorly soluble anesthetic more than that of a soluble anesthetic (Stoelting and Longnecker, 1972). This occurs because uptake of a soluble anesthetic offsets dilutional effects of shunted blood on the Pa. Uptake of a poorly soluble drug is minimal, and dilutional effects on the Pa are relatively unopposed. This impact of solubility in the presence of a right-to-left shunt is opposite to that observed with changes in cardiac output and alveolar ventilation. All factors considered, it seems unlikely that a right-to-left shunt alone will alter the induction rate of anesthesia significantly.

Left-to-right tissue shunts (arteriovenous fistulas, volatile anesthetic-induced increases in cutaneous blood flow) result in delivery to the lungs of blood containing a higher partial pressure of anesthetic than that present in blood that has passed through tissues. As a result, left-to-right tissue shunts offset the dilutional effect of right-to-left shunts on the Pa. Indeed, the effect of a left-to-right shunt on the rate of rise in the Pa is detectable only if there is a concomitant presence of a right-to-left shunt.

Alveolar-to-Venous Partial Pressure Differences

The A-vD reflects tissue uptake of the inhaled anesthetic. Tissue uptake affects uptake at the lung by controlling the rate of rise of the mixed venous partial pressure (Pv) of anesthetic. Factors that determine the fraction of anesthetic removed from blood traversing a tissue parallel those factors that determine uptake at the lungs (tissue solubility, tissue blood flow, and arterial-to-tissue partial pressure differences).

Highly perfused tissues (brain, heart, kidneys) account for less than 10% of body mass but receive about 75% of the cardiac output (Table 1-2). As a result of the small mass and high blood flow, these tissues, known as the vessel-rich group, equilibrate rapidly with the Pa. Indeed,

after about three time constants, approximately 75% of the returning venous blood is at the same partial pressure as the PA. For this reason, uptake of a volatile anesthetic is decreased greatly after about 15 minutes, as reflected by a narrowing of the inspired-to-alveolar partial pressure difference. Continued uptake of anesthetic after saturation of vessel-rich–group tissues reflects principally the entrance of anesthetic into skeletal muscles and fat. Skeletal muscles and fat represent about 70% of the body mass but receive only about 25% of the cardiac output (Table 1-2). As a result of the large tissue mass, sustained tissue uptake of the inhaled anesthetic continues, and the effluent venous blood is at a lower partial pressure than the PA. For this reason, the A-vD difference for anesthetic is maintained and uptake from the lungs continues, even after several hours of continuous administration.

Recovery from Anesthesia

Recovery from anesthesia is depicted by the rate of decrease in the Pbr as reflected by the PA. Although similarities exist between the rate of induction and recovery, as reflected by changes in the PA of the inhaled anesthetic, there are important differences between the two events. For example, failure of certain tissues to reach equilibrium with the PA of the inhaled anesthetic means that the rate of decline of the PA during recovery from anesthesia will be more rapid than the rate of increase of the PA during induction of anesthesia. Indeed, even after a prolonged anesthetic, skeletal muscles probably, and fat almost certainly, will not have equilibrated with the PA of the inhaled anesthetic. Thus, when the PI of an anesthetic is abruptly reduced to zero at the conclusion of an anesthetic, these tissues initially cannot contribute to the transfer of drug back into blood for delivery to the liver for metabolism or to the lungs for exhalation. As long as gradients exist between the Pa and tissues, the tissues will continue to take up anesthetic. Thus, during recovery from anesthesia, the continued passage of anesthetic from blood to tissues, such as fat, acts to speed the rate of decline in the PA of that anesthetic. Continued tissue uptake of anesthetic will depend on the solubility of the inhaled anesthetic and the duration of anesthesia, with the impact most important with soluble anesthetics (Stoelting and Eger, 1969c).

Anesthetic that has been absorbed into the components of the anesthetic breathing system will pass from the components back into the gases of the breathing circuit at the conclusion of anesthesia and retard the rate of decline in the PA of the anesthetic. Likewise, exhaled gases of the patient contain anesthetic that will be rebreathed in the absence of high fresh-gas flows into the anesthetic breathing circuit. For this reason, fresh-gas flow rates of at least 5 L·min^{-1} of oxygen are commonly delivered at the conclusion of anesthesia..

In contrast to the rate of rise of the PA during induction of anesthesia, the rate of decrease in the PA during recovery from anesthesia is not entirely consistent with what might be predicted from the inhaled anesthetic's blood:gas partition coefficient (Fig. 1-15) (Carpenter et al, 1986a). For example, the PA for halothane decreases more rapidly than that for isoflurane and enflurane despite the greater blood solubility of halothane. Similarly, the PA of methoxyflurane decreases below that of enflurane even though methoxyflurane is about six times more soluble in blood than is enflurane. The more rapid decrease in the PA for halothane and methoxyflurane is, in large part, due to the metabolism of these drugs in the liver (Carpenter et al, 1986b) (see Chapter 2). This suggests that metabolism can significantly influence the rate of recovery from halothane and methoxyflurane anesthesia.

Diffusion Hypoxia

Diffusion hypoxia occurs when inhalation of nitrous oxide is discontinued abruptly, leading to a reversal of partial pressure gradients such that nitrous oxide leaves the blood to enter alveoli (Fink, 1955). This initial high-volume outpouring of nitrous oxide from the blood into the alveoli can so dilute the PAO_2 that the PaO_2 decreases. In addition to dilution of the PAO_2 by nitrous oxide, there is also dilution of the $PACO_2$, which decreases the stimulus to breath (Sheffer et al, 1972). This decreased stimulus to breath exaggerates the impact on PaO_2 of the outpouring of nitrous oxide into the alveoli. Outpouring of nitrous oxide into alveoli is greatest during the first 1 to 5 minutes following its discontinuation at the conclusion of anesthesia. For this reason, it is common practice to fill the lungs with oxygen at the end of anesthesia to ensure that arterial hypoxemia will not occur as a result of dilution of the PAO_2 by nitrous oxide.

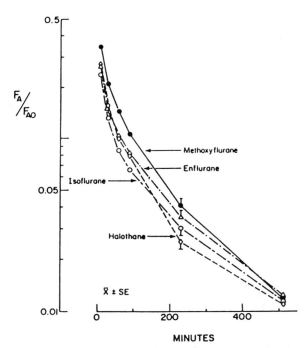

FIGURE 1–15. The decline in the alveolar concentration is expressed as the ratio of the alveolar partial pressure at a given time (F_A) to the alveolar concentration present immediately before discontinuation of the administration of the anesthetic (F_{AO}). Unlike induction of anesthesia (see Fig. 1–12), the rate of decline in anesthetic concentrations during recovery from anesthesia does not precisely follow predictions based on blood:gas partition coefficients of halothane and methoxyflurane owing to the influence of metabolism of these drugs (From Carpenter RL, Eger EI, Johnson BH, Unadkat JD, Sheiner LB. Pharmacokinetics of inhaled anesthetics in humans: Measurements during and after the simultaneous administration of enflurane, halothane, isoflurane, methoxyflurane, and nitrous oxide. Anesth Analg 1986; 65: 575–87; with permission.)

PHARMACODYNAMICS OF INHALED ANESTHETICS

Minimum Alveolar Concentration

MAC of an inhaled anesthetic is defined as that concentration at 1 atmosphere that prevents skeletal muscle movement in response to a supramaximal painful stimulus (surgical skin incision) in 50% of patients (Merkel and Eger, 1963). The fact that the alveolar concentration reflects the partial pressure at the site of anesthetic action (brain) has made MAC the most useful index of anesthetic equal potency. The use of equally potent doses (comparable MAC concentrations) of inhaled anesthetics is mandatory for comparing effects of these drugs not only at the brain but at all other organs (Table 1-8). For example, similar MAC concentrations of inhaled anesthetics produce equivalent depression of the central nervous system, whereas effects on cardiopulmonary parameters may be different for each drug (see Chapter 2). This emphasizes that MAC represents only one point on the dose-response curve of effects produced by inhaled anesthetics and that these dose-response curves for various inhaled anesthetics are not parallel. Use of MAC also allows a quantitative analysis of the effect, if any, of various pharmacologic and physiologic factors on anesthetic requirements (Table 1-9) (Hall and Sullivan, 1990; Quasha et al, 1980).

MAC values for inhaled anesthetics are additive. For example, 0.5 MAC of nitrous oxide plus 0.5 MAC isoflurane has the same effect at the brain as does a 1-MAC concentration of either anesthetic alone. The fact that 1 MAC for nitrous oxide is greater than 100% means that this anesthetic cannot be used alone at 1 atmosphere and still provide an acceptable inhaled concentration of oxygen. Dose-response curves for inhaled anesthetics, although not parallel, are all steep. This is emphasized by the fact that a 1-MAC dose prevents skeletal muscle movement in response to a painful stimulus in 50% of patients, whereas a modest increase to about 1.3 MAC prevents movement in at least 95% of patients.

Table 1–8
Comparative Minimum Alveolar Concentration (MAC) of Inhaled Anesthetics

	MAC (30 to 55 years old 37 C, P_B 760 mmHg)
Nitrous oxide*	104%
Desflurane	4.58%
Sevoflurane	1.71%
Halothane	0.74%
Enflurane	1.68%
Isoflurane	1.15%
Methoxyflurane	0.16%

*Determined in a hyperbaric chamber in males 21 to 35 years old.

Table 1–9
Impact of Physiologic and Pharmacologic Factors on Minimum Alveolar Concentration (MAC)

Increase in MAC
Hyperthermia
Hypernatremia
Drug-induced elevations in CNS catecholamine stores

Decrease in MAC
Hypothermia
Hyponatremia
Pregnancy
Lithium
Lidocaine
Neuraxial opioids
PaO_2 <38 mmHg
Blood pressure <40 mmHg
Increasing age
Preoperative medication
Drug-induced decreases in CNS catecholamine stores
Alpha-2 agonists
Acute alcohol ingestion
Cardiopulmonary bypass

No Change in MAC
Duration of anesthesia
Hyperkalemia or hypokalemia
Anesthetic metabolism
Chronic alcohol abuse
Thyroid gland dysfunction
Gender
$PaCO_2$ 15–95 mmHg
PaO_2 >38 mmHg
Blood pressure >40 mmHg

Mechanism of Anesthesia

The mechanism by which inhaled anesthetics produce progressive and, occasionally, selective depression of the central nervous system is not known (Pocock and Richards, 1991). A single theory, however, to explain the mechanism of anesthesia seems unlikely. Most evidence is consistent with inhibition of synaptic transmission through multineural polysynaptic pathways, especially in the reticular activating system. It is generally thought that peripheral nerves conduct normally during general anesthesia. Speific genes that alter sensitivity to volatile anesthetics have been identified in a nematode model emphasizing the importance of the molecular composition of the site of action of anesthetics (Morgan et al, 1988).

Meyer-Overton Theory (Critical Volume Hypothesis)

Correlation between lipid solubility of inhaled anesthetics (oil:gas partition coefficient) and anesthetic potency (MAC) suggests that anesthesia occurs when a sufficient number of anesthetic molecules dissolve (critical concentration) in crucial hydrophobic sites such as lipid cell membranes. Conceptually, expansion of cell membranes by dissolved anesthetic molecules could distort channels necessary for sodium ion (Na^+) flux and the subsequent development of action potentials necessary for synaptic transmission. Likewise, changes in the lipid matrix produced by dissolved anesthetic molecules could alter the function of proteins in cell membranes, thus reducing Na^+ conductance. Consistent with altered Na^+ conductance is the ability of inhaled anesthetics to increase the threshold of cells to firing so as to reduce the rate of rise in action potentials. Evidence supporting distortion of Na^+ channels by dissolved anesthetic molecules is the observation that high pressures (40 to 100 atmospheres) partially antagonize the action of inhaled anesthetics (pressure reversal) presumably by returning (compressing) lipid membranes and their Na^+ channels to their "awake" contour (Halsey and Smith, 1975). Nevertheless, not all lipid-soluble drugs are anesthetics, and, in fact, some may be convulsants.

Protein Receptor Hypothesis

Evidence of protein receptors in the central nervous system as a site and mechanism of action of inhaled anesthetics is suggested by the steep dose-response curve (MAC) for inhaled anesthetics. Indeed, a crucial degree of receptor occupancy is characteristic of a steep dose-response curve. Receptor specificity is also suggested by conversion of an anesthetic to a nonanesthetic by increasing the molecular weight, despite corresponding increases in lipid solubility.

The dextroisomer, but not the levoisomer, of medetomidine, an alpha-2 agonist, produces dose-dependent reductions in MAC in animals (Segal et al, 1988; Doze et al, 1989). The stereospecificity of the MAC-reducing effects of dexmedetomidine suggests that this hypnotic-anesthetic effect is mediated through a homogenous receptor population. It is speculated that alpha-2 agonists act on postsynaptic alpha-2 receptors in the central nervous system so as to activate an inhibitory G-protein and to increase potassium ion (K^+) conductance. The inhibitory G-protein and hyperpolarization produced by increased K^+ conductance results in depression of neuronal excitability characteristic of general anesthesia. Indeed, pertussis toxin (a specific inactivator of inhibitory G-proteins) and 4-aminopyridine (a blocker of K^+ channels) produce dose-dependent decreases in the hypnotic-anesthetic effects of dexmedetomidine (Doze et al, 1990).

Recognition that there is an endogenous pain suppression system has led to the speculation that inhaled anesthetics could act by evoking the release of endorphins that attach to specific opioid receptors. Although it is possible that inhaled anesthetics may produce some degree of analgesia by stimulating the release of endorphins, it is unlikely these drugs produce unconsciousness characteristic of general anesthesia by the release of endorphins.

Alterations in Neurotransmitter Availability

It is conceivable that inhaled anesthetics could interfere with the formation, release, or breakdown of neurotransmitters in the central nervous system. *In vitro* studies have demonstrated the ability of both inhaled and injected anesthetics to inhibit breakdown of the inhibitory neurotransmitter, gamma-aminobutyric acid (GABA). This inhibition leads to increased brain concentrations of GABA and the speculation that anesthesia could result from accumulation of this inhibitory neurotransmitter in the central nervous system. Inhibition of GABA breakdown is greatest with halothane, followed by enflurane, thiopental, and ketamine (Cheng and Brunner, 1981). Morphine does not influence the breakdown of GABA.

REFERENCES

Avram MJ, Krejcie TC, Henthorn TK. The relationship of age to the pharmacokinetics of early drug distribution: The concurrent disposition of thiopental and indocyanine green. Anesthesiology 1990;72:403–11.

Bentley JB, Borel JD, Nad RE, Gillespie TJ. Age and fentanyl pharmacokinetics. Anesth Analg 1982;61:968–71.

Berman ML, Lowe HJ, Bochantin J, Hagler K. Uptake and elimination of methoxyflurane as influenced by enzyme induction in the rat. Anesthesiology 1973;38:352–7.

Carpenter RL, Eger EI, Johnson BH, Unadkat JD, Sheiner LB. Pharmacokinetics of inhaled anesthetics in humans: Measurements during and after the simultaneous administration of enflurane, halothane, isoflurane, methoxyflurane, and nitrous oxide. Anesth Analg 1986a;65:575–82.

Carpenter RL, Eger EI, Johnson BH, Unadkat JD, Sheiner LB. The extent of metabolism of inhaled anesthetics in humans. Anesthesiology 1986b;65:201–5.

Cheng S-C, Brunner EA. Effects of anesthetic agents on synaptosomal GABA disposal. Anesthesiology 1981;55:34–40.

Doze VA, Chen B-X, Maze M. Dexmedetomidine produces a hypnotic-anesthetic action in rats via activation of central alpha-2 adrenoceptors. Anesthesiology 1989;71:75–9.

Doze VA, Chen B-X, Tinklenberg JA, Segal IS, Maze M. Pertussis toxin and 4-aminopyridine differently affect the hypnotic-anesthetic action of dexmedetomidine and pentobarbital. Anesthesiology 1990;73:304–7.

Eger EI. Effect of inspired anesthetic concentration on the rate of rise of alveolar concentration. Anesthesiology 1963;24:153–7.

Eger EI, Saidman LJ. Hazards of nitrous oxide anesthesia in bowel obstruction and pneumothorax. Anesthesiology 1965;26:61–6.

Ellis DE, Stoelting RK. Individual variations in fluroxene, halothane and methoxyflurane blood-gas partition coefficients, and the effect of anemia. Anesthesiology 1975;42:748–50.

Epstein RM, Rackow H, Salanitre E, Wolf G. Influence of the concentration effect on the uptake of anesthetic mixtures: The second gas effect. Anesthesiology 1964;25:364–71.

Fassoulaki A, Eger EI. Starvation increases the solubility of volatile anaesthetics in rat liver. Br J Anaesth 1986;58:327–9.

Fink BR. Diffusion anoxia. Anesthesiology 1955;16:511–9.

Hall RI, Sullivan JA. Does cardiopulmonary bypass alter enflurane requirements for anesthesia? Anesthesiology 1990;73:249–355.

Halsey MJ, Sawyer DC, Eger EI, Bahlman SH, Impleman DMK. Hepatic metabolism of halothane, methoxyflurane, cyclopropane, Ethrane and Forane in miniature swine. Anesthesiology 1971;35:43–7.

Halsey MJ, Smith B. Pressure reversal of narcosis produced by anesthetics, narcotics and tranquilizers. Nature 1975;257:811–3.

Hug CC. Pharmacokinetics of drugs administered intravenously. Anesth Analg 1978;57:704–23.

Jones RM, Cashman JN, Eger EI, Damask MC, Johnson BH. Kinetics and potency of desflurane (I-653) in volunteers. Anesth Analg 1990;70:3–7.

Jung D, Mayersohn M, Perrie D, Calkins J, Saunders R. Thiopental disposition as a function of age in female patients undergoing surgery. Anesthesiology 1982;56:263–8.

Klotz U, Avant GR, Hoyuma RJ, Schenker S, Wilkinson GR. The effects of age and liver disease on the disposition and elimination of diazepam in adult man. J Clin Invest 1975;55:347–57.

Laasberg HL, Hedley-White J. Halothane solubility in blood and solutions of plasma proteins: Effects of temperature, protein composition and hemoglobin concentration. Anesthesiology 1970;32:351–6.

Merkel G, Eger EI. A comparative study of halothane and halopropane anesthesia: Including method for determining equipotency. Anesthesiology 1963;24:346–57.

Morgan PG, Sedensky MM, Meneely PM, Cascorbi HF. The effect of two genes on anesthetic response in the nematode Caenorhabditis elegans. Anesthesiology 1988;62:246–51.

Munson ES, Eger EI, Tham MK, Embro WJ. Increase in anesthetic uptake, excretion and blood solubility in man after eating. Anesth Analg 1978;57:224–31.

Munson ES, Merrick HC. Effect of nitrous oxide on venous air embolism. Anesthesiology 1966;27:783–7.

Pocock G, Richards CD. Cellular mechanisms in general anesthesia. Br J Anaesth 1991;66:116–78.

Quasha AL, Eger EI, Tinker JH. Determination and application of MAC. Anesthesiology 1980;53:315–34.

Roerig DL, Kotrly KJ, Vucins EJ, Ahlf SB, Dawson CA, Kampine JP. First pass uptake of fentanyl, meperidine, and morphine in the human lung. Anesthesiology 1987;67:466–72.

Salanitre E, Rackow H. The pulmonary exchange of nitrous oxide and halothane in infants and children. Anesthesiology 1969;30:388–94.

Sawyer DC, Eger EI, Bahlman SH, Cullen BF, Impelman D. Concentration dependence of hepatic halothane metabolism. Anesthesiology 1971;34:230–4.

Segal IS, Vickery RG, Walton JK, Doze VA, Maze M. Dexmedetomidine diminishes halothane anesthetic requirements in rats through a postsynaptic alpha-2 adrenergic receptor. Anesthesiology 1988;69:818–23.

Sheffer L, Steffenson JL, Birch AA. Nitrous oxide-induced diffusion hypoxia in patients breathing spontaneously. Anesthesiology 1972;37:436–9.

Stanski DR, Maitre PO. Population pharmacokinetics and pharmacodynamics of thiopental: The effect of age revisited. Anesthesiology 1990;72:412–22.

Stanski DR, Watkins WD. Drug disposition in anesthesia. New York, Grune and Stratton, 1982.

Stoelting RK, Eger EI. An additional explanation for the second gas effect: A concentrating effect. Anesthesiology 1969a;30:273–7.

Stoelting RK, Eger EI. Percutaneous loss of nitrous oxide, cyclopropane, ether and halothane in man. Anesthesiology 1969b;30:278–83.

Stoelting RK, Eger EI. The effects of ventilation and anesthetic solubility on recovery from anesthesia: An *in vivo* and analog analysis before and after equilibration. Anesthesiology 1969c;30:290–6.

Stoelting RK, Longnecker DE. Effect of right-to-left shunt on rate of increase in arterial anesthetic concentration. Anesthesiology 1972;36:352–6.

Vestal RE, Wood AJJ. Influence of age and smoking on drug kinetics in man: Studies using model compounds. Clin Pharmacokinet 1980;5:309–19.

Wilkinson Gr, Shand DG. A physiologic approach to hepatic drug clearance. Clin Pharmacol Ther 1975;18:377–90.

Wood M. Plasma drug binding: Implications for anesthesiologists. Anesth Analg 1986;65:786–804.

Wood M. Variability of human drug response. Anesthesiology 1989;71:631–3.

Wood M, Wood AJJ. Changes in plasma drug binding and alpha$_1$ acid glycoprotein in mother and newborn infant. Clin Pharmacol Ther 1981;29:522–6.

Yasuda N, Targ AC, Eger EI. Solubility of I-653, sevoflurane, isoflurane, and halothane in human tissues. Anesth Analg 1989;69:370–3.

Chapter

2

Inhaled Anesthetics

INTRODUCTION

The discovery of the anesthetic properties of nitrous oxide, diethyl ether, and chloroform in the 1840s was followed by a hiatus of about 80 years before other inhaled anesthetics were introduced (Fig. 2-1) (Eger, 1984a). In 1950, all available inhaled anesthetics were either flammable or potentially toxic to the liver. Recognition that combining carbon with fluorine decreased flammability led to the introduction, in 1951, of the first halogenated hydrocarbon anesthetic, fluroxene. Fluroxene was used clinically for several years before its voluntary withdrawal from the market owing to its potential flammability and increasing evidence that this drug could cause organ toxicity (Johnson et al, 1973).

Halothane was synthesized in 1951 and introduced for clinical use in 1956. However, the tendency for alkane derivatives, such as halothane, to enhance the arrhythmogenic effects of epinephrine led to the search for new inhaled anesthetics derived from ethers. Methoxyflurane, a methyl ethyl ether, was the first such derivative, being introduced for clinical use in 1960. Although this drug does not enhance the arrhythmogenic effects of epinephrine, its extreme solubility in blood and lipids results in a prolonged induction and slow recovery from anesthesia. More important, however, is the extensive hepatic metabolism of methoxyflurane that results in elevations in plasma fluoride concentrations sufficient to produce nephrotoxicity in some patients, especially if the duration of administration exceeds 2.5 MAC hours. Enflurane, the next methyl ethyl ether derivative, was intro-

duced for clinical use in 1973. This anesthetic does not enhance the arrhythmogenic effects of epinephrine and, unlike halothane and methoxyflurane, is resistant to metabolism, thus minimizing the likelihood of hepatotoxicity or nephrotoxicity. Isoflurane, the isomer of enflurane, was introduced for clinical use in 1981. This drug is the most resistant to metabolism of all the clinically available inhaled anesthetics, emphasizing the unlikely occurrence of organ toxicity following its administration.

Commonly administered inhaled anesthetics include the inorganic gas nitrous oxide, and the volatile liquids halothane, enflurane, and iso-

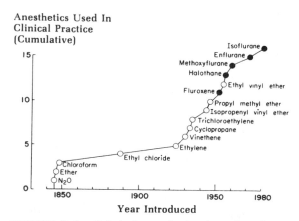

FIGURE 2–1. Inhaled anesthetics introduced into clinical practice. Solid circles are drugs that contain fluorine. (From Eger EL. Isoflurane [Forane]: A compendium and reference. 2nd edition. Madison, WI, Ohio Medical Products, 1985: 1–110; with permission.)

33

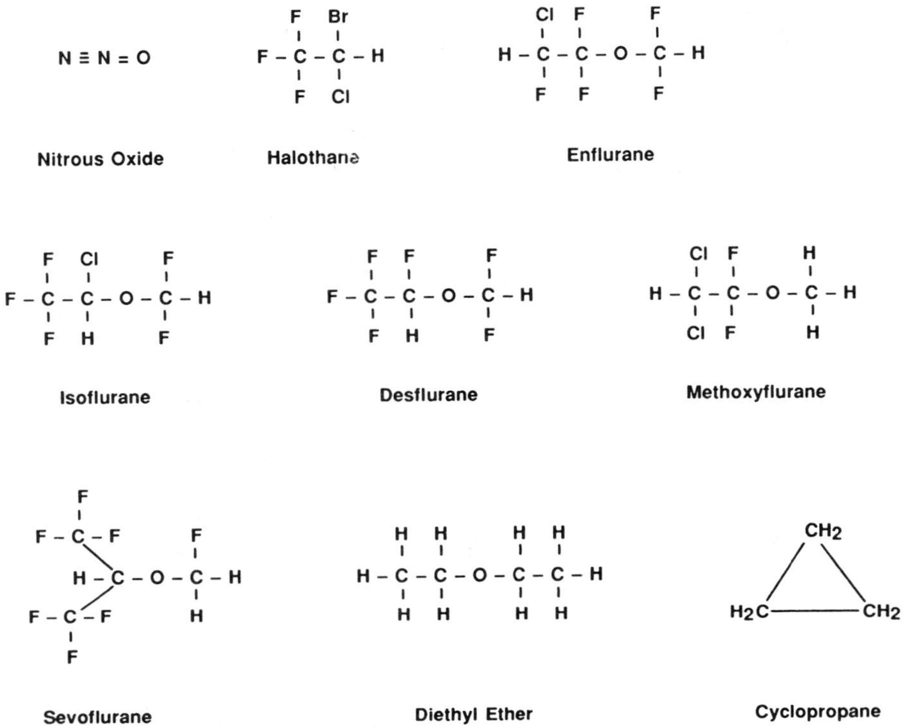

FIGURE 2–2.   Inhaled anesthetics.

flurane (Fig. 2-2; Table 2-1). Potentially useful volatile anesthetics in the future may include desflurane and sevoflurane (Table 2-1) (Jones, 1990). Available but rarely administered inhaled anesthetics include the volatile liquids methoxyflurane and diethyl ether, and the cyclic hydrocarbon gas cyclopropane. Volatile liquids are administered as vapors following their evaporation in devices known as vaporizers.

Nitrous Oxide

Nitrous oxide is a low–molecular-weight, odorless to sweet-smelling, nonflammable gas of low potency and poor blood solubility (0.46) that is most commonly administered in combination with opioids or volatile anesthetics to produce general anesthesia. Although nitrous oxide is nonflammable, it will support combustion. Its poor blood solubility permits rapid achievement of an alveolar and brain partial pressure of the

drug (see Fig. 1-12). Analgesic effects of nitrous oxide are prominent, but skeletal muscle relaxation is minimal. The speculated role of nitrous oxide in postoperative nausea and vomiting is not confirmed by controlled studies (Muir et al, 1987; Hovorka et al, 1989). Nitrous oxide has no effect on polarographic PO_2 measurements but does cause a small increase in the P_{50} (about 1.6 mmHg) that is rapidly inducible and reversible (Kambam and Holiday, 1987). Increasing awareness of the possible adverse effects related to the high-volume absorption of nitrous oxide (see Chapter 1), and appreciation of potential toxic effects on organ function, may lead to a decline in the use of this anesthetic.

Halothane

Halothane is a halogenated alkane derivative that exists as a clear, nonflammable liquid at room temperature. The vapor of this liquid has a sweet, nonpungent odor. An intermediate solubility in blood, combined with a high potency, permits rapid onset and recovery from anesthesia using halothane alone or in combination with nitrous oxide or injected drugs such as opioids.

Halothane was developed on the basis of predictions that its halogenated structure would provide nonflammability, intermediate blood solubility, anesthetic potency, and molecular stability. Specifically, carbon-fluorine decreases flammability and the trifluorocarbon contributes to molecular stability. The presence of a carbon-chlorine and carbon-bromine bond plus the retention of a hydrogen atom ensures anesthetic potency. Despite its chemical stability, halothane is susceptible to decomposition to hydrochloric acid, hydrobromic acid, chloride, bromide, and phosgene. For this reason, halothane is stored in amber-colored bottles, and thymol is added as a preservative to prevent spontaneous oxidative decomposition. Thymol that remains in vaporizers following vaporization of halothane can cause vaporizer turnstiles or temperature-compensating devices to malfunction.

Enflurane

Enflurane is a halogenated methyl ethyl ether that exists as a clear, nonflammable volatile liquid at room temperature and has a pungent,

ethereal odor. Its intermediate solubility in blood combined with a high potency permits rapid onset and recovery from anesthesia using enflurane alone or in combination with nitrous oxide or injected drugs such as opioids.

Isoflurane

Isoflurane is a halogenated methyl ethyl ether that exists as a clear, nonflammable, volatile liquid at room temperature and has a pungent, ethereal odor. Its intermediate solubility in blood combined with a high potency permits rapid onset and recovery from anesthesia using isoflurane alone or in combination with nitrous oxide or injected drugs such as opioids.

Although isoflurane is an isomer of enflurane, the manufacturing processes are not similar. The compounds used at the start of manufacturing are different, with 2,2,2-trifluoroethanol the starting compound for isoflurane and chlorotrifluoroethylene for enflurane. The subsequent purification of isoflurane by distillation is complex and expensive. Isoflurane is characterized by extreme physical stability, undergoing no detectable deterioration during 5 years of storage or on exposure to soda lime or sunlight. The stability of isoflurane negates the need to add preservatives such as thymol to the commercial preparation.

Table 2–1
Physical and Chemical Properties of Inhaled Anesthetics

	Nitrous oxide	Halothane	Enflurane	Isoflurane	Desflurane	Sevoflurane
Molecular weight	44	197	184	184	168	200
Specific gravity (25 C)		1.86	1.52	1.50		
Boiling point (C)		50.2	56.5	48.5	23.5	58.5
Vapor pressure (mmHg, 20 C)	Gas	244	172	240	664	160
Odor	Sweet	Organic	Ethereal	Ethereal		
Pungency	None	None	Moderate	Moderate		
Preservative necessary	No	Yes	No	No	No	No
Stability					Yes	No
Soda lime	Yes	No	Yes	Yes		
Sunlight	Yes	No	Yes	Yes		
Reacts with metal	No	Yes	No	No		

Desflurane

Desflurane is a fluorinated methyl ethyl ether that differs from isoflurane only by substitution of a fluorine atom for the chlorine found on the alpha-ethyl component of isoflurane. Solubility characteristics (blood:gas partition coefficient 0.42 and oil:gas partition coefficient 18.7) and potency (MAC 4.58%) permit rapid achievement of an alveolar partial pressure necessary for anesthesia followed by prompt awakening when desflurane is discontinued (Jones et al, 1990a). The vapor pressure of desflurane at 20 C is 664 mmHg. The ratio of the fatal anesthetic concentration to that preventing movement to a painful stimulation (MAC) for desflurane in animals is 2.45 compared with 3.02 for isoflurane.

Desflurane produces dose-related decreases in blood pressure and cardiac output that range from similar to to somewhat greater than those evoked by equivalent doses of isoflurane (Weiskopf et al, 1989). Infusions of epinephrine that provoke cardiac dysrhythmias during administration of desflurane and isoflurane are similar. Metabolism of desflurane is less than isoflurane, and the likelihood of organ damage from toxic metabolites seems remote. Indeed, plasma fluoride concentrations and renal or hepatic function tests do not change following inhalation of desflurane for about 90 minutes (Jones et al, 1990b).

Sevoflurane

Sevoflurane is a fluorinated methyl ethyl ether with a vapor pressure of 160 mmHg at 20 C. Solubility characteristics (blood:gas partition coefficient 0.59 and oil:gas partition coefficient 55) and potency (MAC 1.71) permit rapid achievement of an alveolar partial pressure necessary for anesthesia followed by a prompt awakening when sevoflurane is discontinued (Katoh and Ikeda, 1987). Inhalation of sevoflurane is not irritating to the airways, and there is a high degree of patient acceptance. Cardiovascular effects of sevoflurane appear to be similar to those of other volatile anesthetics. Defluorination of sevoflurane manifests as plasma fluoride concentrations that average 22 $\mu M \cdot L^{-1}$ after 1 hour of administration. This peak level declines rapidly, often to near normal values in less than 1 hour, reflecting the poor overall lipid solubility of this drug.

COMPARATIVE PHARMACOLOGY

Inhaled anesthetics often evoke differing pharmacologic effects at comparable MAC concentrations, emphasizing that dose-response curves for these drugs are not necessarily parallel. Measurements obtained from normothermic volunteers, exposed to equal potent concentrations of inhaled anesthetics during controlled ventilation of the lungs to maintain normocapnia, have provided the basis of comparison for pharmacologic effects of these drugs on various organ systems (Eger, 1985a). In this regard, it is important to recognize that surgically stimulated patients who have other confounding variables may respond differently than healthy volunteers (Table 2-2).

CENTRAL NERVOUS SYSTEM EFFECTS

Mental impairment is not detectable in volunteers breathing 1600 ppm (0.16%) nitrous oxide or 16 ppm (0.0016%) halothane (Frankhuizen et al, 1978). It is, therefore, unlikely that impairment of mental function in the personnel who work in the operating room can result from inhaling trace concentrations of anesthetics. Reaction times do not increase significantly until 10% to 20% nitrous oxide is inhaled (Garfield et al, 1975).

Volatile anesthetics do not cause retrograde amnesia or prolonged impairment of intellectual function. Cerebral metabolic oxygen require-

Table 2-2
Variables that Influence Pharmacologic Effects of Inhaled Anesthetics

Anesthetic concentration

Spontaneous vs controlled ventilation

Variations from normocapnia

Surgical stimulation

Patient age

Coexisting disease

Concomitant drug therapy

Intravascular fluid volume

Preoperative medication

Injected drugs to induce and/or maintain anesthesia or skeletal muscle relaxation

Alterations in body temperature

ments are reduced in parallel with drug-induced decreases in cerebral activity. Drug-induced increases in cerebral blood flow may increase intracranial pressure in patients with space-occupying intracranial lesions.

Electroencephalogram

Volatile anesthetics in concentrations less than 0.4 MAC similarly increase the frequency and voltage on the electroencephalogram (EEG). At about 0.4 MAC, there is an abrupt shift of high-voltage activity from posterior to anterior portions of the brain (Tinker et al, 1977). Cerebral metabolic oxygen requirements also begin to decrease abruptly at about 0.4 MAC. It is likely that these changes reflect a transition from wakefulness to unconsciousness. Furthermore, amnesia probably occurs at this dose of volatile anesthetic. As the dose of volatile anesthetic approaches 1 MAC, the frequency on the EEG decreases and maximum voltage occurs. During administration of isoflurane, burst suppression appears on the EEG at about 1.5 MAC, and, at 2 MAC, electrical silence predominates (Eger et al, 1971). Electrical silence does not occur with enflurane, and only unacceptably high concentrations of halothane (greater than 3.5 MAC) produce this effect. The effects of nitrous oxide on the EEG are similar to those produced by volatile anesthetics. Slower frequency and higher voltage develop on the EEG as the dose of nitrous oxide is increased or when nitrous oxide is added to a volatile anesthetic to provide a greater total MAC concentration.

Seizure Activity

Enflurane can produce fast-frequency and high-voltage activity on the EEG that often progresses to spike wave activity, which is indistinguishable from changes that accompany a seizure (Neigh et al, 1971). This EEG activity may be accompanied by tonic-clonic twitching of skeletal muscles in the face and extremities. The likelihood of enflurane-induced seizure activity is increased when the concentration of enflurane is greater than 2 MAC or when hyperventilation of the lungs decreases $PaCO_2$ to less than 30 mmHg. Repetitive auditory stimuli can also initiate seizure activity during the administration of enflurane. There is no evidence of anaerobic metabolism in

the brain during seizure activity produced by enflurane. Furthermore, in an animal model, enflurane does not enhance preexisting seizure foci, with the possible exception being certain types of myoclonic epilepsy and photosensitive epilepsy (Oshima et al, 1985).

Isoflurane does not evoke seizure activity on the EEG, even in the presence of deep levels of anesthesia, hypocapnia, or repetitive auditory stimulation. Indeed, isoflurane possesses anticonvulsant properties, being able to suppress seizure activity produced by flurothyl (Koblin et al, 1980). An undocumented speculation is that the greater MAC value for enflurane compared with its isomer, isoflurane, reflects the need for a higher concentration to suppress the stimulating effects of enflurane in the central nervous system.

Animals suspended by their tails may experience seizures in the first 15 to 90 minutes following discontinuation of nitrous oxide but not of volatile anesthetics (Smith et al, 1979). It is possible that these withdrawal seizures reflect acute nitrous oxide dependence. In patients, delirium or excitement during recovery from anesthesia that included nitrous oxide could reflect this phenomenon.

Evoked Potentials

Volatile anesthetics cause dose-related decreases in the amplitude, and increases in the latency, of the cortical component of median nerve somatosensory evoked potentials, visual evoked potentials, and auditory evoked potentials. Reductions in amplitude are more marked than increases in latencies. In the presence of 60% nitrous oxide, wave forms adequate for monitoring cortical somatosensory evoked potentials are present during administration of 0.5 to 0.75 MAC halothane and 0.5 to 1 MAC enflurane and isoflurane (Pathak et al, 1987). Even nitrous oxide alone may decrease the amplitude of cortical somatosensory evoked potentials.

Cerebral Blood Flow

Volatile anesthetics administered during normocapnia in concentrations greater than 0.6 MAC produce dose-dependent increases in cerebral blood flow (Fig. 2-3) (Eger, 1985a). This drug-induced increase in cerebral blood flow occurs despite concomitant reductions in cerebral meta-

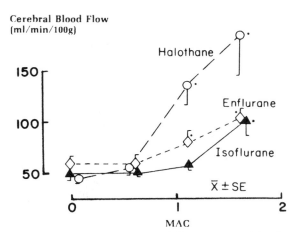

FIGURE 2–3. Cerebral blood flow measured in the presence of normocapnia and absence of surgical stimulation. *P <0.05. (From Eger EI. Isoflurane [Forane]: A compendium and reference. 2nd edition. Madison, WI, Ohio Medical Products, 1985: 1–110; with permission.)

bolic oxygen requirements. The greatest increase in cerebral blood flow occurs with halothane, is intermediate with enflurane, and is least with isoflurane. For example, at 1.1 MAC, cerebral blood flow increases almost 200% during administration of halothane, 30% to 50% with enflurane, and is unchanged with isoflurane. In patients with intracranial space-occupying lesions, the administration of halothane–nitrous oxide in concentrations equivalent to about 1.5 MAC increases regional cerebral blood flow 166%, compared with 35% during enflurane and no change with isoflurane (Eintrei et al, 1985). Nitrous oxide also increases cerebral blood flow, but its restriction to concentrations less than 1 MAC limits the magnitude of this change.

Anesthetic-induced increases in cerebral blood flow occur within minutes of initiating administration of the inhaled drug and whether blood pressure is unchanged or decreased, emphasizing the cerebral-vasodilating effects of these drugs. Animals exposed to halothane demonstrate a time-dependent decrease in the previously elevated cerebral blood flow beginning after about 30 minutes and reaching predrug levels after about 150 minutes (Albrecht et al, 1983). This normalization of cerebral blood flow reflects a concomitant increase in cerebral vascular resistance that is not altered by alpha- or beta-adrenergic blockade and is not a result of

changes in the pH of cerebrospinal fluid (Warner et al, 1985).

In animals, autoregulation of cerebral blood flow in response to changes in blood pressure is retained during administration of 1 MAC isoflurane but not halothane (Fig. 2-4) (Drummond et al, 1982; Eger, 1985a). Indeed, increases in blood pressure produce smaller increases in brain protrusion during administration of isoflurane and enflurane compared with halothane (Drummond et al, 1982). It is speculated that loss of autoregulation during administration of halothane is responsible for the greater brain swelling seen in animals anesthetized with this drug. Inhaled anesthetics do not alter the responsiveness of the cerebral circulation to changes in $PaCO_2$.

Cerebral Metabolic Oxygen Requirements

Inhaled anesthetics produce dose-dependent reductions in cerebral metabolic oxygen requirements that are greater during administration of isoflurane than with an equivalent MAC concentration of halothane (Todd and Drummond, 1984). When the EEG becomes isoelectric, an additional increase in the concentration of volatile anesthetics does not produce further decreases in cerebral metabolic oxygen requirements. The greater decrease in cerebral metabolic oxygen requirements produced by isoflurane may explain

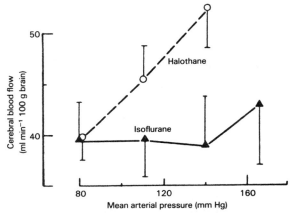

FIGURE 2–4. Autoregulation of cerebral blood flow (mean ± SE) as measured in animals. (From Eger EI. Pharmacology of isoflurane. Br J Anaesth 1984; 56: 71S–99S; with permission.)

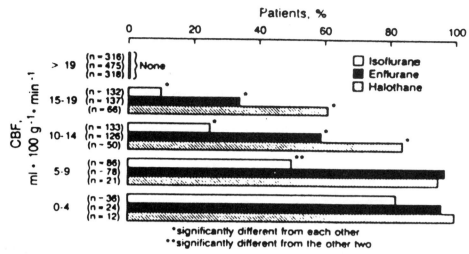

FIGURE 2–5. The number of patients (%) manifesting signs of cerebral ischemia on the electroencephalogram during administration of different volatile anesthetics and various ranges of cerebral blood flow (*CBF*). (From Michenfelder JD, Sundt TM, Fode N, Sharbrough FW. Isoflurane when compared to enflurane and halothane decreases the frequency of cerebral ischemia during carotid endarterectomy. Anesthesiology 1987; 67: 336–40; with permission.)

why cerebral blood flow is not predictably increased by this anesthetic at concentrations of less than 1.1 MAC. For example, decreased cerebral metabolism means less carbon dioxide is produced, which thus opposes any increase in cerebral blood flow. It is conceivable that isoflurane could evoke unexpected increases in cerebral blood flow if administered to a patient in whom cerebral metabolic oxygen requirements were already decreased, as by drugs.

Cerebral Protection

In animals experiencing temporary focal ischemia, there is no difference in neurologic outcome when cerebral function is suppressed by isoflurane or thiopental if blood pressure is equally maintained (Milde et al, 1988). In humans undergoing carotid endarterectomy, the cerebral blood flow at which ischemic changes appear on the EEG is lower during administration of isoflurane than during exposure to enflurane or halothane. (Fig. 2-5) (Michenfelder et al, 1987). Although neurologic outcome is not different based on the volatile anesthetic administered, these data suggest that, relative to enflurane and halothane, isoflurane may offer a degree of cerebral protection for transient incomplete regional cerebral ischemia during carotid endarterectomy. Unchanged cerebral blood flow and decreased cerebral metabolic oxygen requirements during isoflurane-induced controlled hypotension for clipping of cerebral aneurysms indicates that global cerebral oxygen supply-demand balance is favorably altered in patients anesthetized with this anesthetic (Newman et al, 1986).

Intracranial Pressure

Inhaled anesthetics produce elevations in intracranial pressure that parallel increases in cerebral blood flow produced by these drugs. Patients with space-occupying intracranial lesions are most vulnerable to these drug-induced elevations in intracranial pressure. Hyperventilation of the lungs to lower the $PaCO_2$ to about 30 mmHg opposes the tendency for inhaled anesthetics to increase intracranial pressure (Adams et al, 1981). In this regard, isoflurane differs from halothane in that hyperventilation of the lungs can be instituted at the time the anesthetic is administered rather than prior to its introduction.

With enflurane, it must be remembered that hyperventilation of the lungs increases the risk of seizure activity, which could lead to increased cerebral metabolic oxygen requirements and carbon dioxide production. These enflurane-induced changes will tend to increase cerebral blood flow, which could further increase intracranial pressure. The ability of nitrous oxide to increase intracranial pressure is probably less than that of volatile anesthetics, reflecting the restriction of the dose of this drug to less than 1 MAC.

Cerebrospinal Fluid Production

Enflurane increases both the rate of production and the resistance to reabsorption of cerebrospinal fluid, which may contribute to sustained increases in intracranial pressure associated with administration of this drug (Artru, 1984a). Conversely, isoflurane does not alter production of cerebrospinal fluid and, at the same time, decreases resistance to its reabsorption (Artru, 1984b). These observations are consistent with minimal increases in intracranial pressure observed during administration of isoflurane. Increases in intracranial pressure associated with administration of nitrous oxide presumably reflect increases in cerebral blood flow, because enhanced production of cerebrospinal fluid does not occur in the presence of this anesthetic (Artru, 1982).

CIRCULATORY EFFECTS

Inhaled anesthetics produce dose-dependent and drug-specific circulatory effects (Eger, 1985a). These effects manifest on blood pressure, heart rate, cardiac output, stroke volume, right atrial pressure, systemic vascular resistance, cardiac rhythm, and coronary blood flow. Circulatory effects of inhaled anesthetics may be different in the presence of (1) controlled ventilation of the lungs compared with spontaneous breathing, (2) preexisting cardiac disease, or (3) drugs that act directly or indirectly on the heart. Mechanisms of circulatory effects are diverse but often reflect effects of inhaled anesthetics on (1) myocardial contractility, (2) peripheral vascular smooth muscle tone, and (3) autonomic nervous system activity (see the section entitled "Mechanisms of Circulatory Effects").

Blood Pressure

Volatile anesthetics produce dose-dependent decreases in blood pressure, with enflurane and isoflurane producing somewhat greater decreases than halothane (Fig. 2-6) (Calverley et al, 1978b; Eger et al, 1970; Eger 1985a; Stevens et al, 1971). In contrast with volatile anesthetics, nitrous oxide produces either no change or modest increases in blood pressure (Fig. 2-6) (Eger, 1985a; Hornbein et al, 1982). Substitution of nitrous oxide for a portion of the volatile anesthetic reduces the magnitude of blood pressure decrease produced by the same MAC concentration of the volatile anesthetic alone (Fig. 2-7) (Dolan et al, 1974; Eger 1985a). Surgical stimulation also reduces the magnitude of blood pressure decrease produced by volatile anesthetics. The decrease in blood pressure produced by enflurane and halothane is, in part or in whole, a consequence of decreases in myocardial contractility and cardiac output, whereas with isoflurane, the decrease in blood pressure results almost entirely from a decrease in systemic vascular resistance (see the section entitled "Mechanisms of

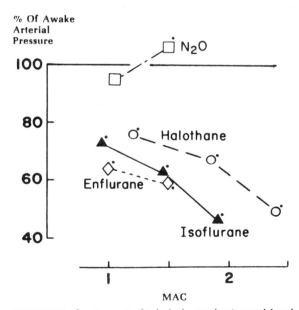

FIGURE 2–6.   Impact of inhaled anesthetics on blood pressure in the presence of normocapnia and absence of surgical stimulation. *P <0.05. (From Eger EI. Isoflurane [Forane]. A compendium and reference. 2nd edition. Madison, WI, Ohio Medical Products, 1985; 1–110; with permission.)

% Of Awake Blood Pressure

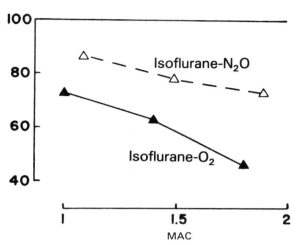

FIGURE 2-7. The substitution of N_2O for a portion of isoflurane produces less depression of blood pressure than the same dose of volatile anesthetics alone. (From Eger EI. Isoflurane [Forane]. A compendium and reference. 2nd edition. Madison, WI, Ohio Medical Products, 1985: 1–110; with permission.)

Circulatory Effects"). It is important to recognize that artificially elevated preoperative levels of blood pressure, as can accompany apprehension, may be followed by decreases in blood pressure that exceed the true pharmacologic effect of the volatile anesthetic.

Heart Rate

The effects of volatile anesthetics on heart rate may be influenced by the awake level of autonomic nervous system activity. For example, increased sympathetic nervous system activity, as accompanies apprehension, may artificially elevate heart rate and alter the magnitude of the true pharmacologic effect of the volatile anesthetic. Likewise, excessive awake parasympathetic nervous system activity may result in unexpected increases in heart rate when anesthesia is established. With this in mind, it is a common observation that heart rate is not substantially altered during administration of halothane despite drug-induced reductions in blood pressure. This unchanged heart rate may reflect depression of the carotid sinus (baroreceptor-reflex response) by halothane, as well as drug-induced decreases in

the rate of sinus node depolarization. Junctional rhythm and associated decreases in blood pressure most likely reflect suppression of sinus node activity by halothane. Halothane also decreases the speed of conduction of cardiac impulses through the atrioventricular node and His-Purkinje system. In contrast to halothane, heart rate tends to increase during isoflurane-induced reductions in blood pressure, suggesting better preservation of the carotid sinus reflex response (Kotrly et al, 1984). Nevertheless, there is evidence that isoflurane and enflurane have similar depressive effects on the carotid sinus control of heart rate with or without the presence of surgical stimulation (Fig. 2-8) (Takeshima and Dohi, 1989). During awakening from anesthesia, the carotid sinus reflex response seems to recover more rapidly in patients exposed to isoflurane than in those receiving enflurane. In neonates, administration of isoflurane is associated with attenuation of carotid sinus reflex responses, as reflected by drug-induced decreases in blood pressure that are not accompanied by increases in heart rate (Murat et al, 1989). Heart rate responses during administration of isoflurane also seem to be blunted in elderly patients, in patients receiving opioids as preoperative medication, or during the induction of anesthesia (Fig. 2-9) (Cahalan et al, 1987; Mallow et al, 1976). Conversely, isoflurane-induced increases in heart rate are more likely to occur in younger patients and may be accentuated by the presence of other drugs (atropine, pancuronium) that exert vagolytic effects. Nitrous oxide also depresses the carotid sinus, but quantitating this effect is difficult because of the limited potency of nitrous oxide and its frequent simultaneous administration with other injected or inhaled drugs.

Cardiac Output and Stroke Volume

Administration of isoflurane during controlled ventilation of the lungs to maintain normocapnia does not greatly reduce the cardiac output from awake levels (Fig. 2-10) (Eger, 1985a). In contrast, halothane and enflurane produce dose-dependent reductions in cardiac output that principally reflect decreases in stroke volume owing to reductions in myocardial contractility (Fig. 2-10) (Eger, 1985a). Isoflurane also decreases stroke volume, but this is largely offset by increases in heart rate such that cardiac output is reduced only minimally. Cardiac output is mod-

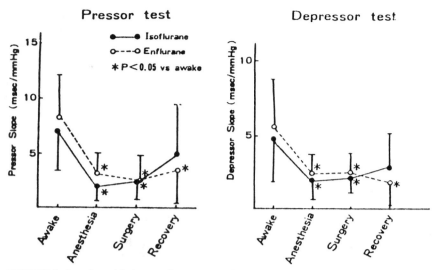

FIGURE 2–8. Carotid sinus reflex activity during administration of phenylephrine (pressor test) or nitroglycerin (depressor test) is similarly decreased during administration of isoflurane or enflurane. (From Takeshima R, Dohi S. Comparison of arterial baroreflex function in humans anesthetized with enflurane or isoflurane. Anesth Analg 1989; 69: 284–90; with permission.)

estly increased by nitrous oxide, possibly reflecting mild sympathomimetic effects of this drug.

In addition to better maintenance of heart rate, isoflurane's minimal depressant effects on cardiac output could reflect activation of homeostatic mechanisms that obscure direct cardiac depressant effects. Indeed, volatile anesthetics, including isoflurane, produce similar dose-dependent depression of myocardial contractility when studied *in vitro* using isolated papillary muscle preparations (Kemmotsu et al, 1973). *In vitro* depression of myocardial contractility produced by nitrous oxide is about one half that produced by comparable concentrations of volatile anesthetics. Direct myocardial depressant effects *in vivo* are most likely offset by mild sympathomimetic effects of nitrous oxide.

Another possible explanation for the lesser impact of isoflurane on myocardial contractility may be a greater anesthetic potency of isoflurane relative to halothane and enflurane (Eger, 1985a). For example, the multiple of MAC times the oil:gas partition coefficient for halothane, enflurane, and isoflurane is 168, 163, and 105, respectively. The implication is that isoflurane may more readily depress the brain and, thus, at a given MAC value, appear to spare the heart.

Indeed, in animals, the lesser myocardial depression associated with administration of isoflurane manifests as a greater margin of safety between the dose that produces anesthesia and that which produces cardiovascular collapse (Wolfson et al, 1978).

Right Atrial Pressure

Inhaled anesthetics produce dose-dependent increases in right atrial pressure, presumably reflecting direct myocardial depression and depressant drug effects on the peripheral vasculature (Fig 2-11) (Eger, 1985a). Consistent with minimal *in vivo* depression of myocardial contractility during administration of isoflurane is failure of the right atrial pressure to increase compared with other inhaled anesthetics. Peripheral vasodilating effects of isoflurane, and to a lesser extent of enflurane, would also minimize the effects of direct myocardial depression on right atrial pressure produced by these drugs. Increased right atrial pressure during administration of nitrous oxide most likely reflects increased pulmonary vascular resistance owing to sympathomimetic effects of this drug (Smith et al, 1970).

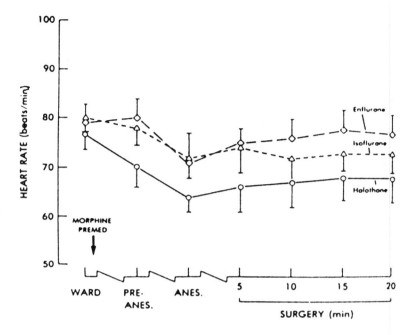

FIGURE 2–9. Morphine premedication is not associated with increases in heart rate (mean ± SE) during administration of volatile anesthetics with or without surgical stimulation. (From Cahalan MK, Lurz FW, Eger EI, Schwartz LA, Beaupre PN, Smith JS. Narcotics decrease heart rate during inhalational anesthesia. Anesth Analg 1987; 66: 166–70; with permission.)

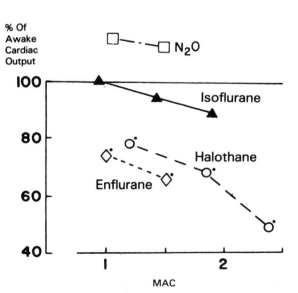

FIGURE 2–10. Impact of inhaled anesthetics on cardiac output in the presence of normocapnia and absence of surgical stimulation. *P <0.05. (From Eger EI. Isoflurane [Forane]. A compendium and reference. 2nd edition. Madison, WI, Ohio Medical Products, 1985: 1–110; with permission.)

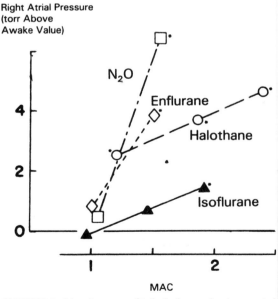

FIGURE 2–11. Impact of inhaled anesthetics on right atrial pressure in the presence of normocapnia and absence of surgical stimulation. *P <0.05. (From Eger EI. Isoflurane [Forane]. A compendium and reference. 2nd edition. Madison, WI, Ohio Medical Products, 1985: 1–110; with permission.)

Systemic (Peripheral) Vascular Resistance

Isoflurane produces dose-dependent decreases in systemic vascular resistance that exceed the decreases produced by enflurane (Fig. 2-12) (Eger, 1985a). Systemic vascular resistance does not change during administration of halothane or nitrous oxide (Fig. 2-12) (Eger, 1985a). Substitution of nitrous oxide for a portion of the isoflurane dose reduces the magnitude of decrease in systemic vascular resistance produced by administration of isoflurane. The effect of isoflurane on calculated systemic vascular resistance is predictable considering this drug's known effects on blood pressure and cardiac output. Likewise, the absence of changes in systemic vascular resistance during administration of halothane emphasizes that reductions in blood pressure produced by this drug parallel decreases in myocardial contractility and cardiac output.

Decreases in systemic vascular resistance during administration of isoflurane principally reflect substantial (up to fourfold) increases in

% Of Awake Peripheral Resistance

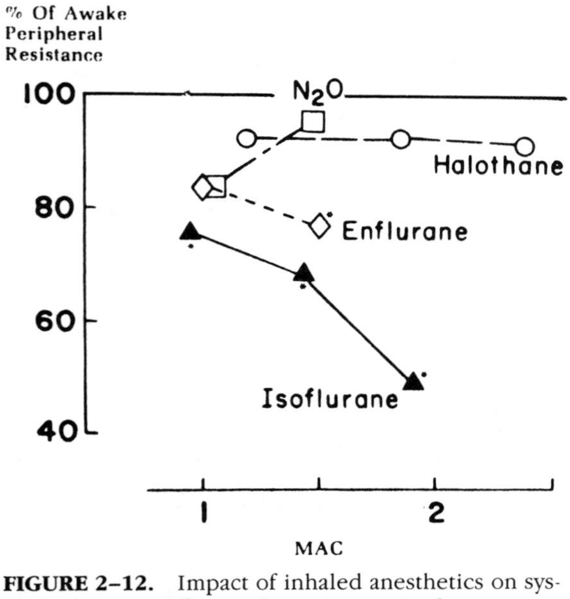

FIGURE 2–12. Impact of inhaled anesthetics on systemic (peripheral) vascular resistance in the presence of normocapnia and absence of surgical stimulation. *P <0.05. (From Eger EI. Isoflurane [Forane]. A compendium and reference. 2nd edition. Madison, WI, Ohio Medical Products, 1985: 1–110; with permission.)

skeletal-muscle blood flow (Stevens et al, 1971). Cutaneous blood flow is also increased by isoflurane. Implications of these alterations in blood flow may include (1) excess (wasted) perfusion relative to oxygen needs, (2) loss of body heat owing to increased cutaneous blood flow, and (3) enhanced delivery of drugs, such as muscle relaxants, to the neuromuscular junction. A beta-agonist effect of isoflurane is consistent with vascular smooth muscle relaxation in skeletal muscles.

Failure of systematic vascular resistance to decrease during administration of halothane does not mean that this drug lacks vasodilating effects on some organ systems. Clearly, halothane is a potent cerebral vasodilator, and cutaneous vasodilation is prominent. These vasodilating effects of halothane, however, are offset by absent changes or vasoconstriction in other vascular beds such that the overall effect is an unchanged calculated systemic vascular resistance.

The increase in cutaneous blood flow produced by all volatile anesthetics arterializes peripheral venous blood, providing an alternative to sampling arterial blood for evaluation of pH and $PaCO_2$ (Fig. 2-13) (Williamson and Munson, 1982). These drug-induced increases in cutaneous blood flow most likely reflect a central inhibitory action of these anesthetics on temperature-regulating mechanisms. In contrast to volatile anesthetics, nitrous oxide may produce constriction of cutaneous blood vessels (Smith et al, 1978).

Pulmonary Vascular Resistance

Volatile anesthetics appear to exert little or no predictable effect on pulmonary vascular smooth muscle. Conversely, nitrous oxide may produce increases in pulmonary vascular resistance that are exaggerated in patients with preexisting pulmonary hypertension (Hilgenberg et al, 1980; Schulte-Sasse et al, 1982). The neonate with or without preexisting pulmonary hypertension may also be uniquely vulnerable to the pulmonary vascular vasoconstricting effects of nitrous oxide (Eisele et al, 1986). In patients with congenital heart disease, these increases in pulmonary vascular resistance may increase the magnitude of right-to-left intracardiac shunting of blood and further jeopardize arterial oxygenation.

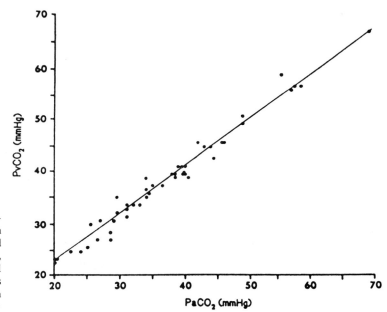

FIGURE 2–13. There is a linear relationship between PCO_2 measured in "arterialized" peripheral venous blood and the $PaCO_2$. (From Williamson DC, Munson ES. Correlation of peripheral venous and arterial blood gas values during general anesthesia. Anesth Analg; 1982: 61: 950–2; with permission.)

Duration of Administration

Administration of a volatile anesthetic for 5 hours or longer is accompanied by recovery from the depressant circulatory effects of these drugs. For example, compared with measurements at 1 hour, the same MAC concentration after 5 hours is associated with a return of cardiac output toward predrug levels (Figs. 2-14 and 2-15) (Bahlman et al, 1972; Calverley et al, 1978b). After 5 hours, heart rate is also increased, but blood pressure is unchanged, as the increase in cardiac output is offset by decreases in systemic vascular resistance. Evidence of recovery with time is most apparent during administration of halothane, is intermediate with enflurane, and is minimal during inhalation of isoflurane. Minimal evidence of recovery during administration of isoflurane is predictable, because this drug does not substantially alter cardiac output even at 1 hour.

The return of cardiac output toward predrug levels with time, in association with increases in heart rate and peripheral vasodilation, resembles a beta-adrenergic agonist response. Indeed, pretreatment with propranolol prevents evidence of recovery with time from the circulatory effects of volatile anesthetics (Price et al, 1970).

Cardiac Dysrhythmias

The ability of volatile anesthetics to reduce the dose of epinephrine necessary to evoke ventricular cardiac dysrhythmias is greatest with halothane. For example, the dose of submucosally injected epinephrine necessary to produce cardiac dysrhythmias in 50% of patients anesthetized with a 1.25 MAC concentration of a volatile anesthetic is 2.1, 6.7, and 10.9 $\mu g \cdot kg^{-1}$ during administration of halothane, isoflurane, and enflurane, respectively (Fig. 2-16) (Johnston et al, 1976). This order of arrhythmogenic potential is consistent with the alkane structure of halothane compared with ether derivatives such as isoflurane and enflurane. In contrast to adults, children tolerate larger doses of subcutaneous epinephrine (7.8 to 10 $\mu g \cdot kg^{-1}$) injected with or without lidocaine during halothane anesthesia (Karl et al, 1983; Ueda et al, 1983). Mechanical stimulation associated with injection of epinephrine for repair of cleft palate has been associated with cardiac dysrhythmias (Ueda et al, 1983).

Inclusion of lidocaine, 0.5%, in the epinephrine solution that is injected submucosally nearly doubles the dose of epinephrine necessary to provoke ventricular cardiac dysrhythmias (Fig. 2-16) (Johnston et al, 1976). A similar response

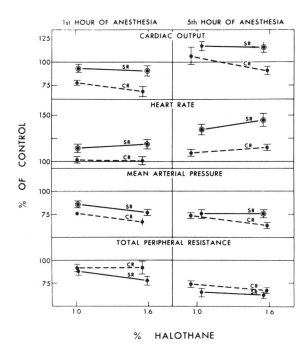

FIGURE 2–14. Comparison of circulatory effects of halothane during spontaneous breathing (*SR*) and controlled ventilation of the lungs (*CR*) after 1 and 5 hours of administration of halothane. (From Bahlman SH, Eger EI, Halsey MJ, et al. The cardiovascular effects of halothane in man during spontaneous ventilation. Anesthesiology 1972; 36: 494–502; with permission.)

occurs when lidocaine is combined with epinephrine injected submucosally during administration of enflurane (Horrigan et al, 1978). Despite this apparent protective effect of lidocaine, the systemic concentrations of the local anesthetic are less than 1 $\mu g \cdot ml^{-1}$ following its subcutaneous injection with epinephrine (Stoelting, 1978).

In animals, enhancement of the arrhythmogenic potential of epinephrine is independent of the dose of halothane between alveolar concentrations of 0.5% and 2% (Metz and Maze, 1985). If true in patients, it is likely that cardiac dysrhythmias owing to epinephrine will persist until the halothane concentration decreases to less than 0.5%. For this reason, therapeutic interventions other than decreasing the inhaled concentration of halothane may be required to treat cardiac dysrhythmias promptly owing to epinephrine.

The explanation for the difference between volatile anesthetics and the arrhythmogenic potential of epinephrine may reflect the effects of these drugs on the transmission rate of cardiac impulses through the heart. Nevertheless, halothane, enflurane, and isoflurane all slow the rate of sinoatrial node discharge and prolong His-Purkinje and ventricular conduction times (Atlee and Bosnjak, 1990) (see Chapter 48). Slow conduction of cardiac impulses through the His-Purkinje system during administration of halothane would increase the likelihood of cardiac dysrhythmias owing to a reentry mechanism (see Chapter 48). A role of alpha- and beta-adrenergic receptors in the heart is suggested by the in-

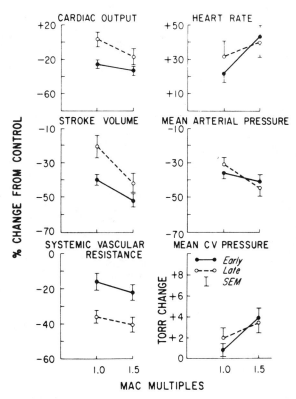

FIGURE 2–15. Comparison of circulatory effects of enflurane after 1 hour (*solid line*) and 6 hours (*broken line*) of administration during controlled ventilation of the lungs to maintain normocapnia. (From Calverley RK, Smith NT, Prys-Roberts C, Eger EI, Jones CW. Cardiovascular effects of enflurane anesthesia during controlled ventilation in man. Anesth Analg 1978; 57: 619–28; with permission.)

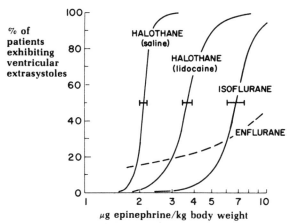

FIGURE 2–16. Number (%) of patients developing ventricular cardiac dysrhythmias (three or more premature ventricular contractions) with increasing doses of submucosal epinephrine injected during administration of 1.25 MAC concentrations of the volatile anesthetic. (From Johnston RR, Eger EI, Wilson C. A comparative interaction of epinephrine with enflurane, isoflurane and halothane in man. Anesth Analg 1976; 55: 709–12; with permission.)

creased dose of epinephrine required to produce cardiac dysrhythmias in dogs anesthetized with halothane and pretreated with droperidol, metoprolol, or prazosin (Fig. 2-17) (Maze and Smith, 1983; Maze et al, 1985).

Coronary Blood Flow

Isoflurane is a more potent coronary artery vasodilator than halothane or enflurane. There is compelling experimental as well as clinical evidence that isoflurane-induced coronary artery vasodilation can cause redistribution of coronary blood flow from diseased areas of myocardium to areas with normally responsive coronary arteries (coronary steal syndrome) (Priebe, 1989). Indeed, evidence of myocardial ischemia (ST segment changes on the electrocardiogram and decreased lactate extraction) has been observed in patients with coronary artery disease who have been anesthetized with nitrous oxide-isoflurane (Reiz et al, 1983). In one report describing patients undergoing coronary artery bypass graft operations, the administration of isoflurane was associated with a higher incidence of myocardial

infarction than was enflurane (Inoue et al, 1990). Because isoflurane (when compared to adenosine) is probably not a potent enough coronary vasodilator, and because of the added negative inotropic effect of isoflurane that will help to counteract the detrimental effects of coronary steal, only a subset of patients with steal-prone coronary artery anatomy are likely to be susceptible for the development of coronary steal syndrome. The anatomic requirements for coronary steal syndrome include total occlusion of a major coronary artery with collateral flow distal to the occlusion via a vessel with significant (greater than 90%) stenosis. An estimated 12% of patients with coronary artery disease have steal-prone anatomy and may be at increased risk for the development of isoflurane-induced myocardial ischemia (Buffington et al, 1987). Nevertheless, the incidence of myocardial ischemia in the presence of steal-prone anatomy is not different in patients receiving isoflurane as the primary anesthetic drug compared with halothane, enflurane, or sufentanil (Slogoff et al, 1991).

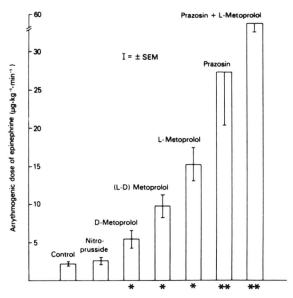

FIGURE 2–17. Arrhythmogenic dose of epinephrine during halothane anesthesia (1.2 MAC) in the dog following different treatments. *P $<$0.05. **P $<$0.01. (From Maze M, Smith CM. Identification of receptor mechanism mediating epinephrine-induced arrhythmias during halothane anesthesia in the dog. Anesthesiology 1983; 59: 322–6; with permission.)

Alterations in blood pressure and heart rate, or the presence or absence of beta-adrenergic blockade, may be more important determinants of the development of myocardial ischemia than the specific volatile anesthetic selected. For example, when isoflurane is administered as the primary or secondary anesthetic (to control blood pressure during opioid anesthetic techniques) to patients undergoing coronary artery bypass graft operations, the incidence of new perioperative ischemia, postoperative myocardial infarction, and mortality is not different from that observed during administration of halothane or enflurane (O'Young et al, 1987; Slogoff and Keats, 1988; Tuman et al, 1989). There is no evidence that nitrous oxide evokes myocardial ischemia in patients with coronary artery disease when administered as an adjuvant to fentanyl (Mitchell et al, 1989). It is estimated that as many as two thirds of the episodes of perioperative myocardial ischemia are unrelated to hemodynamic abnormalities (silent ischemia), suggesting that perioperative ischemia is principally a characteristic of underlying coronary artery disease rather than the consequence of a particular anesthetic drug, especially if sustained increases in heart rate (greater than 110 beats·min^{-1}) are avoided. In this regard, inclusion of opioids or prior treatment with beta-adrenergic antagonists may minimize the occurrence of events that alter the balance between myocardial oxygen requirements and delivery.

Spontaneous Breathing

Circulatory effects produced by volatile anesthetics during spontaneous breathing are different from those observed during normocapnia and controlled ventilation of the lungs. This difference reflects the impact of sympathetic nervous system stimulation owing to accumulation of carbon dioxide (respiratory acidosis) and improved venous return during spontaneous breathing. In addition, carbon dioxide may have direct relaxing effects on peripheral vascular smooth muscle. Indeed, cardiac output, blood pressure, and systemic vascular resistance are decreased and heart rate is increased during spontaneous breathing, compared with measurements during administration of volatile anesthetics in the presence of controlled ventilation of the lungs to maintain normocapnia (Fig. 2-14) (Bahlman et al, 1972; Calverley et al, 1978a; Cromwell et al, 1971).

Preexisting Diseases and Drug Therapy

Preexisting cardiac disease may influence the significance of circulatory effects produced by inhaled anesthetics. For example, volatile anesthetics decrease myocardial contractility of normal and failing cardiac muscle by similar amounts, but the significance is greater in diseased cardiac muscle because contractility is decreased even before administration of depressant anesthetics (Shimosato et al, 1973). In patients with coronary artery disease, administration of 40% nitrous oxide produces evidence of myocardial depression that does not occur in patients without heart disease (Eisele and Smith, 1972). Valvular heart disease may influence the significance of anesthetic-induced circulatory effects. For example, peripheral vasodilation produced by isoflurane is undesirable in patients with aortic stenosis but may be beneficial in those with mitral or aortic regurgitation. Arterial hypoxemia may enhance the cardiac depressant effects of volatile anesthetics (Cullen and Eger, 1970). Conversely, anemia does not alter anesthetic-induced circulatory effects compared with measurements from normal animals (Loarie et al, 1979).

Prior drug therapy that alters sympathetic nervous system activity (antihypertensives, beta-adrenergic antagonists) may influence the magnitude of circulatory effects produced by volatile anesthetics. Calcium entry blockers decrease myocardial contractility and thus render the heart more vulnerable to direct depressant effects of inhaled anesthetics. In animals, depressant effects of verapamil on cardiac output are greater during administration of enflurane than of isoflurane (see Chapter 18).

Mechanisms of Circulatory Effects

There is no single mechanism that explains the depressant circulatory effects of volatile anesthetics in all situations. Proposed mechanisms include (1) direct myocardial depression, (2) inhibition of central nervous system sympathetic outflow, (3) peripheral autonomic ganglion blockade, (4) attenuated carotid sinus reflex activity, (5) decreased formation of cyclic adenosine monophosphate, (6) decreased release of catecholamines from the adrenal medulla, and (7) decreased influx of calcium ions through slow channels. Indeed, negative inotropic, vasodilating, and depressant effects on the sinoatrial node produced by volatile anesthetics are similar to the effects produced by calcium entry blockers (Lynch, 1981). Plasma catecholamine concentrations typically do not increase during administration of volatile anesthetics, which is evidence that these drugs do not activate and may even decrease activity of the central and peripheral sympathetic nervous system.

Isoflurane may be unique among the volatile anesthetics in possessing mild beta-adrenergic agonist properties. This effect is consistent with the maintenance of cardiac output, increased heart rate, and decreased systemic vascular resistance that may accompany administration of isoflurane (Stevens et al, 1971). A beta-agonist effect of isoflurane, however, is not supported by animal data, failing to demonstrate a difference between volatile anesthetics with or without beta-adrenergic blockade (Philbin and Lowenstein, 1976).

Nitrous oxide administered alone or added to unchanging concentrations of volatile anesthetics produces signs of mild sympathomimetic stimulation characterized by (1) increases in the plasma concentrations of catecholamines, (2) mydriasis, (3) increases in body temperature, (4) diaphoresis, (5) increases in right atrial pressure, and (6) evidence of vasoconstriction in the systemic and pulmonary circulations. Evidence of this sympathomimetic effect is more prominent when nitrous oxide is administered in the presence of halothane than of enflurane or isoflurane (Smith et al, 1970). It is presumed that this mild sympathomimetic effect masks any direct depressant effects of nitrous oxide on the heart. Nitrous oxide–induced increases in sympathetic nervous system activity may reflect activation of brain nuclei that regulate beta-adrenergic outflow from the central nervous system (Fukunaga and Epstein, 1973). Sympathetic nervous system stimulation may also result because nitrous oxide can inhibit uptake of norepinephrine by the lungs, thus making more neurotransmitter available to receptors (Naito and Gillis, 1973).

In contrast to sympathomimetic effects observed with the administration of nitrous oxide alone or added to volatile anesthetics, the inhalation of nitrous oxide in the presence of opioids results in evidence of profound circulatory depression characterized by decreases in blood pressure and cardiac output, and increases in left ventricular end-diastolic pressure and systemic vascular resistance (Lappas et al, 1975; McDermott and Stanley, 1974; Stoelting and Gibbs, 1973). It is possible that opioids inhibit the centrally mediated sympathomimetic effects of nitrous oxide, thus unmasking its direct depressant effects on the heart (Flaim et al, 1978).

VENTILATION EFFECTS

Inhaled anesthetics produce dose-dependent and drug-specific effects on (1) the pattern of breathing, (2) the ventilatory response to carbon dioxide, (3) the ventilatory response to hypoxemia, and (4) the airway resistance. The PaO_2 predictably declines during administration of inhaled anesthetics in the absence of supplemental oxygen. Drug-induced inhibition of hypoxic pulmonary vasoconstriction as a mechanism for this decrease in oxygenation has not been confirmed during one-lung ventilation in patients breathing halothane or isoflurane (see Fig. 46-4). Changes in intraoperative PaO_2 and the incidence of postoperative pulmonary complications are not different in patients anesthetized with halothane, enflurane, or isoflurane (Gold et al, 1983).

Pattern of Breathing

Inhaled anesthetics, except for isoflurane, produce dose-dependent increases in the frequency of breathing (Fig. 2-18). (Eger, 1985b) Isoflurane increases the frequency of breathing similarly to other inhaled anesthetics up to a dose of 1 MAC. At a concentration greater than 1 MAC, however, isoflurane does not produce a further increase in the frequency of breathing. Nitrous oxide increases the frequency of breathing more than other inhaled anesthetics at concentrations greater than 1 MAC. The effect of inhaled anesthetics on the frequency of breathing presumably reflects central nervous system stimulation. Activation of pulmonary stretch receptors by inhaled anesthetics has not been demonstrated. The exception may be nitrous oxide,

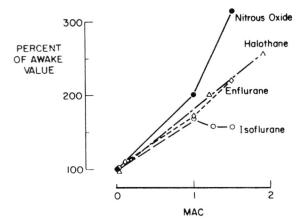

FIGURE 2–18. Impact of inhaled anesthetics on frequency of breathing in the absence of surgical stimulation. (From Eger EI. Nitrous oxide. New York, Elsevier, 1985; with permission.)

which, at anesthetic concentrations greater than 1 MAC, may also stimulate pulmonary stretch receptors (Eger, 1984).

Tidal volume is decreased in association with anesthetic-induced increases in the frequency of breathing. The net effect of these changes is a rapid and shallow pattern of breathing during general anesthesia. The increase in the frequency of breathing is insufficient to offset reductions in tidal volume, leading to decreases in minute ventilation and an increases in $PaCO_2$. The pattern of breathing during general anesthesia is also characterized as regular and rhythmic in contrast to the awake pattern of intermittent deep breaths separated by varying intervals.

Ventilatory Response to Carbon Dioxide

Volatile anesthetics produce dose-dependent depression of ventilation characterized by decreases in the ventilatory response to carbon dioxide and an increases in the $PaCO_2$. In the absence of surgical stimulation or other drugs and at comparable MAC concentrations, enflurane produces the greatest elevations in $PaCO_2$, followed by isoflurane and halothane (Fig. 2-19) (Bahlman et al, 1972; Calverley et al, 1978a; Cromwell et al, 1971; Eger, 1985a). The presence of chronic obstructive airway disease, however, may accentuate the magnitude of increases in

$PaCO_2$ produced by volatile anesthetics (Pietak et al, 1975). Nitrous oxide does not increase the $PaCO_2$, suggesting that substitution of this anesthetic for a portion of the volatile anesthetic would result in less depression of ventilation. Indeed, nitrous oxide combined with a volatile anesthetic produces less depression of ventilation and increase in $PaCO_2$ than does the same MAC concentration of the volatile drug alone (France et al, 1974; Lam et al, 1982). This ventilatory depressant-sparing effect of nitrous oxide is detectable with all three volatile anesthetics, but the greatest impact occurs when nitrous oxide is used to replace an equivalent MAC amount of enflurane (Lam et al, 1982).

Despite the apparent benign effect of nitrous oxide on ventilation, the slope of the carbon dioxide response curve is decreased similarly and shifted to the right by anesthetic concentrations of all inhaled anesthetics (Fig. 2-20) (Eger, 1985a; Fourcade et al, 1971; Knill et al, 1979). Subanesthetic concentrations (0.1 MAC) of inhaled anesthetics, however, do not alter the ventilatory response to carbon dioxide. In addition to nitrous oxide, painful (surgical incision) stimulation and duration of drug administration influence the magnitude of increase in $PaCO_2$ produced by volatile anesthetics.

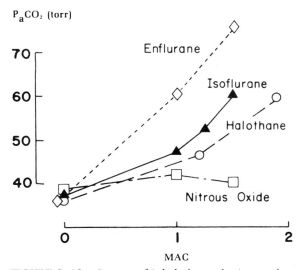

FIGURE 2–19. Impact of inhaled anesthetics on the resting $PaCO_2$ (mmHg) in the absence of surgical stimulation. (From Eger EI. Isoflurane [Forane]. A compendium and reference. 2nd edition. Madison, WI, Ohio Medical Products, 1985: 1–110; with permission.)

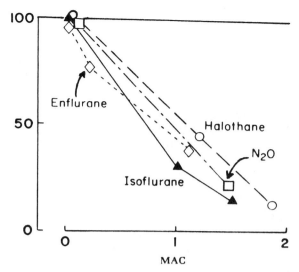

FIGURE 2–20. Impact of inhaled anesthetics on the slope of the line depicting the ventilatory response to CO_2. (From Eger EI. Isoflurane [Forane]. A compendium and reference. 2nd edition. Madison, WI, Ohio Medical Products, 1985: 1–110; with permission.)

Surgical Stimulation

Surgical stimulation increases minute ventilation by about 40% because of increases in tidal volume and frequency of breathing. The $PaCO_2$, however, decreases only about 10% (4 to 6 mmHg) despite the larger increase in minute ventilation (Fig. 2-21) (Eger, 1985a; France et al, 1974). The reason for this discrepancy is speculated to be an increased production of carbon dioxide resulting from activation of the sympathetic nervous system in response to painful surgical stimulation. Increased production of carbon dioxide is presumed to offset the impact of increased minute ventilation on the $PaCO_2$.

Duration of Administration

After about 5 hours of administration, the increase in $PaCO_2$ produced by a volatile anesthetic is less than that present during administration of the same concentration for 1 hour (Table 2-3) (Calverley et al, 1978a). Likewise, the slope and position of the carbon dioxide response curve return toward normal after about 5 hours of administration of the volatile anesthetics (Lam et al, 1982). The reason for this apparent recovery from the ventilatory depressant effects of volatile anesthetics with time is not known.

Mechanism of Depression

Anesthetic-induced depression of ventilation as reflected by increases in the $PaCO_2$ most likely reflects the direct depressant effects of these drugs on the medullary ventilatory center. An additional mechanism may be the ability of halothane and possibly other inhaled anesthetics to interfere selectively with intercostal muscle function, contributing to loss of chest wall stabilization during spontaneous breathing (Tusiewicz et al, 1977). This loss of chest wall stabilization could interfere with expansion of the chest in response to chemical stimulation of ventilation as normally produced by increases in the $PaCO_2$ or arterial hypoxemia. Furthermore, this loss of chest wall stabilization means that descent of the diaphragm tends to cause the chest to collapse inward during inspiration, contributing to reductions in lung volumes, particularly the functional residual capacity. It is thus likely that halothane-induced depression of ventilation reflects both central and peripheral effects of the drug.

Management of Depression

The predictable ventilatory depressant effects of volatile anesthetics are most often managed by institution of mechanical (controlled) ventilation of the lungs. In this regard, the inherent ventilatory depressant effects of volatile anesthetics facilitate the initiation of controlled lung ventilation. Assisted ventilation of the lungs is a questionably effective method for offsetting the ventilatory depressant effects of volatile anesthetics. For example, the apneic threshold (maximal $PaCO_2$ that does not initiate spontaneous breath-

Table 2–3
Evidence for Recovery from the Ventilatory Depressant Effects of Volatile Anesthetics

	Arterial PCO_2	
Enflurane (MAC)	1 Hour of Administration (mmHg)	5 Hours of Administration (mmHg)
1	61	46
2	Apnea	67

(Data from Calverley RK, Smith NT, Jones CW, Prys-Roberts C, Eger EI. Ventilatory and cardiovascular effects of enflurane anesthesia during controlled ventilation in man. Anesth Analg 1978; 57: 610–18.)

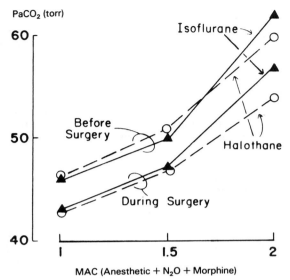

FIGURE 2–21. Impact of surgical stimulation on the resting PaCO$_2$ (mmHg) during administration of isoflurane or halothane. (From Eger EI. Isoflurane [Forane]. A compendium and reference. 2nd edition. Madison, WI, Ohio Medical Products, 1985: 1–110; with permission.)

ing) is only 3 to 5 mmHg lower than the PaCO$_2$ present during spontaneous breathing (Ravin and Olsen, 1972). As a result, a PaCO$_2$ elevated to 50 mmHg by ventilatory-depressant effects of a volatile anesthetic could only be lowered to 45 to 46 mmHg by assisted ventilation of the lungs before apnea occurs.

Ventilatory Response to Hypoxemia

All inhaled anesthetics, including nitrous oxide, profoundly depress the ventilatory response to arterial hypoxemia that is normally mediated by the carotid bodies. For example, 0.1 MAC produces 50% to 70% depression, and 1.1 MAC produces 100% depression of this response (Knill et al, 1982; Yacoub et al, 1976). This contrasts with the absence of significant depression of the ventilatory response to carbon dioxide during administration of 0.1 MAC concentrations of volatile anesthetics. Inhaled anesthetics also attenuate the usual synergistic effect of arterial hypoxemia and hypercapnia on stimulation of ventilation.

Airway Resistance

Volatile anesthetics produce dose-dependent and similar reductions in airway resistance following antigen-induced bronchoconstriction in an animal model (Fig. 2-22) (Hirshman et al, 1982). Clinical concentrations of halothane have direct relaxant effects on airway smooth muscle that most likely reflect drug-induced reductions in afferent (vagal) nerve traffic from the central nervous system. Indeed, the effects of halothane and a beta-2 agonist, albuterol, are additive, emphasizing that the anesthetic acts principally by decreasing vagal tone (Tobias and Hirshman, 1990).

Halothane and enflurane reverse the bronchoconstricting effects of hypocapnia, with halothane being more efficacious at lower doses.

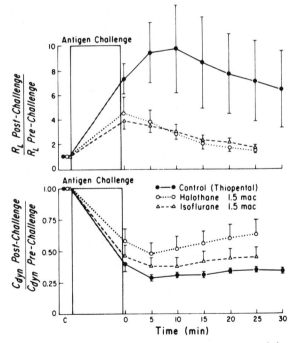

FIGURE 2–22. Increases in airway resistance and decreases in pulmonary compliance following *Ascaris* antigen challenge during anesthesia in dogs. These changes are similarly attenuated by halothane and isoflurane. Mean ± SD. (From Hirshman CA, Edelstein G, Peetz S, Wayne R, Downes H. Mechanism of action of inhalational anesthesia on airways. Anesthesiology 1982; 56: 107–11; with permission.)

Furthermore, halothane prevents and reverses airway constriction in patients with asthma and attenuates histamine-induced bronchoconstriction. d-Tubocurarine–induced histamine release from a human tissue preparation is attenuated in a dose-related manner by halothane but not by nitrous oxide (Fig. 2-23) (Kettlekamp et al, 1987). Despite these observations, it is not documented that bronchodilating effects of volatile anesthetics, specifically halothane, are an effective method for treating status asthmaticus that is unresponsive to more conventional treatments. In the absence of bronchoconstriction, the bronchodilating effects of volatile anesthetics are difficult to demonstrate, because normal bronchomotor tone is low and only minimal additional relaxation is possible. Inhaled anesthetics are not irritating to airways, thus increased secretions or elevations in airway resistance by this mechanism are unlikely. Like other inhaled anesthetics, nitrous oxide decreases functional residual capacity; this may be exaggerated by nitrous oxide–induced skeletal muscle rigidity.

HEPATIC EFFECTS

Hepatic Blood Flow

Portal vein blood flow decreases, whereas hepatic artery blood flow increases, during administration of isoflurane to an animal model (Fig. 2-24) (Gelman et al, 1984). In contrast, decreases in portal vein blood flow are not offset by increases in hepatic artery blood flow during the administration of halothane (Fig. 2-24) (Gelman et al, 1984). As a result, hepatic oxygen delivery is better maintained in the presence of isoflurane than during administration of halothane. In another report, patients receiving 1 MAC isoflurane plus nitrous oxide demonstrated increases in hepatic blood flow and increased hepatic venous

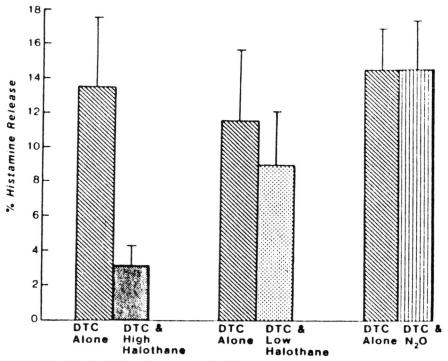

FIGURE 2–23.   Inhibition (mean ± SE) of d-tubocurarine (DTC)-induced histamine release by halothane but not by nitrous oxide. (From Kettlekamp NS, Austin DR, Downes H, Cheek DBC, Hirshman CA. Inhibition of d-tubocurarine-induced histamine release by halothane. Anesthesiology 1987; 66: 666–9; with permission.)

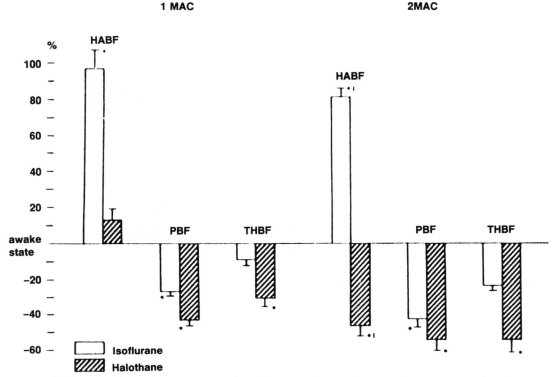

FIGURE 2-24.   Changes (%, mean ± SE) in liver circulation during administration of isoflurane or halothane. HABF-hepatic artery blood flow; PBF-portal vein blood flow; THBF-total hepatic blood flow (From Gelman S, Fowler KC, Smith LR. Liver circulation and function during isoflurane and halothane anesthesia. Anesthesiology 1984; 61: 726–30; with permission.)

oxygen saturation, whereas hepatic blood flow did not change in patients receiving 1 MAC halothane plus nitrous oxide (Goldfarb et al, 1990). Selective hepatic artery vasoconstriction has been reported in otherwise healthy patients during the administration of halothane (Benumof et al, 1976). Maintenance of hepatic oxygen delivery relative to demand during exposure to anesthetics is uniquely important in view of the evidence that hepatocyte hypoxia is a significant mechanism in the multifactorial etiology of postoperative hepatic dysfunction.

Drug Clearance

Volatile anesthetics may interfere with clearance of drugs from the plasma as a result of reductions in hepatic blood flow or inhibition of drug-metabolizing enzymes. Intrinsic clearance by hepatic metabolism of drugs such as propranolol is decreased 54% to 68% by inhaled anesthetics (Whelan et al, 1989). This decreased clearance may be stereoselective, as evidenced by a greater reduction of hepatic metabolism of the dextro than the levo isomer of propranolol in the presence of halothane (Fig. 2-25) (Whelan et al, 1989). Metabolism of drugs whose principal route of metabolism is by oxidation is inhibited by halothane. In contrast, halothane does not inhibit clearance of morphine, whose primary route of metabolism is by glucuronidation, suggesting that inhibition of drug metabolism by inhaled anesthetics may be pathway (enzyme) specific. In the overall hepatic clearance of drugs, reductions in hepatic blood flow seem less important than anesthetic-induced inhibition of hepatic drug-metabolizing enzymes (Reilly et al, 1985).

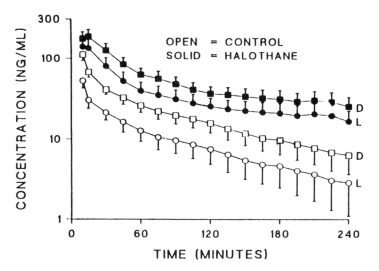

FIGURE 2–25. Mean (± SE) arterial plasma concentration of the D (dextro) and L (levo) isomers of propranolol awake vs during administration of halothane. (From Whelan E, Wood AJJ, Koshakji R, Shay S, Wood M. Halothane inhibition of propranolol metabolism is stereoselective. Anesthesiology 1989; 71: 561–4; with permission.)

Liver Function Tests

Halothane, but not isoflurane or enflurane, is associated with transient elevations of bromsulphalein retention following prolonged administration (8.8 to 11.6 MAC hours) in the absence of surgical stimulation (Eger et al, 1976; Stevens et al, 1973). Transient elevations of liver transaminase enzymes follow prolonged administration of enflurane but not halothane or isoflurane. These changes following prolonged administration of halothane and enflurane are statistically significant but not clinically important. In the presence of surgical stimulation, bromsulphalein retention and elevations of liver transaminase enzymes follow transiently the administration of even isoflurane, suggesting that changes in hepatic blood flow evoked by painful stimulation can adversely alter hepatic function independently of the volatile anesthetic.

Hepatotoxicity

All anesthetics studied in the hypoxic rat model that includes enzyme induction may produce centrilobular necrosis, but the incidence is greatest with halothane (Fig. 2-26) (Shingu et al, 1983). It is likely that inadequate hepatocyte oxygenation (oxygen supply relative to oxygen demand) is the principal mechanism responsible for hepatic dysfunction that follows anesthesia and surgery. Any anesthetic that decreases alveo-

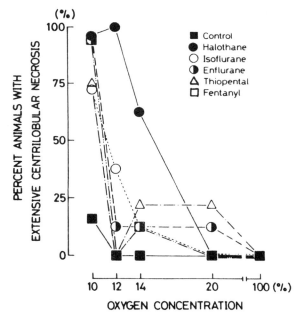

FIGURE 2–26. Hepatic damage may occur in the rat model following administration of inhaled or injected drugs when the inhaled oxygen concentration is 10%. Conversely, hepatic damage occurs following administration of halothane, but not enflurane or isoflurane, when the inhaled concentration of oxygen is 12% or 14%. (From Shingu K, Eger EI, Johnson BH, Van Dyke RA, Lurz FW, Cheng A. Effect of oxygen concentration, hyperthermia, and choice of vendor on anesthetic-induced hepatic injury in rats. Anesth Analg 1983; 62: 146–50; with permission.)

lar ventilation and/or reduces hepatic blood flow could interfere with adequate hepatocyte oxygenation. Enzyme induction increases oxygen demand and could make patients vulnerable to decreased hepatic oxygen supply owing to anesthetic-induced ventilatory or circulatory events that decrease oxygen delivery. Preexisting liver disease, such as cirrhosis, may be associated with marginal hepatocyte oxygenation, which would be further jeopardized by the depressant effects of anesthetics on hepatic blood flow and/or arterial oxygenation. Indeed, liver transaminase enzymes are increased more in cirrhotic than noncirrhotic animals exposed to halothane (Fig. 2-27) (Baden et al, 1987). Hypothermia, which decreases hepatic oxygen demand, may protect the liver from drug-induced events that reduce hepatic oxygen delivery.

Halothane

Halothane is speculated to produce two types of hepatotoxicity. The first is a mild, self-limited postoperative hepatotoxicity that is characterized by transient elevations in plasma levels of liver transaminase enzymes. The rarer and more severe form of hepatotoxicity (halothane hepatitis) occurs in 1 in 10,000 to 30,000 patients exposed to halothane and may lead to massive hepatic necrosis and death. It is likely that the more common self-limited form of hepatic dysfunction following halothane is a nonspecific drug effect owing to changes in hepatic blood flow that impair hepatocyte oxygenation. Conversely, the more rare, life-threatening form of hepatic dysfunction characterized as halothane hepatitis is most likely an immune-mediated hepatotoxicity.

HALOTHANE HEPATITIS. Clinical manifestations of halothane hepatitis that suggest an immune-mediated response include eosinophilia, fever, rash, arthralgia, and prior exposure to halothane. More important, the plasma of many patients with a clinical diagnosis of halothane hepatitis has been found to contain specific antibodies that react with halothane-induced liver antigens (neoantigens), whereas the plasma of patients with other forms of hepatitis do not contain antibodies of this specificity (Hubbard et al, 1988). These neoantigens are formed by the covalent interaction of the reactive oxidative trifluoroacetyl halide metabolite of halothane with hepatic microsomal proteins. This acetylation of liver proteins in effect changes these proteins from self to nonself (neoantigens), resulting in formation of antibodies against this now foreign protein. It is presumed that the subsequent antigen-antibody interaction is responsible for the liver injury associated with halothane hepatitis. The possibility of a genetic susceptibility factor is suggested by case reports of halothane hepatitis in closely related females (Farrell et al, 1985; Gourlay et al, 1981).

Several observations suggest that reductive metabolism is not the primary mechanism in the occurrence of halothane hepatitis. For example, neither enflurane or isoflurane undergoes reductive metabolism, yet these drugs both produce centrilobular necrosis in the hypoxic rate model. Furthermore, metabolites produced by reductive metabolism of halothane do not themselves produce hepatotoxicity. Finally, fasting does not alter metabolism but enhances hepatotoxicity produced by volatile anesthetics.

FIGURE 2–27. Increases (mean ± SE) in liver transaminase enzymes following administration of 1.05% halothane for 3 hours to noncirrhotic or cirrhotic rats. (From Baden JM, Serra M, Fujinaga M, Mazze RI. Halothane metabolism in cirrhotic rats. Anesthesiology 1987; 67: 660–4; with permission.)

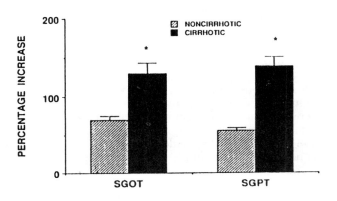

Enflurane and Isoflurane

Mild, self-limited postoperative hepatic dysfunction that is associated with enflurane or isoflurane most likely reflects anesthetic-induced alterations in hepatic oxygen delivery relative to demand that result in inadequate hepatocyte oxygenation. More disturbing, however, is the realization that an oxidative halide metabolite of both these anesthetics is able to acetylate the same liver proteins that are rendered antigenic by the trifluoroacetyl halide metabolite of halothane (Christ et al, 1988). As a result, acetylated liver proteins capable of evoking an antibody response could occur after exposure to halothane, enflurane, or isoflurane. Furthermore, there is cross-sensitivity between halogenated anesthetics such that changing halogenated anesthetics for patients requiring multiple exposures will not necessarily reduce the risk of anesthetic-induced liver injury in susceptible patients. Considering the magnitude of metabolism of these volatile drugs, however, it is predictable that the incidence of anesthetic-induced hepatitis owing to an immune-mediated mechanism would be greatest with halothane, intermediate with enflurane, and lowest with isoflurane. Indeed, based on the estimated use of enflurane and isoflurane, the alleged incidence of hepatic dysfunction produced by these anesthetics as indicated by the number of published reports is less than the spontaneous attack rate of viral hepatitis (Brown and Gandolfi, 1987). Nevertheless, development of a enzyme-linked immunosorbent assay for detection of antibodies evoked by acetylation of liver proteins may help detect those rare patients who have become sensitized owing to a prior exposure to halothane and thus at presumed increased risk for subsequent exposure to enflurane or isoflurane (Martin et al, 1990).

RENAL EFFECTS

Volatile anesthetics produce similar dose-related reductions in renal blood flow, glomerular filtration rate, and urine output (Cousins et al, 1976; Mazze et al, 1974). These changes are not a result of release of antidiuretic hormone, but rather most likely reflect effects of volatile anesthetics on blood pressure and cardiac output. Preoperative hydration attenuates or abolishes many of the changes in renal function associated with volatile anesthetics. Halothane does not alter autoregulation of renal blood flow (see Chapter 53). Renal function following kidney transplantation is not influenced by the volatile anesthetic administered (Cronnelly et al, 1984).

Nephrotoxicity

Fluoride-induced nephrotoxicity is a potential hazard following metabolism of volatile anesthetics, principally enflurane. Peak plasma fluoride concentrations following a 2.5 MAC hour exposure to enflurane are about 20 $\mu M \cdot L^{-1}$, which is about one third the level considered to be potentially nephrotoxic. Metabolism of halothane and isoflurane to inorganic fluoride is insufficient to introduce even a theoretical risk of fluoride-induced nephrotoxicity. Indeed, the ability to concentrate urine remains unaltered following short-term administration of volatile anesthetics including enflurane (Fig. 2–28) (Cousins et al, 1976). Conversely, prolonged administration (greater than 9.6 MAC hours) of enflurane, but not halothane, is associated with detectable decreases in urine-concentrating ability despite plasma fluoride concentrations averaging 15 $\mu M \cdot L^{-1}$ (Fig. 2-29) (Mazze et al, 1977). This observation that even low plasma fluoride concentrations may transiently interfere with renal tubular function suggests that administration of enflurane to patients with preexisting renal disease might be harmful. Nevertheless, there is no detectable reduction in renal function in patients with chronic renal disease who undergo elective operations and receive halothane or enflurane (Mazze et al, 1984). In fact, plasma creatinine concentrations decline and creatinine clearance increases following anesthesia with either anesthetic.

SKELETAL MUSCLE EFFECTS

Enflurane and isoflurane produce skeletal muscle relaxation that is about twofold greater than that associated with a comparable dose of halothane. Nitrous oxide does not relax skeletal muscles, and in doses greater than 1 MAC, it may produce skeletal muscle rigidity (Hornbein et al,

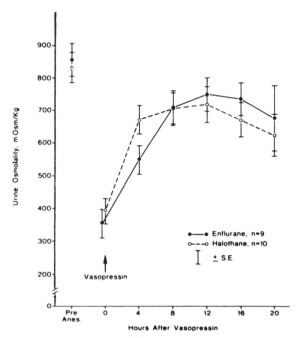

FIGURE 2–28. The ability to concentrate urine in response to administration of vasopressin remains unaltered following short-term administration of halothane (4.1 MAC hours) or enflurane (2.7 MAC hours). (From Cousins MJ, Greenstein LR, Hitt BA, Mazze RI. Metabolism and renal effects of enflurane in man. Anesthesiology 1976; 44: 44–53; with permission.)

1982). This effect of nitrous oxide is consistent with enhancement of skeletal muscle rigidity produced by opioids when low concentrations of nitrous oxide are administered. The ability of skeletal muscles to sustain contractions in response to high-frequency (greater than 120 Hz), continuous stimulation is often impaired in the presence of 1.25 MAC enflurane or isoflurane, but not halothane or nitrous oxide (Fig. 2-30) (Miller et al, 1971). Increased doses of enflurane and isoflurane further impair the ability of skeletal muscles to sustain a contraction in response to high-frequency stimulation.

Volatile anesthetics produce dose-dependent enhancement of the effects of neuromuscular blocking drugs, with the effects of enflurane and isoflurane being similar and greater than halothane (see Chapter 8). *In vitro,* isoflurane and halothane produce similar potentiation of the effects of neuromuscular blocking drugs (Vitez et al, 1974). Nitrous oxide does not significantly potentiate the *in vivo* effects of neuromuscular blocking drugs.

Volatile anesthetics can trigger malignant hyperthermia, but enflurane and isoflurane are less potent in this regard than is halothane. Nitrous oxide compared with volatile anesthetics is a weak trigger for malignant hyperthermia. For example, augmentation of caffeine-induced contractures of frog sartorius muscle by nitrous oxide is 1.3 times, whereas that for isoflurane is 3 times, enflurane 4 times, and halothane 11 times (Reed and Strobel, 1978).

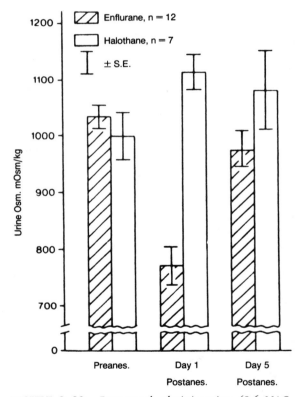

FIGURE 2–29. Prolonged administration (9.6 MAC hours) of enflurane, but not halothane, is associated with transient impairment of the ability of the renal tubules to concentrate urine. (From Mazze RI, Calverley RK, Smith NT. Inorganic fluoride nephrotoxicity: Prolonged enflurane and halothane anesthesia in volunteers. Anesthesiology 1977; 46: 265–71; with permission.)

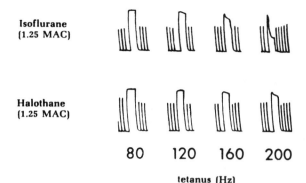

Isoflurane
(1.25 MAC)

Halothane
(1.25 MAC)

80   120   160   200

tetanus (Hz)

FIGURE 2–30. The thenar response to continuous stimulation (tetanus) at increasing frequency (Hz) is less likely to be sustained during administration of isoflurane compared with halothane. (From Miller RD, Eger EI, Way WL, Stevens WC, Dolan WM. Comparative neuromuscular effects of Forane and halothane alone and in combination with d-tubocurarine in man. Anesthesiology 1971; 35: 38–42; with permission.)

OBSTETRIC EFFECTS

Volatile anesthetics produce similar and dose-dependent decreases in uterine smooth muscle contractility and blood flow (Fig. 2-31) (Eger, 1985a; Munson and Embro, 1977; Palahniuk and Shnider, 1974). These changes are modest at 0.5 MAC (analgesic concentrations) but become substantial at concentrations greater than 1 MAC. Nitrous oxide does not alter uterine contractility in doses used to provide analgesia during vaginal delivery.

Anesthetic-induced uterine relaxation may be desirable to facilitate removal of retained placenta. Conversely, uterine relaxation produced by volatile anesthetics may contribute to blood loss owing to uterine atony. Indeed, blood loss during therapeutic abortion is greater in patients anesthetized with a volatile anesthetic compared with that in patients receiving a nitrous oxide–barbiturate–opioid anesthetic (Cullen et al, 1970; Dolan et al, 1972).

In animals, evidence of fetal distress does not accompany anesthetic-induced decreases in maternal uterine blood flow as long as the anesthetic concentration is less than 1.5 MAC (Biehl et al, 1983). Furthermore, volatile anesthetics at about 0.5 MAC concentrations combined with 50% nitrous oxide ensure amnesia during cesar-

ean section and do not produce detectable effects on the neonate (Warren et al, 1983). Inhaled anesthetics rapidly cross the placenta to enter the fetus, but these drugs are likewise rapidly exhaled by the newborn infant. Nitrous oxide-induced analgesia for vaginal delivery develops more rapidly than with volatile anesthetics, but, after about 10 minutes, all inhaled drugs provide comparable analgesia.

RESISTANCE TO INFECTION

Many normal functions of the immune system are depressed after exposure to the combination of anesthesia and surgery (Stevenson et al, 1990). It would seem that many of the immune changes seen in surgical patients are primarily the result of surgical trauma and endocrine responses (increased catecholamines and corticosteroids) rather than the result of the anesthetic exposure itself. Inhaled anesthetics, particularly nitrous oxide, produce dose-dependent inhibition of polymorphonuclear leukocytes and their subsequent migration (chemotaxis) for phagocytosis, which is necessary for the inflammatory response to infection. Nevertheless, decreased resistance

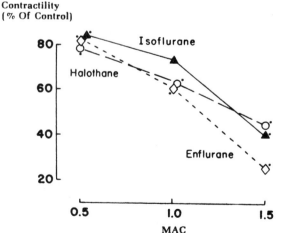

Contractility
(% Of Control)

FIGURE 2–31. Impact of volatile anesthetics on contractility of uterine smooth muscle strips studied *in vitro.* *P <0.05. (From Eger EI. Isoflurane [Forane]. A compendium and reference. 2nd edition. Madison, WI, Ohio Medical Products, 1985: 1–110; with permission.)

to bacterial infection owing to inhaled anesthetics seems unlikely, considering the duration and dose of these drugs. Furthermore, when leukocytes reach the site of infection, their ability to phagocytize bacteria appears to be normal.

Inhaled anesthetics do not have bacteriostatic effects at clinically useful concentrations. Conversely, the liquid form of volatile anesthetics may be bactericidal (Johnson and Eger, 1979). All volatile anesthetics (doses as low as 0.2 MAC) produce dose-dependent inhibition of measles virus replication and reduce mortality in mice receiving intranasal influenza virus (Knight et al, 1983). This inhibition may reflect anesthetic-induced decreases in deoxyribonucleic acid (DNA) synthesis.

GENETIC EFFECTS

The Ames test, which identifies chemicals that act as mutagens and carcinogens, is negative for enflurane, isoflurane, and nitrous oxide, including their known metabolites (Baden et al, 1977). Halothane also results in a negative Ames test, but potential metabolites may be positive (Sachder et al, 1980). In animals, nitrous oxide administered during vulnerable periods of gestation may result in adverse reproductive effects manifesting as an increased incidence of fetal resorptions (abortions) (Bussard et al, 1974; Lane et al, 1980). Conversely, administration of volatile anesthetics during these vulnerable periods does not increase the incidence of fetal resorptions (Mazze et al, 1986). Learning function may be impaired in newborn animals exposed *in utero* to inhaled anesthetics (Chalon et al, 1982; Mazze et al, 1984b).

The increased incidence of spontaneous abortions in operating room personnel may reflect a teratogenic effect from chronic exposure to trace concentrations of inhaled anesthetics, especially nitrous oxide (Lane et al, 1980). Nitrous oxide irreversibly oxidizes the cobalt atom of vitamin B_{12} such that the activity of vitamin B_{12}-dependent enzymes (methionine synthetase and thymidylate synthetase) is reduced. In patients undergoing laparotomy with general anesthesia including 70% nitrous oxide, the half-time for inactivation of methionine synthetase is about 46 minutes (Fig. 2-32) (Nunn et al, 1988). Inactivation of methionine synthetase is more rapid in

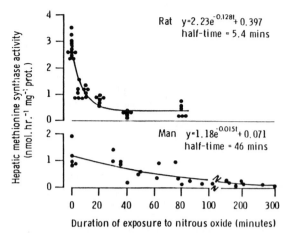

FIGURE 2–32. Time course of inactivation of hepatic methionine synthase (synthetase) activity during administration of 50% nitrous oxide to rats or 70% nitrous oxide to humans. (From Nunn JF, Weinbran HK, Royston D, Cormack RS. Rate of inactivation of human and rodent hepatic methionine synthase by nitrous oxide. Anesthesiology 1988; 68: 213–6; with permission.)

rats exposed to 50% nitrous oxide, with a half-time of 5.4 minutes. Therefore, it is probably not valid to extrapolate time frames established in rodents to humans. Volatile anesthetics do not alter activity of vitamin B_{12}-dependent enzymes.

Methionine synthetase converts homocysteine to methionine, which is necessary for the formation of myelin. Thymidylate synthetase is important in the conversion of DNA to thymidine and the subsequent formation of DNA. Interference with myelin formation and DNA synthesis could have significant effects on the rapidly growing fetus, manifesting as spontaneous abortions or congenital anomalies. Inhibition of these enzymes could also manifest as depression of bone marrow function and neurologic disturbances. The speculated but undocumented role of trace concentrations of nitrous oxide in the production of spontaneous abortions has led to the use of scavenging systems designed to remove anesthetic gases, including nitrous oxide, from the operating room. Nevertheless, animal studies using intermittent exposure to trace concentrations of nitrous oxide, halothane, enflurane, and isoflurane have not revealed harmful reproductive effects (Mazze, 1985).

BONE MARROW FUNCTION

Interference with DNA synthesis is responsible for the megaloblastic changes and agranulocytosis that may follow prolonged administration of nitrous oxide. Megaloblastic changes in bone marrow are consistently found in patients who have been exposed to anesthetic concentrations of nitrous oxide for 24 hours (Nunn, 1987). Exposure to nitrous oxide lasting 4 days or longer results in agranulocytosis. These bone marrow effects occur as a result of nitrous oxide–induced interference with activity of vitamin B_{12}–dependent enzymes, which are necessary for synthesis of DNA and the subsequent formation of erythrocytes (see the section entitled "Genetic Effects").

It is presumed that a healthy surgical patient could receive nitrous oxide for 24 hours without harm. Because the inhibition of methionine synthetase is rapid and its recovery is slow, it is to be expected that exposure repeated at intervals of less than 3 days may result in a cumulative effect. This relationship may be further complicated by other factors influencing levels of methionine synthetase and tetrahydrofolate (necessary for the transmethylation reaction) that might be important in critically ill patients receiving nitrous oxide. Nevertheless, the contradiction between the serious biochemical effects of nitrous oxide and the apparent absence of adverse clinical effects in routine use for anesthesia makes it difficult to draw firm conclusions.

PERIPHERAL NEUROPATHY

Animals exposed to 15% nitrous oxide for up to 15 days develop ataxia and exhibit evidence of spinal cord and peripheral nerve degeneration. Humans who chronically inhale nitrous oxide for nonmedical purposes may develop a neuropathy characterized by sensorimotor polyneuropathy that is often combined with signs of posterior and lateral spinal cord degeneration resembling pernicious anemia (Layzer et al, 1978). The speculated mechanism of this neuropathy is the ability of nitrous oxide to oxidize irreversibly the cobalt atom of vitamin B_{12} such that activity of vitamin B_{12}–dependent enzymes is reduced (see the section entitled "Genetic Effects").

TOTAL BODY OXYGEN REQUIREMENTS

Total body oxygen requirements are reduced similar amounts by volatile anesthetics. Oxygen requirements of the heart decrease more than those of other organs, reflecting drug-induced reductions in cardiac work associated with decreases in blood pressure and myocardial contractility. Theoretically, reduced oxygen requirements would protect tissues from ischemia that might result from decreased oxygen delivery owing to drug-induced decreases in perfusion pressure. Decreases in total body oxygen requirements probably reflect metabolic depressant effects as well as reduced functional needs in the presence of anesthetic-produced depression of organ function.

METABOLISM

Metabolism of inhaled anesthetics is important for two reasons. First, intermediary metabolites or end-metabolites may be toxic to the kidneys, liver, or reproductive organs. Second, the degree of metabolism may influence the rate of decrease in the alveolar partial pressure at the conclusion of an anesthetic. Conversely, the rate of increase in the alveolar partial pressure during induction of anesthesia is unlikely to be influenced by metabolism because inhaled anesthetics are administered in great excess of the amount metabolized.

Assessment of the magnitude of metabolism of inhaled anesthetics is by (1) measurement of metabolites, or (2) comparison of the total amount of anesthetic recovered in the exhaled gases with the amount taken up during administration (mass balance). Advantages of the mass balance technique are that knowledge of metabolite pharmacokinetics and identification and collection of metabolites are not necessary. Indeed, recovery of metabolites may be incomplete, leading to an underestimation of the magnitude of metabolism. A disadvantage of the mass balance approach is that loss of anesthetic through the surgical incision, across the intact skin, in urine, and in feces may prevent complete recovery, and these losses would be construed as due to metabolism. Nevertheless, the error introduced by these losses is likely to be insignificant, with the occasional exception of large and highly perfused wound surfaces.

Comparison of metabolite recovery and mass balance studies results in greatly different estimates of the magnitude of metabolism of volatile anesthetics (Table 2-4) (Carpenter et al, 1986). For example, mass balance estimates of the magnitude of metabolism are 1.5 to 3 times greater than estimates determined by the recovery of metabolites. This is not surprising because recovery of metabolites will underestimate the magnitude of metabolism unless all metabolites are recovered. Based on mass balance studies, it is concluded that alveolar ventilation is principally responsible for elimination of enflurane and isoflurane; alveolar ventilation and metabolism are equally important for elimination of halothane; and metabolism is the most important mechanism for elimination of methoxyflurane (Carpenter et al, 1986).

Determinants of Metabolism

The magnitude of metabolism of inhaled anesthetics is determined by (1) the chemical structure of the anesthetic, (2) hepatic enzyme activity, (3) blood concentration of the anesthetic, and (4) genetic factors. Overall, genetic factors appear to be the most important determinant of drug-metabolizing enzyme activity. In this regard, humans are active metabolizers of drugs compared with lower animal species such as the rat.

Table 2–4
Metabolism of Volatile Anesthetics as Assessed by Metabolite Recovery vs Mass Balance Studies

Anesthetic	Magnitude of Metabolism	
	Metabolite Recovery (%)	Mass Balance (%)
Isoflurane	0.2	0*
Enflurane	2.4	8.5
Halothane	11–25	46.1
Methoxyflurane	48	75.3

*Metabolism of isoflurane assumed to be 0 for this calculation.

(Data adapted from Carpenter RL, Eger EI, Johnson BH, Unadkat JD, Sheiner LB. The extent of metabolism of inhaled anesthetics in humans. Anesthesiology 1986; 65: 201–5.)

Chemical Structure

The ether bond and carbon-halogen bond are the sites in the anesthetic molecule most susceptible to oxidative metabolism. Oxidation of the ether bond is less likely when hydrogen atoms on the carbons surrounding the oxygen atom of this bond are replaced with halogen atoms. Two halogen atoms on a terminal carbon represent the optimal arrangement for dehalogenation, whereas a terminal carbon with three fluorine atoms is very resistant to oxidative metabolism. The bond energy for carbon-fluorine is twice that for carbon-bromine or carbon-chlorine. The absence of ester bonds in inhaled anesthetics negates any role of metabolism by hydrolysis.

Hepatic Enzyme Activity

The activity of hepatic cytochrome P-450 enzymes responsible for metabolism of volatile anesthetics may be increased by a variety of drugs, including the anesthetics themselves. Phenobarbital, phenytoin, and isoniazid may increase defluorination of volatile anesthetics, especially enflurane. There is evidence in patients that brief (1-hour) exposures during surgical stimulation increase hepatic microsomal enzyme activity independently of the anesthetic drug (halothane or isoflurane) or technique (spinal) used (Loft et al, 1985). Conversely, surgery lasting more than 4 hours can lead to depressed microsomal enzyme activity.

Blood Concentrations

The fraction of anesthetic that undergoes metabolism on passing through the liver is influenced by the blood concentration of the anesthetic (Fig. 2-33) (Sawyer et al, 1971; White et al, 1979). For example, a 1-MAC concentration saturates hepatic enzymes and reduces the fraction of anesthetic that is removed (metabolized) during a single passage through the liver. Conversely, subanesthetic concentrations (0.1 MAC or less) undergo extensive metabolism on passage through the liver. Disease states such as cirrhosis of the liver or cardiac failure could theoretically alter metabolism by decreasing hepatic blood flow and drug delivery or reducing the amount of viable liver and thus enzyme activity. Obesity, for unknown reasons, predictably increases defluorination of halothane and enflurane (Bentley et al, 1979; Young et al, 1975).

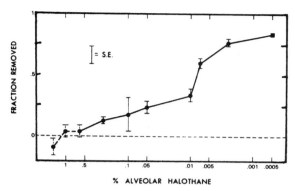

FIGURE 2–33. Fraction of halothane removed during passage through the liver at progressively decreasing alveolar concentrations. (From Sawyer DC, Eger EI, Dahlman SH, Cullen BF, Impelman D. Concentration dependence of hepatic halothane metabolism. Anesthesiology 1971; 34: 230–5; with permission.)

Inhaled anesthetics that are not highly soluble in blood and tissues (nitrous oxide, enflurane, isoflurane) tend to be rapidly exhaled by the lungs at the conclusion of an anesthetic. As a result, less drug is available to pass through the liver continually at low blood concentrations conducive to metabolism. This is reflected in the magnitude of metabolism of these drugs (Table 2-4) (Carpenter et al, 1986). Halothane and methoxyflurane are more soluble in blood and lipids and thus likely to be stored in tissues that act as a reservoir to maintain subanesthetic concentrations conducive to metabolism for prolonged periods of time following discontinuation of their administration.

Nitrous Oxide

An estimated 0.004% of an absorbed dose of nitrous oxide undergoes reductive metabolism to nitrogen in the gastrointestinal tract (Hong et al, 1980a; Trudell, 1985). Anaerobic bacteria, such as pseudomonas, are responsible for this reductive metabolism. Reductive products of some nitrogen compounds include free radicals that could produce toxic effects on cells. The potential toxic role of these metabolites, however, remains undocumented. Oxygen concentrations greater than 10% in the gastrointestinal tract and antibiotics inhibit metabolism of nitrous oxide by anaerobic bacteria. There is no evidence that nitrous oxide undergoes oxidative metabolism in the liver (Hong et al, 1980b).

Halothane

Halothane is uniquely metabolized because it undergoes oxidation when ample oxygen is present but reductive metabolism when hepatocyte PO_2 decreases.

Oxidative Metabolism

The principal oxidative metabolites of halothane are trifluoracetic acid, chloride, and bromide. The energy bond for carbon-fluorine is strong, accounting for the absence of detectable amounts of fluoride as an oxidative metabolite of halothane. It is estimated that the plasma concentrations of bromide increase 0.5 $mEq \cdot L^{-1}$ for every MAC hour of halothane administration (Fig. 2-34) (Johnstone et al, 1975). Because signs of bromide toxicity such as somnolence and confusion do not occur until plasma concentrations of bromide are greater than 6 $mEq \cdot L^{-1}$, the likelihood of symptoms from metabolism of halothane to bromide seems remote. Nevertheless, prolonged halothane anesthesia may more likely be associated with intellectual impairment than a similar dose of an anesthetic that is not metabolized to bromide.

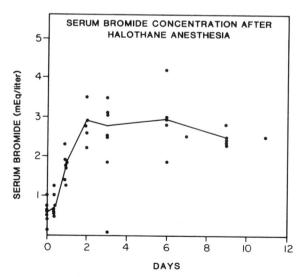

FIGURE 2–34. Serum bromide concentrations in volunteers following prolonged (about 7 hours) exposure to halothane. (From Johnstone RE, Kennell EM, Behar MG, Brummund W, Ebersole RC, Shaw LM. Increased serum bromide concentration after halothane anesthesia in man. Anesthesiology 1975; 42: 598–601; with permission.)

Reductive Metabolism

Reductive metabolism, which, among the volatile anesthetics, has been documented to occur only during breakdown of halothane, is most likely to occur in the presence of hepatocyte hypoxia and enzyme induction. Reductive metabolites of halothane include fluoride and volatile products, some of which result from the reaction of halothane with soda lime. In the past, reductive metabolites of halothane have been considered to be potentially hepatotoxic. Nevertheless, more recent data do not support a predominant role for reductive metabolism in initiation of halothane hepatitis (see the section entitled "Halothane Hepatitis"). Increased plasma fluoride concentrations reflect reductive metabolism of halothane in obese patients and children with cyanotic congenital heart disease (Fig. 2-35) (Moore et al, 1986; Nawaf and Stoelting, 1979). The level of plasma fluoride elevation (less than 10 $\mu M \cdot L^{-1}$) is far below the presumed nephrotoxic concentration of 50 $\mu M \cdot L^{-1}$, and changes in liver transaminase enzymes as evidence of hepatotoxicity owing to reductive metabolism are not seen in these patients.

Enflurane

Enflurane undergoes oxidative metabolism to inorganic fluoride and organic fluoride compounds. Fluoride results from dehalogenation of the terminal carbon atom. Oxidation of the ether bond and release of additional fluoride do not occur, reflecting the chemical stability imparted to this bond by the surrounding halogens. As with isoflurane, the methyl portion of the molecule seems to be resistant to oxidation, and reductive metabolism does not occur. Minimal metabolism of enflurane reflects its chemical stability and low solubility in tissues such that the drug is exhaled unchanged rather than repeatedly passing through the liver at low plasma concentrations conducive to metabolism.

Enzyme induction with phenobarbital or phenytoin increases the liberation of fluoride from enflurane *in vitro* but not *in vivo* (Mazze et al, 1982). This observation is most likely due to low tissue solubility of enflurane such that, *in vivo*, the availability of substrate (enflurane) becomes the rate-limiting factor, whereas *in vitro*, the substrate concentration is controlled and the effect of enzyme induction manifests as increased metabolism of enflurane to fluoride (Greenstein et al, 1975). For these reasons, it seems unlikely that the nephrotoxic potential of enflurane would be increased by enzyme induction. An exception may be patients who are being treated with isoniazid, because this drug can increase defluorination of enflurane in genetically determined patients who are rapid acetylators.

Isoflurane

Isoflurane undergoes minimal oxidative metabolism. Metabolism of isoflurane begins with oxidation of the carbon-halogen link of the alpha

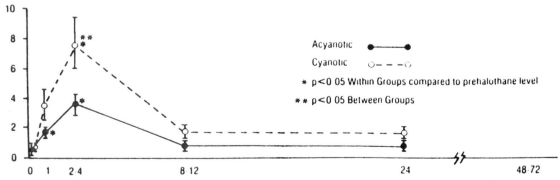

FIGURE 2–35. Plasma concentrations of fluoride are greater following administration of halothane to cyanotic than acyanotic patients. (Modified from Moore RA, McNicholas KW, Gallagher JD, et al. Halothane metabolism in acyanotic and cyanotic patients undergoing open heart surgery. Anesth Analg 1986; 65: 1257–62; with permission.)

carbon atom, leading to an unstable compound that subsequently decomposes to difluoromethanol and trifluoracetic acid. Difluoromethanol breaks down to formic acid and, in the process, releases two fluoride ions. Trifluoracetic acid is the principal organic fluoride metabolite of isoflurane. Reductive metabolism of isoflurane does not occur. Minimal metabolism of isoflurane reflects this drug's chemical stability and low solubility in tissues such that the drug is exhaled unchanged rather than repeatedly passing through the liver at low plasma concentrations conducive to metabolism. Chemical stability of isoflurane is ensured by the trifluorocarbon and the presence of halogen atoms on three sides of the ether bond.

Minimal changes in plasma concentrations of fluoride (peak less than 5 μM·L^{-1}) resulting from metabolism of isoflurane plus the absence of other toxic metabolites render nephrotoxicity or hepatotoxicity following administration of isoflurane unlikely. Enzyme induction with phenobarbital or phenytoin increases the liberation of fluoride from isoflurane *in vitro* but not *in vivo* (Mazze et al, 1982). Even in the presence of enzyme induction, however, the metabolism of isoflurane and resulting plasma concentrations of fluoride remain much less than with enflurane. Likewise, isoniazid, which dramatically increases metabolism of enflurane in susceptible patients, fails to significantly alter metabolism of isoflurane.

REFERENCES

Adams RW, Cucchiari RF, Gronert GA, Messick JM, Michenfelder JD. Isoflurane and cerebrospinal fluid pressure in neurosurgical patients. Anesthesiology 1981;54:97–9.

Albrecht RF, Miletich DJ, Madala LR. Normalization of cerebral blood flow during prolonged anesthesia. Anesthesiology 1983;58:26–31.

Artru AA. Anesthetics produce prolonged alterations of CSF dynamics. Anesthesiology 1982;57:A356.

Artru AA. Effects of halothane, enflurane, isoflurane and fentanyl on resistance to reabsorption of cerebrospinal fluid. Anesth Analg 1984a;63:180.

Artru AA. Isoflurane does not increase the rate of CSF production in the dog. Anesthesiology 1984b;60:193–7.

Atlee JL, Bosnjak ZJ. Mechanisms for cardiac dysrhythmias during anesthesia. Anesthesiology 1990;72:347–74.

Baden JM, Serra M, Fujinaga M, Mazze RI. Halothane metabolism in cirrhotic rats. Anesthesiology 1987;67:660–4.

Bahlman SH, Eger EI, Halsey MJ, et al. The cardiovascular effects of halothane in man during spontaneous ventilation. Anesthesiology 1972;36:494–502.

Bentley JB, Vaughn RW, Miller MS, Calkins JM, Gandolfi AJ. Serum inorganic fluoride levels in obese patients during and after enflurane anesthesia. Anesth Analg 1979;58:409–12.

Benumof JL, Bookstein JJ, Saidman LJ, Harris R. Diminished hepatic arterial flow during halothane administration. Anesthesiology 1976;45:545–51.

Biehl DR, Yarnell R, Wade JG, Sitar D. The uptake of isoflurane by the foetal lamb *in utero:* Effect on regional blood flow. Can Anaesth Soc J 1983;30:581–6.

Brown BR, Gandolfi AJ. Adverse effects of volatile anesthetics. Br J Anaesth 1987;59:14–23.

Buffington CW, Romson JL, Levine A, Duttlinger NC, Huang AH. Isoflurane induces coronary steal in a canine model of chronic coronary occlusion. Anesthesiology 1987;66:280–92.

Bussard DA, Stoelting RK, Peterson C, Ishaq M. Fetal changes in hamsters anesthetized with nitrous oxide and halothane. Anesthesiology 1974;41:275–8.

Cahalan MK, Lurz FW, Eger EI, Schwartz LA, Beaupre PN, Smith JS. Narcotics decrease heart rate during inhalational anesthesia. Anesth Analg 1987;66:166–70.

Calverley RK, Smith NT, Jones CW, Prys-Roberts C, Eger EI. Ventilatory and cardiovascular effects of enflurane anesthesia during spontaneous ventilation in man. Anesth Analg 1978a;57:610–8.

Calverley RK, Smith NT, Prys-Roberts C, Eger EI, Jones CW. Cardiovascular effects of enflurane anesthesia during controlled ventilation in man. Anesth Analg 1978b;57:619–28.

Carpenter RL, Eger EI, Johnson BH, Unadkat JD, Sheiner LB. The extent of metabolism of inhaled anesthetics in humans. Anesthesiology 1986;65:201–5.

Chalon J, Ramanathan S, Turndorf H. Exposure to isoflurane affects learning function of murine progeny. Anesthesiology 1982;57:A360.

Christ DD, Kenna JG, Kammerer W, Satoh H, Pohl LR. Enflurane metabolism produces covalently bound liver adducts recognized by antibodies from patients with halothane hepatitis. Anesthesiology 1988;69:833–8.

Cousins MJ, Greenstein LR, Hitt BA, Mazze RI. Metabolism and renal effects of enflurane in man. Anesthesiology 1976;44:44–53.

Cromwell TH, Stevens WC, Eger EI, et al. The cardiovascular effects of compound 469 (Forane) during spontaneous ventilation and CO$_2$ challenge in man. Anesthesiology 1971;35:17–25.

Cronnelly R, Salvatierra O, Feduska NJ. Renal allograft function following halothane, enflurane, or isoflurane anesthesia. Anesth Analg 1984;63:202.

Cullen DJ, Eger EI. The effects of halothane on respiratory and cardiovascular responses to hypoxia in dogs: A dose response study. Anesthesiology 1970; 33:487–96.

Cullen BF, Margolis AJ, Eger EI. The effects of anesthesia and pulmonary ventilation on blood loss during elective therapeutic abortion. Anesthesiology 1970; 32:108–13.

Dolan WM, Eger EI, Margolis AJ. Forane increases bleeding in therapeutic suction abortion. Anesthesiology 1972;36:96–7.

Dolan WM, Stevens WC, Eger EI, et al. The cardiovascular and respiratory effects of isoflurane-nitrous oxide anesthesia. Can Anaesth Soc J 1974;21:557–68.

Drummond JC, Todd MM, Shapiro HM. CO_2 responsiveness of the cerebral circulation during isoflurane anesthesia and N_2O sedation in cats. Anesthesiology 1982;57:A333.

Eger EI. Pharmacology of isoflurane. Br J Anaesth 1984;56:71S-99S.

Eger EI. Isoflurane (Forane): A Compendium and Reference. 2nd edition. Madison, WI, Ohio Medical Products, 1985a:1–110.

Eger EI. Nitrous Oxide. New York, Elsevier, 1985b.

Eger EI, Calverley RK, Smith NT. Changes in blood chemistries following prolonged enflurane anesthesia. Anesth Analg 1976;55:547–9.

Eger EI, Smith NT, Stoelting RK, Cullen DJ, Kadis LB, Whitcher CE. Cardiovascular effects of halothane in man. Anesthesiology 1970;32:396–409.

Eger EI, Stevens WC, Cromwell TH. The electroencephalogram in man anesthetized with Forane. Anesthesiology 1971;35:504–8.

Eintrei C, Leszniewski W, Carlsson C. Local application of ^{133}Xenon for measurement of regional cerebral blood flow (rCBF) during halothane, enflurane, and isoflurane anesthesia in humans. Anesthesiology 1985;63:391–4.

Eisele JH, Milstein JM, Goetzman BW. Pulmonary vascular responses to nitrous oxide in newborn lambs. Anesth Analg 1986;65:62–4.

Eisele JH, Smith NT. Cardiovascular effects of 40 percent nitrous oxide in man. Anesth Analg 1972; 51:956–63.

Farrell G, Prendergast D, Murray M. Halothane hepatitis: Detection of a constitutional susceptibility factor. N Engl J Med 1985;313:1310–4.

Flaim SF, Zelis R, Eisele JH. Differential effects of morphine on forearm blood flow: Attenuation of sympathetic control of the cutaneous circulation. Clin Pharmacol Ther 1978;23:542–6.

Fourcade HE, Stevens WC, Larson CP. The ventilatory effects of Forane, a new inhaled anesthetic. Anesthesiology 1971;35:26–31.

France CJ, Plumer MH, Eger EI, Wahrenbrock EA. Ventilatory effects of isoflurane (Forane) or halothane when combined with morphine, nitrous oxide and surgery. Br J Anaesth 1974;46:117–20.

Frankhuizen JL, Vlek CAJ, Burm AGL, Rejger V. Failure to replicate negative effects of trace anesthetics on mental performance. Br J Anaesth 1978;50:229–34.

Fukunaga AF, Epstein RM. Sympathetic excitation during nitrous oxide-halothane anesthesia in the cat. Anesthesiology 1973;39:23–36.

Garfield JM, Garfield FB, Sampson J. Effects of nitrous oxide on decision-strategy and sustained attention. Psychopharmacologia 1975;42:5–10.

Gelman S, Fowler KC, Smith LR. Liver circulation and function during isoflurane and halothane anesthesia. Anesthesiology 1984;61:726–30.

Gold MI, Schwam SJ, Goldberg M. Chronic obstructive pulmonary disease and respiratory complications. Anesth Analg 1983;62:975–81.

Goldfarb G, Debaene B, Ang ET, Roulot D, Jolis P, Lebrec D. Hepatic blood flow in humans during isoflurane-N_2O and halothane-N_2O anesthesia. Anesth Analg 1990;71:349–53.

Gourlay GK, Adams JF, Cousins MJ, Hall P. Genetic differences in reductive metabolism and hepatotoxicity of halothane in three rat strains. Anesthesiology 1981;55:96–103.

Greenstein LR, Hitt BA, Mazze RI. Metabolism *in vitro* of enflurane, isoflurane, and methoxyflurane. Anesthesiology 1975;42:420–4.

Hilgenberg JC, McCammon RL, Stoelting RK. Pulmonary and systemic vascular responses to nitrous oxide in patients with mitral stenosis and pulmonary hypertension. Anesth Analg 1980;59:323–6.

Hirshman CA, Edelstein G, Peetz S, Wayne R, Downes H. Mechanism of action of inhalation anesthesia on airways. Anesthesiology 1982;56:107–11.

Hong K, Trudell JR, O'Neil JR, Cohen EN. Metabolism of nitrous oxide by human and rat intestinal contents. Anesthesiology 1980a;52:16–9.

Hong K, Trudell JR, O'Neil JR, Cohen EN. Biotransformation of nitrous oxide. Anesthesiology 1980b;53:354–55.

Hornbein TF, Eger EI, Winter PM, Smith C, Wetstone D, Smith KH. The minimum alveolar concentration of nitrous oxide in man. Anesth Analg 1982;61:553–6.

Horrigan RW, Eger EI, Wilson EI, Wilson C. Epinephrine-induced arrhythmias during enflurane anesthesia in man: A non-linear dose-response relationship and dose-dependent protection from lidocaine. Anesth Analg 1978;57:547–50.

Hovorka J, Korttila K, Erkola O. Nitrous oxide does not increase nausea and vomiting following gynaecological laparoscopy. Can J Anaesth 1989;36:145–8.

Hubbard AK, Roth TP, Gandolfi AJ, Brown BR, Webster NR, Nunn JF. Halothane hepatitis patients generate an antibody response toward a covalently bound metabolite of halothane. Anesthesiology 1988; 68:791–6.

Inoue K, Reichelt W, El-Banayosy A, et al. Does isoflurane lead to a higher incidence of myocardial infarction and perioperative death than enflurane in coronary artery surgery. A clinical study of 1178 patients. Anesth Analg 1990;71:469–74.

Johnson BH, Eger EI. Bactericidal effects of anesthetics. Anesth Analg 1979;58:136–8.

Johnston RR, Cromwell TH, Eger EI, Cullen D, Stevens WC, Joas T. The toxicity of fluroxene in animals and man. Anesthesiology 1973;38:313–9.

Johnston RR, Eger ET, Wilson C. A comparative interaction of epinephrine with enflurane, isoflurane and halothane in Man. Anesth Analg 1976;55:709–12.

Johnstone RE, Kennell EM, Behar MG, Brummund W, Ebersole RC, Shaw LM. Increased serum bromide concentration after halothane anesthesia in man. Anesthesiology 1975;42:598–601.

Jones RM. Desflurane and sevoflurane: Inhalation anesthetics for this decade? Br J Anaesth 1990; 65:527–36.

Jones RM, Cashman JN, Eger EI, Damask MC, Johnson BH. Kinetics and potency of desflurane (I-653) in volunteers. Anesth Analg 1990a;70:3–7.

Jones RM, Koblin DD, Cashman JN, Eger EI, Johnson BH, Damask MC. Biotransformation and hepatorenal function in volunteers after exposure to desflurane (I-653). Br J Anaesth 1990b;64:482–7.

Kambam JR, Holaday DA. Effect of nitrous oxide on the oxyhemoglobin dissociation curve and PO_2 measurements. Anesthesiology 1987;66:208–9.

Karl HW, Swedlow DB, Lee KW, Downes JJ. Epinephrine-halothane interactions in children. Anesthesiology 1983;58:142–5.

Katoh T, Ikeda K. The minimum alveolar concentration (MAC) of sevoflurane in humans. Anesthesiology 1987;66:301–3.

Kemmotsu O, Hashimoto Y, Shimosato S. Inotropic effects of isoflurane on mechanics of contraction in isolated cat papillary muscles from normal and failing hearts. Anesthesiology 1973;39:470–7.

Kettlekamp NS, Austin DR, Downes H, Cheek DBC, Hirshman CA. Inhibition of d-tubocurarine-induced histamine release by halothane. Anesthesiology 1987;66:666–9.

Knight PR, Bedows E, Nahrwold ML, Maassab HF, Smitka CW, Busch MT. Alterations in influenza virus pulmonary pathology induced by diethyl ether, halothane, enflurane and pentobarbital in mice. Anesthesiology 1983;58:209–15.

Knill RL, Clement JL. Variable effects of anaesthetics on the ventilatory response to hypoxaemia in man. Can Anaesth Soc J 1982;29:93–9.

Knill RL, Manninen PH, Clement JL. Ventilation and chemoreflexes during enflurane sedation and anaesthesia in man. Can Anaesth Soc J 1979;26:353–60.

Koblin DD, Eger EI, Johnson BH, Collins P, Terrell RC, Spears L. Are convulsant gases also anesthetics? Anesthesiology 1980;53:S47.

Kotrly KJ, Ebert TJ, Vucins E, Igler FO, Barney JA, Kampine JP. Baroreceptor reflex control of heart rate during isoflurane anesthesia in humans. Anesthesiology 1984;60:173–9.

Lam AM, Clement JL, Chung DC, Knill RL. Respiratory effects of nitrous oxide during enflurane anesthesia in humans. Anesthesiology 1982;56:298–303.

Lane GA, Nahrwold ML, Tait AR. Anesthetics as teratogens: Nitrous oxide is fetotoxic, xenon is not. Science 1980;210:899–901.

Lappas DG, Buckley MJ, Laver MB, Daggett WM, Lowenstein E. Left ventricular performance and pulmonary circulation following addition of nitrous oxide to morphine during coronary-artery surgery. Anesthesiology 1975;43:61–9.

Layzer RB, Fishman RA, Schafer JA. Neuropathy following use of nitrous oxide. Neurology 1978;28:504–6.

Loarie DJ, Wilkinson P, Tyberg J, White A. The hemodynamic effects of halothane in anemic dogs. Anesth Analg 1979;58:195–200.

Loft S, Boel J, Kyst A, Rasmussen B, Hansen SH, Dossing M. Increased hepatic microsomal enzyme activity after surgery under halothane or spinal anesthesia. Anesthesiology 1985;62:11–6.

Lynch C, Vogel S, Sperelakis N. Halothane depression of myocardial slow action potentials. Anesthesiology 1981;55:360–8.

Mallow JE, White RD, Cucchiara RF, Tarhan S. Hemodynamic effects of isoflurane and halothane in patients with coronary artery disease. Anesth Analg 1976;55:135–8.

Martin JL, Kenna JG, Pohl LR. Antibody assays for the detection of patients sensitized to halothane. Anesth Analg 1990;70:154–9.

Maze M, Hayward E, Gaba DM. Alpha-adrenergic blockade raises epinephrine-arrhythmia threshold in halothane-anesthetized dogs in a dose-dependent fashion. Anesthesiology 1985;63:611–5.

Maze M, Smith CM. Identification of receptor mechanism mediating epinephrine-induced arrhythmias during halothane anesthesia in the dog. Anesthesiology 1983;59:322–6.

Mazze RI. Fertility, reproduction, and postnatal survival in mice chronically exposed to isoflurane. Anesthesiology 1985;63:663–7.

Mazze RI, Calverley RK, Smith NT. Inorganic fluoride nephrotoxicity: Prolonged enflurane and halothane anesthesia in volunteers. Anesthesiology 1977; 46:265–71.

Mazze RI, Cousins MJ, Barr GA. Renal effects and metabolism of isoflurane in man. Anesthesiology 1974; 40:536–40.

Mazze RI, Fujinaga M, Rice SA, Harris SB, Baden JM. Reproductive and teratogenic effects of nitrous oxide, halothane, isoflurane and enflurane in Sprague-Dawley rats. Anesthesiology 1986;64:339–44.

Mazze RI, Sievenpiper TS, Stevenson J. Renal effects of isoflurane in patients with abnormal renal function. Anesthesiology 1984a;60:161–3.

Mazze RI, Wilson AI, Rice SA, Baden JM. Effects of isoflurane on reproduction and fetal development in mice. Anesth Analg 1984b;63:249.

Mazze RI, Woodruff RE, Heerdt MD. Isoniazid-induced enflurane defluorination in humans. Anesthesiology 1982;57:5–8.

McDermott RW, Stanley TH. The cardiovascular effects of low concentrations of nitrous oxide during morphine anesthesia. Anesthesiology 1974;41:89–91.

Metz S, Maze M. Halothane concentration does not alter the threshold for epinephrine-induced arrhythmias in dogs. Anesthesiology 1985;62:470–4.

Michenfelder JD, Sundt TM, Fode N, Sharbrough FW. Isoflurane when compared to enflurane and halothane decreases the frequency of cerebral ischemia during carotid endarterectomy. Anesthesiology 1987;67:336–40.

Milde LN, Milde JH, Lanier WL, Michenfelder JD. Comparison of the effects of isoflurane and thiopental on neurologic outcome and neuropathology after temporary focal cerebral ischemia in primates. Anesthesiology 1988;69:905–13.

Miller RD, Eger EI, Way WL, Stevens WC, Dolan WM. Comparative neuromuscular effects of Forane and halothane alone and in combination with d-tubocurarine in man. Anesthesiology 1971;35:38–42.

Mitchell MM, Prakash O, Rulf ENR, vaDaele MERM, Cahalan MK, Roelandt JRTC. Nitrous oxide does not induce myocardial ischemia in patients with ischemic heart disease and poor ventricular function. Anesthesiology 1989;71:526–34.

Moore RA, McNicholas KW, Gallagher JD, et al. Halothane metabolism in acyanotic and cyanotic patients undergoing open heart surgery. Anesth Analg 1986;65:1257–62.

Muir JJ, Warner MA, Offord KP, Buck CF, Harper OV, Kunkel SE. Role of nitrous oxide and other factors in postoperative nausea and vomiting: A randomized and blinded prospective study. Anesthesiology 1987;66:513–8.

Munson ES, Embro WJ. Enflurane, isoflurane and halothane and isolated human uterine muscle. Anesthesiology 1977;46:11–4.

Murat I, Lapeyre G, Saint-Maurice C. Isoflurane attenuates baroreflex control of heart rate in human neonates. Anesthesiology 1989;70:395–400.

Naito H, Gillis CN. Effects of halothane and nitrous oxide on removal of norepinephrine from the pulmonary circulation. Anesthesiology 1973;39:575–80.

Nawaf K, Stoelting RK. SGOT values following evidence of reductive biotransformation of halothane in man. Anesthesiology 1979;51:185–6.

Neigh JL, Garman JK, Harp JR. The electroencephalographic pattern during anesthesia with Ethrane: Effects of depth of anesthesia, $PaCO_2$ and nitrous oxide. Anesthesiology 1971;35:482–7.

Newman B, Gelb AW, Lam AM. The effect of isoflurane-induced hypotension on cerebral blood flow and cerebral metabolic rate for oxygen in humans. Anesthesiology 1986;64:307–10.

Nunn JF. Clinical aspects of the interaction between nitrous oxide and vitamin B_{12}. Br J Anaesth 1987; 59:3–13.

Nunn JF, Weinbran HK, Royston D, Cormack RS. Rate of inactivation of human and rodent hepatic methionine synthase by nitrous oxide. Anesthesiology 1988;68:213–6.

Oshima E, Urabe N, Shingu K, Mori K. Anticonvulsant actions of enflurane on epilepsy models in cats. Anesthesiology 1985;63:29–40.

O'Young, Mastrocostopoulos G, Hilgenberg A, Palacios I, Kyritsis A, Lappas DG. Myocardial circulatory and metabolic effects of isoflurane and sufentanil during coronary artery surgery. Anesthesiology 1987; 66:653–8.

Palahniuk RJ, Shnicer SM. Maternal and fetal cardiovascular and acid base changes during halothane and isoflurane anesthesia in the pregnant ewe. Anesthesiology 1974;41:462–72.

Pathak KS, Ammadio M, Kalamchi A, Scoles PV, Shaffer JW, Mackey W. Effects of halothane, enflurane, and isoflurane on somatosensory evoked potentials during nitrous oxide anesthesia. Anesthesiology 1987; 66:753–7.

Philbin DM, Lowenstein E. Lack of beta-adrenergic activity of isoflurane in the dog: A comparison of circulatory effects of halothane and isoflurane after propranolol administration. Br J Anaesth 1976; 48:1165–70.

Pietak S, Weenig CS, Hickey RF, Fairley HB. Anesthetic effects of ventilation in patients with chronic obstructive pulmonary disease. Anesthesiology 1975; 42:160–6.

Price HL, Skovsted P, Pauca AW, Cooperman L. Evidence for a-receptor activation produced by halothane in normal man. Anesthesiology 1970;32:389–95.

Priebe H-J. Isoflurane and coronary hemodynamics. Anesthesiology 1989;71:690–76.

Ravin MB, Olsen MB. Apneic thresholds in anesthetized subjects with chronic obstructive pulmonary disease. Anesthesiology 1972;37:450–4.

Reed SB, Strobel GE. An *in vitro* model of malignant hyperthermia: Differential effects of inhalation anesthetics on caffeine-induced muscle contractures. Anesthesiology 1978;48:254–9.

Reilly CS, Wood AJJ, Koshaji RP, Wood M. The effect of halothane on drug disposition in intrinsic drug metabolizing capacity and hepatic blood flow. Anesthesiology 1985;63:70–6.

Reiz S, Balfors E, Sorensen MD, Ariola S, Friedman A, Truedsson H. Isoflurane: A powerful coronary vasodilatory in patients with ischemic heart disease. Anesthesiology 1983;59:91–7.

Sachder K, Cohen EN, Simmou VF. Genotoxic and mutagenic assays of halothane metabolites in *Bacillus subtilis* and *Salmonella typhimurium*. Anesthesiology 1980;53:31–9.

Sawyer DC, Eger EI, Bahlman SH, Cullen BF, Impelman D. Concentration dependence of hepatic halothane metabolism. Anesthesiology 1971;34:230–5.

Schulte-Sasse U, Hess W, Tarnow J. Pulmonary vascular responses to nitrous oxide in patients with normal and high pulmonary vascular resistance. Anesthesiology 1982;57:9–13.

Shimosato S, Yasuda I, Kemmotsu O, Shanks C, Gamble C. Effect of halothane on altered contractility of isolated heart muscle obtained from cats with experimentally produced ventricular hypertrophy and failure. Br J Anaesth 1973;45:2–9.

Shingu K, Eger EI, Johnson BH, VanDyke RA, Lurz FW, Cheng A. Effect of oxygen concentration, hyperthermia, and choice of vendor on anesthetic-induced hepatic injury in rats. Anesth Analg 1983;62:146–50.

Slogoff S, Keats AS. Does chronic treatment with calcium entry blocking drugs reduce perioperative myocardial ischemia? Anesthesiology 1988;68:676–80.

Slogoff S, Keats AS, Dear WE, et al. Steal-prone coronary anatomy and myocardial ischemia associated with four primary anesthetic agents in humans. Anesth Analg 1991;72:22–7.

Smith NT, Calverley RK, Prys-Roberts C, Eger EI, Jones CW. Impact of nitrous oxide on the circulation during enflurane anesthesia in man. Anesthesiology 1978;48:345–9.

Smith NT, Eger EI, Stoelting RK, Whayne TF, Cullen D, Kadis LB. The cardiovascular and sympathomimetic responses to the addition of nitrous oxide to halothane in man. Anesthesiology 1970;32:410–21.

Smith RA, Winter PM, Smith M, Eger EI. Convulsions in mice after anesthesia. Anesthesiology 1979;50:501–4.

Stevens WC, Cromwell TH, Halsey MJ, Eger EI, Shakespear TF, Bahlman SH. The cardiovascular effects of a new inhalation anesthetic, Forane, in human volunteers at constant arterial carbon dioxide tension. Anesthesiology 1971;35:8–16.

Stevens WC, Eger EI, Joas TA, Cromwell TH, White A, Dolan WM. Comparative toxicity of isoflurane, halothane, fluroxene and diethyl ether in human volunteers. Can Anaesth Soc J 1973;20:357–68.

Stevenson GW, Hall SC, Rudnick S, Seleny FL, Stevenson HC. The effect of anesthetic agents on the human immune response. Anesthesiology 1990;72:542–52.

Stoelting RK. Plasma lidocaine concentrations following subcutaneous or submucosal epinephrine-lidocaine injection. Anesth Analg 1978;57:724–6.

Stoelting RK, Gibbs PS. Hemodynamic effects of morphine and morphine-nitrous oxide in valvular heart disease and coronary artery disease. Anesthesiology 1973;38:45–52.

Takeshima R, Dohi S. Comparison of arterial baroreflex function in humans anesthetized with enflurane or isoflurane. Anesth Analg 1989;69:284–90.

Tinker JH, Sharbrough FW, Michenfelder JD. Anterior shift of the dominant EEG rhythm during anesthesia in the JAVA monkey: Correlation with anesthetic potency. Anesthesiology 1977;46:252–9.

Tobias JD, Hirshman CA. Attenuation of histamine-induced airway constriction by albuterol during halothane anesthesia. Anesthesiology 1990;72:105–10.

Todd MM, Drummond JC. A comparison of the cerebrovascular and metabolic effects of halothane and isoflurane in the cat. Anesthesiology 1984;60:276–82.

Trudell JR. Metabolism of nitrous oxide. In Eger EI, ed. Nitrous Oxide. New York, Elsevier, 1985.

Tuman KJ, McCarthy RJ, Spiess BD, DaValle M, Dabir R, Ivankorich AD. Does choice of anesthetic agent significantly affect outcome after coronary artery surgery. Anesthesiology 1989;70:189–98.

Tusiewicz K, Bryan AC, Froese AB. Contributions of changing rib cage-diaphragm interactions to the ventilatory depression of halothane anesthesia. Anesthesiology 1977;47:327–37.

Ueda W, Hirakawa M, Mae O. Appraisal of epinephrine administration to patients under halothane anesthesia for closure of cleft palate. Anesthesiology 1983;58:574–6.

Vitez TS, Miller RD, Eger EI, VanNyhuis LS, Way WL. Comparison *in vitro* of isoflurane and halothane potentiation of d-tubocurarine and succinylcholine neuromuscular blockades. Anesthesiology 1974; 41:53–6.

Warner DS, Boarini DJ, Kassell NF. Cerebrovascular adaptation to prolonged halothane anesthesia is not related to cerebrovascular fluid pH. Anesthesiology 1985;63:243–8.

Warren TM, Datta S, Ostheimer GW, Naulty JS, Weiss JB, Morrison JA. Comparison of the maternal and neonatal effects of halothane, enflurane and isoflurane for cesarean delivery. Anesth Analg 1983;62:516–20.

Weiskopf RB, Holmes MA, Rampil IJ, et al. Cardiovascular safety and actions of high concentrations of I-653 and isoflurane in swine. Anesthesiology 1989;70:793–8.

Whelan E, Wood AJJ, Koshakji R, Shay S, Wood M. Halothane inhibition of propranolol metabolism is stereoselective. Anesthesiology 1989;71:561–4.

White AE, Stevens WC, Eger EI, Mazze RI, Hitt BA. Enflurane and methoxyflurane metabolism at anesthetic and subanesthetic concentrations. Anesth Analg 1979;58:221–4.

Williamson DC, Munson ES. Correlation of peripheral venous and arterial blood gas values during general anesthesia. Anesth Analg 1982;61:950–2.

Wolfson B, Hetrick WD, Lake CL, Siker ES. Anesthetic indices: Further data. Anesthesiology 1978;48:187–90.

Yacoub O, Doell D, Kryger MH, Anthonisen NR. Depression of hypoxic ventilatory response by nitrous oxide. Anesthesiology 1976;45:385–9.

Young SR, Stoelting RK, Peterson C, Madura JA. Anesthetic biotransformation and renal function in obese patients during and after methoxyflurane or halothane anesthesia. Anesthesiology 1975;42:451–7.

Chapter

3

Opioid Agonists
and Antagonists

INTRODUCTION

The word *opium* is derived from the Greek word for juice; the juice of the poppy is the source of 20 distinct alkaloids of opium. *Opiate* is the term used to designate drugs derived from opium. Morphine was isolated in 1803, followed by codeine in 1832 and papaverine in 1848. Morphine can be synthesized, but it is more easily derived from opium. The term *narcotic* is derived from the Greek word for stupor and traditionally has been used to refer to potent morphine-like analgesics with the potential to produce physical dependence. The development of synthetic drugs with morphine-like properties has led to use of the term *opioid* to refer to all exogenous substances, natural and synthetic, that bind specifically to any of several subpopulations of opioid receptors and produce at least some agonist (morphine-like) effects. Opioids are unique in producing analgesia without loss of touch, proprioception, or consciousness. A convenient classification of opioids includes opioid agonists, opioid agonist-antagonists, and opioid antagonists (Table 3-1).

STRUCTURE ACTIVITY RELATIONSHIPS

The alkaloids of opium can be divided into two distinct chemical classes: phenanthrenes and benzylisoquinolines. The principal phenanthrene alkaloids present in opium are morphine, codeine, and thebaine (Fig. 3-1). The principal benzylisoquinoline alkaloids present in opium, which lack opioid activity, are papaverine and noscapine (Fig. 3-2).

The three rings of the phenanthrene nucleus are composed of 14 carbon atoms (Fig. 3-1). The fourth piperidine ring includes a tertiary amine nitrogen and is present in most opioid agonists. At pH 7.4, the tertiary amine nitrogen is highly ionized, making the molecule water soluble. A close relationship exists between stereochemical

Table 3–1
Classification of Opioid Agonists and Antagonists

Opioid Agonists	Opioid Agonists–Antagonists
Morphine	Pentazocine
Meperidine	Butorphanol
Fentanyl	Nalbuphine
Sufentanil	Buprenorphine
Alfentanil	Nalorphine
Phenoperidine	Bremazocine
Codeine	Dezocine
Dextromethorphan	
Hydromorphone	
Oxymorphone	**Opioid Antagonists**
Methadone	Naloxone
Heroin	Naltrexone

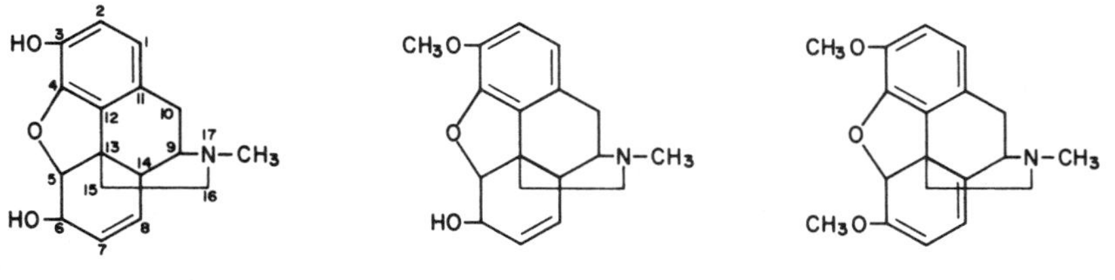

FIGURE 3-1. Phenanthrene alkaloids.

Morphine

Codeine

Thebaine

structure and potency of opioids, with levorotatory isomers being the most active.

Semisynthetic Opioids

Semisynthetic opioids result from relatively simple modification of the morphine molecule (Fig. 3-1). For example, substitution of a methyl group for the hydroxyl group on carbon 3 results in methylmorphine (codeine). Substitution of acetyl groups on carbons 3 and 6 results in diacetylmorphine (heroin). Thebaine has insignificant analgesic activity but serves as the precursor for etorphine (analgesic potency more than 1000 times morphine) and the opioid antagonist naloxone.

Synthetic Opioids

Synthetic opioids contain the phenanthrene nucleus of morphine but are manufactured by synthesis rather than chemical modification of morphine. Morphinan derivatives (levorphanol), methadone derivatives, benzomorphan derivatives (pentazocine), and phenylpiperidine derivatives (meperidine, fentanyl) are examples of groups of synthetic opioids. There are similarities in the molecular weights (236 to 326) and pKs of phenylpiperidine derivatives and amide local anesthetics.

MECHANISM OF ACTION

Opioids act as agonists at stereospecific opioid receptors at presynaptic and postsynaptic sites in the central nervous system (principally brain stem and spinal cord) and other tissues. These same opioid receptors normally are activated by endogenous ligands known as endorphins. Opioids mimic the action of endorphins by binding to opioid receptors, resulting in activation of a pain-modulating system. Receptors responsible for many opioid side effects differ from those producing analgesia, implying that analgesics lacking unwanted effects may be possible.

Existence of the opioid in the ionized state appears to be necessary for strong binding at the anionic opioid receptor site. Only levorotatory forms of the opioid exhibit agonist activity. The affinity of most opioid agonists for receptors correlates well with their analgesic potency. It is assumed that increasing opioid-receptor occupancy parallels opioid effects. Binding of an exogenous opioid agonist or endogenous ligand inhibits adenylate cyclase activity manifesting as hyperpolarization of the neuron, which results in suppression of spontaneous discharge and evoked responses. In addition, opioids may interfere with transmembrane transport of calcium ions and act presynaptically to interfere with the release of neurotransmitters including acetylcholine, dopamine, norepinephrine, and substance P. Depression of cholinergic transmission

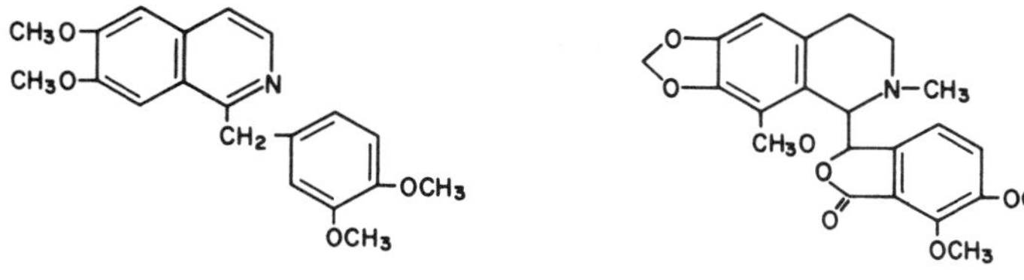

FIGURE 3-2. Benzylisoquinoline alkaloids.

Papaverine

Noscapine

in the central nervous system as a result of opioid-induced inhibition of acetylcholine release from nerve endings may play a prominent role in the analgesic and other side effects of opioid agonists. Opioids do not alter responsiveness of afferent nerve endings to noxious stimulation, nor do they impair conduction of nerve impulses along peripheral nerves.

OPIOID RECEPTORS

There are several types of opioid receptors, each mediating a spectrum of pharmacologic effects in response to activation by an opioid with agonist activity (Table 3-2) (Vaught et al, 1982). Subpopulations of opioid receptors are likely within major classifications. An ideal opioid agonist would have a high specificity for receptors, producing desirable responses (analgesia) and little or no specificity for receptors associated with side effects (hypoventilation, nausea, physical dependence).

Mu or morphine-preferring receptors are principally responsible for supraspinal analgesia. Activation of a subpopulation of mu receptors (mu-1) is speculated to result in analgesia, whereas mu-2 receptors are responsible for hypoventilation, bradycardia, and physical dependence. Beta-endorphin is the endogenous ligand, whereas mu-receptor agonists include morphine, meperidine, fentanyl, sufentanil, and alfentanil. Meptazinol is a relatively selective mu-1 receptor agonist, producing analgesia without undesirable side effects mediated by mu-2 receptors. Naloxone is a specific mu-receptor antagonist, attaching to but not activating the receptor. The role of *delta* receptors is to modulate the activity of mu receptors. Activation of *kappa* receptors results in analgesia with little or no de-

Table 3–2
Classification of Opioid Receptors

	Effect	Agonist	Antagonist
Mu-1	Supraspinal analgesia	Beta endorphin	Naloxone
		Meptazinol*	Pentazocine
		Morphine	Nalbuphine
Mu-2	Hypoventilation	Meperidine	
	Bradycardia	Fentanyl	
	Physical dependence	Sufentanil	
	Euphoria	Alfentanil	
	Ileus		
Delta	Modulate mu receptor activity	Leuenkephalin	Naloxone
			Metenkephalin
Kappa	Analgesia	Dynorphin	Naloxone
	Sedation	Pentazocine	
	Hypoventilation(?)	Butorphanol	
	Miosis	Nalbuphine	
		Buprenorphine	
		Nalorphine	
Sigma	Dysphoria	Pentazocine(?)	Naloxone
	Hypertonia	Ketamine(?)	
	Tachycardia		
	Tachypnea		
	Mydriasis		

*Relatively selective for mu-1 receptors.

pression of ventilation. Opioid agonist-antagonists often act principally on kappa receptors. Activation of *sigma* receptors results in excitatory symptoms such as dysphoria, hypertonia, tachycardia, and tachypnea.

Endorphins

The presence of highly specific opioid receptors is consistent with the demonstration of ligands (alpha, beta, gamma, and delta endorphins; leuenkephalin; and metenkephalin) that activate these receptors. The term *endorphin* is a combination of the words *endogenous* and *morphine* that is applied to all endogenous peptides with opioid activity. The anterior pituitary contains the peptides dynorphin and beta lipotropin that may function as prohormones with their hydrolysis, giving rise to endorphins.

Endogenous Pain-Suppression System

The obvious role of opioid receptors and endorphins is to function as an endogenous pain-suppression system (see Chapter 43). Opioid receptors are located in areas of the brain (periaqueductal gray matter of the brain stem, amygdala, corpus striatum, and hypothalamus) and spinal cord (substantia gelatinosa) that are involved with pain perception, integration of pain impulses, and responses to pain. It is speculated that endorphins inhibit the release of excitatory neurotransmitters from terminals of nerves carrying nociceptive stimuli. As a result, neurons are hyperpolarized, which suppresses spontaneous discharge and evoked responses. Analgesia induced by electrical stimulation of specific sites in the brain or mechanical stimula-

tion of peripheral areas (acupuncture) most likely reflects release of endorphins (Pomeranz and Chiu, 1976). Even the analgesic response to a placebo may also involve the release of endorphins. After about 60 years of age, patients experience a decrease in sensitivity to pain and an increased analgesic response to opioids (Bellville et al, 1971).

Neuraxial Opioids

Placement of opioids in the epidural or subarachnoid space to manage acute and/or chronic pain is based on the knowledge that opioid receptors are present in the substantia gelatinosa of the spinal cord (Cousins and Mather, 1984). Presumably, opioids placed in the epidural space diffuse across the dura to gain access to opioid receptors on the spinal cord. Analgesia is dose related (epidural dose is 5 to 10 times the subarachnoid dose) and specific for visceral rather than somatic pain. Although neuraxial placement of opioids is not adequate for surgical anesthesia, there is evidence that such placement reduces the anesthetic requirements (MAC) for volatile anesthetics (Fig. 3-3) (Drasner et al, 1988). Analgesia produced by neuraxial opioids, in contrast to intravenous administration of opioids or regional anesthesia with local anesthetics, is not associated with sympathetic nervous system denervation, skeletal muscle weakness, or loss of proprioception.

Side effects associated with neuraxial opioids include (1) pruritus, (2) urinary retention, (3) nausea and vomiting, (4) sedation, and (5) early and delayed depression of ventilation or circulation. Early depression of ventilation reflects systemic absorption of opioid from its epidural placement site,

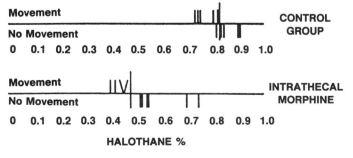

FIGURE 3-3. MAC for halothane is 0.81% in control patients and 0.46% in those receiving 0.75 mg of morphine intrathecally prior to the induction of anesthesia. (Drasner K, Bernards CM, Ozanne GM. Intrathecal morphine reduces the minimum alveolar concentration of halothane in humans. Anesthesiology 1988; 69: 310–2; with permission.)

whereas delayed depression of ventilation (6 to 24 hours after injection) is due to cephalad spread of the opioid in cerebrospinal fluid to medullary centers in the area of the fourth cerebral ventricle. Opioids with high lipid solubility, such as fentanyl or sufentanil, attach to lipid components in the spinal cord; thus, less drug is available to diffuse cephalad, making delayed depression of ventilation less likely than after injection of relatively poorly lipid-soluble morphine. Administration of epidural morphine following cesarean section is associated with an increased likelihood of reactivation of herpes labialis (cold sores) in patients with a prior history of this viral infection (Crone et al, 1990).

OPIOID AGONISTS

Opioid agonists include but are not limited to morphine, meperidine, fentanyl, sufentanil, and alfentanil (Table 3-1). These are the opioids most likely to be used with inhaled anesthetics during general anesthesia. Indeed, large doses of morphine, fentanyl, and sufentanil have been used as the sole anesthetic in critically ill patients.

Morphine

Morphine is the prototype opioid agonist to which all other opioids are compared. In humans, morphine produces analgesia, euphoria, sedation, and diminished ability to concentrate. Other sensations include nausea, a feeling of body warmth, heaviness of the extremities, dryness of the mouth, and pruritus, especially around the nose. The cause of pain persists, but even low doses of morphine increase the threshold to pain and modify the perception of noxious stimulation such that it is no longer experienced as pain. Continuous, dull pain is relieved by morphine more effectively than is sharp, intermittent pain. In contrast to nonopioid analgesics, morphine is effective against pain arising from the viscera as well as from skeletal muscles, joints, and integumental structures. Analgesia is most prominent when morphine is administered before the painful stimulus occurs (Woolf and Wall, 1986). This is a pertinent consideration in administering an opioid to patients prior to the acute surgical stimulus. In the absence of pain, however, morphine may produce excessive sedation and dysphoria rather than euphoria.

Pharmacokinetics

Morphine is well absorbed following intramuscular administration, with onset of effect in 15 to 30 minutes and a peak effect in 45 to 90 minutes. The duration of action is about 4 hours. Absorption of morphine from the gastrointestinal tract is not reliable. Morphine is usually administered intravenously in the perioperative period, thus eliminating the unpredictable influence of drug absorption. The peak analgesic effect of morphine administered intravenously occurs about 20 minutes after injection.

Plasma morphine concentrations following rapid intravenous injections do not correlate closely with the opioid's pharmacologic activity (Aitkenhead et al, 1984). Presumably, this discrepancy reflects a delay in penetration of morphine across the blood-brain barrier. Cerebrospinal fluid concentrations of morphine peak 15 to 30 minutes after intravenous injection and decay more slowly than plasma concentrations (Fig. 3-4) (Hug and Murphy, 1981). As a result, the an-

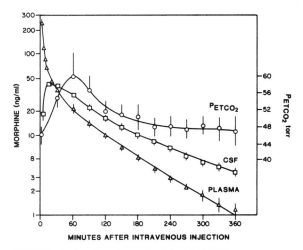

FIGURE 3-4. Cerebrospinal fluid (CSF) concentrations following intravenous administration decay more slowly than plasma concentrations. The end-tidal CO_2 concentration (P_{ETCO_2}) remains elevated despite a decreasing plasma concentration of morphine. Mean ± SE. (From Hug CC, Murphy MR. Tissue redistribution of fentanyl and termination of its effects in rats. Anesthesiology 1981; 55: 369–75; with permission.)

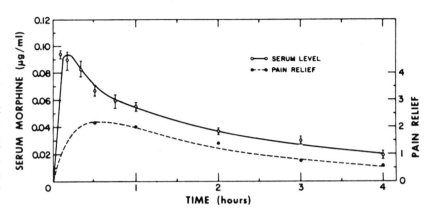

FIGURE 3–5. Moderate analgesia probably requires maintenance of plasma (serum) concentrations of morphine of at least 0.05 μg·ml⁻¹. Mean ± SE. (From Berkowitz BA, Ngai SH, Yang JC, Hempstead J, Spector S. The disposition of morphine in surgical patients. Clin Pharmacol Ther 1975; 17: 629–35; with permission.)

algesic and ventilatory depressant effects of morphine may not be evident during the initial high plasma concentrations following intravenous administration of the opioid. Likewise, these same drug effects persist despite decreasing plasma concentrations of morphine. Moderate analgesia probably requires maintenance of plasma morphine concentrations of at least 0.05 μg·ml⁻¹ (Fig. 3-5) (Berkowitz et al, 1975). Patient-controlled demand delivery systems usually provide acceptable postoperative analgesia, with total doses of morphine ranging from 1.3 to 2.7 mg·h⁻¹ (White, 1985).

Only a small amount of administered morphine gains access to the central nervous system. For example, it is estimated that less than 0.1% of morphine that is administered intravenously has entered the central nervous system at the time of peak plasma concentrations. Reasons for poor penetration of morphine into the central nervous system include (1) relatively poor lipid solubility, (2) high degree of ionization (90%) at physiologic pH, (3) protein binding, and (4) rapid conjugation with glucuronic acid. Alkalinization of the blood, as produced by hyperventilation of the lungs, will increase the nonionized fraction of morphine and thus facilitate its passage into the central nervous system. Nevertheless, respiratory acidosis, which decreases the nonionized fraction of morphine, results in higher brain and plasma concentrations of morphine than are present during normocarbia (Fig. 3-6) (Finck et al, 1977). This suggests that carbon dioxide–induced increases in cerebral blood flow and resulting facilitated delivery of morphine to the brain are more important than the fraction of drug that exists in either the

ionized or nonionized fraction. In contrast to the central nervous system, morphine accumulates rapidly in the kidneys, liver, and skeletal muscles. Morphine, unlike fentanyl, does not undergo significant first-pass uptake into the lungs (Roerig et al, 1987).

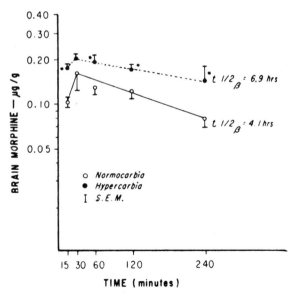

FIGURE 3–6. Hypercarbia, which decreases the nonionized fraction of morphine, results in a higher brain concentration and longer elimination half-life (t1/2$_\beta$) than occurs in the presence of normocarbia. *P <0.05. (From Finck AD, Ngai SH, Berkowitz BA. Antagonism of general anesthesia by naloxone in the rat. Anesthesiology 1977; 46: 241–5; with permission.)

METABOLISM.   The principal pathway of metabolism of morphine is conjugation with glucuronic acid in hepatic and extrahepatic sites, especially the kidneys. About 75% to 85% of a dose of morphine appears as morphine-3-glucuronide, and 5% to 10% is morphine-6-glucuronide. Morphine-3-glucuronide is detectable in the plasma within 1 minute following intravenous injection, and its concentration exceeds that of unchanged drug by almost tenfold within 90 minutes (Fig. 3-7) (Murphy and Hug, 1981). An estimated 5% of morphine is demethylated to normorphine, and a small amount of codeine may also be formed. Metabolites of morphine are eliminated principally in the urine, with only 7% to 10% undergoing biliary excretion. Morphine-3-glucuronide is detectable in the urine for up to 72 hours after administration of morphine. A small fraction (usually less than 5%) of injected morphine can be recovered unchanged in the urine.

Morphine-3-glucuronide is pharmacologically inactive, whereas morphine-6-glucuronide produces analgesia and depression of ventilation (Pelligrins et al, 1989). In fact, it is possible that the majority of analgesic activity is derived from morphine-6-glucuronide (Hanna et al, 1990). Elimination of morphine glucuronides may be impaired in patients with renal failure, causing an accumulation of metabolites and unexpected ventilatory depressant effects of small doses of opioids (Fig. 3-8) (Chauvin et al, 1987a). Indeed, prolonged depression of ventilation (up to 7 days) has been observed in patients in renal failure following administration of morphine (Don et al, 1975). Formation of glucuronide conjugates may be impaired by monoamine oxidase inhibitors, which is consistent with exaggerated effects of morphine when administered to patients being treated with these drugs.

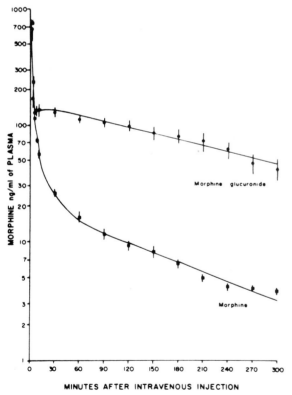

FIGURE 3-7.   Morphine glucuronide is detectable in the plasma within 1 minute following intravenous injection and its concentration exceeds that of unchanged morphine by almost tenfold within 90 minutes. Mean ± SE. (From Murphy MR, Hug CC. Pharmacokinetics of intravenous morphine in patients anesthetized with enflurane-nitrous oxide. Anesthesiology 1981; 54: 187–92; with permission.)

ELIMINATION HALF-TIME.   Following intravenous administration, the elimination half-time is 114 minutes for morphine and 173 minutes for morphine-3-glucuronide (Table 3-3; Fig. 3-7) (Murphy and Hug, 1981). The decrease in the plasma concentration of morphine following initial distribution of the drug is principally due to metabolism, because only a small amount of unchanged opioid is excreted by the kidneys. Plasma morphine concentrations are greater in elderly than in young adults (Fig. 3-9) (Berkowitz et al, 1975). In the first 4 days of life, the clearance of morphine is reduced and its elimination half-time is prolonged compared with that found in older infants (Lynn and Slattery, 1987). This is consistent with the clinical observation that neonates are more sensitive than older children to the ventilatory depressant effects of morphine. Patients with renal failure exhibit higher plasma concentrations of morphine than do normal patients, reflecting a smaller volume of distribution (Vd) as the elimination of unchanged drug is not altered compared with normal patients (Aitkenhead et al, 1984). Anesthesia alone does not alter the elimination half-time of morphine.

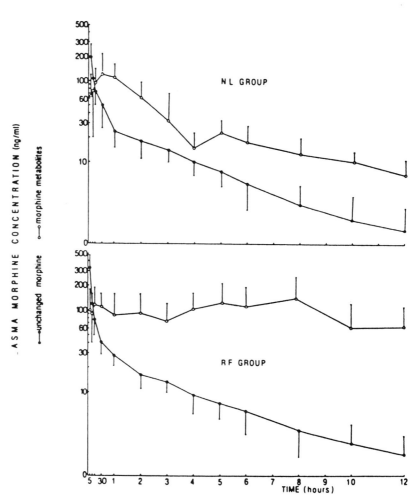

FIGURE 3–8. Plasma concentrations of unchanged morphine (closed circles) and morphine metabolites (open circles) in normal (NL) and renal failure (RF) patients. (From Chauvin M, Sandouk P, Scherrman JM, Farinotti R, Strumga P, Duvaldestin P. Morphine Pharmacokinetics in renal failure. Anesthesiology 1987; 66: 327–31; with permission.)

Side Effects

Side effects described for morphine are also characteristic for other opioid agonists, although the incidence or magnitude may vary.

CARDIOVASCULAR SYSTEM. Administration of morphine even in large doses (1 $mg \cdot kg^{-1}$ IV) to supine and normovolemic patients is unlikely to cause direct myocardial depression or hypotension. The same patients changing from a supine to a standing position, however, may manifest orthostatic hypotension and syncope, presumably reflecting morphine-induced impairment of compensatory sympathetic nervous system responses. For example, morphine reduces sympathetic nervous system tone to peripheral veins, resulting in venous pooling and subsequent decreases in venous return, cardiac output, and blood pressure (Lowenstein et al, 1972).

Morphine can also evoke reductions in blood pressure due to drug-induced bradycardia or histamine release. Morphine-induced bradycardia results from increased activity over the vagal nerves, which probably reflects stimulation of the vagal nucleus in the medulla. This opioid may also exert a direct depressant effect on the sinoatrial node and acts to slow conduction of cardiac impulses through the atrioventricular node. These actions may, in part, explain reduced vulnerability to ventricular fibrillation with morphine. Administration of opioids (morphine) in

Table 3-3
Pharmacokinetics of Opioid Agonists and Antagonists

Opioid	pK	Protein Binding (%)	Volume of Distribution (L·kg⁻¹)	Clearance (ml·kg⁻¹· min⁻¹)	Elimination Half-Time (min)
Morphine	7.93	26–36	3.2–3.4	15–23	114
Meperidine	8.5	64–82	2.8–4.2	10–17	180–264
Fentanyl	8.43	79–87	3.2–5.9	11–21	185–219
Sufentanil	8.01	92.5	2.86	13	148–164
Alfentanil	6.5	89–92	0.5–1	5–7.9	70–98
Naloxone			1.8	30	60–90

the preoperative medication or before the induction of anesthesia (fentanyl) tends to slow heart rate during exposure to volatile anesthetics with or without surgical stimulation (see Fig. 2-9) (Cahalan et al, 1987).

Opioid induced histamine release and associated hypotension are variable in both incidence and degree. The magnitude of morphine induced histamine release and subsequent reduction in blood pressure can be minimized by (1) limiting the rate of morphine infusion to 5 mg·min⁻¹ IV, (2) keeping the patient in a supine to a slightly head-down position, and (3) optimizing intravascular fluid volume. Conversely, administration of morphine, 1 mg·kg⁻¹ IV, over a 10-minute period produces substantial increases in plasma concentrations of histamine that are paralleled by significant decreases in blood pressure and systemic vascular resistance (Figs. 3-10 and 3-11) (Rosow et al, 1982). It is important to recognize, however, that not all patients respond to this rate of morphine infusion with the release of histamine, emphasizing the individual variability associated with the administration of this drug (Fig. 3-10) (Rosow et al, 1982). In contrast to morphine, the infusion of fentanyl, 50 μg·kg⁻¹ IV, over a 10-minute period, does not evoke release of histamine in any patient (Fig. 3-10) (Rosow et al, 1982). Sufentanil, like fentanyl, does not evoke the release of histamine (Flacke et al, 1987). Pretreatment of patients with H-1 and H-2 receptor antagonists does not alter release of histamine evoked by morphine but does prevent changes in blood pressure and systemic vascular resistance (Philbin et al, 1981).

Morphine does not sensitize the heart to catecholamines or otherwise predispose to car-

diac dysrhythmias as long as hypercarbia or arterial hypoxemia does not result from ventilatory depressant effects of the opioid. Tachycardia and hypertension that occur during anesthesia with morphine are not pharmacologic effects of the opioid, but rather are responses to painful surgical stimulation that are not suppressed by morphine. Both the sympathetic nervous system and the renin-angiotensin mechanism contribute to these cardiovascular responses (Bailey et al, 1975). Large doses of morphine or other opioid

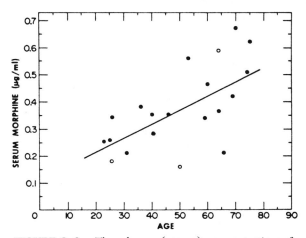

FIGURE 3-9. The plasma (serum) concentration of morphine increases progressively with advancing age. (From Berkowitz BA, Ngai SH, Yang JC, Hempstead J, Spector S. The disposition of morphine in surgical patients. Clin Pharmacol Ther 1975; 17; 629–35; with permission.)

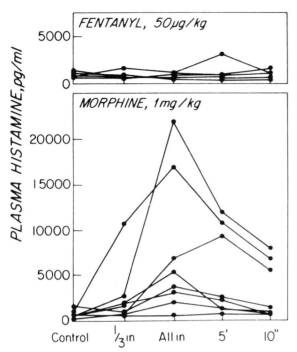

FIGURE 3-10. Intravenous administration of morphine, but not fentanyl, is associated with an unpredictable increase in the plasma concentration of histamine. (From Rosow CE, Moss J, Philbin DM, Savarese JJ. Histamine release during morphine and fentanyl anesthesia. Anesthesiology 1982; 56: 93-6; with permission.)

agonists may reduce the likelihood that tachycardia and hypertension will occur in response to painful stimulation, but once the response has occurred, administration of additional opioid is unlikely to be effective. During anesthesia, opioid agonists are commonly administered with inhaled anesthetics to ensure complete amnesia for the painful surgical stimulus. The combination of an opioid agonist such as morphine or fentanyl with nitrous oxide results in cardiovascular depression (decreased cardiac output and blood pressure plus elevated filling pressures), which does not occur when either drug is administered alone (Stoelting and Gibbs, 1973). Likewise, decreases in systemic vascular resistance and blood pressure may accompany the combination of an opioid and benzodiazepine, whereas these effects do not accompany the administration of either drug alone (Fig. 3-12) (Tomicheck et al, 1983).

VENTILATION. All opioid agonists produce dose-dependent depression of ventilation primarily through a direct depressant effect on brain stem ventilation centers (see Chapter 49). This depression of ventilation is characterized by reduced responsiveness of these ventilation centers to carbon dioxide as reflected by an increase in the resting $PaCO_2$ and displacement of the carbon dioxide response curve to the right. Opioid agonists also interfere with pontine and medullary ventilatory centers that regulate rhythm of breathing, leading to prolonged pauses between breaths and periodic breathing. It is possible that opioid agonists diminish sensitivity to carbon dioxide by reducing the release of acetylcholine from neurons in the area of the medullary ventilatory center in response to hypercarbia. In this re-

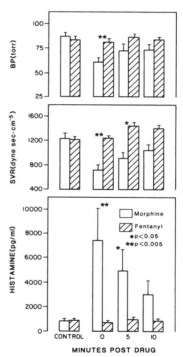

FIGURE 3-11. Morphine-induced decreases in blood pressure (*BP*) and systemic vascular resistance (*SVR*) are accompanied by increases in the plasma concentration of histamine. Similar changes do not accompany the intravenous administration of fentanyl. Mean ± SE. (From Rosow CE, Moss J, Philbin DM, Savarese JJ. Histamine release during morphine and fentanyl anesthesia. Anesthesiology 1982; 56: 93-6; with permission.)

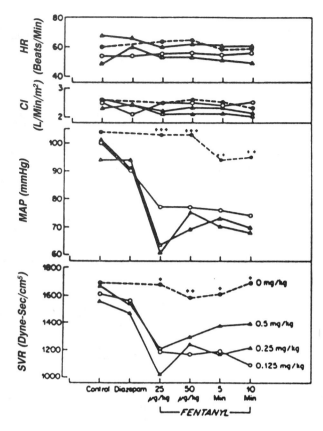

FIGURE 3–12. Administration of fentanyl (50 $\mu g \cdot kg^{-1}$ IV at 400 $\mu g \cdot min^{-1}$) following injection of diazepam (0.125–0.5 $mg \cdot kg^{-1}$ IV) is associated with significant decreases in mean arterial pressure (MAP) and systemic vascular resistance (*SVR*), whereas heart rate (HR) and cardiac index (CI) do not change. Administration of fentanyl in the absence of prior injection of diazepam is devoid of circulatory effects. (From Tomicheck RC, Rosow CE, Philbin DM, Moss J, Teplick RS, Schneider RC. Diazepam-fentanyl interaction: Hemodynamic and hormonal effects in coronary artery surgery. Anesth Analg 1983; 62: 881–4; with permission).

gard, physostigmine, which elevates central nervous system levels of acetylcholine, may antagonize depression of ventilation but not analgesia produced by morphine (see Chapter 9).

Depression of ventilation produced by opioid agonists is rapid and persists for several hours, as demonstrated by decreased ventilatory responses to carbon dioxide. High doses of opioids may result in apnea, but the patient remains conscious and able to initiate a breath if asked to do so. Death from an opioid overdose is almost invariably attributable to depression of ventilation.

Clinically, depression of ventilation produced by opioid agonists manifests as a decreased frequency of breathing that is often accompanied by a compensatory increase in tidal volume. The incompleteness of this compensatory increase in tidal volume is evidenced by predictable increases of the $PaCO_2$. Many factors influence the magnitude and duration of depression of ventilation produced by opioid agonists. For example, elderly patients and patients who are sleeping are usually more sensitive to ventilatory depressant effects of opioids. Conversely, pain from surgical stimulation counteracts depression of ventilation produced by opioids. Likewise, the analgesic effect of opioids slows breathing that has been rapid and shallow owing to pain.

Opioids produce dose-dependent depression of ciliary activity in the airways. Increases in airway resistance following administration of an opioid are probably due to a direct effect on bronchial smooth muscle and an indirect action owing to release of histamine.

NERVOUS SYSTEM. Opioids in the absence of hypoventilation decrease cerebral blood flow and intracranial pressure (Larson et al, 1974). These drugs must be used with caution in patients with head injury because of their (1) associated effects on wakefulness, (2) production of miosis, and (3) depression of ventilation with associated increases in intracranial pressure if the $PaCO_2$ becomes elevated. Furthermore, head injury may impair the integrity of the blood-brain barrier, with resultant increased sensitivity to opioids.

The effect of morphine on the electroencephalogram (EEG) resembles changes associated with sleep. For example, there is replacement of rapid alpha waves by slower delta waves. Recording of the EEG fails to reveal any evidence of seizure activity following administration of large doses of opioids (see the section entitled "Fentanyl"). Opioids do not alter the responses to neuromuscular blocking drugs. Skeletal muscle rigidity, especially of the thoracic and abdominal muscles, is common when large doses of opioid agonists are administered rapidly intravenously. This rigidity may be related to actions at opioid receptors and involve interactions with dopaminergic and gamma-aminobutyric acid–responsive neurons. Decreased thoracic compliance associated with skeletal muscle rigidity may interfere with adequate ventilation of the lungs and lead to impairment of venous return because of the high mechanical inflation pressures necessary to ventilate the lungs.

Miosis is due to an excitatory action of opioids on the autonomic nervous system component of the Edinger-Westphal nucleus of the oculomotor nerve. Tolerance to the miotic effect of morphine is not prominent. Miosis can be antagonized by atropine, and profound arterial hypoxemia can still result in mydriasis.

BILIARY TRACT. Opioids can cause spasm of biliary smooth muscle, resulting in increases in intrabiliary pressure that may be associated with epigastric distress or biliary colic. This pain may be confused with angina pectoris. Naloxone will relieve pain caused by biliary spasm but not myocardial ischemia. Conversely, nitroglycerin will relieve pain owing to biliary spasm or myocardial ischemia. Equal analgesic doses of fentanyl, morphine, meperidine, and pentazocine increase common bile duct pressure 99%, 53%, 61%, and 15% above predrug levels, respectively (Radnay et al, 1980). During surgery, opioid-induced spasm of the sphincter of Oddi may appear radiologically as a sharp constriction at the distal end of the common bile duct and be misinterpreted as a common bile duct stone (McCammon

et al, 1978). It may be necessary to reverse opioid-induced biliary smooth muscle spasm with naloxone so as to correctly interpret the cholangiogram (Lang and Pilon, 1980). Glucagon, 2 mg IV, also reverses opioid-induced biliary smooth muscle spasm and, unlike naloxone, does not antagonize the analgesic effects of the opioid (Jones et al, 1980). Nevertheless, biliary muscle spasm does not occur in most patients who receive opioids. Indeed, the incidence of spasm of the sphincter of Oddi is about 3% in patients receiving fentanyl as a supplement to inhaled anesthetics (Jones et al, 1981).

Contraction of the smooth muscles of the pancreatic ducts is probably responsible for increases in plasma amylase and lipase concentrations that may be present following the administration of morphine. Such elevations may confuse the diagnosis when acute pancreatitis is a possibility.

GASTROINTESTINAL TRACT. The use of opium to treat diarrhea preceded its use for analgesia. Morphine reduces the propulsive peristaltic contractions of the small and large intestine and enhances the tone of the pyloric sphincter, ileocecal valve, and anal sphincter. The delayed passage of intestinal contents through the colon allows increased absorption of water to take place. As a result, constipation often accompanies therapy with opioids. Minimal tolerance to the constipating effects of opioids occurs.

NAUSEA AND VOMITING. Opioid-induced nausea and vomiting are caused by direct stimulation of the chemoreceptor trigger zone in the floor of the fourth ventricle (see Fig. 41-16). This may reflect the role of opioid agonists as partial dopamine agonists at dopamine receptors in the chemoreceptor trigger zone. Indeed, apomorphine is a profound emetic and is also the most potent of the opioids at dopamine receptors. Stimulation of dopamine receptors as a mechanism for opioid-induced nausea and vomiting is consistent with the antiemetic efficacy of butyrophenones. Morphine may also cause nausea and vomiting by increasing gastrointestinal secretions and delaying passage of intestinal contents towards the colon.

Morphine depresses the vomiting center in the medulla (see Fig. 41-16). As a result, the intravenous administration of morphine produces less nausea and vomiting than the intramuscular administration of morphine, presumably because opioid administered intravenously reaches the vomiting center as rapidly as it reaches the chemoreceptor trigger zone. Nausea and vomiting are relatively uncommon in recumbent patients given morphine. This suggests that a vestibular component may be contributing to opioid-induced nausea and vomiting.

GENITOURINARY. Morphine can increase the tone and peristaltic activity of the ureter. In contrast to similar effects on biliary tract smooth muscle, the same opioid-induced effects on the ureter can be reversed by an anticholinergic drug such as atropine. Urinary urgency is produced by opioid-induced augmentation of detrusor muscle tone, but, at the same time, the tone of the vesicle sphincter is enhanced, making voiding difficult.

Antidiuresis that accompanies administration of morphine to animals has been attributed to opioid-induced release of antidiuretic hormone. In humans, however, administration of morphine in the absence of painful surgical stimulation does not evoke the release of antidiuretic hormone (Philbin et al, 1976). Furthermore, when morphine is administered in the presence of an adequate intravascular fluid volume, there is no change in urine output (Stanley et al, 1974).

CUTANEOUS CHANGES. Morphine causes cutaneous blood vessels to dilate. The skin of the face, neck, and upper chest frequently becomes flushed and warm. These changes in cutaneous circulation are in part caused by the release of histamine. Histamine release probably accounts for urticaria and erythema commonly seen at the morphine injection site. In addition, morphine-induced histamine release probably accounts for conjunctival erythema and pruritus.

Localized cutaneous evidence of histamine release, especially along the vein into which morphine is injected, does not represent an allergic reaction. Overall, the incidence of true allergy to opioids is uncommon, although documented cases have been reported (Bennett et al, 1986; Levy and Rockoff, 1982; Zucker-Pinchoff and Ramanathan, 1989). More often, predictable side effects of opioids such as localized histamine release, orthostatic hypotension, and nausea and vomiting are misinterpreted as an allergic reaction.

PLACENTA. The placenta offers no real barrier to transfer of opioids from mother to fetus. Therefore, depression of the neonate can occur as a consequence of administration of opioids to the mother during labor. In this regard, maternal administration of morphine may produce greater neonatal depression than meperidine (Way et al, 1965). This may reflect immaturity of the neonate's blood-brain barrier. Chronic maternal use of an opioid can result in the development of physical dependence (intrauterine addiction) in the fetus. Subsequent administration of naloxone to the neonate can precipitate a life-threatening neonatal abstinence syndrome.

DRUG INTERACTIONS. Ventilatory depressant effects of some opioids may be exaggerated by amphetamines, phenothiazines, monoamine oxidase inhibitors, and tricyclic antidepressants. For example, patients receiving monoamine oxidase inhibitors may experience exaggerated central nervous system depression and hyperpyrexia following administration of an opioid agonist, especially meperidine. This exaggerated response may reflect alterations in the rate or pathway of metabolism of the opioid. Sympathomimetic drugs appear to enhance analgesia produced by opioids. The cholinergic nervous system seems to be a positive modulator of opioid-induced analgesia in that physostigmine enhances and atropine antagonizes analgesia.

TOLERANCE AND PHYSICAL DEPENDENCE. Tolerance and physical dependence with repeated opioid administration are characteristic features of all opioid agonists and are among the major limitations to their clinical use. Cross-tolerance develops between all the opioids. Tolerance can occur without physical dependence, but the reverse does not seem to occur.

Tolerance is the development of the need to increase the dose of opioid agonist to achieve the same analgesic effect previously achieved with a lower dose. Such acquired tolerance usually takes 2 to 3 weeks to develop with analgesic doses of morphine. The miotic and constipating actions of morphine persist, whereas tolerance to depression of ventilation develops.

The potential for physical dependence (addiction) is an agonist effect of opioids. Indeed, physical dependence does not occur with opioid antagonists and is unlikely with opioid agonist-antagonists. When opioid agonist actions predominate, there often develops, with repeated use, a compulsive desire (psychological) and continuous need (physiologic) for the drug. Physical dependence on morphine usually requires about 25 days to develop but may occur sooner in emotionally unstable persons. Some degree of physical dependence, however, occurs after only 48 hours of continuous medication. When physical dependence is established, discontinuation of the opioid agonist produces a typical withdrawal abstinence syndrome within 15 to 20 hours, with a peak in 2 to 3 days, and remission in 10 to 14 days. Initial symptoms of withdrawal include yawning, diaphoresis, lacrimation, or coryza. Insomnia and restlessness are prominent. Abdominal cramps, nausea, vomiting, and diarrhea reach their peak in 72 hours and then decline over the next 7 to 10 days. During withdrawal, tolerance to morphine is rapidly lost, and the syndrome can be terminated by a modest dose of opioid agonist. The longer the period of abstinence, the smaller the dose of opioid agonist that will be required.

Mechanisms responsible for development of tolerance or physical dependence to opioid agonists have not been conclusively determined. In many respects, symptoms of opioid withdrawal resemble a denervation hypersensitivity that might reflect an increase (up-regulation) in the number of responding opioid receptors in the brain. This increase in opioid receptors could reflect chronic opioid-induced inhibition of acetylcholine release. Opioid agonists are also known to inhibit adenylate cyclase activity and cyclic adenosine monophosphate (cyclic AMP) production. Abrupt withdrawal of opioids leads to a marked increase in both the level of cyclic AMP and brain sympathetic nervous system activity. Indeed, clonidine, a centrally acting alpha-2 adrenergic agonist that diminishes transmission in sympathetic pathways in the central nervous system, is an effective drug in suppressing withdrawal signs in persons who are physically dependent on opioids (Gold et al, 1980). Tolerance and physical dependence are often attributed to cellular adaptation, but the proof for this premise is lacking. Tolerance is not due to enzyme induction, because no increase in the rate of metabolism of opioid agonists occurs.

OVERDOSE. The principal manifestation of opioid overdose is depression of ventilation manifesting as a slow breathing frequency that may progress to apnea. Pupils are symmetric and miotic unless severe arterial hypoxemia is present, which results in mydriasis. Skeletal muscles are flaccid, and upper airway obstruction may occur. Pulmonary edema commonly occurs, but the mechanism is not known. Hypotension and seizures develop if arterial hypoxemia persists. The triad of miosis, hypoventilation, and coma should suggest overdose with an opioid. Treatment of opioid overdose is mechanical ventilation of the lungs with oxygen and administration of an opioid antagonist, naloxone. Administration of naloxone to treat an opioid overdose in a physically dependent patient may precipitate acute withdrawal.

Meperidine

Meperidine is a synthetic opioid agonist derived from phenylpiperidine (Fig. 3-13). There are several analogues of meperidine, including fentanyl, sufentanil, alfentanil, and phenoperidine (Fig. 3-13). Structurally, meperidine is similar to atropine, and it possesses a mild atropine-like antispasmodic effect. Nevertheless, the principal pharmacologic effects of meperidine resemble morphine.

Pharmacokinetics

Meperidine is about one tenth as potent as morphine, with 80 to 100 mg IM being equivalent to about 10 mg of morphine IM. The duration of action of meperidine is 2 to 4 hrs, making it a shorter-acting opioid agonist than morphine. In equal analgesic doses, meperidine produces as much sedation, euphoria, nausea, vomiting, and depression of ventilation as does morphine. Unlike morphine, meperidine is well absorbed from the gastrointestinal tract, but nevertheless it is only about one half as effective orally as when administered intramuscularly.

METABOLISM. Metabolism of meperidine in the liver is extensive, with about 90% of the drug initially undergoing demethylation to normeperidine and hydrolysis to meperidinic acid.

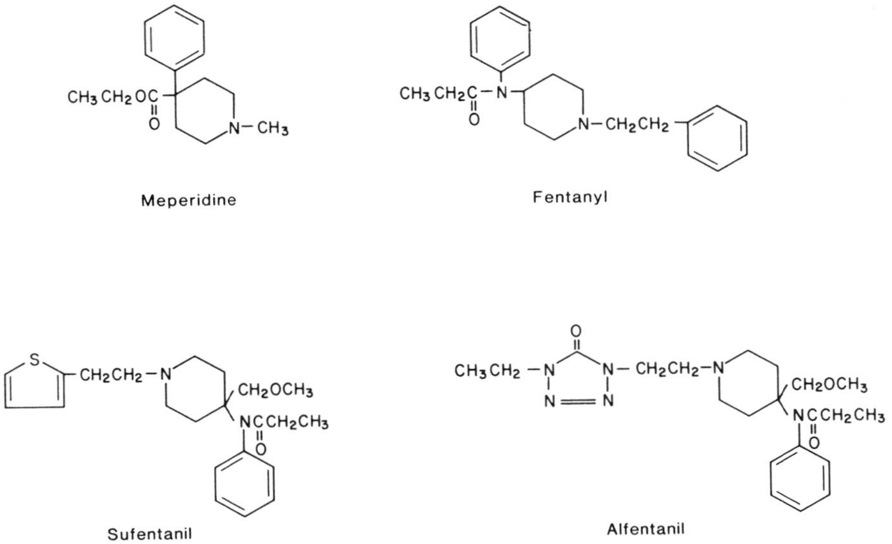

FIGURE 3–13.   Synthetic opioid agonists.

Normeperidine may subsequently be hydrolyzed to normeperidic acid. Urinary excretion of meperidine is pH dependent. For example, if the urinary pH is less than 5, as much as 25% of the opioid is excreted unchanged. Indeed, acidification of the urine can be considered in an attempt to speed elimination of meperidine.

Normeperidine has an elimination half-time of 15 to 40 hours and can be detected in the urine for as long as 3 days following administration of meperidine. This metabolite, in addition to having stimulant effects on the central nervous system, is about one half as active as the parent compound as an analgesic. Normeperidine toxicity manifesting as myoclonus and seizures is most likely during prolonged administration of meperidine, especially to patients with impaired renal function (Armstrong and Berston, 1986). Normeperidine may also be important in meperidine-induced delirium (confusion, hallucinations), which has been observed in patients receiving the drug for more than 3 days, corresponding to the accumulation of this active metabolite (Eisendrath et al, 1987).

ELIMINATION HALF-TIME.   The elimination half-time of meperidine is 180 to 264 minutes (Table 3-3). Since clearance of meperidine primarily depends on hepatic metabolism, it is possible that large doses of opioid would saturate enzyme sys-

tems and result in prolonged elimination half-time. Nevertheless, elimination half-time is not altered by doses of meperidine up to 5 mg·kg^{-1} IV (Koska et al, 1981). About 60% of meperidine is bound to plasma proteins. Elderly patients manifest decreased plasma protein binding of meperidine, resulting in increased plasma concentrations of free drug and an apparent increased sensitivity to the opioid. Increased tolerance of alcoholics to meperidine and other opioids presumably reflects an increased Vd, resulting in lower plasma concentrations of meperidine.

Clinical Uses

The principal use of meperidine is for analgesia during labor and delivery and following surgery. An intramuscular injection of meperidine to provide postoperative analgesia results in peak plasma concentrations that vary three- to fivefold as well as times required to achieve peak concentrations that vary three- to sevenfold among patients (Austin et al, 1980a). The minimum analgesic plasma concentration of meperidine is highly variable among patients; however, in the same patient, differences in concentrations as small as 0.05 µg·ml^{-1} can represent a margin between no relief and complete analgesia. A plasma meperidine concentration of 0.7 µg·ml^{-1} would be expected to provide postoperative analgesia in about 95% of patients (Austin et al, 1980b). Patient-controlled analgesia delivery systems usually provide acceptable postoperative analgesia, with total doses of meperidine ranging from 12 to 36 mg·h^{-1} (White, 1985).

Oral absorption may make meperidine more useful than morphine for the treatment of many forms of pain. Unlike morphine, meperidine is not useful for the treatment of diarrhea and is not an effective antitussive. During bronchoscopy, the relative lack of antitussive activity of meperidine makes it less useful. Meperidine is not used in high doses because of significant negative inotropic effects plus histamine release in a substantial number of patients (Flacke et al, 1987; Priano and Vatner, 1981).

Side Effects

(For additional discussion, see the section entitled "Morphine, Side Effects"). In therapeutic doses, meperidine is associated with orthostatic hypotension. In fact, hypotension after meperidine injection is more frequent and more profound than after comparable doses of morphine. Orthostatic hypotension suggests that meperidine, like morphine, interferes with compensatory sympathetic nervous system reflexes. Meperidine, in contrast to morphine, rarely causes bradycardia but instead may increase heart rate, reflecting its modest atropine-like qualities. Large doses of meperidine result in reductions in myocardial contractility that, among opioids, is unique for this drug. Delirium and seizures, when they occur, presumably reflect accumulation of normeperidine, which has stimulating effects on the central nervous system.

Meperidine readily impairs ventilation and may be even more of a ventilatory depressant than morphine. This opioid promptly crosses the placenta, and concentrations of meperidine in umbilical cord blood at birth may exceed maternal plasma concentrations (Morgan et al, 1978). Nevertheless, meperidine produces less depression of ventilation in the neonate than does morphine (Way et al, 1965). Meperidine may produce less constipation and urinary retention than morphine. After equal analgesic doses, biliary tract spasm is less after meperidine injection than after morphine injection but greater than that caused by codeine (Radnay et al, 1980). Meperidine does not cause miosis but rather tends to cause mydriasis, reflecting its modest atropine-like ac-

tions. A dry mouth and an increase in heart rate are further evidence of the atropine-like effects of meperidine.

The pattern of withdrawal symptoms after abrupt discontinuation of meperidine differs from that of morphine in that there are few autonomic nervous system effects. In addition, symptoms of withdrawal develop more rapidly and are of a shorter duration compared with those of morphine.

Fentanyl

Fentanyl is a synthetic opioid agonist that is related to the phenylpiperidines. As an analgesic, fentanyl is 75 to 125 times more potent than morphine.

Pharmacokinetics

A single dose of fentanyl administered intravenously has a more rapid onset (less than 30 seconds) and shorter duration of action than morphine. The greater potency and more rapid onset of action reflect the greater lipid solubility of fentanyl compared with that of morphine, which facilitates its passage across the blood-brain barrier. Likewise, the short duration of action of a single dose of fentanyl reflects its rapid redistribution to inactive tissue sites such as fat and skeletal muscles, with an associated decline in the plasma concentration of the drug (Fig. 3-14) (Hug and Murphy, 1981). The lungs also serve as a large, inactive storage site, with an estimated 75% of the initial fentanyl dose undergoing first-pass pulmonary uptake (Roerig et al, 1987). This nonrespiratory function of the lung limits the initial amount of drug that reaches the systemic circulation and may play an important role in determining the pharmacokinetic profile of fentanyl. When multiple intravenous doses of fentanyl are administered or when there is continuous infusion of the drug, progressive saturation of these inactive tissue sites occurs. As a result, the plasma concentration of fentanyl does not decline rapidly, and the duration of analgesia, as well as depression of ventilation, may be prolonged (Murphy et al, 1979).

METABOLISM. Fentanyl is extensively metabolized by dealkylation, hydroxylation, and amide hydrolysis to inactive metabolites, including

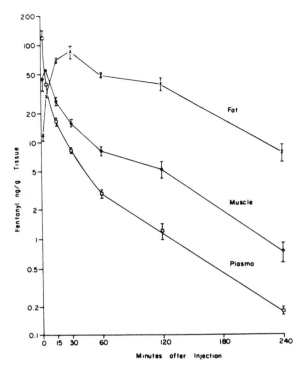

FIGURE 3–14. The short duration of action of a single intravenous dose of fentanyl reflects its rapid redistribution to inactive tissue sites such as fat and skeletal muscles with associated decreases in the plasma concentration of drug. Mean ± SE. (From Hug CC, Murphy MR. Tissue redistribution of fentanyl and termination of its effects in rats. Anesthesiology 1981; 55: 369–75; with permission.)

norfentanyl and desproprionylnorfentanyl, that are excreted in the bile and urine (McClain and Hug, 1980). For example, 85% of an injected dose of fentanyl appears in the urine and feces over 72 hours as metabolites, whereas less than 8% is recovered as unchanged drug in the urine. A high degree of metabolism to more polar and inactive metabolites is predictable for a highly lipid-soluble drug such as fentanyl.

ELIMINATION HALF-TIME. Despite the clinical impression that fentanyl has a short duration of action, its elimination half-time of 185 to 219 minutes is greater than that for morphine (Table 3-3). This longer elimination half-time reflects a larger Vd of fentanyl because clearance of both opioids is similar (Table 3-3). The larger Vd of

fentanyl is due to its greater lipid solubility and thus more rapid passage into tissues compared with the less lipid-soluble morphine. Plasma concentrations of fentanyl are maintained by its slow reuptake from inactive tissues sites, which accounts for persistent drug effects that parallel the prolonged elimination half-time. In animals, the elimination half-time, Vd, and clearance of fentanyl are independent of the dose of opioid between 6.4 and 640 µg·kg^{-1} IV (Murphy et al, 1983). This suggests that saturation of clearance or tissue uptake mechanisms do not occur.

A prolonged elimination half-time for fentanyl in elderly patients is due to decreased clearance of the opioid because Vd is not changed in comparison with younger adults (Bentley et al, 1982). This change may reflect age-related reductions in hepatic blood flow, microsomal enzyme activity, or albumin production, as fentanyl is highly bound (79% to 87%) to protein. For these reasons, it is likely that a given dose of fentanyl will be effective for a longer period of time in elderly patients than in younger patients. A prolonged elimination half-time of fentanyl has also been observed in patients undergoing abdominal aortic surgery requiring infrarenal aortic cross-clamping (Hudson et al, 1986). Somewhat surprising, however, is the failure of cirrhosis of the liver to prolong significantly the elimination half-time of fentanyl (Haberer et al, 1982).

Clinical Uses

Fentanyl is administered clinically in a wide range of doses. For example, low doses of fentanyl, 1 to 2 µg·kg^{-1} IV, are injected to provide analgesia. Fentanyl, 2 to 10 µg·kg^{-1} IV, may be administered as an adjuvant to inhaled anesthetics in an attempt to blunt circulatory responses to (1) direct laryngoscopy for intubation of the trachea, or (2) sudden changes in the level or surgical stimulation. Injection of an opioid such as fentanyl before painful surgical stimulation may decrease the subsequent amount of opioid required in the postoperative period to provide analgesia (Woolf and Wall, 1986). Large doses of fentanyl, 50 to 150 µg·kg^{-1} IV, have been used alone to produce surgical anesthesia. Large doses of fentanyl as the sole anesthetic have the advantage of stable hemodynamics owing principally to (1) the lack of direct myocardial depressant effects, (2) the absence of histamine release, and (3) the suppression of the stress responses to surgery. Disadvantages of using fentanyl as the sole anesthetic include (1) failure to prevent responses to painful stimulation reliably at any dose, especially in patients with good left ventricular function, (2) possible patient awareness, and (3) postoperative depression of ventilation (Hilgenberg, 1981; Sprigge et al, 1982; Wynands et al, 1983).

Fentanyl may be administered as a transmucosal preparation (oral transmucosal fentanyl citrate, or a lollipop containing the equivalent of 5 to 20 $\mu g \cdot kg^{-1}$ of fentanyl) to decrease anxiety in the preoperative period and to facilitate induction of anesthesia, especially in children (Feld et al, 1989; Stanley et al, 1989)

Transdermal fentanyl preparations delivering 75 to 100 $\mu g \cdot h^{-1}$ result in sustained plasma concentrations of opioid during their presence and a decreasing plasma concentration for several hours after removal of the delivery system, reflecting continued absorption from the cutaneous depot (Varvel et al, 1989). Transdermal fentanyl systems applied before the induction of anesthesia and left in place for 24 hours reduce the amount of parenteral opioid required for postoperative analgesia (Caplan et al, 1989; Rowbotham et al, 1989).

In dogs, maximal analgesic, ventilatory, and cardiovascular effects are present when the plasma concentration of fentanyl is about 30 $ng \cdot ml^{-1}$ (Arndt et al, 1984). This confirms that analgesic actions of fentanyl cannot be separated from its effects on ventilation and heart rate. The fact that all receptor-mediated effects are similar at the same plasma concentration of fentanyl suggests saturation of the opioid receptors.

Side Effects

(For additional discussion, see also the section entitled "Morphine, Side Effects.") Persistent or recurrent depression of ventilation owing to fentanyl is a potential postoperative problem (Fig. 3-15) (Becker et al, 1976). Secondary peaks in plasma concentrations of fentanyl and morphine have been attributed to sequestration of fentanyl in acidic gastric fluid (ion trapping). Sequestered fentanyl could then be absorbed from the more alkaline small intestine back into the circulation to increase the plasma concentration of opioid and cause depression of ventilation to recur (Stoeckel et al, 1979). This, however, may not be the mechanism for the secondary peak of

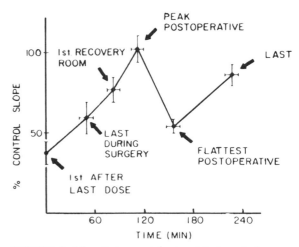

FIGURE 3–15. Recurrent fentanyl-induced depression of ventilation is evidenced by changes in the slope of the carbon dioxide ventilatory-response curve. Mean ± SE. (From Becker LD, Paulson BA, Miller RD, Severinghaus JW, Eger EI. Biphasic respiratory depression after fentanyl-droperidol or fentanyl alone used to supplement nitrous oxide anesthesia. Anesthesiology 1976; 44: 291–6; with permission.)

fentanyl, because any of the absorbed opioid from the gastrointestinal tract or skeletal muscles as evoked by movement associated with transfer to the recovery room would be subject to first-pass hepatic metabolism. An alternative explanation for the secondary peak of fentanyl is washout of the opioid from the lung as ventilation to perfusion relationships are reestablished in the postoperative period.

In comparison with morphine, fentanyl even in large doses (50 $\mu g \cdot kg^{-1}$ IV) does not evoke the release of histamine (Fig. 3-10) (Rosow et al, 1982). As a result, dilatation of venous capacitance vessels leading to hypotension is unlikely. Carotid sinus baroreceptor reflex control of heart rate is markedly depressed by fentanyl, 10 $\mu g \cdot kg^{-1}$ IV, administered to neonates (Fig. 3-16) (Murat et al, 1988). Therefore, changes in blood pressure occurring during fentanyl anesthesia have to be carefully considered because cardiac output is principally rate dependent in neonates. Bradycardia is more prominent with fentanyl than morphine and may lead to occasional decreases in blood pressure and cardiac output. Allergic reactions occur rarely in response to administration of fentanyl (Bennett et al, 1986; Zucker-Pinchoff and Ramanathan, 1989).

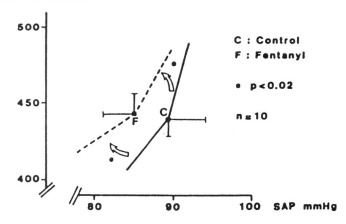

FIGURE 3-16. Fentanyl depresses the carotid sinus reflex-mediated heart rate response to changes in blood pressure in neonates. (From Murat I, Levron J-B, Berg A, Saint-Maurice C. Effects of fentanyl on baroreceptor reflex control of heart rate in newborn infants. Anesthesiology 1988; 68: 717-22; with permission.)

Seizure activity has been described following rapid intravenous administration of fentanyl, sufentanil, and alfentanil (Molbegott et al, 1987; Safwat and Daniel, 1983; Strong and Matson, 1989). In the absence of EEG evidence of seizure activity, however, it is difficult to distinguish opioid-induced skeletal muscle rigidity from seizure activity. Indeed, recording of the EEG during periods of opioid-induced skeletal muscle rigidity fails to reveal evidence of seizure activity in the brain (Smith et al, 1990). Even plasma concentrations as high as 1750 ng·ml^{-1} following rapid administration of fentanyl 150 µg·kg^{-1} IV do not produce EEG evidence of seizure activity (Murkin et al, 1984). Conversely, opioids might produce a form of myoclonus secondary to depression of inhibitory neurons that would produce a clinical picture of seizure activity in the absence of EEG changes. Fentanyl in doses exceeding 30 µg·kg^{-1} IV produces changes in somatosensory evoked potentials that, although detectable, do not interfere with the use and interpretation of this monitor during anesthesia (Schubert et al, 1987).

Sufentanil

Sufentanil is a thienyl analogue of fentanyl. The analgesic potency of sufentanil is five to ten times that of fentanyl, which parallels the greater affinity of sufentanil for opioid receptors compared with that of fentanyl. An important distinction from fentanyl is the 1000-fold difference between the analgesic dose of sufentanil and the dose that produces seizures in animals (deCastro et al, 1979). This difference is 160-fold for fentanyl and may be important when large doses of opioid agonists are used to produce anesthesia.

Pharmacokinetics

The elimination half-time of sufentanil (148 to 164 minutes) is intermediate between that of fentanyl and alfentanil (Table 3-3) (Bovill et al, 1984). A single intravenous dose of sufentanil has a similar elimination half-time in patients with or without cirrhosis of the liver (Chauvin et al, 1989). A prolonged elimination half-time has been observed in elderly patients receiving sufentanil for abdominal aortic surgery (Hudson et al, 1989). A high tissue affinity is consistent with the lipophilic nature of sufentanil, which permits rapid penetrance of the blood-brain barrier and onset of central nervous system effects. A rapid redistribution to inactive tissue sites terminates the effect of small doses, but a cumulative drug effect can accompany large or repeated doses of sufentanil.

Extensive protein binding of sufentanil (92.5%) compared with fentanyl (79% to 87%) contributes to a smaller Vd, which is characteristic of sufentanil. Binding to alpha-1 acid glycoprotein constitutes a principal proportion of the total plasma protein binding of sufentanil. Levels of alpha-1 acid glycoprotein vary over a threefold range in healthy volunteers and are increased after surgery, which would result in a decrease in the plasma-free fraction of sufentanil. Lower concentrations of alpha-1 acid glycoprotein in neonates and infants probably account for decreases in protein binding of sufentanil in these age groups compared with that in older children and adults (Meistelman et al, 1990). The resulting increased free fraction of sufentanil in the neonate might contribute to enhanced effects of this opioid in neonates. Indeed, fentanyl and its derivatives produce anesthesia and depression of ventilation at lower doses in neonates than in adults (Greeley et al, 1987; Yaster, 1987).

METABOLISM. Sufentanil is rapidly metabolized by N-dealkylation at the piperidine nitrogen and by O-demethylation (Weldon et al, 1985). The products of N-dealkylation are pharmacologically inactive, whereas desmethyl sufentanil from O-demethylation has about 10% of the activity of sufentanil. Less than 1% of an administered dose of sufentanil appears unchanged in the urine. Indeed, high lipid solubility of sufentanil results in maximal renal tubular reabsorption of free drug as well as its enhanced access to hepatic microsomal enzymes. Extensive hepatic extraction means that clearance of sufentanil will be sensitive to changes in hepatic blood flow but not to alterations in drug-metabolizing capacity of the liver. Sufentanil metabolites are excreted almost equally in urine and feces, with about 30% appearing as conjugates. The production of a weakly active metabolite and the substantial amount of conjugated metabolite formation imply the possible importance of normal renal function for the clearance of sufentanil. Indeed, prolonged depression of ventilation in association with an abnormally elevated plasma concentration of sufentanil has been observed in a patient with chronic renal failure (Waggum et al, 1985).

Clinical Uses

In volunteers, a single dose of sufentanil, 0.1 to 0.4 $\mu g \cdot kg^{-1}$ IV, produces a longer period of analgesia and less depression of ventilation than does a comparable dose of fentanyl (1 to 4 $\mu g \cdot kg^{-1}$ IV) (Bailey et al, 1990). Compared with large doses of morphine or fentanyl, sufentanil, 18.9 $\mu g \cdot kg^{-1}$ IV, results in more rapid induction of anesthesia, earlier emergence from anesthesia, and earlier extubation of the trachea (Fig. 3-17) (Sanford et al, 1986). The time for return of spontaneous ventilation is not significantly

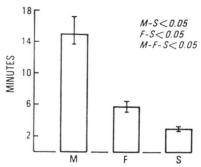

FIGURE 3–17. The time between the beginning of opioid administration and the patient's inability to respond to a verbal command was defined as induction time. Sufentanil resulted in a significantly more rapid induction of anesthesia than did morphine or fentanyl. M, morphine. F, fentanyl. S, sufentanil. Mean ± SE. (From Sanford TJ, Smith NT, Dee-Silver H, Harrison WK. A comparison of morphine, fentanyl, and sufentanil anesthesia for cardiac surgery: Induction, emergence, and extubation. Anesth Analg 1986; 65: 259–66; with permission.)

different between the three opioids. As observed with other opioids, sufentanil causes a decrease in cerebral metabolic requirements for oxygen, and cerebral blood flow is reduced (Keykhah et al, 1985). Bradycardia produced by sufentanil may be sufficient to decrease cardiac output (Sebel and Bovill, 1982). As observed with fentanyl, delayed depression of ventilation has also been described following the administration of sufentanil (Chang and Fish, 1985). Sufentanil does not increase cerebral blood flow in humans (Mayer et al, 1990).

Although large doses of sufentanil (10 to 30 $\mu g \cdot kg^{-1}$ IV) or fentanyl (50 to 150 $\mu g \cdot kg^{-1}$ IV) produce minimal hemodynamic effects in patients with good left ventricular function, the blood pressure and hormonal (catecholamine) responses to painful stimulation such as median sternotomy are not predictably prevented (Philbin et al, 1990; Sonntag et al, 1989). It seems unlikely that any clinically useful dose of sufentanil or fentanyl will abolish such responses in all patients. On theoretical grounds, it is a remote possibility that the further introduction of even more potent synthetic opioids will result in less hemodynamic responsiveness when these drugs are administered as the sole anesthetic (Philbin et al, 1990).

Alfentanil

Alfentanil is an analogue of fentanyl that is less potent (one fifth to one tenth) and has one third the duration of action of the parent opioid. The onset of action of alfentanil after intravenous administration is 1 to 2 minutes, in contrast to 5 to 6 minutes for fentanyl. This rapid onset of action is a result of the low pK of alfentanil such that nearly 90% of the drug exists in the nonionized form at physiologic pH. It is the nonionized fraction that readily crosses the blood-brain barrier. The brief duration of action of alfentanil is a result of redistribution to inactive tissue sites and hepatic metabolism. This termination of effect by redistribution of alfentanil is similar to the redistribution responsible for lowering the plasma concentrations of fentanyl and thiopental. Unlike thiopental or fentanyl, however, continuous intravenous infusion or repeated doses of alfentanil do not result in a significant cumulative drug effect.

Pharmacokinetics

The Vd of alfentanil is four to six times smaller than that of fentanyl (Table 3-3) (Camu et al, 1982; Stanski and Hug, 1982). This reduced Vd compared with that of fentanyl reflects lower lipid solubility and greater protein binding. Despite this lesser lipid solubility, penetration of the blood-brain barrier by alfentanil is rapid because of its high degree of nonionization at physiologic pH. Alfentanil is principally bound to alpha-1 acid glycoprotein, a protein whose plasma concentration is not altered by liver disease.

ELIMINATION HALF-TIME. The elimination half-time of alfentanil is 70 to 98 minutes compared with 185 to 219 minutes for fentanyl (Table 3-3) (Camu et al, 1982). Cirrhosis of the liver, but not cholestatic disease, prolongs the elimination half-time of alfentanil (Davis et al, 1989; Ferrier et al, 1985). Renal failure does not alter the clearance or elimination half-time of alfentanil (Chauvin et al, 1987b). Elimination half-time for alfentanil is shorter in children (4 to 8 years old) than adults, reflecting a smaller Vd in these younger patients (Meistelman et al, 1987). Because protein binding is similar, it is likely that a decreased percentage of adipose tissue in children is responsible for the short elimination half-time.

METABOLISM. The principal pathway for metabolism of alfentanil to inactive metabolites is N-dealkylation at the piperidine nitrogen with formation of noralfentanil (Meuldermans et al, 1988). Conjugation with glucuronic acid is another important metabolic pathway. Less than 0.5% of an administered dose of alfentanil is excreted unchanged in the urine. Efficiency of hepatic metabolism is emphasized by elimination of about 96% of alfentanil from the plasma within 60 minutes following its injection. Erythromycin can inhibit the metabolism of alfentanil and can result in a prolonged opioid effect (Bartkowski and McDonnell, 1990).

Clinical Uses

Alfentanil, 150 to 300 $\mu g \cdot kg^{-1}$ IV, administered rapidly, produces unconsciousness in about 45 seconds. Following this induction, maintenance of anesthesia can be provided with a continuous infusion of alfentanil, 25 to 150 $\mu g \cdot kg^{-1} \cdot h^{-1}$ IV, combined with an inhaled drug (Ausems et al, 1983). Cumulative drug effects are unlikely even with prolonged infusions of alfentanil. Indeed, the small Vd and short elimination half-time preclude significant accumulation and render alfentanil a useful drug for continuous intravenous infusion. Unlike other opioids, supplemental doses of alfentanil seem to be more likely to decrease blood pressure that is elevated following painful stimulation. Alfentanil increases biliary tract pressures similarly to fentanyl, but the duration of this increase is shorter than that produced by fentanyl (Hynyen et al, 1986).

Phenoperidine

Phenoperidine is chemically related to meperidine, being about 100 times more potent as an analgesic. Side effects include nausea, vomiting, and depression of ventilation. About 50% of an administered dose of phenoperidine appears unchanged in the urine. The remainder is metabolized to meperidine and then to meperidinic acid, which appears in the urine.

Codeine

Codeine is the result of the substitution of a methyl group for the hydroxyl group on carbon

3 of morphine (Fig. 3-1). The presence of this methyl group limits first-pass hepatic metabolism and accounts for the efficacy of codeine when administered orally. The elimination half-time of codeine after oral or intramuscular administration is 3 to 3.5 hours. About 10% of administered codeine is demethylated in the liver to morphine, which may be responsible for the analgesic effect of codeine. Any remaining codeine is demethylated to inactive norcodeine, which is conjugated or excreted unchanged by the kidneys.

Codeine is an effective antitussive at oral doses of 15 mg. Maximal analgesia, equivalent to that produced by 650 mg of aspirin, occurs with 60 mg of codeine. When administered intramuscularly, codeine, 120 mg, is equivalent in analgesic effect to 10 mg of morphine. Most often, codeine is included in medications as an antitussive or is combined with nonopioid analgesics for the treatment of mild to moderate pain. Physical dependence liability of codeine appears to be less than that of morphine and occurs only rarely after oral analgesic use. Codeine produces minimal sedation, nausea, vomiting, and constipation. Dizziness may occur in ambulatory patients. Codeine even in large doses is unlikely to produce apnea. Administration of codeine intravenously is not recommended, because histamine-induced hypotension is likely.

Dextromethorphan

Dextromethorphan is equal in potency to codeine as an antitussive but lacks analgesic or physical dependence properties. Unlike codeine, this drug rarely produces sedation or gastrointestinal disturbances.

Hydromorphone

Hydromorphone is a derivative of morphine that is about eight times as potent as morphine but has a slightly shorter duration of action. This opioid produces somewhat more sedation and evokes less euphoria than morphine. Administered orally, the analgesic potency of hydromorphone is about one fifth that observed after intramuscular injection. The uses and side effects of hydromorphone are the same as those of morphine.

Oxymorphone

Oxymorphone is the result of the addition of a hydroxyl group to hydromorphone. It is about 10 times as potent as morphine and seems to cause more nausea and vomiting. Physical dependence liability is great.

Methadone

Methadone is a synthetic opioid agonist that produces analgesia and is highly effective by the oral route (Fig. 3-18). Efficient oral absorption and prolonged duration of action of methadone render this an attractive drug for suppression of withdrawal symptoms in physically dependent persons such as heroin addicts. Methadone can substitute for morphine in addicts at about one fourth the dosage. Controlled withdrawal using methadone is milder and less acute than that from morphine. Methadone, 20 mg IV, produces postoperative analgesia lasting more than 24 hours, reflecting its prolonged (35-hour) elimination half-time (Gourlay et al, 1982). This drug is metabolized in the liver to inactive substances that are excreted in the urine and bile with small amounts of unchanged drug.

Side effects of methadone (depression of ventilation, miosis, constipation, biliary tract spasm) resemble those of morphine. Its sedative and euphoric actions seem to be less than those produced by morphine. Methadone-induced miosis is less prominent than that caused by morphine, and the addict develops complete tolerance to this action.

Propoxyphene

Propoxyphene is structurally similar to methadone and binds to opioid receptors as reflected

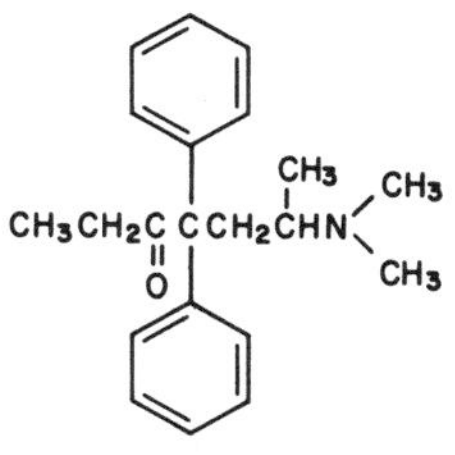

FIGURE 3-18. Methadone.

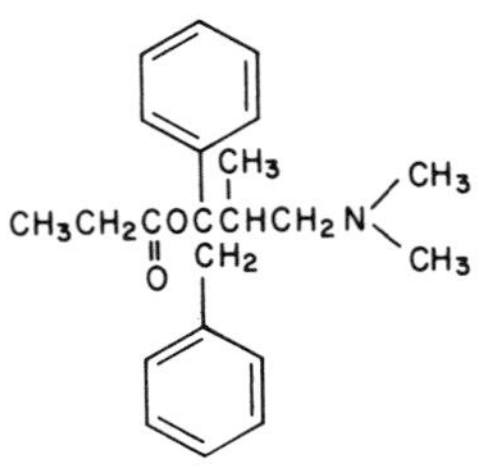

FIGURE 3–19.   Propoxyphene.

by antagonism of its pharmacologic effects by naloxone (Fig. 3-19). Oral doses of 90 to 120 mg of propoxyphene produce analgesia and central nervous system effects similar to those produced by 60 mg of codeine and 60 mg of aspirin. The only clinical use of propoxyphene is treatment of mild to moderate pain that is not adequately relieved by aspirin. Propoxyphene does not possess antipyretic or anti-inflammatory effects, and antitussive activity is not significant.

Propoxyphene is completely absorbed after oral administration, but, because of extensive first-pass hepatic metabolism (demethylation to norpropoxyphene), the systemic availability is greatly reduced. The elimination half-time following oral administration is about 14.6 hours. The most common side effects following propoxyphene administration are vertigo, sedation, nausea, and vomiting. Propoxyphene is about one third as potent as codeine in depressing ventilation. Overdose, however, is complicated by seizures and depression of ventilation.

Abrupt discontinuation of chronically administered propoxyphene results in a mild withdrawal syndrome. The incidence of abuse of propoxyphene is similar to that of codeine. Administration of this drug intravenously produces severe damage to veins and limits abuse by this route. Administration of propoxyphene in combination with alcohol and other central nervous system depressants may result in excessive drug depression.

Heroin

Heroin (diacetylnorphene) is a synthetic opioid produced by acetylation of morphine. When administered parenterally, heroin acts in a markedly different way from morphine. For example, there is rapid penetration of heroin into the brain, where it is hydrolyzed to the active metabolites, monoacetylmorphine and morphine. This unique rapid entrance into the central nervous system is most likely caused by the lipid solubility and chemical structure of heroin. Compared with morphine, parenteral heroin has (1) a more rapid onset, (2) a lack of nauseating effect, and (3) greater potential for physical dependency. This great liability for physical dependency is the reason that heroin is not available in the United States (Angell, 1984; Mondzac, 1984).

OPIOID AGONIST-ANTAGONISTS

Opioid agonist-antagonists include, but are not limited to, pentazocine, butorphanol, nalbuphine, buprenorphine, nalorphine, bremazocine, and dezocine (Fig. 3-20). These drugs bind to mu receptors, where they produce limited responses (partial agonists) or no effect (competitive antagonists). In addition, these drugs often exert partial agonist actions at other receptors, including kappa and delta receptors. Antagonist properties of these drugs can attenuate the efficacy of subsequently administered opioid agonists. Side effects are similar to those of opioid agonists, and, in addition, these drugs may cause dysphoric reactions. Advantages of opioid agonist-antagonists are the ability to produce analgesia with limited depression of ventilation and a low potential to produce physical dependence. Furthermore, these drugs have a ceiling effect such that increasing doses do not produce additional responses. This ceiling effect on depression of ventilation, however, is often accompanied by an equally modest ability to decrease anesthetic requirements.

Pentazocine

Pentazocine is a benzomorphan derivative that possesses opioid agonist actions as well as weak antagonist actions. It is presumed to exert its agonist effects at delta and kappa receptors. Concomitant opioid antagonist activity is weak, being only about one fifth as potent as nalorphine. Nevertheless, antagonist effects of pentazocine

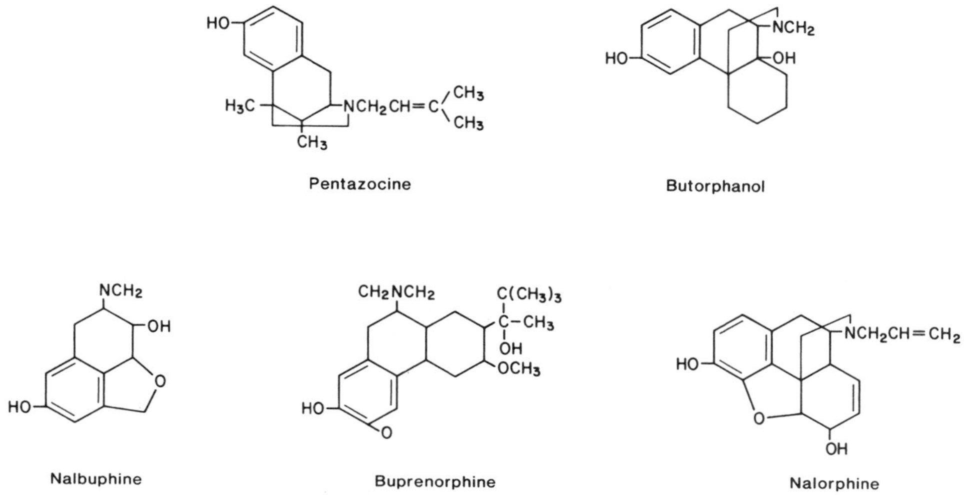

FIGURE 3–20. Opioid agonist-antagonists.

are sufficient to precipitate withdrawal symptoms when administered to patients who have been receiving opioids on a regular basis. The agonist effects of pentazocine are antagonized by naloxone. Indeed, physical dependence to pentazocine can be demonstrated by abrupt withdrawal precipitated by naloxone.

Pharmacokinetics

Pentazocine is well absorbed after oral or parenteral administration. First-pass hepatic metabolism is extensive, with only about 20% of an oral dose entering the circulation. Metabolism of pentazocine occurs by oxidation of terminal methyl groups, and resulting inactive glucuronic conjugates are excreted in the urine. An estimated 5% to 25% of an administered dose of pentazocine is excreted unchanged in the urine, and less than 2% undergoes biliary excretion. The elimination half-time is 2 to 3 hours.

Clinical Uses

Pentazocine, 10 to 30 mg IV or 50 mg orally, is used most often for the relief of moderate pain. An oral dose of 50 mg is equivalent in analgesic potency to 60 mg of codeine. Pentazocine is useful for treatment of chronic pain when there is a high risk of physical dependence. Placement in the epidural space produces a rapid onset of anal-gesia that is shorter lasting than that produced by morphine (Kalia et al, 1983).

Side Effects

The most common side effect of pentazocine is sedation, followed by diaphoresis and dizziness. Sedation is prominent following epidural placement of pentazocine, presumably reflecting activation of kappa receptors. Nausea and vomiting are less common than with morphine. Dysphoria, including fear of impending death, is associated with high doses of pentazocine. This tendency to dysphoria limits the physical dependence liability of pentazocine. Pentazocine produces an increase in plasma concentrations of catecholamines, which may account for increases in heart rate, systemic blood pressure, pulmonary artery blood pressure, and left ventricular end-diastolic pressure that accompany administration of this drug (Lee et al, 1976). Pentazocine, 20 to 30 mg IM, produces analgesia, sedation, and depression of ventilation similar to 10 mg of morphine. Increasing the intramuscular dose above 30 mg does not produce proportionate increases in these responses. Elevation of biliary tract pressure is less than that produced by equal analgesic doses of morphine, meperidine, or fentanyl (Radnay et al, 1980). Pentazocine crosses the placenta and may cause fetal depression. In contrast to morphine, miosis does not occur after administration of pentazocine.

Butorphanol

Butorphanol is an agonist-antagonist opioid that resembles pentazocine. Compared with pentazocine, the agonist effects of butorphanol are about 20 times greater, whereas antagonist actions are 10 to 30 times greater. It is speculated that butorphanol has (1) a low affinity for mu receptors to produce antagonism, (2) a moderate affinity for kappa receptors to produce analgesia, and (3) a minimal affinity for sigma receptors, so the incidence of dysphoria is low.

Butorphanol is rapidly and almost completely absorbed after intramuscular injection. In postoperative patients, 2 to 3 mg IM produces analgesia and depression of ventilation similar to 10 mg of morphine. Since butorphanol is available only in the parenteral form, it is better suited for the relief of acute rather than chronic pain. The intraoperative use of butorphanol, like pentazocine, seems to be limited. The elimination half-time of butorphanol is 2.5 to 3.5 hours. Metabolism is principally to inactive hydroxybutorphanol, which is eliminated largely in the bile and to a lesser extent in the urine.

Side Effects

Common side effects of butorphanol include sedation, nausea, and diaphoresis. Dysphoria, reported frequently with other opioid agonist-antagonists, is infrequent following administration of butorphanol. Depression of ventilation is similar to that produced by similar doses of morphine. Like pentazocine, analgesic doses of butorphanol increase systemic blood pressure, pulmonary artery blood pressure, and cardiac output. Also, similar to pentazocine, the effects of butorphanol on the biliary and gastrointestinal tract seem to be milder than those produced by morphine. Finally, it may be difficult to use an opioid agonist effectively as an analgesic in the presence of butorphanol. This must be remembered when considering the use of butorphanol or any other opioid agonist-antagonist for preoperative medication. Withdrawal symptoms do occur after acute discontinuation of chronic therapy with butorphanol, but symptoms are mild.

Nalbuphine

Nalbuphine is an agonist-antagonist opioid that is related chemically to oxymorphone and naloxone. It is equal in potency as an analgesic to morphine, and is about one fourth as potent as nalorphine as an antagonist. Nalbuphine is metabolized in the liver and has an elimination half-time of 3 to 6 hours. Naloxone reverses the agonist effects of nalbuphine. Nalbuphine, 10 mg IM, produces analgesia with an onset of effect and duration of action similar to those of morphine. Depression of ventilation is similar to that of morphine until 30 mg IM of nalbuphine is exceeded, after which no further depression of ventilation occurs (ceiling effect) (Gal et al, 1982). Sedation is the most common side effect, occurring in about one third of patients treated with nalbuphine. The incidence of dysphoria is less than that with pentazocine or butorphanol but is qualitatively similar and increases in frequency as the dose of nalbuphine is increased. In contrast to pentazocine and butorphanol, nalbuphine does not increase systemic blood pressure, pulmonary artery blood pressure, heart rate, or atrial filling pressures (Lee et al, 1976). For this reason, nalbuphine may be useful to provide sedation and analgesia in patients with heart disease as during cardiac catheterization. Abrupt withdrawal of nalbuphine after chronic administration produces withdrawal symptoms that are milder than those of morphine and more severe than those of pentazocine. The abuse potential of nalbuphine is low.

The antagonist effects of nalbuphine are speculated to occur at mu receptors. As a result, the subsequent use of morphine-like drugs for anesthesia after preoperative medication with nalbuphine may not provide adequate analgesia. Likewise, the efficacy of opioid agonists to provide analgesia may be compromised by nalbuphine, which has previously been administered and found to be inadequate in controlling postoperative pain. Conversely, antagonist effects of nalbuphine at mu receptors could be used to advantage in the postoperative period to reverse lingering ventilatory depressant effects of opioid agonists while still maintaining analgesia. Nalbuphine, 10 to 20 mg IV, reverses postoperative depression of ventilation caused by fentanyl but maintains analgesia (Bailey et al, 1987; Moldenhauer et al, 1985). Evidence of recurrent hypoventilation often occurs 2 to 3 hours following administration of nalbuphine to antagonize the effects of fentanyl.

Buprenorphine

Buprenorphine is an agonist-antagonist opioid derived from the opium alkaloid thebaine. Its analgesic potency is great, with 0.3 mg IM being equivalent to 10 mg of morphine. Following intramuscular administration, the onset of buprenorphine effect occurs in about 30 minutes, and the duration of action is at least 8 hours. It is estimated that the affinity of buprenorphine for mu receptors is 50 times greater than that of morphine, and subsequent slow dissociation from these receptors accounts for its prolonged duration of action and resistance to antagonism with naloxone. After intramuscular administration, nearly two thirds of the drug appears unchanged in the bile and the remainder is excreted in the urine as inactive metabolites.

Buprenorphine is effective in relieving moderate to severe pain such as that present in the postoperative period and that associated with cancer, renal colic, or myocardial infarction. Placed in the epidural space, the high lipid solubility (five times that of morphine) and affinity for opioid receptors limits cephalad spread and the likelihood of delayed depression of ventilation (Lanz et al, 1984). Antagonist effects of buprenorphine reflect the ability of this drug to displace opioid agonists from mu receptors.

Side effects of buprenorphine include drowsiness, nausea, vomiting, and depression of ventilation that are similar in magnitude to the side effects of morphine but may be prolonged and resistant to antagonism with naloxone. In contrast to other opioid agonist-antagonists, dysphoria is unlikely to occur in association with administration of this drug. Because of its antagonist properties, buprenorphine can precipitate withdrawal in patients who are physically dependent on morphine. Conversely, withdrawal symptoms in patients who are physically dependent on buprenorphine develop slowly and are of lesser intensity than those associated with morphine. In this respect, withdrawal from buprenorphine resembles that from other opioid agonist-antagonists, and the risk of abuse is low.

Nalorphine

Nalorphine is equally potent with morphine as an analgesic but is not chemically useful because of a high incidence of dysphoria. The high incidence of dysphoria may reflect activity of this drug at sigma receptors. Antagonist actions of nalorphine reflect its ability to displace opioid agonists from mu receptors.

Bremazocine

Bremazocine is a benzomorphan derivative that is twice as potent an analgesic as morphine but, in animals, does not produce depression of ventilation or evidence of physical dependence (Freye et al, 1983). It is speculated that bremazocine interacts selectively with kappa receptors. Failure of naloxone to reverse sedation produced by bremazocine is further evidence that this drug is acting at other than mu receptors.

Dezocine

Dezocine, 0.15 mg·kg-1 is an opioid agonist-antagonist with analgesic potency, onset, and duration of action in the relief of postoperative pain comparable to morphine. Absorption of dezocine, 10 to 15 mg after intramuscular administration, is rapid and complete with analgesia occurring after about 30 minutes. Following intravenous administration of dezocine, 5 to 10 mg, the onset of analgesia occurs in about 15 minutes. Elimination of dezocine is principally in the urine as a glucuronide conjugate. Like other opioid agonist-antagonists, dezocine exhibits a ceiling effect for depression of ventilation that parallels its analgesic activity (Gal and DiFazio, 1984). Large doses of dezocine, administered intravenously to humans, do not produce significant changes in blood pressure, pulmonary artery pressure, or cardiac output.

Dezocine has a high affinity for mu receptors and a moderate affinity for delta receptors (Rowlingson et al, 1983). The interaction at delta receptors serves to facilitate the effect of agonist activity at mu receptors. The incidence of dysphoria is minimal after administration of dezocine, presumably reflecting the low affinity of this drug for sigma receptors.

Meptazinol

Meptazinol is a partial opioid agonist with relative selectivity at mu-1 receptors. As a result, depression of ventilation does not occur with analgesic doses of meptazinol (100 mg IM equivalent to morphine 8 mg). The onset of analgesia is rapid, but the duration of action is less than 2 hours. Bioavailability after oral administration is less than 10%. Metabolism is to inactive glucuronide conjugates that are excreted by the kidneys. Protein binding is 20% to 25%, and the elimination half-time is about 2 hours. Physical dependence does not occur, miosis is slight, and constipation is absent. Nausea and vomiting are common side effects. Meptazinol cannot be substituted for an opioid agonist in patients physically dependent on opioids.

OPIOID ANTAGONISTS

Minor changes in the structure of an opioid agonist can convert the drug into an opioid antagonist at one or more of the opioid receptor sites. The most common change is substitution of an allyl group for the methyl group on an opioid agonist. For example, naloxone is the N-alkyl derivative of oxymorphone (Fig. 3-21).

Naloxone and naltrexone are pure opioid antagonists with no agonist activity that have replaced nalorphine and levorphanol, each of which possesses opioid agonist as well as antagonist activity. Both naloxone and naltrexone have a high affinity for mu and, to a lesser extent, delta and kappa receptors and can displace opioid agonists from these receptors. Following this displacement, the binding of naloxone or naltrexone does not activate opioid receptors, and antagonism occurs.

Naloxone

Naloxone is selective when used to (1) treat opioid-induced depression of ventilation as may be present in the postoperative period; (2) treat opioid-induced depression of ventilation in the neonate owing to maternal administration of opioid; (3) facilitate treatment of deliberate opioid overdose; and (4) detect suspected physical dependence. Naloxone, 1 to 4 μg·kg^{-1} IV, promptly reverses opioid-induced analgesia and depression of ventilation. The short duration of action of naloxone (30 to 45 minutes) is presumed to be due to its rapid removal from the brain. This emphasizes that supplemental doses of naloxone will likely be necessary for sustained antagonism of opioid agonists. In this regard, a continuous intravenous infusion of naloxone, 5 μg·kg^{-1}·h^{-1}, prevents depression of ventilation without altering analgesia produced by neuraxial opioids (Rawal et al, 1986).

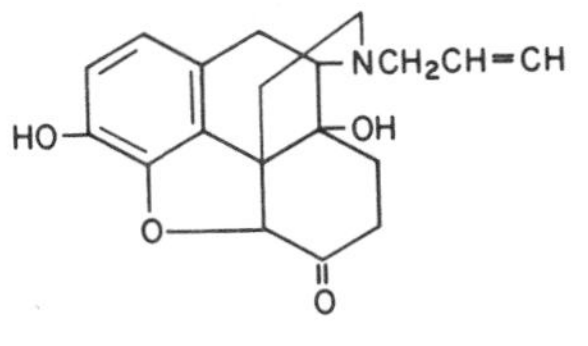

Naloxone is metabolized primarily in the liver by conjugation with glucuronic acid to form naloxone-3-glucuronide. The elimination half-time is 60 to 90 minutes (Table 3-3). Naloxone is absorbed orally, but metabolism during its first pass through the liver renders it only one fifth as potent as when administered parenterally.

Side Effects

Antagonism of opioid-induced depression of ventilation is accompanied by an inevitable reversal of analgesia. It may be possible, however, to titrate the dose of naloxone such that depression of ventilation is partially but acceptably antagonized so as to also maintain partial analgesia.

Nausea and vomiting appear to be closely related to the dose and speed of injection of naloxone (Kripke et al, 1976; Longnecker et al, 1973). Administration of naloxone slowly over 2 to 3 minutes rather than as a bolus seems to reduce the incidence of nausea and vomiting. Fortunately, awakening occurs either before or simultaneously with vomiting, which ensures that the patient's protective upper airway reflexes have returned and the likelihood of pulmonary aspiration is minimized.

Cardiovascular stimulation following administration of naloxone manifests as increased sympathetic nervous system activity, presumably reflecting the abrupt reversal of analgesia and the sudden perception of pain. This increased sympathetic nervous system activity may manifest as tachycardia, hypertension, pulmonary edema, and cardiac dysrhythmias (Flacke et al, 1977; Michaelis et al, 1974; Tanaka, 1974). Even ventricular fibrillation has occurred following the intravenous administration of naloxone and the

FIGURE 3-21.   Naloxone.

associated sudden increase in sympathetic nervous system activity (Andree, 1980; Azar and Turndorf, 1979).

Naloxone can easily cross the placenta. For this reason, administration of naloxone to an opioid-dependent parturient may produce acute withdrawal in the neonate.

Role in Treatment of Shock

Naloxone produces a dose-related improvement in myocardial contractility and survival in animals subjected to hypovolemic shock and, to a lesser extent, in those subjected to septic shock (Faden, 1984). The beneficial effects of naloxone in the treatment of shock occur only with doses greater than 1 mg·kg⁻¹ IV, suggesting that beneficial effects of this drug are not opioid-receptor mediated or alternatively, are mediated by opioid receptors other than mu receptors, possibly delta and kappa receptors.

Antagonism of General Anesthesia

The occasional observation that high doses of naloxone seem to antagonize the depressant effect of inhaled anesthetics may represent drug-induced activation of the cholinergic arousal system in the brain, independently of any interaction with opioid receptors (Kraynack and Gintautas, 1982). A role of endorphins in the production of general anesthesia is not supported by data demonstrating a failure of naloxone to alter anesthetic requirements (MAC) in animals (Harper et al, 1978).

Naltrexone

Naltrexone, like naloxone, is a relatively pure mu receptor antagonist. In contrast to naloxone, naltrexone is highly effective orally, producing sustained antagonism of the effects of opioid agonists for as long as 24 hours.

ANESTHETIC REQUIREMENTS

The contribution of opioids to total anesthetic requirements can be quantitated by determining the decrease in MAC of a volatile anesthetic in the presence of opioids. Maximal decreases in enflurane MAC of 65% are produced by mor-

phine, 5 mg·kg⁻¹ IV, or a dose of fentanyl that produces a plasma concentration of 30 ng·kg⁻¹ (Murphy and Hug, 1982a; Murphy and Hug, 1982b). In rats, sufentanil reduces halothane MAC by 90%, whereas in dogs the decrease in enflurane MAC (about 70%) is similar to fentanyl (Fig. 3-22) (Hall et al, 1987; Hecker et al, 1983). These data cast doubt on the ability of opioid agonists, including sufentanil, to provide total amnesia reliably in every patient, even with high doses. Opioid agonist-antagonists are less effective in decreasing MAC than are opioid agonists. For example, butorphanol, nalbuphine, and pentazocine maximally decrease MAC 11%, 8%, and 20%, respectively, even when the dose of these drugs is increased 40-fold (Hoffman and DeFazio, 1970; Murphy and Hug, 1982b). The ceiling effect for MAC parallels the ceiling effect for depression of ventilation and is consistent with the clinical impression that even large doses of opioid agonist-antagonists do not produce unconsciousness or prevent patient movement in response to painful stimulation. For this reason, the use of large doses of opioid agonist-antagonists for anesthesia does not seem logical.

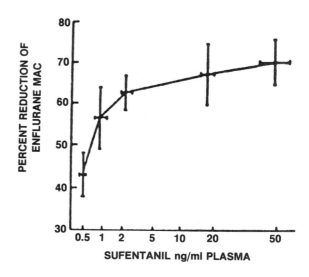

FIGURE 3–22. The reduction in enflurane MAC was determined during continuous intravenous infusion of sufentanil to maintain an unchanging plasma concentration of opioid. Mean ± SE. (From Hall RI, Murphy MR, Hug CC. The enflurane sparing effect of sufentanil in dogs. Anesthesiology 1987; 67: 518–25; with permission.)

The exception among the opioid agonist-antagonists may be dezocine, which decreases MAC more than 50% in animals. This effect of dezocine, however, is limited by drug-induced hypotension, which seems to be due to direct myocardial depression.

REFERENCES

Aitkenhead AR, Vater M, Acholas K, Cooper CMS, Smith G. Pharmacokinetics of single-dose IV morphine in normal volunteers and patients with end-stage renal failure. Br J Anaesth 1984;56:813–8.

Andree RA. Sudden death following naloxone administration. Anesth Analg 1980;59:782–4.

Angell M. Should heroin be legalized for the treatment of pain? N Engl J Med 1984;311:529–30.

Armstrong PJ, Berston A. Normeperidine toxicity. Anesth Analg 1986;65:536–8.

Arndt JO, Mikat M, Parasher C. Fentanyl's analgesic, respiratory, and cardiovascular actions in relation to dose and plasma concentration in unanesthetized dogs. Anesthesiology 1984;61:355–61.

Ausems ME, Hug CC, deLange S. Variable rate infusion of alfentanil as a supplement to nitrous oxide anesthesia for general surgery. Anesth Analg 1983;62:982–6.

Austin KL, Stapleton JV, Mather LE. Multiple intramuscular injections—A major source of variability in analgesic response to meperidine. Pain 1980a;8:47–62.

Austin KL, Stapleton JV, Mather LE. Relationship between blood meperidine concentrations and analgesic response. Anesthesiology 1980b;53:460–6.

Azar I, Turndorf H. Severe hypertension and multiple atrial premature contractions following naloxone administration. Anesth Analg 1979;58:524–5.

Bailey DR, Miller ED, Kaplan JA, Rogers PW. The renin-angiotensin-aldosterone system during cardiac surgery with morphine-nitrous oxide anesthesia. Anesthesiology 1975;42:538–44.

Bailey PL, Clark NJ, Pace NL, et al. Antagonism of postoperative opioid-induced respiratory depression: Nalbuphine versus naloxone. Anesth Analg 1987;66:1109–14.

Bailey PL, Streisand JB, East KA, et al. Differences in magnitude and duration of opioid-induced respiratory depression and analgesia with fentanyl and sufentanil. Anesth Analg 1990;70:8–15.

Bartkowski RR, McDonnell TE. Prolonged alfentanil effect following erythromycin administration. Anesthesiology 1990;73:566–8.

Becker LD, Paulson BA, Miller RD, Severinghaus JW, Eger EI. Biphasic respiratory depression after fentanyl-droperidol or fentanyl alone used to supplement nitrous oxide anesthesia. Anesthesiology 1976;44:291–6.

Bellville JW, Forrest WH, Miller E, Brown BW. Influence of age on pain relief from analgesics. JAMA 1971;217:1835–41.

Bennett MJ, Anderson LK, McMillan JC, Ebertz JM, Hanifin JM, Hirshman CA. Anaphylactic reaction during anaesthesia associated with positive intradermal skin test to fentanyl. Can Anaesth Soc J 1986;33:75–8.

Bentley JB, Borel JD, Nenad RE, Gillespie TJ. Age and fentanyl pharmacokinetics. Anesth Analg 1982;61:968–71.

Berkowitz BA, Ngai SH, Yang JC, Hempstead J, Spector S. The disposition of morphine in surgical patients. Clin Pharmacol Ther 1975;17:629–35.

Bovill JG, Sebel PS, Blackburn CL, Oei-Lim V, Heykants JJ. The pharmacokinetics of sufentanil in surgical patients. Anesthesiology 1984;61:502–6.

Cahalan MK, Lurz FW, Eger EI, Schwartz LA, Beaupre PN, Smith JS. Narcotics decrease heart rate during inhalational anesthesia. Anesth Analg 1987;66:166–70.

Camu F, Gepts E, Rucquoi M, Heykants J. Pharmacokinetics of alfentanil in man. Anesth Analg 1982;61:657–61.

Caplan RA, Ready LB, Oden RV, Matsen FA, Nessly ML, Olsson GL. Transdermal fentanyl for postoperative pain management. A double-blind placebo study. JAMA 1989;260:1036–9.

Chang J, Fish KJ. Acute respiratory arrest and rigidity after anesthesia with sufentanil: A case report. Anesthesiology 1985;63:710–1.

Chauvin M, Sandouk P, Scherrman JM, Farinotti R, Strumga P, Duvaldestin P. Morphine pharmacokinetics in renal failure. Anesthesiology 1987a;66:327–31.

Chauvin M, Lebrault C, Levron JC, Duvaldestin P. Pharmacokinetics of alfentanil in chronic renal failure. Anesth Analg 1987b;66:53–6.

Chauvin M, Ferrier C, Haberer JP, et al. Sufentanil pharmacokinetics in patients with cirrhosis. Anesth Analg 1989;68:1–4.

Cousins MJ, Mather LE. Intrathecal and epidural administration of opioids. Anesthesiology 1984;61:276–310.

Crone L-AL, Conly JM, Storgard C, et al. Herpes labialis in parturients receiving morphine following cesarean section. Anesthesiology 1990;73:208–13.

Davis PJ, Stiller RL, Cook DR, Brandom BW, David JE, Scierka AM. Effects of cholestatic hepatic disease and chronic renal failure on alfentanil pharmacokinetics in children. Anesth Analg 1989;68:579–83.

deCastro J, van de Water A, Wouters L, Xhonneux R, Reneman R, Kay B. Comparative study of cardiovascular, neurological and metabolic side effects of eight narcotics in dogs. Acta Anaesthesiol Belg 1979;30:5–99.

Don HF, Dieppa RD, Taylor P. Narcotic analgesics in anuric patients. Anesthesiology 1975;42:745–7.

Drasner K, Bernards CM, Ozanne GM. Intrathecal morphine reduces the minimum alveolar concentration of halothane in humans. Anesthesiology 1988;69:310–2.

Eisendrath SJ, Goldman B, Douglas J, Dimatteo L, Van-Dyke C. Meperidine-induced delirium. Am J Psychiatry 1987;144:1062–5.

Faden AI. Opiate antagonists and thyrotropin-releasing hormone. I. Potential role in the treatment of shock. JAMA 1984;252:1177–80.

Feld LH, Champeau MW, vanSteennis C, Scott JC. Preanesthetic medication in children: A comparison of oral transmucosal fentanyl citrate versus placebo. Anesthesiology 1989;71:374–7.

Ferrier C, Marty J, Bouffard Y, Haberer JP, Levron JC, Duvaldestin P. Alfentanil pharmacokinetics in patients with cirrhosis. Anesthesiology 1985;62:480–4.

Finck AD, Ngai SH, Berkowitz BA. Antagonism of general anesthesia by naloxone in the rat. Anesthesiology 1977;46:241–5.

Flacke JW, Flacke WE, Bloor BC, VanEtten AP, Kripke BJ. Histamine release by four narcotics: A double-blind study in humans. Anesth Analg 1987;66:723–30.

Flacke JW, Flacke WE, Williams GD. Acute pulmonary edema following naloxone reversal of high-dose morphine anesthesia. Anesthesiology 1977;47:376–8.

Freye E, Hartung E, Schenk GK. Bremazocine: An opiate that induces sedation and analgesia without respiratory depression. Anesth Analg 1983;62:483–8.

Gal TJ, DiFazio CA. Ventilatory and analgesic effects of dezocine in humans. Anesthesiology 1984;61:716–22.

Gal TJ, DiFazio CA, Moscicki J. Analgesic and respiratory depressant activity of nalbuphine: A comparison with morphine. Anesthesiology 1982;57:367–74.

Gold MS, Pottash AC, Sweeney Dr, Kleber HD. Opiate withdrawal using clonidine: A safe, effective and rapid non-opiate treatment. JAMA 1980;243:343–6.

Gourlay GK, Wilson PR, Glynn CJ. Pharmacodynamics and pharmacokinetics of methadone during the perioperative period. Anesthesiology 1982;57:458–67.

Greeley WJ, DeBruijn NP, Davis DP. Sufentanil pharmacokinetics in pediatric cardiovascular patients. Anesth Analg 1987;66:1067–72.

Haberer JP, Schoeffler P, Couderc E, Duvaldestin P. Fentanyl pharmacokinetics in anaesthetized patients with cirrhosis. Br J Anaesth 1982;54:1267–70.

Hall RI, Murphy MR, Hug CC. The enflurane sparing effect of sufentanil in dogs. Anesthesiology 1987;67:518–25.

Hanna MH, Peat SJ, Woodham M, Knibb A. Fung C. Analgesic efficacy and CSF pharmacokinetics of intrathecal morphine-6-glucuronide: Comparison with morphine. Br J Anaesth 1990;64:547–50.

Harper MH, Winter PM, Johnson BH, Eger EI. Naloxone does not antagonize general anesthesia in the rat. Anesthesiology 1978;49:3–5.

Hecker BR, Lake CL, DiFazio CA, Moscicki JC, Engle JS. The decrease of the minimum alveolar anesthetic concentration produced by sufentanil in rats. Anesth Analg 1983;62:987–90.

Hilgenberg JC. Intraoperative awareness during high-dose fentanyl-oxygen anesthesia. Anesthesiology 1981;54:341–3.

Hoffman JC, DiFazio CA. The anesthesia-sparing effect of pentazocine, meperidine, and morphine. Arch Int Pharmacodyn 1970;186:261–8.

Hudson RJ, Bergstrom RG, Thomson IR, Sabourin MA, Rosenbloom M, Strunin L. Pharmacokinetics of sufentanil in patients undergoing abdominal aortic surgery. Anesthesiology 1989;70:426–31.

Hudson RJ, Thomson IR, Cannon JE, Friesen RM, Meatherall RC. Pharmacokinetics of fentanyl in patients undergoing abdominal aortic surgery. Anesthesiology 1986;64:334–8.

Hug CC, Murphy MR. Tissue redistribution of fentanyl and termination of its effects in rats. Anesthesiology 1981;55:369–75.

Hynyen MJ, Turunen MT, Korttila KT. Effects of alfentanil and fentanyl on common bile duct pressure. Anesth Analg 1986;65:370–2.

Jones RM, Detmer M, Hill AB, Bjoraker DG, Pandit U. Incidence of choledochoduodenal sphincter spasm during fentanyl-supplemented anesthesia. Anesth Analg 1981;60:638–40.

Jones RM, Fiddian-Green R, Knight PR. Narcotic-induced choledochoduodenal sphincter spasm reversed by glucagon. Anesth Analg 1980;59:946–7.

Kalia PK, Madan R, Saksema R, Batra RK, Gode GR. Epidural pentazocine for postoperative pain relief. Anesth Analg 1983;62:949–50.

Keykhah MM, Smith DS, Carlsson C, Safo Y, Engleback I, Harp JR. Influence of sufentanil on cerebral metabolism and circulation in the rat. Anesthesiology 1985;63:274–7.

Koska AJ, Kramer WG, Romagnoli A, Keats AS, Sabawala PB. Pharmacokinetics of high-dose meperidine in surgical patients. Anesth Analg 1981;60:8–11.

Kraynack BJ, Gintautas JG. Naloxone: Analeptic action unrelated to opiate receptor antagonism? Anesthesiology 1982;56:251–3.

Kripke BJ, Finck AJ, Shah N, Snow JC, Naloxone antagonism after narcotic supplemented-anesthesia. Anesth Analg 1976;55:800–5.

Lang DW, Pilon RN. Naloxone reversal of morphine-induced biliary colic. Anesth Analg 1980;59:619–20.

Lanz E, Simko G, Theiss D, Glocke MH. Epidural buprenorphine: A double-blind study of postoperative analgesia and side effects. Anesth Analg 1984;63:593–8.

Larson CP, Mazze RI, Cooperman LH, Wollman H. Effects of anesthetics on cerebral, renal, and splanchnic circulations: Recent developments. Anesthesiology 1974;41:169–81.

Lee G, DeMaria A, Amsterdam EA, et al. Comparative effects of morphine, meperidine and pentazocine on cardiocirculatory dynamics in patients with acute myocardial infarction. Am J Med 1976;60:949–55.

Levy JH, Rockoff MA. Anaphylaxis to meperidine. Anesth Analg 1982;61:301–3.

Longnecker DE, Grazis PA, Eggers GWN. Naloxone for antagonism of morphine induced respiratory depression. Anesth Analg 1973;52:447–53.

Lowenstein E, Whiting RB, Bittar DA, Sanders CA, Powell WJ. Locally and neurally mediated effects of morphine on skeletal muscle vascular resistance. J Pharmacol Exp Ther 1972;180:359–67.

Lynn AM, Slattery JT. Morphine pharmacokinetics in early infancy. Anesthesiology 1987;66:136–9.

Mayer N, Weinstabl C, Podreka I, Spiss CK. Sufentanil does not increase cerebral blood flow in healthy human volunteers. Anesthesiology 1990;73:240–3.

McCammon RL, Viegas OJ, Stoelting RK, Dryden GE. Naloxone reversal of choledochoduodenal sphincter spasm associated with narcotic administration. Anesthesiology 1978;48:437.

McClain DA, Hug CC. Intravenous fentanyl kinetics. Clin Pharmacol Ther 1980;22:106–14.

Meistelman C, Benhamou D, Barre J, et al. Effects of age on plasma protein binding of sufentanil. Anesthesiology 1990;72:470–3.

Meistelman C, Saint-Maurice C, Lepaul M, Levron J-C, Loose J-P, Gee KM. A comparison of alfentanil pharmacokinetics in children and adults. Anesthesiology 1987;66:13–6.

Meuldermans W, VanPeer A, Hendrickx J. Alfentanil pharmacokinetics and metabolism in humans. Anesthesiology 1988;69:527–534.

Michaelis LL, Hickey PR, Clark TA, Dixon WM. Ventricular irritability associated with the use of naloxone. Ann Thorac Surg 1974;18:608–14

Molbegott LP, Flaskburg MH, Karasic HL, Karlin BL. Probable seizures after sufentanil. Anesth Analg 1987;66:91–3.

Moldenhauer CC, Roach GW, Finlayson DC, et al. Nalbuphine antagonism of ventilatory depression following high-dose fentanyl anesthesia. Anesthesiology 1985;62:647–50.

Mondzac AM. Compassionate pain relief: Is heroin the answer? N Engl J Med 1984;311:530–5.

Morgan D, Moore G, Thomas J, Triggs E. Disposition of meperidine in pregnancy. Clin Pharmacol Ther 1978;23:288–95.

Murat I, Levron J-B, Berg A, Saint-Maurice C. Effects of fentanyl on baroreceptor reflex control of heart rate in newborn infants. Anesthesiology 1988;68:717–22.

Murkin JM, Moldenhauer CC, Hug CC, Epstein CM. Absence of seizures during induction of anesthesia with high dose fentanyl. Anesth Analg 1984;63:489–94.

Murphy MR, Hug CC. Pharmacokinetics of intravenous morphine in patients anesthetized with enflurane-nitrous oxide. Anesthesiology 1981;54:187–92.

Murphy MR, Hug CC. The anesthetic potency of fentanyl in terms of its reduction of enflurane MAC. Anesthesiology 1982a;57:485–8.

Murphy MR, Hug CC. The enflurane sparing effect of morphine, butorphanol, and nalbuphine. Anesthesiology 1982b;57:489–92.

Murphy MR, Hug CC, McClain DD. Dose-dependent pharmacokinetics of fentanyl. Anesthesiology 1983;59:537–40.

Murphy MR, Olson WA, Hug CC. Pharmacokinetics of ^{3}H-fentanyl in the dog anesthetized with enflurane. Anesthesiology 1979;50:13–9.

Pelligrino DA, Riegler FX, Albrecht RF. Ventilatory effects of fourth cerebroventricular infusions of morphine-6- or morphine-3-glucuronide in the awake dog. Anesthesiology 1989;71:936–40.

Philbin DM, Moss J, Akins CW, et al. The use of H_1 and H_2 histamine antagonists with morphine anesthesia: A double blind study. Anesthesiology 1981;55:292–6.

Philbin DM, Rosow CE, Schneider RC, Koski G. D'Ambra MND. Fentanyl and sufentanil anesthesia revisited: How much is enough? Anesthesiology 1990;73:5–11.

Philbin DM, Wilson NE, Sokoloshi I, Coggins C. Radioimmunoassay of antidiuretic hormone during morphine anesthesia. Can Anaesth Soc J 1976;23:290–5.

Pomeranz B, Chiu D. Naloxone blockade of acupuncture analgesia: Endorphin implicated. Life Sci 1976;19:1757–62.

Priano LL, Vatner SF. Generalized cardiovascular and regional hemodynamic effects of meperidine in conscious dogs. Anesth Analg 1981;60:649–54.

Radnay PA, Brodman E, Mankikar D, Duncalf D. The effect of equi-analgesic doses of fentanyl, morphine, meperidine, and pentazocine on common bile duct pressure. Anaesthetist 1980;29:26-9.

Rawal N, Schott U, Dahlstrom B, et al. Influence of naloxone infusion on analgesia and respiratory depression following epidural morphine. Anesthesiology 1986;64:194–201.

Roerig DL, Kotrly KJ, Vucins EJ, Ahlf SB, Dawson CA, Kampine JP. First pass uptake of fentanyl, meperidine, and morphine in the human lung. Anesthesiology 1987;67:466–72.

Rosow CE, Moss J, Philbin DM, Savarese JJ. Histamine release during morphine and fentanyl anesthesia. Anesthesiology 1982;56:93–6.

Rowbotham DJ, Wyld R, Peacock JE, Duthie DJR, Nimmo WS. Transdermal fentanyl for the relief of pain after upper abdominal surgery. Br J Anaesth 1989;63:56–9.

Rowlingson JC, Moscicki JC, DiFazio CA. Anesthetic potency of dezocine and its interaction with morphine in rats. Anesth Analg 1983; 62:899–902.

Safwat AM, Daniel D. Grand mal seizure after fentanyl administration. Anesthesiology 1983;59:78.

Sanford TJ, Smith NT, Dec-Silver H, Harrison WK. A comparison of morphine, fentanyl, and sufentanil anesthesia for cardiac surgery: Induction, emergence and extubation. Anesth Analg 1986;65:259–66.

Schubert A, Drummond JC, Peterson DO, Saidman LJ. The effect of high-dose fentanyl on human median nerve somatosensory-evoked responses. Can J Anaesth 1987;34:35–40.

Sebel PS, Bovill JG. Cardiovascular effects of sufentanil anesthesia. Anesth Analg 1982;61:115–9.

Smith NT, Benthuysen JL, Bickford RG, et al. Seizures during opioid anesthetic induction: Are they opioid-induced rigidity? Anesthesiology 1989;71:852–62.

Sonntag H, Stephen H, Lange H, Rieke H, Kettler D, Martschausky N. Sufentanil does not block sympathetic response to surgical stimuli in patients having coronary artery revascularization surgery. Anesth Analg 1989;68:584–92.

Sprigge JS, Wynands JE, Whalley DG, et al. Fentanyl infusion anesthesia for aortocoronary bypass surgery: Plasma levels and hemodynamic response. Anesth Analg 1982;61:972–8.

Stanley TH, Gray NH, Bidwai AV, Lordon R. The effects of high dose morphine and morphine plus nitrous oxide on urinary output in man. Can Anaesth Soc J 1974;21:379–84.

Stanley TH, Hague B, Mock DL, et al. Oral tansmucosal fentanyl citrate (lollipop) premedication in human volunteers. Anesth Analg 1989;69:21–7.

Stanski DR, Hug CC. Alfentanil: A kinetically predictable narcotic analgesic. Anesthesiology 1982; 57:435–8.

Stoeckel H, Hengstmann JH, Schuttler J. Pharmacokinetics of fentanyl as a possible explanation for recurrence of respiratory depression. Br J Anaesth 1979;51:741–5.

Stoelting RK, Gibbs PS. Hemodynamic effects of morphine and morphine-nitrous oxide in valvular heart disease and coronary artery disease. Anesthesiology 1973;38:45–52.

Strong WE, Matson M. Probable seizure after alfentanil. Anesth Analg 1989;68:692–3.

Tanaka GY. Hypertensive reaction to naloxone. JAMA 1974;228:25–6.

Tomicheck RC, Rosow CE, Philbin DM, Moss J, Teplick RS, Schneider RC. Diazepam-fentanyl interaction: Hemodynamic and hormonal effects in coronary artery surgery. Anesth Analg 1983;62:881–4.

Varvel JR, Shafer SL, Hwang SS, Coen PA, Stanski DR. Absorption characteristics of transdermally administered fentanyl. Anesthesiology 1989;70:928–34.

Vaught JL, Rothman RB, Westfall TC. Mu and delta receptors: Their role in analgesia and in the differential effects of opioid peptides on analgesia. Life Sci 1982;30:1443–55.

Waggum DC, Cork RC, Weldon ST, Gandolfi AJ, Perry DS. Postoperative respiratory depression and elevated sufentanil levels in a patient in chronic renal failure. Anesthesiology 1985;63:708–10.

Way WL, Costley EC, Way EL. Respiratory sensitivity of the newborn infant to meperidine and morphine. Clin Pharmacol Ther 1965;6:454–61.

Weldon ST, Perry DF, Cork RC, Gandolfi AJ. Detection of picogram levels of sufentanil by capillary gas chromatography. Anesthesiology 1985;63:684–7.

White PF. Patient-controlled analgesia: A new approach to the management of postoperative pain. Semin Anesth 1985;4:255–66.

Woolf CJ, Wall PD. Morphine sensitive and morphine insensitive actions of C-fibers input on the rat spinal cord. Neurosci Lett 1986;64:221–5.

Wynands JE, Wong P, Whalley DG, Sprigge JS, Townsend GE, Patel Y. Oxygen-fentanyl anesthesia in patients with poor left ventricular function: Hemodynamics and plasma fentanyl concentrations. Anesth Analg 1983;62:476–82.

Yaster M. The dose response of fentanyl in neonatal anesthesia. Anesthesiology 1987;66:433–5.

Zucker-Pinhoff B, Ramanathan S. Anaphylactic reaction to epidural fentanyl. Anesthesiology 1989; 71:599–601.

4

Barbiturates

INTRODUCTION

Classification of barbiturates as long, intermediate, short, and ultrashort acting is not recommended, as it falsely implies that the action of these drugs ends abruptly after specified time intervals. This is clearly not the case for barbiturates; residual plasma concentrations and drug effects persist for several hours, even following administration of "ultrashort-acting" drugs for induction of anesthesia.

COMMERCIAL PREPARATIONS

Barbiturates are prepared commercially as sodium salts that are readily soluble in water or saline to form highly alkaline solutions. For example, the pH of a 2.5% solution of thiopental is 10.5. These highly alkaline solutions are incompatible for mixture with drugs such as opioids, catecholamines, and neuromuscular blocking drugs, which are acidic in solution. The bacteriostatic properties of commercial solutions of barbiturates are due to their highly alkaline pH. Commercial preparations of barbiturates often contain a mixture of six parts anhydrous sodium carbonate to prevent precipitation of the insoluble free-acid form of the barbiturate by atmospheric carbon dioxide .

Thiopental and thiamylal are usually prepared for clinical use in 2.5% solutions. A 5% solution is not recommended. Methohexital is used most often as a 1% solution. Solutions of barbiturates remain stable at room temperature for up to 2 weeks.

STRUCTURE ACTIVITY RELATIONSHIPS

Barbiturates are defined as any drug derived from barbituric acid. Barbituric acid, which lacks central nervous system activity, is a cyclic compound obtained by the combination of urea and malonic acid (Fig. 4-1). Barbiturates with sedative-hypnotic properties result from substitutions at the number 2 and 5 carbon atoms of barbituric acid (Fig. 4-2). A barbiturate with a branched-chain substitution on the number 5 carbon atom usually has greater hypnotic activity than the corresponding drug with a straight chain. Drugs with a phenyl group in the number 5 carbon position, such as phenobarbital, have enhanced anticonvulsant activity. Sedative and anticonvulsant activities are separate effects of barbiturates. A methyl radical on the number 5 carbon atom, as is present with methohexital, confers convulsive activity manifesting as involuntary skeletal muscle movement.

Barbiturates that retain an oxygen atom on the number 5 carbon of the barbituric acid ring are designated *oxybarbiturates*. Replacement of this oxygen atom with a sulfur atom results in *thiobarbiturates*, which are more lipid soluble than oxybarbiturates. In general, a structural change such as sulfuration that increases lipid solubility is associated with greater hypnotic potency and a more rapid onset but shorter duration of action. For example, thiopental has a more rapid onset and a shorter duration of action than its oxybarbiturate analogue, pentobarbital. Thiamylal is the thioanalogue of the oxybarbiturate, secobarbital. Addition of a methyl group to the nitrogen atom of the barbituric acid ring, as with

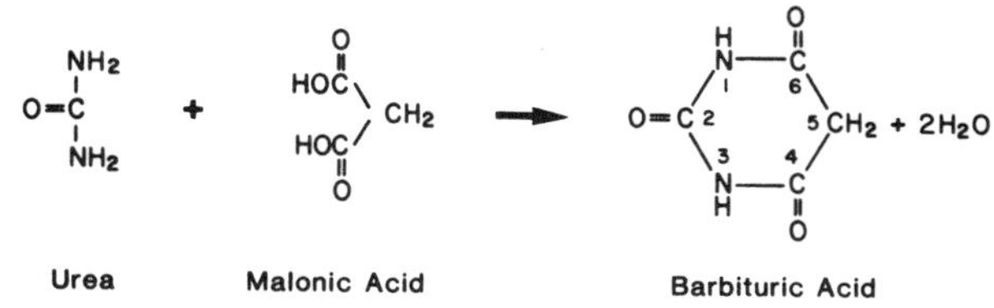

FIGURE 4–1. Barbituric acid is formed by the combination of urea and malonic acid.

Urea   Malonic Acid   Barbituric Acid

methohexital, results in a compound with a short duration of action.

MECHANISM OF ACTION

Barbiturates seem to be uniquely capable of depressing the reticular activating system, which is presumed to be important in the maintenance of wakefulness. This response may reflect the ability of barbiturates to decrease the rate of dissociation of the inhibitory neurotransmitter gamma-aminobutyric acid from its receptors. Gamma-aminobutyric acid causes an increase in chloride conductance through ion channels, resulting in hyperpolarization and, consequently, inhibition of postsynaptic neurons.

Barbiturates selectively depress transmission in sympathetic nervous system ganglia in concentrations that have no detectable effect on nerve conduction. This effect may contribute to decreases in blood pressure that can accompany intravenous injections of barbiturates or that occur in association with a barbiturate overdose. At the neuromuscular junction, high doses of barbiturates reduce sensitivity of postsynaptic membranes to the depolarizing actions of acetylcholine.

PHARMACOKINETICS

Prompt awakening following intravenous administration of thiopental, thiamylal, and methohexital reflects redistribution of these drugs from the brain to inactive tissues (Fig. 4-3) (Saidman, 1974). Ultimately, however, elimination from the body depends almost entirely on metabolism, because less than 1% of these drugs are recovered unchanged in the urine (Saidman and Eger, 1966).

Protein Binding

Protein binding of barbiturates parallels lipid solubility. The lipid solubility of a barbiturate is de-

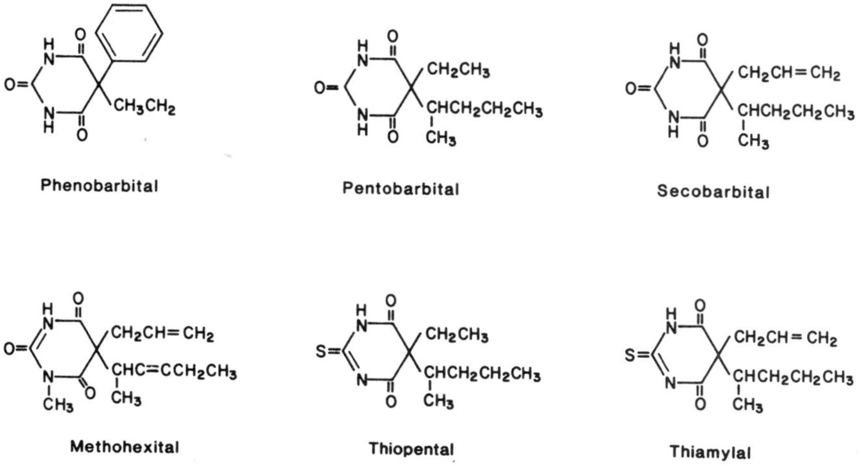

Phenobarbital   Pentobarbital   Secobarbital

Methohexital   Thiopental   Thiamylal

FIGURE 4–2. Barbiturates with sedative-hypnotic properties result from substitutions at the number 2 and 5 carbon atoms of barbituric acid (see Fig. 4–1).

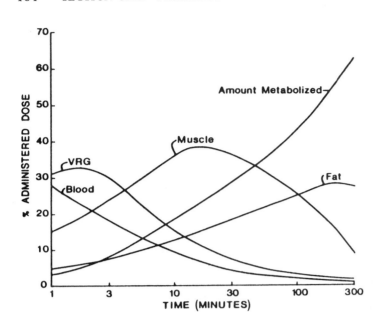

FIGURE 4–3.   Following an intravenous bolus, the percentage of thiopental remaining in blood rapidly decreases as drug moves from blood to tissues. Time to achievement of peak tissue levels is a direct function of tissue capacity for barbiturate relative to blood flow. Initially, most thiopental is taken up by the vessel-rich–group (*VRG*) tissues because of their high blood flow. Subsequently, drug is redistributed to skeletal muscles and, to a lesser extent, to fat. The rate of metabolism equals the early rate of removal by fat, and the sum of these two events is similar to uptake of drug by skeletal muscles. (From Saidman LJ. Uptake, distribution, and elimination of barbiturates. In: Eger EL, ed. Anesthetic Uptake and Action. Baltimore, Williams and Wilkins, 1974; with permission.)

termined almost entirely by the solubility of the nonionized molecule; the ionized molecule is poorly soluble in lipid. Thiobarbiturates are bound to a greater extent than their oxybarbiturate analogues. This difference probably relates to the effect of the sulfur substitution on the affinity for a hydrophobic portion of the protein.

Thiopental, as a highly lipid-soluble barbiturate, is the most avidly bound to plasma proteins, with binding to albumin ranging from 72% to 86% (Ghoneim et al, 1976). The higher percentage of protein binding occurs at lower plasma concentrations of thiopental. Changes in pH between 7.35 to 7.5 do not alter the degree of protein binding. Decreased protein binding of thiopental owing to displacement from binding sites by other drugs, such as aspirin and phenylbutazone, can lead to enhanced drug effects. Decreased protein binding of thiopental may explain, in part, increased drug sensitivity demonstrated by patients with uremia or cirrhosis of the liver (Ghoneim and Pandya, 1975). Decreased protein binding in patients with uremia may be partially due to competitive binding inhibitors such as nitrogenous waste products. Hypoalbuminemia may account for decreased protein binding of barbiturates in patients with cirrhosis of the liver. Protein binding of thiopental in neonatal plasma (placental blood) is about half that measured in adults, suggesting a possible increased sensitivity to thiopental in neonates (Kingston et al, 1990). This unbound fraction of thiopental could be increased further by fetal acidosis that may accompany a stressful delivery.

Distribution

Distribution of barbiturates in the body is determined by their lipid solubility, protein binding, and degree of ionization. Of the factors that influence distribution of thiopental, thiamylal, and methohexital, lipid solubility is most important. Tissue blood flow is a major determinant in delivery of barbiturates to tissues and their ultimate distribution in the body. Alterations in blood volume or distribution of blood flow to tissues may alter the distribution of thiopental or similar drugs. For example, hypovolemia may decrease blood flow to skeletal muscles, whereas blood flow to the brain and heart are maintained. Thiopental plasma concentrations are increased because of less dilution, resulting in the potential for exaggerated cerebral and cardiac depression in the presence of hypovolemia.

Brain

Thiopental, thiamylal, and methohexital undergo maximal brain uptake within 30 seconds, accounting for the rapid onset of central nervous system depression (Fig. 4-3) (Saidman, 1974). The brain receives about 10% of the total dose in the first 30 to 40 seconds. This maximal brain concentration is followed by a decrease over the next 5 minutes to one half the initial peak concentration, owing to redistribution of drug from the brain to other tissues. Indeed, redistribution is the principal mechanism, accounting for early awakening following a single dose of these drugs. After about 30 minutes, the barbiturate has been further redistributed and as little as 10% remains in the brain. Redistribution occurs promptly because initial high uptake of lipid-soluble drug into the brain and other highly perfused tissues causes the plasma concentration of barbiturate to decrease, resulting in reversal of the concentration gradient for the movement of drug between blood and tissues.

Skeletal Muscles

Skeletal muscles are the most prominent sites for initial distribution of highly lipid-soluble barbiturates, such as thiopental (Fig. 4-3) (Saidman, 1974). Indeed, the initial decrease in the plasma concentration of thiopental is principally due to uptake of drug into skeletal muscles, with only a modest contribution from metabolism. Equilibrium with skeletal muscles is reached in about 15 minutes following intravenous injection of thiopental.

Fat

Fat is the only compartment in which thiopental content continues to increase 30 minutes after injection (Fig. 4-3) (Saidman, 1974). With a fat:blood partition coefficient of about 11, thiopental will move from blood to fat as long as the concentration in fat is less than 11 times that in blood. Despite this affinity for fat, the initial uptake of drug into adipose tissue is slow, emphasizing the role of low fat blood flow in limiting delivery of barbiturate to this tissue. Indeed, redistribution of drug to fat will not significantly affect early awakening from a single intravenous dose of barbiturate. Maximal deposition of thiopental in fat is present after about 2.5 hours, and this tissue becomes a potential reservoir for maintaining plasma concentrations of the drug. For example, large or repeated doses of lipid-soluble barbiturates produce a cumulative drug effect because of the storage capacity of fat. When this occurs, the usual rapid awakening, characteristic of

these drugs, is absent. For this reason, the dose of thiopental is best calculated according to lean body mass so as to avoid overdose.

Ionization

The distribution of thiopental from blood to tissues will be influenced by the state of ionization of the drug and its binding to plasma proteins. Since the pK of thiopental (7.6) is near blood pH, acidosis will favor the nonionized fraction of drug, whereas alkalosis has the opposite effect. The nonionized form of drug has greater access to the central nervous system because of its greater lipid solubility. Acidosis will thus increase and alkalosis will decrease the intensity of barbiturate effects. Evidence of increased brain penetration of barbiturate is the decrease in plasma concentration of thiopental associated with an acute reduction in blood pH (Brodie et al, 1950).

Metabolic-induced alterations in pH produce more pronounced effects on drug distribution than do respiratory alterations. For example, in the presence of metabolic changes, the intracellular pH in the brain may remain relatively unchanged, reflecting the inability of hydrogen ions to cross lipid barriers easily. As a result, movement of drug across the blood-brain barrier is favored. In contrast, respiratory-induced changes in pH are associated with rapid diffusion of carbon dioxide and similar changes in intracellular and extracellular pH, resulting in less net movement of drug.

Metabolism

Oxybarbiturates are metabolized only in hepatocytes, whereas thiobarbiturates also break down to a small extent in extrahepatic sites such as the kidneys and possibly the central nervous system. Metabolites are usually inactive and are always more water soluble than the parent compound, thus facilitating renal excretion. Side chain oxidation at the number 5 carbon atom of the benzene ring to yield carboxylic acid is the most important initial step in terminating pharmacologic activity of barbiturates by metabolism. This oxidation occurs primarily in the endoplasmic reticulum of hepatocytes. The reserve capacity of the liver to carry out oxidation of barbiturates is great, and hepatic dysfunction must be extreme before a prolonged duration of action of barbiturates owing to reduced metabolism occurs.

Thiopental

Metabolism of thiopental, along with redistribution to inactive tissue sites, is an important determinant of early awakening. Data based on measurements obtained several hours after injection of thiopental suggest that metabolism of thiopental occurs at a slow rate, with 10% to 24% being metabolized by the liver each hour (Mark et al, 1965). These data do not reflect the magnitude of metabolism early after drug administration and thus underestimate the role of metabolism of thiopental in prompt awakening following a single intravenous injection of the drug (Fig. 4-3) (Saidman, 1974). For example, after several hours, most of the thiopental body stores are in fat and the fraction of drug delivered to the liver is far less than in the first few minutes following injection. Ultimately, metabolism of thiopental is almost complete (99%), with the principal sites of metabolism being oxidation of substituents on the number 5 carbon atom, desulfuration on the number 2 carbon atom, and hydrolytic opening of the barbituric acid ring.

Hepatic clearance of thiopental is characterized by a low hepatic extraction ratio and a capacity-dependent elimination influenced by hepatic enzyme activity but not hepatic blood flow. Nevertheless, enzyme induction or inhibition does not modify the duration of action of thiopental observed in animals. In patients with cirrhosis of the liver, clearance of thiopental from the plasma is not different from that in normal patients (Pandele et al, 1983). Therefore, it is unlikely that a prolonged effect of a single dose of thiopental will occur in patients with cirrhosis of the liver. Conversely, enzyme induction from chronic exposure to environmental pollution is presumed to be the explanation for increased thiopental dose requirements in patients from urban compared with rural areas.

Methohexital

Methohexital is metabolized to a greater extent than thiopental, reflecting its lesser lipid solubility; thus, more methohexital remains in the plasma to become available to the liver for metabolism (Whitwam, 1976). Side chain oxidation of methohexital results in the formation of an inactive metabolite, hydroxymethohexital. Overall, the hepatic clearance of methohexital is three to four times that of thiopental. Despite this greater

hepatic clearance, early awakening from a single dose of methohexital depends primarily on its redistribution to inactive tissue sites (Hudson et al, 1983). Nevertheless, metabolism will exert a greater role in terminating the effect of methohexital than for thiopental. For example, metabolism may be an important determinant of the time required for complete psychomotor recovery. Indeed, many psychomotor functions recover more quickly after administration of methohexital compared with thiopental (Korttila et al, 1975). Recovery from methohexital is predictably more rapid than that from thiopental when repeated doses of drug are administered, reflecting the greater role of metabolism in the clearance of methohexital from the plasma. The hepatic clearance of methohexital is more dependent on changes in cardiac output and hepatic blood flow than is the hepatic clearance of thiopental.

Renal Excretion

All barbiturates are filtered by the renal glomeruli, but the high degree of protein binding limits the magnitude of filtration, whereas high lipid solubility favors reabsorption of any filtered drug back into the circulation. Indeed, less than 1% of administered thiopental, thiamylal, or methohexital is recovered unchanged in the urine. Among the barbiturates, phenobarbital is the only one that undergoes significant renal excretion in the unchanged form, reflecting the lesser protein binding and lipid solubility of this barbiturate compared with that of thiopental. Renal excretion of phenobarbital can be significantly increased by osmotic diuresis. Alkalinization of the urine also hastens renal excretion of phenobarbital because of the shift toward the ionized state caused by this pH change.

Elimination Half-Time

Distribution half-time and volume of distribution (Vd) of thiopental and methohexital are similar (Table 4-1) (Hudson et al, 1983). Conversely, elimination half-time and clearance of these two drugs differ (Table 4-1; Fig. 4-4) (Hudson et al, 1983). The shorter elimination half-time of methohexital compared with that of thiopental

Table 4–1
Comparative Pharmacokinetics

	Thiopental	*Methohexital*
Rapid distribution half-time (min)	8.5	5.6
Slow distribution half-time (min)	62.7	58.3
Elimination half-time (h)	11.6	3.9*
Clearance (ml·kg⁻¹·min⁻¹)	3.4	10.9*
Volume of distribution (L·kg⁻¹)	2.5	2.2

*Significantly different from thiopental.
(Data from Hudson RJ, Stanski DR, Burch PG. Pharmacokinetics of methohexital and thiopental in surgical patients. Anesthesiology 1983; 59: 215–9.)

results entirely from the greater hepatic clearance of methohexital.

The elimination half-time of thiopental is prolonged in obese patients compared with non-obese patients, reflecting an increased Vd resulting from excess fat stores (Jung et al, 1982). Increasing age is associated with a slower passage of thiopental from the central compartment to peripheral compartments (approximately 30% slower in 80-year-old patients compared with young adults), whereas the initial Vd is unchanged (Fig. 4-5) (Avram et al, 1990; Stanski and Maitre, 1990). This slower rate of intercompartmental clearance results in higher plasma concentrations of thiopental for distribution into the brain to create a greater anesthetic effect in the elderly. Evidence that pharmacokinetics (intercompartmental clearance) is responsible for the decreased thiopental dose requirements in elderly patients is the similar plasma concentration of thiopental in all adult-age patients required to suppress the electroencephalogram (EEG) to a similar degree (Fig. 4-6) (Avram et al, 1990; Homer and Stanski, 1985; Stanski and Maitre, 1990).

In pediatric patients, the elimination half-time of thiopental is shorter than in adults (Sorbo et al, 1984). This shorter elimination half-time is due to more rapid hepatic clearance of thiopental by pediatric patients. Therefore, recovery after large or repeated doses of thiopental may be more rapid for infants and children than for adults. Protein binding and Vd of thiopental are

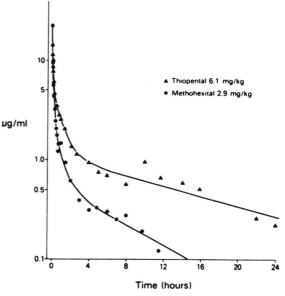

FIGURE 4–4. The rate of decline of the plasma concentration and thus the elimination half-time is shorter following the intravenous administration of methohexital than following thiopental. (From Hudson RJ, Stanski DR, Bureh PG. Pharmacokinetics of methohexital and thiopental in surgical patients. Anesthesiology 1983; 59: 215–9; with permission.)

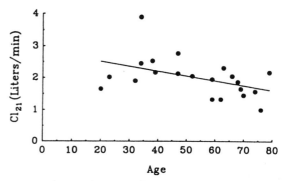

FIGURE 4–5. The rate of intercompartmental clearance of thiopental from the central compartment to the peripheral compartment (V₂) slows with increasing age. (From Avram MJ, Krejcie TC, Henthorn TK. The relationship of age to the pharmacokinetics of early drug distribution: The concurrent disposition of thiopental and indocyanine green. Anesthesiology 1990; 72: 403–11; with permission.)

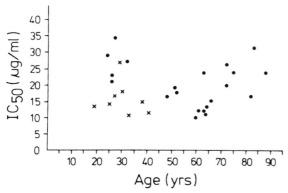

FIGURE 4–6. The plasma concentration of thiopental needed to slow activity on the electroencephalogram 50% (IC_{50}) is independent of age. Blood sampling was either arterial (X) or venous (O). (From Homer TD, Stanski DR. The effect of increasing age on thiopental disposition and anesthetic requirement. Anesthesiology 1985; 62: 714–24; with permission.)

not different in pediatric and adult patients. Elimination half-time is prolonged during pregnancy because of increased protein binding of thiopental.

CLINICAL USES

The principal clinical uses of barbiturates are (1) induction of anesthesia and (2) treatment of elevated intracranial pressure. Use of phenobarbital to treat hyperbilirubinemia and kernicterus reflects barbiturate-induced increases in hepatic glucuronyl transferase enzyme activity. Other clinical uses of barbiturates are declining because these drugs (1) lack specificity of effect in the central nervous system, (2) have a lower therapeutic index than do benzodiazepines, (3) result in tolerance more often than do benzodiazepines, (4) have greater liability for abuse, and (5) have a high risk for drug interactions. Other undesirable features of barbiturates include paradoxical excitement instead of sedation, especially in elderly patients or in the presence of pain. Barbiturate-induced paradoxical excitement suggests depression of central nervous system inhibitory centers as the mechanism. Small doses of barbiturates seem to lower the pain threshold, accounting for the perception that these drugs are antianalgesic. Therefore, bar-

biturates cannot be relied on to produce sedation in the presence of pain. Skeletal muscle relaxation does not occur, and there is no clinically significant effect of barbiturates on the neuromuscular junction. Drowsiness may last for only a short time after a sedative-hypnotic dose of a barbiturate administered orally, but residual central nervous system effects characterized as "hangover" may persist for several hours. Barbiturates have been replaced by benzodiazepines for preanesthetic medication. The rapid onset of action of barbiturates renders these drugs useful for treatment of grand mal seizures, but, again, benzodiazepines are probably superior, providing a more specific site of action in the central nervous system.

Induction of Anesthesia

The supremacy of the barbiturates for intravenous induction of anesthesia has remained virtually unchallenged since the introduction of thiopental by Lundy in 1934. Thiamylal is indistinguishable from thiopental as used for intravenous induction of anesthesia. The oxybarbiturate methohexital is the only barbiturate with actions sufficiently different to offer an alternative to thiopental for intravenous induction of anesthesia. The most important advantage of methohexital compared with thiopental is a more rapid recovery of consciousness, making it useful for outpatient procedures. The principal disadvantage of methohexital is the increased incidence of excitatory phenomena, such as involuntary skeletal muscle movements, including hiccough. The incidence of these excitatory phenomena is dose dependent and may be decreased by inclusion of opioids in the preoperative medication and by use of optimum doses of methohexital (1 to 1.5 mg·kg^{-1}). Indeed, high doses of methohexital, as administered in a continuous intravenous infusion for neuroanesthesia, are associated with postoperative seizures in about one third of patients (Todd et al, 1984).

The relative potency of barbiturates used for intravenous induction of anesthesia, assuming that thiopental is 1, is thiamylal, 1.1, and methohexital is 2.5. At a blood pH of 7.4, methohexital is 76% nonionized compared with 61% for thiopental, which is consistent with the greater potency of methohexital. The central nervous system is exquisitely sensitive to intravenous doses of these barbiturates that produce minimal to no effect on skeletal, cardiac, or smooth muscle. For example, thiopental, 3 to 5 mg·kg⁻¹ IV, rapidly enters the central nervous system and produces unconsciousness within 30 seconds. The dose of thiopental required to induce anesthesia decreases with age, reflecting a slower passage of the barbiturate from the central compartment to peripheral compartments (Fig. 4–5) (Avram et al, 1990; Stanski and Maitre, 1990). Thiopental requirements, for unknown reasons, seem to be increased in children more than 1 year after thermal injury (Cote and Petkau, 1985). Despite a contrary clinical impression, thiopental dose requirements (EEG suppression as the end point) are not different between nonalcoholics and alcoholics with abstinence of 9 to 17 days and 30 days (Fig. 4-7) (Swerdlow et al, 1990).

Rectal administration of barbiturates, especially methohexital, 20 to 30 mg·kg⁻¹, has been used to induce anesthesia in uncooperative or young patients. Loss of consciousness after rectal administration of methohexital correlates with a plasma concentration greater than 2 µg·ml⁻¹ (Liu et al, 1985).

Occasionally, intravenous administration of a barbiturate is used as a supplement to inhaled anesthetics or as the sole anesthetic for brief and usually pain-free procedures such as cardioversion or electroshock therapy. Methohexital, but not thiopental, is effective in inducing seizure activity in patients with psychomotor epilepsy undergoing cortical resection of seizure-producing areas (Ford et al, 1982; Rockoff and Goudsouzian, 1981).

Treatment of Elevated Intracranial Pressure

Barbiturates are administered to decrease intracranial pressure, which remains elevated despite deliberate hyperventilation of the lungs and drug-induced diuresis (Shapiro et al, 1973). Barbiturates decrease intracranial pressure by decreasing cerebral blood volume through drug-induced cerebral vascular vasoconstriction and an associated decrease in cerebral blood flow. The reduction in cerebral blood flow and associated increase in the perfusion-to-metabolism ratio render thiopental an attractive drug for induction of anesthesia in patients with increased intracranial pressure (Fig. 4-8) (Bedford et al, 1980). An isoelectric EEG confirms the presence of maximal barbiturate-induced depression of cerebral metabolic oxygen requirements. Improved outcome following head trauma has not, however, been demonstrated in patients treated with barbiturates despite the ability of these drugs to decrease and control intracranial pressure (Ward et al, 1985).

A hazard of high-dose barbiturate therapy as used to lower intracranial pressure is hypotension, which can jeopardize the maintenance of an adequate cerebral perfusion pressure. Doses of

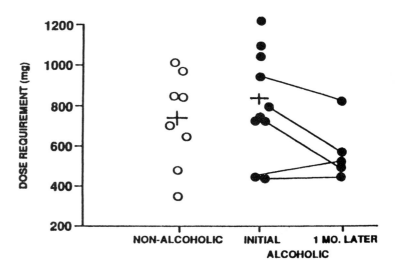

FIGURE 4–7. Thiopental doses needed to achieve burst suppression with 3 seconds of isoelectric electroencephalogram are similar in nonalcoholics and alcoholic patients with abstinence of 9–17 days (initial) and 30 days (1 month later). (From Swerdlow BN, Holley FO, Maitre PO, Stanski DR. Chronic alcohol intake does not change thiopental anesthetic requirements, pharmacokinetics, or pharmacodynamics. Anesthesiology 1990; 72: 455–61, with permission.)

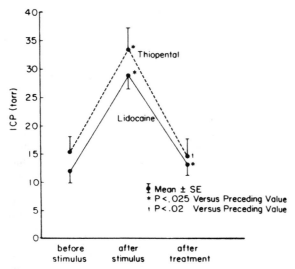

FIGURE 4-8. The administration of thiopental, 3 mg·kg^{-1} IV, is as effective as lidocaine, 1.5 mg·kg^{-1} IV, in lowering intracranial pressure (*ICP*) following surgical stimulation in patients with brain tumors. (From Bedford RF, Persing JA, Pobereskin L, Butler A. Lidocaine or thiopental for rapid control of intracranial hypertension. Anesth Analg 1980; 59: 435–7; with permission.)

thiopental sufficient to suppress EEG activity in animals are more likely than pentobarbital to lead to hypotension and ventricular fibrillation (Roesch et al, 1983). In patients, doses of thiopental (37.5 mg·kg^{-1}) and methohexital sufficient to produce an isoelectric EEG result in peripheral vasodilation and myocardial depression (Todd et al, 1984; Todd et al, 1985). Nevertheless, these cardiovascular effects are smaller in magnitude than those produced by the dose of isoflurane (2 MAC) required to produce an equivalent degree of depression of the EEG. This suggests that barbiturates may be hemodynamically preferable to isoflurane if profound EEG depression is desired.

Cerebral Protection

The ability of barbiturate therapy to improve brain survival following global cerebral ischemia owing to cardiac arrest is unlikely, since these drugs are effective only when the EEG remains active and metabolic suppression is possible (Michenfelder, 1986). During cardiac arrest, the EEG becomes flat in 20 to 30 seconds, and barbiturates would not be expected to improve outcome. Indeed, administration of thiopental, 30 mg·kg^{-1} IV, as a single injection to comatose survivors of cardiac arrest does not increase survival or improve neurologic outcome (Brain Resuscitation Clinical Trial Study Group, 1986).

In contrast to global cerebral ischemia, animal studies consistently show improved outcome with barbiturate therapy of incomplete (focal) cerebral ischemia that permits drug-induced metabolic suppression (Todd et al, 1982). In this regard, barbiturate-induced decreases in cerebral metabolic oxygen requirements exceed decreases in cerebral blood flow, which may provide protection to poorly perfused areas of the brain. Consistent with these animal data showing protection against focal ischemic effects is the observation that neuropsychiatric complications, following cardiopulmonary bypass and presumably due to embolism, clear more rapidly in patients treated prospectively with thiopental (average dose 39.5 mg·kg^{-1}) to maintain an isoelectric EEG (Nussmeier et al, 1986). This beneficial effect is accompanied by an increased need for inotropic support at the conclusion of cardiopulmonary bypass and a delayed awakening. Other patients at risk for incomplete cerebral ischemia who might benefit from prior production of an isoelectric EEG (metabolic suppression) with barbiturates include those scheduled for carotid endarterectomy or thoracic aneurysm resection, and those treated with profound controlled hypotension.

SIDE EFFECTS

Barbiturates are administered almost exclusively to produce depressant effects on the central nervous system. Side effects, especially on the cardiovascular system, inevitably accompany the clinical use of barbiturates.

Cardiovascular System

Oral sedative doses of barbiturates do not produce cardiovascular effects different from the slight decrease in blood pressure and heart rate that accompany physiologic sleep. Hemodynamic effects of equivalent doses of methohexital, thiamylal, and thiopental as administered for the intravenous induction of anesthesia are similar (Todd et al, 1984). In normovolemic subjects, thiopental, 5 mg·kg^{-1} IV, produces a transient 10- to 20-mmHg decrease in blood pressure that is offset by a compensatory 15- to 20-beat·min^{-1} increase in heart rate (Fig. 4-9) (Filner and Karliner, 1976). This dose of thiopental produces minimal to no evidence of myocardial depression. When reductions in myocardial contractility are demonstrated after induction of anesthesia with barbiturates, the magnitude of this decrease is far less than that produced by volatile anesthetics (Becker and Tonnesen, 1978; Kaplan et al, 1976). Cardiac dysrhythmias following induction of anesthesia with barbiturates are unlikely in the presence of adequate ventilation and oxygenation.

The most likely explanation for compensatory tachycardia and unchanged myocardial contractility associated with intravenous administration of thiopental is a carotid sinus baroreceptor–mediated increase in peripheral sympathetic nervous system activity. In the absence of compensatory increases in sympathetic nervous system activity, as in isolated heart preparations, a negative inotropic effect of barbiturates is readily demonstrated. Direct myocardial depression may also accompany overdoses of barbiturates or the large doses of barbiturates administered to lower intracranial pressure.

The mild and transient decrease in blood pressure that accompanies induction of anesthesia with barbiturates is principally due to peripheral vasodilatation, reflecting depression of the medullary vasomotor center and decreased sympathetic nervous system outflow from the central nervous system. The resulting dilatation of peripheral capacitance vessels leads to pooling of

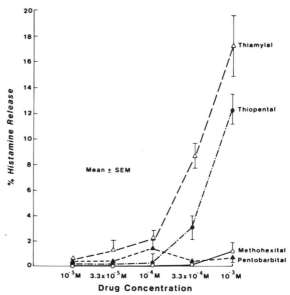

FIGURE 4-10. Thiamylal and thiopental produce dose-dependent release of histamine from human skin mast cell preparations, whereas methohexital and pentobarbital are devoid of this effect. (From Hirshman CA, Edelstein RA, Ebertz JM, Hanifin JM. Thiobarbiturate-induced histamine release in human skin mast cells. Anesthesiology 1985; 63: 353–6; with permission.)

blood, decreased venous return, and the potential for decreases in cardiac output and blood pressure (Yamamura et al, 1983). Histamine release can occur in response to rapid intravenous administration of barbiturates, but this is rarely of clinical significance. In an *in vitro* model, thiopental and thiamylal, but not methohexital, evoke histamine release (Fig. 4-10) (Hirshman et al, 1985).

Vasodilatation of cutaneous and skeletal muscle blood vessels may also contribute to heat loss and reductions in body temperature. The fact that blood pressure and cardiac output are minimally altered by the intravenous induction of anesthesia with barbiturates reflects the ability of carotid sinus–mediated baroreceptor reflex responses to offset the effects of peripheral vasodilatation. In the absence of compensatory baroreceptor-mediated increases in peripheral sympathetic nervous system activity, peripheral pooling of blood can result in sustained decreases in venous return, cardiac output, and blood pressure. Indeed, hypovolemic patients, who are less able

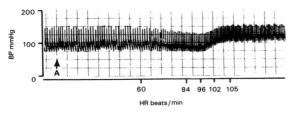

FIGURE 4-9. In normovolemic patients, the rapid administration of thiopental, 5 mg·kg^{-1} IV (*A*), is followed by a modest decrease in blood pressure, which is subsequently offset by a compensatory increase in heart rate (*HR*). (From Filner BF, Karliner JS. Alterations of normal left ventricular performance by general anesthesia. Anesthesiology 1976; 45: 610–20; with permission.)

to compensate for peripheral-vasodilating effects of barbiturates, are highly vulnerable to marked reductions in blood pressure when these drugs are administered rapidly for the intravenous induction of anesthesia. Treatment with beta-adrenergic antagonists or centrally acting antihypertensive drugs could theoretically accentuate blood pressure decreases evoked by barbiturates by impairing the activity of compensatory baroreceptor responses.

Conceptually, the slow intravenous administration of thiopental should be more likely to permit compensatory reflex responses and thus minimize blood pressure reductions compared with rapid intravenous injection. This would be most important in the presence of hypovolemia. Nevertheless, rapid or slow intravenous administration of thiopental to normovolemic patients produces similar decreases in blood pressure and increases in heart rate (Table 4-2) (Seltzer et al, 1980). Furthermore, the dose administered slowly in 50-mg increments to achieve a predetermined endpoint was more than the single dose administered intravenously (Table 4-2) (Seltzer et al, 1980).

Ventilation

Barbiturates, as administered intravenously for the induction of anesthesia, produce dose-dependent depression of medullary and pontine ventilatory centers. For example, thiopental decreases the sensitivity of the medullary ventilatory center to stimulation by carbon dioxide. Apnea is especially likely in the presence of other depressant drugs as used for preoperative medication. Resumption of spontaneous ventilation following a single intravenous induction dose of barbiturate is characterized by a slow frequency of breathing and a decreased tidal volume. Laryngeal reflexes and the cough reflex are not depressed until large doses of barbiturates have been administered. Stimulation of the upper airway as by laryngoscopy, intubation of the trachea, or secretions in the presence of inadequate depression of laryngeal reflexes by barbiturates may result in laryngospasm or bronchospasm. Increased irritability of the larynx because of a parasympathomimetic action of thiopental is an unlikely explanation for laryngospasm or bronchospasm. Indeed, thiopental is not likely to selectively alter parasympathetic nervous system

Table 4–2
Incremental versus Rapid Injection of Thiopental

	Incremental (50 mg every 15 seconds until loss of lash reflex)	Rapid
Total dose (mg·kg⁻¹)	5.58	4
Systolic blood pressure decrease (mmHg)	14	16
Diastolic blood pressure decrease (mmHg)	6	9
Heart rate increase (beats·min⁻¹)	12	16
Measure of myocardial contractility	17.5	22.5

(Data from Seltzer JL, Gerson JI, Allen FB. Comparison of the cardiovascular effects of bolus vs. incremental administration of thiopentone. Br J Anaesth 1980; 52: 527–9.)

activity, although depression of sympathetic nervous system outflow from the central nervous system could theoretically result in a predominance of vagal tone.

Electroencephalogram

Small intravenous doses of barbiturates increase low-voltage, fast-wave activity (1 to 5 cycles·sec⁻¹) on the EEG. This activation of the EEG is accompanied by clouding of consciousness. As the dose of barbiturate is increased, high-voltage, slow-wave activity (less than 4 cycles·sec⁻¹) similar to physiologic sleep appears on the EEG and consciousness is lost, although arousal may accompany strong painful stimulation. A further increase in the dose of barbiturate causes the frequency of activity on the EEG to decrease to 1 to 3 cycles·sec⁻¹, followed by electrical silence on the EEG if the plasma concentration of barbiturate continues to increase. A continuous intravenous infusion of thiopental, 4 mg·kg⁻¹, produces an isoelectric EEG that is consistent with near-maximal reductions in cerebral metabolic oxygen requirements (Turcant et al, 1985). Alternatively, pentobarbital administered as a continuous infusion to maintain the plasma concentration between 3 and 6 mg·dl⁻¹ is also associated with an isoelectric EEG (Rockoff et al, 1979). Barbiturate-induced depression of cerebral metabolic oxygen requirements when the EEG is isoelectric is about 50%, reflecting a decrease in neuronal, but not metabolic, needs for oxygen. Hypothermia is the only reliable method for decreasing the basal cellular requirements for oxygen.

Somatosensory Evoked Responses

Thiopental produces dose-dependent changes in median nerve somatosensory evoked responses and brain stem auditory evoked responses. Nevertheless, even doses of thiopental sufficient to produce an isoelectric EEG fail to render any component of these responses unobtainable (Drummond et al, 1985). Therefore, thiopental is an acceptable drug to administer when the ability to monitor somatosensory evoked potentials is desirable.

Liver

Thiopental, in the absence of other drugs, produces only modest decreases in hepatic blood flow. Induction doses of thiopental do not alter postoperative liver function tests. Continuous intravenous infusion of methohexital for up to 4 hours does not produce laboratory evidence of hepatocellular damage (Prys-Roberts et al, 1983). In the hypoxic rat model, thiopental has a detectable but minimal potential to produce hepatocellular damage (Shingu et al, 1983).

Enzyme Induction

Barbiturates stimulate an increase in liver microsomal protein content (enzyme induction) after 2 to 7 days of sustained drug administration. Phenobarbital is the most potent of the barbiturates for producing enzyme induction, leading to a 20% to 40% increase in the protein content of hepatic microsomal enzymes. At maximal induction of enzyme activity, rates of metabolism are approximately doubled. After discontinuation of a barbiturate, enzyme induction may persist for up to 30 days.

Altered drug responses and drug interactions may reflect barbiturate-induced enzyme induction, resulting in accelerated metabolism of (1) other drugs, such as oral anticoagulants, phenytoin, and tricyclic antidepressants; or (2) endogenous substances, including corticosteroids, bile salts, and vitamin K. Indeed, glucuronyl transferase activity is increased by barbiturates. Barbiturates also stimulate the activity of a mitochondrial enzyme (in contrast to a microsomal enzyme) known as d-aminolevulinic acid synthetase. As a result, the production of heme is accelerated, and acute intermittent porphyria may be exacerbated in susceptible patients who receive barbiturates. Barbiturates can also enhance their own metabolism, which contributes to tolerance.

Kidneys

Renal effects of thiopental may include modest reductions in renal blood flow and glomerular filtration rate. The most likely explanation is drug-induced reductions in blood pressure and cardiac output. Histologic evidence of renal damage is not detectable after use of barbiturates for induction of anesthesia.

Placental Transfer

Barbiturates used for intravenous induction of anesthesia readily cross the placenta, as evidenced by peak umbilical vein concentrations within 1 minute after administration. Nevertheless, plasma fetal concentrations of barbiturates are substantially less than those in maternal plasma (Christensen et al, 1981; Kosaka et al, 1969; Mark and Poppers, 1982). Clearance by the fetal liver and dilution by blood from the viscera and extremities result in the fetal brain being exposed to lower barbiturate concentrations than are measured in the umbilical vein. Indeed, maternal doses of thiopental up to 4 mg·kg^{-1} IV probably do not result in excessive concentrations of barbiturate in the fetal brain (Kosaka et al, 1969).

The elimination half-time of thiopental in neonates following maternal administration at cesarean section is 11 to 42.7 hours (Christensen et al, 1981). Nevertheless, these residual drug concentrations seem to be innocuous, as evidenced by unchanged neurobehavioral scores measured 48 hours after delivery (Hodgkinson et al, 1978).

Tolerance and Physical Dependence

Acute tolerance to barbiturates occurs earlier than does barbiturate-induced induction of microsomal enzymes. When barbiturate tolerance becomes maximal, the required effective dose of barbiturate may be increased sixfold. This magnitude of increase is at least double that which could be accounted for by increased metabolism resulting from enzyme induction. The observation that plasma concentrations of thiopental present on awakening are higher after a single large sleep dose than after a single small sleep dose may be an artifact of rapid intravenous injection, resulting in a transient distortion of drug distribution between the brain and peripheral circulation (Brodie et al, 1951).

Tolerance to sedative effects of barbiturates occurs sooner and is greater than that which occurs for the anticonvulsant and lethal effects. Thus, as tolerance to barbiturate-induced sedation increases, the therapeutic index decreases. Acute tolerance also applies to the effect of barbiturates on metabolic oxygen consumption, with supplemental doses of thiopental having less effect than the initial dose. The development of tolerance may be less for barbiturates that produce short-term depression of the central nervous system.

Tolerance and physical dependence on barbiturates are closely related. The severity of the withdrawal syndrome relates to the degree of tolerance and the rate of elimination of the barbiturates. Slow elimination of the barbiturate allows time for the central nervous system to diminish its compensatory excitatory responses more nearly in phase with the diminution in barbiturate-induced depression of the central nervous system. For example, persons who are physiologically dependent on barbiturates may be withdrawn more safely if long-acting phenobarbital is substituted for the shorter-acting barbiturate on which the individual is dependent. Nevertheless, abrupt discontinuation of phenobarbital in patients being treated for epilepsy may result in status epilepticus, even when the patient has been taking relatively small doses of the drug.

Intraarterial Injection

Intraarterial injection of thiopental usually results in immediate, intense vasoconstriction and excruciating pain that radiates along the distribution of the artery (Stone and Donnelly, 1961). Vasoconstriction may obscure distal arterial pulses, and blanching of the extremity is followed by cyanosis. Gangrene and permanent nerve damage may occur. The mechanism of these changes is not fully understood. Possible explanations include (1) formation of thiopental crystals in the artery that evoke intense vasoconstriction or that are carried distally to occlude end-arterioles, (2) hemolysis of erythrocytes and aggregation of platelets that occlude distal arterioles, and (3) local release of norepinephrine (Brown et al, 1968; Burn, 1960; Burn and Hobbs, 1959). The adverse response is not due to the alkalinity of the solution. Instead, the formation of thiopental crystals may occur because the pH becomes too low for the barbiturate to remain in solution (Waters, 1966). In this regard, crystal-forming ability is less likely to occur with dilute solutions of thiopental (2.5% rather than 5%). Nevertheless, accidental intraarterial injection of 2.5% concentrations of thiopental or thiamylal can still cause vascular insufficiency (Dohi and Naito, 1983). Likewise, methohexital can result in changes similar to those produced by thiopental. Ultimately, the damage produced by an intraarterial injection of a barbiturate is related to the dose and concentration of drug injected. All vessels examined pathologically demonstrate a severe endoarteritis.

Treatment of accidental intraarterial injection of a barbiturate includes immediate attempts to dilute the drug, prevention of arterial spasm, and general measures to sustain adequate blood flow. Dilution of the barbiturate is best accomplished by injection of saline through the needle that still remains in the artery. At the same time, injection of lidocaine, papaverine, or phenoxybenzamine may be considered to produce vasodilation (Guerra, 1980). If the needle has been removed from the artery prior to recognition of the accidental intraarterial injection, the injection of vasodilator drug may be made into a more proximal artery because the affected artery will be in spasm. Direct injection of heparin into the artery may be considered (O'Donnell et al, 1969). Sympathectomy of the upper extremity produced by a stellate ganglion block or brachial plexus block may relieve vasoconstriction. Urokinase may improve distal blood flow following accidental intraarterial injection of thiopental (Vangerven et al, 1989). Despite aggressive treatment, gangrene may still occur.

Venous Thrombosis

Venous thrombosis following intravenous administration of a barbiturate for induction of anesthesia presumably reflects deposition of barbiturate crystals in the vessel. Crystal formation in veins, however, is less hazardous than in arteries because of the ever-increasing diameter of the veins. The importance of administering a dilute solution of barbiturate for intravenous induction of anesthesia is suggested by the decreased incidence of venous thrombosis after use of 2.5% thiopental and 1% methohexital, compared with 5% and 2% solutions, respectively (O'Donnell et al, 1969).

Allergic Reactions

Allergic reactions in association with intravenous administration of barbiturates for induction of anesthesia most likely represent anaphylaxis (antigen-antibody interaction) (Watkins, 1979). Nevertheless, thiopental can also produce signs of an allergic reaction in the absence of a prior exposure, suggesting an anaphylactoid response (Hirshman et al, 1982). The incidence of allergic reactions to thiopental is estimated to be 1 per 30,000 patients (Clarke, 1981). The majority of reported cases are in patients with a history of chronic atopy, who often have received thiopental previously without adverse responses (Etter et al, 1980; Hirshman et al, 1982; Lilly and Hoy, 1980). Treatment of an allergic reaction following intravenous administration of thiopental, thiamylal, or methohexital must be aggressive, including epinephrine and prompt intravascular fluid replacement. Despite appropriate therapy, mortality following an allergic reaction to drugs such as thiopental seems unusually high (Stoelting, 1983).

REFERENCES

Avram MJ, Krejcie TC, Henthorn TK. The relationship of age to the pharmacokinetics of early drug distribution: The concurrent disposition of thiopental and indocyanine green. Anesthesiology 1990;72:403–11.

Becker KE, Tonnesen AS. Cardiovascular effects of plasma levels of thiopental necessary for anesthesia. Anesthesiology 1978; 49:197–208.

Bedford RF, Persing JA, Pobereskin L, Butler A. Lidocaine or thiopental for rapid control of intracranial hypertension. Anesth Analg 1980;59:435–7.

Brain Resuscitation Clinical Trial I Study Group. Randomized clinical study of thiopental loading in comatose survivors of cardiac arrest. N Engl J Med 1986;314:397–403.

Brodie BB, Mark CL, Lief PA, Bernstein E. Acute tolerance to thiopental. J Pharmacol Exp Ther 1951; 102:215–8.

Brodie BB, Mark LC, Papper EM, Bernstein E, Papper EM. The fate of thiopental in man and a method for its estimation in biological material. J Pharmacol Exp Ther 1950;98:85–96.

Brown SS, Lyons SM, Dundee JW. Intra-arterial barbiturates: A study of some factors leading to intravascular thrombosis. Br J Anaesth 1968;40:13–9.

Burn JH. Why thiopentone injected into an artery may cause gangrene. Br Med J 1960;2:414–6.

Burn JH, Hobbs R. Mechanism of arterial spasm following intra-arterial injection of thiopentone. Lancet 1959;1:1112–5.

Christensen JH, Andreasen F, Jansen JA. Pharmacokinetics of thiopental in cesarean section. Acta Anaesthesiol Scand 1981;25:174–9.

Clarke RSJ. Adverse effects of intravenously administered drugs in anaesthetic practice. Drugs 1981; 22:26–41.

Cote CJ, Petkau AJ. Thiopental requirements may be increased in children reanesthetized at least one year after recovery from extensive thermal injury. Anesth Analg 1985;64:1156–60.

Dohi S, Naito H. Intraarterial injection of 2.5% thiamylal does cause gangrene (letter). Anesthesiology 1983;59:154.

Drummond JC, Todd MM, U HS. The effect of high-dose sodium thiopental on brain stem auditory and median nerve somatosensory evoked responses in humans. Anesthesiology 1985;63:249–54.

Etter MS, Helrich M, Mackenzie CF. Immunoglobulin E fluctuation in thiopental anaphylaxis. Anesthesiology 1980;52:181–3.

Filner BF, Karliner JS. Alterations of normal left ventricular performance by general anesthesia. Anesthesiology 1976;45:610–20.

Ford FW, Morrell F, Whisler WW. Methohexital anesthesia in the surgical treatment of uncontrollable epilepsy. Anesth Analg 1982;61:997–1001.

Ghoneim MM, Pandya H. Plasma protein binding of thiopental in patients with impaired renal or hepatic function. Anesthesiology 1975;42:545–9.

Ghoneim MM, Pandya HB, Kelly SE, Fischer LJ, Corry RJ. Binding of thiopental to plasma proteins: Effects of distribution in the brain and heart. Anesthesiology 1976;45:635–9.

Guerra F. Thiopental forever after. In Aldrete JA, Stanley TH, eds. Trends in Intravenous Anesthesia. Chicago. Year Book Medical Publishers 1980:143.

Hirshamn CA, Peters J, Cartwright-Lee I. Leukocyte histamine release of thiopental. Anesthesiology 1982;56:64–7.

Hirshman CA, Edelstein RA, Ebertz JM, Hanifin JM. Thiobarbiturate-induced histmaine release in human skin mast cells. Anesthesiology 1985;63:353–6.

Hodgkinson R, Bhatt M, Kim SS, Grewal G, Marx GF. Neonatal neurobehavioral tests following cesarean section under general and spinal anesthesia. Am J Obstet Gynecol 1978;132:670–4.

Homer TD, Stanski DR. The effect of increasing age on thiopental disposition and anesthetic requirement. Anesthesiology 1985;62:714–24.

Hudson RJ, Stanski DR, Burch PG. Pharmacokinetics of methohexital and thiopental in surgical patients. Anesthesiology 1983;59:215–9.

Jung D, Mayersohn M, Perrier D, Calkins J, Saunders R. Thiopental disposition in lean and obese patients undergoing surgery. Anesthesiology 1982;56:269–74.

Kaplan JA, Miller ED, Bailey DR. A comparative study of enflurane and halothane using systolic time intervals. Anesth Analg 1976;55:263–8.

Kingston HGG, Kendrick A, Sommer KM, Olsen GD, Downes H. Binding of thiopental in neonatal serum. Anesthesiology 1990;72:428–31.

Korttila K, Linnoila M, Ertama P, Hakknien S. Recovery and simulated driving after intravenous anesthesia with thiopental, methohexital, propanidid or alphadione. Anesthesiology 1975;43:291–9.

Kosaka Y, Takahashi T, Mark LC. Intravenous thiobarbiturate anesthesia for cesarean section. Anesthesiology 1969;31:489–506.

Lilly JK, Hoy RH. Thiopental anaphylaxis and reagin involvement. Anesthesiology 1980;53:335–7.

Liu LMP, Gaudreault P, Friedman PA, Goudsouzian NG, Liu PL. Methohexital plasma concentrations in children following renal administration. Anesthesiology 1985;62:567–70.

Mark LC, Poppers PJ. The dilemma of general anesthesia for cesarean section: Adequate fetal oxygenation vs. maternal awareness during operation. Anesthesiology 1982;56:405–6.

Mark LC, Brand L, Kamvyssi S, Britton RC. Thiopental metabolism by human liver *in vivo* and *in vitro*. Nature 1965;206:1117–9.

Michenfelder JD. A valid demonstration of barbiturate-induced brain protection in man—at last. Anesthesiology 1986;64:140–2.

Nussmeier NA, Arlund C, Slogoff S. Neuropsychiatric complications after cardiopulmonary bypass: Cerebral protection by a barbiturate. Anesthesiology 1986;64:165–70.

O'Donnell JF, Hewitt JC, Dundee JW. Clinical studies of induction agents XXVIII: A further comparison of venous complications following thiopentone, metho-

hexitone and propanidid. Br J Anaesth 1969;41:681–3.

Pandele G, Chaux F, Salvadori C, Farinotti M, Duvaldestin P. Thiopental pharmacokinetics in patients with cirrhosis. Anesthesiology 1983;59:123–6.

Prys-Roberts C, Sear JW, Low JM, Phillips KC, Dagnino J. Hemodynamic and hepatic effects of methohexital infusion during nitrous oxide anesthesia in humans. Anesth Analg 1983;62:317–23.

Rockoff MA, Goudsouzian NG. Seizures induced by methohexital. Anesthesiology 1981;54:333–5.

Rockoff MA, Marshall LF, Shapiro HM. High dose barbiturate therapy in humans: A clinical review of 60 patients. Ann Neurol 1979;6:194–9.

Roesch C, Haselby KA, Paradise RP, et al. Comparison of cardiovascular effects of thiopental and pentobarbital at equivalent levels of CNS depression. Anesth Analg 1983;62:749–53.

Saidman LJ. Uptake, distribution, and elimination of barbiturates. In Eger EI ed. Anesthetic Uptake and Action. Baltimore. Williams and Wilkins, 1974.

Saidman LJ, Eger EI. The effect of thiopental metabolism on duration of anesthesia. Anesthesiology 1966;27:118–26.

Seltzer JL, Gerson JI, Allen FB. Comparison of the cardiovascular effects of bolus vs. incremental administration of thiopentone. Br J Anaesth 1980;52:527–9.

Shapiro HR, Galindo A, Whyte JR, et al. Rapid intraoperative reduction in intracranial pressure with thiopentone. Br J Anaesth 1973;45:1057–62.

Shingu K, Eger EI, Johnson BH, et al. Hepatic injury induced by anesthetic agents in rats. Anesth Analg 1983;62:140–5.

Sorbo S, Hudson RJ, Loomis JC. The pharmacokinetics of thiopental in pediatric surgical patients. Anesthesiology 1984;61:666–70.

Stanski DR, Maitre PO. Population pharmacokinetics and pharmacodynamics of thiopental: The effect of age revisited. Anesthesiology 1990;72:412–22.

Stoelting RK. Allergic reactions during anesthesia. Anesth Analg 1983;62:341–56.

Stone HH, Donnelly CC. The accidental intra-arterial injection of thiopental. Anesthesiology 1961;22:995–1006.

Swerdlow BN, Holley FO, Maitre PO, Stanski DR. Chronic alcohol intake does not change thiopental anesthetic requirements, pharmacokinetics, or pharmacodynamics. Anesthesiology 1990;72:455–61.

Todd MM, Chadwick HS, Shapiro HM, Dunlop BJ, Marshall LF, Dueck R. The neurologic effects of thiopental therapy following experimental cardiac arrest in cats. Anesthesiology 1982;57:76–86.

Todd MM, Drummond JC, Sang H. The hemodynamic consequences of high-dose methohexital anesthesia in humans. Anesthesiology 1984;61:495–501.

Todd MM, Drummond JC, Sang H. The hemodynamic consequences of high-dose thiopental anesthesia. Anesth Analg 1985;64:681–7.

Turcant A, Delhumeau A, Premel-Cabic A, et al. Thiopental pharmacokinetics under conditions of long-term infusion. Anesthesiology 1985;63:50–4.

Vangerven M, Delrue G, Brugman E, Cosaert P. A new therapeutic approach to accidental intra-arterial injection of thiopentone. Br J Anaesth 1989;62:98–100.

Ward JD, Becker DP, Miller DJ, et al. Failure of prophylactic barbiturate coma in the treatment of severe head trauma. J Neurosurg 1985;62:383–8.

Waters DJ. Intra-arterial thiopentone: A physico-chemical phenomenon. Anaesthesia 1966;21:346–56.

Watkins J. Anaphylactoid reactions to IV substances. Br J Anaesth 1979;51:51–60.

Whitwam JG. Methohexitone. Br J Anaesth 1976; 48:617–9.

Yamamura T, Kimura T, Furukawa K. Effects of halothane, thiamylal, and ketamine on central sympathetic and vagal tone. Anesth Analg 1983;62:129–34.

5

Benzodiazepines

INTRODUCTION

Benzodiazepines were initially observed to exert taming effects in animals; this led to the subsequent evaluation of these drugs in humans. In many situations, benzodiazepines have replaced barbiturates because of their favorable pharmacologic characteristics. Favorable pharmacologic characteristics of benzodiazepines include (1) production of anterograde amnesia, (2) minimal depression of ventilation or the cardiovascular system, (3) specific site of action as anticonvulsants, (4) relative safety if taken in overdose, and (5) rarity of abuse or development of significant physical dependence. Benzodiazepines unequivocally impair acquisition or encoding of new information (anterograde amnesia), whereas stored information (retrograde amnesia) is not altered (Ghoneim and Mewaldt, 1990). Like barbiturates, benzodiazepines have a rapid onset and short duration of action and lack analgesic effects. Among the many benzodiazepines available, there are both similarities and differences in potency and selectivity for producing specific effects. The central nervous system effects of benzodiazepines are rapidly reversed by intravenous administration of flumazenil, a selective benzodiazepine antagonist (see the section entitled "Flumazenil").

STRUCTURE ACTIVITY RELATIONSHIPS

Structurally, benzodiazepines are similar and share many active metabolites (Fig. 5-1). The term *benzodiazepine* refers to the portion of the structure composed of a benzene ring fused to a seven-membered diazepam ring. Because all important benzodiazepines contain a 5-aryl substituent and a 1, 4-diazepine ring, the term has come to mean the 5-aryl–1, 4-benzodiazepine structure.

MECHANISM OF ACTION

Benzodiazepine receptors are modulatory sites located on the alpha subunits of gamma-aminobutyric acid (GABA) receptors in the central nervous system (Fig. 5-2) (Mohler and Richards, 1988). Benzodiazepines enhance the chloride-channel gating function of GABA by facilitating the binding of this inhibitory neurotransmitter to its receptors. The resulting enhanced opening of chloride channels leads to hyperpolarization of cell membranes, making them more resistant to neuronal excitation. This resistance to excitation is presumed to be the mechanism by which benzodiazepine exert their therapeutic (anxiolytic, hypnotic, anticonvulsant, muscle-relaxant) effects. The existence of endogenous ligands for benzodiazepines receptors remains an undocumented hypothesis.

Benzodiazepine receptors occur almost exclusively on postsynaptic nerve endings in the central nervous system. This anatomic distribution of receptors is consistent with the minimal effects of these drugs outside the central nervous system (minimal circulatory effects). The highest density of benzodiazepine receptors is in the cerebral cortex, followed in decreasing order by the hypothalamus, cerebellum, midbrain, hippocampus, medulla, and spinal cord. Those central nervous system structures thought to be most involved in memory trace formation also contain the highest concentration of GABA-benzodiazepine receptors.

Electroencephalogram

The effects of benzodiazepines that appear on the electroencephalogram (EEG) resemble those of barbiturates in that alpha activity is decreased and low-voltage rapid beta activity is increased. This shift from alpha to beta activity occurs more in the frontal and rolandic areas with the benzodiazepines, which, unlike the barbiturates, do not cause posterior spread. In common with the barbiturates, however, tolerance to the effects of benzodiazepines on the EEG does occur.

The effects of benzodiazepines on the reticular activating system are especially interesting because of the importance of this region for the maintenance of wakefulness. In humans, cortical somatosensory evoked potentials, thought to be modulated by the reticular activating system, are diminished in amplitude by diazepam, the latency of the early potential is shortened, and that of the late peak is prolonged (Saletu et al, 1972).

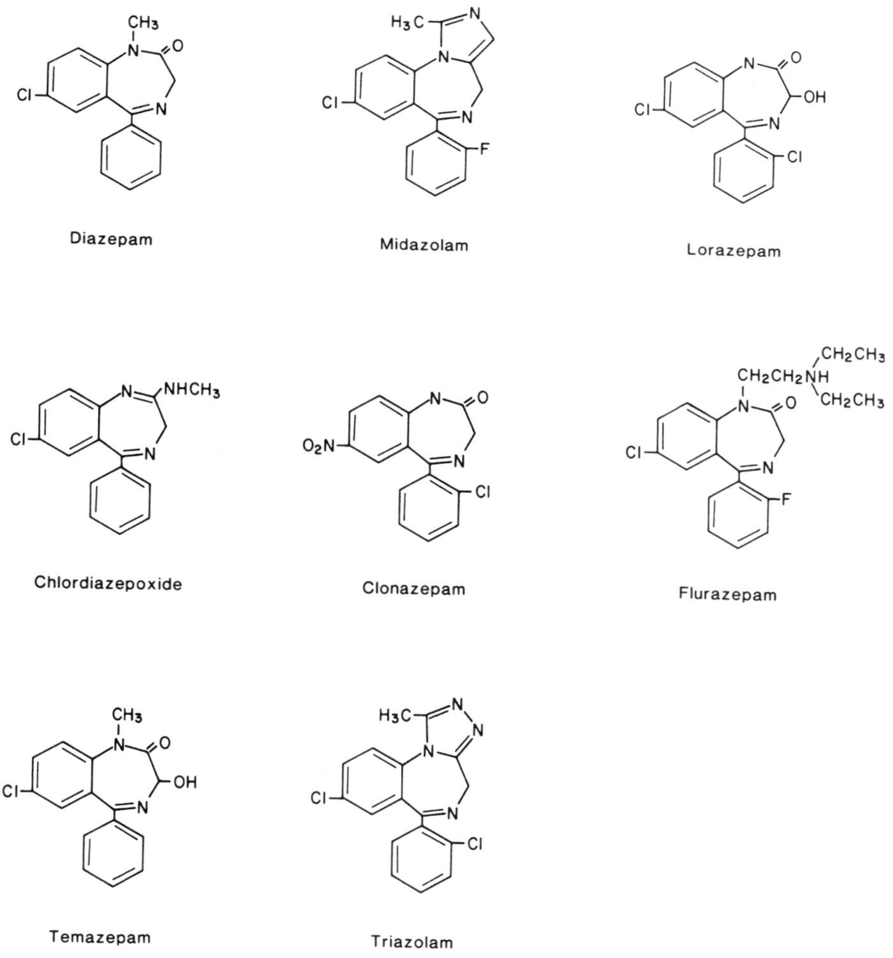

Diazepam   Midazolam   Lorazepam

Chlordiazepoxide   Clonazepam   Flurazepam

Temazepam   Triazolam

FIGURE 5-1. Benzodiazepines.

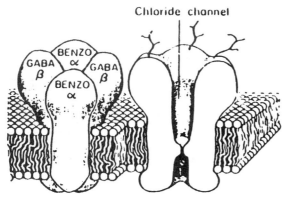

Chloride channel

FIGURE 5–2. Model of the gamma-aminobutyric acid (*GABA*) receptor forming a chloride channel. Benzodiazepines (*BENZO*) attach selectively to α subunits and are presumed to facilitate the action of the inhibitory neurotransmitter, GABA, on the α subunits. (From Mohler H, Richards JG. The benzodiazepine receptor: A pharmacologic control element of brain function. Eur J Anesthesiol 1988; 2: 15–24; with permission.)

Antagonism

The central nervous system actions of benzodiazepines are promptly reversed following the intravenous administration of a specific benzodiazepine antagonist (see the section entitled "Flumazenil"). Antagonism of benzodiazepine-induced central nervous system effects with physostigmine is both nonspecific and inconsistent (Caldwell and Gross, 1982). Aminophylline, 1 mg·kg^{-1} IV, may also antagonize benzodiazepine-induced sedation (Meyer et al, 1984; Wangler and Kilpatrick, 1985). Presumably, aminophylline acts by antagonizing the sedative effects of adenosine that accumulate in the central nervous system in response to administration of benzodiazepines.

DIAZEPAM

Diazepam is the standard with which all benzodiazepines are compared.

Commercial Preparation

Diazepam is dissolved in organic solvents (propylene glycol, sodium benzoate) because it is insoluble in water. The solution is viscid with a pH of 6.6 to 6.9. Dilution with water or saline causes cloudiness but does not alter the potency of the drug. Injection by either the intramuscular or intravenous route may be painful.

Pharmacokinetics

Diazepam is rapidly absorbed from the gastrointestinal tract after oral administration, reaching peak concentrations in about 1 hour in adults but as quickly as 15 to 30 minutes in children. There is rapid uptake of diazepam into the brain followed by redistribution to inactive tissue sites, especially fat, as this benzodiazepine is highly lipid soluble. Volume of distribution (Vd) of diazepam is large, reflecting extensive tissue uptake of this lipid-soluble drug (Table 5-1). Females, with a greater body content of fat are likely to have a larger Vd for diazepam than males. Diazepam rapidly crosses the placenta, achieving fetal concentrations equal to and sometimes greater than those present in the maternal circulation (Dawes, 1973). The duration of action of benzodiazepines is not linked to receptor events but rather is determined by the rate of metabolism and elimination.

Protein Binding

Protein binding of benzodiazepines parallels their lipid solubility. As such, highly lipid-soluble diazepam is extensively bound, presumably to albumin (Table 5-1). Cirrhosis of the liver or renal insufficiency with associated reductions in plasma concentrations of albumin may manifest as decreased protein binding of diazepam and an increased incidence of drug-related side effects (Greenblatt and Koch-Weser, 1974). The high degree of protein binding limits the efficacy of hemodialysis in the treatment of diazepam overdose.

Metabolism

Diazepam is principally metabolized by hepatic microsomal enzymes using an oxidative pathway of N-demethylation. The two principal metabolites of diazepam are desmethyldiazepam and oxazepam (Fig. 5-3). Desmethyldiazepam is metabolized more slowly and is only slightly less potent than diazepam. Therefore, it is likely that this metabolite contributes to the return of drowsiness that manifests 6 to 8 hours after administration of diazepam, as well to as sustained effects usually attributed to the parent drug. Alternatively, enterohepatic recirculation may contrib-

Table 5-1
Comparative Pharmacology of Benzodiazepines

	Equivalent Dose ($mg \cdot kg^{-1}$)	Volume of Distribution ($L \cdot kg^{-1}$)	Protein Binding (percent)	Clearance ($ml \cdot kg^{-1} \cdot min^{-1}$)	Elimination Half-Time (h)
Diazepam	0.3–0.5	1–1.5	96–98	0.2–0.5	21–37
Midazolam	0.15–0.3	1–1.5	96–98	6–8	1–4
Lorazepam	0.05	0.8–1.3	96–98	0.7–1	10–20

ute to the recurrence of sedation (Eustace et al, 1975). The plasma concentration of oxazepam after a single injection of diazepam is clinically insignificant and probably reflects its rapid removal as a conjugate of glucuronic acid. Ultimately, desmethyldiazepam is excreted in the urine in the form of oxidized and glucuronide conjugated metabolites. Unchanged diazepam is not appreciably excreted in the urine. Benzodiazepines do not produce enzyme induction.

Elimination Half-Time

The elimination half-time of diazepam is prolonged, ranging from 21 to 37 hours in healthy volunteers (Table 5-1). Cirrhosis of the liver is accompanied by up to fivefold increases in the elimination half-time of diazepam (Klotz et al, 1975). Likewise, the elimination half-time of diazepam increases progressively with increasing age, which is consistent with the increased sensitivity of these patients to the drug's sedative effects (Fig. 5-4) (Klotz et al, 1975). Prolongation of the elimination half-time of diazepam in the presence of cirrhosis of the liver is due to decreased protein binding of the drug, leading to an increased Vd. In addition, hepatic clearance of diazepam is likely to be reduced, reflecting decreased hepatic blood flow characteristic of cirrhosis of the liver. The explanation for prolonged elimination half-time of diazepam in elderly patients is also an increased Vd. Presumably, increased total body fat content that accompanies aging results in an increased Vd of a highly lipid-soluble drug, such as diazepam. Hepatic clearance of diazepam is not changed by aging.

Desmethyldiazepam, the principal metabolite of diazepam, has a elimination half-time of 48 to 96 hours. As such, the elimination half-time of the metabolite may exceed that of the parent drug. Indeed, plasma concentrations of diazepam often decline more rapidly than plasma con-

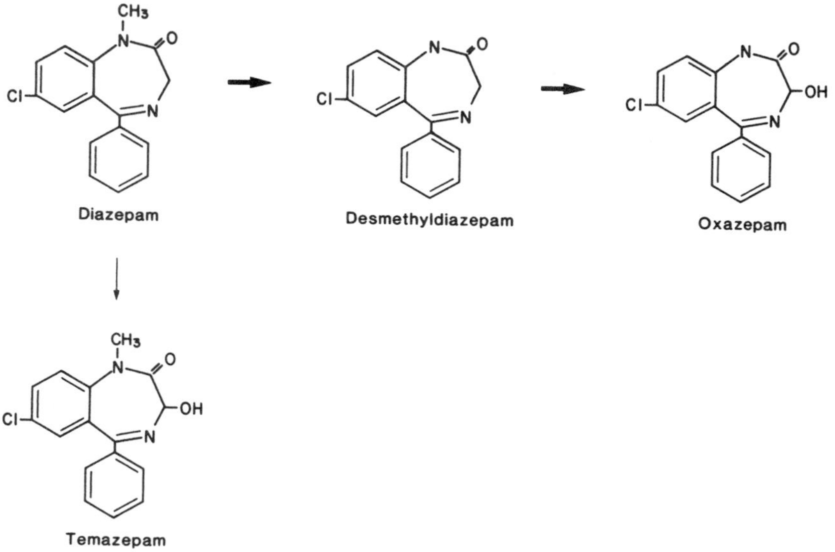

FIGURE 5-3. The principal metabolites of diazepam are desmethyldiazepam and oxazepam. A lesser amount of diazepam is metabolized to temazepam.

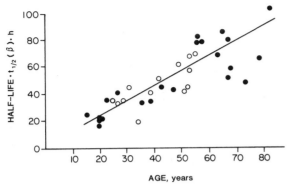

FIGURE 5–4.   The elimination half-time of diazepam increases progressively with increasing age. (From Klotz U, Avant GR, Hoyumpa A, Schender S, Wilkinson GR. The effects of age and liver disease on the deposition and elimination of diazepam in adult man. J Clin Invest 1975; 55: 347–59; with permission.)

centrations of desmethyldiazepam. This pharmacologically active metabolite can accumulate in plasma and tissues during chronic use of diazepam. Prolonged somnolence associated with high doses of diazepam is likely to be caused by sequestration of the parent drug and its active metabolite, desmethyldiazepam, in tissues, presumably fat, for subsequent release back into the circulation. A week or more is often required for elimination of these compounds from plasma following discontinuation of chronic diazepam therapy.

Effects on Organ Systems

Benzodiazepines, as represented by diazepam, produce minimal depressant effects on ventilation and circulation. Hepatic and renal function are not noticeably depressed by benzodiazepines. Diazepam does not increase the incidence of nausea and vomiting. There is no change in the circulatory concentrations of stress-responding hormones (catecholamines, antidiuretic hormone, cortisol).

Ventilation

Diazepam produces minimal depressant effects on ventilation, with detectable increases in $PaCO_2$, typically not occurring until 0.2 mg·kg^{-1} IV is administered. This slight increase in $PaCO_2$

is due primarily to a decrease in tidal volume. Nevertheless, rarely, small doses of diazepam (less than 10 mg IV) have produced apnea (Braunstein, 1979). Combination of diazepam with other central nervous system depressants (opioids, alcohol) or administration of this drug to patients with chronic obstructive airway disease may result in exaggerated or prolonged depression of ventilation.

The slope of the line depicting the ventilatory response to carbon dioxide is decreased nearly 50% within 3 minutes following the administration of diazepam, 0.4 mg·kg^{-1} IV (Fig. 5-5) (Gross et al, 1982). This depression of the slope persists for about 25 minutes and parallels the level of consciousness. Despite the decrease in slope, the carbon dioxide response curve is not shifted to the right as observed with depression of ventilation produced by opioids. These depressant effects on ventilation seem to be a cen-

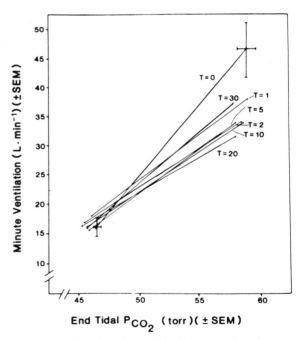

FIGURE 5–5.   The slope of the line depicting the ventilatory response to carbon dioxide is decreased following (*T*=minutes) administration of diazepam, 0.4 mg·kg^{-1} IV. (From Gross JB, Smith L, Smith TC. Time course of ventilatory response to carbon dioxide after intravenous diazepam. Anesthesiology 1982; 57: 18–21; with permission.)

tral nervous system effect, because the mechanics of respiratory muscles are unchanged. The ventilatory depressant effects of benzodiazepines are reversed by surgical stimulation but not by naloxone.

Cardiovascular System

Diazepam administered in doses of 0.5 to 1 mg·kg^{-1} IV for induction of anesthesia typically produces minimal decreases in blood pressure, cardiac output, and systemic vascular resistance that are similar in magnitude to those observed during natural sleep (10% to 20% decreases) (Table 5-2) (McCammon et al, 1980). There is a transient depression of baroreceptor-mediated heart rate responses that is less than the depression evoked by volatile anesthetics but that could, in hypovolemic patients, interfere with optimal compensatory changes (Marty et al, 1986). Increased coronary blood flow has been observed following the administration of diazepam (Ikran et al, 1973). The significance, if any, of this effect on coronary blood flow is questionable, because it is not known whether the increased flow is diverted to ischemic areas of the myocardium. In patients with elevated left ventricular end-diastolic pressures, a small dose of diazepam significantly decreases this pressure. Diazepam appears to have no direct action on the sympathetic nervous system, and it does not cause orthostatic hypotension.

The incidence and magnitude of blood pressure reductions produced by diazepam seem to be less than those associated with barbiturates as administered intravenously for the induction of anesthesia (Knapp and Dubow, 1970). Nevertheless, occasionally, a patient may unpredictably experience hypotension with even small doses of diazepam (Falk et al, 1978). The addition of nitrous oxide following induction of anesthesia with diazepam is not associated with adverse cardiac changes (Table 5-2) (McCammon et al, 1980). Therefore, nitrous oxide can be administered in the presence of diazepam to ensure adequate anesthesia. This contrasts with direct myocardial depression and decreases in blood pressure that occur when nitrous oxide is administered in the presence of opioids (see Chapter 3). Likewise, prior administration of diazepam, 0.125 to 0.5 mg·kg^{-1} IV, followed by injection of fentanyl, 50 μg·kg^{-1} IV, is associated with decreases in systemic vascular resistance and blood pressure that do not accompany administration of the opioid alone (see Fig. 3-12).

Skeletal Muscle

Skeletal muscle relaxant effects reflect actions of diazepam on spinal internuncial neurons and not

Table 5–2
Cardiovascular Effects of Diazepam (0.5 mg·kg^1 IV) and Diazepam-N$_2$O (50%)

	Awake	Diazepam	Diazepam-N$_2$O
Systolic blood pressure (mmHg)	144	125*	121*
Diastolic blood pressure (mmHg)	81	74	75
Mean arterial pressure (mmHg)	102	91*	91*
Heart rate (beats·min^{-1})	66	68	65
Pulmonary artery pressure (mmHg)	18.4	16.3	17.2
Pulmonary artery occlusion pressure (mmHg)	11.5	10.6	11.9
Cardiac output (L·min^{-1})	5.3	5.1	4.8*
Systemic vascular resistance (dyne·s·cm^{-5})	1391	1344	1377

*P <0.05 compared with the awake value.
(Data from McCammon RL, Hilgenburg JC, Stoelting RK. Hemodynamic effects of diazepam-nitrous oxide in patients with coronary artery disease. Anesth Analg 1980; 59: 438–41.)

actions at the neuromuscular junction (Dretchen et al, 1971). Presumably, diazepam diminishes the tonic facilitory influence on spinal gamma neurons, and, thus skeletal muscle tone is decreased. Benzodiazepines do not produce adequate relaxation for surgical procedures, nor does their use influence the dose requirements for neuromuscular blocking drugs. Tolerance occurs to the skeletal muscle relaxant effects of benzodiazepines.

Overdose

Central nervous system intoxication can be expected at diazepam plasma concentrations greater than 1000 ng·ml^{-1}. Despite massive overdoses of diazepam (up to 700 mg), serious sequelae (coma) are unlikely to occur if cardiac and pulmonary function are supported and other drugs such as alcohol are not present.

Drug Interactions

Alcohol

Depressant effects of benzodiazepines may be greatly enhanced by alcohol, perhaps reflecting a common site of action of both drugs on GABA receptors so as to enhance ion flux through chloride channels. This speculated common site of action is consistent with cross-tolerance between benzodiazepines and alcohol as well as the effectiveness of diazepam in treating the alcohol withdrawal syndrome (delirium tremens). Alcohol may also enhance the systemic absorption of benzodiazepines from the gastrointestinal tract and inhibit subsequent metabolism of the drug.

Cimetidine

Cimetidine delays the hepatic clearance and thus prolongs the elimination half-time of both diazepam and desmethyldiazepam (Fig. 5-6) (Greenblatt et al, 1984a). Indeed, sedation is increased when diazepam is administered with cimetidine compared with that when diazepam is administered alone. Presumably, this delayed clearance reflects cimetidine-induced inhibition of microsomal enzymes necessary for the oxidation of diazepam and desmethyldiazepam.

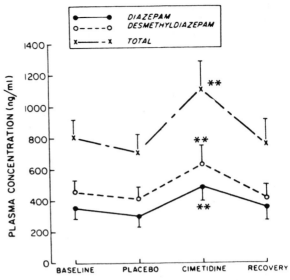

FIGURE 5–6. The plasma concentrations of diazepam and its active metabolite, desmethyldiazepam, are increased when the parent drug is administered during cimetidine therapy. Mean ± SE. (From Greenblatt DJ, Abernathy DR, Morse DS, Harmatz JS, Shader RI. Clinical importance of the interaction of diazepam and cimetidine. N Engl J Med 1984; 310: 1639–43; with permission.)

Anesthetics

The dose of thiopental required for induction of anesthesia is decreased by diazepam (Gyermek, 1975). Diazepam, 0.2 mg·kg^{-1} IV, decreases anesthetic requirements (MAC) for halothane from 0.73% to 0.475%, and doubling the dose of diazepam produces only minimal additional reductions as a reflection of a ceiling effect (Fig. 5-7) (Perisho et al, 1971). Halothane decreases the disappearance rate of diazepam from the plasma but has no significant effect on plasma concentrations of metabolites (Kanto and Isalo, 1973).

Abuse and Dependence Liability

The abuse and dependence liability of benzodiazepines is modest in comparison to opioids. Physiologic dependence can develop in patients who take therapeutic doses of benzodiazepines for prolonged periods. Such dependence may contribute to continued use but is not usually accompanied by a desire to increase the dose. Withdrawal symptoms may be uncomfortable (anxiety, restlessness, insomnia) but are rarely severe (seizures) and can be minimized by gradual reductions in dosage. Withdrawal symptoms may not appear for as long as 7 days following abrupt discontinuation. Psychological addiction is not regarded as a substantial risk of benzodiazepine therapy.

Clinical Uses

Clinical uses of diazepam include (1) preoperative medication, (2) induction of anesthesia, (3) intravenous sedation, (4) anticonvulsant activity, (5) treatment of delirium tremens, and (6) production of skeletal muscle relaxation, which is important in the management of lumbar disc disease and rare diseases such as tetanus.

Preoperative Medication

The anxiolytic, amnesic, and hypnotic effects of benzodiazepines are the basis for the use of these

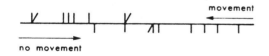

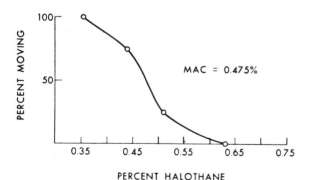

FIGURE 5–7. Diazepam, 0.2 mg·kg⁻¹ IV, reduces anesthetic requirements for halothane (MAC) in adult patients from 0.73% to 0.475%. (From Perisho JA, Buechel DR, Miller RD. The effect of diazepam [Valium] on minimum alveolar anesthetic requirements [MAC] in man. Can Anaesth Soc J 1971; 18: 536–40; with permission.)

drugs, especially diazepam, in preoperative medication. Preoperative medication with diazepam is preferably accomplished with oral administration rather than with intramuscular injection. The intramuscular injection of diazepam is painful because of the vehicle in which the drug is dissolved. Furthermore, absorption after intramuscular injection of diazepam, although usually complete, may be unpredictable in some patients (Divoil et al, 1983).

Diazepam, 0.1 to 0.2 mg·kg⁻¹ administered orally with water, is rapidly absorbed from the gastrointestinal tract. Peak plasma concentrations of diazepam occur after about 55 minutes, with the estimated systemic absorption of the orally administered drug being 94%. The anterograde amnesic effect of diazepam is modest but is greatly increased when scopolamine is also included in the preoperative medication (Frumin et al, 1976).

Induction of Anesthesia

The popularity of diazepam for intravenous induction of anesthesia is related to its minimal depressant effects on ventilation and on the cardiovascular system. Nevertheless, in most patients, diazepam has not represented a serious challenge to thiopental, because diazepam is slow to produce an effect, whereas recovery is prolonged compared with the effects of barbiturates. Furthermore, thrombophlebitis may follow the intravenous injection of diazepam. The potential for diazepam to produce prolonged sedation must be appreciated, especially when dealing with outpatients. Patients probably should not be allowed to drive for up to 24 hours after large doses of diazepam have been administered; after even small doses, patients should probably avoid alcohol for 24 hours.

Anticonvulsant Activity

The prior administration of diazepam, 0.25 mg·kg⁻¹ IM, to monkeys protects against the occurrence of systemic toxicity produced by lidocaine. Evidence for this protection is an increased convulsant dose of lidocaine in the benzodiazepine-pretreated animals (Fig. 5-8) (deJong and Heavner, 1974). Diazepam, 0.1 mg·kg⁻¹ IV, is effective in abolishing seizure ac-

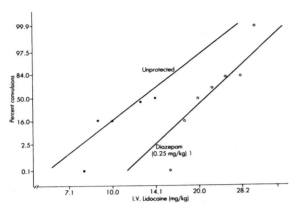

FIGURE 5–8. Prior administration of diazepam, 0.25 mg·kg^{-1} IM, increases the intravenous dose of lidocaine required to produce seizures compared with untreated (unprotected animals). (From deJong RH, Heavner JE. Diazepam prevents and aborts lidocaine convulsions in monkeys. Anesthesiology 1974; 49: 226–30; with permission.)

tivity produced by lidocaine, delirium tremens, and status epilepticus.

The efficacy of diazepam as an anticonvulsant may reflect its ability to facilitate the actions of the inhibitory neurotransmitter, GABA. In contrast with barbiturates, which inhibit seizures by nonselective depression of the central nervous system, diazepam selectively inhibits activity in the limbic system, particularly the hippocampus. The duration of anticonvulsant activity exceeds the elimination half-time of diazepam, suggesting a role for the pharmacologically active metabolite desmethyldiazepam.

MIDAZOLAM

Midazolam is a water-soluble benzodiazepine with an imidazole ring in its structure that accounts for stability in aqueous solutions and rapid metabolism (Fig. 5-1) (Reves et al, 1985). Like other benzodiazepines, midazolam produces anxiolytic, amnesic, hypnotic, anticonvulsant, and skeletal muscle relaxant effects. The anticonvulsant activity of midazolam is similar to that of diazepam. Neuromuscular transmission is not affected, and the dose requirements for neuromuscular blocking drugs are not altered. Compared with diazepam, midazolam is two to three times as potent. Indeed, midazolam has an

affinity for the benzodiazepine receptor that is approximately twice that of diazepam (Mohler and Okada, 1977).

Commercial Preparation

The pK of midazolam is 6.15, which permits the preparation of salts that are water soluble. The parenteral solution of midazolam used clinically is buffered to an acidic pH of 3.5. This is important because midazolam is characterized by a pH-dependent ring-opening phenomenon in which the ring remains open at pH values less than 4, thus maintaining water solubility of the drug (Fig. 5-9). The ring closes at pH greater than 4 as occurs when the drug is exposed to physiologic pH, thus converting midazolam to a highly lipid-soluble drug (Fig. 5-9).

Water solubility of midazolam obviates the need for a solubilizing preparation, such as propylene glycol, that can produce venoirritation or interfere with absorption after intramuscular injection. Indeed, midazolam causes minimal to no irritation after intravenous or intramuscular injection. Midazolam is compatible with lactated Ringer's solution and can be mixed with the acidic salts of other drugs, including opioids and anticholinergics.

Pharmacokinetics

Midazolam undergoes rapid absorption from the gastrointestinal tract and prompt passage across the blood-brain barrier. Only about 50% of an

Midazolam

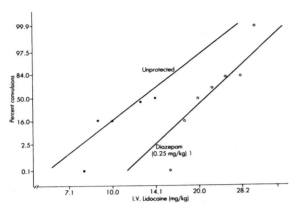

FIGURE 5–9. Reversible ring opening of midazolam above and below a pH of 4. The ring closes at a pH >4, converting midazolam from a water-soluble to a lipid-soluble drug.

orally administered dose of midazolam reaches the circulation, reflecting a substantial first-pass hepatic effect. As with most benzodiazepines, midazolam is bound extensively to plasma proteins; this binding is independent of the plasma concentration of midazolam (Table 5-1) (Greenblatt et al, 1984b). The short duration of action of a single dose of midazolam is due to its lipid solubility, leading to rapid redistribution from the brain to inactive tissue sites as well as rapid hepatic clearance.

There are important pharmacokinetic differences between midazolam and diazepam (Table 5-1) (Reves et al, 1985). For example, the elimination half-time of midazolam is 1 to 4 hours, which is much shorter than that of diazepam. The elimination half-time may be doubled in elderly patients, reflecting age-related decreases in hepatic blood flow and possibly enzyme activity. The Vds of midazolam and diazepam are similar, probably reflecting their similar lipid solubility and high degree of protein binding. Elderly and morbidly obese patients have an increased Vd of midazolam resulting from enhanced distribution of the drug into peripheral adipose tissues. The clearance of midazolam is more rapid than that of diazepam. As a result of these differences, the central nervous system effects of midazolam would be expected to be shorter than those of diazepam. Indeed, tests of mental function return to normal within 4 hours after the administration of midazolam (Reves et al, 1985).

Metabolism

Midazolam undergoes hydroxylation by hepatic microsomal oxidative mechanisms to 1-hydroxymidazolam (Fig. 5-10) (Reves et al, 1985). Smaller amounts of 4-hydroxymidazolam are formed in parallel. These metabolites are excreted in the urine as glucuronide conjugates. Very little unchanged midazolam is excreted by the kidneys. The 1- and 4-hydroxy metabolites of midazolam have pharmacologic activity, although this is less than that of the parent compound. Neither the contribution of these metabolites to the overall clinical effects of midazolam nor their potency or duration of action has been established (Reves et al, 1985). In contrast to diazepam, H-2 receptor antagonists do not interfere with the metabolism of midazolam (Greenblatt et al, 1986). Conversely, hepatic clearance of midazolan may be decreased by con-

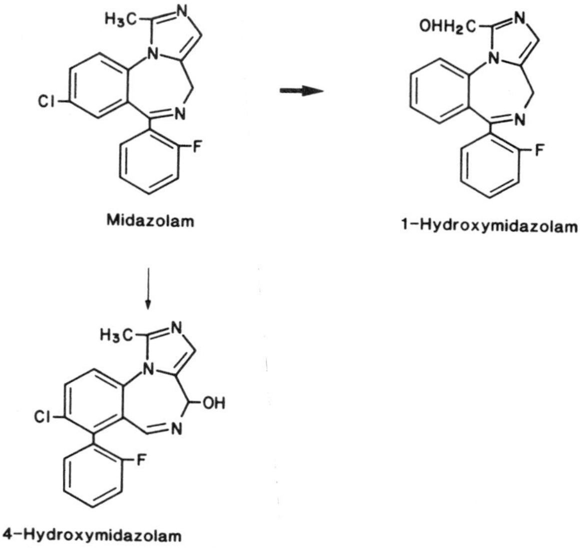

FIGURE 5-10. The principal metabolite of midazolam is 1-hydroxymidazolam. A lesser amount of midazolam is metabolized to 4-hydroxymidazolam.

comitant administration of any enzyme inhibiting drug, such as erythromycin, resulting in unexpected central nervous system depression (Hiller, et al, 1990).

Renal Clearance

The elimination half-time, Vd, and clearance of midazolam are not altered by renal failure (Vinik et al, 1983). This is consistent with the extensive metabolism of midazolam.

Effects on Organ Systems

Cerebral Blood Flow

Midazolam produces dose-related reductions in cerebral blood flow and cerebral oxygen utilization. For example, administration of midazolam, 0.15 mg·kg^{-1} IV, induces sleep, decreases cerebral blood flow 39%, and increases cerebral vascular resistance 52% (Forster et al, 1982). Patients with decreased intracranial compliance show little or no change in intracranial pressure when given midazolam in doses of 0.15 to 0.27 mg·kg^{-1} IV. Thus, midazolam is an acceptable alternative to barbiturates for induction of anesthesia in patients with intracranial pathology. Furthermore, midazolam may protect the brain more than diazepam, but less than thiopental, against the adverse effects of ischemia (Nugent et al, 1982). Similar to thiopental, induction of anesthesia with midazolam does not prevent increases in intracranial pressure associated with direct laryngoscopy for intubation of the trachea (Giffin et al, 1984).

Ventilation

Midazolam, 0.15 mg·kg^{-1} IV, depresses ventilation similar to diazepam, 0.3 mg·kg^{-1}IV (Forster et al, 1980). Patients with chronic obstructive airway disease experience even greater midazolam-induced depression of ventilation (Gross et al, 1983). Transient apnea may occur following rapid injection of high doses of midazolam (greater than 0.15 mg·kg^{-1} IV), especially in the presence of preoperative medication that includes opioids (Kanto et al, 1982).

Cardiovascular System

Midazolam, 0.2 mg·kg^{-1} IV, for induction of anesthesia produces a greater increase in heart rate and decrease in blood pressure than does diazepam, 0.5 mg·kg^{-1} IV (Samuelson et al, 1981). These midazolam-induced hemodynamic changes are similar to changes produced by thiopental, 3 to 4 mg·kg^{-1} IV (Lebowitz et al, 1982). Cardiac output is not altered by midazolam. Midazolam, like diazepam, produces transient depression of baroreceptor-mediated heart rate responses following intravenous administration in doses appropriate for induction of anesthesia (Marty et al, 1986). In the presence of hypovolemia, administration of midazolam results in enhanced blood pressure-lowering effects similar in magnitude to those produced by other intravenous induction drugs (Adams et al, 1985). Midazolam does not prevent blood pressure and heart rate responses evoked by intubation of the trachea.

Clinical Uses

Clinical uses of midazolam are similar to those for diazepam and include preoperative medication, induction of anesthesia, and intravenous sedation.

Preoperative Medication

Midazolam, like diazepam, is useful for preoperative medication because of its anxiolytic, amnesic, and hypnotic effects. Onset of these effects is rapid after administration of midazolam, 0.05 to 0.1 mg·kg^{-1} IM. Scopolamine administered concurrently with midazolam enhances its anxiolytic and amnesic effects. Anterograde amnesia, produced by midazolam as by other benzodiazepines, is dose related and often parallels the degree of sedation. Prolonged amnesia could interfere with recall of instructions provided to outpatients, but in this regard, midazolam is not different than thiopental (Kothary et al, 1981).

Intravenous Sedation

Midazolam in doses of 1 to 2.5 mg IV is effective for sedation during regional anesthesia as well as for brief therapeutic procedures. Compared with diazepam, midazolam produces a more rapid onset with greater amnesia and less postoperative sedation, but the time to complete recovery is no shorter (McClure et al, 1983). Pain on injection and subsequent venous thrombosis are less likely following administration of midazolam than diazepam.

Induction of Anesthesia

Induction of anesthesia can be produced by administration of midazolam, 0.1 to 0.2 mg·kg^{-1} IV, over 30 to 60 seconds. Nevertheless, thiopental usually produces induction of anesthesia 50% to 100% faster than midazolam (Fig. 5-11) (Sarnquist et al, 1980). Onset of unconsciousness is facilitated when a small dose of opioid (fentanyl, 50 to 100 µg IV) precedes the injection of midazolam by 1 to 3 minutes. The dose of midazolam required for intravenous induction of anesthesia is also less when preoperative medication is used. Elderly patients require less midazolam for the intravenous induction of anesthesia than do young adults (Gamble et al, 1981). The explanation for this is not clear, because prolonged elimination half-time should not alter the acute hypnotic effect of a single intravenous dose of midazolam. A possible explanation is the increased sensitivity of the central nervous system to the effects of midazolam with increasing age (Greenblatt et al, 1982).

Midazolam may be administered to supplement opioids or inhaled anesthetics during main-

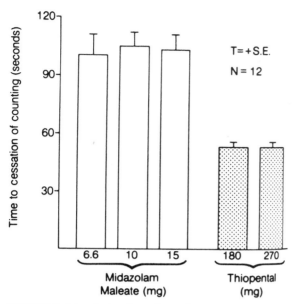

FIGURE 5–11. Induction of anesthesia as depicted by time to cessation of counting occurs in about 110 seconds following the intravenous administration of midazolam compared with about 50 seconds following injection of thiopental. (From Sarnquist FH, Mathers WD, Brock-Utne J, Carr B, Canup C, Brown CR. A bioassay of a water-soluble benzodiazepine against sodium thiopental. Anesthesiology 1980; 52: 149–53; with permission.)

tenance of anesthesia. Anesthetic requirements (MAC) for halothane are reduced in a dose-related manner by midazolam (Fig. 5-12) (Melvin et al, 1982). Awakening following general anesthesia that includes induction of anesthesia with midazolam is 1 to 2.5 times longer than that observed when thiopental is used for the intravenous induction of anesthesia (Jensen et al, 1982). Gradual awakening in patients who receive midazolam is rarely associated with nausea, vomiting, or emergence excitement. One hour after surgery, patients are equally alert with either midazolam or thiopental, and discharge time from an outpatient recovery room is similar with both anesthetics (Crawford et al, 1984).

LORAZEPAM

Lorazepam resembles oxazepam, differing only in the presence of an extra chlorine atom on the ortho position of the 5-phenyl moiety (Figs. 5-1

and 5-4). Lorazepam is a more potent amnesic than diazepam. The effects of lorazepam on ventilation, the cardiovascular system, and skeletal muscles resemble those of diazepam.

Pharmacokinetics

Lorazepam is conjugated with glucuronic acid to form pharmacologically inactive metabolites. This contrasts with formation of pharmacologically active metabolites following administration of diazepam. The elimination half-time is 10 to 20 hours, with urinary excretion of lorazepam glucuronide accounting for greater than 80% of the injected dose (Table 5-1). This shorter elimination half-time compared with that of diazepam probably reflects lesser lipid solubility of lorazepam. Nevertheless, clinical effects of diazepam

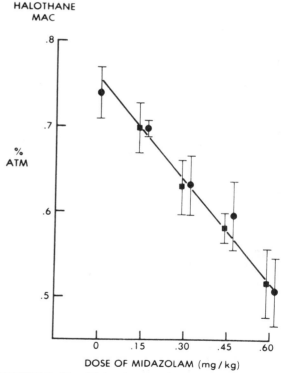

FIGURE 5–12. Midazolam produces dose-dependent decreases in halothane anesthetic requirements (MAC) in patients. Mean ± SE. (From Melvin MA, Johnson BH, Quasha AL, Eger EI. Induction of anesthesia with midazolam decreases halothane MAC in humans. Anesthesiology 1982; 57: 238–41; with permission.)

may be shorter because it dissociates more rapidly than lorazepam from benzodiazepine receptors, thus permitting its more rapid redistribution to inactive tissue sites. Because formation of glucuronide metabolites of lorazepam is not entirely dependent on hepatic microsomal enzymes, the metabolism of lorazepam is less likely than diazepam to be influenced by alterations in hepatic function, increasing age, or drugs such as cimetidine. Indeed, the elimination half-time of lorazepam is not prolonged in elderly patients or in those treated with cimetidine.

Clinical Uses

Lorazepam undergoes reliable absorption after oral and intramuscular injection, which contrasts with diazepam. Following oral administration, maximal plasma concentrations of lorazepam occur in 2 to 4 hours and persist at therapeutic levels for up to 24 to 48 hours. The recommended oral dose of lorazepam for preoperative medication is 50 $\mu g \cdot kg^{-1}$, not to exceed 4 mg (Fragen and Caldwell, 1976). With this dose, maximal anterograde amnesia lasting up to 6 hours occurs, and sedation is not excessive. Larger oral doses produce addition sedation without increasing amnesia. The prolonged duration of action of lorazepam limits its usefulness for preoperative medication when rapid awakening at the end of surgery is desirable.

A slow onset of effects limits the usefulness of lorazepam for (1) intravenous induction of anesthesia, (2) intravenous sedation during regional anesthesia, or (3) use as an anticonvulsant. Like diazepam, lorazepam is effective in limiting the incidence of emergence reactions following administration of ketamine. Although insoluble in water and thus requiring use of solvents such as polyethylene glycol or propylene glycol, lorazepam is alleged to be less painful on injection and to produce less venous thrombosis than diazepam (Hegarty and Dundee, 1977).

OXAZEPAM

Oxazepam, a pharmacologically active metabolite of diazepam, is commercially available (Fig. 5-4). Its duration of action is slightly shorter than that of diazepam because oxazepam is converted to pharmacologically inactive metabolites by conjugation with glucuronic acid. Indeed, the elimination half-time is relatively short, being 5 to 15 hours. Like lorazepam, the duration of action of oxazepam is unlikely to be influenced by hepatic dysfunction or administration of cimetidine.

Oral absorption of oxazepam is relatively slow. As a result, this drug may not be useful for the treatment of insomnia characterized by difficulty in falling asleep. Conversely, oxazepam may be used for treatment of insomnia characterized by nightly awakenings or shortened total sleep time.

CHLORDIAZEPOXIDE

Chlordiazepoxide was the first benzodiazepine introduced into clinical practice (Fig. 5-1). It is less potent than diazepam as an anxiolytic and less active as an anticonvulsant and skeletal muscle relaxant. An active metabolite, desmethylchlordiazepoxide has an elimination half-time of 24 to 96 hours. Physical dependence and withdrawal symptoms may occur on discontinuation of chronic therapy.

CLONAZEPAM

Clonazepam is a highly lipid-soluble benzodiazepine that is well absorbed after oral administration. Metabolism of clonazepam is to inactive conjugated and unconjugated metabolites that appear in the urine. The elimination half-time is 24 to 48 hours. Clonazepam is particularly effective in the control and prevention of seizures, especially myoclonic and infantile spasms.

FLURAZEPAM

Flurazepam is chemically and pharmacologically similar to other benzodiazepines but is used exclusively to treat insomnia (Fig. 5-1). Following administration of 15 to 30 mg orally to adults, a hypnotic effect occurs in 15 to 25 minutes and lasts 7 to 8 hours. The period of rapid-eye-movement sleep is decreased by this drug. The principal metabolite of flurazepam is desalkyl-flurazepam. This metabolite is pharmacologically active and has a prolonged elimination half-time that may manifest as daytime sedation (hangover). Furthermore, slow elimination of this same metabolite on termination of flurazepam therapy probably accounts for rebound insomnia.

TEMAZEPAM

Temazepam is an orally active benzodiazepine administered exclusively for the treatment of insomnia (Fig. 5-1). Oral absorption is complete, but peak plasma concentrations do not reliably occur until about 2.5 hours after its administration. Metabolism in the liver results in weakly active to inactive metabolites that are conjugated with glucuronic acid. The elimination half-time is about 15 hours. Temazepam, 15 to 30 mg orally, does not alter the proportion of rapid-eye-movement sleep to total sleep in adults. Despite the relatively long elimination half-time, temazepam, as used to treat insomnia, is unlikely to be accompanied by residual drowsiness the following morning. Tolerance or signs of withdrawal do not occur, even after nightly administration for 30 consecutive days.

TRIAZOLAM

Triazolam is an orally absorbed benzodiazepine that is effective in the treatment of insomnia (Fig. 5-1). Peak plasma concentrations following oral administration of 0.25 to 0.5 mg to adults occur in about 1 hour. The elimination half-time is 1.7 to 5.2 hours, rendering triazolam one of the shortest-acting benzodiazepines. The two principal metabolites of triazolam have little if any hypnotic activity, and their elimination half-time is less than 4 hours. Cumulative effects or tolerance does not seem to occur. Triazolam does not change the proportion of rapid-eye-movement to total sleep time. Rebound insomnia, however, may occur when this drug is discontinued. Marked anterograde amnesia has developed when this drug has been self-administered in attempts to facilitate sleep when traveling through several time zones.

QUAZEPAM

Quazepam, 7.5 to 15 mg orally, is an effective treatment of insomnia, producing a rapid onset of sedation. Tolerance does not occur, patients wake easily and are alert, and rebound insomnia is not observed. There does not seem to be an increased risk of amnesia.

FLUMAZENIL

Flumazenil is a specific and exclusive benzodiazepine antagonist with a high affinity for benzodiazepine receptors, where it exerts minimal agonist activity (Fig. 5-13) (Haefely, 1988). As a competitive antagonist, flumazenil prevents or reverses, in a dose-dependent manner, all the agonist effects of benzodiazepines. For example, flumazenil, 8 to 15 $\mu g \cdot kg^{-1}$ IV, reverses the central nervous system effects of benzodiazepine agonists within about 2 minutes. This antagonism is not followed by acute anxiety, hypertension, tachycardia, or neuroendocrine evidence of a stress response in postoperative patients (White et al, 1989; Kaukinen et al, 1990). The weak intrinsic agonist activity of flumazenil most likely attenuates the evidence of abrupt reversal of agonist effects. This weak agonist activity may also be the reason flumazenil does not precipitate withdrawal seizures when administered to patients being treated for seizure disorders. In addition to reversing lingering depressant effects of benzodiazepines in the postoperative period, flumazenil is useful in the differential diagnosis of patients who self-administer an overdose of an unknown drug and become comatose. The duration of antagonism provided by flumazenil is relatively brief, and return of benzodiazepine agonist effects may require repeated doses of the antagonist. Flumazenil does not alter anesthetic requirements (MAC) for volatile anesthetics, suggesting that these drugs do not exert any of their depressant effects on the central nervous system at benzodiazepine receptors (Schwieger et al, 1989).

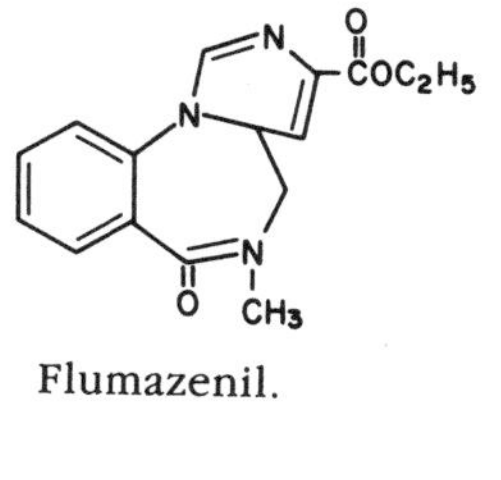

FIGURE 5–13. Flumazenil.

REFERENCES

Adams P, Gelman S, Reves JG, Greenblatt DJ, Alvis JM, Bradley E. Midazolam pharmacodynamics and pharmacokinetics during acute hypovolemia. Anesthesiology 1985;63:140–6.

Braunstein MC. Apnea with maintenance of consciousness following intravenous diazepam. Anesth Analg 1979;58:52–3.

Caldwell CB, Gross JB. Physostigmine reversal of midazolam-induced sedation. Anesthesiology 1982;57:125–7.

Crawford ME, Carl P, Andersen RS, Mikkelsen BO. Comparison between midazolam and thiopentone-based balanced anaesthesia for day-care surgery. Br J Anaesth 1984;56:165–9.

Dawes GS. The distribution and action of drugs on the fetus *in utero.* Br J Anaesth 1973;45:766–9.

deJong RH, Heavner JE. Diazepam prevents and aborts lidocaine convulsions in monkeys. Anesthesiology 1974;41:226–30.

Divoll M. Greenblatt DJ, Ochs HR, Shader RI. Absolute bioavailability of oral and intramuscular diazepam: Effects of age and sex. Anesth Analg 1983;62:1–8.

Dretchen K, Ghoneim MM, Long JP. The interaction of diazepam with myoneural blocking agents. Anesthesiology 1971;34:463–8.

Eustace PW, Hailey DM, Cox AG, Baired ES. Biliary excretion of diazepam in man. Br J Anaesth 1975;47:983–5.

Falk RB, Denlinger JK, Nahrwold ML, Todd RA. Acute vasodilation following induction of anesthesia with intravenous diazepam and nitrous oxide. Anesthesiology 1978;49:149–50.

Forster A, Gardaz J-P, Suter PM, Gemperele M. Respiratory depression of midazolam and diazepam. Anesthesiology 1980;53:494–9.

Forster A, Juge O, Morel D. Effects of midazolam on cerebral blood flow in human volunteers. Anesthesiology 1982;56:453–5.

Fragen RJ, Caldwell N. Lorazepam premedication; Lack of recall and relief of anxiety. Anesth Analg 1976;55:792–6.

Frumin MJ, Herekar VR, Jarvik ME. Amnesic actions of diazepam and scopolamine in man. Anesthesiology 1976;45:406–12.

Gamble JAS, Kawar P, Dundee JW, Moore J, Briggs LP. Evaluation of midazolam as an intravenous induction agent. Anesthesia 1981;36:868–73.

Ghoneim MM, Mewaldt SP. Benzodiazepines and human memory: A review. Anesthesiology 1990;72:926–38.

Giffin JP, Cottrell JE, Shwiry B, Hartung J, Epstein J, Lim K. Intracranial pressure, mean arterial pressure, and heart rate following midazolam or thiopental in humans with brain tumors. Anesthesiology 1984;60:491–4.

Greenblatt DJ, Abernathy DR, Morse DS, Harmatz JS, Shader RI. Clinical importance of the interaction of diazepam and cimetidine. N Engl J Med 1984a;310:1639–43.

Greenblatt DJ, Abernathy DR, Locniskar A, Harmatz JS, Limjuco RA, Shader RI. Effect of age, gender, and obesity on midazolam kinetics. Anesthesiology 1984b;61:27–35.

Greenblatt DJ, Koch-Weser J. Clinical toxicity of chlordiazepoxide and diazepam in relation to serum albumin concentration: A report from the Boston Collaborative Drug Surveillance Program. Eur J Clin Pharmacol 1974;7:259–62.

Greenblatt DJ, Locniskar A, Scavone JM, et al. Absence of interaction of cimetidine and ranitidine with intravenous and oral midazolam. Anesth Analg 1986;65:176–80.

Greenblatt DJ, Sellers EM, Shader RI. Drug disposition in old age. N Engl J Med 1982;306:1081–8.

Gross JB, Smith L, Smith TC. Time course of ventilatory response to carbon dioxide after intravenous diazepam. Anesthesiology 1982;57:18–21.

Gross JB, Zebrowski ME, Carel WD, Gardner S, Smith TC. Time course of ventilatory depression after thiopental and midazolam in normal subjects and in patients with chronic obstructive pulmonary disease. Anesthesiology 1983;58:540–4.

Gyermek L. Clinical effects of diazepam prior to and during general anesthesia. Curr Ther Res 1975;17:175–88.

Haefely W. The preclinical pharmacology of flumazenil. Eur J Anesthesiol 1988;2:25–36.

Hegarty JE, Dundee JW. Sequelae after the intravenous injection of three benzodiazepines: Diazepam, lorazepam and flunitrozepam. Br Med J 1977;2:1384–5.

Hiller A, Olkkola KT, Isohanni P, Saarvivaara L. Unconsciousness associated with midazolam and erythromycin. Br J Anaesth 1990;65:826–8.

Ikran H, Rubin AP, Jewkes RF. Effect of diazepam on myocardial blood flow of patients with and without coronary artery disease. Br Heart J 1973;35:626–30.

Jensen S, Schou-Olesen A, Huttel MS. Use of midazolam as an induction agent: Comparison with thiopental. Br J Anaesth 1982;54:605–7.

Kanto J, Isalo EUM. Diazepam as an inductive agent in two kinds of combination anaesthesia: The disappearance of diazepam and its metabolites from the plasma. Ann Chir Gynaecol Fenn 1973;62:251–5.

Kanto J, Sjovall S, Vuori A. Effect of different kinds of premedication of the induction properties of midazolam. Br J Anaesth 1982;54:507–11.

Kaukinen S, Kataja J, Kaukinen L. Antagonism of benzodiazepine-fentanyl anesthesia with flumazenil. Can J Anaesth 1990;37:40–5.

Klotz U, Avant GR, Hoyumpa A, Schender S, Wilkinson GR. The effects of age and liver disease on the disposition and elimination of diazepam in adult man. J Clin Invest 1975;55:347–59.

Knapp RB, Dubow H. Comparison of diazepam with thiopental as an induction agent in cardiopulmonary disease. Anesth Analg 1970;49:722–6.

Kothary SP, Brown ACD, Pandit UA, Samra SK. Time course of antirecall effect of diazepam and lorazepam following oral administration. Anesthesiology 1981;55:641–4.

Lebowitz PW, Cote ME, Daniels AL, et al. Comparative cardiovascular effects of midazolam and thiopental in healthy patients. Anesth Analg 1982;61:661–5.

Marty J, Gauzit R, Lefevre P, et al. Effects of diazepam and midazolam on baroreflex control of heart rate and on sympathetic activity in humans. Anesth Analg 1986;65:113–9.

McCammon RL, Hilgenberg JC, Stoelting RK. Hemodynamic effects of diazepam-nitrous oxide in patients with coronary artery disease. Anesth Analg 1980;59:438–41.

McClure JH, Brown DT, Wildsmith JAW. Comparison of the IV administration of midazolam and diazepam as sedation during spinal anaesthesia. Br J Anaesth 1983;55:1089–93.

Melvin MA, Johnson BH, Quasha AL, Eger EI. Induction of anesthesia with midazolam decreases halothane MAC in humans. Anesthesiology 1982;57:238–41.

Meyer BH, Weis OF, Muller FO. Antagonism of diazepam of aminophylline in healthy volunteers. Anesth Analg 1984;63:900–2.

Mohler H, Okada T. Benzodiazepine receptor: Demonstration of the central nervous system. Science 1977;198:849–51.

Mohler H, Richards JG. The benzodiazepine receptor: A pharmacological control element of brain function. Eur J Anesthesiology 1988;2:15–24.

Nugent M, Artru AA, Michenfelder JD. Cerebral metabolic, vascular, and protective effects of midazolam maleate: Comparison to diazepam. Anesthesiology 1982;56:172–6.

Perisho JA, Buechel DR, Miller RD. The effect of diazepam (Valium) on minimum alveolar anesthetic requirements (MAC) in man. Can Anaesth Soc J 1971;18:536–40.

Reves JG, Fragen RJ, Vinik HR, Greenblatt DJ. Midazolam: Pharmacology and uses. Anesthesiology 1985;62:310–24.

Saletu B, Saletu M, Ital T. Effect of minor and major tranquilizers on somatosensory evoked potentials. Psychopharmacologia 1972;24:347–58.

Samuelson PN, Reves JG, Kouchoukos NT, Smith LR, Dole KM. Hemodynamic responses to anesthetic induction with midazolam or diazepam in patients with ischemic heart disease. Anesth Analg 1981; 60:802–9.

Sarnquist FH, Mathers WD, Brock-Utne J, Carr B, Canup C, Brown CR. A bioassay of a water-soluble benzodiazepine against sodium thiopental. Anesthesiology 1980;52:149–53.

Schwieger IM, Szlam F, Hug CC. Absence of agonistic or antagonistic effect of flumazenil (Ro 15-1788) in dogs anesthetized with enflurane, isoflurane, or fentanyl-enflurane. Anesthesiology 1989;70:477–80.

Vinik HR, Reves JG, Greenblatt DJ, Abernathy DR, Smith LR. The pharmacokinetics of midazolam in chronic renal failure patients. Anesthesiology 1983;59:390–4.

Wangler MA, Kilpatrick DS. Aminophylline is an antagonist of lorazepam. Anesth Analg 1985;64:834–6.

White PF, Shafer A, Boyle WA, Doze VA, Duncan S. Benzodiazepine antagonism does not provoke a stress response. Anesthesiology 1989;70:636–9.

Chapter 6

Nonbarbiturate Induction Drugs

KETAMINE

Ketamine is a phencyclidine derivative that produces "dissociative anesthesia," which is characterized by evidence on the electroencephalogram (EEG) of dissociation between the thalamocortical and limbic systems (Reich and Silvay, 1989). Dissociative anesthesia resembles a cataleptic state in which the eyes remain open with a slow nystagmic gaze. The patient is noncommunicative, although wakefulness may appear to be present. Varying degrees of hypertonus and purposeful skeletal muscle movements often occur independently of surgical stimulation. The patient is amnesic, and analgesia is intense. The possibility of emergence delirium may limit the clinical usefulness of ketamine. Ketamine must be considered a drug that is vulnerable to abuse, emphasizing the need to take appropriate precautions against its unauthorized use.

Structure Activity Relationships

Ketamine is a water-soluble molecule that structurally resembles phencyclidine (Fig. 6-1). The presence of an asymmetric carbon atom results in the existence of two optical isomers of ketamine. Only the racemic mixture containing equal amounts of the two ketamine isomers is available for clinical use. When studied separately, the positive isomer produces (1) more intense analgesia, (2) more rapid recovery, and (3) a lower incidence of emergence reactions than the nega-

tive isomer (White et al, 1980). Both isomers of ketamine appear able to inhibit uptake of catecholamines back into postganglionic sympathetic nerve endings (a cocaine-like effect). The fact that individual optical isomers of ketamine differ in their pharmacologic properties suggests that this drug interacts with specific receptors.

Mechanism of Action

Ketamine is a potent analgesic at subanesthetic plasma concentrations, and its analgesic and anesthetic effects may be mediated by different mechanisms. Specifically, analgesia may be due to an interaction between ketamine and opioid receptors in the central nervous system (Reich and Silvay, 1989).

Opioid Receptor Theory

N-methyl-aspartate is an excitatory amine speculated to act on receptors that are a subgroup on opioid receptors. Ketamine may act as an antagonist at these receptors to block spinal nociceptive reflexes (Yamamura et al, 1990). Interaction of

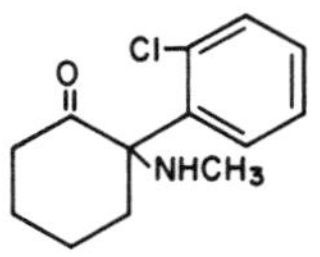

FIGURE 6–1.   Ketamine.

ketamine with sigma opioid receptors may be a plausible theory to explain dysphoric emergence reactions.

Cross-tolerance between ketamine and opioids suggests a common receptor for ketamine-induced analgesia. An opioid receptor theory would be further supported by reversal of the effects of ketamine with naloxone. To date, studies on the effect of naloxone or responses to ketamine have been inconclusive (Reich and Silvay, 1989).

Miscellaneous Receptor Theory

Other neuronal systems may be involved in the antinociceptive action of ketamine, since blockade of norepinephrine and serotonin receptors attenuates the analgesic action of ketamine. Ketamine also interacts with muscarinic cholinergic receptors in the central nervous system, suggesting that centrally acting anticholinesterase agents such as physostigmine might reverse ketamine anesthesia (Toro-Matos et al, 1980).

Pharmacokinetics

The pharmacokinetics of ketamine resembles that of thiopental in rapid onset of action, relatively short duration of action, and high lipid solubility (Table 6-1). Ketamine has a pK of 7.5 at physiologic pH. Peak plasma concentrations of ketamine occur within 1 minute following intravenous administration and within 5 minutes following intramuscular injection. Ketamine is not significantly bound to plasma proteins and leaves the blood rapidly to be distributed into tissues. Initially, ketamine is distributed to highly perfused tissues such as the brain, where the peak

concentration may be four to five times that present in plasma. The extreme lipid solubility of ketamine (5 to 10 times that of thiopental) ensures its rapid transfer across the blood-brain barrier. Furthermore, ketamine-induced increases in cerebral blood flow could facilitate delivery of drug and thus enhance rapid achievement of high brain concentrations. Subsequently, ketamine is redistributed from the brain and other highly perfused tissues to less well-perfused tissues. The elimination half-time of ketamine is 1 to 2 hours.

Failure of impaired renal function or enzyme induction to alter the duration of action of a single dose of ketamine suggests that redistribution of drug from the brain to inactive tissue sites is primarily responsible for termination of unconsciousness. Hepatic metabolism, as with thiopental, is important for ultimate clearance of ketamine from the body. Ketamine stored in tissues may contribute to cumulative drug effects with repeated or continuous administration.

Metabolism

Ketamine is metabolized extensively by hepatic microsomal enzymes. An important pathway of metabolism is demethylation of ketamine by cytochrome P-450 enzymes to form norketamine (Fig. 6-2) (White et al, 1982). In animals, norketamine is one fifth to one third as potent as ketamine. This active metabolite may contribute to prolonged effects of ketamine. Norketamine is eventually hydroxylated and then conjugated to more water-soluble and inactive glucuronide metabolites. Following intravenous administration, less than 4% of a dose of ketamine can be recovered from the urine as unchanged drug. Fecal excretion accounts for less than 5% of an injected dose of ketamine. Halothane or diazepam slows

Table 6–1
Comparative Characteristics of Nonbarbiturate Induction Drugs

	Elimination Half-Time (h)	Volume of Distribution (L·kg⁻¹)	Clearance (ml·kg⁻¹·min⁻¹)	Blood Pressure	Heart Rate
Ketamine	1–2	2.5–3.5	16–18	Increased	Increased
Etomidate	2–5	2.2–4.5	10–20	No change	No change
Propofol	0.5–1.5	3.5–4.5	30–60	Decreased	Decreased

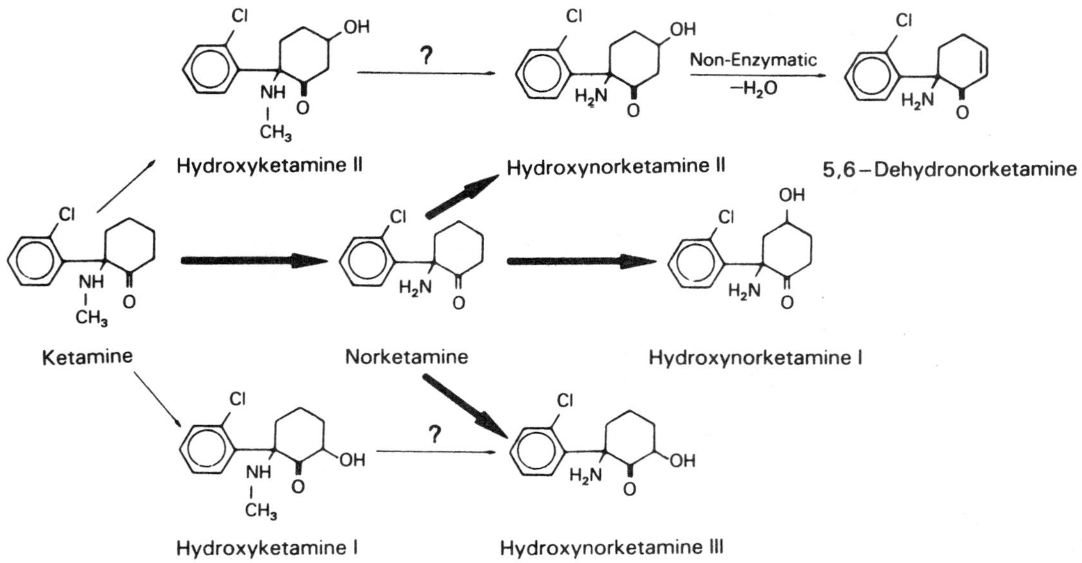

FIGURE 6–2. Metabolism of ketamine. (From White PF, Way WL, Trevor AJ. Ketamine: Its pharmacology and therapeutic uses. Anesthesiology 1982; 56: 119–36; with permission.)

the metabolism of ketamine and prolongs the drug's effects (Borondy and Glazko, 1977; White et al, 1976).

Chronic administration of ketamine stimulates the activity of enzymes responsible for its metabolism. Accelerated metabolism of ketamine as a result of enzyme induction could explain, in part, the observation of tolerance to the analgesic effects of ketamine that occurs in patients receiving repeated doses of this drug. Indeed, tolerance may occur in burn patients receiving more than two short-interval exposures to ketamine (Demling et al, 1978). Development of tolerance is also consistent with reports of ketamine dependence (White et al, 1982).

Clinical Uses

Ketamine is a unique drug evoking intense analgesia at subanesthetic doses and producing prompt induction of anesthesia when administered intravenously at higher doses. Inclusion of an antisialagogue in the preoperative medication is often recommended to avoid coughing and laryngospasm owing to ketamine-induced salivary secretions. Glycopyrrolate may be preferable, as atropine or scopolamine could theo-retically increase the incidence of emergence delirium (see the section entitled "Emergence Delirium").

Analgesia

Intense analgesia can be achieved with subanesthetic doses of ketamine, 0.2 to 0.5 mg·kg^{-1} IV. Analgesia is alleged to be greater for somatic than for visceral pain. Analgesia can be produced during labor without associated depression of the neonate (Akamatsu et al, 1974; Janeczko et al, 1974). Neonatal neurobehavioral scores of infants born by vaginal delivery with ketamine analgesia are lower than those of infants born with epidural anesthesia, but higher than the scores in infants delivered with thiopental-nitrous oxide (Hodgkinson et al, 1977). Epidural or intrathecal administration of ketamine produces analgesia without depression of ventilation (Islas et al, 1985).

Induction of Anesthesia

Induction of anesthesia is produced by administration of ketamine, 1 to 2 mg·kg^{-1} IV or 5 to 10 mg·kg^{-1} IM. Injection of ketamine intravenously does not produce pain or venous irritation. The need for large intramuscular doses reflects a significant first-pass hepatic effect for ketamine. Consciousness is lost in 30 to 60 seconds after intravenous administration and in 2 to 4 minutes after intramuscular injection. Unconsciousness is associated with maintenance of normal or only slightly depressed pharyngeal and laryngeal reflexes. Return of consciousness usually occurs in 10 to 15 minutes following an intravenous induction dose of ketamine, but complete recovery is delayed. Amnesia persists for about 1 hour after recovery of consciousness, but ketamine does not cause retrograde amnesia.

Because of its rapid onset of action, ketamine has been used as an intramuscular induction drug in children and difficult-to-manage mentally retarded patients regardless of age. Ketamine has been used extensively for burn dressing changes, debridements, and skin-grafting procedures. The excellent analgesia and ability to maintain spontaneous ventilation in an airway that may otherwise be altered by burn-scar contractures are important advantages of ketamine in these patients. Tolerance may develop, however, in burn patients undergoing repeated, short-interval anesthetics with ketamine (Demling et al, 1978). Induction of anesthesia in acutely hypovolemic patients is often accomplished with ketamine, taking advantage of the drug's cardiovascular-stimulating effects. Beneficial effects of ketamine on airway resistance make this a potentially useful drug for rapid intravenous induction of anesthesia in patients with asthma (Hirshman et al, 1979).

The administration of ketamine to patients with coronary artery disease has been questioned because of increased myocardial oxygen requirements that may accompany this drug's sympathomimetic effects on the heart (Reves et al, 1978). Nevertheless, induction of anesthesia with administration of diazepam, 0.5 mg·kg^{-1} IV, and ketamine, 0.5 mg·kg^{-1} IV, followed by a continuous intravenous infusion of ketamine, 15 to 30 µg·kg^{-1}·min^{-1}, has been proposed for anesthesia in patients with coronary artery disease (White et al, 1982). Ketamine should be used cautiously or avoided in patients with systemic or pulmonary hypertension or increased intracranial pressure, although this concern may deserve reevaluation based on more recent information (see the sections entitled "Cardiovascular System" and "Central Nervous System"). Nystagmus associated with administration of ketamine may be undesirable in operations or examinations of the eye performed under anesthesia.

Ketamine has been administered safely to patients with malignant hyperthermia and does not trigger the syndrome in susceptible swine (Dershwitz et al, 1989). This drug has also been administered without incident to a patient with acute intermittent porphyria, but caution is recommended because ketamine can increase ALA synthetase activity in animals (Kostrzewski and Gregor, 1978). Extensive experience with ketamine for pediatric cardiac catheterization has shown the drug to be useful, but its possible cardiac-stimulating effects must be considered in the interpretation of catheterization data.

Side Effects

Central Nervous System

Ketamine is reported to be a potent cerebral vasodilator capable of increasing cerebral blood flow by 60% in the presence of normocapnia (Takeshita et al, 1972). As a result, patients with intracranial pathology may be vulnerable to sustained elevations in intracranial pressure following administration of ketamine. Nevertheless, in mechanically ventilated animals with intracranial hypertension, there is no further increase in intracranial pressure following administration of ketamine, 0.5 or 2 mg·kg^{-1} IV (Pfenninger et al, 1985). Furthermore, anterior fontanelle pressure, an indirect monitor of intracranial pressure, declines in mechanically ventilated preterm neonates following injection of ketamine, 2 mg·kg^{-1} IV (Friesen et al, 1987). Prior administration of thiopental, diazepam, or midazolam has been shown to blunt ketamine-induced increases in cerebral blood flow (Reich and Silvay, 1989; Thorsen and Gran, 1980).

Ketamine's effects on the EEG are characterized by abolition of alpha rhythm and dominance of theta activity. Onset of delta activity coincides with loss of consciousness. Ketamine-induced excitatory activity occurs in both the thalamus and limbic system without evidence of subsequent spread of seizure activity to cortical areas (Ferrer-Allado et al, 1973). As such, ketamine would be unlikely to precipitate generalized convulsions in patients with seizure disorders.

Indeed, ketamine does not alter the seizure threshold in epileptic patients (Celsia et al, 1975).

Ketamine increases the cortical amplitude of somatosensory evoked potentials (Schubert et al, 1990). This ketamine-induced increase in amplitude is attenuated by nitrous oxide. Auditory and visual evoked responses are decreased by ketamine.

Cardiovascular System

Ketamine produces cardiovascular effects that resemble sympathetic nervous system stimulation. Systemic and pulmonary arterial blood pressure, heart rate, cardiac output, cardiac work, and myocardial oxygen requirements increase (Table 6-2) (Tweed et al, 1972). The increase in systolic blood pressure in adults receiving clinical doses of ketamine is 20 to 40 mmHg, with a slightly smaller increase in diastolic blood pressure. Typically, blood pressure increases progressively during the first 3 to 5 minutes following intravenous injection of ketamine and then decreases to normal limits over the next 10 to 20 minutes. The cardiovascular-stimulating effects on the systemic and pulmonary circulation are blunted or prevented by prior administration of benzodiazepines or concomitant administration of inhaled anesthetics, including nitrous oxide (Balfors et al, 1983; Reich and Silvay, 1989). Likewise, ketamine administered to mildly sedated infants fails to produce hemodynamic changes in either the systemic or pulmonary circulations (Hickey et al, 1985).

In shocked animals, ketamine is associated with a higher survival rate than in animals anesthetized with halothane (Longnecker and Sturgill, 1976). Blood pressure may be better maintained in hemorrhaged animals anesthetized with ketamine, but greater increases in arterial lactate concentrations occur than in animals with lower arterial blood pressures anesthetized with a volatile anesthetic (Weiskopf et al, 1981). This suggests inadequate tissue perfusion despite maintenance of blood pressure by ketamine. Presumably, ketamine-induced vasoconstriction maintains blood pressure at the expense of tissue perfusion. Critically ill patients occasionally respond to ketamine with unexpected decreases in blood pressure and cardiac output, which may reflect depletion of catecholamine stores and exhaustion of sympathetic nervous system compensating mechanisms, leading to an unmasking of ketamine's direct myocardial-depressant effects.

The effect of ketamine on cardiac rhythm is inconclusive. There is evidence that ketamine enhances the arrhythmogenicity of epineph-

Table 6–2
Circulatory Effects of Ketamine

	Control	Ketamine ($2\ mg \cdot kg^{-1}\ IV$)	Percent Change
Heart rate (beats$\cdot$min^{-1})	74	98	+33
Mean arterial pressure (mmHg)	93	119	+28
Cardiac index (L$\cdot$min$^{-1}\cdot$m^{-2})	3.0	3.8	+29
Stroke volume index (ml$\cdot$m^{-2})	43	44	
Systemic vascular resistance (units)	16.2	15.9	
Right atrial pressure (mmHg)	7	8.9	
Left ventricular end-diastolic pressure (mmHg)	13	13.1	
Pulmonary artery pressure (mmHg)	17	24.5	+44
Minute work index (kg-m$\cdot$m^{-2})	5.4	8.9	+40
Tension-time index (mmHg$\cdot$sec)	2700	4640	+68

(Data from Tweed WA, Minuck MS, Mymin D. Circulatory response to ketamine anesthesia. Anesthesiology 1972; 37: 613–9.)

rine (Koehntop et al, 1977). Conversely, ketamine may abolish epinephrine-induced cardiac dysrhythmias.

MECHANISMS OF CARDIOVASCULAR EFFECTS. The mechanisms for ketamine-induced cardiovascular effects are complex. Direct stimulation of the central nervous system leading to increased sympathetic nervous system outflow seems to be the most important mechanism (Wong and Jenkins, 1974). Evidence for this mechanism is the ability of inhaled anesthetics, ganglionic blockade, cervical epidural anesthesia, and spinal cord transection to prevent ketamine-induced increases in blood pressure and heart rate (Stanley, 1973; Traber et al, 1970). Furthermore, increases in plasma concentrations of epinephrine and norepinephrine occur as early as 2 minutes after intravenous administration of ketamine and return to control levels 15 minutes later (Baraka et al, 1973). *In vitro,* ketamine produces direct myocardial depression, emphasizing the importance of an intact sympathetic nervous system for the cardiac-stimulating effects of this drug (Schwartz and Horwitz, 1975). Depression of baroreceptor reflex activity leading to activation of the sympathetic nervous system has not been confirmed as the mechanism responsible for ketamine's cardiovascular effects. The role of ketamine-induced inhibition of norepinephrine uptake into postganglionic sympathetic nerve endings and associated elevations of plasma catecholamine concentrations on the drugs cardiac-stimulating effects are not known. (Koehntop et al, 1977).

Ventilation and Airway

Ketamine does not produce significant depression of ventilation. The ventilatory response to carbon dioxide is maintained during ketamine anesthesia, and the $PaCO_2$ is unlikely to increase more than 3 mmHg (Soliman et al, 1975). Breathing frequency typically decreases for 2 to 3 minutes following administration of ketamine. Apnea, however, can occur if the drug is administered rapidly intravenously or an opioid is included in the preoperative medication.

Upper airway skeletal muscle tone is well maintained, and upper airway reflexes remain relatively intact (Taylor and Towey, 1971). Despite continued presence of upper airway reflexes, ketamine anesthesia does not negate the need for protection of the lungs against aspiration by placement of a cuffed tube in the trachea. Salivary and tracheobronchial mucous gland secretions are increased by intramuscular or intravenous administration of ketamine, leading to the frequent recommendation that an antisialagogue be included in the preoperative medication when the use of this drug is anticipated.

Ketamine is as effective as halothane or enflurane in preventing experimentally induced bronchospasm in dogs (Hirshman et al, 1979). This bronchodilating action of ketamine is related to its sympathomimetic properties. For this reason, ketamine may be a useful drug in the perioperative management of patients with asthma.

Hepatic or Renal Function

Ketamine does not significantly alter laboratory tests that reflect hepatic or renal function.

Allergic Reactions

Ketamine does not evoke the release of histamine and rarely, if ever, causes allergic reactions.

Drug Interactions

The importance of an intact and normally functioning central nervous system in determining the cardiovascular effects of ketamine is emphasized by hemodynamic depression rather than stimulation that occurs when ketamine is administered in the presence of inhaled anesthetics. For example, depression by inhaled anesthetics of sympathetic outflow from the central nervous system prevents the typical increases in blood pressure and heart rate that occur when ketamine is administered alone (Stanley, 1973). Ketamine administered in the presence of halothane may result in hypotension (Bidwai et al, 1975). Presumably, halothane, by depressing sympathetic nervous system outflow from the central nervous system, unmasks direct cardiac-depressant effects of ketamine. Furthermore, halothane, by decreasing endogenous release of norepinephrine, could allow direct depressant effects of ketamine on the heart to manifest. Diazepam, 0.3 to 0.5 mg·kg^{-1} IV, or an equivalent dose of midazolam, is also effective in preventing the cardiac-stimulating effects of ketamine. In the presence of verapamil, the blood pressure-elevating effects of ketamine may be attenuated, whereas drug-induced elevations in heart rate are enhanced (Fragen and Avram, 1986).

In animals, ketamine causes a dose-dependent decrease in halothane anesthetic requirements (MAC) (Fig. 6-3) (White et al, 1975). This decrease in anesthetic requirement persists for several hours. Halothane, and presumably other volatile anesthetics, prolongs the duration of action of ketamine by delaying both its redistribution to inactive tissue sites and its metabolism (White et al, 1976).

Ketamine-induced enhancement of nondepolarizing neuromuscular blocking drugs may reflect interference by ketamine with calcium ion binding or its transport (Johnston et al, 1974). Alternatively, ketamine may decrease sensitivity of postjunctional membranes to neuromuscular blocking drugs. The duration of apnea following administration of succinylcholine is prolonged, possibly reflecting inhibition of plasma cholinesterase activity by ketamine. Pancuronium may enhance the cardiac-stimulating effects of ketamine.

Seizures have been described in asthmatic patients receiving aminophylline followed by administration of ketamine (Hirshman et al, 1982). Furthermore, in animals, aminophylline or ketamine alone does not alter the seizure threshold, but the combination of these two drugs reduces the seizure threshold.

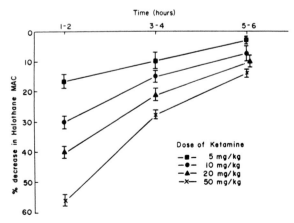

FIGURE 6–3. Ketamine produces dose-dependent decreases in halothane anesthetic requirements (MAC) in animals. Mean ± SE. (From White PF, Johnston RR, Rudwill CR. Interaction of ketamine and halothane in rats. Anesthesiology 1975; 42: 179–86; with permission.)

Emergence Delirium

Emergence from ketamine anesthesia in the postoperative period may be associated with visual, auditory, proprioceptive, and confusional illusions, which may progress to delirium. Cortical blindness may be transiently present. Dreams and hallucinations can occur up to 24 hours after administration of ketamine. The dreams frequently have a morbid content and are often experienced in vivid technicolor. Dreams and hallucinations usually disappear within a few hours.

MECHANISMS. Emergence delirium probably occurs secondary to ketamine-induced depression of the inferior colliculus and medial geniculate nucleus, leading to misinterpretation of auditory and visual stimuli (White et al, 1982). Furthermore, the loss of skin and musculoskeletal sensations results in decreased ability to perceive gravity, thereby producing a sensation of bodily detachment or floating in space.

INCIDENCE. The observed incidence of emergence delirium following ketamine ranges from 5% to 30% (White et al, 1982). Factors associated with an increased incidence of emergence delirium include (1) age greater than 16 years, (2) female sex, (3) doses of ketamine greater than 2 mg·kg^{-1} IV, and (4) a history of personality problems or frequent dreaming (White et al, 1982). It is possible that the incidence of dreaming is similar in children, but this age group is often unable to communicate the dream occurrence. Indeed, there are reports of recurrent hallucinations in children as well as in adults receiving ketamine (Fine and Finestone, 1973; Meyers and Charles, 1978). Nevertheless, psychological changes in children following anesthesia with ketamine or inhaled drugs are not different (Modvig and Nielsen, 1977). Likewise, no significant long-term personality differences are present in adults receiving ketamine compared with thiopental (Moretti et al, 1984).

Emergence delirium occurs less frequently when ketamine is used repeatedly. For example, it is rare for emergence delirium to occur after the third or more anesthetics with ketamine. Finally, inhaled anesthetics can also produce auditory, visual, proprioceptive, and confusional illusions, but the incidence of such phenomena, especially unpleasant experiences, is indeed greater following anesthesia that includes administration of ketamine.

PREVENTION. A variety of drugs used in preoperative medication or as adjuvants during maintenance of anesthesia have been evaluated in attempts to prevent emergence delirium following administration of ketamine. Benzodiazepines have proven the most effective in the prevention of this phenomenon, with midazolam being more effective than diazepam (Cartwright and Pingel, 1984; Toft and Romer, 1987). A common approach is to administer the benzodiazepine intravenously about 5 minutes prior to induction of anesthesia with ketamine. Inclusion of thiopental or inhaled anesthetics may decrease the incidence of emergence delirium attributed to ketamine. Conversely, the inclusion of atropine or droperidol in the preoperative medication may increase the incidence of emergence delirium (Erbguth et al, 1972).

Despite contrary opinions, there is no evidence that permitting patients to awaken from ketamine anesthesia in quiet areas alters the incidence of emergence delirium (Hejja and Galloon, 1975). Prospective discussion with the patient of the common side effects of ketamine (dreams, floating sensations, blurred vision) is likely to reduce the incidence of emergence delirium as much as any other approach (White et al, 1982).

ETOMIDATE

Etomidate is a carboxylated imidazole-containing compound that is chemically unrelated to any other drug used for the induction of anesthesia (Fig. 6-4). The imidazole nucleus renders etomidate, like midazolam, water soluble at an acidic pH and lipid soluble at physiologic pH. Following an induction dose of 0.3 mg·kg^{-1} IV, the onset of unconsciousness occurs within one arm-to-brain circulation time. As with thiopental,

FIGURE 6–4. Etomidate.

an age-related pharmacokinetic change and not an alteration in brain responsiveness is the most likely explanation for the decrease in dose requirements for etomidate observed in elderly patients (Arden et al, 1986). Central nervous system depression may reflect a gamma-aminobutyric acid–like action of etomidate. Awakening following a single intravenous dose of etomidate is more rapid than after barbiturates, and there is little or no evidence of a hangover or cumulative drug effect. Recovery of psychomotor function after administration of etomidate is intermediate between methohexital and thiopental. Duration of action is prolonged by increasing the dose of etomidate or administering the drug as a continuous intravenous infusion. As with barbiturates, analgesia is not produced by etomidate. For this reason, administration of an opioid prior to induction of anesthesia with etomidate may be useful so as to blunt the hemodynamic responses evoked by direct laryngoscopy and intubation of the trachea.

Etomidate may be an alternative to barbiturates for intravenous induction of anesthesia in the presence of an unstable cardiovascular system or decreased intravascular fluid volume. Another use of etomidate is induction of anesthesia for brief outpatient surgical procedures. Continuous intravenous infusion of etomidate with intermittent injections of opioid can be used for more prolonged surgical procedures. Etomidate does not trigger malignant hyperthermia in susceptible swine (Suresh and Nelson, 1985).

The principal limiting factor in the clinical use of etomidate for induction of anesthesia is the unknown significance of the ability of this drug to depress adrenocortical function transiently (see the section entitled "Adrenocortical Suppression"). Nausea and vomiting are more common after induction of anesthesia with etomidate than with thiopental (Holdcroft et al, 1976). Etomidate does not evoke the release of histamine, and the incidence of allergic reactions is infrequent.

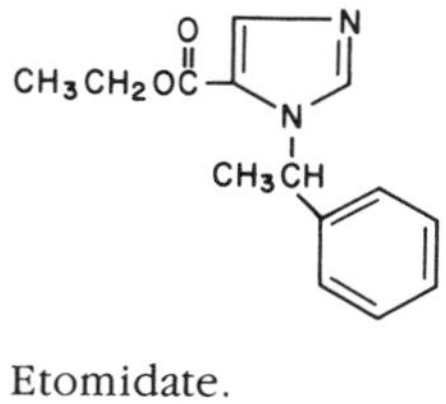

Pharmacokinetics

The volume of distribution of etomidate is larger than body weight, suggesting considerable tissue uptake (Table 6-1). Distribution of etomidate throughout body water is favored by its moderate lipid solubility and existence as a weak base (pK

4.2). Etomidate penetrates the brain rapidly, reaching peak levels within 1 minutes after intravenous injection. About 76% of etomidate is bound to albumin independently of the plasma concentration of drug. Reductions in plasma albumin concentrations, however, result in dramatic increases in the free plasma concentrations of etomidate. Prompt awakening after a single intravenous dose of etomidate reflects principally the redistribution of the drug from brain to inactive tissue sites. Rapid metabolism is also likely to contribute to prompt recovery.

Metabolism

Etomidate is rapidly metabolized by hydrolysis of the ethyl ester side chain to its carboxylic acid ester, resulting in a pharmacologically inactive compound. Hepatic microsomal enzymes and plasma esterases are responsible for this hydrolysis. Hydrolysis is nearly complete, as evidenced by recovery of less than 3% of an administered dose of etomidate as unchanged drug in the urine. About 85% of a single intravenous dose of etomidate can be accounted for as carboxylic acid ester metabolite in the urine, whereas another 10% to 13% is present as this metabolite in the bile. Overall, the clearance for etomidate is five times that for thiopental; this is reflected as a shorter elimination half-time of 2 to 5 hours.

Side Effects

Central Nervous System

Etomidate is a potent direct cerebral vasoconstrictor that decreases cerebral blood flow and cerebral metabolic oxygen requirements 35% to 45% (Milde et al, 1985). As a result, previously elevated intracranial pressure is lowered by etomidate. These changes are similar to those changes produced by similar doses of thiopental.

Etomidate, like methohexital, may activate seizure foci manifesting as fast activity on the EEG (Ebrahim et al, 1986). For this reason, etomidate should be used with caution in patients with focal epilepsy. Conversely, this characteristic of etomidate may be used to facilitate location of a seizure focus in patients undergoing cortical resection of epileptogenic tissue. Etomidate has been observed to augment the ampli-

tude of somatosensory evoked potentials, making monitoring of these responses more reliable (Sloan et al, 1988).

Cardiovascular System

Cardiovascular stability is characteristic in patients receiving etomidate. Administration of etomidate, 0.3 mg·kg^{-1} IV, evokes minimal changes in heart rate, stroke volume, or cardiac output, whereas mean arterial pressure may decrease up to 15% because of reductions in systemic vascular resistance. In animals, etomidate decreases myocardial contractility less than equally potent doses of thiopental (Kissin et al, 1983). Etomidate does not result in detrimental effects when accidentally injected into an artery. In contrast to other intravenous anesthetics and volatile anesthetics, etomidate does not decrease renal blood flow. Hepatic and renal function tests are not altered by etomidate. Intraocular pressure is lowered by etomidate to a similar degree as by thiopental.

Ventilation

The depressant effects of etomidate on ventilation seem to be less than those of barbiturates, although apnea may occasionally accompany a rapid intravenous injection of the drug (Choi et al, 1985). In the majority of patients, etomidate-induced reductions in tidal volume are offset by compensatory increases in the frequency of breathing. These effects on ventilation are transient, lasting only 3 to 5 minutes. Etomidate may stimulate ventilation independently of the medullary centers that normally respond to carbon dioxide. For this reason, etomidate may be useful when maintenance of spontaneous ventilation is desirable. Depression of ventilation may be exaggerated when etomidate is combined with inhaled anesthetics or opioids during continuous intravenous infusion techniques.

Pain on Injection

Pain occurring during intravenous injection of etomidate is frequent, manifesting in up to 80% of patients (Holdcroft et al, 1976). Pain is most likely to occur when etomidate is injected into small veins. Preparation of etomidate without the addition of propylene glycol reduces the incidence of pain, as does inclusion of an opioid in the preoperative medication and injection of etomidate into a large vein.

Myoclonus

Involuntary muscle movements characterized as myoclonus occur in about one third of patients during induction of anesthesia with etomidate. These involuntary skeletal muscle movements associated with etomidate occur with a greater frequency than with methohexital, whereas the incidence of hiccough is similar for both drugs. Prior administration of an opioid (fentanyl, 1 to 2 μg·kg^{-1} IV) or a benzodiazepine may reduce the incidence of myoclonus associated with administration of etomidate.

Although myoclonus may resemble seizures, it is not considered hazardous and is not associated with epileptiform discharges on the EEG. The mechanism of etomidate-induced myoclonus appears to be disinhibition of subcortical structures that normally suppress extrapyramidal motor activity. It is possible that myoclonus could occur on awakening if the extrapyramidal system emerged more quickly than the cortex that inhibits it (Laughlin and Newberg, 1985).

Adrenocortical Suppression

Etomidate causes adrenocortical suppression by producing a dose-dependent inhibition of the conversion of cholesterol to cortisol (Fig. 6-5) (Fragen et al, 1984; Wagner et al, 1984). The specific enzyme inhibited by etomidate appears to be 11-beta-hydroxylase as evidenced by the accumulation of 11-deoxycorticosterone (Owen and Spence, 1984). This enzyme inhibition lasts 4 to 8 hours after an induction dose of etomidate. Conceivably, patients experiencing sepsis or hemorrhage that might require an adequate cortisol response would be at a disadvantage should etomidate be administered (Longnecker, 1984). Conversely, suppression of adrenocortical function could be considered desirable from the standpoint of "stress-free" anesthesia. Nevertheless, in at least one report, it was not possible to demonstrate a difference in the plasma concentrations of cortisol, corticosterone, or adrenocorticotrophic in patients receiving a single dose of etomidate or thiopental (Duthie et al, 1985).

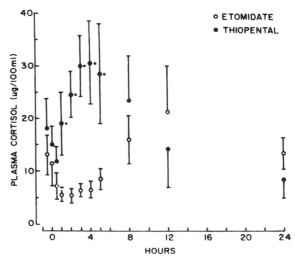

FIGURE 6–5. Etomidate, but not thiopental, is associated with decreases in the plasma concentrations of cortisol. *P <0.05 compared with thiopental. Mean ± SD. (From Fragen RJ, Shanks CA, Molteni A, Abram MJ. Effects of etomidate on hormonal responses to surgical stress. Anesthesiology 1984; 61: 652–6; with permission.)

PROPOFOL

Propofol is a substituted isopropylphenol that is administered intravenously as a 1% solution in an aqueous solution of 10% soybean oil, 2.25% glycerol, and 1.2% purified egg phosphatide (Fig. 6-6) (Sebel and Lowdon, 1989; Shafer et al, 1988). Administration of propofol, 2 to 2.5 mg·kg^{-1} IV (equivalent to thiopental, 4 to 5 mg·kg^{-1} IV, or methohexital, 1.5 mg·kg^{-1} IV) over 15 seconds or less produces unconsciousness within about 30 seconds. Awakening is more rapid and complete than that following induction of anesthesia with thiopental or methohexital. This more rapid return to consciousness with minimal residual central nervous system effects seems to be the most important advantage of propofol over other drugs used to produce induction of anesthesia.

Pharmacokinetics

Clearance of propofol, from the plasma exceeds hepatic blood flow, emphasizing that tissue up-

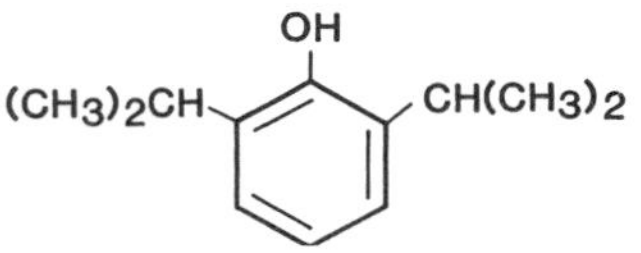

FIGURE 6–6.   Propofol.

take as well as metabolism is important in removal of this drug from the plasma (Table 6-1). Less than 0.3% of a dose is excreted unchanged in the urine along with inactive glucuronide and sulfate conjugates. The elimination half-time is 0.5 to 1.5 hours.

Despite the rapid clearance of propofol by metabolism, there is no evidence of impaired elimination in patients with cirrhosis. Renal dysfunction does not influence the clearance of propofol. Patients older than 60 years of age exhibit a reduced rate of plasma clearance of propofol compared with younger adults. The rapid clearance of propofol from the plasma suggests this drug could be administered as a continuous intravenous infusion without an excessive cumulative effect. Continuous intravenous infusion rates decrease with long operations, suggesting a modest cumulative effect, especially in elderly patients. Propofol readily crosses the placenta but is rapidly cleared from the neonatal circulation (Dailland et al, 1989).

Clinical Uses

Propofol, because of its rapid onset and prompt recovery without residual sedation, is a useful drug for intravenous induction of anesthesia, especially for outpatient surgery or otherwise brief procedures (cardioversion, electroconvulsive therapy) requiring a short period of unconsciousness. Propofol does not alter the effects of succinylcholine. The efficient clearance of propofol from the plasma minimizes the likelihood of cumulative drug effects, permitting continuous intravenous infusions of propofol during maintenance of anesthesia as the sole anesthetic or as adjuvant to inhaled or injected (opioids, benzodiazepines) drugs. In the presence of nitrous oxide (67%), the continuous intravenous infusion rate of propofol necessary to prevent skeletal muscle movement in 95% of patients (ED_{95}) is about 112 $\mu g \cdot kg^{-1} \cdot min^{-1}$ (Spelina et al, 1986). Continuous intravenous infusions of propofol, 1 to 2.8 $mg \cdot kg^{-1} \cdot h^{-1}$ does not produce evidence of

adrenocortical suppression when administered to produce sedation in critically ill patients.

Side Effects

Central Nervous System

In brain-injured patients, propofol, 2 $mg \cdot kg^{-1}$ IV, followed by 150 $\mu g \cdot kg^{-1} \cdot min^{-1}$ IV, results in decreased cerebral perfusion pressure, cerebral blood flow, and intracranial pressure (Pinaud et al, 1990). In these same patients, propofol did not exert a consistent effect on cerebral vascular resistance and the cerebral arteriovenous oxygen content difference was unchanged. The reactivity of cerebral vessels to changes in $PaCO_2$ seems to be maintained during anesthesia with propofol. Propofol increases the latency and decreases the amplitude of somatosensory evoked potentials.

Cardiovascular System

Propofol produces reductions in blood pressure that are greater than those evoked by comparable doses of thiopental. These decreases in blood pressure are often accompanied by corresponding changes in cardiac output or systemic vascular resistance. Stimulation produced by direct laryngoscopy and intubation of the trachea reverses the blood pressure effects of propofol, although this drug is more effective than thiopental in blunting the magnitude of this pressor response. Blood pressure effects of propofol may be exaggerated in hypovolemic patients, elderly patients, and in patients with compromised left ventricular function owing to coronary artery disease. Addition of nitrous oxide does not alter the cardiovascular effects of propofol.

Despite decreases in blood pressure, heart rate often remains unchanged in contrast to the modest increases that typically accompany the rapid intravenous injection of thiopental. This stable heart rate in spite of drug-induced decreases in blood pressure is speculated to reflect a sympatholytic or vagotonic effect of propofol. Bradycardia and/or heart block has been observed following induction of anesthesia with propofol, resulting in the occasional recommendation that anticholinergic drugs be given when vagal stimulation is likely to occur in association with use of this drug (James et al, 1989). Baroreceptor reflex sensitivity does not appear to be altered by propofol.

Ventilation

Propofol is a profound depressant of ventilation, causing many patients to become transiently apneic following rapid intravenous injection of the drug. Opioids administered with the preoperative medication may enhance this ventilatory depressant effect. Painful surgical stimulation is likely to counteract the ventilatory depressant effects of propofol.

Hepatic or Renal Function

Propofol does not adversely affect hepatic or renal function as reflected by measurement of liver transaminase enzymes or creatinine concentrations. Prolonged intravenous infusions of propofol may result in excretion of green urine, reflecting the presence of phenols in the urine. This discoloration does not alter renal function.

Coagulation

Propofol does not alter tests of coagulation or platelet function. This is reassuring since the emulsion in which propofol is dispensed resembles Intralipid, which has been associated with alterations in blood coagulation.

Allergic Reactions

The emulsion formulation of propofol appears to be devoid of allergic potential. Changes in plasma histamine concentrations do not follow the intravenous administration of propofol.

Site of Injection

Pain on injection of propofol occurs in fewer than 10% of patients if intravenous injection is into a large arm vein vs the dorsum of the hand. The incidence of thrombosis or phlebitis after intravenous injection of propofol is usually less than 1%. An accidental injection of propofol into the radial artery was accompanied by severe pain in the hand but no evidence of vascular compromise or sequelae (Holley and Cuthrell, 1990).

Miscellaneous Effects

Propofol does not block the secretion of cortisol following single doses for intravenous induction of anesthesia or as a continuous intravenous infu-sion for as long as 24 hours to provide sedation in the intensive care unit. Excitatory responses such as hypertonus, tremor, hiccough, or spontaneous movement with induction of anesthesia with propofol are rare. Nausea and vomiting are infrequent in patients receiving propofol. Nevertheless, an antiemetic effect of the lipid emulsion portion of propofol has not been documented (Ostman et al, 1990). Intraocular pressure is decreased by propofol. Propofol does not trigger malignant hyperthermia in susceptible swine, and exacerbation of intermittent porphyria is reported not to occur when propofol is used as the sole anesthetic (Raff and Harrison, 1989; Sebel and Lowdon, 1989). The vehicle for propofol does not contain antibacterial preservatives, emphasizing the importance of maintaining strict asepsis when handling the drug and the need to discard any unused drug at the conclusion of single patient use. Postoperative temperature elevations have been attributed to failure to observe aseptic techniques, leading to bacterial contamination of propofol.

REFERENCES

Akamatsu TJ, Bonica JJ, Rehmet R. Experiences with the use of ketamine for parturition. I. Primary anesthetic for vaginal delivery. Anesth Analg 1974; 53;284–7.

Arden JR, Holley FO, Stanski DR. Increased sensitivity to etomidate in the elderly: Initial distribution versus altered brain response. Anesthesiology 1986; 65:19–27.

Balfors E, Haggmark S, Nyhman H, et al. Droperidol inhibits the effects of intravenous ketamine on central hemodynamics and myocardial O_2 consumption in patients with generalized atherosclerotic disease. Anesth Analg 1983;62:193–7.

Baraka A, Harrison T, Kachachi T. Catecholamine levels after ketamine anesthesia in man. Anesth Analg 1973;52:198–200.

Bidwai AV, Stanley TH, Graves CL, Kawamura R, Sentker CR. The effects of ketamine on cardiovascular dynamics during halothane and enflurane anesthesia. Anesth Analg 1975;54:588–92.

Borondy PE, Glasko AJ. Inhibition of ketamine metabolism by diazepam. Fed Proc 1977;36:938.

Cartwright PD, Pingel SM. Midazolam and diazepam in ketamine anaesthesia. Anaesthesia 1984;59:439–42.

Celesia GG, Chen R-C, Bamforth BJ. Effects of ketamine in epilepsy. Neurology 1975;25:169–72.

Choi SD, Spaulding BC, Gross JB, Apfelbaum JL. Comparison of the ventilatory effects of etomidate and methohexital. Anesthesiology 1985;62:442–7.

Dailland P, Cockshott ID, Lirzin JD, et al. Intravenous propofol during cesarean section: Placental transfer, concentrations in breast milk, and neonatal effects. A preliminary study. Anesthesiology 1989;71:827–34.

Demling RH, Ellerbee S, Jarrett F. Ketamine anesthesia for tangential excision of burn eschar: A burn unit procedure. J Trauma 1978;18:269–70.

Dershwitz M, Sreter FA, Ryan JF. Ketamine does not trigger malignant hyperthermia in susceptible swine. Anesth Analg 1989;69:501–3.

Duthie DJR, Fraser R, Nimmo WS. Effect of induction of anaesthesia with etomidate on corticosteroid synthesi in man. Br J Anaesth 1985;57:156-9.

Ebrahim ZY, DeBoer GE, Luders H, Hahn JF, Lesser RP. Effect of etomidate on the electroencephalogram of patients with epilepsy. Anesth Analg 1986;65:1004–6.

Erbguth PH, Reiman B, Klein RL. The influence of chlorpromazine, diazepam and droperidol on emergence from ketamine. Anesth Analg 1972;51:693–700.

Ferrer-Allado T, Brechner VL, Diamond A, Cozen H, Crandall P. Ketamine-induced electroconvulsive phenomena in the human limbic and thalamic regions. Anesthesiology 1973;38:333–44.

Fine J, Finestone SC. Sensory disturbances following ketamine anesthesia: Recurrent hallucinations. Anesth Analg 1973;52:428–30.

Fragen RJ, Avram MJ. Comparative pharmacology of drugs used for the induction of anesthesia. In: Stoelting RK, Barash PG, Gallagher TJ, eds. Advances in Anesthesia. Chicago, Year Book Medical Publishers, 1986:103–32.

Fragen RJ, Shanks CA, Molteni A, Abram MJ. Effects of etomidate on hormonal responses to surgical stress. Anesthesiology 1984;61:652–6.

Friesen RH, Thieme RE, Honda AT, Morrison JE. Changes in anterior fontanel pressure in preterm neonates receiving isoflurane, halothane, fentanyl, or ketamine. Anesth Analg 1987;66:431–4.

Hejja P, Galloon S. A consideration of ketamine dreams. Can Anaesth Soc J 1975;22:100–5.

Hickey PR, Hansen DD, Cramolini GM, Vincent RN, Lang P. Pulmonary and systemic hemodynamic responses to ketamine in infants with normal and elevated pulmonary vascular resistance. Anesthesiology 1985;62:287–93.

Hirshman CA, Downes H, Farbood A, Bergman NA. Ketamine block of bronchospasm in experimental canine asthma. Br J Anaesth 1979;51:713–8.

Hirshman CA, Krieger W, Littlejohn G, Lee R, Julien R. Ketamine-aminophylline–induced decreased in seizure threshold. Anesthesiology 1982;56:464–7.

Hodgkinson K, Marx GF, Kim SS, Miclat NM. Neonatal neurobehavioral tests following vaginal delivery under ketamine, thiopental, and extradural anesthesia. Anesth Analg 1977;56:548–53.

Holdcroft A, Morgan M, Whitman JG, Lumley J. Effect of dose and premedication on induction complications with etomidate. Br J Anaesth 1976;48:199–205.

Holley HS, Cuthrell L. Intraarterial injection of propofol. Anesthesiology 1990;73:183–4.

Islas J-A, Astorga J, Larado M. Epidural ketamine for control of postoperative pain. Anesth Analg 1985; 4:1161–2.

James MFM, Reyneke CJ, Whiffler K. Heart block following propofol: A case report. Br J Anaesth 1989;62:213–5.

Janeczko GF, El-Etr AA, Younes S. Low-dose ketamine anesthesia for obstetrical delivery. Anesth Analg 1974;53:828–31.

Johnston RR, Miller RD, Way WL. The interaction of ketamine with d-tubocurarine, pancuronium, and succinylcholine in man. Anesth Analg 1974; 53:496–501.

Kissin I, Motomura S, Aultman BS, Reves JG. Inotropic and anesthetic potencies of etomidate and thiopental in dogs. Anesth Analg 1983;62:961–5.

Koehntop DE, Liao J-C, Van Bergen FH. Effects of pharmacologic alterations of adrenergic mechanisms by cocaine, tropolene, aminophylline and ketamine on epinephrine-induced arrhythmias during halothane-nitrous oxide anesthesia. Anesthesiology 1977;46:83–93.

Kostrzewski E, Gregor A. Ketamine in acute intermittent porphyria—dangerous or safe? Anesthesiology 1978;49:376–7.

Laughlin TP, Newberg LA. Prolonged myoclonus after etomidate anesthesia. Anesth Analg 1985;64:80–2.

Longnecker DE. Stress free: To be or not to be? Anesthesiology 1984;61:643–4.

Longnecker DE, Sturgill BC. Influence of anesthetic agents on survival following hemorrhage. Anesthesiology 1976;45:516–21.

Meyers EF, Charles P. Prolonged adverse reactions to ketamine in children. Anesthesiology 1978;49:39–40.

Milde LN, Milde JH, Michenfelder JD. Cerebral functional, metabolic, and hemodynamic effects of etomidate in dogs. Anesthesiology 1985;63:371–7.

Modvig KM, Nielsen SF. Psychological changes in children after anesthesia: A comparison between halothane and ketamine. Acta Anaesthesol Scand 1977;21:541–4.

Moretti RJ, Hassan SZ, Goodman LI, Meltzer HY. Comparison of ketamine and thiopental in healthy volunteers: Effects on mental status, mood, and personality. Anesth Analg 1984;63:1087–96.

Ostman PL, Gaure E, Glosten B, Kemen M, Robert MK, Bedwell S. Is the antiemetic effect of the emulsion formulation of propofol due to the lipid emulsion? Anesth Analg 1990;71:536–40.

Owen H, Spence AA. Etomidate. Br J Anaesth 1984;56:555–7.

Pfenninger E, Dick W, Ahnefeld FW. The influence of ketamine on both normal and raised intracranial pressure of artificially ventilated animals. Eur J Anesthesiol 1985;2:297–307.

Pinaud M, Leausque J-N, Chetanneau A, Fauchoux N, Menegalli D, Souron R. Effects of propofol on cerebral hemodynamics and metabolism in patients with brain trauma. Anesthesiology 1990;73:404–9.

Raff M, Harrison GG. The screening of propofol in MHS swine. Anesth Analg 1989;68:750–1.

Reich DL, Silvay G. Ketamine: An update on the first twenty-five years of clinical experience. Can J Anaesth 1989;36:186–97.

Reves JG, Lell WA, McCracken LE, Kravetz RA, Prough DS. Comparison of morphine and ketamine. Anesthetic techniques for coronary surgery: A randomized study. South Med J 1978;71:33–6.

Schubert A, Licine MG, Lineberry PJ. The effect of ketamine on human somatosensory evoked potentials and its modification by nitrous oxide. Anesthesiology 1990;72:33–9.

Schwartz DA, Horwitz LD. Effects of ketamine on left ventricular performance. J Pharmacol Exp Ther 1975;194:410–4.

Sebel PS, Lowdon JD. Propofol: A new intravenous anesthetic. Anesthesiology 1989;71:260–77.

Shafer A, Doze VA, Shafer SF, White PF. Pharmacokinetics and pharmacodynamics of propofol infusions during general anesthesia. Anesthesiology 1988;69:348–56.

Sloan TB, Ronai AK, Toleikis R, et al. Improvement of intraoperative somatosensory evoked potentials by etomidate. Anesth Analg 1988;67:582–5.

Soliman MG, Brinale GF, Kuster G. Response to hypercapnia under ketamine anesthesia. Can Anaesth Soc J 1975;22:486–94.

Spelina KR, Coates DP, Monk CR, Prys-Roberts C, Morley I, Turtle MJ. Dose requirements of propofol by infusion during nitrous oxide anesthesia in man. I: Patients premedicated with morphine sulfate. Br J Anaesth 1986;58:1080–4.

Stanley TH. Blood pressure and pulse rate responses to ketamine during general anesthesia. Anesthesiology 1973;39:648–9.

Suresh MS, Nelson TE. Malignant hyperthermia: Is etomidate safe? Anesth Analg 1985;64:420–4.

Takeshita H, Okuda Y, Sari A. The effects of ketamine on cerebral circulation and metabolism in man. Anesthesiology 1972;36:69–75.

Takeyasu Y, Harada K, Okamura A, Kemmotsu O. Is the site of action of ketamine anesthesia the N-methyl-D-aspartate receptor? Anesthesiology 1990;72:704–10.

Taylor PA, Towey RM. Depression of laryngeal reflexes during ketamine anesthesia. Br Med J 1971;2:688–9.

Thorsen T, Gran L. Ketamine/diazepam infusion anesthesia with special attention to the effect on cerebral spinal fluid pressure and arterial blood pressure. Acta Anaesthesiol Scand 1980;24:1–4.

Toft P, Romer U. Comparison of midazolam and diazepam to supplement total intravenous anaesthesia with ketamine for endoscopy. Can J Anaesth 1987; 34:466–9.

Toro-Matos A, Rendon-Platas AM, Avila-Valdez E, Villarrel-Guzman RA. Physostigmine antagonizes ketamine. Anesth Analg 1980;59:764–7.

Traber DL, Wilson RD, Priano LL. Blockade of the hypertensive response to ketamine. Anesth Analg 1970;49:420–6.

Tweed WA, Minuck MS, Mymin D. Circulatory response to ketamine anesthesia. Anesthesiology 1972; 37:613–9.

Wagner RL, White PF, Kan PB, Rosenthal MH, Feldman D. Inhibition of adrenal steroidogenesis by the anesthetic etomidate. N Engl J Med 1984;310:1415–21.

Weiskopf RB, Townley MI, Riordan KK, Baysinger M, Mahoney E. Comparison of cardiopulmonary responses to graded hemorrhage during enflurane, halothane, isoflurane and ketamine anesthesia. Anesth Analg 1981;60:481–92.

White PF, Ham J, Way WL, Trevor AJ. Pharmacology of ketamine isomers in surgical patients. Anesthesiology 1980;52:231–9.

White PF, Johnston RR, Rudwill CR. Interaction of ketamine and halothane in rats. Anesthesiology 1975;42:179–86.

White PF, Marietta MP, Pudwill CR, Way WL, Trevor AJ. Effects of halothane anesthesia on the biodisposition of ketamine in rats. J Pharmacol Exp Ther 1976;196:545–55.

White PF, Way WL, Trevor AJ. Ketamine: Its pharmacology and therapeutic uses. Anesthesiology 1982; 56:119–36.

Wong DHW, Jenkins LC. An experimental study of the mechanism of action of ketamine on the central nervous system. Can Anaesth Soc J 1974;21:57–67.

Yamamura T, Harada K, Okamura A, Kemmotsu O. Is the site of action of ketamine anesthesia the N-Methyl-D-aspartate receptor? Anesthesiology 1990; 72:704–10.

Chapter

7

Local Anesthetics

Local anesthetics are drugs that produce reversible conduction blockade of impulses along central and peripheral nerve pathways following regional anesthesia. With progressive increases in concentrations of local anesthetics, the transmission of autonomic, somatic sensory, and somatic motor impulses is interrupted, producing autonomic nervous system blockade, sensory anesthesia, and skeletal muscle paralysis in the area innervated by the affected nerve. Removal of the local anesthetic is followed by spontaneous and complete return of nerve conduction with no evidence of structural damage to nerve fibers as a result of the drug's effects.

Cocaine was introduced as the first local anesthetic in 1884 by Kollar for use in ophthalmology. Halsted recognized the ability of injected cocaine to interrupt nerve impulse conduction leading to the introduction of peripheral nerve block anesthesia and spinal anesthesia. As an ester of benzoic acid, cocaine is present in large amounts in the leaves of *Erythroxylon coca,* a tree growing in the Andes mountains, where its cerebral stimulating qualities are well known. Another unique feature of cocaine is its ability to produce localized vasoconstriction, making it popular to use in rhinolaryngologic procedures and nasotracheal intubation to shrink the nasal mucosa. Abuse potential of cocaine limits its legitimate medical uses, whereas irritant properties of cocaine preclude its use for topical anesthesia of the cornea or any form of injection to produce anesthesia (see the section entitled "Cocaine Toxicity").

The first synthetic local anesthetic was the ester derivative, procaine, introduced by Einhorn in 1905. Lidocaine was synthesized as an amide local anesthetic by Lofgren in 1943. It produces more rapid, intense, and long-lasting conduction blockade than procaine. Unlike procaine, lidocaine is effective topically and is a highly efficacious cardiac antidysrhythmic drug. For these reasons, lidocaine is the standard to which all other local anesthetics are compared.

COMMERCIAL PREPARATIONS

Local anesthetics are poorly soluble in water and, therefore, are marketed most often as water-soluble hydrochloride salts. These hydrochloride salt solutions are acidic (pH 6), contributing to the stability of the local anesthetic. An acidic pH is also important if epinephrine is present in the local anesthetic solution, because this catecholamine is unstable at an alkaline pH. Sodium bisulfite, which is strongly acidic, may be added to commercially prepared local anesthetic–epinephrine solutions (pH 4) to prevent oxidative decomposition of epinephrine.

Carbonated local anesthetic solutions (pH 6.5) have been suggested as an alternative to hydrochloride preparations. An alleged more rapid onset of action and intensity of blockade produced by carbonated lidocaine is attributed to diffusion of carbon dioxide into tissues to reduce pH and create a more favorable distribution of local anesthetic (Bromage et al, 1974). Conceptually, carbon dioxide more readily converts the local anesthetic amide to the more active ammonium ion by lowering the pH inside the membrane. Despite these perceived advantages, some studies have failed to document a more rapid onset of blockade with carbonated local anes-

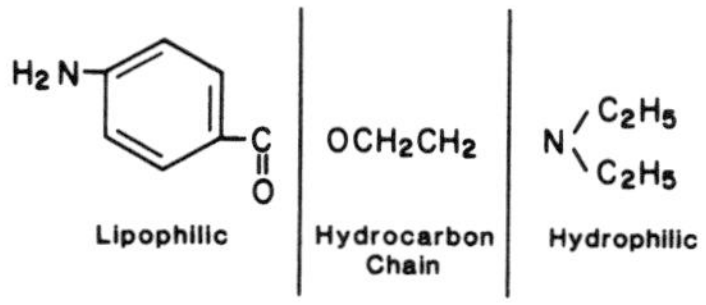

FIGURE 7–1. Local anesthetics consist of a lipophilic and hydrophilic portion separated by a connecting hydrocarbon chain.

thetic solutions, and this form of commercial preparation has not achieved widespread popularity.

STRUCTURE ACTIVITY RELATIONSHIPS

Local anesthetics consist of a lipophilic and a hydrophilic portion separated by a connecting hydrocarbon chain (Fig. 7-1). The hydrophilic group is usually a tertiary amine, such as diethylamine, whereas the lipophilic portion is usually an unsaturated aromatic ring, such as para-amino-

benzoic acid. The lipophilic portion is essential for anesthetic activity, and therapeutically useful local anesthetics require a delicate balance between lipid solubility and water solubility. In almost all instances, an ester (-CO-) or an amide (-NHC-) bond links the hydrocarbon chain to the lipophilic aromatic ring. The nature of this bond is the basis for classifying drugs that produce conduction blockade of nerve impulses as ester local anesthetics or amide local anesthetics (Fig. 7-2). The important differences between ester and amide local anesthetics relate to the site of metabolism and the potential to produce allergic reactions.

Modifying the chemical structure of a local anesthetic alters its pharmacologic effects. For example, lengthening the connecting hydrocarbon chain or increasing the number of carbon atoms on the tertiary amine or aromatic ring often results in a drug with a different lipid solubility, potency, rate of metabolism, and duration of action (Table 7-1; Fig. 7-1). Indeed, substituting a

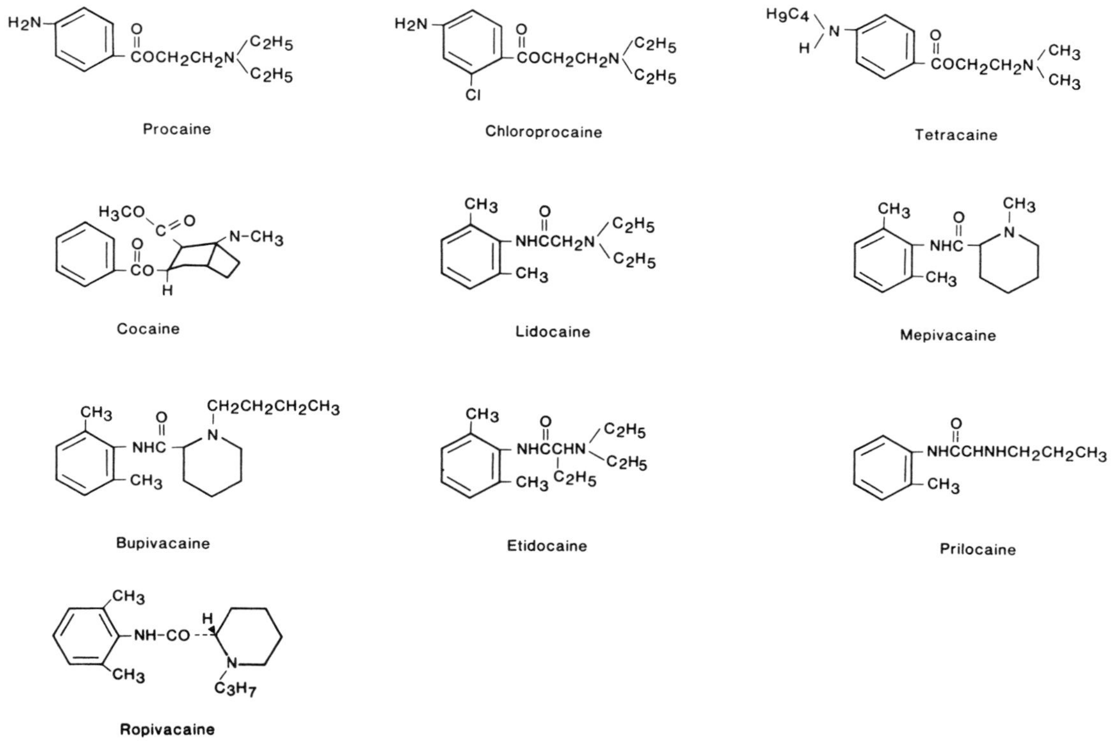

FIGURE 7–2. Ester and amide local anesthetics.

Table 7–1

Comparative Pharmacology of Local Anesthetics

Classification	Potency	Onset	Duration After Infiltration (min)	Maximum Single Dose For Infiltration (adult, mg)*
Esters				
Procaine	1	Slow	45–60	500
Chloroprocaine	4	Rapid	30–45	600
Tetracaine	16	Slow	60–180	100 (topical)
Amides				
Lidocaine	1	Rapid	60–120	300
Mepivacaine	1	Slow	90–180	300
Bupivacaine	4	Slow	240–480	175
Etidocaine	4	Slow	240–480	300
Prilocaine	1	Slow	60–120	400
Ropivacaine[†]				

Classification	Toxic Plasma Concentration ($\mu g \cdot ml^{-1}$)	pK	Fraction Nonionized (percent) pH 7.2	pH 7.4	pH 7.6	Protein Binding (percent)
Esters						
Procaine		8.9	2	3	5	6
Chloroprocaine		8.7	3	5	7	
Tetracaine		8.5	5	7	11	76
Amides						
Lidocaine	>5	7.9	17	25	33	70
Mepivacaine	>5	7.6	28	39	50	77
Bupivacaine	~1.5	8.1	11	15	24	95
Etidocaine	~2	7.7	24	33	44	94
Prilocaine	>5	7.9	17	24	33	55
Ropivacaine[†]	>4	8.1		94		

Classification	Lipid Solubility	Volume of Distribution (L)	Clearance ($L \cdot min^{-1}$)	Elimination Half-Times (min)
Esters				
Procaine	0.6			
Chloroprocaine				
Tetracaine	80			
Amides				
Lidocaine	2.9	91	0.95	96
Mepivacaine	1.0	84	9.78	114
Bupivacaine	28	73	0.47	210
Etidocaine	141	133	1.22	156
Prilocaine	0.9			
Ropivacaine[†]				

*Use only as guideline; dose may be increased if solution contains epinephrine.
[†]Resembles bupivacaine
(Reprinted from Covino BG, Vassallo, HL. Local anesthetics: Mechanisms of Action and Clinical Use. New York, Grune and Stratton, 1976, p. 73, with permission.)

butyl group for the amine group on the benzene ring of procaine results in tetracaine. Compared with procaine, tetracaine is more lipid soluble, is 10 times more potent, and has a longer duration of action corresponding to a four- to fivefold decrease in the rate of metabolism. Halogenation of procaine to chloroprocaine results in a three- to fourfold increase in the hydrolysis rate of chloroprocaine by plasma cholinesterase. This rapid hydrolysis rate of chloroprocaine limits the duration of action and systemic toxicity of this local anesthetic. Addition of a butyl group to the amine end of mepivacaine results in bupivacaine, which is 35 times more lipid soluble and has a potency and duration of action three to four times that of mepivacaine. Etidocaine resembles lidocaine, but substituting a propyl group for an ethyl group at the amine end and adding an ethyl group on the alpha carbon of the connecting hydrocarbon chain produces a 50-fold increase in lipid solubility and a two- to threefold increase in the duration of action. Ropivacaine structurally resembles bupivacaine and mepivacaine but is prepared as a specific isomer rather than as a racemic mixture such as bupivacaine (see the section entitled "Ropivacaine"). Systemic toxicity as reflected by cardiac depression may be less with the isomer than with the racemic preparations of local anesthetics.

PHARMACOKINETICS

Local anesthetics are weak bases that have pH values somewhat above physiologic pH (Table 7-1). As a result, less than 50% of the local anesthetic exists in a lipid-soluble nonionized form at physiologic pH. For example, at pH 7.4, only 5% of tetracaine exists in a nonionized form. Acidosis in the environment into which the local anesthetic is injected—as is present with tissue infection—further increases the ionized fraction of drug. This is consistent with the poor quality of local anesthesia that often results when a local anesthetic is injected into an acidic infected area. Local anesthetics with pKs nearest to physiologic pH have the most rapid onset of action, reflecting the presence of an optimal ratio of ionized to nonionized drug fraction (Table 7-1).

Intrinsic vasodilator activity will also influence apparent potency and duration of action.

For example, the enhanced vasodilator action of lidocaine compared with mepivacaine results in greater vascular absorption and shorter duration of action of lidocaine. Bupivacaine and etidocaine produce similar vasodilation but plasma concentrations of bupivacaine after epidural placement exceed those of etidocaine. Presumably, greater lipid solubility of etidocaine results in tissue sequestration and less available drug for systemic absorption. Occasional prolonged sensory blockade following injection of etidocaine has been attributed to tissue sequestration.

Absorption and Distribution

Absorption of a local anesthetic from its site of injection into the systemic circulation is influenced by the site of injection and dosage, use of epinephrine, and pharmacologic characteristics of the drug (Fig. 7-3) (Covino and Vassallo,

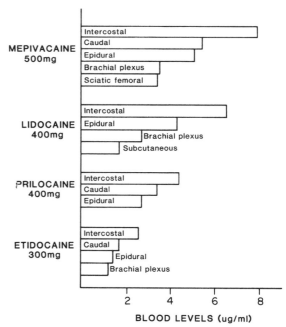

FIGURE 7-3. Peak plasma concentrations of local anesthetic are influenced by the site of injection for accomplishment of regional anesthesia. (From Covino BG, Vassallo HL. Local Anesthetics: Mechanisms of Action and Clinical Use. New York: Grune and Stratton, 1976; with permission.)

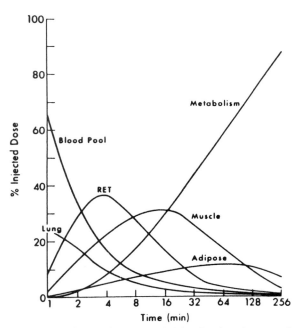

FIGURE 7–4. Perfusion model for the distribution of lidocaine in various tissues and its elimination after an intravenous infusion for 1 minute. RET, rapidly equilibrating (highly perfused) tissues. (From Benowitz N, Forsyth RP, Melmon KL, et al. Lidocaine disposition kinetics in monkey and man. I: Prediction by a perfusion model. Clin Pharmacol Ther: 1974; 16: 87–92; with permission.)

1976). The ultimate plasma concentration of a local anesthetic is determined by the rate of tissue distribution and the rate of clearance of the drug. For example, the intravenous infusion of lidocaine for 1 minute is followed by a rapid decline in the drug's plasma concentration that is paralleled by an initial high uptake into the lungs and distribution of the local anesthetic to highly perfused tissues, that is, the brain, heart, and kidneys (Fig. 7-4) (Benowitz et al, 1974). Lipid solubility of the local anesthetic is important in this redistribution as well as being a primary determinant of intrinsic local anesthetic potency. After distribution to highly perfused tissues, the local anesthetic is redistributed to less well perfused tissues including skeletal muscles and fat. Finally, the local anesthetic is eliminated from the plasma by metabolism and excretion.

In addition to tissue blood flow and lipid solubility of the local anesthetic, patient-related factors such as age, cardiovascular status, and hepatic function will also influence the absorption and resultant plasma concentrations of local anesthetics. Protein binding of local anesthetics will influence their distribution and excretion. In this regard, protein binding parallels lipid solubility of the local anesthetic and is inversely related to the plasma concentration of drug (Table 7-1; Fig. 7-5) (Tucker et al, 1970). Overall, amide local anesthetics are more widely distributed in tissues than ester local anesthetics following systemic absorption.

Lung Extraction

The lungs are capable of extracting local anesthetics such as lidocaine, bupivacaine, and prilocaine from the circulation (Jorfeldt et al, 1980). Following rapid entry of local anesthetics into the venous circulation, this pulmonary extraction will limit the concentration of drug that reaches the systemic circulation for distribution to the coronary and cerebral circulations. For bupivacaine, this first-pass pulmonary extraction is dose depen-

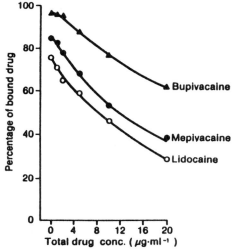

FIGURE 7–5. The percentage of local anesthetic bound to protein is inversely related to the plasma concentration of drug. (From Tucker GT, Boyes RN, Bridenbaugh PO, Binding of anilide-type local anesthetics in human plasm: I. Relationships between binding, physiochemical properties, and anesthetic-activity. Anesthesiology 1970; 33: 287–93; with permission.)

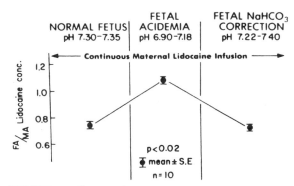

| NORMAL FETUS pH 7.30-7.35 | FETAL ACIDEMIA pH 6.90-7.18 | FETAL NaHCO₃ CORRECTION pH 7.22-740 |

FIGURE 7–6. Fetal–maternal arterial (FA/MA) lidocaine ratios are greater during fetal acidemia compared with a normal pH. Mean ± SE. (From Biehl D, Shnider SM, Levinson G, Callender K. Placental transfer of lidocaine: Effects of fetal acidosis. Anesthesiology 1978; 48: 409–12; with permission.)

dent, suggesting that the uptake process becomes saturated rapidly (Rothstein et al, 1984). Propranolol impairs bupivacaine extraction by the lung, perhaps reflecting a common receptor site for the two drugs (Rothstein and Pitt, 1983). Furthermore, propranolol decreases plasma clearance of lidocaine and bupivacaine, presumably reflecting propranolol-induced reductions in hepatic blood flow or inhibition of hepatic metabolism (Bowdle et al, 1987).

Placental Transfer

A clinically significant tissue distribution of local anesthetics involves the placental transfer of local anesthetics. Plasma protein binding influences the rate and degree of diffusion of local anesthetics across the placenta (Table 7-1). Bupivacaine, which is highly protein bound (approximately 95%), has an umbilical vein–maternal arterial concentration ratio of about 0.32 compared with a ratio of 0.73 for lidocaine (approximately 70% protein bound) and a ratio of 0.85 for prilocaine (approximately 55% protein bound) (Thomas et al, 1976). Ester local anesthetics, because of their rapid hydrolysis, are not available to cross the placenta in significant amounts. Acidosis in the fetus, which occurs during prolonged labor, can result in accumulation of local anesthetic in the fetus (ion trapping) (Fig. 7-6) (Biehl et al, 1978).

Clearance

Clearance values and elimination half-times for amide local anesthetics probably represent mainly hepatic metabolism, since renal excretion of unchanged drug is minimal (Table 7-1). Pharmacokinetic studies of ester local anesthetics are limited because of a short elimination half-time due to their rapid hydrolysis in the plasma and liver.

Metabolism of Amide Local Anesthetics

Amide local anesthetics undergo varying rates of metabolism by microsomal enzymes located primarily in the liver. Prilocaine undergoes the most rapid metabolism; lidocaine and mepivacaine are intermediate; and bupivacaine and etidocaine undergo the slowest metabolism among the amide local anesthetics. The initial step is conversion of the amide base to aminocarboxylic acid and a cyclic aniline derivative. Complete metabolism usually involves additional steps, such as hydroxylation of the aniline moiety and N-dealkylation of the aminocarboxylic acid.

Compared with ester local anesthetics, the metabolism of amide local anesthetics is more complex and slower. This slower metabolism means that sustained elevations of the plasma concentrations of amide local anesthetics, and thus systemic toxicity, are more likely than with ester local anesthetics. Furthermore, cumulative drug effects of amide local anesthetics are more likely than with ester local anesthetics.

LIDOCAINE. The principal metabolic pathway of lidocaine is oxidative dealkylation in the liver to monoethylglycinexylidide followed by hydrolysis of this metabolite to xylidide (Fig. 7-7). Monoethylglycinexylidide has approximately 80% of the activity of lidocaine for protecting against cardiac dysrhythmias in an animal model. This metabolite has a prolonged elimination half-time accounting for its efficacy in controlling cardiac dysrhythmias after the infusion of lidocaine is discontinued. Xylidide has only approximately 10% of the cardiac antidysrhythmic activity of lidocaine. In humans, approximately 75% of xylidide is excreted in the urine as 4-hydroxy-2,6-dimethylaniline.

Hepatic disease or decreases in hepatic blood flow, which may occur during anesthesia, can reduce the rate of metabolism of lidocaine.

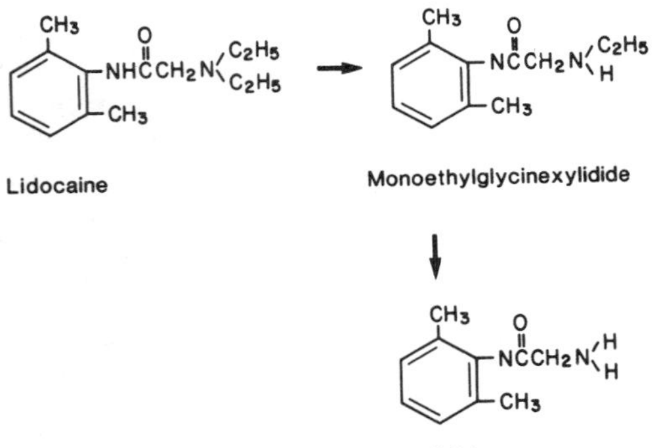

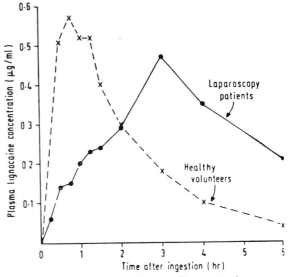

FIGURE 7–7.   Metabolism of lidocaine.

For example, the elimination half-time of lidocaine is increased more than fivefold in patients with liver dysfunction compared with normal patients. Decreased hepatic metabolism of lidocaine should be anticipated when patients are anesthetized with volatile anesthetics (Fig. 7-8) (Adejepon-Yamoah et al, 1973). Maternal clearance of lidocaine is prolonged in toxemia of pregnancy, and repeated administration of lidocaine can result in higher plasma concentrations than in normotensive patients (Ramanathan et al, 1986).

MEPIVACAINE.   Mepivacaine resembles the structure and pharmacologic properties of lidocaine. The duration of action of mepivacaine is somewhat longer than that of lidocaine. Clearance of mepivacaine is decreased in neonates, leading to a prolonged elimination half-time. In contrast to lidocaine, mepivacaine lacks vasodilator activity. As such, mepivacaine is an alternate selection when addition of epinephrine to the local anesthetic solution is not recommended.

BUPIVACAINE.   Despite the popularity of bupivacaine, its metabolic pathways have not been elucidated fully (Pihlajamaki et al, 1990). Proposed pathways include aromatic hydroxylation, N-dealkylation, amide hydrolysis, and conjugation. Only the N-dealkylated metabolite, N-desbutylbupivacaine, has been determined in blood or urine following epidural or spinal anesthesia. The mean total urinary excretion of bupivacaine and its dealkylation and hydroxylation metabolites account for less than 40% of the total local anesthetic dose, indicating a minor role for the metabolic pathways in humans (Pihlajamaki et al, 1990).

ETIDOCAINE.   A small amount (less than 1%) of etidocaine is excreted unchanged in the urine. Despite its structural similarity to lidocaine, the metabolites of etidocaine differ from those of lidocaine.

PRILOCAINE.   Prilocaine is an amide local anesthetic that is metabolized to ortho-toluidine. Ortho-toluidine is an oxidizing compound capable of converting hemoglobin to methemoglobin. When the dose of prilocaine is greater than 600 mg, there may be sufficient methemoglobin present ($3–5$ g·dl^{-1}) to cause the patient to appear cyanotic and oxygen-carrying capacity is decreased. Methemoglobinemia is readily reversed by the administration of methylene blue, 1 to 2 mg·kg^{-1} IV, over 5 minutes. This therapeutic effect, however, is short-lived because methylene blue may be cleared before conversion of all the methemoglobin to hemoglobin. The unique ability of prilocaine to cause dose-related methemoglobinemia limits the clinical usefulness of this local anesthetic with the exception being intravenous regional anesthesia.

FIGURE 7–8.   Plasma lidocaine (lignocaine) concentrations are higher during general anesthesia (laparoscopy patients) than in the absence of general anesthesia (healthy volunteers). (From Adejepon-Yamoah KK, Scott DB, Prescott LF. Impaired absorption and metabolism of oral lignocaine in patients undergoing laparoscopy. Br J Anaesth 1973; 143–7; with permission.)

DIBUCAINE. Dibucaine is a quinoline derivative with an amide bond in the connecting hydrocarbon chain. This local anesthetic is metabolized in the liver and is the most slowly eliminated of all the amide derivatives.

Metabolism of Ester Local Anesthetics

Ester local anesthetics undergo hydrolysis by cholinesterase enzyme principally in the plasma and to a lesser extent in the liver. The rate of hydrolysis varies with chloroprocaine being most rapid; procaine, intermediate; and tetracaine, the slowest. The resulting metabolites are pharmacologically inactive, although para-aminobenzoic acid may be an antigen responsible for subsequent allergic reactions. The exception to hydrolysis of ester local anesthetics in the plasma is cocaine, which undergoes significant metabolism in the liver.

Systemic toxicity is inversely proportional to the rate of hydrolysis; thus, tetracaine is more likely than chloroprocaine to result in excessive plasma concentrations. Because cerebrospinal fluid contains little or no cholinesterase enzyme, anesthesia produced by subarachnoid placement of tetracaine will persist until the drug has been absorbed into the circulation. Plasma cholinesterase activity and the hydrolysis rate of ester local anesthetics are slowed in the presence of liver disease or an elevated blood urea nitrogen concentration (Reidenberg et al, 1972). Plasma cholinesterase activity may be decreased in parturients and in patients being treated with certain chemotherapeutic drugs (Finster, 1976; Kaniaris et al, 1979). Patients with atypical plasma cholinesterase may be at increased risk for developing excess systemic concentrations of an ester local anesthetic due to absent or limited plasma hydrolysis.

PROCAINE. Procaine is hydrolyzed to para-aminobenzoic acid, which is excreted unchanged in the urine, and to diethylaminoethanol, which is further metabolized because only 30% is recovered in the urine. Overall, less than 50% of procaine is excreted unchanged in the urine. Increased plasma concentrations of para-aminobenzoic acid do not produce symptoms of systemic toxicity.

CHLOROPROCAINE. Addition of a chlorine atom to the benzene ring of procaine to form chloro-procaine increases by 3.5 times the rate of hydrolysis of the local anesthetic by plasma cholinesterase as compared with procaine. Resulting pharmacologically inactive metabolites of chloroprocaine are 2-chloroaminobenzoic acid and 2-diethylaminoethanol. Maternal and neonatal plasma cholinesterase activity may be decreased up to 40% at term, but minimal placental passage of chloroprocaine confirms that even this decreased activity is adequate to hydrolyze most of the chloroprocaine absorbed from the maternal epidural space (Kuhnert et al, 1980). The maternal elimination half-time of chloroprocaine following epidural administration is 1.5 to 6.4 minutes (Kuhnert et al, 1986a).

TETRACAINE. Tetracaine undergoes hydrolysis by plasma cholinesterase, but the rate is slower than for procaine.

COCAINE. Cocaine is metabolized by plasma and liver cholinesterases to water-soluble metabolites that are excreted in the urine. Plasma cholinesterase activity is decreased in parturients, neonates, the elderly, and patients with severe underlying liver disease. Cocaine may be present in the urine for 24 to 36 hours depending on the route of administration and cholinesterase activity. Absorption of cocaine across mucous membranes is slow and the elimination half-time is 60 to 90 minutes. Assays for the metabolites of cocaine in urine are useful markers of cocaine use or abstention.

Renal Elimination

Poor water solubility of local anesthetics usually limits renal excretion of unchanged drug to less than 5% of the injected dose (Tucker and Mather, 1979). The exception is cocaine, where 10% to 12% of unchanged drug can be recovered in the urine. Water-soluble metabolites of local anesthetics, such as para-aminobenzoic acid resulting from metabolism of ester local anesthetics are readily excreted in the urine.

Use of Vasoconstrictors

The duration of action of a local anesthetic is proportional to the time the drug is in contact with nerve fibers. For this reason, epinephrine (1:200,000) may be added to local anesthetic solutions to produce vasoconstriction, which limits systemic absorption and maintains the drug concentration in the vicinity of the nerve fibers to be anesthetized. Indeed, addition of epinephrine to a lidocaine solution prolongs the duration of conduction blockade by approximately 50% and decreases systemic absorption of local anesthetics by approximately one third (Fig. 7-9) (Scott et al, 1972).

The impact of adding epinephrine to the local anesthetic solution is influenced by the specific local anesthetic selected and the level of sensory blockade required if a spinal or epidural anesthetic is chosen. For example, the impact of epinephrine in prolonging the duration of conduction blockade and decreasing systemic absorption of bupivacaine and etidocaine is less than observed with lidocaine presumably because the greater lipid solubility of bupivacaine and etidocaine causes them to bind avidly to tissues. The duration of sensory anesthesia in the lower extremities but not the abdominal region is extended when epinephrine (0.2 mg) or phenylephrine (2 mg) is added to local anesthetic solutions of bupivacaine or lidocaine injected into the subarachnoid space. Vasoconstrictors prolong the effect of tetracaine for spinal anesthesia. Epinephrine added to a low dose (6 mg) of tetracaine increases the success rate of spinal anesthesia, whereas the success rate is not altered by epinephrine when the subarachnoid dose of tetracaine is 10 mg (Carpenter et al, 1989). In addition to reducing systemic absorption to prolong conduction blockade, epinephrine may also enhance conduction blockade by

increasing neuronal uptake of the local anesthetic. The addition of epinephrine to local anesthetic solutions has little, if any, effect on the onset rate of local anesthesia.

Decreased systemic absorption of local anesthetic due to vasoconstriction produced by epinephrine increases the likelihood that the rate of metabolism will match that of absorption, thus reducing the possibility of systemic toxicity. Whenever local anesthetic solutions containing epinephrine are administered in the presence of inhaled anesthetics, the possibility of enhanced cardiac irritability should be considered. Systemic absorption of epinephrine may accentuate hypertension in vulnerable patients.

Low–molecular-weight dextran added to local anesthetic solutions, as used for peripheral nerve block anesthesia, prolongs the duration of action of the anesthetic. Presumably, dextran decreases the systemic absorption rate of the local anesthetic (Kaplan et al, 1975).

Combinations of Local Anesthetics

Local anesthetics may be combined in an effort to produce a rapid onset (chloroprocaine) and prolonged duration (bupivacaine) of action. Nevertheless, placement of chloroprocaine in the epidural space may decrease the efficacy of subsequent epidural bupivacaine-induced analgesia during labor. It is speculated the low pH of the chloroprocaine solution could decrease the nonionized pharmacologically active fraction of bupivacaine. Tachyphylaxis to the local anesthetic mixture could also reflect local acidosis due to the low pH of the bathing solution. For these reasons, adjustment of the pH of the chloroprocaine solution with the addition of 1 ml of 8.4% sodium bicarbonate added to 30 ml of chloroprocaine solution just before placement into the epidural space may improve the efficacy of the chloroprocaine-bupivacaine combination (Chestnut et al, 1989). Local anesthetic toxicity of combinations of drugs is additive rather than synergistic (Munson et al, 1977).

MECHANISM OF ACTION

Local anesthetics prevent transmission of nerve impulses (conduction blockade) by inhibiting

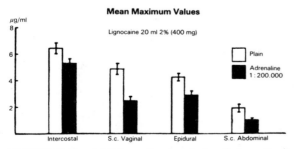

FIGURE 7–9. Addition of epinephrine (adrenaline) to the solution containing lidocaine (lignocaine) or prilocaine reduces systemic absorption of the local anesthetic by about one third. (From Scott DB, Jebson PJR, Braid B, Ortengren B, Frisch P. Factors affecting plasma levels of lignocaine and prilocaine. Br J Anaesth 1972; 44: 1040–9; with permission.)

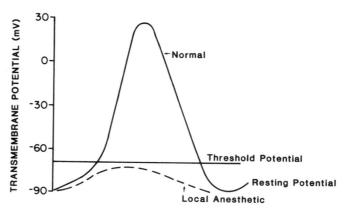

FIGURE 7–10.   Local anesthetics slow the rate of depolarization of the nerve action potential such that threshold potential is not reached. As a result, an action potential cannot be propagated in the presence of local anesthetic, and conduction blockade results.

passage of sodium ions (Na^+) through ion-selective Na^+ channels in nerve membranes (Butterworth and Strichartz, 1990). The Na^+ channel itself is a specific receptor for local anesthetic molecules. Occlusion of open Na^+ channels by local anesthetic molecules contributes little to overall inhibition of Na^+ permeability. Failure of ion channel permeability to Na^+ to increase slows the rate of depolarization such that threshold potential is not reached and, thus, an action potential is not propagated (Fig. 7-10). Local anesthetics do not alter the resting transmembrane potential or threshold potential.

Sodium Channels

Na^+ channels exist in activated-open, inactivated-closed, and rested-closed states during various phases of the action potential. In the resting nerve membrane, Na^+ channels are distributed in equilibrium between the rested-closed and inactivated-closed states. By selectively binding to Na^+ channels in inactivated-closed states, local anesthetic molecules stabilize these channels in this configuration and prevent their change to the rested-closed and activated-open states in response to nerve impulses. Na^+ channels in the inactivated-closed state are not permeable to Na^+ and thus conduction of nerve impulses in the form of propagated action potentials cannot occur. It is speculated that local anesthetics bind to specific sites located on the inner portion of Na^+ channels (internal gate or H gate) as well as obstructing Na^+ channels near their external openings to maintain these channels in inactiv-

ated-closed states (Butterworth and Strichartz, 1990).

Frequency-Dependent Blockade

Na^+ channels tend to recover from local anesthetic-induced conduction blockade between action potentials and to develop additional conduction blockade each time Na^+ channels open during an action potential (frequency-dependent blockade). Therefore, local anesthetic molecules can gain access to receptors only when Na^+ channels are in activated-open states. For this reason, selective conduction blockade of nerve fibers by local anesthetics may be related to the nerve's characteristic frequencies of activity as well as to its anatomical properties, such as its diameter. Indeed, a resting nerve is less sensitive to local anesthetic–induced conduction blockade than is a nerve that has been repetitively stimulated. Etidocaine characteristically blocks motor nerves before sensory nerves because of frequency-dependent blockade (Bromage et al, 1974). In addition to local anesthetics, the pharmacologic effects of other drugs, including anticonvulsants and barbiturates, may reflect frequency-dependent blockade.

MINIMUM CONCENTRATION

The minimum concentration of local anesthetic necessary to produce conduction blockade of nerve impulses is termed the *Cm*. The Cm is analogous to the minimum alveolar concentration

(MAC) for inhaled anesthetics. Nerve fiber diameter influences Cm with larger nerve fibers requiring higher concentrations of local anesthetic for production of conduction blockade. An increased tissue pH or high frequency of nerve stimulation decreases Cm.

Each local anesthetic has a unique Cm reflecting differing potencies for each drug. The Cm of motor fibers is approximately twice that of sensory fibers; thus, sensory anesthesia may not always be accompanied by skeletal muscle paralysis. Despite an unchanged Cm, less local anesthetic is needed for subarachnoid than epidural anesthesia, reflecting greater access of local anesthetics to unprotected nerves in the subarachnoid space.

Peripheral nerves comprise myelinated A and B fibers and unmyelinated C fibers (see Chapter 41). A minimal length of myelinated nerve fiber must be exposed to an adequate concentration of local anesthetic for conduction blockade of nerve impulses to occur. For example, if only one node of Ranvier is blocked (site of change in Na^+ permeability), then the nerve impulse can jump (skip) across this node and conduction blockade does not occur. For conduction blockade to occur in an A fiber, it is necessary to expose at least two and preferably three successive nodes of Ranvier (approximately 1 cm) to an adequate concentration of local anesthetic. Both types of pain-conducting fibers (myelinated A-delta and non-myelinated C fibers) are blocked by similar concentrations of local anesthetics despite the differences in the diameters of these fibers. Preganglionic B fibers are more readily blocked by local anesthetics than any fiber even though these fibers are myelinated.

Differential Conduction Blockade

Differential conduction blockade is illustrated by selective blockade of preganglionic sympathetic nervous system B fibers with low concentrations of local anesthetics. Slightly higher concentrations of local anesthetics interrupt conduction in small C fibers and small and medium-sized A fibers with loss of sensation for pain and temperature. Nevertheless, touch, proprioception, and motor function are still present such that the patient will sense pressure but not pain with surgical stimulation . In an anxious patient, however,

any sensation may be misinterpreted as failure of the local anesthetic.

Changes During Pregnancy

Increased sensitivity (more rapid onset of conduction blockade) may be present during pregnancy (Datta et al, 1983). Alterations in protein-binding characteristics of bupivacaine may result in increased concentrations of pharmacologically active unbound drug in the parturient's plasma (Denson et al, 1984a). Nevertheless, progesterone, which binds to the same alpha-1 acid glycoprotein as bupivacaine, does not influence protein binding of this local anesthetic (Denson et al, 1984b). This evidence suggests that bupivacaine and progesterone bind to discrete but separate sites on protein molecules.

SIDE EFFECTS

The principal side effects related to the use of local anesthetics are allergic reactions and systemic toxicity.

Allergic Reactions

Allergic reactions to local anesthetics are rare despite the frequent use of these drugs. It is estimated that fewer than 1% of all adverse reactions to local anesthetics are due to an allergic mechanism (Brown et al, 1981). Instead, the overwhelming majority of adverse responses that are often attributed to an allergic reaction are, instead, manifestations of excess plasma concentrations of the local anesthetic.

Ester local anesthetics that produce metabolites related to para-aminobenzoic acid are more likely than amide local anesthetics, which are not metabolized to para-aminobenzoic acid, to evoke an allergic reaction. An allergic reaction following the use of a local anesthetic may be due to methylparaben or similar substances used as preservatives in commercial preparations of ester and amide local anesthetics. These preservatives are structurally similar to para-aminobenzoic acid. As a result, an allergic reaction may reflect prior stimulation of antibody production by the preservative and not the local anesthetic.

Cross-Sensitivity

Cross-sensitivity between ester local anesthetics reflects the common metabolite, para-amino-benzoic acid. A similar cross-sensitivity, however, does not exist between classes of local anesthetics. Therefore, a patient with a known allergy to an ester local anesthetic can receive an amide local anesthetic without an increased risk of an allergic reaction. Likewise, an ester local anesthetic can be administered to a patient with a known allergy to an amide local anesthetic. It is important that the "safe" local anesthetic be preservative-free.

Documentation of Allergy

Documentation of allergy to a local anesthetic is based on the clinical history and perhaps the use of intradermal testing (Incaudo et al, 1978). The occurrence of rash, urticaria, and laryngeal edema, with or without hypotension and bronchospasm, is highly suggestive of a local anesthetic–induced allergic reaction. Conversely, hypotension associated with syncope or tachycardia when an epinephrine-containing local anesthetic solution is administered suggests an accidental intravascular injection of drug. Use of an intradermal test requires injection of preservative-free preparations of local anesthetic solutions to eliminate the possibility that the allergic reaction was caused by a substance other than the local anesthetic.

Systemic Toxicity

Systemic toxicity of a local anesthetic is due to an excess plasma concentration of the drug. Plasma concentrations of local anesthetics are determined by the rate of drug entrance into the circulation relative to its redistribution to inactive tissue sites and clearance by metabolism. Accidental direct intravascular injection of local anesthetic solutions during performance of peripheral nerve block anesthesia or epidural anesthesia is the most common mechanism for production of excess plasma concentrations of local anesthetics. Less often, excess plasma concentrations of local anesthetics result from absorption of the local anesthetic from the injection site. The magnitude of this systemic absorption de-

pends on (1) the dose administered into the tissues, (2) the vascularity of the injection site, (3) the presence of epinephrine in the solution, and (4) the physicochemical properties of the drug (Table 7-1). For example, systemic absorption of local anesthetics is greatest following injection for an intercostal nerve block, intermediate for epidural anesthesia, and least for a brachial plexus block (Fig. 7-3) (Covino and Vassallo, 1976). Addition of 5 µg of epinephrine to every ml of local anesthetic solution (a 1:200,000 dilution) reduces systemic absorption of local anesthetics by approximately one third (Scott et al, 1972) (see the section entitled "Use of Vasoconstrictors"). Systemic toxicity of local anesthetics involves the central nervous system and cardiovascular system.

Central Nervous System

Low plasma concentrations of local anesthetics are likely to produce numbness of the tongue and circumoral tissues, presumably reflecting delivery of drug to these highly vascular areas. As the plasma concentrations continue to increase, local anesthetics readily cross the blood-brain barrier and produce a predictable pattern of central nervous system changes. Restlessness, vertigo, tinnitus, and difficulty in focusing occur initially. Further increases in the central nervous system concentration of a local anesthetic result in slurred speech and skeletal muscle twitching. This skeletal muscle twitching is often first evident in the face and extremities and signals the imminence of tonic-clonic seizures. Lidocaine and other amide local anesthetics may cause drowsiness before the onset of seizures. Seizures are classically followed by central nervous system depression, which may also be accompanied by hypotension and apnea. The onset of seizures may reflect selective depression of inhibitory cortical neurons by local anesthetics, leaving excitatory pathways unopposed. An alternative explanation for seizures is local anesthetic–induced inhibition of the release of neurotransmitters, particularly gamma-aminobutyric acid. The precise site of local anesthetic–induced seizures is not known, although it appears to be in the temporal lobe or the amygdala.

Plasma concentrations of local anesthetics producing signs of central nervous system toxicity depend on the specific drug involved. Lidocaine, mepivacaine, and prilocaine demonstrate effects on the central nervous system at plasma concentrations of 5 to 10 $\mu g \cdot ml^{-1}$, whereas bupivacaine and etidocaine show effects on the central nervous system at venous plasma concentrations of 1.5 $\mu g \cdot ml^{-1}$. Furthermore, the active metabolites of lidocaine, including monoethylglycinexylidide, may exert an additive effect in causing systemic toxicity following epidural administration of lidocaine. For this reason, it has been recommended that the plasma concentration of lidocaine be monitored when the cumulative epidural dose of lidocaine is greater than 900 mg (Inoue et al, 1985). The seizure threshold for lidocaine may be related to central nervous system levels of serotonin (5-hydroxytryptophan). For example, accumulation of serotonin decreases the seizure threshold of lidocaine and prolongs the duration of seizure activity.

There is an inverse relationship between the $PaCO_2$ and seizure thresholds of local anesthetics, presumably reflecting variations in cerebral blood flow and resultant delivery of drugs to the brain. For unknown reasons, gallamine elevates the seizure threshold for lidocaine in animals (see Chapter 8). Increases in the serum potassium (K^+) concentration can facilitate depolarization and thus markedly increase local anesthetic toxicity. Conversely, hypokalemia, by creating hyperpolarization, can greatly decrease local anesthetic toxicity.

TREATMENT. Treatment of local anesthetic-induced seizures includes ventilation of the lungs with oxygen because arterial hypoxemia and metabolic acidosis occur within seconds (Moore et al, 1980). Equally important is the delivery of supplemental oxygen at the earliest sign of local anesthetic toxicity. Hyperventilation of the lungs seems logical in an attempt to reduce the delivery of local anesthetic to the brain. Conversely, this maneuver could theoretically slow removal of local anesthetic from the brain. Diazepam is effective in suppressing local anesthetic-induced seizures.

Cardiovascular System

The cardiovascular system is more resistant to the toxic effects of high plasma concentrations of local anesthetics than is the central nervous system. For example, lidocaine in plasma concentrations less than 5 $\mu g \cdot ml^{-1}$ is devoid of adverse cardiac effects, producing only a decrease in the rate of spontaneous phase 4 depolarization (automaticity). Nevertheless, plasma lidocaine concentrations of 5 to 10 $\mu g \cdot ml^{-1}$ and equivalent plasma concentrations of other local anesthetics may produce profound hypotension due to relaxation of arteriolar vascular smooth muscle and direct myocardial depression. As a result, hypotension reflects both decreased systemic vascular resistance and cardiac output.

Part of the cardiac toxicity that results from high plasma concentrations of local anesthetics occurs because these drugs also block cardiac Na^+ channels. At low concentrations of local anesthetics, this effect on Na^+ channels probably contributes to cardiac antidysrhythmic properties of these drugs. However, when the plasma concentrations of local anesthetics are excessive, sufficient cardiac Na^+ channels become blocked so that conduction and automaticity become adversely depressed. For example, excessive plasma concentrations of lidocaine may slow conduction of cardiac impulses through the heart, manifesting as prolongation of the P–R interval and QRS complex on the electrocardiogram. Effects of local anesthetics on calcium ion and K^+ channels may also contribute to cardiac toxicity.

SELECTIVE CARDIAC TOXICITY. Accidental intravenous injection of bupivacaine may result in precipitous hypotension, cardiac dysrhythmias, and atrioventricular heart block (Albright, 1979). Indeed, intravenous injection of bupivacaine or lidocaine to awake animals produces serious cardiac dysrhythmias only in animals receiving bupivacaine (Table 7-2) (Kotelko et al, 1984). Furthermore, pregnancy may increase sensitivity to cardiotoxic effects, as emphasized by occurrence of cardiopulmonary collapse with a smaller dose of bupivacaine in pregnant compared with nonpregnant animals (Fig. 7-11) (Morishima et al, 1985). Likewise, cardiac toxicity of bupivacaine in animals is enhanced by preexisting arterial hypoxemia, acidosis, or hypercarbia.

Local anesthetics depress the maximal depolarization rate of the cardiac action potential (V_{max}), which reflects an effect on Na^+ movement. In isolated papillary muscle preparations, V_{max} is depressed more by bupivacaine than by lidocaine (Fig. 7-12) (Clarkson and Hondeghem, 1985). Dissociation of highly lipid-soluble bupivacaine from Na^+ channel receptor sites is slow, accounting for this drug's persistent depressant

Table 7–2

Animals Manifesting Adverse Cardiac Changes Following Administraiton of Bupivacaine or Lidocaine

Cardiac Change	Bupivacaine (percent of animals)	Lidocaine (percent of animals)
Sinus tachycardia	0	100
Supraventricular tachycardia	60	9
Atrioventricular heart block	60	0
Ventricular tachycardia	80	0
Premature ventricular contractions	100	0
Wide QRS complexes	100	0
ST–T wave changes	60	40

(Reprinted from Kotelko DM, Shnider SM, Dailey PA, et al. Bupivacaine-induced cardiac arrhythmias in sheep. Anesthesiology 1984; 60: 10–18, with permission.)

effect on V_{max} and subsequent cardiac toxicity (Atlee and Bosnjak, 1990). In contrast, less lipid-soluble lidocaine dissociates rapidly from cardiac Na^+ channels and cardiac toxicity is low. Tachycardia can enhance frequency-dependent blockade of cardiac Na^+ channels by bupivacaine, further contributing to its selective cardiac toxicity (Kendig, 1985). Conversely, a low degree of frequency-dependent blockade may contribute to the antidysrhythmic properties of lidocaine. In anesthetized dogs, bretylium, 20 mg·kg^{-1} IV, reverses bupivacaine-induced cardiac depression and elevates the threshold for ventricular tachycardia (Kasten and Martin, 1985). In an effort to decrease the potential for cardiotoxicity should accidental intravascular injection occur, it may be prudent to limit the concentration of bupivacaine to be used for epidural anesthesia to no greater than 0.5%.

Ventilatory Response to Hypoxia

Lidocaine in clinically useful plasma concentrations depresses the ventilatory response to hypoxemia (Gross et al, 1984). In this regard, patients with carbon dioxide retention whose resting ventilation depends on hypoxic drive may be at risk of ventilatory failure when lidocaine is administered for treatment of cardiac dysrhythmias. Conversely, systemic absorption of bupivacaine, such as follows a brachial plexus block, stimulates the ventilatory response to carbon dioxide (Negre et al, 1985).

USES OF LOCAL ANESTHETICS

Local anesthetics are most often used to produce regional anesthesia. Less common reasons to select local anesthetics are to prevent or treat cardiac dysrhythmias (see Chapter 17); prevent or treat increases in intracranial pressure; provide analgesia; and treat grand mal seizures.

Regional Anesthesia

Regional anesthesia is classified according to the following six sites of placement of the local anesthetic: (1) topical or surface anesthesia, (2) local infiltration, (3) peripheral nerve block, (4) intravenous regional anesthesia (Bier block), (5) epidural anesthesia, and (6) spinal (subarachnoid) anesthesia (Table 7-3). "Spinal anesthesia" rather than "subarachnoid anesthesia" or "spinal block" is the preferred terminology because it is understood by even nonanesthesiologists. Furthermore, the term "block" implies an obstruction. Maximum doses of local anesthetics (based on body weight) as recommended for topical or peripheral nerve block anesthesia must be viewed as imprecise guidelines that often do not consider the pharmacokinetics of the drugs (Scott, 1989).

Topical Anesthesia

Local anesthetics are used to produce topical anesthesia by placement on the mucous membranes

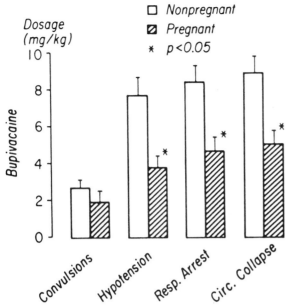

FIGURE 7–11. The dose of bupivacaine required to evoke toxic effects is less in pregnant than in nonpregnant ewes. Mean ± SE. (From Morishima HO, Pederson H, Finster M, et al. Bupivacaine toxicity in pregnant and nonpregnant ewes. Anesthesiology 1985; 63: 134–9; with permission.)

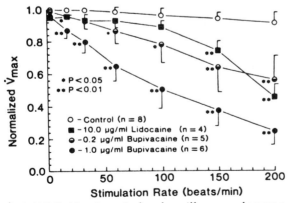

FIGURE 7–12. In an isolated papillary muscle preparation, $\dot{V}_{max}$ is depressed more by bupivacaine than by lidocaine. (From Clarkson CW, Hondeghem LM. Mechanism for bupivacaine depression of cardiac conduction: Fast block of sodium channels during the action potential with slow recovery from block during diastole. Anesthesiology 1985; 62: 396–405.

of the nose, mouth, tracheobronchial tree, esophagus, or genitourinary tract. Cocaine (4% to 10%), tetracaine (1% to 2%), and lidocaine (2% to 4%) are most often used. It is estimated that topical cocaine anesthesia is used in more than 50% of the 370,000 rhinolaryngologic procedures performed annually in the United States (Lange et al, 1989) (see the section entitled "Cocaine Toxicity"). Cocaine's popularity for topical anesthesia reflects its unique ability to produce localized vasoconstriction, thus decreasing blood loss and improving surgical visualization. Procaine and chloroprocaine penetrate mucous membranes poorly and are ineffective for topical anesthesia.

Pramoxine is applied topically to the skin or mucous membranes to relieve pain caused by minor burns or pruritus due to dermatoses or hemorrhoids. It also may be used to facilitate sigmoidoscopic examinations and to anesthetize the upper airway prior to direct laryngoscopy. This local anesthetic is not recommended for application to nasal or tracheal mucosa because it may cause irritation. Structurally, pramoxine is unrelated to ester or amide local anesthetics, therefore minimizing the likelihood of cross-sensitivity with other local anesthetics (Fig. 7-13). Dyclonine, hexylcaine, and piperocaine are effective topically for producing anesthesia of the mucous membranes (onset in approximately 5 minutes) such as prior to direct laryngoscopy (Fig. 7-13).

Topical anesthesia inhibits ciliary activity; this may impair removal of secretions. Local anesthetics are absorbed into the systemic circulation following topical application to mucous membranes. Systemic absorption of tetracaine, and to a lesser extent lidocaine, following placement on the tracheobronchial mucosa produces plasma concentrations similar to those present after intravenous injection of the local anesthetic. For example, plasma lidocaine concentrations 15 minutes following laryngotracheal spray of the local anesthetic are similar to those concentrations present at the same time after an intravenous injection of lidocaine (Viegas and Stoelting, 1975). This systemic absorption reflects the high vascularity of the tracheobronchial tree and the injection of the local anesthetic as a spray that spreads the solution over a wide surface area.

Local Infiltration

Local infiltration anesthesia is extravascular placement of local anesthetic in the area to be an-

Table 7–3
Uses of Local Anesthetics to Produce Regional Anesthesia

	Topical Anesthesia	Local Infiltration	Peripheral Nerve Block	Intravenous Regional Anesthesia	Epidural Anesthesia	Spinal Anesthesia
Procaine	No	Yes	Yes	No	No	Yes
Chloroprocaine	No	Yes	Yes	No	Yes	No
Tetracaine	Yes	No	No	No	No	Yes
Lidocaine	Yes	Yes	Yes	Yes	Yes	Yes
Mepivacaine	No	Yes	Yes	No	Yes	No
Bupivacaine	No	Yes	Yes	Yes(?)*	Yes	Yes
Etidocaine	No	Yes	Yes	No	Yes	No
Prilocaine	No	Yes	Yes	Yes	Yes	No
Pramoxine	Yes	No	No	No	No	No
Dyclonine	Yes	No	No	No	No	No
Hexylcaine	Yes	No	No	No	No	No
Piperocaine	Yes	No	No	No	No	No

*?, Potential for cardiotoxicity must be considered.

esthetized. Subcutaneous injection of the local anesthetic in the area to be traversed for placement of an intravascular cannula is an example of infiltration anesthesia. Lidocaine is the topical anesthetic most often selected for infiltration anesthesia.

The duration of infiltration anesthesia can be approximately doubled by adding 1:200,000 epinephrine to the local anesthetic solution. Epinephrine-containing solutions, however, should not be injected intracutaneously or into tissues supplied by end-arteries (fingers, ears, nose) because resulting vasoconstriction can produce ischemia and even gangrene.

Peripheral Nerve Block Anesthesia

Peripheral nerve block anesthesia is achieved by injection of local anesthetic into the tissues surrounding individual peripheral nerves or nerve plexuses such as the brachial plexus. When local anesthetic is deposited around a peripheral nerve, it diffuses from the outer surface (mantle) toward the center (core) of the nerve along a concentration gradient (Winnie et al, 1977b). Consequently, nerve fibers located in the mantle of the mixed nerve are anesthetized first. These mantle fibers usually are distributed to more proximal anatomical structures in contrast to distal struc-

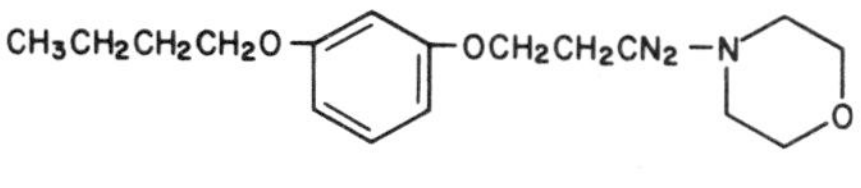

Pramoxine

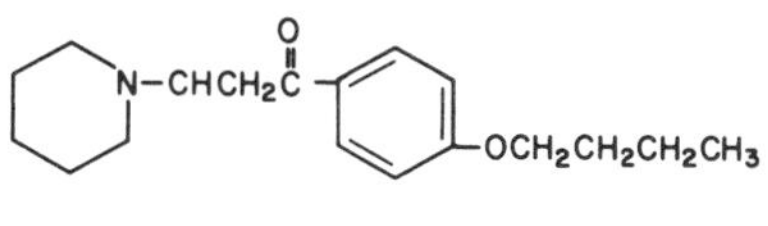

Dyclonine

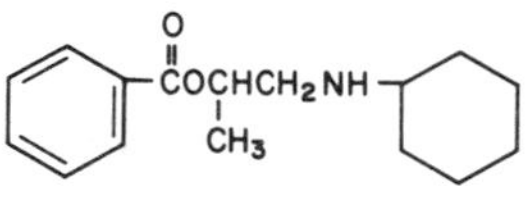

Hexylcaine

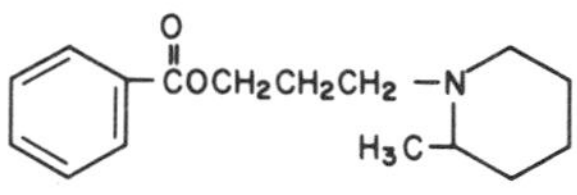

Piperocaine

FIGURE 7–13.   Local anesthetics used to produce topical anesthesia.

tures innervated by nerve fibers near the core of the nerve. This explains the initial development of analgesia proximally, with subsequent distal spread as local anesthetic diffuses to reach more central core nerve fibers. Conversely, recovery of sensation occurs in a reverse direction: nerve fibers in the mantle that are exposed to extraneural fluid are the first to lose local anesthetic such that sensation returns initially to the proximal and last to the distal parts of the limb.

Skeletal muscle paralysis may precede the onset of sensory anesthesia if motor nerve fibers are distributed peripheral to sensory fibers in the mixed peripheral nerve (Winnie et al, 1977a). Indeed, the sequence of onset and recovery from blockade of sympathetic, sensory, and motor nerve fibers in a mixed peripheral nerve depend as much on anatomical location of the nerve fibers within the mixed nerve as on their sensitivity to local anesthetics. This differs from results of *in vitro* studies on single nerve fibers where diffusion distance does not play a role. In an *in vitro* model, nerve fiber size is most important, with the onset of conduction blockade being inversely proportional to fiber size. For example, the smallest sensory and autonomic nervous system fibers are anesthetized first, followed by larger motor and proprioceptive axons.

The rapidity of onset of sensory anesthesia following injection of a local anesthetic into tissues around a peripheral nerve depends on the pK of the drug. The pK determines the amount of local anesthetic that exists in the active nonionized form at the pH of the tissue (Table 7-1). For example, the onset of action of lidocaine occurs in approximately 3 minutes, whereas onset after bupivacaine injection requires approximately 15 minutes, reflecting the greater fraction of lidocaine that exists in the lipid-soluble nonionized form. Tetracaine, with a slow onset of anesthesia and a high potential to cause systemic toxicity, is not recommended for local infiltration or peripheral nerve block anesthesia.

Duration of peripheral nerve block anesthesia depends on the dose of local anesthetic, its lipid solubility, its degree of protein binding, and concomitant use of a vasoconstrictor such as epinephrine. The duration of action is prolonged more safely by epinephrine than by increasing the dose of local anesthetic, which also increases the likelihood of systemic toxicity. Bupivacaine combined with epinephrine may produce pe-

ripheral nerve block anesthesia lasting up to 24 hours.

Intravenous Regional Anesthesia (Bier Block)

The intravenous injection of a local anesthetic into an extremity isolated from the rest of the circulation by a tourniquet produces a rapid onset of anesthesia and skeletal muscle relaxation. The duration of the anesthesia is independent of the specific local anesthetic, being determined by how long the tourniquet is kept inflated. The mechanism by which local anesthetics produce intravenous regional anesthesia is unknown but probably reflects action of the drug on nerve endings as well as nerve trunks. Normal sensation and skeletal muscle tone return promptly on release of the tourniquet, which allows blood flow to dilute the concentration of local anesthetic.

Ester and amide local anesthetics produce satisfactory effects when used for intravenous regional anesthesia. Lidocaine and prilocaine are the most frequently selected amide local anesthetics for producing this type of regional anesthesia. The onset, duration, and quality of intravenous regional anesthesia produced by 50 ml of a 0.5% solution of lidocaine or prilocaine is similar, but plasma concentrations of prilocaine are lower than those of lidocaine following tourniquet deflation (Fig. 7-14) (Bader et al, 1988). The associated degree of methemoglobinemia (3% of hemoglobin as methemoglobin) seen with prilocaine is far below the level needed to produce cyanosis (10% of hemoglobin as methemoglobin). The significantly lower plasma prilocaine concentrations following tourniquet deflation may indicate a greater margin of safety for prilocaine as compared to lidocaine in terms of potential systemic toxicity. Chloroprocaine is not selected for intravenous regional anesthesia because of a high incidence of associated thrombophlebitis, whereas bupivacaine is a questionable selection considering its greater likelihood than other local anesthetics for producing cardiotoxicity.

Epidural Anesthesia

Local anesthetic placed in the lumbar epidural or sacral caudal space produces epidural anesthesia by two presumed mechanisms. First, local anesthetic diffuses across the dura to act on nerve

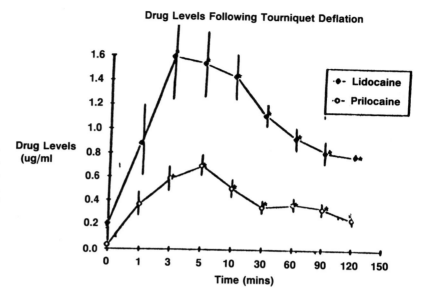

Drug Levels Following Tourniquet Deflation

FIGURE 7–14. Following tourniquet deflation, plasma concentrations of lidocaine exceed concentrations of prilocaine. Mean ± SE. *P < 0.05. (From Bader AM, Concepcion M, Hurley RJ, Arthur GR. Comparison of lidocaine and prilocaine for intravenous regional anesthesia. Anesthesiology 1988; 69: 409–12; with permission.)

roots and the spinal cord as it does when injected directly into the lumbar subarachnoid space to produce spinal anesthesia. Second, local anesthetic also diffuses into the paravertebral area through the intervertebral foramina, producing multiple paravertebral nerve blocks. These slow diffusion processes account for the 15- to 30-minutes, delay in onset of sensory anesthesia following placement of local anesthetics in the epidural space. Lidocaine is commonly used for epidural anesthesia because of its good diffusion capabilities through tissues. Bupivacaine is often selected when prolonged epidural anesthesia is desired, as during labor. Chloroprocaine is often selected when rapid onset and short duration of sensory anesthesia are appropriate.

In contrast to spinal anesthesia, during epidural anesthesia there often is not a zone of differential sympathetic nervous system blockade, and the zone of differential motor blockade may average up to four rather than two segments below the sensory level. Another difference from spinal anesthesia is the larger dose required to produce epidural anesthesia, leading to substantial systemic absorption of local anesthetic. For example, peak plasma concentrations of lidocaine are 3 to 4 $\mu g \cdot ml^{-1}$ following placement of 400 mg into the epidural space. Peak plasma concentrations of bupivacaine following epidural injection of 150 mg average 1 $\mu g \cdot ml^{-1}$. Addition of

1:200,000 epinephrine to the lidocaine solution decreases systemic absorption of the local anesthetic by approximately one third. Systemic absorption of epinephrine produces beta-adrenergic stimulation characterized by peripheral vasodilation with resultant decreases in blood pressure even though cardiac output is increased by the inotropic and chronotropic effects of epinephrine.

Increased plasma concentrations of local anesthetics following epidural anesthesia are of special importance when this technique is used to provide anesthesia to the parturient. Local anesthetics cross the placenta and may produce detectable, although not necessarily adverse, effects on the fetus for 24 to 48 hours. The fetus and neonate are less able to metabolize mepivacaine, resulting in a prolonged elimination half-time compared with adults. Use of a more lipid-soluble and protein-bound local anesthetic, such as bupivacaine, may limit passage across the placenta to the fetus. Even low doses of lidocaine such as are used for spinal anesthesia during labor result in some systemic absorption as reflected by the presence of lidocaine and its metabolites in neonatal urine for more than 36 hours (Kuhnert et al, 1986b). Conversely, bupivacaine is undetectable in neonatal plasma 24 hours after cesarean delivery using bupivacaine-induced spinal anesthesia (Kuhnert et al, 1987).

Indeed, maternal plasma concentrations of bupivacaine in mothers of these neonates is approximately 5% of that level present after epidural anesthesia, and plasma umbilical vein concentrations are approximately 7% of those present after epidural anesthesia.

Spinal Anesthesia.

Spinal anesthesia is produced by injection of local anesthetic into the lumbar subarachnoid space. Local anesthetics placed in the lumbar cerebrospinal fluid act on superficial layers of the spinal cord, but the principal site of action is the preganglionic fibers as they leave the spinal cord in the anterior rami. Because the concentration of local anesthetics in cerebrospinal fluid decreases as a function of distance from the site of injection and because different types of nerve fibers differ in their sensitivity to effects of local anesthetics, zones of differential anesthesia develop. Because preganglionic sympathetic nervous system fibers are anesthetized by concentrations of local anesthetics that are inadequate to affect sensory or motor fibers, the level of sympathetic nervous system denervation during spinal anesthesia extends approximately two spinal segments cephalad to the level of sensory anesthesia. For the same reasons, the level of motor anesthesia averages two segments below sensory anesthesia.

Dosages of local anesthesia used for spinal anesthesia vary according to (1) the height of the patient, which determines the volume of the subarachnoid space; (2) the segmental level of anesthesia desired; and (3) the duration of anesthesia desired. The total dose of local anesthetic administered for spinal anesthesia is more important than the concentration of drug or the volume of the solution injected. Tetracaine, lidocaine, and bupivacaine are the local anesthetics most frequently used for spinal anesthesia. Bupivacaine used for spinal anesthesia is more effective than tetracaine in preventing lower extremity tourniquet pain during orthopedic surgery (Stewart et al, 1988). This effectiveness may reflect the ability of bupivacaine to produce greater frequency-dependent conduction blockade of C fibers than does tetracaine. Dibucaine is 1.5 to 2 times as potent as tetracaine when used for spinal anesthesia. Chloroprocaine is not placed in the subarachnoid space because of potential neuro-toxicity (Covino et al, 1980; Ravindran et al, 1980; Reisner, Hochman, and Plumer, 1980).

Specific gravity of local anesthetic solutions injected into the lumbar cerecrospinal fluid is important in determining spread of the drugs. Addition of glucose to local anesthetic solutions increases specific gravity of the solutions above that of cerebrospinal fluid (hyperbaric). Addition of distilled water lowers the specific gravity of local anesthetic solutions below that of cerebrospinal fluid (hypobaric). Cerebrospinal fluid does not contain significant amounts of cholinesterase enzyme; therefore, the duration of action of ester local anesthetics as well as of amides placed in the subarachnoid space depends on vascular absorption of the drug. Duration of anesthesia can be extended up to 100% by addition of epinephrine to the solution.

PHYSIOLOGIC EFFECTS. The goal of spinal anesthesia is to provide sensory anesthesia and skeletal muscle relaxation. It is the accompanying level of sympathetic nervous system blockade, however, that produces physiologic alterations. Plasma concentrations of local anesthetics following subarachnoid injection are too low to produce physiologic changes.

Sympathetic nervous system blockade results in arteriolar dilatation, but blood pressure does not decline proportionally because of compensatory vasoconstriction in areas with intact sympathetic nervous system innervation. Compensatory vasoconstriction occurs principally in the upper extremities and does not involve the cerebral vasculature. Even with total sympathetic nervous system blockade produced by spinal anesthesia, the decrease in systemic vascular resistance is less than 15%. This change is minimal because smooth muscles of arterioles retain intrinsic tone and do not dilate maximally.

The most important cardiovascular responses produced by spinal anesthesia are those that result from changes in the venous circulation. Unlike arterioles denervated by sympathetic nervous system blockade, venules do not maintain intrinsic tone and thus dilate maximally during spinal anesthesia. The resulting increased vascular capacitance decreases venous return to the heart, leading to decreases in cardiac output and blood pressure. The physiologic effect of spinal anesthesia on venous return emphasizes the risk of extreme hypotension if this technique is used in a hypovolemic patient. Prompt augmentation of venous return through administration of a drug with alpha agonist activity, as well as a slightly head-down position, may minimize the likelihood of unexpected cardiac arrest during spinal anesthesia (Caplan et al, 1988; Keats, 1988).

Blockade of preganglionic cardiac accelerator fibers (T1 to T4) results in heart rate slowing, particularly if decreased venous return and central venous pressure reduce the stimulation level of intrinsic stretch receptors in the right atrium. For example, heart rate will increase with a head-down position that increases venous return and central venous pressure to stimulate these receptors. During spinal anesthesia, myocardial oxygen requirements are decreased as a result of decreased heart rate, venous return, and blood pressure.

Apnea that occurs with an excessive level of spinal anesthesia probably reflects ischemic paralysis of the medullary ventilatory centers due to profound hypotension and associated decreases in cerebral blood flow. Concentrations of local anesthetics in ventricular cerebrospinal fluid are usually too low to produce pharmacologic effects on the ventilatory centers. Rarely is the cause of apnea due to phrenic nerve paralysis.

Analgesia

Lidocaine and procaine have been demonstrated to produce intense analgesia when injected intravenously. Use of local anesthetics for this purpose, however, is limited by the small margin of safety between intravenous analgesic doses and those that produce systemic toxicity. Nevertheless, continuous low-dose intravenous infusion of lidocaine to maintain a plasma concentration of 1 to 2 $\mu g \cdot ml^{-1}$ decreases the severity of postoperative pain and reduces requirements for opioids without producing systemic toxicity (Cassuto et al, 1985). Lidocaine administered intravenously also decreases anesthetic requirements for volatile drugs. For example, halothane MAC in rats is decreased 40% by lidocaine, sufficient to produce plasma concentrations of 1 $\mu g \cdot ml^{-1}$ (Fig. 7-15) (DiFazio et al, 1976). A ceiling effect occurs above this plasma concentration, reflected by the absence of a further reduction in MAC despite more than fivefold increases in the lidocaine concentration. Lidocaine may also be

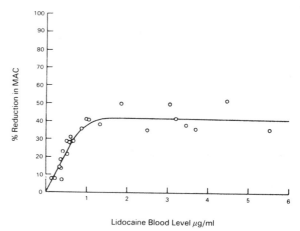

FIGURE 7-15. Halothane anesthetic requirements (MAC) are decreased in animals by approximately 40% when the plasma lidocaine concentration is 1 $\mu g \cdot ml^{-1}$. Further increases in the plasma lidocaine concentration do not decrease MAC an additional amount as evidence of a ceiling effect. (From DiFazio CA, Niederlehner JR, Burney RG. The anesthetic potency of lidocaine in the rat. Anesth Analg 1976; 55: 818–21; with permission.)

administered intravenously in the perioperative period as a cough suppressant. In this regard, the cough reflex during intubation of the trachea is suppressed by plasma concentrations of lidocaine greater than 3 $\mu g \cdot ml^{-1}$ (Yukioka et al, 1985).

Prevention or Treatment of Increases in Intracranial Pressure

Lidocaine, 1.5 $mg \cdot kg^{-1}$ IV, is as effective as thiopental in preventing increases in intracranial pressure evoked by intubation of the trachea (see Fig. 4–7) (Bedford et al, 1980). The antitussive effect of lidocaine may account in part for this effect. More likely, however, is the ability of lidocaine, like barbiturates, to decrease cerebral blood flow by increases in cerebral vascular resistance (Sakabe et al, 1974). Presumably, intracranial pressure declines in response to decreases in cerebral blood volume associated with decreases in cerebral blood flow. An advantage of using lidocaine rather than barbiturates to lower intracranial pressure is a lesser likelihood of drug-induced hypotension.

Lidocaine, 1.5 mg·kg^{-1} IV, which is used to prevent increases in intracranial pressure, is also effective in attenuating blood pressure but not heart rate responses associated with direct laryngoscopy for intubation of the trachea (Stoelting, 1977). Reflex-induced bronchospasm may also be attenuated by intravenous administration of lidocaine.

Suppression of Grand Mal Seizures

Suppression of grand mal seizures has been produced by intravenous administration of low doses of lidocaine or mepivacaine (Berry et al, 1961). Presumably, these and perhaps other local anesthetics when present at low plasma concentrations are effective in suppressing seizures through initial depression of hyperexcitable cortical neurons. Nevertheless, inhibitory neurons are usually more sensitive to depressant actions of local anesthetics than are excitatory neurons, and excitatory phenomena predominate.

COCAINE TOXICITY

Cocaine produces sympathetic nervous system stimulation by blocking the presynaptic uptake of norepinephrine and dopamine, thus increasing their postsynaptic concentrations. Intranasal administration of cocaine near the dose used for topical anesthesia in rhinolaryngologic procedures causes vasoconstriction of the coronary arteries with a decrease in coronary blood flow despite increases in myocardial oxygen requirements due to hypertension and tachycardia (Lange et al, 1989). It is presumed these effects would be more pronounced with the recreational use of cocaine. There is a temporal association between the recreational use of cocaine and cerebrovascular accidents (Levine et al, 1990). Cocaine-induced cardiovascular effects may manifest as myocardial ischemia, myocardial infarction, or cardiac dysrhythmias, including ventricular fibrillation. Administration of topical cocaine plus epinephrine, or in the presence of volatile anesthetics that sensitize the myocardium, may exaggerate the cardiac stimulating effects of cocaine. Cocaine should be used with caution, if at all, in patients with hypertension or coronary artery disease and in patients receiving drugs that potentiate the effects of catecholamines such as

monoamine oxidase inhibitors. Cardiovascular toxicity due to cocaine may be treated with esmolol to maintain a heart rate of less than 100 beats·min^{-1}, whereas seizures respond to diazepam (Pollan and Tadjziechy, 1989). The selective beta-1 effects of esmolol reduce the likelihood that unopposed cocaine-induced alpha stimulation will produce coronary artery and peripheral vascular vasospasm.

Cocaine produces dose-dependent reductions in uterine blood flow that result in fetal hypoxemia (Woods et al, 1987). Cocaine may produce hyperpyrexia, which could contribute to seizures.

ROPIVACAINE

Ropivacaine is an amide local anesthetic with a chemical structure, pK, and protein binding that resemble bupivacaine (Table 7-1; Fig. 7-1) (Concepcion et al, 1990; Moller and Covino, 1990). This drug is unique among local anesthetics because it is prepared as the S-isomer rather than as a racemic mixture. Previous studies involving the isomers of local anesthetics suggest that cardiac toxicity of the S-isomer may be less than that of racemic preparations. Indeed, ropivacaine's lipid solubility and depressant effect on cardiac excitation and conduction are intermediate between lidocaine and bupivacaine (Moller and Covino, 1990; Scott et al, 1989). In contrast to bupivacaine, ropivacaine produces less motor blockade and has a greater tendency to block A-delta and C fibers (Feldman and Covino, 1988). These characteristics of ropivacaine may be advantageous for obstetric patients in labor and for those experiencing acute and chronic pain. In humans, 20 ml of 0.5% ropivacaine or bupivacaine placed in the epidural space produces similar sensory and motor blocking characteristics, with the exception that bupivacaine produces a blockade of slightly longer duration (Fig. 7-16) (Brown et al, 1990). Ropivacaine, 33 ml of a 0.5% solution used for performance of a subclavian perivascular block, produces a rapid onset of sensory anesthesia (averaging less than 4 minutes) with prolonged sensory (averaging more than 13 hours) and motor blockade (Hickey et al, 1990). Systemic toxicity in animals occurs when venous plasma concentrations of ropivacaine are greater than 4 µg·kg^{-1}. In humans, the peak venous plasma concentration of ropivacaine is 1.3

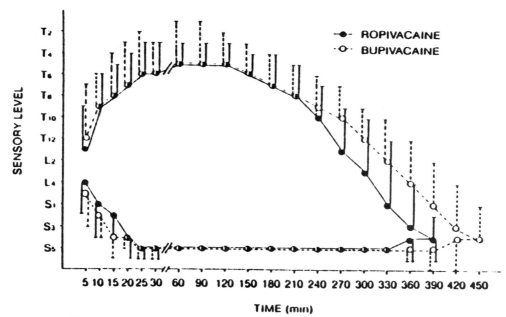

FIGURE 7–16. The characteristics of motor and sensory blockade produced by 0.5% ropivacaine or bupivacaine placed in the epidural space are similar except for a more rapid regression of the upper level of sensory blockade in patients receiving ropivacaine. (From Brown DL, Carpenter RL, Thompson GE. Comparison of 0.5% ropivacaine and 0.5% bupivacaine for epidural anesthesia in patients undergoing lower extremity surgery. Anesthesiology 1990; 72: 633–6; with permission.)

$\mu g \cdot ml^{-1}$ following epidural placement of 200 mg of the local anesthetic.

REFERENCES

Adejepon-Yamoah KK, Scott DB, Prescott LF. Impaired absorption and metabolism of oral lignocaine in patients undergoing laparoscopy. Br J Anaesth 1973;45:143–7.

Albright GA. Cardiac arrest following regional anesthesia with etidocaine or bupivacaine (editorial). Anesthesiology 1979;51:285–7.

Atlee JL, Bosnjak ZJ. Mechanisms for dysrhythmias during anesthesia. Anesthesiology 1990;72:347–74.

Bader AM, Concepcion M, Hurley RJ, Arthur GR. Comparison of lidocaine and prilocaine for intravenous regional anesthesia. Anesthesiology 1988;69:409–12.

Bedford RF, Persing JA, Roberskin L, Butler A. Lidocaine or thiopental for rapid control of intracranial hypertension. Anesth Analg 1980;59:435–7.

Benowitz N, Forsyth RP, Melmon KL, et al. Lidocaine disposition kinetics in monkey and man. I: Prediction by a perfusion model. Clin Pharmacol Ther 1974;16:87–92.

Berry CA, Sanner JH, Keasling HH. A comparison of the anticonvulsant activity of mepivacaine and lidocaine. J. Pharmacol Exp Ther 1961;133:357–63.

Biehl D, Shnider SM, Levinson G, Callender K. Placental transfer of lidocaine: Effects of fetal acidosis. Anesthesiology 1978;48:409–12.

Bowdle TA, Freund PR, Slattery JT. Propranolol reduces bupivacaine clearance. Anesthesiology 1987;66:36–8.

Bromage PR, Datta S. Dunford LA. Etidocaine: An evaluation in epidural analgesia for obstetrics. Can Anaesth Soc J 1974;21:535–45.

Brown DL, Carpenter RL, Thompson GE. Comparison of 0.5% ropivacaine and 0.5% bupivacaine for epidural anesthesia in patients undergoing lower extremity surgery. Anesthesiology 1990;72:633–6.

Brown DT, Beamish D, Wildsmith JAW. Allergic reaction to an amide local anaesthetic. Br J Anaesth 1981;53:435–7.

Butterworth JF, Strichartz GR. Molecular mechanisms of local anesthesia: A review. Anesthesiology 1990;72:722–34.

Caplan RA, Ward RJ, Psoner K, Cheney FW. Unexpected cardiac arrest during spinal anesthesia: A closed claims analysis of predisposing factors. Anesthesiology 1988;68:5–11.

Chang-Hyon Y. The half-life of 2-chloroprocaine. Anesth Analg 1986a;65:273–9.

Carpenter RL, Smith HS, Bridenbaugh LD. Epinephrine increases the effectiveness of tetracaine spinal anesthesia. Anesthesiology 1989;71:33–6.

Cassuto J, Wallin G, Hogstrom S, Faxes A, Rimback G. Inhibition of postoperative pain by continuous low-dose intravenous infusion of lidocaine. Anesth Analg 1985;64:971–4.

Chestnut DH, Geiger M, Bates JN, Choi WW. The influence of pH-adjusted 2-chloroprocaine on the quality and duration of subsequent epidural bupivacaine analgesia during labor: A randomized, double blind study. Anesthesiology 1989;70:437–11.

Clarkson CW, Hondeghem LM. Mechanism for bupivacaine depression of cardiac conduction: Fast block of sodium channels during the action potential with slow recovery from block during diastole. Anesthesiology 1985;62:396–405.

Concepcion M, Arthur GR, Steele SM, Bader AM, Covino BG. A new local anesthetic, ropivacaine. Its epidural effects in humans. Anesth Analg 1990;70:80–5.

Covino BG, Marx GF, Finster M, Zsigmond EK. Prolonged sensory/motor deficits following inadvertent spinal anesthesia (editorial). Anesth Analg 1980;59:399–400.

Covino BG, Vassallo HL. Local anesthetics: Mechanisms of Action and Clinical Use. New York, Grune and Stratton, 1976.

Datta S, Lambert DH, Gergus J, Gissen AJ, Covino BJ. Differential sensitivities of mammalian nerve fibers during pregnancy. Anesth Analg 1983;62:1070–2.

Denson DD, Coyle DE, Santos D, Turner PA, Myers JA, Knapp R. Bupivacaine protein binding in the term parturient. Effects of lactic acidosis. Clin Pharmacol Ther 1984a;35:409–15.

Denson DD, Santos DJ, Coyle DE. The effect of elevated progesterone on the serum protein binding of bupivacaine. Anesthesiology 1984b:61:A235.

DiFazio CA, Niederlehner JR, Burney RG. The anesthetic potency of lidocaine in the rat. Anesth Analg 1976;55:818–21.

Feldman HS, Covino BG. Comparative motor-blocking effects of bupivacaine and ropivacaine, a new amino amide local anesthetic in the rat and dog. Anesth Analg 1988;67:1047–52.

Finster M. Toxicity of local anesthetics in the fetus and the newborn. Bull NY Acad Med 1976;52:222–5.

Gross JB, Caldwell CB, Shaw LM, Apfelbaum JL. The effect of lidocaine infusion on the ventilatory response to hypoxia. Anesthesiology 1984;61:662–5.

Hickey R, Candido KD, Ramamurthy S, et al. Brachial plexus block with a new local anaesthetic: 0.5 percent ropivacaine. Can J Anaesth 1990;37:732–8.

Incaudo G, Schatz M, Patterson R, Rosenberg M, Yamamoto F, Hamburger RN. Administration of local anesthetics to patients with a prior adverse reaction. J Allergy Clin Immunol 1978;61:339–45.

Inoue R, Suganuma T, Echizen H, Ishizaki T, Kushida K, Tomona Y. Plasma concentrations of lidocaine and its principal metabolites during intermittent epidural anesthesia. Anesthesiology 1985;63:304–10.

Jorfeldt L, Lewis DH, Lofstrom JB, Post C. Lung uptake of lidocaine in man. Regional Anesthesia 1980;5:6–7.

Kaniaris P, Fassoulaki A, Liarmakopoulou K, Dermitzakis E. Serum cholinesterase levels in patients with cancer. Anesth Analg 1979;58:82–4.

Kaplan JA, Miller ED, Gallagher EG. Postoperative analgesia for thoracotomy patients. Anesth Analg 1975;54:773–7.

Kasten GW, Martin ST. Bupivacaine cardiovascular toxicity: Comparison of treatment with bretylium and lidocaine. Anesth Analg 1985;64:911–6.

Keats AS. Anesthesia mortality—A new mechanism. Anesthesiology 1988;68:2–4.

Kendig JJ. Clinical implications of the modulated receptor hypothesis: Local anesthetics and the heart (editorial). Anesthesiology 1985;62:382–4.

Kotelko DM, Shnider SM, Dailey PA, et al. Bupivacaine-induced cardiac arrhythmias in sheep. Anesthesiology 1984;60:10–18.

Kuhnert BR, Kuhnert PM, Philipson EH, Syracuse CD, Kaine CJ, Chang-Hyon Y. The half-life of 2-chloroprocaine. Anesth Analg 1986a;65:273–8.

Kuhnert BR, Kuhnert PM, Prochaska BS, Gross TL. Plasma levels of 2-chloroprocaine in obstetric patients and their neonates after epidural anesthesia. Anesthesiology 1980;53:21–5.

Kuhnert BR, Philipson EH, Pimental R, Kuhnert PM, Zuspan KJ, Syracuse CD. Lidocaine disposition in mother, fetus, and neonate after spinal anesthesia. Anesth Analg 1986b;65:139–44.

Kuhnert BR, Zuspan KJ, Kuhnert PM, Syracuse CD, Brown DE. Bupivacaine disposition in mother, fetus, and neonate after spinal anesthesia for caesarean section. Anesth Analg 1987;66:407–12.

Lange RA, Cigarroa RG, Yancy CW, et al. Cocaine-induced coronary artery vasoconstriction. N Engl J Med 1989;321:1557–62.

Levine RA, Brust JCM, Futrell N, et al. Cocaine-induced coronary artery vasoconstriction. N Engl J Med 1989;323:699–704.

Moller R, Covino BG. Cardiac electrophysiologic properties of bupivacaine and lidocaine compared with those of ropivacaine, a new amide local anesthetic. Anesthesiology 1990;72:322–9.

Moore DC, Crawford RD, Scurlock JE. Severe hypoxia and acidosis following local anesthetic-induced convulsions. Anesthesiology 1980;53:259–60.

Morishima HO, Pederson H, Finster M, et al. Bupivacaine toxicity in pregnant and nonpregnant ewes. Anesthesiology 1985;63:134–9.

Munson ES, Paul WL, Embro WJ. Central-nervous system toxicity of local anesthetic mixtures in monkeys. Anesthesiology 1977;46:179–83.

Negre I, Labaille T, Samili K, Noviant Y. Ventilatory response to carbon dioxide following axillary blockade with bupivacaine. Anesthesiology 1985;63:401–3.

Pihlajamaki K, Kantro J, Lindberg R, Karanko M, Kiiholma P. Extradural administration of bupivacaine: Pharmacokinetics and metabolism in pregnant and non-pregnant women. Br J Anaesth 1990;64:556–62.

Pollan S, Tadjziechy M. Esmolol in the management of epinephrine and cocaine-induced cardiovascular toxicity. Anesth Analg 1989;69:663–4.

Ramanathan J, Bottorff M, Jeter JN, Khalil M, Sibai BM. The pharmacokinetics and maternal and neonatal effects of epidural lidocaine in preeclampsia. Anesth Analg 1986;65:120–6.

Ravindran RS, Bond VK, Tasch MD, Gupta CD. Luerssen TG. Prolonged neural blockade following regional analgesia with 2-chloroprocaine. Anesth Analg 1980;59:447–51.

Reidenberg MM, James M, Drign LG. The rate of procaine hydrolysis in serum of normal subjects and diseased patients. Clin Pharmacol Ther 1972;13:279–84.

Reisner LS, Hochman BN, Plumer MH. Persistent neurologic deficit and adhesive arachnoiditis following intrathecal 2-chloroprocaine injection. Anesth Analg 1980;59:452–4.

Rothstein P, Cole J, Pitt BR. Pulmonary extraction of bupivacaine is dose dependent. Anesthesiology 1984;61:A236.

Rothstein P, Pitt BR. Pulmonary extraction of bupivacaine and its modification by propranolol. Anesthesiology 1983;59:A189.

Sakabe T, Maekawa T, Ishikawa T, Takeshita H. The effects of lidocaine on canine cerebral metabolism and circulation related to the electroencephalogram. Anesthesiology 1974;40:433–41.

Scott DB. Maximum recommended doses of local anaesthetic drugs. Br J Anaesth 1989;63:373–4.

Scott DB, Jebson PJR, Braid B, Ortengren B, Frisch P. Factors affecting plasma levels of lignocaine and prilocaine. Br J Anaesth 1972;44:1040–9.

Scott DB, Lee A, Fagan D, Bowler GMR, Bloomfield P, Lundh R. Acute toxicity of ropivacaine compared with that of bupivacaine. Anesth Analg 1989;69:563–9.

Stewart A, Lambert DH, Concepcion MA, et al. Decreased incidence of tourniquet pain during spinal anesthesia with bupivacaine. A possible explanation. Anesth Analg 1988;67:833–7.

Stoelting RK. Circulatory changes during direct laryngoscopy and tracheal intubation: Influence of duration of laryngoscopy with or without prior lidocaine. Anesthesiology 1977;47:381–3.

Thomas J, Long G, Moore G, Morgan D. Plasma protein binding and placental transfer of bupivacaine. Clin Pharmacol 1976;19:426–34.

Tucker GT, Boyes RN, Bridenbaugh PO, et al. Binding of anilide-type local anesthetics in human plasma: I. Relationships between binding, physicochemical properties, and anesthetic activity. Anesthesiology 1970;33:287–93.

Tucker GT, Mather LE. Clinical pharmacokinetics of local anesthetics. Clin Pharmacokinet 1979;4:241–78.

Viegas O, Stoelting RK. Lidocaine in arterial blood after laryngotracheal administration. Anesthesiology 1975;43:491–3.

Winnie AP, LaValley DA, DeSosa B, Mazud KZ. Clinical pharmacokinetics of local anesthetics. Can Anaesth Soc J 1977a;24:252–62.

Winnie AP, Tay C-H, Patel KP, Ramamurthy S, Durrani Z. Pharmacokinetics of local anesthetics during plexus blocks. Anesth Analg 1977b;56:852–61.

Woods JR, Plessinger MA, Clark KE. Effect of cocaine on uterine blood flow and fetal oxygenation. JAMA 1987;257:957–61.

Yukioka H, Yoshimoto N, Nishimura K, Fujimori M. Intravenous lidocaine as a suppressant of coughing during tracheal intubation. Anesth Analg 1985;64:1189–92.

Chapter

8

Neuromuscular Blocking Drugs

The principal pharmacologic effect of neuromuscular blocking drugs is to interrupt transmission of nerve impulses at the neuromuscular junction. On the basis of distinct electrophysiologic differences in their mechanisms of action and durations of action, these drugs can be classified as depolarizing neuromuscular blocking drugs and nondepolarizing neuromuscular blocking drugs which are further subdivided into long-acting, and intermediate-acting drugs (Table 8-1). Neuromuscular blocking drugs produce phase I depolarizing neuromuscular blockade, phase II depolarizing neuromuscular blockade, or nondepolarizing neuromuscular blockade.

Clinically, the most reliable method for determining the type and degree of neuromuscular blockade present is to observe or record the skeletal muscle response that is evoked by a supramaximal electrical stimulus delivered from a peripheral nerve stimulator. Most often, contraction of the adductor pollicis muscle (twitch response) following electrical stimulation of the ulnar nerve is used to assess the effect of neuromuscular blocking drugs. It is important to recognize that the dose of neuromuscular blocking drug necessary to produce a given degree of neuromuscular blockade at the diaphragm is approximately twice the dose required to produce similar blockade of the adductor pollicis muscle (Donati et al, 1986). A single twitch response evoked using a peripheral nerve stimulator reflects events at the postjunctional membrane.

Conversely, the response to continuous stimulation or train-of-four stimulation reflects events at the presynaptic membrane. The differences in effects of nondepolarizing neuromuscular drugs on responses to single stimulus vs multiple or continuous stimulation most likely reflect differences in the magnitude of presynaptic and postsynaptic effects of these drugs (Bowman, 1980). The electromyogram serves the same purpose as the peripheral nerve stimulator.

Table 8–1
Classification of Neuromuscular Blocking Drugs

Depolarizers
　Succinylcholine
　Decamethonium

Nondepolarizers
　Long-acting
　　d-Tubocurarine
　　Metocurine
　　Gallamine
　　Pancuronium
　　Doxacurium
　　Pipecuronium
　Intermediate-acting
　　Atracurium
　　Vecuronium
　　Mivacurium

HISTORY

Modern clinical use of neuromuscular blocking drugs dates from 1932 when purified fractions of d-tubocurarine (dTc) were administered to control skeletal muscle spasms in patients with tetanus. In 1940, dTc was administered as an adjuvant to drug-induced electroshock therapy. The first use of dTc to produce skeletal muscle relaxation during surgery and general anesthesia was reported in 1942 (Griffith and Johnson, 1942). The use of curarized animals in experiments conducted on succinylcholine in 1906 masked the neuromuscular blocking properties of this drug. Indeed, the neuromuscular blocking effects of succinylcholine were not recognized until 1949.

CLINICAL USES

Currently, the principal uses of neuromuscular blocking drugs are to provide skeletal muscle relaxation to facilitate intubation of the trachea and to provide optimal surgical working conditions. However, neuromuscular blocking drugs lack central nervous system depressant and analgesic effects. Therefore, these drugs cannot substitute for anesthetic drugs. Furthermore, ventilation of the lungs must be provided mechanically whenever substantial neuromuscular blockade is produced by these drugs. Clinically, the degree of neuromuscular blockade is typically evaluated by monitoring the evoked skeletal muscle responses produced by an electrical stimulus delivered from a peripheral nerve stimulator. Other indicators of residual neuromuscular blockade include grip strength, ability to sustain head lift, vital capacity measurement, and generation of negative inspiratory pressure.

Drug Selection

The choice between depolarizing and nondepolarizing neuromuscular blocking drugs is influenced by speed of onset, duration of action, and possibility of drug-induced side effects owing to the actions of these drugs at sites other than the neuromuscular junction. A rapid onset and brief duration of neuromuscular blockade, as provided by succinylcholine and to a lesser extent by mivacurium, is useful when intubation of the trachea is the reason for administering a neuromuscular blocking drug. When sustained periods of neuromuscular blockade are needed, nondepolarizing neuromuscular blocking drugs are selected for injection as intermittent doses or as a continuous intravenous infusion. Succinylcholine may also be administered as a continuous intravenous infusion to provide sustained paralysis. When a rapid onset of neuromuscular blockade is not considered necessary, skeletal muscle relaxation to facilitate intubation of the trachea can be provided by nondepolarizing neuromuscular blocking drugs.

Sequence of Onset of Neuromuscular Blockade

Neuromuscular blocking drugs affect small, rapidly moving muscles such as those of the eyes and digits before those of the trunk and abdomen. Ultimately, intercostal muscles and finally the diaphragm are paralyzed. Recovery of skeletal muscles usually occurs in the reverse order to that of paralysis such that the diaphragm is the first to regain function.

Intravenous injection of a nondepolarizing neuromuscular blocking drug to a person who is awake initially produces difficulty in focusing and weakness in the mandibular muscles followed by ptosis, diplopia, and dysphagia. Relaxation of the small muscles of the ears improves acuity of hearing. Consciousness and sensorium remain undistributed even in the presence of complete neuromuscular blockade.

STRUCTURE ACTIVITY RELATIONSHIPS

Neuromuscular blocking drugs have structural similarities to the endogenous neurotransmitter acetylcholine (Fig. 8-1). For example, succinylcholine is two molecules of acetylcholine linked through acetate methyl groups. The long, slender, and flexible structure of succinylcholine allows it to bind to and activate cholinergic receptors. Bulky and rigid molecules that are characteristic of nondepolarizing neuromuscular drugs, although containing portions similar to acetylcholine, cannot activate the cholinergic receptor. Pancuronium is most closely related structurally to acetylcholine. The acetylcholine-like fragments of pancuronium give the steroidal molecule its high degree of neuromuscular

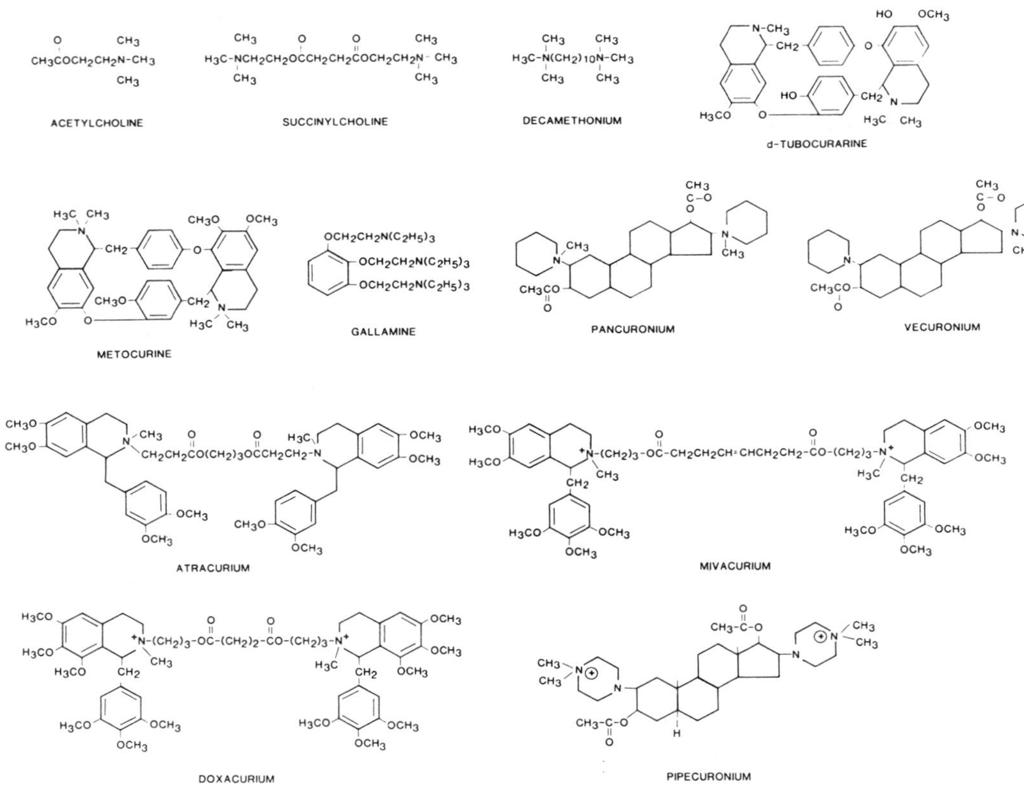

FIGURE 8–1. Acetylcholine and neuromuscular blocking drugs.

blocking activity and its plasma cholinesterase-inhibiting action.

Acetylcholine has a positively charged quaternary ammonium group (four carbon atoms attached to one nitrogen atom) that attaches to the negatively charged cholinergic receptor (Fig. 8-1). The same feature is common to neuromuscular blocking drugs, which all contain one or more positively charged quaternary ammonium groups. For example, dTc and vecuronium are monoquaternary; metocurine, pancuronium, and atracurium are bisquaternary; and gallamine is triquaternary (Fig. 8-1). Pancuronium is an aminosteroid with no hormonal activity. The bisquaternary ammonium structure of most of these drugs suggests that an electrostatic association occurs between two ionized cationic centers of the drug and anionic groups on the cholinergic receptor. It is no longer tenable to propose that nondepolarizing neuromuscular blocking activity depends on an optimal distance between quaternary ammonium groups. Indeed, dTc and vecuronium contain only one quaternary ammonium group. It is likely, however, that an interquaternary distance of 1.25 nm confers optimal neuromuscular blocking activity.

The electrostatic attraction of the negatively charged cholinergic receptor for the positively charged quaternary ammonium group occurs at cholinergic sites other than the neuromuscular junction, including cardiac muscarinic receptors and autonomic ganglia nicotinic receptors. This lack of specificity for the neuromuscular junction means that neuromuscular blocking drugs could produce cardiovascular effects, particularly as reflected by changes in blood pressure and heart rate.

The specificity of a drug for the autonomic ganglia nicotinic receptor vs the neuromuscular junction is influenced by the length of the carbon chain separating the two positively charged ammonium groups. Maximal autonomic ganglion blockade occurs when the positive charges are separated by six carbon atoms (hexamethonium), whereas neuromuscular blockade occurs when 10 carbon atoms are present (decamethonium). As a bulky monoquaternary molecule, dTc is more likely to produce autonomic ganglion blockade than is a bisquaternary drug. Indeed, methylation of dTc to the bisquaternary ammonium drug metocurine dramatically decreases the autonomic blocking properties associated with production of neuromuscular blockade. Likewise, bisquaternary ammonium neuromuscular blocking drugs such as metocurine and pancuronium are less likely than the monoquaternary dTc to evoke the release of histamine. Presumably, the histamine-releasing properties of dTc are due to the presence of the tertiary amine. The increased efficacy of dTc in the presence of acidosis most likely reflects increased ionization of the tertiary amino group as the plasma pH decreases. Gallamine possesses marked vagolytic effects presumably due to the presence of three quaternary ammonium nitrogen atoms.

NEUROMUSCULAR JUNCTION

A neuromuscular junction consists of a prejunctional motor nerve ending separated from a highly folded postjunctional membrane of the skeletal muscle fiber by a synaptic cleft that is 20 to 30 nm wide and filled with extracellular fluid (Fig. 8-2) (Drachman, 1978) (see Chapter 55). The nonmyelinated nerve ending contains mitochondria, endoplasmic reticulum, and synaptic vesicles necessary to synthesize the neurotransmitter acetylcholine. The resting transmembrane potential of approximately −90 mV across nerve and skeletal muscle membranes is maintained by the unequal distribution of potassium (K^+) and sodium (Na^+) ions across the membrane. Nicotinic cholinergic receptors are situated on both the presynaptic and postsynaptic membranes.

Acetylcholine

The neurotransmitter at the neuromuscular junction is the quaternary ammonium ester acetylcholine. Acetylcholine in motor nerve endings is synthesized by the acetylation of choline under the control of the enzyme choline acetylase. This acetylcholine is stored in synaptic vesicles in motor nerve endings and released into the synaptic cleft as packets (quanta), each of which contains at least 1000 molecules of acetylcholine. Arrival of a nerve impulse causes the release of hundreds of quanta of acetylcholine that bind to nicotinic cholinergic receptors on postsynaptic membranes, causing a change in membrane permeability to ions. This change in permeability causes a decline in the transmembrane potential from approximately −90 mV to −45 mV (threshold potential). At that point, a propagated action potential spreads over the surfaces of skeletal muscle fibers leading to their contraction. In the absence of action potentials, quanta of acetylcholine are released randomly, producing miniature endplate potentials of less than 1 mV that are insufficient to trigger depolarization. Calcium ions (Ca^{2+}) must be present for the release of acetylcholine from synaptic vesicles into the synaptic cleft. It is speculated that a nerve action potential activates adenylate cyclase in membranes of nerve terminals leading to the forma-

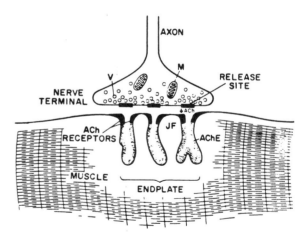

FIGURE 8–2. Schematic depiction of the neuromuscular junction. Acetylchloride (ACh) is present in vesicles (V) of the axon for release in response to nerve impulses. The neurotransmitter diffuses across the synaptic cleft to attach to receptors that are concentrated on the junctional folds (JF) of the skeletal muscle endplate. Acetylcholinesterase (AChE) is present in the JF to facilitate rapid hydrolysis of ACh. (From Drachman DA. Myasthenia gravis. N Engl J Med 1978; 298: 136–42; with permission.)

tion of cyclic adenosine monophosphate (cyclic AMP). Cyclic AMP subsequently opens Ca^{2+} channels, causing synaptic vesicles to fuse with the nerve membrane and to release acetylcholine (Standaert and Dretchen, 1981). Indeed, drugs such as aminophylline that stimulate formation of cyclic AMP facilitate neuromuscular transmission, and calcium entry blocking drugs such as verapamil interfere with neuromuscular transmission.

Situated in close proximity to cholinergic receptors is the enzyme acetylcholinesterase. This enzyme is responsible for the rapid hydrolysis (less than 15 ms) of acetylcholine to acetic acid and choline. Choline can reenter motor nerve endings to again participate in the synthesis of new acetylcholine. The rapid hydrolysis of acetylcholine prevents sustained depolarization of the neuromuscular junction.

Postjunctional Nicotinic Receptors

Postjunctional membranes possess two types of receptors that respond to neuromuscular blocking drugs (Standaert, 1984). Nicotinic cholinergic receptors are present in large numbers on postjunctional membranes. Extrajunctional cholinergic receptors appear throughout skeletal muscles whenever there is deficient stimulation of the skeletal muscle by the nerve.

Nicotinic Cholinergic Receptors

Postjunctional nicotinic cholinergic receptors are glycoproteins with a molecular weight of approximately 250,000 daltons. Each receptor consists of five subunits designated alpha, beta, gamma, and delta (Fig. 8-3) (Taylor, 1985). There are two alpha subunits weighing approximately 40,000 daltons each; the other subunits weigh 50,000 to 65,000 daltons. Electron micrographs of nicotinic cholinergic receptors show these receptors to be particularly concentrated on the shoulders of the postjunctional membrane folds, which places them precisely opposite prejunctional release sites for acetylcholine.

Nicotinic cholinergic receptors extend through the entire cell membrane and continue for approximately 2 nm into the cytoplasm (Stroud, 1983). The subunits of the receptor are arranged to form a channel that allows the flow of ions along a concentration gradient (Fig. 8-3) (Taylor, 1985). For example, Na^+ and Ca^{2+} move

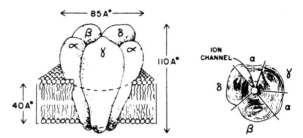

FIGURE 8–3. The postjunctional nicotinic cholinergic receptor consists of five subunits designated alpha (two subunits), beta, gamma, and delta. (From Taylor P. Are neuromuscular blocking agents more efficacious in pairs? Anesthesiology 1985; 63: 1–3; with permission.)

into skeletal muscles, whereas K^+ exit by way of these channels. These channels are open (in the active state) only when an acetylcholine molecule occupies each of the alpha subunits, causing the subunits to rotate into an open conformation that allows the flow of ions (Fig. 8-3) (Taylor, 1985). This flow of ions is the basis of normal neuromuscular transmission.

The two alpha subunits, in addition to being the binding sites for acetylcholine, are the sites occupied by neuromuscular blocking drugs. For example, occupation of one or both alpha subunits by a nondepolarizing neuromuscular blocking drug causes the channel to remain closed. As a result, ions do not flow in these channels, and depolarization cannot occur at these sites. If enough channels remain closed, there is blockade of neuromuscular transmission. A nondepolarizing neuromuscular blocking drug may show preference for one of the two alpha subunits. This may result in synergism if two nondepolarizing neuromuscular blocking drugs with different selective preferences for each alpha subunit are administered simultaneously. Succinylcholine, by binding to each alpha subunit, causes the channel to remain open, causing sustained depolarization that prevents propagation of an action potential. Large doses of nondepolarizing muscle relaxants may also prevent normal flow of ions by entering the channels formed by the nicotinic cholinergic receptors to produce channel blockade. Similar blockade of Na^+ channels is produced by local anesthetics.

Extrajunctional Cholinergic Receptors

Extrajunctional cholinergic receptors are normally not present in large numbers because their synthesis is suppressed by neural activity. Whenever motor nerves are less active due to traumatized skeletal muscle or denervation, these extrajunctional cholinergic receptors proliferate rapidly (Pumplin and Fambrough, 1982). These extrajunctional cholinergic receptors appear over the entire postjunctional membrane rather than being confined to the area of the neuromuscular junction.

Extrajunctional cholinergic receptors are highly responsive to agonists such as acetylcholine or succinylcholine. Because extrajunctional cholinergic receptors are formed rapidly after slackening of neural influence on skeletal muscles and are degraded soon after the neural influence returns, mixtures of nicotinic cholinergic receptors and extrajunctional cholinergic receptors are present in many clinical situations and may account for differences in responses to neuromuscular blocking drugs among individuals and various disease states.

Prejunctional Nicotinic Receptors

Prejunctional nicotinic cholinergic receptors on motor nerve endings influence the release of neurotransmitters. These prejunctional receptors seem to be different from postjunctional nicotinic cholinergic receptors in (1) their chemical binding characteristics, (2) the nature of the ion channel they control, and (3) their preferential blockade during high-frequency stimulation. Some nondepolarizing neuromuscular blocking drugs block prejunctional Na^+ but not Ca^{2+} channels. As a result, these drugs may interfere with mobilization of acetylcholine from synthesis sites to release sites. Interference with release of acetylcholine, which is Ca^{2+} dependent, does not occur.

DEPOLARIZING NEUROMUSCULAR BLOCKING DRUGS

Depolarizing neuromuscular blocking drugs are represented by succinylcholine and decamethonium (Fig. 8-1). Succinylcholine, 0.5 to 1 $mg\cdot kg^{-1}$ IV, has a rapid onset (30 to 60 seconds) and short duration of action (3 to 5 minutes). These characteristics make succinylcholine a useful drug for providing skeletal muscle relaxation to facilitate intubation of the trachea. In adult patients, the ED_{90} for succinylcholine as de-

termined following administration of thiopental and while breathing nitrous oxide is 0.27 $mg\cdot kg^{-1}$ IV (Smith et al, 1988). Succinylcholine has several associated adverse side effects that can limit or even contraindicate its use. Decamethonium is available but rarely used.

Mechanism of Action

Succinylcholine attaches to each of the alpha subunits of the nicotinic choligenic receptor and mimics the action of acetylcholine, thus depolarizing the postjunctional membrane. Compared with acetylcholine, the hydrolysis of succinylcholine is slow, resulting in sustained depolarization (opening) of the receptor channels. Neuromuscular blockade develops because a depolarized postjunctional membrane cannot respond to subsequent release of acetylcholine (depolarizing neuromuscular blockade). Depolarizing neuromuscular blockade is also referred to as phase I blockade. Succinylcholine has presynaptic effects, but these are considered minor when compared with postsynaptic actions (Standaert and Adams, 1965). Sustained opening of receptor channels and resulting depolarization of postjunctional membranes produced by succinylcholine is associated with leakage of K^+ from the interior of cells sufficient to produce an average 0.5 $mEq\cdot L^{-1}$ increase in serum K^+ concentrations.

A single large dose of succinylcholine (more than 2 $mg\cdot kg^{-1}$ IV), repeated doses, or a prolonged continuous intravenous infusion of succinylcholine may result in postjunctional membranes that do not respond normally to acetylcholine even when postjunctional membranes have become repolarized (desensitization neuromuscular blockade). The mechanism for the development of desensitization neuromuscular blockade is unknown and, for this reason, phase II blockade, which does not imply a mechanism, is the preferred terminology (Hunter and Feldman, 1976). It is likely that combinations of receptor desensitization, channel blockade, and entrance of succinylcholine into the cytoplasm of skeletal muscles are responsible for the events that manifest as phase II blockade.

Characteristics of Phase I Blockade

Electrically evoked mechanical responses, using a peripheral nerve stimulator, that are characteristic of phase I blockade are (1) decreased contraction in response to a single twitch stimulus, (2) decreased amplitude but sustained response to continuous stimulation, (3) train-of-four ratio more than 0.7, (4) absence of posttetanic facilitation, and (5) augmentation of neuromuscular blockade by anticholinesterase drugs. In addition, the onset of phase I blockade is accompanied by skeletal muscle fasciculations that reflect the generalized depolarization of postjunctional membranes produced by succinylcholine.

Characteristics of Phase II Blockade

Electrically evoked mechanical responses, using a peripheral nerve stimulator, that are characteristic of phase II blockade resemble those considered typical of neuromuscular blockade produced by nondepolarizing neuromuscular blocking drugs. Furthermore, phase II blockade can be reversed with anticholinesterase drugs. Despite these similarities, it is likely that mechanisms of nondepolarizing neuromuscular blockade and succinylcholine-induced phase II blockade differ.

The transition between phase I and phase II blockade is fairly abrupt, occurring with a succinylcholine dose of 2 to 4 mg·kg^{-1} IV (Fig. 8-4) (Lee, 1975). Clinically, the onset of phase II blockade is often manifested initially as tachyphylaxis and the need to increase the infusion rate of succinylcholine or to administer progressively larger incremental doses. At a single moment, varying degrees of phase I and phase II blockade may be present (Ali and Savarese, 1976). When neuromuscular blockade is predominantly phase I, administering an anticholinesterase drug will enhance neuromuscular blockade. Conversely, an anticholinesterase drug will antagonize a predominant phase II blockade. An acceptable approach is to observe the mechanical responses evoked by a peripheral nerve stimulator after administering a small dose of anticholinesterase drug such as edrophonium, 0.1 to 0.2 mg·kg^{-1} IV. If this small dose of anticholinesterase drug improves neuromuscular transmission, it is likely that an additional dose of anticholinesterase drug will antagonize, rather than enhance, neuromuscular blockade produced by succinylcholine.

Duration of Action

The brief duration of action of succinylcholine (3 to 5 minutes) is principally due to its hydrolysis

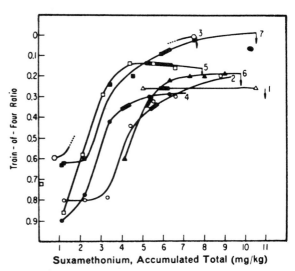

FIGURE 8–4. The transition between phase I and phase II blockade as depicted by the train-of-four ratio is fairly abrupt, occurring at a total dose of succinylcholine (suxamethonium) of 2 to 4 mg·kg^{-1} IV. (From Lee C. Dose relationship of phase II, tachyphylaxis and train-of-four fade on suxamethonium-induced dual neuromuscular block in man. Br J Anaesth 1975; 47: 841–5; with permission.)

by plasma cholinesterase (pseudocholinesterase) enzyme (Fig. 8-5). The initial metabolite, succinylmonocholine, is a much weaker neuromuscular blocker (1/20 to 1/80 as potent) than the parent drug. Succinylmonocholine is subsequently hydrolyzed to succinic acid and choline. Rapid hydrolysis makes it difficult to obtain pharmacokinetic data for succinylcholine. Nevertheless, based on isolated tourniquet techniques, it seems likely that significant amounts of succinylcholine are still circulating even 3 minutes after injection (Holst-Larsen, 1976).

Plasma cholinesterase has an enormous capacity to hydrolyze succinylcholine at a rapid rate such that only a small fraction of the original intravenous dose of drug actually reaches the neuromuscular junction. Because plasma cholinesterase is not present in significant amounts at the neuromuscular junction, neuromuscular blockade produced by succinylcholine is terminated by its diffusion away from the neuromuscular junction into extracellular fluid. Therefore, plasma cholinesterase influences the duration of action of succinylcholine by controlling the amount of neuromuscular blocking drug that is hydrolyzed before reaching the neuromuscular junction.

Plasma Cholinesterase Activity

Reductions in the hepatic production of plasma cholinesterase, drug-induced decreases in plasma cholinesterase activity, or the genetically determined presence of atypical plasma cholinesterase result in slow to absent hydrolysis of succinylcholine and corresponding prolongation of the neuromuscular blockade produced by this drug (Fig. 8-6) (Viby-Mogensen, 1980). Liver disease must be severe before reductions in plasma cholinesterase production sufficient to prolong succinylcholine-induced neuromuscular blockade occur (Foldes et al, 1956). Potent anticholinesterase drugs, used in insecticides and occasionally in the treatment of glaucoma and myasthenia gravis, as well as chemotherapeutic drugs (nitrogen mustard and cyclophosphamide), may decrease plasma cholinesterase activity so that prolonged neuromuscular blockade follows administration of succinylcholine. The duration of action of succinylcholine administered after injecting metoclopramide 10 mg IV is prolonged, presumably reflecting inhibition of plasma cholinesterase by metoclopramide (Kao and

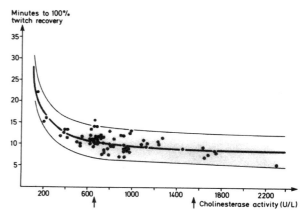

FIGURE 8-6. The duration of succinylcholine-induced neuromuscular blockade parallels activity of plasma cholinesterase enzyme. (From Viby-Mogensen J. Correlation of succinylcholine duration of action with plasma cholinesterase activity in subjects with the genotypically normal enzyme. Anesthesiology 1980; 53: 517–20; with permission.)

Turner, 1989). High estrogen levels, as observed in parturients at term, are associated with up to 40% decreases in plasma cholinesterase activity. Paradoxically, the duration of action of succinylcholine-induced skeletal muscle paralysis is not prolonged, presumably reflecting an increased volume of distribution (Vd) of the drug at term (Leighton et al, 1986).

Atypical Plasma Cholinesterase

The presence of atypical plasma cholinesterase is often recognized only after an otherwise healthy patient experiences prolonged neuromuscular blockade (1 to 3 hours) following a conventional dose of succinylcholine. There are several genetically determined variants of plasma cholinesterase, although dibucaine-related variants are most important (Table 8-2). Dibucaine, a local anesthetic with an amide linkage, inhibits the activity of normal plasma cholinesterase approximately 80% compared with only approximately 20% inhibition of the activity of the atypical enzyme. A dibucaine number of 80, which reflects 80% inhibition of enzyme activity, confirms the presence of normal plasma cholinesterase, whereas approximately 1 in every 3200 patients is homozygous for the atypical plasma cholinesterase and has a dibucaine number of 20. Ap-

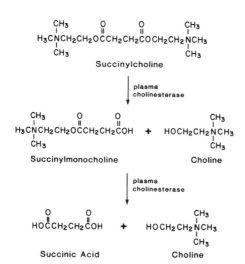

FIGURE 8-5. The brief duration of action of succinylcholine is principally due to its rapid hydrolysis in the plasma by cholinesterase enzyme to inactive metabolites.

Table 8–2
Hereditary Variants of Plasma Cholinesterase

Genotype	Dibucaine Number	Fluoride Number	Response to Succinylcholine	Frequency
E^uE^u	80	60	Normal	96%
E^aE^a	20	20	Greatly prolonged	1 in 3200
E^uE^a	60	45	Slightly prolonged	1 in 480
E^uE^f	75	50	Slightly prolonged	1 in 200
E^fE^a	45	35	Greatly prolonged	1 in 20,000

E^u, normal enzyme gene; E^a, atypical enzyme gene; E^f, fluoride sensitive gene.

proximately 1 in every 480 patients is heterozygous for atypical plasma cholinesterase enzyme and has a dibucaine number of 40 to 60. These heterozygous patients may manifest a modestly prolonged duration of neuromuscular blockade following administration of succinylcholine.

It is important to recognize that the dibucaine number reflects the quality of plasma cholinesterase (ability to metabolize succinylcholine) and not the quantity of the enzyme that is circulating in the plasma. For example, reductions in plasma cholinesterase activity due to liver disease or anticholinesterase drugs are associated with a normal (near 80) dibucaine number. A small number of patients have an isoenzyme of plasma cholinesterase that is associated with an accelerated rate of hydrolysis and a shorter duration of action of succinylcholine (Sugimori, 1986).

Adverse Side Effects

Adverse side effects that may accompany the administration of succinylcholine include (1) cardiac dysrhythmias, (2) hyperkalemia, (3) myalgia, (4) myoglobinuria, (5) increased intragastric pressure, (6) increased intraocular pressure, (7) increased intracranial pressure (ICP), and (8) sustained skeletal muscle contraction. These side effects may limit or even contraindicate the administration of succinylcholine.

Administration of nonparalyzing doses of a nondepolarizing neuromuscular blocking drug (pretreatment) may attenuate or prevent the occurrence of cardiac dysrhythmias, myalgia, and elevations in intragastric and intraocular pressure following injection of succinylcholine (Miller

and Way, 1971; Miller et al, 1968; Stoelting, 1977; Stoelting and Peterson, 1975). Pretreatment, however, does not influence the magnitude of K^+ release evoked by succinylcholine (Stoelting and Peterson, 1975).

Cardiac Dysrhythmias

Sinus bradycardia, junctional rhythm, and even sinus arrest may follow the administration of succinylcholine. These cardiac effects reflect the actions of succinylcholine at cardiac muscarinic cholinergic receptors where the drug mimics the normal effects of acetylcholine. Cardiac dysrhythmias are most likely to occur when a second intravenous dose of succinylcholine is administered approximately 5 minutes after the first dose. This relationship to the second dose suggests a possible role of the metabolites of succinylcholine (succinylmonocholine and choline) in producing bradycardia (Schoenstadt and Whitcher, 1963). Administration of gallamine, 0.3 $mg \cdot kg^{-1}$ IV, approximately 3 minutes before the first dose of succinylcholine greatly reduces the incidence of heart rate slowing after the first or second intravenous dose of succinylcholine (Table 8-3) (Stoelting, 1977). A similar protective effect is not provided by atropine, 6 $\mu g \cdot kg^{-1}$ IV (Table 8-3) (Stoelting, 1977).

In contrast to actions at cardiac muscarinic cholinergic receptors, effects of succinylcholine at autonomic nervous system ganglia may produce ganglionic stimulation and associated increases in heart rate and blood pressure. This ganglionic stimulation reflects an effect of succinylcholine on autonomic ganglia that resembles that of the normal neurotransmitter acetylcholine.

Table 8–3

Succinylcholine (SCh)–induced Cardiac Rhythm Changes with Prior Injection of Gallamine or Atropine

	Gallamine (0.3 mg·kg⁻¹)	Atropine (6 μg·kg⁻¹)
Heart rate 15% less than control 1 min after SCh		
First SCh injection	1 of 40 patients	1 of 40 patients
Second SCh injection*	1 of 39 patients	14 of 40 patients
Junctional rhythm present 1 min after SCh		
First SCh injection	1 of 40 patients	1 of 40 patients
Second SCh injection*	0 of 39 patients	0 of 40 patients

*Second injection 5 min after first injection.
(Data from Stoelting RK. Comparison of gallamine and atropine as pretreatment before anesthetic induction and succinylcholine administration. Anesth Analg 1977; 56: 493–5, with permission.)

Hyperkalemia

Hyperkalemia may occur following administration of succinylcholine to patients with unhealed third-degree burns, denervation leading to skeletal muscle atrophy, severe skeletal muscle trauma, and upper motor neuron lesions (Cooperman et al, 1970; Gronert and Theye, 1975; Tobey, 1970). Severe abdominal infections have been associated with succinylcholine-induced K⁺ release (Kohlschutter et al, 1976). The potential for excessive K⁺ release following denervation may develop within 96 hours and may persist for an indefinite period up to 6 months or longer (Fig. 8-7) (John et al, 1976). There is no evidence of succinylcholine-induced hyperkalemia in patients with Parkinson's disease, cerebral palsy, or myelomeningocele, or in those undergoing cerebral aneurysm surgery (Dierdorf et al, 1985; Dierdorf et al, 1986; Manninen et al, 1990; Muzzi et al, 1989). Pretreatment with a subparalyzing dose of a nondepolarizing neuromuscular blocking drug does not influence the magnitude of K⁺ release evoked by succinylcholine (Stoelting and Peterson, 1975).

Proliferation of extrajunctional cholinergic receptors providing more sites for K⁺ to leak outward from cells during depolarization is the presumed explanation for hyperkalemia that follows administration of succinylcholine to patients with denervation injury. This mechanism has not been confirmed in burn injury patients (see the section entitled "Thermal [Burn] Injury").

Myalgia

Postoperative skeletal muscle myalgia, which is particularly prominent in the muscles of the neck, back, and abdomen, can occur after administration of succinylcholine, especially to young adults undergoing minor surgical procedures that permit early ambulation. Myalgia localized to neck muscles may be perceived as a sore throat by the patient and attributed to tracheal intubation by the anesthesiologist. It is speculated that unsynchronized contractions of skeletal muscle fibers associated with generalized depolarization produced by succinylcholine lead to myalgia. Indeed, prevention of succinylcholine-induced skeletal muscle fasciculations with the prior administration of a subparalyzing dose of dTc prevents or attenuates the incidence of myalgia following administration of succinylcholine (Table 8-4) (Stoelting and Peterson, 1975). Surprisingly, use of vecuronium in place of succinylcholine does not decrease the occurrence of myalgia following laparoscopy (Zahl and Apfelbaum, 1989).

Myoglobinuria.

Damage to skeletal muscles is suggested by the occurrence of myoglobinuria following administration of succinylcholine, especially to pediatric patients (Ryan et al, 1971). Presumably, myoglobinuria reflects skeletal muscle damage associated with succinylcholine-induced fasciculations.

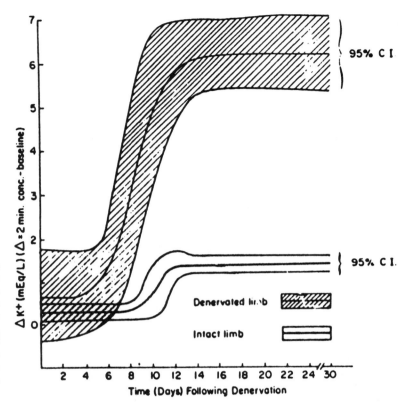

FIGURE 8–7. Changes in plasma potassium (K⁺) concentrations begin as early as 4 days after denervation injury in animals, whereas peak increases occur 14 days after injury. (From John DA, Tobey RE, Homer LD, Rice CL. Onset of succinylcholine-induced hyperkalemia following denervation. Anesthesiology 1976; 45: 294–9; with permission.)

For reasons that are not clear, myoglobinuria rarely occurs in adults receiving succinylcholine.

Increased Intragastric Pressure

Succinylcholine produces inconsistent elevations in intragastric pressure (Fig. 8-8) (Miller and Way, 1971). When intragastric pressure increases, it seems to be related to the intensity of skeletal muscle fasciculations induced by succinylcholine. Indeed, prevention of skeletal muscle fasciculations by prior administration of a subparalyzing dose of a nondepolarizing neuromuscular blocking drug prevents increases in intragastric pressure produced by the subsequent administration of succinylcholine (Miller and Way, 1971). The risk of increased intragastric pressure (the gastroesophageal sphincter can open spontaneously at pressures of more than 28 cm H₂O) is passage of gastric fluid into the esophagus and pharynx and subsequent inhalation into the lungs. Minimal to absent skeletal muscle fasciculations in children are consistent

with the absence of appreciable increases in intragastric pressure that accompany administration of succinylcholine to this age group (Salem, Wong, and Lin, 1972).

Increased Intraocular Pressure

Succinylcholine causes a maximum increase in intraocular pressure 2 to 4 minutes after its administration (Pandey et al, 1972). This increase in the intraocular pressure is transient, lasting only 5 to 10 minutes. The mechanism by which succinylcholine increases intraocular pressure has not been clearly defined, but presumably involves contraction of tonic myofibrils or transient dilation of choroidal blood vessels. For these reasons, administration of succinylcholine is usually avoided in patients with an open eye injury or a recent ocular incision. Intraocular pressure may decrease following administration of nondepolarizing neuromuscular blocking drugs, presumably reflecting the effects of paralysis of extraocular muscles.

Table 8–4
Skeletal Muscle Myalgia Following Intravenous Administration of Succinylcholine (SCh) with or without d-Tubocurarine (dTc) Pretreatment

	Number of Patients Complaining of Myalgia 24 Hours After Administration of SCh
Control	0 of 20 patients
SCh (1 mg·kg⁻¹)	8 of 20 patients
dTc (0.04 mg·kg⁻¹) SCh (1 mg·kg⁻¹)	0 of 20 patients
dTc (0.04 mg·kg⁻¹) SCh (2 mg·kg⁻¹)	5 of 20 patients

Data from Stoelting RK, Peterson C. Adverse effects of increased succinylcholine dose following d-tubocurarine pretreatment. Anesth Analg 1975; 54: 282–8, with permission.)

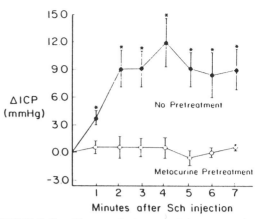

FIGURE 8–9. Changes in intracranial pressure (ICP) after administration of succinylcholine (SCh) 1 mg·kg⁻¹ IV to anesthetized patients with intracranial tumors. Pretreatment was with metocurine 0.03 mg·kg⁻¹ IV. (From Stirt JA, Grosslight KR, Bedford RF, Vollmer D. "Defasciculation" with metocurine prevents succinylcholine-induced increases in intracranial pressure. Anesthesiology 1987; 67: 50–3; with permission.)

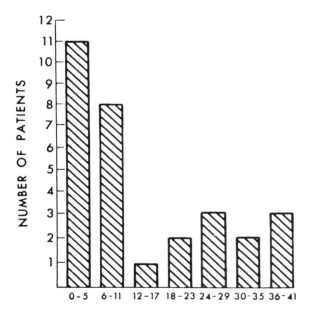

FIGURE 8–8. Succinylcholine produces inconsistent and unpredictable increases of intragastric pressure. (From Miller RD, Way WL. Inhibition of succinylcholine induced increased intragastric pressure by nondepolarizing muscle relaxants and lidocaine. Anesthesiology 1971; 34: 185–8; with permission.)

Increased Intracranial Pressure

Succinylcholine may evoke increases in intracranial pressure in anesthetized patients with intracranial mass lesions (Fig. 8-9) (Stirt et al, 1987). These increases in ICP are prevented by preceding succinylcholine with a subparalyzing dose of metocurine. In halothane anesthetized animals, succinylcholine, 1 mg·kg⁻¹ IV, produces evidence of arousal on the electroencephalogram (EEG) that is associated with substantial increases in cerebral blood flow and corresponding increases in ICP (Lanier et al, 1986).

Sustained Skeletal Muscle Contraction

Skeletal muscle contraction that is sustained may accompany the administration of succinylcholine to patients with myotonia congenita or myotonia dystrophica (Mitchell et al, 1978). This sustained skeletal muscle contraction may interfere with ventilation of the lungs and become life-threatening.

Masseter spasm occurs in approximately 1% of children anesthetized with halothane who received succinylcholine. This incidence increases to 2.8% in children with strabismus (Carroll, 1987). Masseter spasm may be an early manifestation of succinylcholine-induced malignant hyperthermia.

LONG-ACTING NONDEPOLARIZING NEUROMUSCULAR BLOCKING DRUGS

Long-acting nondepolarizing neuromuscular blocking drugs are characterized by an onset of maximum neuromuscular blockade in 3 to 5 minutes and a duration of action of 60 to 90 minutes (Tables 8-1 and 8-5). Dose response curves for these drugs in adult patients do not deviate from parallelism (Fig. 8-10) (Savarese et al, 1977). The dose of neuromuscular blocking drug necessary to depress twitch is derived from such curves. For example, the dose of nondepolarizing neuromuscular blocking drug necessary to depress twitch 50% (ED_{50}) and 95% (ED_{95}) is frequently used as an index of equal potency for comparisons between drugs (Table 8-5).

Mechanism of Action

Nondepolarizing neuromuscular blocking drugs are classically thought to act by combining with nicotinic cholinergic receptors without causing any activation of these receptor channels. Specifically, these drugs can act competitively with acetylcholine at the alpha subunits of postjunctional nicotinic cholinergic receptors without causing a receptors change in the configuration (Fig. 8-8) (see the section entitled "Postjunctional Nicotinic Receptors"). In addition, these drugs, especially at high doses, may act by blocking the receptor channels. For example, dTc at low concentrations is relatively selective for the alpha subunits, whereas high doses also block the channels. Nondepolarizing neuromuscular blocking drugs also act at prejunctional nicotinic receptors. Nevertheless, it is the actions at postjunctional sites that are most important.

Occupation of as many as 70% of the nicotinic cholinergic receptors by a neuromuscular blocking drug does not produce evidence of neuromuscular blockade as reflected by the twitch response to a single stimulus (Fig. 8-11) (Waud and Waud, 1971). Neuromuscular transmission, however, fails when 80% to 90% of the receptors are blocked. This confirms the wide safety margin of neuromuscular transmission and is the basis for the techniques of clinical monitoring of neuromuscular blockade.

Characteristics of Nondepolarizing Neuromuscular Blockade

Characteristic skeletal muscle responses in the presence of nondepolarizing neuromuscular blockade, as evoked by electrical stimulation from a peripheral nerve stimulator, include (1) decreased twitch response to a single stimulus, (2) unsustained response (fade) during continuous stimulation, (3) train-of-four ratio less than 0.7, (4) posttetanic potentiation, (5) potentiation by other nondepolarizing neuromuscular blocking drugs, and (6) antagonism by anticholinesterase drugs. In addition, skeletal muscle fasciculations do not accompany the onset of nondepolarizing neuromuscular blockade.

Skeletal muscle contraction is an all-or-nothing phenomenon. Each muscle fiber either contracts maximally or does not contract at all. Therefore, when twitch response is reduced, some fibers are contracting normally, whereas others are completely blocked. Fade of skeletal muscle contraction in response to continuous electrical stimulation suggests that some fibers are more susceptible to being blocked by neuromuscular blocking drugs and need a greater sustained release of acetylcholine to trigger their responses.

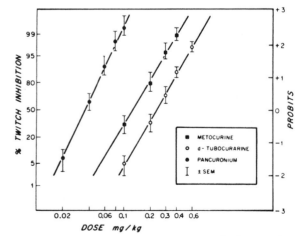

FIGURE 8–10. Dose-response curves for long-acting nondepolarizing neuromuscular blocking drugs do not deviate from parallelism. (From Savarese JJ, Ali HH, Antonio RP. The clinical pharmacology of metocurine: Dimethyltubocurarine revisited. Anesthesiology 1977; 47: 277–84; with permission.)

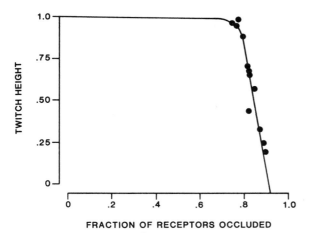

FIGURE 8–11. Schematic depiction of the number of receptors that must be occupied (receptor occupancy theory) before the existence of neuromuscular blockade is evident as a decrease in twitch height.

Pharmacokinetics

Nondepolarizing neuromuscular blocking drugs, because of their quaternary ammonium groups, are highly ionized at physiologic pH and possess limited lipid solubility (Shanks, 1986). As a result of these two characteristics, the Vd of neuromuscular blocking drugs is small (80 to 140 ml·kg^{-1}), being limited principally to the extracellular fluid (Table 8-5). In addition, neuromuscular blocking drugs cannot easily cross lipid membrane barriers such as the blood-brain barrier, renal tubular epithelium, gastrointestinal epithelium, or placenta. Therefore, neuromuscular blocking drugs do not produce central nervous system effects, renal tubular reabsorption is minimal, oral administration is ineffective, and maternal administration does not affect the fetus.

The rate of disappearance of long-acting nondepolarizing neuromuscular blocking drugs from the plasma is characterized by an initial rapid decline followed by a slower decline. Distribution of neuromuscular blocking drugs to highly perfused tissues including the lungs is the major cause of the initial rapid decrease in the plasma concentration, whereas the slower decrease after approximately 15 minutes is entirely due to clearance mechanisms. Renal and hepatic elimination are aided by access to a large fraction of the administered dose owing to the high de-

gree of ionization, which maintains high plasma concentrations of drug and also prevents renal reabsorption of excreted drug. Pharmacokinetics of nondepolarizing neuromuscular blocking drugs are calculated following bolus intravenous injection of the drug. If the Vd is reduced, as by increased protein binding, dehydration, or acute hemorrhage, the same dose of drug produces a greater plasma concentration and the apparent potency of the drug is augmented.

Pharmacokinetic factors that should be considered in predicting the response to nondepolarizing neuromuscular blocking drugs include (1) size of the initial dose, (2) renal disease, (3) biliary and hepatic disease, (4) protein binding, (5) anesthetic drugs, and (6) advanced age. The relative impact of these different factors varies among the neuromuscular blocking drugs. Indeed, many of the variable patient responses evoked by neuromuscular blocking drugs can be explained by differences in pharmacokinetics.

Size of the Initial Dose

The size of the initial dose of dTc, and presumably other nondepolarizing neuromuscular blocking drugs, does not influence the pharmacokinetics or pharmacodynamics of the drug. For example, there is no significant difference in the dose of dTc required to maintain the same degree of neuromuscular blockade whether the drug is administered intravenously as a single bolus, intermittently, or as a continuous intravenous infusion. (Ham et al, 1979). Clearly, the size of the initial dose or supplemental doses of nondepolarizing neuromuscular blocking drugs determines the resulting plasma concentration of drug. The magnitude of neuromuscular blockade, as characterized by twitch response, is proportional to the plasma concentration of the neuromuscular blocking drug (Matteo et al, 1974; Shanks et al, 1979). For example, twitch response begins to reappear at a plasma dTc concentration of approximately 0.7 µg·ml^{-1}; twitch response is 50% when the plasma concentration is 0.45 µg·ml^{-1}; and recovery of twitch response is complete at a plasma concentration of 0.2 µg·ml^{-1} (Fig. 8-12) (Matteo et al, 1974).

Renal Disease

Renal disease can greatly alter the pharmacokinetics of long-acting nondepolarizing neuro-

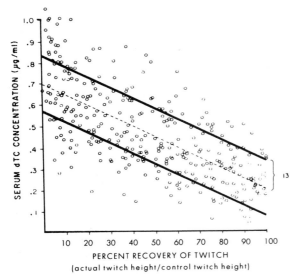

FIGURE 8–12. d-Tubocurarine (dTc)-induced neuromuscular blockade parallels the plasma (serum) concentration of the drug. (From Matteo RS, Spector S, Horowitz PE. Relation of serum d-tubocurarine concentration to neuromuscular blockade in man. Anesthesiology 1974; 41: 440–3; with permission.)

muscular blocking drugs. The rate at which the plasma concentration of pancuronium decreases is more influenced by renal failure than is the rate of decrease in the plasma concentrations of dTc or metocurine (Fig. 8-13) (Brotherton and Matteo, 1981; McLeod et al, 1976; Miller et al, 1977). Indeed, an estimated 80% of a single dose of pancuronium is eliminated unchanged in the urine. Conversely, approximately 45% of an administered dose of dTc is recovered unchanged in the urine during the first 24 hours following its administration, whereas only an additional 7% of drug is recovered in the urine after 96 hours. Therefore, it is likely that dTc is stored in inactive tissue sites, perhaps for prolonged periods. Similarly, approximately 43% of metocurine is recovered unchanged in the urine. Because biliary excretion and metabolism of metocurine are not significant, it is presumed this drug, like dTc, is stored for prolonged periods in inactive tissue sites.

Renal failure does not alter the distribution half-time of nondepolarizing neuromuscular blocking drugs because this phase reflects passage of drug to tissues independent of clearance mechanisms. Likewise, plasma concentrations of neuromuscular blocking drugs necessary to produce a given degree of neuromuscular blockade

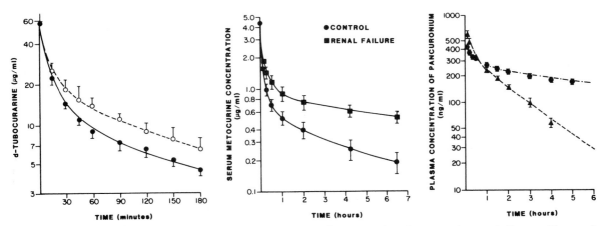

FIGURE 8–13. The rate at which the plasma concentration of pancuronium decreases is more influenced by renal failure than is the rate of decline in the plasma concentrations of d-tubocurarine or metocurine. Mean ± SE. (From Brotherton WP, Matteo RS. Pharmacokinetics and pharmacodynamics of metocurine in humans with and without renal failure. Anesthesiology 1981;55:273–6; McLeod K, Watson MJ, Rawlings MD. Pharmacokinetics of pancuronium in patients with normal and impaired renal function. Br J Anaesth 1976;48:341–5; and Miller RD, Matteo R, Benet LZ, Sohn YJ. Influence of renal failure on the pharmacokinetics of d-tubocurarine in man. J Pharmacol Exp Ther 1977; 202: 1–7; with permission.)

Table 8-5

Comparative Pharmacology of Nondepolarizing Muscle Relaxants

	ED_{95} $(mg \cdot kg^{-1})$	Onset to Maximum Twitch Suppression (min)	Duration to Return Control Twitch Height (min)
d-Tubocurarine	0.51	3–5	60–90
Metocurine	0.28	3–5	60–90
Gallamine	1*	3–5	60–90
Pancuronium	0.07	3–5	60–90
Pipecuronium	0.05–0.06	3–5	60–90
Doxacurium	0.03–0.04	4–6	60–90
Atracurium	0.20	3–5	20–35
Vecuronium	0.05	3–5	20–35
Mivacurium	0.08	2–3	12–20

	Volume of Distribution	Renal Excretion (percent unchanged)	Biliary Excretion (percent unchanged)	Hepatic Degradation
d-Tubocurarine	0.30	45	10–40	NS
Metocurine	0.51	43	<2	NS
Gallamine	0.21	>95	0	NS
Pancuronium	0.26	80	5–10	10%–40%
Pipecuronium		70	20	10%
Doxacurium		70	Unknown	Unknown
Atracurium		NS	NS	Modest (?)
Vecuronium		15–25	40–75	20%–30%
Mivacurium		NS	NS	NS

	Hydrolysis in Plasma	Elimination Half-Time (h)	Intubating Dose $(mg \cdot kg^{-1})$	Supplemental Doses $(mg \cdot kg^{-1})$ N_2O	Volatile
d-Tubocurarine	0	2.0	0.6	0.1	0.05
Metocurine	0	5.8	0.4	0.07	0.04
Gallamine	0	2.3			
Pancuronium	0	2.4	0.1	0.015	0.007
Pipecuronium	0		0.14		
Doxacurium	Minimal		0.5–0.8		
Atracurium	Spontaneous and enzymatic		0.4–0.5	0.1	0.07
Vecuronium	0		0.08–0.1	0.02	0.015
Mivacurium	Enzymatic		0.16		

*Estimate.

NS, Not significant.

are not altered by renal failure. Predictably, the elimination half-time of these drugs is prolonged in the presence of renal failure, paralleling the magnitude of drug normally eliminated unchanged in the urine.

Biliary and Hepatic Disease

Patients with total biliary obstruction and hepatic cirrhosis have increased Vd, decreased plasma clearance, and a prolonged elimination half-time of pancuronium (Table 8-6) (Duvaldestin et al, 1978). The large Vd means a large initial dose of pancuronium will be required to produce the same plasma concentration but the resulting neuromuscular blockade may be prolonged because of decreased clearance.

An estimated 10% to 40% of a dose of pancuronium undergoes hepatic deacetylation to 3-hydroxypancuronium, 17-hydroxypancuronium, and 3,17-hydroxypancuronium (Agoston et al, 1973). The 3-hydroxypancuronium metabolite is approximately 50% as potent as pancuronium at the neuromuscular junction, whereas the other metabolites have only minimal activity (Miller et al, 1978a).

In normal patients, an estimated 10% of dTc is eliminated unchanged in the bile. The amount of biliary elimination may increase to approximately 40% in the presence of renal failure. Therefore, dTc disappears from the neuromuscular junction and plasma even in the absence of renal function. Biliary excretion of metocurine is minimal (estimated at less than 2% of an injected dose) regardless of the state of renal function. Unlike pancuronium, dTc and metocurine do not undergo significant hepatic metabolism (Stanski et al, 1979).

Protein Binding

The extent and importance of protein binding of the various nondepolarizing neuromuscular blocking drugs are not clearly defined. Various studies demonstrate binding to both albumin and gamma globulin (Skivington, 1972). Protein binding of dTc is not altered by renal or hepatic disease even though these diseases are known to be associated with altered protein binding to other drugs (Ghoneim et al, 1973). Previously, it had been speculated that increased binding of dTc to gamma globulin was responsible for resis-

tance to the effects of this drug in patients with severe cirrhosis of the liver.

Anesthetic Drugs

Despite changes in the distribution of blood flow, inhaled anesthetics have little or no effect on the pharmacokinetics of neuromuscular blocking drugs. For example, the distribution and elimination half-time of dTc, and presumably the other nondepolarizing neuromuscular blocking drugs, are not significantly different during nitrous oxide–opioid or nitrous oxide–halothane anesthesia (Ramzan et al, 1981). Enhancement of neuromuscular blockade by volatile anesthetics reflects a pharmacodynamic action as manifested by decreased plasma concentrations of neuromuscular blocking drugs required to produce a given degree of neuromuscular blockade in the presence of volatile anesthetics.

Advanced Age

Aging is associated with a decreased clearance rate for dTc, metocurine, and pancuronium from the plasma (Fig. 8-14) (Duvaldestin et al, 1982; Matteo et al, 1985). The resulting prolonged elimination half-time reflects declining renal function in the elderly manifesting as a prolonged duration of neuromuscular blockade. The absence of age-related changes in responsiveness of the neuromuscular junction (changes in pharmacodynamics) is confirmed by similar dose-response curves in elderly and young adults for all three of the long-acting nondepolarizing neuromuscular blocking drugs (Fig. 8-15) (Duvaldestin et al, 1982; Matteo et al, 1985).

Central Nervous System

Despite being highly ionized, detectable amounts of dTc are present in cerebrospinal fluid (Fig. 8-16) (Matteo et al, 1977). Gallamine and dTc have been shown to increase the dose of lidocaine administered to animals that is necessary to evoke a seizure (Munson and Wagman, 1973). Previously reported pancuronium-induced decreases in halothane anesthetic requirements (MAC) in patients have not been reproducible following administration of paralyzing doses of pancuronium, atracurium, or vecuronium (Fig. 8-17) (Fahey et al, 1989; Forbes et al, 1979).

Response of Pediatric Patients

Plasma concentrations of dTc necessary to decrease twitch response 50% during nitrous oxide–halothane anesthesia are age dependent, being lowest in neonates and highest in adults (Table 8-7) (Fisher et al, 1982b). Conversely, elimination half-time is longer in neonates than adults. Since plasma clearance is not different between pediatric and adult patients, the prolonged elimination half-time of dTc reflects the larger Vd in younger patients. Based on these observations, it is clear that neonates and infants are more sensitive to dTc and presumably other nondepolarizing neuromuscular blocking drugs. This increased sensitivity to nondepolarizing neuromuscular blocking drugs demonstrated by neonates is an example of age-related differences in pharmacodynamics. Nevertheless, the initial dose administered to achieve the same plasma concentration of neuromuscular blocking drug is similar in both age groups because the large Vd in neonates offsets the impact of increased sensitivity of the neuromuscular junction (Fisher et al, 1982b).

Cardiovascular Effects

Neuromuscular blocking drugs may exert cardiovascular effects through drug-induced re-

Table 8–6
Pharmacokinetics of Pancuronium and Hepatic Dysfunction

	Normal Hepatic Function	Cirrhosis
Volume of distribution (ml·kg⁻¹)	279	416*
Clearance (ml·kg⁻¹·min⁻¹)	1.9	1.5*
Elimination half-time (min)	114	208*

*,P < 0.05 compared with normal hepatic function.
(Data from Duvaldestin P, Agoston S, Henzel E, Kersten UW, Desmonts JM. Pancuronium pharmacokinetics in patients with liver cirrhosis. Br J Anaesth 1978; 50: 131–6, with permission.)

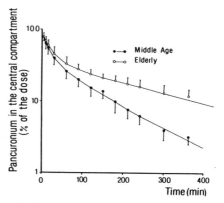

FIGURE 8–14. Aging is associated with a decreased rate of decline in the plasma concentrations of long-acting nondepolarizing neuromuscular blocking drugs such as pancuronium. (From Duvaldestin P, Saada J, Berger JL, D'Hollander A, Desmonts JM. Pharmacokinetics, pharmacodynamics, and dose-response relationship of pancuronium in control and elderly subjects. Anesthesiology 1982; 56: 36–40; with permission.)

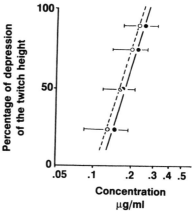

FIGURE 8–15. Absence of age-related changes in the responsiveness of the neuromuscular junction to long-acting nondepolarizing neuromuscular blocking drugs, such as pancuronium, is confirmed by the similarity of plasma concentrations necessary to produce comparable responses in young adults (●) and elderly individuals (○). (From Duvaldestin P, Saada J, Berger JL, D'Hollander A, Desmonts JM. Pharmacokinetics, pharmacodynamics, and dose-response relationship of pancuronium in control and elderly subjects. Anesthesiology 1982; 56: 36–40; with permission.)

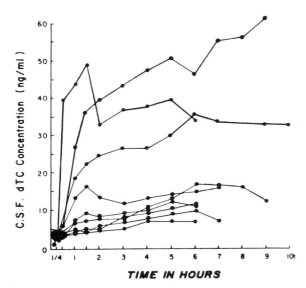

FIGURE 8–16. Following intravenous administration, d-tubocuraine (dTc) is detectable in the cerebrospinal fluid (CSF). (From Matteo RS, Pua EK, Khambatta HJ, Spector S. Cerebrospinal fluid levels of d-tubocurarine in man. Anesthesiology 1977; 46: 396–9; with permission.)

lease of histamine or other vasoactive substances such as prostacyclin from circulating mast cells, effects at cardiac muscarinic receptors, or effects on nicotinic receptors at autonomic ganglia (Table 8-8). Considerable species difference exists with respect to mechanisms responsible for circulatory effects of neuromuscular blocking drugs. It is likely that the relative magnitude of circulatory effects varies from patient to patient according to factors such as underlying autonomic nervous system activity, preoperative medication, drugs administered for maintenance of anesthesia, and concurrent drug therapy. Despite the frequent reference to the cardiovascular effects of nondepolarizing neuromuscular blocking drugs, it is rare that these changes achieve clinical significance.

The difference between the dose of neuromuscular blocking drug that produces neuromuscular blockade and circulatory effects is defined as the *autonomic margin of safety* (Hughes and Chapple, 1976). An ED_{95} dose of dTc that produces neuromuscular blockade also produces circulatory changes, and the autonomic margin of safety is narrow. Conversely, metocurine, atracurium, and vecuronium have wide autonomic margins of safety because the ED_{95} dose necessary to produce neuromuscular blockade is less than the dose that evokes circulatory changes.

d-Tubocurarine

Rapid intravenous injection of an ED_{95} dose of dTc can evoke sufficient histamine release and, to a lesser extent, blockade of sympathetic and parasympathetic nervous system ganglia, to cause significant (more than 20%) decreases in mean arterial pressure (Fig. 8-18) (Stoelting, 1972). Decreased venous return owing to loss of skeletal muscle tone and the effects of positive airway pressure also contribute to decreases in blood pressure. The maximum decrease in mean arterial pressure following administration of dTc occurs at a time when the cardiac output is unchanged, confirming that blood pressure reductions parallel decreases in systemic vascular resistance (Fig. 8-18) (Stoelting, 1972). This peripheral vasodilation is most likely caused by dTc-induced release of histamine, whereas blockade of autonomic ganglia occurs at higher doses. Indeed, dTc produces dose-dependent increases in plasma concentrations of histamine that parallel decreases in blood pressure (Fig. 8-19) (Moss et al, 1981). Alternatively, bolus administration of dTc may evoke the release of prostacyclin from vascular endothelium, resulting in profound peripheral vasodilation and decreases in blood pressure previously attributed to histamine (Fig. 8-20) (Hatano et al, 1990). In this regard, prostacyclin acts by stimulating H-1 receptors. Prior administration of aspirin prevents dTc-induced release of prostacyclin and associated decreases in blood pressure (Fig. 8-20) (Hatano et al, 1990). Direct cardiac depressant effects of dTc do not occur.

The magnitude of blood pressure decrease depends on the dose of dTc administered as well as the depth of anesthesia (Fig. 8-21) (Munger et al, 1974; Stoelting and Longnecker, 1972a). Furthermore, the injection of dTc over 90 seconds rather than as a bolus minimizes the subsequent decrease in blood pressure (Fig. 8-22) (Stoelting et al, 1980). This rate-related phenomenon is consistent with histamine (possibly prostacyclin) re-

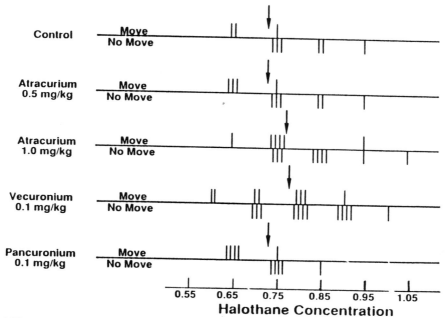

FIGURE 8–17. Minimum alveolar concentration (MAC) of halothane as depicted by the vertical arrow is not altered by nondepolarizing neuromuscular blocking drugs administered to adults. (From Fahey MR, Sessler DI, Cannon JE, Brady K, Stoen R, Miller RD. Atracurium, vecuronium and pancuronium do not alter the minimum alveolar concentration of halothane in humans. Anesthesiology 1989; 71: 53–6; with permission.)

Table 8–7
Pharmacokinetics and Pharmacodynamics of d-Tubocurarine (dTc)

	Volume of Distribution (L·kg⁻¹)	*Clearance (ml·kg⁻¹· min⁻¹)*	*Elimination Half-Time (min)*	*Plasma Concentration Necessary to Maintain 50% Twitch Suppression (µg·ml⁻¹)*
	0.74[*]	3.7	174[**]	0.18[***]
Infants	0.52	3.3	130	0.27[***]
Children	0.41	4.0	90	0.42
Adults	0.31	3.0	89	0.53

[*],$P < 0.05$ compared with infants, children, and adults.
[**],$P < 0.05$ compared with children and adults.
[***],$P < 0.05$ compared with children and adults.
(Data from Fisher DM, O'Keefe C, Stanski DR, Cronnelly R, Miller RD, Gregory GA. Pharmacokinetics and pharmacodynamics of d-tubocurarine in infants, children, and adults. Anesthesiology 1982; 57: 203–8.)

Table 8-8

Mechanisms of Neuromuscular Blocking Drug-Induced Cardiovascular Effects

ED_{95} Dose	Histamine (Protacyclin?) Release	Cardiac Muscarinic Receptors	Nicotinic Receptors at Autonomic Ganglia
Succinylcholine	Slight	Modest stimulation	Modest stimulation
d-Tubocurarine	Moderate	None	Moderate blockade
Metocurine	Modest	None	Modest blockade
Gallamine	None	Moderate blockade	None
Pancuronium	None	Modest blockade	None
Pipecuronium	None	None	None
Doxacurium	None	None	None
Atracurium	Slight	None	None
Vecuronium	None	None	None
Mivacurium	Slight	None	None

lease evoked by a rapid, but not a slow, injection of dTc. In addition, pretreatment with an antihistamine drug, such as promethazine, attenuates blood pressure decreases evoked by dTc in some patients (Stoelting and Longnecker, 1972b). The dependence of blood pressure changes on the dose of dTc and concentration of volatile anesthetic (specifically halothane) most likely reflects drug-induced production of ganglionic blockade or cardiac depression.

Metocurine

In the presence of a volatile anesthetic, such as halothane, an ED_{95} dose of metocurine decreases mean arterial pressure approximately one half as much (10%) as an equivalent dose of dTc (Fig. 8-23) (Stoelting, 1974). During nitrous oxide–thiopental–opioid anesthesia, the administration of metocurine produces minimal dose-related decreases in mean arterial pressure and heart rate (Fig. 8-24) (Savarese et al, 1977). These lesser circulatory effects compared with dTc are consistent with a reduced ability of the bisquaternary ammonium structure of metocurine to evoke the release of histamine (possibly also prostacyclin) or to produce autonomic ganglion blockade.

Pancuronium

Pancuronium, in contrast to dTc, produces a modest 10% to 15% increase in heart rate, mean arterial pressure, and cardiac output (Fig. 8-18) (Stoelting, 1972). These cardiovascular effects are attributed to selective cardiac vagal blockade (atropine-like effect limited to cardiac muscarinic receptors) and activation of the sympathetic nervous system (Domenech et al, 1976). Both release of norepinephrine from adrenergic nerve endings and blockade of uptake of norepinephrine back into postganglionic nerve endings have been proposed as mechanisms for the activation of the sympathetic nervous system by pancuronium (Ivankovich et al, 1975; Vercruyse et al, 1979). Pancuronium may also interfere with activity of muscarinic receptors that normally inhibit the release of norepinephrine. Likewise, pancuronium may produce blockade at muscarinic receptors that normally release dopamine, thus facilitating transmission through autonomic ganglia by inactivating the inhibitory influence of the dopaminergic cell loop (Scott and Savarese, 1985). The increase in circulating plasma concentrations of catecholamines following intravenous administration of pancuronium supports a drug-induced activation of the sympathetic nervous system (Domenich et al, 1976).

Pancuronium increases heart rate principally by blocking vagal muscarinic receptors in the sinoatrial node as evidenced by the ability of prior administration of atropine to block this response. A sympathomimetic effect of pancuronium apparently plays a minor role in heart rate

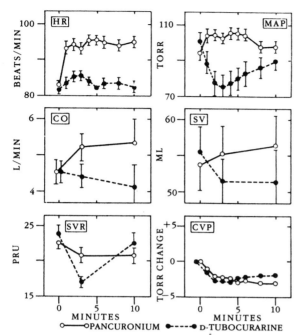

FIGURE 8–18. Rapid administration of d-tubocurarine (0.4 mg·kg⁻¹ IV) during halothane anesthesia results in a decrease in mean arterial pressure (MAP) and a corresponding reduction in systemic vascular resistance (SVR). Under the same conditions, pancuronium causes an increase in MAP, heart rate (HR), and cardiac output (CO). SV, stroke volume. CVP, central venous pressure. (From Stoelting RK. The hemodynamic effects of pancuronium and d-tubocurarine in anesthetized patients. Anesthesiology 1972;36:612–5; with permission.)

responses. Indeed, heart rate responses evoked by pancuronium still occur in patients treated with beta-adrenergic antagonists (Morris et al, 1983). The magnitude of heart rate increase evoked by pancuronium seems more dependent on the preexisting heart rate (an inverse relationship) than the dose or rate of drug administration. Marked increases in heart rate seem more likely to occur in patients with altered atrioventricular conduction of cardiac impulses, such as occur in atrial fibrillation.

The modest increase in blood pressure following the administration of pancuronium reflects the effect of heart rate on cardiac output in the absence of changes in systemic vascular resistance. Positive inotropic effects of pancuronium

have not been demonstrated (Scott and Savarese, 1985).

An increased incidence of cardiac dysrhythmias has been observed following administration of pancuronium, but not succinylcholine, to patients being chronically treated with digitalis. Cardiac dysrhythmias may reflect sudden changes in the balance of autonomic nervous system activity in favor of the sympathetic nervous system. Cardiac stimulating effects of pancuronium may also increase the incidence of myocardial ischemia in patients with coronary artery disease (Thomson and Putnins, 1985). Histamine release and autonomic ganglion blockade are not produced by pancuronium.

Gallamine

Gallamine produces selective cardiac vagal blockade as a reflection of an atropine-like effect limited to cardiac muscarinic receptors. Heart rate increases are dose dependent with the maximum effect being a 30% to 40% increase following administration of paralyzing doses of gallamine (1 mg·kg⁻¹ IV or greater) (Fig. 8-25) (Stoelting, 1973). Paralyzing doses of gallamine, however, do not produce complete vagal block-

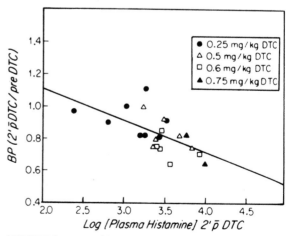

FIGURE 8–19. Blood pressure (BP) decreases following intravenous administration of d-tubocurarine parallel to the plasma concentration of histamine. (From Moss J, Rosow CE, Savarese JJ, Philbin DM, Kniffen KJ. Role of histamine in the hypotensive action of d-tubocurarine in humans. Anesthesiology 1981; 55: 19–25; with permission.)

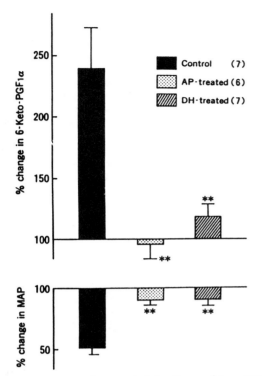

FIGURE 8–20. Changes (%) in plasma 6-keto-PGF$_{1\alpha}$ concentrations (nonenzymatic metabolite of prostacyclin) and in mean arterial pressure (MAP) 2 minutes following d-tubocurarine (dTc) administration in control, aspirin (AP)-treated and diphenhydramine (DH)-treated patients. The values just before dTc administration are considered 100%. Figures in parentheses indicate the number of patients studied. *P <0.01 compared with control. (From Hatano Y, Arai T, Noda J, et al. Contribution of postacyclin to d-tubocurarine-induced hypotension in humans. Anesthesiology 1990; 72: 28–32; with permission.)

ade because atropine can still increase heart rate. Nevertheless, nonparalyzing doses of gallamine (0.3 mg·kg^{-1} IV) used for pretreatment prior to administration of succinylcholine increase heart rate as much as or more than atropine administered intravenously (Stoelting, 1977). Gallamine-induced heart rate increases persist even when effects at the neuromuscular junction are waning or absent. Heart rate increases evoked by gallamine result in modest increases in cardiac output and mean arterial pressure (Fig. 8-25) (Stoelting, 1973).

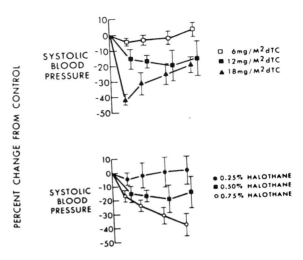

FIGURE 8–21. The magnitude of blood pressure decrease produced by d-tubocurarine (dTc) parallels the dose of drug administered and the depth of anesthesia. Mean ± SE. (From Munger WL, Miller RD, Stevens WC. The dependence of d-tubocurarine-induced hypotension on alveolar concentration of halothane, dose of d-tubocurarine, and nitrous oxide. Anesthesiology 1974; 40: 442–8; with permission.)

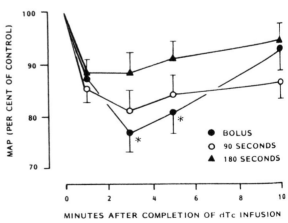

FIGURE 8–22. The rate of injection of d-tubocurarine (dTc) influences the magnitude of drug-induced decreases in mean arterial pressure (MAP). Mean ± SE. (From Stoelting RK, McCammon RL, Hilgenberg JC. Changes in blood pressure with varying rates of administration of d-tubocurarine. Anesth Analg 1980; 59: 697–9; with permission.)

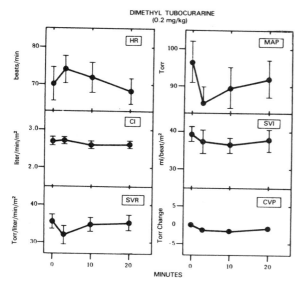

DIMETHYL TUBOCURARINE
(0.2 mg/kg)

FIGURE 8–23. Rapid intravenous administration of metocurine (dimethyl tubocurarine) during halothane anesthesia decreases mean arterial pressure (MAP) approximately one half the magnitude produced by a comparable dose of d-tubocurarine. (see Fig. 8–18) Mean ± SE. HR, heart rate. CI, cardiac index. SVR, systemic vascular resistance. SVI, stroke volume index. CVP, central venous pressure. (From Stoelting RK. Hemodynamic effects of dimethyltubocurarine during nitrous oxide-halothane anesthesia. Anesth Analg 1974; 53: 513–5; with permission.)

Like pancuronium, gallamine may activate the sympathetic nervous system (Brown and Crout, 1970). Cardiac dysrhythmias following administration of gallamine may reflect sudden changes in the balance of autonomic nervous system activity in favor of the sympathetic nervous system. Gallamine does not alter activity of autonomic ganglia or evoke the release of histamine.

Causes of Altered Responses

Drugs administered in the perioperative period may enhance the effects of long-acting nondepolarizing neuromuscular blocking drugs at the neuromuscular junction. Examples of drugs that can enhance neuromuscular blockade include (1) volatile anesthetics, (2) aminoglycoside anti-

biotics, (3) local anesthetics, (4) cardiac antidysrhythmic drugs, (5) diuretics, and (6) magnesium, lithium, and ganglionic blocking drugs. Changes unrelated to concurrent drug, therapy such as (1) hypothermia, (2) acid-base alterations, (3) changes in serum K^+ concentrations, (4) adrenocortical dysfunction, (5) thermal (burn) injury, and (6) allergic reactions, may also influence the characteristics of neuromuscular blockade produced by nondepolarizing neuromuscular blocking drugs. Finally, combinations of nondepolarizing neuromuscular blocking drugs may produce a degree of neuromuscular blockade that is different from the degree that would be produced by either drug alone.

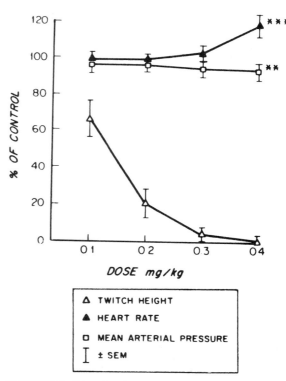

FIGURE 8–24. During nitrous oxide-thiopental-opioid anesthesia, the intravenous administration of metocurine produces minimal, although statistically significant changes in heart rate and mean arterial pressure. **P <0.01; ***P <0.001. (From Savarese JJ, Ali HH, Antonio RP. The clinical pharmacology of metocurine: Dimethyltubocurarine revisited. Anesthesiology 1977; 47: 277–84; with permission.)

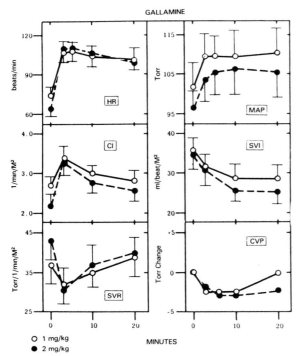

FIGURE 8–25. Circulatory effects following administration of gallamine 1 mg·kg⁻¹ IV (○) or 2 mg·kg⁻¹ IV (●) to patients anesthetized with N₂O-halothane. HR, heart rate. MAP, mean arterial pressure. CI, cardiac index. SVI stroke volume index. SVR, systemic vascular resistance. CVP, central venous pressure. (From Stoelting RK. Hemodynamic effects of gallamine during halothane-nitrous oxide anesthesia. Anesthesiology 1973; 39: 645-7; with permission.)

Volatile Anesthetics

Volatile anesthetics produce dose-dependent enhancement of the magnitude and duration of neuromuscular blockade owing to nondepolarizing neuromuscular blocking drugs (Fogdall and Miller, 1975; Miller et al, 1971). This enhancement of neuromuscular blockade is greatest with enflurane and isoflurane, intermediate with halothane, and least with nitrous oxide–opioid combinations (Fig. 8-26) (Ali and Savarese, 1976). For example, 1.25 MAC halothane decreases dTc dose requirements approximately 50% compared with the dose necessary to produce the same degree of neuromuscular blockade during a nitrous oxide–opioid anesthetic. A

1.25 MAC dose of enflurane and isoflurane decreases dTc dose requirements approximately 70%. These same volatile anesthetics also decrease atracurium and vecuronium dose requirements, but the magnitude (10% to 30%) is less than observed with the long-acting neuromuscular blocking drugs.

Enhancement of neuromuscular blockade produced by halothane does not depend on the duration of halothane administration as measured between 10 and 160 minutes of inhalation of the drug (Fig. 8-27) (Miller et al, 1976; Stanski et al, 1980). In contrast, the ability of enflurane to enhance neuromuscular blockade is time-dependent as reflected by an approximately 10% increase every hour in the magnitude of neuromuscular blockade despite a constant plasma concentration of dTc (Fig. 8-27) (Stanski et al, 1980). It is speculated that halothane acts on the highly perfused neuromuscular junction, accounting for its early onset of maximal effect. In addition to this action at the neuromuscular junction, it is

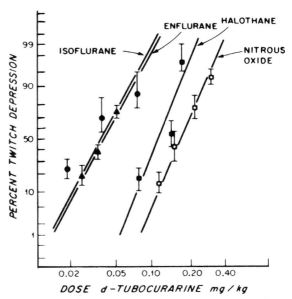

FIGURE 8–26. Volatile anesthetics cause dose-dependent and drug-specific enhancement of neuromuscular blockade produced by long-acting nondepolarizing neuromuscular blocking drugs. Mean ± SE. (From Ali HH, Savarese JJ. Monitoring of neuromuscular function. Anesthesiology 1976; 45: 216–49; with permission.)

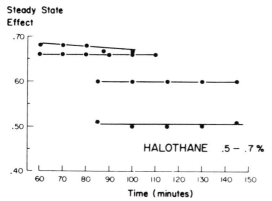

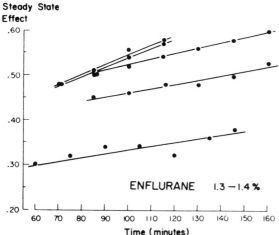

FIGURE 8–27. Enhancement of neuromuscular blockade produced by halothane does not change with time, whereas the magnitude of neuromuscular blockade produced by enflurane increases with time. (From Stanski DR, Ham J, Miller RD, Sheiner LB. Time-dependent increase in sensitivity to d-tubocurarine during enflurane anesthesia in man. Anesthesiology 1980; 52: 483–7; with permission.)

speculated that enflurane also acts directly on skeletal muscles where blood flow is less. As a result, a longer time is required for enflurane to achieve its maximal enhancement of nondepolarizing neuromuscular blockade.

MECHANISM. Volatile anesthetics most likely enhance the effects of nondepolarizing neuromuscular blocking drugs by virtue of anesthetic-induced depression of the central nervous system,

which reduces the tone of skeletal muscles (Waud and Waud, 1975). In addition, volatile anesthetics may decrease sensitivity of postjunctional membranes to depolarization (Waud, 1979). This decrease in end-plate sensitivity depends on the specific volatile anesthetic and the dose administered. Twitch response is decreased by volatile anesthetics alone when the concentration is sufficient to depress depolarization by 50% (1.25 to 1.75 MAC enflurane or 2.83 to 3.67 MAC halothane) (Waud and Waud, 1979). Increased skeletal muscle blood flow as a means to deliver more drug to the neuromuscular junction is probably important only for the enhanced neuromuscular blockade seen in the presence of isoflurane (Vitez et al, 1974). Inhaled anesthetics do not enhance neuromuscular blockade by decreasing the release of acetylcholine from the motor nerve ending or by altering the configuration of cholinergic receptors (Waud and Waud, 1973).

Antibiotics

Several types of antibiotics have been shown to enhance neuromuscular blockade produced by nondepolarizing neuromuscular blocking drugs. Prominent among the antibiotics that produce this enhancement are the aminoglycoside antibiotics. Antagonism of antibiotic-potentiated neuromuscular blockade by an anticholinesterase drug or Ca^{2+} is unpredictable. Antibiotics devoid of neuromuscular blocking effects are the penicillins and cephalosporins.

MECHANISM. Antibiotics may exert effects on the prejunctional membranes similar to magnesium, resulting in decreased release of acetylcholine (Sokoll and Gergis, 1981). Likewise, the same antibiotics may stabilize postjunctional membranes; thus, attempts to propose a common mechanism for antibiotic-induced enhancement of neuromuscular blockade probably are impossible.

Inhibition of the presynaptic release of acetylcholine by antibiotics may reflect competition of these drugs with Ca^{2+}. Indeed, intravenous injection of Ca^{2+} may at least transiently reverse the enhanced neuromuscular blockade associated with administration of antibiotics. Nevertheless, in addition to facilitating the prejunctional release of acetylcholine, Ca^{2+} at the same time stabilizes postjunctional membranes to the effects of acetylcholine. These different effects of Ca^{2+} at the neuromuscular junction are consistent with the unpredictable effects of Ca^{2+} in antagonizing antibiotic-induced enhancement of neuromuscular blockade produced by nondepolarizing neuromuscular blocking drugs.

Local Anesthetics

Small doses of local anesthetics can enhance neuromuscular blockade produced by nondepolarizing neuromuscular blocking drugs, whereas in large doses local anesthetics can block neuromuscular transmission. Depending on the dose, local anesthetics interfere with the prejunctional release of acetylcholine, stabilize postjunctional membranes, and directly depress skeletal muscle fibers. In addition, ester local anesthetics compete with other drugs for plasma cholinesterase, thus introducing the possibility of a prolonged drug effect produced by succinylcholine.

Cardiac Antidysrhythmic Drugs

Lidocaine, as administered intravenously to treat cardiac dysrhythmias, could augment preexisting neuromuscular blockade (Harrah et al, 1970). This potential drug interaction should be considered when administering lidocaine to patients recovering from general anesthesia that included use of a nondepolarizing neuromuscular blocking drug.

Quinidine potentiates neuromuscular blockade produced by nondepolarizing and depolarizing neuromuscular blocking drugs presumably by interfering with the prejunctional release of acetylcholine (Miller et al, 1967). As with lidocaine, this drug interaction may manifest when quinidine is administered to treat cardiac dysrhythmias in patients who previously have received neuromuscular blocking drugs during general anesthesia.

Diuretics

Furosemide, 1 mg·kg⁻¹ IV, enhances neuromuscular blockade produced by nondepolarizing neuromuscular blocking drugs (Miller et al, 1976b). This effect most likely reflects furosemide-induced inhibition of cyclic AMP production, leading to decreased prejunctional output

of acetylcholine. Conversely, large doses of furosemide may inhibit phosphodiesterase, making more cyclic AMP available and leading to antagonism of nondepolarizing neuromuscular blocking drugs (Azar et al, 1980). Azathioprine also antagonizes nondepolarizing neuromuscular blockade presumably by inhibiting phosphodiesterase (Dretchen et al, 1976). This same drug augments neuromuscular blockade produced by succinylcholine.

Mannitol does not influence the degree of neuromuscular blockade produced by nondepolarizing neuromuscular blocking drugs even in the presence of diuresis (Matteo et al, 1980). This emphasizes that renal clearance of neuromuscular blocking drugs depends on glomerular filtration. Osmotic diuretics increase urine output independent of glomerular filtration rate.

Chronic hypokalemia owing to treatment with diuretics reduces dose requirements for pancuronium and increases the dose of neostigmine necessary to reverse neuromuscular blockade (Miller and Roderick, 1978a).

Magnesium

Magnesium enhances neuromuscular blockade produced by nondepolarizing neuromuscular blocking drugs and, to a lesser extent, enhances neuromuscular blockade produced by succinylcholine (Fig. 8-28) (Ghoneim and Long, 1970). It has been suggested that the interaction between magnesium and vecuronium is more pronounced than the interaction between magnesium and dTc (Sinatra et al, 1985). Speculated mechanisms for this interaction include decreased prejunctional release of acetylcholine and decreased sensitivity (stabilization) of postjunctional membranes to acetylcholine. The effects of magnesium are consistent with the enhancement of neuromuscular blockade produced by nondepolarizing neuromuscular blocking drugs as administered to patients with pregnancy-induced hypertension (toxemia of pregnancy) who are being treated with magnesium. The mechanism by which these effects of magnesium enhance neuromuscular blockade produced by succinylcholine is not apparent. It is possible that phase II blockade occurs more readily when succinylcholine is administered in the presence of elevated plasma concentrations of magnesium.

Lithium

Lithium, as used to treat psychiatric depression, may enhance the neuromuscular blocking effects of depolarizing and nondepolarizing neuromuscular blocking drugs (Havdala et al, 1979).

Phenytoin

Patients treated chronically with phenytoin are resistant to the neuromuscular blocking effects of nondepolarizing neuromuscular blocking drugs (Ornstein et al, 1987). This resistance seems to be related to a pharmacodynamic mechanism, since plasma concentrations of drug needed to produce a given level of neuromuscular blockade are increased compared with the plasma level necessary to produce the same response in untreated patients.

Cyclosporine

Cyclosporine may prolong the duration of neuromuscular blockade produced by nondepolarizing neuromuscular blocking drugs (Wood, 1989).

Corticosteroids

Cortisol or adrenocorticotrophic hormone can improve neuromuscular function in patients with myasthenia gravis. Conversely, the intravenous administration of corticosteroids does not alter the characteristics of neuromuscular blockade produced by nondepolarizing neuromuscular blocking drugs (Schwartz et al, 1986).

Ganglionic Blocking Drugs

Ganglionic blocking drugs, such as trimethaphan, can influence responses produced by neuromuscular blocking drugs through (1) decreases in skeletal muscle blood flow, (2) inhibition of plasma cholinesterase activity, and (3) decreased sensitivity of postjunctional membranes (Sklar and Lanks, 1977). Theoretically, a decrease in skeletal muscle blood flow would delay the onset and prolong the duration of neuromuscular blockade.

Hypothermia

Hypothermia prolongs neuromuscular blockade produced by dTc and pancuronium, reflecting delayed biliary and urinary excretion (Ham et al,

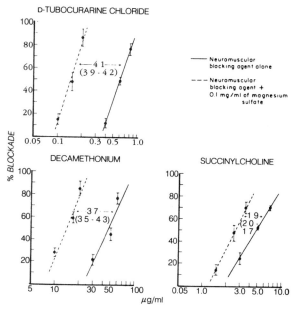

FIGURE 8–28. Magnesium enhances neuromuscular blockade produced by nondepolarizing neuromuscular blocking drugs and to a lesser extent that produced by succinylcholine. Mean ± SE. (From Ghoneim MM, Long JP. The interaction between magnesium and other neuromuscular blocking agents. Anesthesiology 1970; 32: 23–7; with permission.)

1978; Miller et al, 1978b). Pancuronium-induced neuromuscular blockade is enhanced further by hypothermia-induced reductions in the hepatic enzyme activity responsible for metabolizing the drug. Finally, hypothermia also appears to increase sensitivity of the neuromuscular junction to pancuronium but not to dTc.

Acid-Base Changes

Respiratory acidosis enhances dTc and pancuronium-induced neuromuscular blockade and opposes their reversal with neostigmine (Miller and Roderick, 1978b). Changes produced by metabolic acidosis and respiratory and metabolic alkalosis have been inconsistent.

Serum Potassium Concentration

An acute decrease in the extracellular concentration of K^+ will increase the transmembrane potential, causing hyperpolarization of cell membranes. This change manifests as resistance to the effects of depolarizing neuromuscular blocking drugs and increased sensitivity to nondepolarizing neuromuscular blocking drugs. Conversely, hyperkalemia lowers the resting transmembrane potential and thus partially depolarizes cell membranes. This change increases the effects of depolarizing neuromuscular blocking drugs and opposes the action of nondepolarizing neuromuscular blocking drugs.

Thermal (Burn) Injury

Thermal injury causes resistance to nondepolarizing neuromuscular blocking drugs that manifests approximately 10 days after injury, peaks at approximately 40 days, and declines after approximately 60 days (Fig. 8-29) (Dwersteg et al, 1986; Martyn et al, 1982. Martyn et al, 1983). Despite this typical time sequence, one report describes prolonged resistance to metocurine lasting 463 days (Fig. 8-30) (Martyn et al, 1982). Approxi-

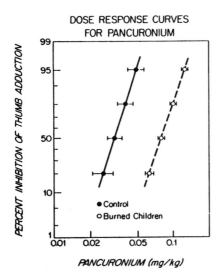

FIGURE 8–29. Dose response curves for pancuronium are shifted to the right in thermal (burn) injured patients indicating a resistance to the neuromuscular blocking effects of the drug. (Martyn JAJ, Liu LMP, Szyfelbein SK, Ambalavankar ES, Goudsouzian NG. The neuromuscular effects of pancuronium in burned children. Anesthesiology 1983; 59: 561–4; with permission.)

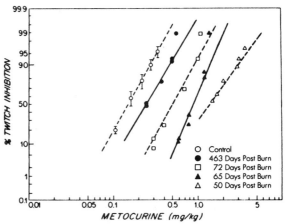

FIGURE 8–30. Resistance to the effects of drug-induced neuromuscular blockade in burn patients, as reflected by rightward displacement of the dose-response curve, may persist for several months. (From Martyn JAJ, Matteo RS, Szyfelbein SK, Kaplan RF. Unprecedented resistance to neuromuscular blocking effects of metocurine, with persistence and complete recovery in a burned patient. Anesth Analg 1982; 61: 614–7; with permission.)

mately 30% or more of the body must be burned to produce resistance. A pharmacodynamic explanation as the principal mechanism for this resistance is documented by the need to achieve higher plasma drug concentrations to produce a given degree of twitch suppression in thermal injury vs nonthermal injury patients (Fig. 8-31) (Marathe et al, 1989a; Martyn et al, 1982). In contrast to denervation injury and an associated increase in extrajunctional cholinergic receptors that respond to acetylcholine, resistance to the effects of nondepolarizing neuromuscular blocking drugs in patients with thermal injury is not associated with changes in density of these receptors (Marathe et al, 1989b). An altered affinity of the cholinergic receptors for acetylcholine or nondepolarizing neuromuscular blocking drugs may be the basis for thermal-induced resistance to these drugs.

Paresis or Hemiplegia

Monitoring neuromuscular blockade with a peripheral nerve stimulator attached to the arm on the side affected by a cerebral vascular accident reveals resistance (decreased sensitivity) to the effects of the neuromuscular blocking drug compared with responses observed on the unaffected side (Iwasaki et al, 1985; Moorthy and Hilgenberg, 1980). Furthermore, even the unaffected arm shows resistance to the effects of neuromuscular blocking drugs compared with responses observed in normal patients (Fig. 8-32) (Shayevitz and Matteo, 1985). As a result, monitoring neuromuscular blockade with a peripheral nerve stimulator following a cerebral vascular accident may underestimate the degree of neuromuscular blockade present at the muscles of ventilation. Resistance to neuromuscular blocking drugs in the affected arm may reflect proliferation of extrajunctional cholinergic receptors that respond to acetylcholine.

Allergic Reactions

Anaphylactic and anaphylactoid reactions occur occasionally following the intravenous administration of nondepolarizing neuromuscular blocking drugs and succinylcholine. There may be cross-sensitivity among all neuromuscular blocking drugs, reflecting the presence of quaternary ammonium groups that act as antigenic stimulants (Didier et al, 1987). A drug with a single quaternary ammonium group, such as vecuronium, may be less likely to cause cross-sensitivity. Anaphylactic reactions following the first exposure to a neuromuscular blocking drug may reflect sensitization from prior contact with cosmetics and soaps that also contain antigenic quaternary ammonium groups.

Succinylcholine Followed by a Nondepolarizing Neuromuscular Blocking Drug

Following administration of a dose of succinylcholine for intubation of the trachea, the subsequent onset of nondepolarizing neuromuscular blockade is faster and recovery is delayed (Ono et al, 1989). This is unexpected because succinylcholine and a nondepolarizing neuromuscular blocking drug should be antagonistic. Presumably, postjunctional membranes remain desensitized by succinylcholine, resulting in prolonged effects produced by nondepolarizing neuromuscular blocking drugs.

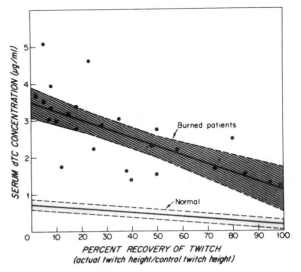

FIGURE 8–31. The plasma (serum) concentration of d-tubocurarine (dTc) associated with a given level of twitch recovery is greater in burned patients than in nonburned patients. (From Martyn JA, Szyfelbein SK, Ali HH, Matteo RS, Savarese JJ. Increased d-Tubocurarine requirement following major thermal injury. Anesthesiology 1980;52:352–5; with permission.)

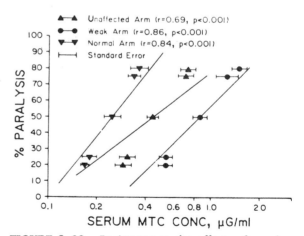

FIGURE 8–32. Resistance to the effects of nondepolarizing neuromuscular blocking drugs is detectable in both the paretic and unaffected arms of patients following a cerebral vascular accident compared with normal patients. Mean ± SE. (From Shayevitz JR, Matteo RS. Decreased sensitivity to metocurine in patients with upper motorneuron disease. Anesth Analg 1985; 64: 767–72; with permission.)

Combinations of Neuromuscular Blocking Drugs

The combination of pancuronium with metocurine or dTc produces neuromuscular blockade that is greater than the additive effects of the individual drugs (Fig. 8-33) (Lebowitz et al, 1980). This greater than additive neuromuscular blocking effect does not occur when metocurine is combined with dTc. Despite the enhancement of neuromuscular blockade by combining pancuronium with metocurine or dTc, the duration of neuromuscular blockade is shorter than that produced by pancuronium alone. It is possible that this enhancement of neuromuscular blockade reflects simultaneous prejunctional and postjunctional receptor blockade (Taylor, 1985). Two neuromuscular blocking drugs (dTc and metocurine) that act principally at the same prejunctional site would not be expected to produce more than additive effects when administered in combination (Bowman, 1980; Robbins et al, 1984). Presumably, decreased release of acetylcholine from prejunctional sites owing to these drugs would increase the potency of neuromuscular blocking drugs that act principally at postjunctional sites (Duncalf et al, 1983). Nevertheless, there is also evidence that this enhancement can be entirely due to postjunctional actions of the neuromuscular blocking drugs (Waud and Waud, 1985).

The combination of nondepolarizing neuromuscular blocking drugs permits achievement of the same degree of neuromuscular blockade with a smaller dose of each drug, which results in fewer dose-related side effects (Lebowitz et al, 1981). Indeed, blood pressure and heart rate effects of the combination of pancuronium and metocurine are less than with pancuronium alone (Fig. 8-34) (Lebowitz et al, 1981).

SECOND GENERATION LONG-ACTING NONDEPOLARIZING NEUROMUSCULAR BLOCKING DRUGS

Second generation long-acting nondepolarizing neuromuscular blocking drugs differ from pancuronium principally because they are devoid of cardiovascular side effects.

Doxacurium

Doxacurium is a long-acting bisquaternary ammonium nondepolarizing neuromuscular blocking drug that is devoid of histamine-releasing or cardiovascular side effects (Fig. 8-1) (Basta et al, 1988). Pharmacokinetics of doxacurium resemble pancuronium with respect to elimination

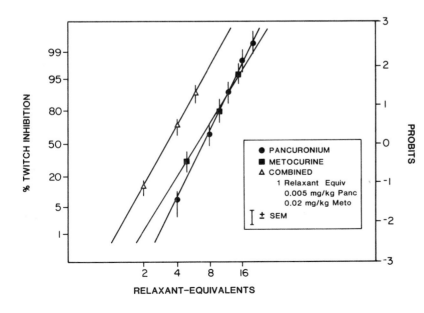

FIGURE 8–33. The combination of pancuronium with metocurine produces neuromuscular blockade that is greater than the additive effects of the individual drugs. (From Lebowitz PW, Ramsey FM, Savarese JJ, Ali HH. Potentiation of neuromuscular blockade in man produced by combinations of pancuronium and metocurine or pancuronium and d-tubocurarine. Anesth Analg 1980; 59: 604–9; with permission.)

half-time and dependence on renal clearance mechanisms. The ED_{95} is 30 $\mu g \cdot kg^{-1}$ IV with spontaneous recovery to 25% of twitch height occurring in approximately 76 minutes following administration of approximately 40 $\mu g \cdot kg^{-1}$ IV. Conditions for intubation of the trachea are considered excellent within 4 minutes after administration of 80 $\mu g \cdot kg^{-1}$ IV of doxacurium (Lennon et al, 1989). Volatile anesthetics decrease doxacurium dose requirements by 20% to 40% compared with doses required during nitrous oxide—fentanyl anesthesia (Katz et al, 1989). Doxacurium does not trigger malignant hyperthermia in susceptible swine (Sufit et al, 1990).

Pipecuronium

Pipecuronium is a long-acting steroidal nondepolarizing neuromuscular blocking drug that is devoid of histamine-releasing or cardiovascular side effects (Fig. 8-1) (Larijani et al, 1989). Pharmacokinetics of pipecuronium resemble pancuronium with respect to elimination half-time and dependence on renal clearance mechanisms (Fig. 8-35) (Caldwell et al, 1989; Wierda et al, 1990). The principal metabolite excreted in the urine is 3-desacetyl pipecuronium. The ED_{95} is 50 to 60 $\mu g \cdot kg^{-1}$ IV with 2 × ED_{95}, producing adequate conditions for intubation of the trachea in 2.5 to 3 minutes and a clinical duration of 80 to 120 minutes (Wierda et al, 1989). The potency of pipecuronium is increased and its duration of action shortened in infants compared with children and adults (Pittet et al, 1990a).

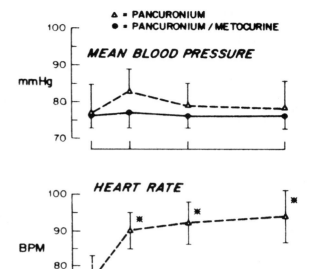

FIGURE 8–34. Blood pressure and heart rate effects of the combination of pancuronium and metocurine are less than with pancuronium alone. (From Lebowitz PW, Ramsey FM, Savarese JJ, Ali HH, deBros FM. Combination of pancuronium and metocurine: Neuromuscular and hemodynamic advantages over pancuronium alone. Anesth Analg 1981; 60: 12–7; with permission.)

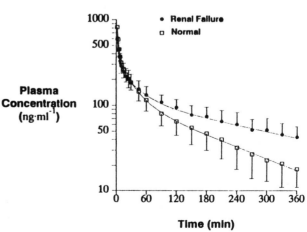

FIGURE 8–35. Clearance of pipecuronium from the plasma is slowed in patients with renal failure compared with normal patients. (From Caldwell JE, Canfell PC, Castagnoli KP, et al. The influence of renal failure on the pharmacokinetics and duration of action of pipecuronium bromide in patients anesthetized with halothane and nitrous oxide. Anesthesiology 1989; 70: 7–12; with permission.)

INTERMEDIATE-ACTING NONDEPOLARIZING NEUROMUSCULAR BLOCKING DRUGS

Atracurium and vecuronium are intermediate-acting nondepolarizing neuromuscular blocking drugs with efficient clearance mechanisms that minimize the likelihood of significant cumulative effects with repeated injections or continuous infusions of these drugs. As such, atracurium and vecuronium are useful alternatives to succinylcholine and long-acting nondepolarizing neuromuscular blocking drugs, especially when intubation of the trachea or skeletal muscle relaxation are needed for short operations, such as outpatient procedures. Compared with long-acting nondepolarizing neuromuscular blocking drugs, these drugs have (1) a similar onset rate of maximum neuromuscular blockade; (2) approximately one third the duration of action (hence, the designation "intermediate-acting"); (3) a 30% to 50% more rapid rate of recovery; (4) minimal to absent cumulative effects; and (5) minimal to absent cardiovascular effects (Basta et al, 1982a; Fahey et al, 1981b). The intermediate duration of action of these drugs is due to their rapid clearance from the circulation. Because of their slow onset, atracurium or vecuronium are usually not acceptable substitutes for succinylcholine when intubation of the trachea must be accomplished within 60 seconds of rendering the patient unconscious. Neuromuscular blockade produced by intermediate-acting neuromuscular blocking drugs is reliably antagonized by anticholinesterase drugs often within 20 minutes of administering a paralyzing dose of these drugs (Gencarelli and Miller, 1982).

Chemical Structure

Atracurium

Atracurium is a bisquaternary ammonium nondepolarizing neuromuscular blocking drug with a bulky structure unlike that of any other neuromuscular blocking drug (Fig. 8-1). This drug was designed specifically to undergo spontaneous *in vivo* degradation (Hofmann elimination) at normal body temperature and pH (Stenlake et al, 1983). The iodide salt, besylate, provides water solubility, and adjusting the pH of the commercial solution to 3.25 to 3.65 minimizes the likelihood of spontaneous *in vitro* degradation. In view of its acid pH *in vitro,* atracurium probably should not be mixed with alkaline drugs such as barbiturates or exposed to solutions with more alkaline pHs, as are present in delivery tubing used for infusion of intravenous fluids. Exposure of atracurium to an increased pH before its entrance into the circulation could theoretically result in premature breakdown of the drug. The potency of atracurium stored at room temperature decreases approximately 5% every 30 days.

Vecuronium

Vecuronium is a monoquaternary steroidal analogue of pancuronium (Fig. 8-1). Structurally, vecuronium is pancuronium without the quaternary methyl group in the A-ring of the steroid nucleus. The absence of this quaternary methyl group reduces the acetylcholine-like character of vecuronium as compared with pancuronium. Indeed, the vagolytic property of vecuronium is decreased approximately 20-fold. The monoquaternary structure of vecuronium increases its lipid solubility compared with pancuronium. Vecuronium is unstable in solution and for this reason is supplied as a lyophilized powder that must be dissolved in sterile water prior to its use.

Metabolism

Atracurium

Atracurium undergoes spontaneous degradation at normal body temperature and pH by a base-catalyzed reaction termed "Hofmann elimination" (Fig. 8-36) (Stenlake et al, 1983). A second and simultaneously occurring route of metabolism is ester hydrolysis (Fig. 8-36) (Stenlake et al, 1983). Hofmann elimination represents a chemical mechanism of elimination whereas ester hydrolysis is a biologic mechanism. These two routes of metabolism are independent of hepatic and renal function as well as plasma cholinesterase activity (Merrett et al, 1983). As such, the duration of atracurium-induced neuromuscular blockade is similar in normal patients and those with absent or impaired renal or hepatic function or those with atypical plasma cholinesterase. Hofmann elimination and ester hydrolysis also

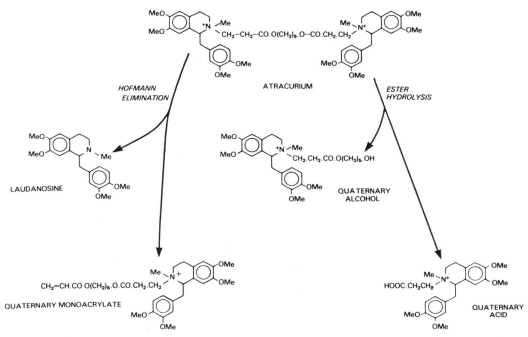

FIGURE 8–36. Atracurium undergoes spontaneous metabolism at normal body temperature and pH by Hofmann elimination and ester hydrolysis. (From Stenlake JB, Waigh RD, Urwin J, Dewar GH, Coker GG. Atracurium: Conception and inception. Br J Anaesth 1983; 55: 3S–10S; with permission.)

account for the lack of cumulative drug effects with repeated doses or continuous infusions of atracurium.

HOFMANN ELIMINATION. Hofmann elimination begins to occur immediately after atracurium enters the circulation. In the presence of physiologic pH, Hofmann elimination occurs at the quaternary nitrogen of the alpha side chain of atracurium to yield laudanosine as the primary metabolite (Fig. 8-36) (Stenlake et al, 1983). Electrophilic acrylates also may be formed by Hofmann elimination. These acrylates are reactive and when studied *in vitro* are capable of damaging cells by alkylating nucleophiles present in cellular membranes (Nigrovic et al, 1989). The clinical significance, if any, of these acrylates is unknown; however, the concentrations of atracurium used for the *in vitro* studies are as much as 1600 times that required to produce neuromuscular blockade *in vivo*. The rate of Hofmann elimination is slowed by acidosis

(pH less than 7.4) or decreases in body temperature to less than 37° C. The reverse changes will speed clearance of atracurium by Hofmann elimination.

ESTER HYDROLYSIS. Ester hydrolysis of atracurium occurs by nonspecific esterases that are unrelated to plasma cholinesterase. It is likely that ester hydrolysis is less important than Hofmann elimination in the total clearance of atracurium from the plasma. As with Hofmann elimination, laudanosine is also a metabolite of ester hydrolysis.

Prolonged neuromuscular blockade does not follow administration of atracurium to patients with atypical plasma cholinesterase, emphasizing the dependence of ester hydrolysis of atracurium on nonspecific esterases that are unrelated to plasma cholinesterase (Baraka, 1987). In contrast to Hofmann elimination, the rate of ester hydrolysis of atracurium is enhanced by decreases in blood pH to less than 7.4.

LAUDANOSINE. Peak plasma concentrations of laudanosine in humans occur 2 minutes after a rapid intravenous injection of atracurium and remain at approximately 75% of peak levels for nearly 15 minutes (Fahey et al, 1985). Laudanosine is cleared principally from the plasma by the kidneys with an elimination half-time of 113 minutes in animals (Hennis et al, 1986). Hepatic cirrhosis in humans does not alter the clearance of laudanosine, whereas excretion of this metabolite is impaired in patients with biliary obstruction (Parker and Hunter, 1989). In animals, plasma concentrations of laudanosine increase during the anhepatic phase of liver transplantation, suggesting the liver is important for clearance of laudanosine in this model (Pittet et al, 1990b). Laudanosine is inactive at the neuromuscular junction. The principal theoretical concern introduced by laudanosine is the capability of this metabolite to cause peripheral vasodilation and central nervous system stimulation. For example, a transient and modest (14%) decrease in blood pressure follows the administration of laudanosine, 1 mg·kg^{-1} IV, to halothane anesthetized dogs (Hennis et al, 1986). Laudanosine crosses the blood-brain barrier and is detectable in the cerebrospinal fluid (2 to 14 ng·ml^{-1}) of patients receiving atracuium (Fahey et al, 1990; Gwinnutt et al, 1990). It seems unlikely that administration of atracurium to patients will result in plasma concentrations of laudanosine capable of producing cardiovascular or central nervous system disturbances. For example, in anesthetized animals, laudanosine plasma concentrations of more than 6 μg·ml^{-1} cause hypotension; laudanosine concentrations of more than 10 μg·ml^{-1} induce epileptic spiking on the EEG; and plasma concentrations of more than 17 μg·ml^{-1} produce seizures (Chapple et al, 1987). In patients receiving a full paralyzing dose of atracurium, the resulting peak plasma concentrations of laudanosine are approximately 0.3 μg·ml^{-1}, which is approximately 20 times less than the plasma concentration producing cardiovascular effects in animals. Anesthetic requirements are not changed in patients receiving as much as 1 mg·kg^{-1} IV (5 × ED$_{95}$) of atracurium, suggesting that any central nervous system stimulating effect from the resulting laudanosine would not be apparent clinically (Fig. 8-17) (Fahey et al, 1989). Nevertheless, there is evidence of increased anesthetic requirements in animals receiving infusions of laudanosine and that administration of atracurium may

produce arousal EEG changes in dogs breathing subanesthetic concentrations of halothane (Fahey et al, 1985; Lanier et al, 1985; Shi et al, 1985). Arousal changes on the EEG observed in these dogs are not associated with increases in cerebral blood flow or intracranial pressure (Lanier et al, 1985).

Clearly, laudanosine resulting from metabolism of atracurium probably will not produce evidence of seizure activity in anesthetized patients because skeletal muscle paralysis from atracurium would preclude movement. Furthermore, inhaled anesthetics (with the possible exception of enflurane) or injected drugs such as thiopental would tend to suppress evidence of laudanosine-evoked central nervous system stimulation. In the absence of central nervous system depression produced by anesthetics, as in the critical care unit, it is theoretically possible that laudanosine-induced evidence of central nervous system stimulation could occur. Nevertheless, in patients receiving continuous infusions of atracurium for as long as 6 days, the plasma concentrations of laudanosine remain below those levels in animals associated with cardiovascular or central nervous system effects (Fig. 8-37) (Chapple et al, 1987; Yate et al, 1987). Furthermore, in an animal model of epilepsy, laudanosine does not alter the incidence of seizure activity (Tateishi et al, 1989).

Vecuronium

Increased lipid solubility of vecuronium as compared with pancuronium facilitates entrance of vecuronium into hepatocytes where it undergoes deacetylation to 3-hydroxyvecuronium, 17-hydroxyvecuronium, and 3,17-dihydroxyvecuronium (Savage et al, 1980). The 3-hydroxyvecuronium derivative is approximately one half as potent as the parent compound but is rapidly converted to the 3,17-dihydroxyvecuronium derivative. The 3,17-dihydroxyvecuronium and 17-hydroxyvecuronium derivatives have less than one tenth the neuromuscular blocking potencies of vecuronium.

Increased lipid solubility also facilitates biliary excretion of vecuronium. For example, in patients, an estimated 50% of the intravenous dose of vecuronium may be present in the liver 30 minutes after injection, and approximately 40% of the drug is excreted unchanged in the bile in the first 24 hours (Bencini et al, 1986a). Approximately 30% of an administered dose of vecu-

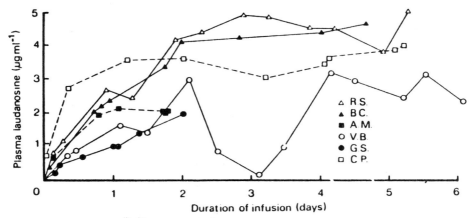

FIGURE 8–37. Plasma laudanosine concentrations in six patients during atracurium infusion. (From Yate PM, Flynn PJ, Arnold RW, Weatherly BC, Simmonds RJ, Dopson T. Clinical experience and plasma laudanosine concentrations during the infusion of atracurium in the intensive therapy unit. Br J Anaesth 1987; 59: 211–7; with permission.)

ronium appears in the urine as unchanged drug and metabolites in the first 24 hours (Bencini et al, 1986b). The extensive hepatic uptake of vecuronium may account for the rapid decrease in vecuronium plasma concentrations and the drug's short duration of action.

Onset and Duration of Action

Atracurium and vecuronium, like the long-acting nondepolarizing neuromuscular blocking drugs, manifest a dose-dependent onset and duration of action with a rate of spontaneous recovery that is independent of the total dose of neuromuscular blocking drug (Table 8-9). The onset of action of atracurium and vecuronium is similar to the long-acting nondepolarizing neuromuscular blocking drugs, but the duration of action is approximately one third that of the long-acting drugs. Increasing the dose of vecuronium from 0.1 mg·kg^{-1} IV to 0.4 mg·kg^{-1} IV decreases the time to zero twitch response from 208 seconds to 106 seconds and prolongs the time to recovery to 25% twitch height from 37 minutes to 138 minutes (Ginsberg et al, 1989). This may be an alternative to succinylcholine when a rapid onset of skeletal muscle paralysis is deemed important.

Priming Principle

The priming principle is based on the concept that the onset of neuromuscular blockade con-

sists of two steps: (1) initial binding of spare receptors during which no clinical effect is observed and (2) subsequent deepening of the blockade. The onset time of nondepolarizing neuromuscular blockade is accelerated if spare receptors are occupied by a small subparalyzing dose (approximately 10% of the drug's ED$_{95}$) followed in approximately 4 minutes by the larger dose of the drug (2 to 3 × ED$_{95}$). For example, the onset of neuromuscular blockade produced by intermediate-acting drugs can be made similar to succinylcholine by administering 0.1 × ED$_{95}$ of atracurium or vecuronium followed in 3 to 6 minutes by the larger remaining portion of the dose (Gergis et al, 1983; Mehta et al, 1985; Schwarz et al, 1985). Administration of vecuronium, 0.01 mg·kg^{-1} IV 4 minutes before 0.1 mg·kg^{-1} IV seems to be the optimal dose and time interval for speeding the onset of neuromuscular blockade produced by this drug (Taboada et al, 1986).

This divided dose technique is known as the priming principle and may serve as a useful alternative when administration of succinylcholine is best avoided. Conceptually, the initial subparalyzing dose is presumed to decrease the safety margin of neuromuscular transmission, allowing a more rapid onset of effect after the second larger dose. A similar more rapid onset occurs with divided doses of long-acting nondepolarizing neuromuscular blocking drugs or the combination of long- and intermediate-acting neuromuscular blocking drugs (Mehta et al, 1985).

Table 8-9

Comparative Pharmacology of Intermediate-Acting Nondepolarizing Neuromuscular Blocking Drugs

	Atracurium	Vecuronium
ED_{95} (mg·kg^{-1})	0.15–0.30	0.04–0.07
Onset to maximum twitch suppression (min)	3–5	3–5
Time to 25% recovery of twitch height (min)	20–35	20–35
Recovery index (min)*	15–25	15–25
Continuous infusion (μg·kg^{-1}·min^{-1})	6.2	1
Volume of distribution (L·kg^{-1})	0.20	0.27
Clearance (ml·kg^{-1}·min^{-1})	5.5	5.2
Active metabolites at neuromuscular junction	No	Slight
Degradation dependent on		
Body temperature	Yes	Yes
Blood pH	Yes	No
Renal function	No	Yes
Hepatic function	No	Yes

*Recovery of twitch height from 25% to 75% of control.

Rate of Recovery

The rate of recovery from 10% to 25% of control twitch response is more rapid with intermediate-acting than long-acting nondepolarizing neuromuscular blocking drugs. This rate of recovery is clinically important because abdominal musculature is adequately relaxed at 10% but not 25% of control twitch response. Typically, neuromuscular blockade can be antagonized 20 to 30 minutes after initial injection of $2 \times ED_{95}$ of atracurium or vecuronium. Supplemental doses of these drugs (usually approximately one third the initial dose) usually can be antagonized 10 to 30 minutes later, providing spontaneous recovery of twitch response has begun.

Atracurium

The elimination half-time and clearance of atracurium in anesthetized patients are consistent with the drug's intermediate duration of action (Table 8-9) (Ward and Wright, 1983). The elimination half-time of approximately 22 minutes reflects rapid metabolism and is approximately one third the elimination half-time for long-acting nondepolarizing neuromuscular blocking drugs.

An estimated 82% of atracurium is bound to plasma proteins, presumably albumin (Foldes and Deery, 1983).

The site of action of atracurium, like that of other nondepolarizing neuromuscular blocking drugs, is on both presynaptic and postsynaptic nicotinic cholinergic receptors (Hughes and Payne, 1983). Atracurium may also produce neuromuscular blockade by directly interfering with passage of ions through channels of nicotinic cholinergic receptors.

During thiopental–fentanyl–nitrous oxide anesthesia, the ED_{95} of atracurium is 0.2 mg·kg^{-1} IV (Basta et al, 1982a). Spontaneous recovery to 95% twitch response after the ED_{95} is 44 minutes compared with 137 minutes for dTc. The onset of maximum twitch depression after the ED_{95} is similar to long-acting neuromuscular blocking drugs.

Vecuronium

The elimination half-time and clearance of vecuronium in anesthetized patients are consistent with the drug's intermediate duration of action, reflecting rapid hepatic metabolism and biliary excretion of vecuronium. (Table 8-9) (Cronnelly et al, 1983) Even though the elimination half-time (71 minutes) of vecuronium is greater than that (22 minutes) for atracurium, the two drugs have similar durations of action. The onset of maximum neuromuscular blockade following administration of vecuronium is similar to pancuronium, but the duration of neuromuscular blockade is shorter and the rate of recovery is more rapid after administration of vecuronium (Fahey et al, 1981). Despite its greater lipid solubility, the Vd of vecuronium does not differ from pancuronium, perhaps explaining the similar onset of action of both drugs (Table 8-5) (Cronnelly et al, 1983).

The plasma concentration of vecuronium necessary to decrease twitch response 50% is similar to the plasma concentration of pancuronium producing the same degree of twitch depression (Cronnelly et al, 1983). This observation suggests that pancuronium and vecuronium are equally potent and, by extrapolation, the ED_{95} for vecuronium would be similar to pancuronium (0.07 mg·kg^{-1}). Nevertheless, other studies have described vecuronium as being 15% to 50% more potent than pancuronium (Fahey et al, 1981; Miller et al, 1984). The reasons for these discrepancies may reflect failure to control precisely the depth of anesthesia or the use of cumulative dose response curves to determine the ED_{95} (Gramstad and Lilleaasen, 1982). For example, the rapid clearance of intermediate-acting nondepolarizing neuromuscular blocking drugs makes it difficult to derive valid ED_{95} values from dose-response techniques based on repeated dose regimens (Fisher et al, 1982a; Gibson et al, 1985).

Cumulative Effects

Consistency of onset to recovery intervals after repeated supplemental doses of atracurium is a unique characteristic of this drug that reflects the absence of a significant cumulative drug effect (Fig. 8-38) (Ali et al, 1983). The absence of a significant cumulative drug effect is due to rapid elimination of atracurium from the plasma that is independent of hepatic or renal clearance mechanisms. Lack of drug cumulation minimizes the likelihood of persistent neuromuscular blockade when prolonged surgical procedures require repeated doses or a sustained continuous intravenous infusion.

Repeated supplemental doses of vecuronium produce slight but detectable increases in the duration of neuromuscular blockade (Fig. 8-39) (Fahey et al, 1981). This cumulative effect is more than that observed with atracurium but much less than that produced by pancuronium. Following a single dose of vecuronium or pancuronium, plasma concentrations decrease rapidly because of redistribution from central to peripheral compartments. With subsequent doses, any drug in the peripheral compartment limits the distribution phase and thus also the rate of decrease in the plasma concentrations of neuromuscular blocking drugs. As a result, pancuronium and, to a lesser extent, vecuronium can be demonstrated to have cumulative effects.

Overall, the lack of significant cumulative drug effect permits continuous intravenous infusion of atracurium or vecuronium with little likelihood of unexpected prolonged neuromuscular blockade. It is important to recognize, however,

FIGURE 8–38. Repeated doses of atracurium (BW33A) do not produce a cumulative drug effect as evidenced by the unchanging time intervals between doses for the same degree of recovery from neuromuscular blockade to occur. (From Ali HH, Savarese JJ, Basta SJ, Sunder N, Gionfriddo M. Evaluation of cumulative properties of three new nondepolarizing neuromuscular blocking drugs: BW A444U, atracunum and vecuronium. Br J Anaesth 1983; 55: 107S–11S; with permission.)

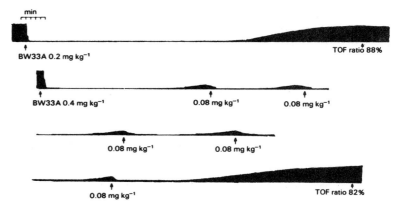

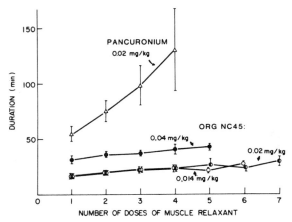

FIGURE 8–39. Repeated doses of vecuronium produce slight evidence of a cumulative drug effect that is greater than that observed after administration of atracurium but less than that associated with pancuronium. (From Fahey MR, Morris RB, Miller RD, Sohn YJ, Cronnelly R, Gencarelli P. Clinical pharmacology of ORG NC45 (Norcuron): A new nondepolarizing muscle relaxant. Anesthesiology 1981; 55: 6–11; with permission.)

ronium, but the potentiation seems to be less than that produced for the long-acting nondepolarizing neuromuscular blocking drugs (Figs. 8-40 and 8-41) (Rupp et al, 1984; Rupp et al, 1985). Furthermore, changes in the alveolar concentration of volatile anesthetic has less impact on neuromuscular blockade produced by intermediate-acting compared with long-acting neuromuscular blocking drugs. The advantage of lessened augmentation of intermediate-acting neuromuscular blocking drugs by volatile anesthetics is a more predictable degree of neuromuscular blockade, without precise knowledge of the alveolar (brain) partial pressure of the anesthetic. Conversely, a disadvantage is that existing neuromuscular blockade is not easily enhanced by increasing the delivered concentration of volatile anesthetic. The reasons for atracurium and vecuronium being less influenced by the specific volatile anesthetic and its concentration are not known.

As evidence of augmentation of neuromuscular blocking effects, the continuous intravenous infusion rate of vecuronium necessary to maintain 90% depression of twitch response during administration of enflurane, isoflurane, or fentanyl, each

that noncumulative effects of these drugs depend on the size of the supplemental doses. Whenever supplemental doses of atracurium or vecuronium exceed the rate of plasma clearance, cumulative drug effects are possible.

Pharmacologic and Physiologic Interactions

Drugs (volatile anesthetics, succinylcholine, and antibiotics) and physiologic changes known to enhance neuromuscular blockade produced by long-acting neuromuscular blocking drugs also interact in a similar manner with intermediate-acting neuromuscular blocking drugs. The magnitude of these interactions, however, may differ between long-acting and intermediate-acting nondepolarizing neuromuscular blocking drugs.

Volatile Anesthetics

Volatile anesthetics enhance neuromuscular blockade produced by atracurium and vecu-

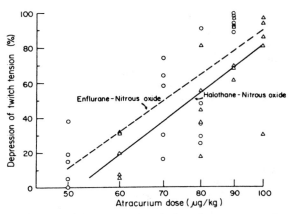

FIGURE 8–40. Atracurium-induced neuromuscular blockade is enhanced by volatile anesthetics, but the magnitude of this enhancement is less than observed with long-acting nondepolarizing neuromuscular blocking drugs (see Fig. 8–26). (From Rupp SM, McChristian JW, Miller RD. Neuromuscular effects of atracurium during halothane-nitrous oxide and enflurane-nitrous oxide anesthesia in humans. Anesthesiology 1985; 63: 16–9; with permission.)

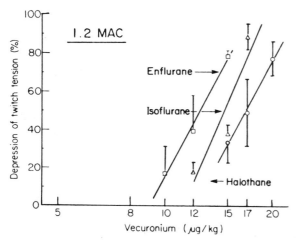

FIGURE 8–41. Vecuronium-induced neuromuscular blockade is enhanced by volatile anesthetics, but the magnitude of this enhancement is less than observed with long-acting nondepolarizing neuromuscular blocking drugs (see Fig. 8–26). (From Rupp SM, Miller RD, Gencarelli P. Vecuronium-induced neuromuscular blockade during enflurane, isoflurane, and halothane anesthesia in humans. Anesthesiology 1984; 60: 102–5; with permission.)

in combination with 60% nitrous oxide, is 0.28, 0.30, and 0.92 $\mu g \cdot kg^{-1} \cdot min^{-1}$, respectively (Fig. 8-42) (Cannon et al, 1987). Plasma concentrations of vecuronium present with 90% twitch suppression in patients receiving enflurane and isoflurane are similar (71 and 72 $ng \cdot ml^{-1}$, respectively) but significantly higher in patients receiving fentanyl (165 $ng \cdot ml^{-1}$), thus confirming that potentiation of vecuronium-induced neuromuscular blockade by volatile anesthetics represents a change in pharmacodynamics rather than a change in pharmacokinetics.

Succinylcholine

As with long-acting nondepolarizing neuromuscular blocking drugs, the prior administration of succinylcholine, 1 $mg \cdot kg^{-1}$ IV, enhances the magnitude of twitch response suppression produced by subsequently administering atracurium or vecuronium even when evidence of neuromuscular blockade produced by succinylcholine has waned (Krieg et al, 1981; Stirt et al, 1983). Despite this initial enhancement, the subsequent duration of action of neuromuscular blockade produced by atracurium or vencuronium is not prolonged by the prior administration of succinylcholine. A smaller dose of succinylcholine, 0.5 $mg \cdot kg^{-1}$ IV, does not enhance subsequent neuromuscular blocking effects of vecuronium (Fisher and Miller, 1983a).

Combination with Long-Acting Neuromuscular Blocking Drugs

The combination of vecuronium with dTc is significantly more potent than would be expected from a simple additive effect of these drugs administered individually (Mirakhur et al, 1985). This response is similar to the enhancement of neuromuscular blockade produced when combinations of long-acting nondepolarizing neuromuscular blocking drugs are administered. Enhancement of neuromuscular blockade produced by combinations of neuromuscular blocking drugs is presumed to reflect different principal sites of action (prejunctional vs postjunctional).

Antibiotics

Aminoglycoside antibiotics prolong neuromuscular blockade produced by atracurium or vecuronium (Chapple et al, 1983).

FIGURE 8–42. Vecuronium infusion rates necessary to maintain 90% depression of twitch response are less during anesthesia with volatile anesthetics compared with fentanyl. ●, mean infusion rates; ■, SD values; □, range of infusion rates. (From Cannon JE, Fahey MR, Castagnoli KP. Continuous infusion of vecuronium: The effect of anesthetic agents. Anesthesiology 1987; 67: 503–6; with permission.)

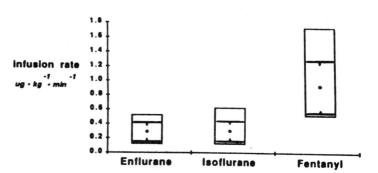

Hypothermia

Hypothermia prolongs the duration of action of atracurium and decreases the rate of continuous intravenous infusion necessary to maintain a constant degree of neuromuscular blockade (Flynn et al, 1983). Presumably, this enhanced neuromuscular blocking effect of atracurium reflects decreased degradation of atracurium by Hofmann elimination and decreased metabolism by ester hydrolysis. Hypothermia also increases the duration of action of vecuronium, presumably reflecting temperature-induced slowing of hepatic and renal clearance mechanisms (Buzello et al, 1985a).

Acid-Base Changes

Atracurium

Despite pH-dependent Hofmann elimination (accelerated by alkalosis and slowed by acidosis), it is unlikely that the range of pH changes encountered clinically is sufficiently great to alter the rate of Hofmann elimination and thus the duration of atracurium-induced neuromuscular blockade (Payne and Hughes, 1981). Furthermore, pH changes influence the rate of ester hydrolysis in a direction opposite to the change in the rate of Hofmann elimination such that slowed Hofmann elimination in the presence of acidosis is theoretically offset by an accelerated rate of ester hydrolysis.

Vecuronium

The impact of acid-base changes on vecuronium-induced neuromuscular blockade depends on whether the changes in blood pH precede or follow the administration of vecuronium (Gencarelli et al, 1983). For example, changes in $PaCO_2$ that precede the administration of vecuronium do not alter the magnitude of neuromuscular blockade. Conversely, hypercarbia introduced after the establishment of vecuronium-induced neuromuscular blockade significantly enhances the effects of the neuromuscular blocking drug. For this reason, the onset of hypoventilation, which may occur in the early postoperative period, could enhance residual neuromuscular blockade. A similar enhancement can occur when respiratory acidosis occurs in the presence of residual dTc neuromuscular blockade.

Histamine

It is estimated that the plasma concentration of histamine must double before cardiovascular changes manifest. This degree of histamine release occurs with the ED_{95} of dTc and $2 \times ED_{95}$ of metocurine (Basta et al, 1982b) Atracurium does not evoke sufficient histamine release to cause cardiovascular changes until a $3 \times ED_{95}$ is administered (Basta et al, 1982b). Histamine release and thus cardiovascular changes do not occur with even a $3.5 \times ED_{95}$ of vecuronium (Basta et al, 1983).

Histamine release evoked by neuromuscular blocking drugs does not occur repeatedly because histamine stores are not replenished for several days. Therefore, a decrease in blood pressure due to drug-induced histamine release is less likely to occur to the same magnitude on repeat dosing. Cardiovascular effects previously attributed to drug-induced histamine release may reflect release of prostacyclin and its vasodilating effects on peripheral vasculature mediated via H-1 receptors (Fig. 8-20) (Hatano et al, 1990).

Renal Dysfunction

The duration of long-acting nondepolarizing neuromuscular blocking drugs can be greatly enhanced by renal dysfunction. In contrast, the impact of renal failure on the duration of action of atracurium is predictably absent with even large doses ($2.5 \times ED_{95}$) of this drug (Hunter et al, 1984). The elimination half-time of vecuronium is prolonged in patients with renal failure, reflecting a decreased clearance of the drug (Lynam et al, 1988). It is estimated that approximately 30% of an administered dose of vecuronium appears in the urine as unchanged drug and metabolites in the first 24 hours (Bencini et al, 1986b). An apparent tolerance to vecuronium in patients with renal failure is suggested by higher plasma concentrations of vecuronium at 25% and 75% recovery compared to patients with normal renal function (Bencini et al, 1986b). This tolerance is consistent with a slower onset of action of vecuronium in patients with renal failure. A similar but less prominent degree of tolerance also may occur following administration of atracurium to patients in renal failure (Hunter et al, 1984). Plasma concentrations of laudanosine following single doses of atracurium, 0.5 mg·kg^{-1}

IV, are higher in patients in renal failure compared with normal patients (Fahey et al, 1985).

Hepatic Dysfunction

Hepatic failure does not alter the elimination half-time of atracurium compared with normal patients (Ward and Neill, 1983). Likewise, the elimination half-time of vecuronium, 0.1 mg·kg⁻¹ IV, administered to patients with alcoholic liver disease is not different than in patients without liver disease (Arden et al, 1988). In contrast, vecuronium, 0.2 mg·kg⁻¹ IV, is associated with a prolonged elimination half-time and thus duration of action in patients with hepatic cirrhosis (Fig. 8-43) (Lebrault et al, 1985). It is possible that other clearance mechanisms such as renal clearance or diffusion of drug into inactive tissues such as cartilage offset the effect of impaired hepatic function when lower doses of vecuronium are administered. In patients with cholestasis who are undergoing biliary surgery, the administration of vecuronium, 0.2 mg·kg⁻¹ IV, results in a prolonged elimination half-time and increased duration of action of the drug (Lebrault et al, 1986).

Circulatory Effects

Long-acting nondepolarizing neuromuscular blocking drugs produce predictable and often clinically significant decreases in blood pressure and systemic vascular resistance (dTc) or increases in heart rate (gallamine, pancuronium). These circulatory effects may be undesirable in the presence of hypovolemia, valvular heart disease, or coronary artery disease. In this regard, a major advantage of vecuronium, and to a lesser extent atracurium, is the unlikely occurrence of drug-induced circulatory effects. Conversely, bradycardia associated with opioid-based anesthetics, which is masked to some extent by heart-rate-accelerating effects of pancuronium, will not be offset by intermediate-acting nondepolarizing neuromuscular blocking drugs.

Atracurium

Blood pressure and heart rate changes do not accompany the rapid intravenous administration of

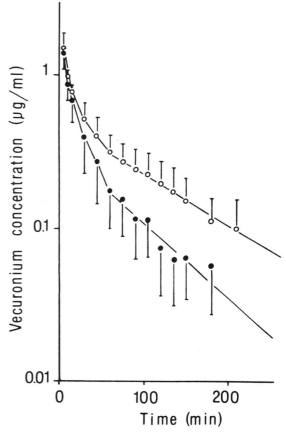

FIGURE 8–43. Disappearance of vecuronium (0.2 mg·kg⁻¹ IV) from the plasma is slowed in patients with hepatic cirrhosis (O) compared with normal patients (●). Mean ± SD. (From Lebrault C, Berger JL, D'Hollander AA, Gomeni R, Henzel D, Duvaldestin P. Pharmacokinetics and pharmacodynamics of vecuronium (ORG NC45) in patients with cirrhosis. Anesthesiology 1985; 62: 601–5; with permission.)

atracurium in doses up to 2 × ED₉₅ with background anesthetics including nitrous oxide, fentanyl, halothane, enflurane, and isoflurane (Fig. 8-44) (Basta et al, 1982a; Hilgenberg et al, 1983; Rupp et al, 1983a; Sokoll et al, 1983). During nitrous oxide–fentanyl anesthesia, the rapid intravenous administration of 3 × ED₉₅ of atracurium increases heart rate 8.3% and decreases mean arterial pressure 21.5% (Fig. 8-44) (Basta et al, 1982a). These circulatory changes are transient, occurring 60 to 90 seconds after administra-

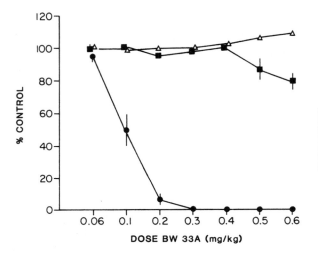

THUMB TWITCH
△ HEART RATE (BPM)
■ MEAN ARTERIAL
   PRESSURE (TORR)
I ± SE

FIGURE 8–44. Heart rate and blood pressure changes do not occur following the rapid intravenous administration of atracurium (BW 33A) up to doses equivalent to $2 \times ED_{95}$ (0.4 $mg \cdot kg^{-1}$ IV). Larger doses of atracurium may produce transient increases in heart rate and decreases in blood pressure. (From Basta SJ, Ali HH, Savarese JJ, et al. Clinical pharmacology of atracurium besylate (BW 33A): A new nondepolarizing muscle relaxant. Anesth Analg 1982; 61:723–9; with permission.)

tion of atracurium and disappearing within 5 minutes. Facial and truncal flushing in some patients suggests release of histamine as the mechanism for the circulatory changes accompanying the rapid administration of high doses of atracurium. Indeed, plasma histamine concentrations increase transiently and parallel heart rate and blood pressure changes when atracurium, 0.6 $mg \cdot kg^{-1}$ IV, is administered rapidly. Conversely, the same dose of atracurium administered slowly (over 30 to 75 seconds) or rapidly but in patients pretreated with H-1 and H-2 receptor antagonists does not evoke circulatory changes despite similar increases in plasma concentrations of histamine as are present in those receiving the same dose rapidly without pretreatment (Scott et al, 1984).

There is evidence that patients treated chronically with H-2 receptor antagonists may experience exaggerated circulatory changes in response to histamine-releasing drugs (Hosking et al, 1988). In this regard, it is speculated that H-2 receptor antagonists exert a partial antagonist effect on H-3 receptors, thus removing the usual negative feedback role of this H-3 receptor in modulating histamine release. As a result, there may be enhanced and sustained release of histamine. Animal evidence also suggests that laudanosine may contribute to transient blood pressure decreases associated with rapid intravenous administration of large doses of atracurium (Hennis et al, 1986).

Vecuronium

Vecuronium is typically devoid of circulatory effects even with rapid intravenous administration of doses that exceed $3 \times ED_{95}$ of the drug, emphasizing the lack of vagolytic effects or histamine release associated with administration of this drug (Morris et al, 1983). Nevertheless, occasional increases in plasma concentrations of histamine without associated blood pressure changes have been reported following administration of vecuronium (Cannon et al, 1988). A modest vagotonic effect of vecuronium is suggested by an increased incidence of bradycardia in patients receiving this drug in the absence of prior administration of an anticholinergic drug or in close association with the injection of a potent opioid such as sufentanil (Cozanitis et al, 1987; Inoue et al, 1988; Salmenpera et al, 1983; Starr et al, 1986). Sinus node exit block and even cardiac arrest has been described in association with vecuronium injection (Milligan and Beers, 1985; Yeaton and Teba, 1988).

Obstetric Patients

The short duration of action of atracurium and vecuronium makes these drugs attractive selections for producing skeletal muscle relaxation during general anesthesia for cesarean section.

The slow onset of action, however, compared with succinylcholine, detracts from their use when rapid intubation of the trachea is considered important. Like the long-acting nondepolarizing neuromuscular blocking drugs, insufficient amounts of atracurium and vecuronium cross the placenta to produce significant effects in the fetus (Dailey et al, 1984; Frank et al, 1983). For example, the maternal-to-fetal ratio of vecuronium following administration of 0.04 to 0.08 mg·kg^{-1} IV to the mother is 0.11. Concentrations of atracurium in umbilical venous blood are below the sensitivity limits of the assay. The clearance of vecuronium may be accelerated during late pregnancy, possibly reflecting stimulation of hepatic microsomal enzymes by progesterone as well as by cardiovascular changes and fluid shifts that occur during pregnancy. Conversely, the duration of action of vecuronium-induced neuromuscular blockade is prolonged in the immediate postpartum period (Hawkins et al, 1989).

Pediatric Patients

Atracurium

Effective doses of atracurium are similar in adults and children (aged 2 to 16 years) when differences in extracellular fluid volume are minimized by calculating the dose on an mg·m^{-2} rather than mg·kg^{-1} basis (Brandom et al, 1984). Conversely, infants aged 1 to 6 months require approximately one half the dose of atracurium given to older children to achieve the same degree of neuromuscular blockade (Brandom et al, 1983). Likewise, the continuous intravenous infusion rate of atracurium required to maintain a steady state neuromuscular blockade is 25% less during the first 30 days of life (0.4 mg·kg^{-1}·h^{-1}) compared with patients more than 1 month old (0.53 mg·kg^{-1}·h^{-1}) (Kalli and Meretoja, 1988). These data imply that infants are more sensitive than children or adults to the neuromuscular blocking effects of atracurium. A similar sensitivity occurs in infants receiving dTc (Fisher et al, 1982b). Recovery from atracurium-induced neuromuscular blockade, however, is more rapid in infants (23 minutes) than adolescents (29 minutes) (Brandom et al, 1983).

Vecuronium

The potency of vecuronium in infants (aged 7 to 45 weeks), children (aged 1 to 8 years), and adults (aged 18 to 38 years) is similar during nitrous oxide–halothane anesthesia (Table 8-10) (Fisher and Miller, 1983b). Onset of action is more rapid in infants than in adults, whereas duration of action is longest in infants and shortest in children (Table 8-10) (Fisher and Miller, 1983b; Meretoja, 1989). Presumably, a high cardiac output in infants speeds the onset of vecuronium-induced neuromuscular blockade, whereas the longer duration of action reflects im-

Table 8–10

Comparison of Vecuronium-Induced Neuromuscular Blockade in Pediatric and Adult Patients

	Vecuronium (mg·kg^{-1})	Onset of Maximum Twitch Suppression (min)	Duration (min to 90% twitch recovery)	Recovery Index (min for twitch response to recover from 25% to 75% of control)
Infants	0.07	1.5[*]	73[*]	20[**]
Children	0.07	2.4	35	9
Adults	0.07	2.9	54	13

[*] P < 0.05 compared with adults.
[**] P < 0.05 compared with children.
(Data from Fisher DM, Miller RD. Neuromuscular effects of vecuronium (ORG NC45) in infants and children during N$_2$O, halothane anesthesia. Anesthesiology 1983; 58: 519–23, with permission.)

the neonate's liver or an increased Vd. An increased Vd means more drug is sequestered in peripheral compartments and unaccessible to hepatic and renal clearance mechanisms. Age-related changes in biliary clearance also may contribute to a longer duration of vecuronium-induced neuromuscular blockade in infants.

Elderly Patients

Atracurium

Increasing age has no effect on the continuous rate of intravenous infusion of atracurium necessary to maintain a constant degree of neuromuscular blockade (D'Hollander et al, 1983). Likewise, the rate of recovery and thus the duration of neuromuscular blockade is similar in young adults and the elderly. This lack of influence of aging on dose requirements of atracurium most likely reflects the independence of Hofmann elimination and ester hydrolysis from age-related effects on renal and hepatic function. Furthermore, changes in Vd that occur with aging will not influence the clearance of atracurium from the plasma. Failure of aging to alter responsiveness of the neuromuscular junction is documented by similar plasma concentrations of atracurium necessary to depress twitch 50% in elderly patients and young adults (Kitts et al, 1990).

Vecuronium

Increasing age is associated with decreases in the continuous rate of intravenous infusion of vecuronium necessary to maintain a constant degree of neuromuscular blockade (D'Hollander et al, 1982). Presumably, this reflects decreased plasma clearance of vecuronium due to age-related decreases in hepatic blood flow and renal blood flow and possibly decreased hepatic microsomal enzyme activity. Furthermore, when the continuous infusion of vecuronium is discontinued, the rate of recovery of twitch response is prolonged in the elderly compared with young adults. This delayed rate of recovery could manifest as a prolonged duration of vecuronium-induced neuromuscular blockade in the elderly. In contrast to the detectable impact of aging during and following the continuous intravenous in-

fusion of vecuronium, the elimination half-time and dose response curves as determined from twitch responses produced by single intravenous doses of vecuronium are not influenced by increasing age (O'Hara et al, 1985; Rupp et al, 1987).

In patients aged 70 to 80 years, the Vd and plasma clearance of vecuronium are decreased compared with younger patients (Rupp et al, 1983b). The decrease in Vd is consistent with age-related reductions in skeletal muscle mass and total body water, whereas reductions in plasma clearance most likely reflect decreased hepatic blood flow in the elderly. Evidence of unchanged responsiveness of the neuromuscular junction despite increasing age is the similarity of the plasma concentration of vecuronium necessary to depress twitch response 50% in elderly patients and young adults patients (Rupp et al, 1983b).

Obesity

The duration of action of vecuronium, but not atracurium, is prolonged in obese (more than 130% of ideal body weight) compared with nonobese adults (Fig. 8-45) (Weinstein et al, 1988).

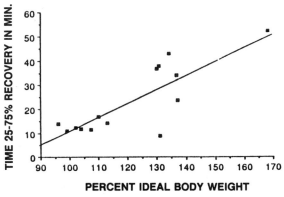

FIGURE 8–45. The rate of recovery following administration of vecuronium 0.1 mg·kg⁻¹ IV is delayed in obese compared with nonobese adults. (From Weinstein JA, Matteo RS, Ornstein E, Schwartz AE, Goldstoff M, Thal G. Pharmacodynamics of vecuronium and atracurium in the obese surgical patient. Anesth Analg 1988; 67: 1149–53; with permission.)

Intracranial Pressure

Intracranial pressure is not changed following the administration of atracurium or vecuronium to anesthetized patients undergoing surgery for expansive brain lesions (Rosa et al, 1986a; Rosa et al, 1986b). These data suggest that atracurium may be used for skeletal muscle relaxation during neurosurgical operations despite its potential for histamine release and stimulation of the central nervous system.

Intraocular Pressure

Administration of paralyzing doses of atracurium or vecuronium following induction of anesthesia with thiopental does not change intraocular pressure (Schneider et al, 1986). Furthermore, neuromuscular blockade produced by these drugs does not prevent increases in intraocular pressure in response to intubation of the trachea.

Malignant Hyperthermia

Malignant hyperthermia does not follow the administration of atracurium or vecuronium to sensitive swine (Buzello et al, 1985b; Ording and Fonsmark, 1988; Rorvik et al, 1988; Skarpa et al, 1983). Prolonged vecuronium-induced neuromuscular blockade has been reported in a malignant hyperthermia-susceptible patient pretreated with dantrolene (Driessen et al, 1985). This response could reflect dantrolene-induced decreases in neurotransmitter mobilization at the neuromuscular junction due to impaired release of Ca^{2+} from storage sites within cholinergic nerve terminals (Durant et al, 1980). It seems likely that similar prolongation of neuromuscular blockade could occur with other neuromuscular blocking drugs administered in the presence of dantrolene.

MIVACURIUM

Mivacurium is an intermediate to short-acting nondepolarizing neuromuscular blocking drug that is hydrolyzed by plasma cholinesterase at a rate equivalent to 88% that of succinylcholine (Figs. 8-1 and 8-46) (Savarese et al, 1988). The ED_{95} of mivacurium is 0.08 mg·kg^{-1} with an onset of 3.8 minutes and spontaneous recovery to 95% twitch height occurring in 24.5 minutes. At 2 × ED_{95}, the onset is 2.5 minutes, and recovery to

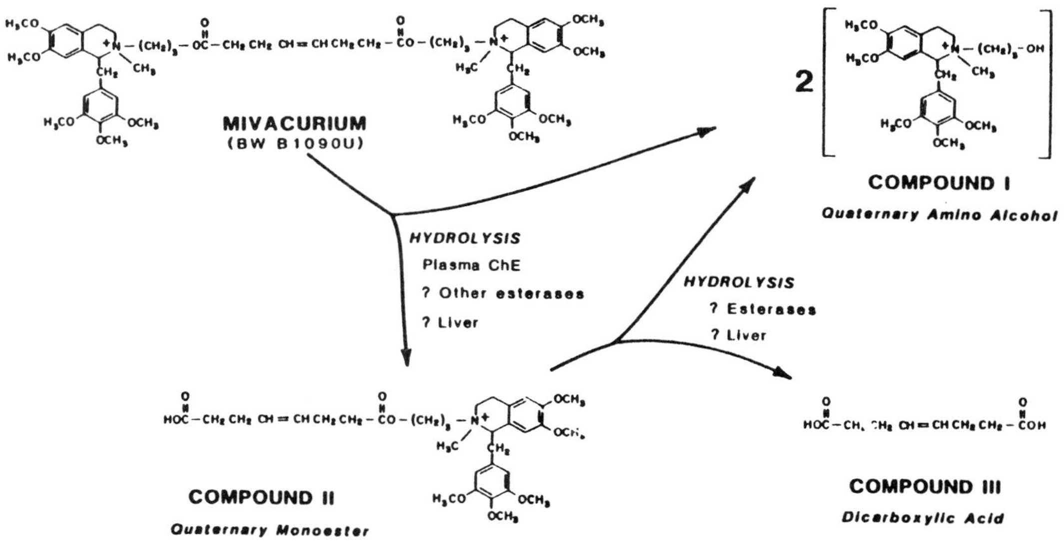

FIGURE 8–46. Proposed metabolic pathway of mivacurium. (From Savarese JJ, Ali HH, Basta SJ, et al. The clinical neuromuscular pharmacology of mivacurium chloride (BW B1090U). A short-acting nondepolarizing ester neuromuscular blocking drug. Anesthesiology 1988; 68: 723–32; with permission.)

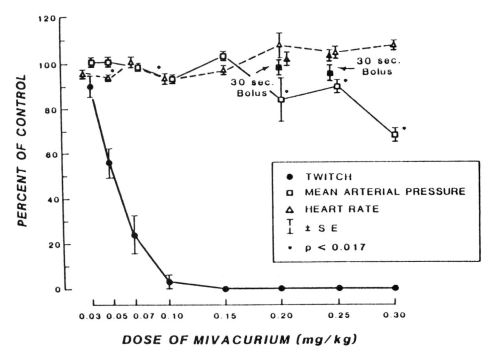

FIGURE 8–47. Neuromuscular and cardiovascular dose-response of mivacurium after injection over 10–15 seconds except where indicated as 30 seconds. (From Savarese JJ, Ali HH, Basta SJ, et al. The cardiovascular effects of mivacurium chloride (BW B1090U) in patients receiving nitrous oxide-opiate-barbiturate anesthesia. Anesthesiology 1989; 70: 386–94; with permission.)

95% twitch height occurs in 30.6 minutes. As such, the duration of action of mivacurium is approximately twice that of succinylcholine and 30% to 40% that of atracurium and vecuronium. The duration of action of mivacurium does not correlate with plasma cholinesterase activity, perhaps reflecting other routes of metabolism or excretion of mivacurium. The cardiovascular response to mivacurium is minimal at doses up to 2 × ED$_{95}$ (Fig. 8-47) (Savarese et al, 1989). Administration of 3 × ED$_{95}$ of mivacurium over 10 to 15 seconds evokes sufficient histamine release to transiently lower mean arterial pressure 13% to 18% (Fig. 8-47) (Savarese et al, 1989). The effect of anticholinesterase drugs is additive to the rapid rate of spontaneous recovery from mivacurium-induced neuromuscular blockade. Therefore, reversal of mivacurium is more rapid than is reversal of long-acting nondepolarizing neuromuscular blocking drugs. Mivacurium does not trigger malignant hyperthermia in susceptible swine (Sufit et al, 1990).

REFERENCES

Agoston S, Vermeer GA, Kersten UW, Meijer DKF. The fate of pancuronium bromide in man. Acta Anaesthesiol Scand 1973;17:267–75.

Ali HH, Savarese JJ. Monitoring of neuromuscular function. Anesthesiology 1976;45:216–49.

Ali HH, Savarese JJ, Basta SJ, Sunder N, Gionfriddo M. Evaluation of cumulative properties of three new nondepolarizing neuromuscular blocking drugs: BW A444U, atracurium and vecuronium. Br J Anaesth 1983;55:107S–11S.

Arden JR. Lynam DP, Castagnoli KP, Canfell PC, Cannol JC, Miller RD. Vecuronium in alcoholic liver disease: A pharmacokinetic and pharmacodynamic analysis. Anesthesiology 1988;68:771–6.

Azar I, Cottrell J. Gupta B. Turndorf H. Furosemide facilitates recovery of evoked twitch response after pancuronium. Anesth Analg 1980;59:55–7.

Baraka A. Neuromuscular blockade of atracurium versus succinylcholine in a patient with complete absence of plasma cholinesterase activity. Anesthesiology 1987;66:80–1.

Basta SJ, Ali HH, Savarese JJ, et al. Clinical pharmacology of atracurium besylate (BW 33A): A new nondepolarizing muscle relaxant. Anesth Analg 1982a;61:723–9.

Basta SJ, Savarese JJ, Ali HH, et al. Vecuronium does not alter serum histamine within the clinical dose range. Anesthesiology 1983;59:A273.

Basta SJ, Savarese JJ, Ali HH, Moss J, Gionfriddo BA. Histamine-releasing potencies of atracurium besylate (BW 33A), Dimethyltubocurarine and d-tubocurarine. Anesthesiology 1982b;57:A261

Basta SJ, Savarese JJ, Ali HH, et al. Clinical pharmacology of doxacurium chloride. A new long-acting nondepolarizing muscle relaxant. Anesthesiology 1988;69:478–86.

Bencini AF, Scaf AHJ, Sohn YJ, Kersten-Kleff UW, Agoston S. Hepatobiliary disposition of vecuronium bromide in man. Br J Anaesth 1986a; 58:988–95.

Bencini AF, Scaf AHJ, Sohn YJ, et al. Disposition and urinary excretion of vecuronium bromide in anesthetized patients with normal renal function or renal failure. Anesth Analg 1986b;65:245–51.

Bowman WC. Prejunctional and post-junctional cholinoceptors at the neuromuscular junction. Anesth Analg 1980;59:935–43.

Brandom BW, Rudd GD, Cook DR. Clinical pharmacology of atracurium in paediatric patients. Br J Anaesth 1983;55:117S–21S.

Brandom BW, Woelfel SK, Cook DR, Fehr BL, Rudd GD. Clinical pharmacology of atracurium in infants. Anesth Analg 1984;63:309–12.

Brotherton WP, Matteo RS. Pharmacokinetics and pharmacodynamics of metocurine in humans with and without renal failure. Anesthesiology 1981; 55:273–6.

Brown BB, Crout JR. The sympathomimetic effect of gallamine on the heart. J Pharmacol Exp Ther 1970;172:216–23.

Buzello W, Schluermann D, Schindler M, Spillner F. Hypothermic cardiopulmonary bypass and neuromuscular blockade by pancuronium and vecuronium. Anesthesiology 1985a;62:201–4.

Buzello W, Williams CH, Chandra P, Watkins ML, Dozier SE. Vecuronium and porcine malignant hyperthermia. Anesth Analg 1985;64:515–9.

Caldwell JE, Canfell PC, Castagnoli KP, et al. The influence of renal failure on the pharmacokinetics and duration of action of pipecuronium bromide in patients anesthetized with halothane and nitrous oxide. Anesthesiology 1989;70:7–12.

Cannon JE, Fahey MR, Castagnoli KP. Continuous infusion of vecuronium: The effect of anesthetic agents. Anesthesiology 1987;67:503–6.

Cannon JE, Fahey MR, Moss J, Miller RD. Large doses of vecuronium and plasma concentrations. Can J Anaesth 1988;35:350–3.

Carroll JB. Increased incidence of masseter spasm in children with strabismus anesthetized with halothane and succinylcholine. Anesthesiology 1987; 67:559–61.

Chapple DJ, Clark JS, Hughes R. Interaction between atracurium and drugs used in anaesthesia. Br J Anaesth 1983;55:17S–22S.

Chapple DJ, Miller AA, Ward JB, Wheatley PL. Cardiovascular and neurological effects of laudanosine. Studies in mice and rats, and in conscious and anaesthetized dogs. Br J Anaesth 1987;59:218–25.

Cooperman LH, Strobel GE, Kennell EM. Massive hyperkalemia after administration of succinylcholine. Anesthesiology 1970;32:161–4.

Cozanitis DA, Pouttu J, Rosenberg PH. Bradycardia associated with the use of vecuronium. A comparative study with pancuronium with and without glycopyrronium. Anaesthesia 1987;42:192–4.

Cronnelly R, Fisher DM, Miller RD, Gencarelli P, Nguyen-Gruenka L, Castagnoli N. Pharmacokinetics and pharmacodynamics of vecuronium (ORG NC45) and pancuronium in anesthetized humans. Anesthesiology 1983;58:405–8.

Dailey PA, Fisher DM, Shnider SM, et al. Pharmacokinetics, placental transfer, and neonatal effects of vecuronium and pancuronium administered during cesarean section. Anesthesiology 1984; 60:569–74.

D'Hollander AA, Luyckx C, Barvais L, Deville A. Clinical evaluation of atracurium besylate requirement for a stable muscle relaxation during surgery: Lack of age-related effects. Anesthesiology 1983; 59:237–40.

D'Hollander AA, Massaux F, Nevelsteen M, Agoston S. Age-dependent dose response relationship of ORG NC45 in anaesthetized patients. Br J Anaesth 1982;54:653–7.

Didier A, Benzarti M, Senft M, et al. Allergy to suxamethonium: Persisting abnormalities in skin tests, specific IgE antibodies and leucocyte histamine release. Clin Allergy 1987;17:385–92.

Dierdorf SF, McNiece WL, Rao CC. Effect of succinylcholine on plasma potassium in children with cerebral palsy. Anesthesiology 1985;62:88–90.

Dierdorf SF, McNiece WL, Rao CC, Wolfe TM, Means LJ. Failure of succinylcholine to alter plasma potassium in children with myelomeningocoele. Anesthesiology 1986;64:272–3.

Domenech JS, Garcia RC, Sasiain JMR, Loyola AQ, Oroz JS. Pancuronium bromide: An indirect sympathomimetic agent. Br J Anaesth 1976;48:1143–8.

Donati F, Antzaka C, Bevan DR. Potency of pancuronium at the diaphragm and the adductor pollicis muscle in humans. Anesthesiology 1986;65:1–5.

Drachman DA, Myasthenia gravis. N Engl J Med 1978;298:136–42.

Dretchen KL, Morgenroth VH, Standaert FG, Walts LF. Azathioprine: Effects on neuromuscular transmission. Anesthesiology 1976;45:604–9.

Driessen JJ, Wuis EW, Gielen JM. Prolonged vecuronium neuromuscular blockade in a patient receiving orally administered dantrolene. Anesthesiology 1985;62:523–4.

Duncalf D, Chaudry I, Aoki T, Nagashima H, Foldes FF. Potentiation of pancuronium, vecuronium and atracurium by d-tubocurarine or metocurine. Anesthesiology 1983;59:A292

Durant NN, Lee C, Katz RL. The action of dantrolene on transmitter mobilization at the rate NMJ. Eur J Pharmacol 1980;68:403–8.

Duvaldestin P, Agoston S, Henzel E, Kersten UW, Desmonts JM. Pancuronium pharmacokinetics in patients with liver cirrhosis. Br J Anaesth 1978; 50:1131–6.

Duvaldestin P, Saada J, Berger JL, D'Hollander A, Desmonts JM. Pharmacokinetics, pharmacodynamics, and dose-response relationship of pancuronium in control and elderly subjects. Anesthesiology 1982;56:36–40.

Dwersteg JF, Pavlin EG, Heimbach DM. Patients with burns are resistant to atracurium. Anesthesiology 1986;65:517–20.

Fahey MR, Canfell PC, Taboada T, Hosobuchi Y, Miller RD. Cerebrospinal fluid concentrations of laudanosine after administration of atracurium. Br J Anaesth 1990;64:105–6.

Fahey MR, Morris RB, Miller RD, Sohn YJ, Cronnelly R, Gencarelli P. Clinical pharmacology of ORG NC45 (Norcuron): A new nondepolarizing muscle relaxant. Anesthesiology 1981;55:6–11.

Fahey MR, Rupp SM, Canfell C, et al. Effect of renal function on laudanosine excretion in man. Br J Anaesth 1985;57:1049–51.

Fahey MR, Sessler DI, Cannon JE, Brady K, Stoen R, Miller RD. Atracurium, vecuronium and pancuronium do not alter the minimum alveolar concentration of halothane in humans. Anesthesiology 1989;71:53–6.

Fisher DM, Fahey MR, Cronnelly R, Miller RD. Potency determination for vecuronium (ORG NC45). Comparison of cumulative and single dose techniques. Anesthesiology 1982a;57:309–10.

Fisher DM, Miller RD. Interaction of succinylcholine and vecuronium during N_2O-halothane anesthesia. Anesthesiology 1983a;59:A278

Fisher DM, Miller RD. Neuromuscular effects of vecuronium (ORG NC45) in infants and children during N_2O, halothane anesthesia. Anesthesiology 1983b;58:519–23.

Fisher DM, O'Keefe C, Stanski DR, Cronnelly R, Miller RD, Gregory GA. Pharmacokinetics and pharmacodynamics of d-tubocurarine in infants, children, and adults. Anesthesiology 1982b;57:203–8.

Flynn PJ, Hughes P, Walton B. The use of atracurium in cardiopulmonary bypass with induced hypothermia. Anesthesiology 1983;59:A262

Fogdall RP, Miller RD. Neuromuscular effects of enflurane, alone and combined with d-tubocurarine, pancuronium, and succinylcholine, in man. Anesthesiology 1975;42:173–7.

Foldes FF, Deery A. Protein binding of atracurium and other short acting neuromuscular blocking agents and their interaction with human cholinesterase. Br J Anaesth 1983;55:31S–4S.

Foldes FF, Rendell-Baker L, Birch JH. Causes and prevention of prolonged apnea with succinylcholine. Anesth Analg 1956;35:609–13.

Forbes AR, Cohen NH, Eger EI. Pancuronium reduces halothane requirement in man. Anesth Analg 1979;58:497–9.

Frank M, Flynn PJ, Hughes R. Atracurium in obstetric anaesthesia. Br J Anaesth 1983;55:113S–14S.

Gencarelli PJ, Miller RD. Antagonism of ORG NC45 (vecuronium) and pancuronium neuromuscular blockade by neostigmine. Br J Anaesth 1982;54:53–6.

Gencarelli PJ, Siven J, Koot HWJ, Miller RD. The effects of hypercarbia and hypocarbia on pancuronium and vecuronium neuromuscular blockades in anesthetized humans. Anesthesiology 1983;59:376–80.

Gergis SD, Sokoll MD, Mehta M, Kemmotsuo O, Rudd GD. Intubation conditions after atracurium and suxamethonium. Br J Anaesth 1983;55:83S.

Ghoneim MM, Kramer E, Bannow R, Pandya H, Routh JI. Binding of d-tubocurare to plasma proteins in normal man and in patients with hepatic or renal disease. Anesthesiology 1973;39:410–5.

Ghoneim MM, Long JP. The interaction between magnesium and other neuromuscular blocking agents. Anesthesiology 1970;32:23–7.

Gibson FM, Mirakhur RK, Lavery GG, Clarke RSJ. Potency of atracurium: A comparison of single dose and cumulative dose techniques. Anesthesiology 1985;62:657–9.

Ginsberg B, Glass PS, Quill T, Shafron D, Ossey KD. Onset and duration of neuromuscular blockade following high-dose vecuronium administration. Anesthesiology 1989;71:201–5.

Gramstad L, Lilleaasen P. Dose-response relation of atracurium, ORG NC45 and pancuronium. Br J Anaesth 1982;54:647–51.

Griffith HR, Johnson GE. The use of curare in general anaesthesia. Anesthesiology 1942;3:418–20.

Gronert GA, Theye RA. Pathophysiology of hyperkalemia induced by succinylcholine. Anesthesiology 1975;43:89–99.

Gwinnutt CL, Eddleston JM Edwards D, Pollard BJ. Concentrations of atracurium and laudanosine in cerebrospinal fluid and plasma in three intensive care patients. Br J Anaesth 1990;65:829–32.

Ham J, Miller RD, Benet LZ, Matteo RS, Roderick LL. Pharmacokinetics and pharmacodynamics of d-tubocurarine during hypothermia in the cat. Anaesthesiology 1978;49:324–9.

Ham J, Miller RD, Sheiner LB, Matteo RS. Dosage-schedule independence of d-tubocurarine pharmacokinetics and pharmacodynamics, and recovery of neuromuscular function. Anesthesiology 1979; 50:528–33.

Harrah MD, Way WL, Katzung BG. The interaction of d-tubocurarine with antiarrhythmic drugs. Anesthesiology 1970;33:406–10.

Hatano Y, Arai T, Noda J, et al. Contribution of prostacyclin to d-tubocurarine-induced hypotension in humans. Anesthesiology 1990;72:28–32.

Havdala HS, Borison RL, Diamond BI. Potential hazards and applications of lithium in anesthesiology. Anesthesiology 1979;50:534–7.

Hawkins JL, Adenwala J, Camp C, Joyce TH. The effect of H_2-receptor antagonist premedication on the duration of vecuronium-induced neuromuscular blockade in postpartum patients. Anesthesiology 1989; 71:175–7.

Hennis PJ, Fahey MR, Canfell PC, Shi W-Z, Miller RD. Pharmacology of laudanosine in dogs. Anesthesiology 1986;65:56–60.

Hilgenberg JC, Stoelting RK, Harris WA. Systemic vascular responses to atracurium during enflurane-nitrous oxide anesthesia in humans. Anesthesiology 1983;58:242–4.

Holst-Larsen H. The hydrolysis of suxamethonium in human blood. Br J Anaesth 1976;48:887–91.

Hosking MP, Lennon RL, Gronert GA. Combined H_1 and H_2 receptor blockade attenuates the cardiovascular effects of high-dose atracurium for rapid sequence endotracheal intubation. Anesth Analg 1988;67:1089–92.

Hughes R, Chapple DJ. Effects of non-depolarizing neuromuscular blocking agents on peripheral autonomic mechanisms in cats. Br J Anaesth 1976; 48:59–67.

Hughes R, Payne JP. Clinical assessment of atracurium using the single twitch and tetanic responses of the adductor pollicis muscles. Br J Anaesth 1983; 55:47S–52S.

Hunter AR, Feldman SA. Muscle relaxants (editorial). Br J Anaesth 1976;48:277–8.

Hunter JM, Jones RS, Utting JE. Comparison of vecuronium, atracurium and tubocurarine in normal patients and in patients with no renal function. Br J Anaesth 1984;56:941–50.

Inoue K, El-Banayosy, Stolarski L, Reichelt W. Vecuronium induced bradycardia following induction of anaesthesia with etomidate or thiopentone, with or without fentanyl. Br J Anaesth 1988;60:10–7.

Ivankovich AD, Miletich DJ, Albrecht RF, Zahed B. The effect of pancuronium on myocardial contraction and catecholamine metabolism. J Pharm Pharmacol 1975;27:837–41.

Iwasaki H, Namiki A, Omote K, Omote T, Takahashi T. Response differences of paretic and healthy extremities to pancuronium and neostigmine in hemiplegic patients. Anesth Analg 1985;64:864–6.

John DA, Tobey RE, Homer LD, Rice CL. Onset of succinylcholine-induced hyperkalemia following denervation. Anesthesiology 1976;45:294–9.

Kalli I, Meretoja OA. Infusion of atracurium in neonates, infants and children. A study of dose requirements. Br J Anaesth 1988;60:651–4.

Kao YJ, Turner DR. Prolongation of succinylcholine block by metoclopramide. Anesthesiology 1989; 70:905–8.

Katz JA, Fragen RJ, Shanks CA, Dunn K, McNulty B, Rudd GD. Dose-response relationships of doxacurium chloride in humans during anesthesia with nitrous oxide and fentanyl, enflurane, isoflurane, or halothane. Anesthesiology 1989;70:432–6.

Kitts JB, Fisher DM, Canfell PC, et al. Pharmacokinetics and pharmacodynamics of atracurium in the elderly. Anesthesiology 1990;72:272–5.

Kohlschutter B, Bauer H, Roth F. Suxamethonium-induced hyperkalemia in patients with severe intra-abdominal infections. Br J Anaesth 1976;48:557–62.

Krieg N, Hendrick HH, Crul JF. Influence of suxamethonium on the potency of ORG NC45 in anesthetized patients. Br J Anaesth 1981;53:259–62.

Lanier WL, Milde JH, Michenfelder JD. The cerebral effects of pancuronium and atracurium in halothane-anesthetized dogs. Anesthesiology 1985;63:589–97.

Lanier WL, Milde JH, Michenfelder JD. Cerebral stimulation following succinylcholine in dogs. Anesthesiology 1986;64:551–9.

Larijani GE, Bartkowski RR, Azad SS, et al. Clinical pharmacology of pipecuronium bromide. Anesth Analg 1989;68:734–9.

Lebowitz PW, Ramsey FM, Savarese JJ, Ali HH. Potentiation of neuromuscular blockade in man produced by combinations of pancuronium and metocurine or pancuronium and d-tubocurarine. Anesth Analg 1980;59:604–9.

Lebowitz PW, Ramsey FM, Savarese JJ, Ali HH, deBros FM. Combination of pancuronium and metocurine: Neuromuscular and hemodynamic advantages over pancuronium alone. Anesth Analg 1981;60:12–7.

Lebrault C, Berger JL, D'Hollander AA, Gomeni R, Henzel D, Duvaldestin P. Pharmacokinetics and pharmacodynamics of vecuronium (ORG NC45) in patients with cirrhosis. Anesthesiology 1985; 62:601–5.

Lebrault C, Duvaldestin P, Henzel D, Chauvin M. Guesnon P. Pharmacokinetics and pharmacodynamics of vecuronium in patients with cholestasis. Br J Anaesth 1986;58:983–7.

Lee C. Dose relationship of phase II, tachyphylaxis and train-of-four fade on suxamethonium-induced dual neuromuscular block in man. Br J Anaesth 1975; 47:841–5.

Leighton BL, Cheek TG, Gross JB, et al. Succinylcholine pharmacodynamics in peripartum patients. Anesthesiology 1986;64:202–5.

Lennon RL, Hosking MP, Houck PC, et al. Doxacurium chloride for neuromuscular blockade before tracheal intubation and surgery during nitrous oxide-oxygen-narcotic-enflurance anesthesia. Anesth Analg 1989;68:255–60.

Lynam DP, Cronnelly R, Castagnoli KP, et al. The pharmacodynamics and pharmacokinetics of vecuronium in patients anesthetized with isoflurane with normal renal function or with renal failure. Anesthesiology 1988;69:227–31.

Manninen PH, Mahendran B, Gelb AW, Merchant RN. Succinylchloride does not increase serum potassium levels in patients with acutely ruptured cerebral ancurysms. Anesth Analg 1900;70:172–5.

Marathe PH, Dwersteg JF, Pavlin EG, Haschke RH, Heimbach DM, Slattery JT. Effect of thermal injury on the pharmacokinetics and pharmacodynamics of atracurium in humans. Anesthesiology 1989a; 70:752–5.

Marathe PH, Haschke RH, Slattery JT, Zucker JR, Pavlin EG. Acetylcholine receptor density and acetylcholinesterase activity in skeletal muscle of rats following thermal injury. Anesthesiology 1989b;70:654–9.

Martyn JAJ, Liu LMP, Szyfelbein SK, Ambalavankar ES, Goudsouzian NG. The neuromuscular effects of pancuronium in burned children. Anesthesiology 1983;59:561–4.

Martyn JAJ, Matteo RS, Szyfelbein SK, Kaplan RF. Unprecedented resistance to neuromuscular blocking effects of metocurine, with persistence and complete recovery in a burned patient. Anesth Analg 1982;61:614–7.

Martyn JJ, Szyfelbein SK, Ali HH, Matteo RS, Savarese JJ. Increased d-Tubocurarine requirement following major thermal injury. Anesthesiology 1980;52:352–5.

Matteo RS, Backus WW, McDaniel DD, Brotherton WP, Abraham R, Diaz J. Pharmacokinetics and pharmacodynamics of d-tubocurarine and metocurine in the elderly. Anesth Analg 1985;64:23–9.

Matteo RS. Nishitateno K, Pua E, Spector S. Pharmacokinetics of d-tubocurarine in man: Effect of an osmotic diuretic on urinary excretion. Anesthesiology 1980;52:335–8.

Matteo RS, Pua EK, Khambatta HJ, Spector S. Cerebrospinal fluid levels of d-tubocurarine in man. Anesthesiology 1977;46:396–9.

Matteo RS, Spector S, Horowitz PE. Relation of serum d-tubocurarine concentration to neuromuscular blockade in man. Anesthesiology 1974;41:440–3.

McLeod K. Watson MJ, Rawlings MD. Pharmacokinetics of pancuronium in patients with normal and impaired renal function. Br J Anaesth 1976;48:341–5.

Mehta MP, Choi WW, Gergis SD, Sokoll MD, Adolphson AJ. Facilitation of rapid endotracheal intubations with divided doses of nondepolarizing neuromuscular blocking drugs. Anesthesiology 1985;62:392–5.

Meretoja AA. Is vecuronium a long-acting neuromuscular blocking agent in neonates and infants. Br J Anaesth 1989;62:184–7.

Merrett RA, Thompson CW, Webb FW. In vitro degradation of atracurium in human plasma. Br J Anaesth 1983;55:61–6.

Miller RD, Agoston S, Booij LHDJ, Kersten U, Crul JF, Ham J. The comparative potency and pharmacokinetics of pancuronium and its metabolites in anesthetized man. J Pharmacol Exp Ther 1978a; 207:539–43.

Miller RD, Agoston S, van der Pol F, Booij LHDJ, Crul JF, Ham J. Hypothermia and pharmacokinetics and pharmacodynamics of pancuronium in the cat. J Pharmacol Exp Ther 1978b;207:532–8.

Miller RD, Criqui M, Eger EI. The influence of duration of anesthesia on a d-tubocurarine neuromuscular blockade. Anesthesiology 1976a;44:207–10.

Miller RD, Matteo R, Benet LZ, Sohn YJ. Influence of renal failure on the pharmacokinetics of d-tubocurarine in man. J Pharmacol Exp Ther 1977;202:1–7.

Miller RD, Roderick L. Diuretic-induced hypokalaemic pancuronium neuromuscular blockade and its antagonism by neostigmine. Br J Anaesth 1978a;50:541–4.

Miller RD, Roderick LL. Acid-base balance and neostigmine antagonism of pancuronium neuromuscular blockade. Br J Anaesth 1978b;50:317–24.

Miller RD, Rupp SM, Fisher DM, Cronnelly R, Fahey MR, Sohn YJ. Clinical pharmacology of vecuronium and atracurium. Anesthesiology 1984;61:444–53.

Miller RD, Sohn YJ, Matteo RS. Enhancement of d-tubocurarine neuromuscular blockade by diuretics in man. Anesthesiology 1976b;45:442–5.

Miller RD, Way WL. Inhibition of succinylcholine induced increased intragastric pressure by nondepolarizing muscle relaxants and lidocaine. Anesthesiology 1971;34:185–8.

Miller RD, Way WL, Dolan WM, Stevens WC, Eger EI. Comparative neuromuscular effects of pancuronium, gallamine, and succinylcholine during Forane and halothane anesthesia in man. Anesthesiology 1971; 35:509–14.

Miller RD, Way WL, Hickey RL. Inhibition of succinylcholine induced increased intraocular pressure by nondepolarizing muscle relaxants. Anesthesiology 1968;29:123–6.

Miller RD, Way WL, Katzung BG. The potentiation of neuromuscular blocking agents by quinidine. Anesthesiology 1967;28:1036–41.

Milligan KR, Beers HT. Vecuronium-associated cardiac arrest. Anesthesia 1985;40:385.

Mirakhur RK, Gibson FM, Ferres CJ. Vecuronium and d-tubocurarine combination: Potentiation of effect. Anesth Analg 1985;64:711–4.

Mitchell MM, Ali HH, Savarese JJ. Myotonia and neuromuscular blocking agents. Anesthesiology 1978; 49:44–8.

Moorthy SS, Hilgenberg JC. Resistance to nondepolarizing muscle relaxants in paretic upper extremities of patients with residual hemiplegia. Anesth Analg 1980;59:624–7.

Morris RB, Cahalan MK, Miller RD, Wilkinson PL, Quasha AL, Robinson SL. The cardiovascular effects of vecuronium (ORG NC45) and pancuronium in patients undergoing coronary artery bypass grafting. Anesthesiology 1983;58:438–40.

Moss J, Rosow CE, Savarese JJ, Philbin DM, Kniffen KJ. Role of histamine in the hypotensive action of d-tubocurarine in humans. Anesthesiology 1981;55:19–25.

Munger WL, Miller RD, Stevens WC. The dependence of d-tubocurarine-induced hypotension on alveolar concentration of halothane, dose of d-tubocurarine, and nitrous oxide. Anesthesiology 1974;40:442–8.

Munson ES, Wagman IH. Elevation of lidocaine seizure threshold by gallamine. Arch Neurol 1973; 28:329–33.

Muzzi DA, Black S, Cucchiara RF. The lack of effect of succinylcholine on serum potassium in patients with Parkinson's disease. Anesthesiology 1989;71:322.

Nigrovic V, Pandya JB, Klaunig JE, Fry K. Reactivity and toxicity of atracurium and its metabolites in vitro. Can J Anaesth 1989;36:262–8.

O'Hara DA, Fragen RJ, Shanks CA. The effects of age on the dose-response curves for vecuronium in adults. Anesthesiology 1985;63:542–4.

Ono K, Manabe N, Ohta Y, Morita K, Kosaka F. Influence of suxamethonium on the action of subsequently administered vecuronium or pancuronium. Br J Anaesth 1989;62:324–6.

Ording H, Fonsmark L. Use of vecuronium and doxapram in patients susceptible to malignant hyperthermia. Br J Anaesth 1988;60:445–9.

Ornstein E, Matteo RS, Schwartz AE, Silverberg PA, Young WL, Diaz J. The effect of phenytoin on the magnitude and duration of neuromuscular block following atracurium or vecuronium. Anesthesiology 1987;67:191–6.

Pandey K, Badola RP, Kumar S. Time course of intraocular hypertension produced by suxamethonium. Br J Anaesth 1972;44:191–6.

Parker CJR, Hunter JM. Pharmacokinetics of atracurium and laudanosine in patients with hepatic cirrhosis. Br J Anaesth 1989;62:177–83.

Payne JP, Hughes R. Evaluation of atracurium in anesthetized man. Br J Anaesth 1981;53:45–56.

Pittet J-F, Tassonju E, Morel DR, Gemperle G, Rouge J-C. Neuromuscular effect of pipecuronium bromide in infants and children during nitrous oxide-alfentanil anesthesia. Anesthesiology 1990a;72:432–5.

Pittet J-F, Tassonji E, Schopfer C, et al. Plasma concentrations of laudanosine, but not atracurium, are increased during the anhepatic phase of orthotopic liver transplantation in pigs. Anesthesiology 1990b; 72:145–52.

Pumplin DW, Fambrough DM. Turnover of acetyl-

choline receptors in skeletal muscle. Ann Rev Physiol 1982;44:319–35.

Ramzan IM, Somogyi AA, Walker JS, Shanks CA, Triggs EJ. Clinical pharmacokinetics of the non-depolarizing muscle relaxants. Clin Pharmacokinet 1981; 6:25–60.

Robbins R, Donati F, Bevan DR, Veban JC. Differential effects of myoneural blocking drugs on neuromuscular transmission in infants. Br J Anaesth 1984;56:1095–9.

Rorvik K, Husby P, Gramstad L, Vamnes JS, Bitsch-Larsen L, Koller M-E. Comparison of large dose of vecuronium with pancuronium for prolonged neuromuscular blockade. Br J Anaesth 1988;61:180–5.

Rosa G, Orfei P, Sanfilippo M, Vilardi V, Gasparetto A. The effects of atracurium besylate (Tracrium) on intracranial pressure and cerebral perfusion pressure. Anesth Analg 1986a;65:381–4.

Rosa G, Sanfilippo M. Vilardi V, Orfei P, Gasparetto A. Effects of vecuronium bromide on intracranial pressure and cerebral perfusion pressure. Br J Anaesth 1986b;58:437–40.

Rupp SM, Castagnoli KP, Fisher DM, Miller RD. Pancuronium and vecuronium pharmacokinetics and pharmacodynamics in younger and elderly adults. Anesthesiology 1987;67:45–9.

Rupp SM, Fahey MR, Miller RD. Neuromuscular and cardiovascular effects of atracurium during nitrous oxide-isoflurane anaesthesia. Br J Anaesth 1983a; 55:67S–70S.

Rupp SM, Fisher DM, Miller RD, Castagnoli K. Pharmacokinetics and pharmacodynamics of vecuronium in the elderly. Anesthesiology 1983b;59:A270.

Rupp SM, McChristian JW, Miller RD. Neuromuscular effects of atracurium during halothane-nitrous oxide and enflurane-nitrous oxide anesthesia in humans. Anesthesiology 1985;63:16–9.

Rupp SM, Miller RD, Gencarelli P. Vecuronium-induced neuromuscular blockade during enflurane, isoflurane, and halothane anesthesia in humans. Anesthesiology 1984;60:102–5.

Ryan JF, Kagen LJ, Hyman, AI. Myoglobinemia after a single dose of succinylcholine. N Engl J Med 1971;285:824–7.

Salem MR, Wong AY, Lin YH. The effect of suxamethonium on the intragastric pressure in infants and children. Br J Anaesth 1972;44:166–70.

Salmenpera M, Peltola K, Takkumen O, Heinonen J. Cardiovascular effects of pancuronium and vecuronium during high-dose fentanyl anesthesia. Anesth Analg 1983;62:1059–64.

Savage DS, Sleigh T, Carlyle I. The emergence of ORG NC45, 1...(2 beta, 3 alpha, 5 alpha, 16 beta, 17 beta) -3,-17 bis (acetylogy)-2-(1-piperidinyl)-androstan-16 y1) ... .1-methyl piperidinium bromide from the pancuronium series. Br J Anaesth 1980;52:3S–10S.

Savarese JJ, Ali HH, Antonio RP. The clinical pharmacology of metocurine: Dimethyltubocurarine revisited. Anesthesiology 1977;47:277–84.

Savarese JJ, Ali HH, Basta SJ, et al. The clinical neuromuscular pharmacology of mivacurium chloride (BW B1090U). A short-acting nondepolarizing ester neuromuscular blocking drug. Anesthesiology 1988;68:723–32.

Savarese JJ, Ali HH, Basta SJ, et al. The cardiovascular effects of mivacurium chloride (BW B1090U) in patients receiving nitrous oxide–opiate–barbiturate anesthesia. Anesthesiology 1989;70:386–94.

Schneider MJ, Stirt JA, Finholt DA. Atracurium, vecuronium, and intraocular pressure in humans. Anesth Analg 1986;65:877–82.

Schoenstadt DA, Whitcher CE. Observations on the mechanism of succinylcholine-induced cardiac arrhythmias. Anesthesiology 1963;24:358–62.

Schwartz AE, Matteo RS, Ornstein E, Silverberg PA. Acute steroid therapy does not alter nondepolarizing muscle relaxant effects in humans. Anesthesiology 1986;65:326–7.

Schwarz S, Ilias W, Lackner F, Mayrhofer O, Foldes FF. Rapid tracheal intubation with vecuronium: The priming principle. Anesthesiology 1985;62:388–93.

Scott RPF, Savarese JJ. The cardiovascular and autonomic effects of neuromuscular blocking agents. Semin Anesth 1985;3:319–34.

Scott RPF, Savarese JJ, Ali HH, et al. Atracurium: Clinical strategies for preventing histamine release and attenuating the hemodynamic response. Anesthesiology 1984;61:A287.

Shanks CA. Pharmacokinetics of the nondepolarizing neuromuscular relaxants applied to calculation of bolus and infusion dosage regimens. Anesthesiology 1986;64:72–86.

Shanks CA, Somogyi AA, Triggs EJ. Dose-response and plasma concentration–response relationships of pancuronium in man. Anesthesiology 1979;51:111–8.

Shayevitz JR, Matteo RS. Decreased sensitivity to metocurine in patients with upper motorneuron disease. Anesth Analg 1985;64:767–72.

Shi W-Z, Fahey MR, Fisher DM, Miller RD, Canfell C, Eger EI. Laudanosine (a metabolite of atracurium) increases the minimal alveolar concentration of halothane in rabbits. Anesthesiology 1985;63:584–8.

Sinatra RS, Philip BK, Naulty JS. Osthheimer GW. Prolonged neuromuscular blockade with vecuronium in a patient treated with magnesium sulfate. Anesth Analg 1985;64:1220–2.

Skarpa M, Dayan AD, Follenfant M, et al. Toxicity testing of atracurium. Br J Anaesth 1983;55:27S–9S.

Skivington MA. Protein binding of three titrated muscle relaxants. Br J Anaesth 1972;44:1030–4.

Sklar GS, Lanks KW. Effects of trimethaphan and sodium nitroprusside on hydrolysis of succinylcholine in vitro. Anesthesiology 1977;47:31–3.

Smith CE, Donati F, Bevan DR. Dose-response curves

for succinylcholine: Single versus cumulative techniques. Anesthesiology 1988;69:338–42.

Sokoll MD, Gergis SD. Antibiotics and neuromuscular function. Anesthesiology 1981;55:148–59.

Sokoll MD, Gergis SD, Mehta M, Ali HH, Lineberry C. Safety and efficacy of atracurium (BW 33A) in surgical patients receiving balanced or isoflurane anesthesia. Anesthesiology 1983;58:450–5.

Standaert FG. Donuts and holes: Molecules and muscle relaxants. Semin Anes 1984;3:251–61.

Standaert FG, Adams JE. The actions of succinylcholine on the mammalian motor nerve terminal. J Pharmacol Exp Ther 1965;149:113–23.

Standaert FG, Dretchen KL. Cyclic nucleotides in neuromuscular transmission. Anesth Analg 1981;60:91–9.

Stanski DR, Ham J, Miller RD, Sheiner LB. Pharmacokinetics and pharmacodynamics of d-tubocurarine during nitrous oxide-narcotic and halothane anesthesia in man. Anesthesiology 1979;51:235–41.

Stanski DR, Ham J, Miller RD, Sheiner LB. Time-dependent increase in sensitivity to d-tubocurarine during enflurane anesthesia in man. Anesthesiology 1980;52:483–7.

Starr NK, Sethna DH, Estafanous FG. Bradycardia and asystole following the rapid administration of sufentanil with vecuronium. Anesthesiology 1986;64:521–3.

Stenlake JB, Waigh RD, Urwin J, Dewar GH, Coker GG. Atracurium: Conception and inception. Br J Anaesth 1983;55:3S–10S.

Stirt JA, Grosslight KR, Bedford RF, Vollmer D. "Defasciculation" with metocurine prevents succinylcholine-induced increases in intracranial pressure. Anesthesiology 1987;67:50–3.

Stirt JA, Katz RL, Murray AL, Guillot JP, Evreux JC. Modification of atracurium blockade by halothane and by suxamethonium. Br J Anaesth 1983;55:71S–7S.

Stoelting RK. The hemodynamic effects of pancuronium and d-tubocurarine in anesthetized patients. Anesthesiology 1972;36:612–5.

Stoelting RK. Hemodynamic effects of gallamine during halothane-nitrous oxide anesthesia. Anesthesiology 1973;39:645–7.

Stoelting RK. Hemodynamic effects of dimethyltubocurarine during nitrous oxide-halothane anesthesia. Anesth Analg 1974;53:513–5.

Stoelting RK. Comparison of gallamine and atropine as pretreatment before anesthetic induction and succinylcholine administration. Anesth Analg 1977;56:493–5.

Stoelting RK, Longnecker DE. Influence of end-tidal halothane concentration of d-tubocurarine hypotension. Anesth Analg 1972a;51:364–7.

Stoelting RK, Longnecker DE. Effects of promethazine on hypotension following d-tubocurarine use in anesthetized patients. Anesth Analg 1972b;51:509–13.

Stoelting RK, McCammon RL, Hilgenberg JC. Changes

in blood pressure with varying rates of administration of d-tubocurarine. Anesth Analg 1980; 59:697–9.

Stoelting RK, Peterson C. Adverse effects of increased succinylcholine dose following d-tubocurarine pretreatment. Anesth Analg 1975;54:282–8.

Stroud RM. Acetylcholine receptor structure. Neurosci Comm 1983;1:124–38.

Sufit RL, Kreul JK, Bellay YM, Helmer P, Brunson DB, Will J. Doxacurium and mivacurium do not trigger malignant hyperthermia in susceptible value. Anesth Analg 1990;71:285–7.

Sugimori T. Shortened action of succinylcholine in individuals with cholinesterase C_5 isozyme. Can Anaesth Soc J 1986;33:321–7.

Taboada JA, Rupp SM, Miller RD. Refining the priming principle for vecuronium during rapid-sequence induction of anesthesia. Anesthesiology 1986; 64:243–7.

Tateishi A, Zornow MH, Scheller MS, Canfell PC. Electroencephalographic effects of laudanosine in an animal model of epilepsy. Br J Anaesth 1989; 62:548–52.

Taylor P. Are neuromuscular blocking agents more efficacious in pairs? Anesthesiology 1985;63:1–3.

Thomson IR, Putnins CL. Adverse effects of pancuronium during high-dose fentanyl anesthesia for coronary artery bypass grafting. Anesthesiology 1985; 62:708–13.

Tobey RE. Paraplegia, succinylcholine, and cardiac arrest. Anesthesiology 1970;32:359–64.

Vercruyse P, Bossuyt P, Hanegreffs G, Verbeuren TJ, Van Houtte PM. Gallamine and pancuronium inhibit pre- and post-junctional muscarinic receptors in canine saphenous veins. J Pharmacol Exp Ther 1979; 209:225–30.

Viby-Mogensen J. Correlation of succinylcholine duration of action with plasma cholinesterase activity in subjects with the genotypically normal enzyme. Anesthesiology 1980;53:517–20.

Vitez TS, Miller RD, Eger EI, Van Hyhuis LS, Way WL. Comparison in vitro of isoflurane and halothane potentiation of d-tubocurarine and succinylcholine neuromuscular blockades. Anesthesiology 1974; 41:53–6.

Ward S, Neill EAM. Pharmacokinetics of atracurium in acute hepatic failure (with acute renal failure). Br J Anaesth 1983;55:1169–72.

Ward S, Wright D. Combined pharmacokinetic and pharmacodynamic study of a single bolus dose of atracurium. Br J Anaesth 1983;55:35S–8S.

Waud BE. Decrease in dose requirements of d-tubocurarine by volatile anesthetics. Anesthesiology 1979;51;298–302.

Waud BE, Waud DR. The relation between tetanic fade and receptor occlusion in the presence of competitive neuromuscular block. Anesthesiology 1971; 35:456–64.

Waud BE, Waud DR. Comparison of drug-receptor dissociation constants at the mammalian neuromuscular junction in the presence and absence of halothane. J Pharmacol Exp Ther 1973;187:40–6.

Waud BE, Waud DR. The effects of diethyl ether, enflurane and isoflurane at the neuromuscular junction. Anesthesiology 1975;42:275–80.

Waud BE, Waud DR. Effects of volatile anesthetics on directly and indirectly stimulated muscle. Anesthesiology 1979;50:103–10.

Waud BE, Waud DR. Interaction among agents that block end-plate depolarization competitively. Anesthesiology 1985;63:4–15.

Weinstein JA, Matteo RS, Ornstein E, Schwartz AE, Goldstoff M, Thal G. Pharmacodynamics of vecuronium and atracurium in the obese surgical patient. Anesth Analg 1988;67:1149–53.

Wierda JMKH, Richardson FJ, Agoston S. Dose-response relation and time course of action of pipecuronium bromide in humans anesthetized with nitrous oxide isoflurane, halothane, or droperidol and fentanyl. Anesth Analg 1989;68:208–13.

Wierda JMKH, Karliczek GF, Vandenbrom RHG, et al. Pharmacokinetics and cardiovascular dynamics of pipecuronium bromide during coronary artery surgery. Can J Anaesth 1990;37:183–91.

Wood GG. Cyclosporine-vecuronium interaction. Can J Anaesth 1989;36:358–66.

Yate PM, Flynn PJ, Arnold RW, Weatherly BC, Simmonds RJ, Dopson T. Clinical experience and plasma laudanosine concentrations during the infusion of atracurium in the intensive therapy unit. Br J Anaesth 1987;59:211–7.

Yeaton P, Teba, L. Sinus node exit block following administration of vecuronium. Anesthesiology 1988; 68:177–8.

Zahl K, Apfelbaum JL. Muscle pain occurs after outpatient laparoscopy despite the substitution of vecuronium for succinylcholine. Anesthesiology 1989; 70:408–11.

Chapter

9

Anticholinesterase Drugs and Cholinergic Agonists

Anticholinesterase drugs inhibit the enzyme acetylcholinesterase (true cholinesterase), which is normally responsible for the hydrolysis of acetylcholine to choline and acetic acid. Acetylcholinesterase is one of the most efficient enzymes known, with a single molecule able to hydrolyze an estimated 300,000 molecules of acetylcholine every minute. Acetylcholinesterase is widely distributed in the body, being present wherever acetylcholine is the neurotransmitter.

CLASSIFICATION

Anticholinesterase drugs are classified according to the mechanism by which they inhibit the activity of acetylcholinesterase (Fig. 9-1). Acetylcholinesterase is inhibited through (1) reversible inhibition, (2) formation of carbamyl esters, and (3) irreversible inactivation by organophosphates.

Reversible Inhibition

Edrophonium is a quaternary ammonium anticholinesterase drug that lacks a carbamyl group, producing reversible inhibition of acetylcholin-

esterase through its electrostatic attachment to the anionic site on the enzyme (Fig. 9-2). This binding is stabilized further by hydrogen bonding at the esteratic site on the enzyme (Fig. 9-2). The edrophonium–acetylcholinesterase enzyme complex prevents the natural substrate acetylcholine from approximating correctly with the enzyme. Because a true chemical (covalent) bond is not formed, acetylcholine can easily compete with edrophonium for access to acetylcholinesterase, making the inhibition truly reversible. Indeed, the duration of action of edrophonium is considered to be brief, reflecting its reversible binding with acetylcholinesterase.

The predominant site of action of edrophonium appears to be presynaptic. This site of action may explain differences in dose-response relationships compared with longer-acting anticholinesterase drugs that presumably act principally at postsynaptic sites (Cronnelly et al, 1982).

Muscarinic effects of edrophonium are mild compared with longer-acting anticholinesterase drugs. Edrophonium is used to (1) antagonize the effects of nondepolarizing neuromuscular blocking drugs, (2) diagnose and assess therapy of myasthenia gravis and cholinergic crisis, and (3) evaluate the presence of dual blockade produced by succinylcholine.

226

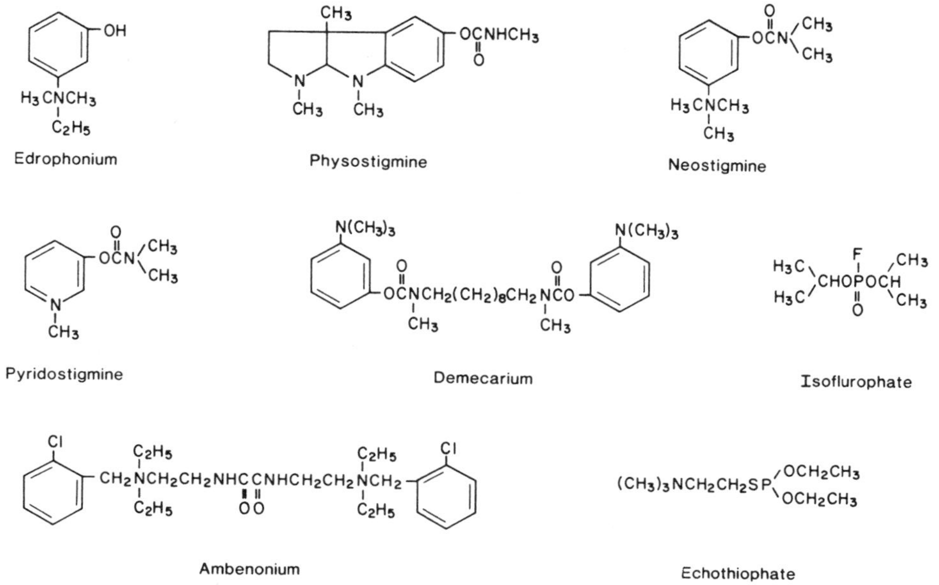

FIGURE 9-1. Anticholinesterase drugs.

Formation of Carbamyl Esters

Drugs such as physostigmine, neostigmine, and pyridostigmine produce reversible inhibition of acetylcholinesterase by formation of a carbamyl ester complex at the esteratic site of the enzyme (Fig. 9-3). In contrast to edrophonium, these drugs act as competitive substrate substitutes for acetylcholine in the normal interaction with acetylcholinesterase. Indeed, the initial formation of the drug-enzyme complex proceeds in the same way as the initial reaction between acetylcholine and acetylcholinesterase. Likewise, the next stage of formation of an intermediate acid-enzyme compound and first split product also proceeds normally. At this stage, there is transfer of a carbamate group to acetylcholinesterase at the esteratic site. This carbamylated acetylcholinesterase cannot hydrolyze acetylcholine until the carbamate–enzyme bond dissociates. Neostigmine also has presynaptic actions as manifested by an increased rate of repetitive firing following a single impulse. This repetitive firing also contributes to the buildup of acetylcholine at the neuromuscular junction.

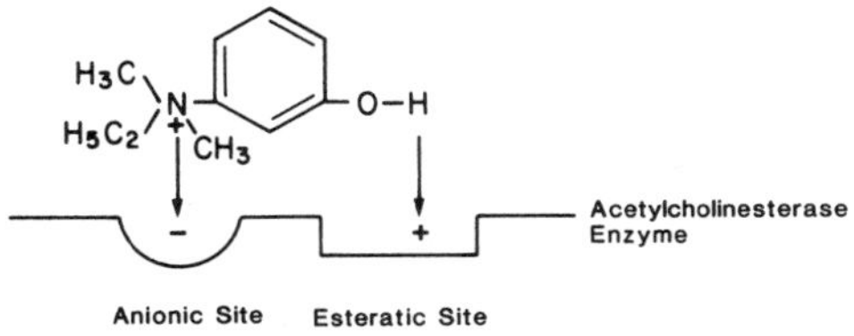

FIGURE 9-2. Edrophonium produces reversible inhibition of acetylcholinesterase by electrostatic attachment to the anionic site and hydrogen bonding at the esteratic site of the enzyme.

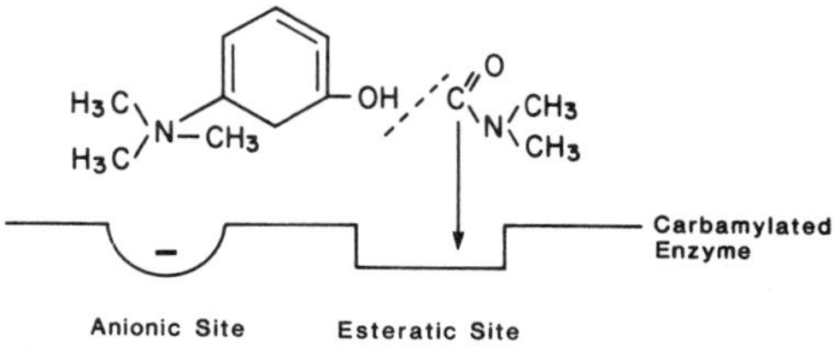

FIGURE 9-3. Drugs, such as physostigmine, neostigmine, and pyridostigmine, produce reversible inhibition of acetylcholinesterase by forming a carbamyl-ester complex at the esteratic site of the enzyme.

Table 9–1
Comparative Characteristics of Anticholinesterase Drugs Administered to Antagonize Nondepolarizing Neuromuscular Blockade

	Elimination Half-Time (min)		Volume of Distribution (L·kg⁻¹)		Clearance (ml·kg⁻¹·min⁻¹)		Renal Contribution to Total Clearance (%)	Speed of Onset	Duration (min)	Principal Site of Action	Dose of Atropine (µg·kg⁻¹)
	Normal	Anephric	Normal	Anephric	Normal	Anephric					
Edrophonium (0.5 mg·kg⁻¹)	110	206	1.1	0.7	9.6	2.7	66	Rapid	60	Presynaptic	7
Neostigmine (0.043 mg·kg⁻¹)	80	183	0.7	0.8	9.0	3.4	54	Intermediate	60	Postsynaptic	15
Pyridostigmine (0.35 mg·kg⁻¹)	112	379	1.1	1.0	8.6	2.1	76	Delayed	90	Postsynaptic	15

(Data from Cronnelly R, Stanski, DR, Miller RD, Sheiner LB, Sohn YJ. Renal function and the pharmacokinetics of neostigmine in anesthetized patients. Anesthesiology 1979; 51: 222–6; Cronnelly R, Stanski DR, Miller RD, Sheirer LB. Pyridostigmine kinetics with and without renal function. Clin Pharmacol Ther 1980; 28: 78–81; Cronnelly R, Morris RB. Antagonism of neuromuscular blockade. Br J Anaesth 1982; 54: 183–93; Morris RB, Cronnelly R, Miller RD, Stanski DR, Fahey MR. Pharmacokinetics of edrophonium and neostigmine when antagonizing d-tubocurarine neuromusular blockade in man. Anesthesiology 1981; 54:399–402; with permission.)

Irreversible Inactivation

Organophosphate anticholinesterase drugs combine with acetylcholinesterase at the esteratic site to form a stable inactive complex that does not undergo hydrolysis (Fig. 9-4). Echothiophate interacts with both the esteratic and anionic subsites, thus accounting for its extreme potency. Spontaneous regeneration of acetylcholinesterase either requires several hours or does not occur, thus requiring synthesis of new enzyme.

Echothiophate is the only organophosphate anticholinesterase drug used clinically (Fig. 9-1). Other drugs such as parathion and malathion are used as insecticides. Malathion is a selective insecticide because enzymes necessary for its metabolism are absent in insects. In mammals and birds, malathion undergoes extensive hydrolysis by enzymes known as phosphoryl-phosphatases before excretion in the urine. Nerve gases such as tabum, saran, and soman are extremely lipid-soluble organophosphate inhibitors, and absorption can occur even through intact skin.

STRUCTURE ACTIVITY RELATIONSHIPS

Acetylcholinesterase consists of an anionic and an esteratic site which are so arranged that they are complementary to the natural substrate acetylcholine (Fig. 9-5). The anionic site of the enzyme binds the quaternary nitrogen of acetylcholine. This binding serves to orient the ester linkage of acetylcholine to the esteratic site of acetylcholinesterase (Fig. 9-5). Thus, acetylcholinesterase has an optimum substrate concentration and is less effective against longer chain substrates.

Neostigmine is a quaternary ammonium derivative of physostigmine, having a greater stability and equal or greater potency (Fig. 9-1).

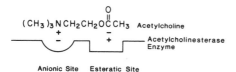

FIGURE 9–4. Organophosphate anticholinesterase drugs produce irreversible inhibition of acetylcholinesterase by forming a phosphorylate complex at the esteratic site of the enzyme.

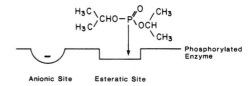

FIGURE 9–5. The anionic and esteratic sites of acetylcholinesterase are arranged so that they are complimentary to the quaternary nitrogen and ester linkage of acetylcholine, respectively.

Pyridostigmine is a closely related congener of neostigmine (Fig. 9-1). An increase in anticholinesterase potency and duration of action occurs from linking two quaternary ammonium nuclei by a chain of appropriate structure and length. For example, the potent anticholinesterase drug demecarium is two molecules of neostigmine connected at the carbamate nitrogen atoms by a series of 10 methylene groups (Fig. 9-1). Another bisquaternary compound is ambenonium, which binds strongly to acetylcholinesterase and exerts direct effects at both prejunctional and postjunctional membranes (Fig. 9-1).

PHARMACOKINETICS

In patients with normal renal and hepatic function, there are no significant pharmacokinetic differences among the anticholinesterase drugs (Table 9-1; Fig. 9-6) (Cronnelly et al, 1979; Cronnelly et al, 1980; Cronnelly and Morris 1982; Morris et al, 1981; Cronnelly, 1985). The similarity in pharmacokinetics among these anticholinesterase drugs means that differences in potency are most likely explained in terms of pharmacodynamics. Affinity for acetylcholinesterase is probably of major importance in determining the relative anticholinesterase potency of these drugs. The fact that edrophonium dose response curves are not parallel to those for neostigmine and pyridostigmine suggests that different mechanisms of action may be involved for the different anticholinesterase drugs (Fig. 9-7) (Cronnelly et al, 1982).

Lipid Solubility

Anticholinesterase drugs containing a quaternary ammonium group (edrophonium, neostigmine,

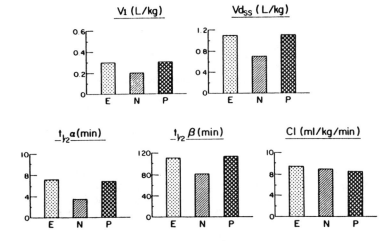

FIGURE 9–6. Pharmacokinetics of edrophonium (*E*), pyridostigmine (*P*), and neostigmine (*N*) in patients with normal renal and hepatic function. (From Cronnelly R. Muscle relaxant antagonists. Semin Anesth 1985; 4: 31–40; with permission.)

or pyridostigmine) are poorly lipid soluble and thus do not easily penetrate lipid cell membrane barriers such as the gastrointestinal tract or blood-brain barrier. Lipid-soluble drugs, such as tertiary amines (physostigmine) and organophosphates, are readily absorbed from the gastrointestinal tract or across mucous membranes and have predictable effects on the central nervous system.

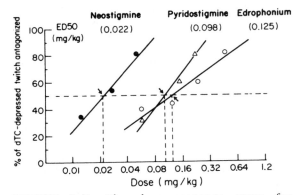

FIGURE 9–7. The dose response curve for edrophonium is not parallel to the curves for neostigmine and pyridostigmine, suggesting different mechanisms of action for the various anticholinesterase drugs. (From Cronnelly R, Morris RB, Miller RD. Edrophonium: Duration of action and atropine requirement in humans during halothane anesthesia. Anesthesiology 1982; 57: 261–6; with permission.)

Volume of Distribution

The large volume of distribution (Vd) of quaternary ammonium anticholinesterase drugs compared with nondepolarizing neuromuscular blocking drugs is surprising because these drugs would not be expected to cross lipid membranes easily (Table 9-1). Presumably, this large Vd reflects extensive tissue storage in organs such as the liver or kidneys. The liver, as a site of this tissue uptake, is suggested by the presence of unchanged Vds in anephric patients (Table 9-1).

Onset of Action

Because the pharmacokinetics of anticholinesterase drugs are similar, it is likely that differences in onset of action reflect a pharmacodynamic mechanism. For example, the more rapid onset of action of edrophonium may reflect a presynaptic (acetylcholine release) rather than a postsynaptic (acetylcholinesterase inhibition) action, whereas the postsynaptic action is predominant for neostigmine and pyridostigmine (Fig. 9-8) (Cronnelly et al, 1982; Miller et al, 1974). It also is possible that onset times could reflect differences in rate constants at presynaptic and postsynaptic sites of action. The slower onset of action of neostigmine and pyridostigmine compared with edrophonium is not related to the need to form active metabolites (Hennis et al, 1984).

Renal Clearance

Renal clearance accounts for approximately 50% of the elimination of neostigmine and approximately 75% of the elimination of edrophonium and pyridostigmine. This large proportion of renal clearance suggests a role for renal tubular secretory mechanisms as well as glomerular filtration. The elimination half-times of these anticholinesterase drugs are greatly prolonged by renal failure (Table 9-1) (Cronnelly et al, 1979; Cronnelly et al, 1980). As a result, plasma clearance of anticholinesterase drugs will be delayed as long as, if not longer than, the nondepolarizing neuromuscular blocking drugs, making the occurrence of recurarization unlikely. In anesthetized patients receiving a functioning renal transplant, the pharmacokinetics of anticholinesterase drugs are similar to those in patients with normal renal function.

Metabolism

In the absence of renal function, hepatic metabolism accounts for 50% of a dose of neostigmine, 30% of edrophonium, and 25% of pyridostigmine. The principal metabolite of neostigmine is 3-hydroxyphenyl trimethylammonium, which has approximately one tenth the antagonist activity of the parent compound (Hennis et al, 1984). The principal metabolite of pyridostigmine is 3-hydroxy-*N*-methylpyridinium, which lacks pharmacologic activity. Edrophonium undergoes conjugation to edrophonium glucuronide, which is presumed to be pharmacologically inactive. Physostigmine is hydrolyzed at its ester linkage, and renal excretion is of minor importance. It can be concluded that metabolites of anticholinesterase drugs do not contribute significantly to the effects of these drugs, including antagonism of neuromuscular blockade.

Influence of Patient Age

The time course of onset and duration of antagonism produced by equipotent doses of neostigmine are similar in infants, children, and adults (Fisher et al, 1983). However, the dose of neostigmine required to produce 50% antagonism of d-tubocurarine–induced neuromuscular block-

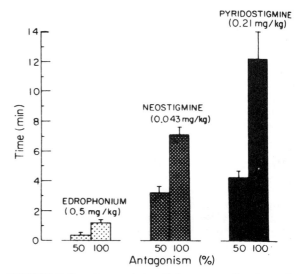

FIGURE 9–8. Comparison of the onset of action of anticholinesterase drugs as reflected by antagonism of drug-induced neuromuscular blockade. Mean ± SE. (From Cronnelly R, Morris RB, Miller RD. Endrophonium: Duration of action and atropine requirement in humans during halothane anesthesia. Anesthesiology 1982; 57: 261–6; with permission.)

ade is less in neonates and children (Fisher et al, 1983). Conversely, dose requirements for edrophonium are not different for infants, children, and adults (Fisher et al, 1984). This difference between edrophonium and neostigmine further supports the concept that these drugs antagonize neuromuscular blockade by different mechanisms (Cronnelly and Morris, 1982).

It is likely that the age-related differences for dose requirements of neostigmine are related to pharmacodynamic mechanisms, since the pharmacokinetics are similar in pediatric and young adult age groups (Fisher et al, 1983). Conversely, the duration of the maximum response produced by neostigmine and pyridostigmine is prolonged in elderly compared with younger patients, reflecting a smaller extracellular fluid volume in elderly patients (Young et al, 1988). Pharmacodynamics are not altered, as emphasized by similar responses evoked by neostigmine at the same plasma concentration in middle-aged and elderly adults. In contrast to neostigmine and pyridostigmine, the duration of action of edrophonium is not prolonged in elderly patients (Matteo et al,

1990). A higher concentration of edrophonium is required to produce the same effects in elderly patients as in younger adults. Explanations for the observed differences between edrophonium and other anticholinesterase drugs may relate to differences in chemical structure and to the possibility that edrophonium produces antagonism of neuromuscular blockade by a different mechanism than do neostigmine or pyridostigmine.

PHARMACOLOGIC EFFECTS

Pharmacologic effects of anticholinesterase drugs are predictable and reflect the accumulation of acetylcholine at muscarinic and nicotinic cholinergic receptor sites. Depending on the reason for administration of anticholinesterase drugs, these effects may be considered therapeutic or undesirable.

Muscarinic cholinergic effects, such as bradycardia, salivation, miosis, and hyperperistalsis, are evoked by lower concentrations of acetylcholine than are required for production of nicotinic effects at autonomic ganglia and the neuromuscular junction. For this reason, using an anticholinesterase drug to reverse nondepolarizing neuromuscular blocking drugs also includes administering an anticholinergic drug to prevent adverse muscarinic cholinergic effects that would otherwise be associated with the high dose of anticholinesterase drug. The anticholinergic drug selectively blocks the effects of acetylcholine at muscarinic cholinergic receptors and leaves intact the responses to acetylcholine at nicotinic cholinergic receptors. Neostigmine and pyridostigmine, but not edrophonium, produce marked and prolonged inhibition of plasma cholinesterase activity (Mirakhur, 1986). Indeed, prolonged effects of succinylcholine that is administered shortly following reversal of nondepolarizing neuromuscular blockade may reflect this enzyme inhibition.

Cardiovascular System

Cardiovascular effects of anticholinesterase drugs reflect effects of accumulated acetylcholine at the heart, blood vessels, autonomic ganglia, and postganglionic cholinergic nerve fibers. The predominant effect on the heart from the peripheral actions of accumulated acetylcholine is bradycardia owing to slowed conduction velocity of cardiac impulses through the atrioventricular node. Typically, blood vessels are dilated, although the coronary and pulmonary circulations may manifest an opposite response. Decreases in blood pressure that accompany accumulation of acetylcholine presumably reflect decreases in systemic vascular resistance.

Gastrointestinal and Genitourinary Tract

Anticholinesterase drugs enhance gastric fluid secretion by parietal cells and increase motility of the entire gastrointestinal tract, particularly the large intestine. The lower portion of the esophagus is stimulated by neostigmine, resulting in a beneficial increase in tone and peristalsis in patients with achalasia. Neostigmine, 0.5 to 1 mg subcutaneously, is often effective in the treatment of paralytic ileus or atony of the urinary bladder. This treatment, however, should not be used when there is mechanical obstruction of the gastrointestinal tract or urinary bladder. Actions of anticholinesterase drugs on gastrointestinal motility most likely reflect effects of accumulated acetylcholine on the ganglion cells of Auerbach's plexus and on smooth muscle fibers. Neostigmine and presumably other anticholinesterase drugs may increase the incidence of postoperative nausea and vomiting even when administered with atropine, which has its own antiemetic properties.

Eye

Anticholinesterase drugs applied topically to the cornea cause constriction of the sphincter of the iris (miosis) and ciliary muscle. Constriction of the ciliary muscle manifests as inability to focus for near vision. This spasm of accommodation is usually shorter in duration than is miosis. Intraocular pressure declines because the outflow of aqueous humor is facilitated.

Salivary Glands

Anticholinesterase drugs augment production of secretions of glands that are innervated by postganglionic cholinergic fibers. Such glands include the bronchial, lacrimal, sweat, salivary, gastric, intestinal, and acinar pancreatic glands. Smooth muscle fibers of bronchioles and ureters are contracted by anticholinesterase drugs.

Beta-Adrenergic Blockade

Theoretically, beta-adrenergic blockade would result in a predominance of parasympathetic nervous system activity at the heart, which might be exaggerated by the subsequent administration of an anticholinesterase drug to reverse nondepolarizing neuromuscular blockade (Sprague, 1975; Prys-Roberts, 1979). Nevertheless, bradycardia does not accompany mixtures of atropine and neostigmine or pyridostigmine administered to animals with acutely produced beta-adrenergic blockade using propranolol (Wagner et al, 1982).

CLINICAL USES

The principal clinical uses of anticholinesterase drugs are (1) antagonist-assisted reversal of neuromuscular blockade produced by nondepolarizing neuromuscular blocking drugs; (2) treatment of central nervous system effects produced by certain drugs; (3) treatment of myasthenia gravis; (4) treatment of glaucoma; and (5) treatment of paralytic ileus and atony of the urinary bladder. A centrally active anticholinesterase drug, tetrahydroaminoacridine, may be useful in the palliative treatment of patients with Alzheimer's disease (Summers et al, 1986).

Antagonist-Assisted Reversal of Neuromuscular Blockade

Antagonist-assisted reversal of neuromuscular blockade using neostigmine, pyridostigmine, or edrophonium reflects increased availability of acetylcholine at the neuromuscular junction by inhibiting acetylcholinesterase, which is needed to hydrolyze acetylcholine. Physostigmine is not used to reverse neuromuscular blockade because the dose required is excessive. Increased amounts of acetylcholine in the region of the neuromuscular junction improve the chances that two acetylcholine molecules will bind to the alpha subunits of the nicotinic cholinergic receptor.

This tips the balance of the competition between acetylcholine and a nondepolarizing neuromuscular blocking drug in favor of the neurotransmitter (acetylcholine) and restores neuromuscular transmission. In addition, anticholinesterase drugs may generate antidromic action potentials and repetitive firing of motor nerve endings (presynaptic effects) (Donati et al, 1983). Postsynaptic and presynaptic mechanisms are dose related and operate simultaneously to restore neuromuscular transmission in the presence of nondepolarizing neuromuscular blocking drugs.

Anticholinesterase drugs typically are administered during the time when spontaneous recovery from neuromuscular blockade is occurring such that the effect of the antagonist adds to the rate of spontaneous recovery from the neuromuscular blocking drug. For this reason, antagonism of neuromuscular blockade induced by an intermediate-acting drug that undergoes rapid spontaneous recovery is much faster than antagonism of a slowly recovering long-acting nondepolarizing neuromuscular blocking drug. This difference is most obvious when reversal is compared at deep levels (more than 90% twitch depression) of neuromuscular blockade.

At equivalent degrees of spontaneous reversal of twitch height, the train-of-four ratio is greater following the administration of edrophonium than with neostigmine or pyridostigmine (Donati et al, 1983). If the train-of-four ratio reflects only presynaptic events, then these results would support a presynaptic predominance for edrophonium compared with neostigmine or pyridostigmine. Conceivably, matching the principal site of action of the anticholinesterase drug with that of the neuromuscular blocking drug (presynaptic vs postsynaptic) would result in more selective antagonism with a minimum dose of anticholinesterase drug. Despite this logic, there is no evidence that anticholinesterase drugs act by different mechanisms when administered to anesthetized patients to antagonize neuromuscular blockade. For example, combinations of edrophonium with neostigmine or pyridostigmine result in only additive effects with respect to the degree of antagonism of neuromuscular blockade achieved, suggesting a similar mechanism of action for these anticholinesterase drugs (Donati et al, 1983; Jones et al, 1984). Thus, mixtures of anticholinesterase drugs offer no clinical advantage over the use of adequate doses of the individual drugs alone (Cronnelly and Miller, 1984).

Onset and Duration of Action

Edrophonium, 0.5 mg·kg[-1] IV, produces antagonism of neuromuscular blockade that is equal in magnitude to that produced by neostigmine, 0.043 mg·kg[-1] IV, or pyridostigmine, 0.21 mg·kg[-1] IV (Fig. 9-9) (Cronnelly et al, 1982; Miller et al, 1974). Edrophonium has the most rapid onset of action, followed by neostigmine and pyridostigmine (Fig. 9-8) (Cronnelly et al, 1982; Miller et al, 1974). When twitch height is depressed 90% or greater, the dose of edrophonium may need to be increased to 1 mg·kg[-1] IV to produce as rapid an onset as neostigmine (Rupp et al, 1986). Although edrophonium in the past has been considered a short-acting drug, controlled studies in anesthetized patients have documented that the duration of action of edrophonium does not differ from neostigmine (Cronnelly et al, 1982). Because neostigmine, pyridostigmine, and edrophonium have similar elimination half-times, but pyridostigmine has a 40% longer duration of action, the time course of reversal of neuromuscular blockade may be unrelated to the clearance of anticholinesterase drugs from the plasma.

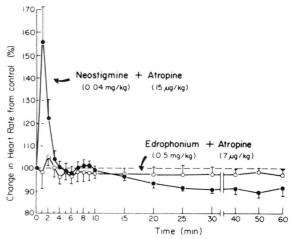

FIGURE 9-10. Heart rate changes are less following the administration of edrophonium-atropine than following administration of neostigmine-atropine. Mean ± SE. (From Cronnelly R, Morris RB, Miller RD. Edrophonium: Duration of action and atropine requirement in humans during halothane anesthesia. Anesthesiology 1982; 57: 261–6; with permission.)

Mixture with Anticholinergic Drugs

Reversal of neuromuscular blockade requires only the nicotinic cholinergic effects of the anticholinesterase drug. Therefore, muscarinic cholinergic effects of the anticholinesterase drug are attenuated or prevented by the concurrent administration of an anticholinergic drug such as atropine or glycopyrrolate (Table 9-1). For example, neostigmine and pyridostigmine both require atropine, 15 µg·kg[-1] IV, to prevent bradycardia and excessive salivation (Fogdall and Miller, 1973). Initial tachycardia observed when atropine is administered simultaneously with neostigmine or pyridostigmine reflects the slower onset of these anticholinesterase drugs relative to atropine. The lesser muscarinic stimulant effects of edrophonium and its more rapid onset of action result in less variation in heart rate when administered with atropine (Fig. 9-10) (Cronnelly et al, 1982). Indeed, edrophonium requires less atropine (7 µg·kg[-1] IV) to prevent associated heart rate changes.

The more delayed onset of cardiac vagal effects of glycopyrrolate is appropriately matched for the slower onset of action of neostigmine and pyridostigmine, whereas the more rapid onset of

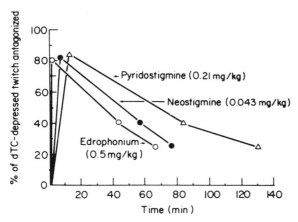

FIGURE 9-9. Edrophonium produces antagonism of drug-induced neuromuscular blockade that is similar in magnitude to that produced by neostigmine or pyridostigmine. (From Cronnelly R, Morris RB, Miller RD. Edrophonium: Duration of action and atropine requirement in humans during halothane anesthesia. Anesthesiology 1982; 57: 261–6; with permission.)

vagolytic activity provided by atropine more closely parallels the onset of activity produced by edrophonium (Azar et al, 1983; Ramamurthy et al, 1972). Indeed, a mixture of neostigmine and glycopyrrolate (7 $\mu g \cdot kg^{-1}$ IV) results in less tachycardia than a mixture of neostigmine and atropine. Conversely, bradycardia is likely following administration of an edrophonium–glycopyrrolate mixture but not an edrophonium–atropine mixture (Fig. 9-11) (Azar et al, 1983). A mixture of edrophonium and atropine also is superior to a mixture of edrophonium and glycopyrrolate because edrophonium and atropine have similar durations of action. Indeed, late bradycardia is more likely when short-acting atropine rather than long-acting glycopyrrolate is combined with neostigmine. This emphasizes the value of matching both the onset and the duration of action of the anticholinergic drug to the anticholinesterase drug.

Excessive Neuromuscular Blockade

Once acetylcholinesterase is maximally inhibited, administering additional anticholinesterase drug does not further antagonize nondepolarizing neuromuscular blockade. For this reason, persistence of neuromuscular blockade despite large doses of anticholinesterase drugs (neo-

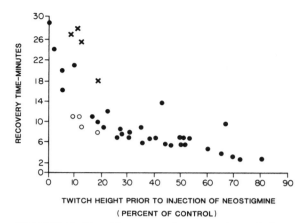

FIGURE 9–12. The rate of antagonism of drug-induced neuromuscular blockade parallels the magnitude of blockade present just before administration of the anticholinesterase drug. (From Katz RL. Clinical neuromuscular pharmacology of pancuronium. Anesthesiology 1971; 34: 550–6; with permission.)

stigmine, 70 $\mu g \cdot kg^{-1}$ IV, or equivalent doses of the other anticholinesterase drugs) is often an indication to ventilate the lungs mechanically until neuromuscular blockade dissipates with time.

Events that Influence Reversal of Neuromuscular Blockade

The speed and extent to which neuromuscular blockade is reversed by anticholinesterase drugs are influenced by a number of factors, including the intensity of the preexisting neuromuscular blockade and the nondepolarizing neuromuscular blocking drug being antagonized. For example, the rate of antagonism directly parallels the magnitude of neuromuscular blockade present just before administration of the anticholinesterase drug (Fig. 9-12) (Katz, 1971). Comparable degrees of neuromuscular blockade due to gallamine are reversed less rapidly by neostigmine than is neuromuscular blockade produced by d-tubocurarine or pancuronium (Miller et al, 1972).

Some data suggest that edrophonium is less effective than neostigmine in antagonizing deep neuromuscular blockade (twitch height 10% of control) produced by continuous infusions of atracurium, vecuronium, or pancuronium (Engbaek et al, 1985; Kopman, 1986). Edrophonium and neostigmine are not equally effective against atracurium and vecuronium. For example, atracur-

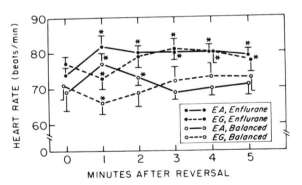

FIGURE 9–11. Bradycardia is more likely to occur following the administration of edrophonium-glycopyrrolate (*EG*) than following administration edrophonium-atropine (*EA*). Mean ± SE. *P <0.05 compared with heart rate at zero time just before administration of the drug combination. (From Azar I, Pham AN, Karambelkar DJ, Lear E. The heart rate following edrophoniam-atropine and edrophonium-glycopyrrolate mixtures. Anesthesiology 1983; 59: 139–41; with permission.)

ium-induced train-of-four fade is antagonized more easily with edrophonium, whereas that of vecuronium is more easily antagonized by neostigmine (Smith et al, 1989). Likewise, pyridostigmine and edrophonium are more effective against pancuronium than d-tubocurarine-induced neuromuscular blockade (Donati et al, 1987).

Antagonism of neuromuscular blockade by anticholinesterase drugs may be inhibited or even prevented by (1) certain antibiotics, (2) hypothermia, (3) respiratory acidosis associated with a $PaCO_2$ greater than 50 mmHg, or (4) hypokalemia and metabolic alkalosis (Fig. 9-13) (Miller et al, 1975).

4-Aminopyridine

The drug 4-aminopyridine has advantages over neostigmine and pyridostigmine for reversing neuromuscular blockade. These advantages include longer duration of action, absence of muscarinic effects, and effectiveness in antagonizing antibiotic-potentiated neuromuscular blockade. This drug is presumed to enhance the presynaptic release of acetylcholine by facilitating the entry of calcium ions into nerve endings. The dose of 4-aminopyridine necessary to antagonize neuromuscular blockade (1 mg·kg^{-1} IV), however, produces central nervous system stimulation. For this reason, 4-aminopyridine has been combined with anticholinesterase drugs in an at-

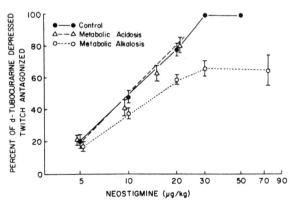

FIGURE 9–13. Antagonism of drug-induced neuromuscular blockade by anticholinesterase drugs is impaired by metabolic alkalosis. Mean ± SE. (From Miller RD, Van Nyhuis LS, Eger EI, Way NL. The effect of acid-base balance on neostigmine antagonism of d-tubocurarine–induced neuromuscular blockade. Anesthesiology 1975; 42: 377–83; with permission.)

tempt to reduce the dose of both drugs and thus minimize side effects. Indeed, 0.35 mg·kg^{-1} IV of 4-aminopyridine reduces by 68% to 75% the amount of anticholinesterase drug required to reliably antagonize nondepolarizing neuromuscular blockade (Fig. 9-14) (Miller et al, 1979). The drug 4-aminopyridine has also been used to treat Eaton-Lambert syndrome, botulism, and myasthenia gravis.

Treatment of Central Nervous System Effects of Certain Drugs

Physostigmine, a tertiary amine, crosses the blood-brain barrier and thus is effective in antagonizing adverse central nervous system effects of certain drugs.

Anticholinergic Drugs

Physostigmine, 15 to 60 µg·kg^{-1} IV, is effective in antagonizing restlessness and confusion (central anticholinergic syndrome) due to atropine or scopolamine (see Chapter 10). Presumably, physostigmine increases concentrations of acetylcholine in the brain, making more neurotransmitter available for interaction with cholinergic receptors. The duration of action of physostigmine is shorter than that of anticholinergic drugs. For this reason, it may be necessary to repeat the dose of physostigmine used in the treatment of central anticholinergic syndrome.

Opioids

Physostigmine may reverse the depression of the ventilatory response to carbon dioxide but not analgesia produced by prior administration of morphine (Snir-Mor et al, 1983; Weinstock et al, 1982). It is speculated that opioids diminish the ventilatory response to carbon dioxide by reducing the amounts of acetylcholine in the area of the respiratory center that would normally be released in response to hypercarbia. Other data, however, do not support an antagonist effect of physostigmine on opioid-induced depression of ventilation (Bourke et al, 1984).

Benzodiazepines

Physostigmine may increase the state of consciousness in patients sedated by diazepam

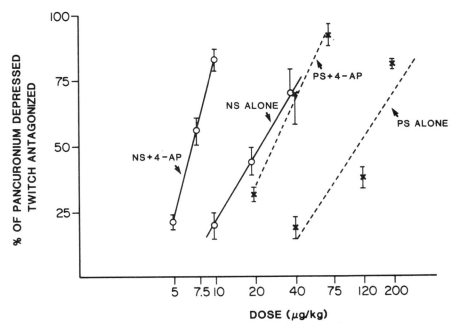

FIGURE 9–14. Dose-response curves for reversal of pancuronium-induced neuromuscular blockade with neostigmine (NS) or pyridostigmine (PS) alone or combined with 4-aminopyridine (4-AP). Mean ± SE. (From Miller RD, Booij LDHJ, Agoston S, Crul JF. Aminopyridine potentiates neostigmine and pyridostigmine in man. Anesthesiology 1979; 50: 416–20; with permission.)

(Bidwai et al, 1979). The development of a specific benzodiazepine receptor antagonist (flumazenil) negates the need for administration of a nonspecific antagonist such as physostigmine.

Anesthetics

Physostigmine reduces postoperative somnolence following anesthesia with a volatile anesthetic (Hill et al, 1977). Furthermore, physostigmine produces electroencephalographic evidence of arousal during administration of halothane (Roy and Stullken, 1981). Perhaps physostigmine acts by permitting acetylcholine to accumulate at muscarinic cholinergic receptors in the ascending reticular activating system. Reversal of the adverse central nervous system effects of ketamine by physostigmine while analgesia remains intact have been described (Balmer and Wyte, 1977). Sedative effects of other drugs, including phenothiazines and tricyclic antidepressants, may also be antagonized by physostigmine.

Treatment of Myasthenia Gravis

Neostigmine, pyridostigmine, and ambenonium are the standard anticholinesterase drugs used in the symptomatic treatment of myasthenia gravis. These drugs increase the response of skeletal muscles to repetitive impulses, presumably by increasing the availability of endogenous acetylcholine.

The quaternary ammonium structure of neostigmine and pyridostigmine limits the oral absorption of these drugs. For example, the oral dose of neostigmine is approximately 30 times greater than the intravenous dose. The interval between oral doses is usually 2 to 4 hours for neostigmine and 3 to 6 hours for pyridostigmine or ambenonium. Muscarinic, cardiovascular, and gastrointestinal side effects are controlled as necessary with anticholinergic drugs.

In assessing the anticholinesterase drug therapy of myasthenia gravis, edrophonium, 1 mg IV, is administered every 1 to 2 minutes until a change in symptoms is observed. Inadequate anticholinesterase drug therapy is diagnosed if there is a decrease in myasthenic symptoms. Conversely, patients with excess anticholinesterase drug therapy experiencing a cholinergic crisis develop increased skeletal muscle weakness with administration of edrophonium. Bromide intoxication has been described in a patient with myasthenia gravis being treated with pyridostigmine bromide (Rothenberg et al, 1990).

Treatment of Glaucoma

Anticholinesterase drugs reduce intraocular pressure in patients with narrow-angle and wide-angle glaucoma, reflecting a decrease in the resistance to outflow of aqueous humor. Treatment of glaucoma with long-acting anticholinesterase drugs (echothiophate, demecarium, isofluro-phate) for 6 months or longer carries the risk of cataract formation. For this reason, short-acting miotic anticholinesterase drugs are used initially, with introduction of long-acting miotic anticholinesterase drugs only when the therapeutic response to the short-acting drugs is not effective. Beta-adrenergic antagonists, such as timolol, do not produce miosis, but do reduce intraocular pressure by decreasing the secretion of aqueous humor.

OVERDOSE OF ANTICHOLINESTERASE DRUGS

Effects of acute intoxication by anticholinesterase drugs manifest as muscarinic and nicotinic symptoms on peripheral and central nervous system sites (Karalliedde and Senanayake, 1989). Muscarinic symptoms include miosis, difficulty focusing, salivation, bronchoconstriction, bradycardia, abdominal cramps, and loss of bladder and rectal control. Nicotinic actions at the neuromuscular junction range from skeletal muscle weakness to overt paralysis with resulting apnea. Central nervous system actions include confusion, ataxia, seizures, coma, and depression of ventilation.

The diagnosis of anticholinesterase drug overdose is made by the history of exposure and characteristic signs and symptoms. Organophosphate anticholinesterases, such as are present in insecticides, are absorbed rapidly by the lungs, skin, and gastrointestinal tract and may be the

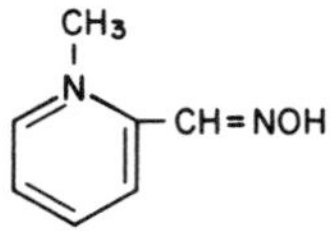

FIGURE 9–15.   Pralidoxime.

cause of toxic symptoms. Accidental poisoning from these drugs most often occurs by inhalation or dermal absorption. The high lipid solubility of organophosphate anticholinesterases ensures that these drugs will cross the blood-brain barrier easily and produce intense effects on the central nervous system.

Treatment

Treatment of anticholinesterase drug overdose is with atropine, occasionally supplemented by an acetylcholinesterase reactivator, pralidoxime (Fig. 9-15). Atropine, 35 to 70 $\mu g \cdot kg^{-1}$ IV, administered every 3 to 10 minutes until muscarinic symptoms disappear, is specific for antagonizing the muscarinic effects of excess acetylcholine but has no impact on nicotinic actions at the neuromuscular junction. Effects of excess acetylcholine at the neuromuscular junction and, to a lesser extent, effects at autonomic ganglia can be reversed by administration of pralidoxime, 15 $mg \cdot kg^{-1}$ IV, over 2 minutes. This dosage is repeated after 20 minutes if skeletal muscle weakness is not reversed. Central nervous system effects are not antagonized by pralidoxime. Pralidoxime is more effective in countering the effects of drugs that phosphorylate acetylcholinesterase than against drugs that carbamylate the enzyme. Furthermore, pralidoxime may be ineffective unless it is administered within minutes after exposure to the potent anticholinesterase drug.

In addition to specific pharmacologic antagonism, treatment of anticholinesterase drug overdose includes supportive measures such as intubation of the trachea and mechanical ventilation of the lungs. Seizures may require suppression with drugs such as thiopental or diazepam.

SYNTHETIC CHOLINERGIC AGONISTS

Synthetic cholinergic agonist drugs have as their primary action the activation of cholinergic receptors that are innervated by postganglionic parasympathetic nerves. Additional actions are exerted on ganglia and on cells that do not receive extensive parasympathetic innervation but, nevertheless, possess cholinergic receptors.

Acetylcholine has no therapeutic application because of its diffuse sites of action and rapid hydrolysis by acetylcholinesterase and to a lesser extent by plasma cholinesterase. Derivatives of acetylcholine have been synthesized that have more selective effects and prolonged durations of action. Of the synthetic acetylcholine derivatives, only methacholine, carbachol, and bethanechol have clinical usefulness (Fig. 9-16). The muscarinic actions of all these drugs are blocked selectively by atropine.

These drugs are administered orally, subcutaneously, or topically to the eye. Asthma, coronary artery disease, and peptic ulcer disease are examples of diseases that could be exacerbated by cholinergic agonists. For example, bronchoconstriction produced by these drugs could produce an asthmatic attack. Vasodilation and resulting decreases in diastolic blood pressure may reduce coronary blood flow sufficiently to evoke myocardial ischemia in vulnerable patients. Finally, enhanced secretion of acidic gastric fluid may aggravate the symptoms of peptic ulcer.

Methacholine

Methacholine has a longer duration of action than acetylcholine because its rate of hydrolysis by acetylcholine is slower than by acetylcholinesterase. Furthermore, methacholine is almost totally resistant to hydrolysis by plasma cholinesterase. Its greater selectivity than acetylcholine is manifested by a lack of significant nicotinic and predominance of muscarinic actions. This drug is rarely used clinically because of the unpredictable nature of its muscarinic effects, especially on the cardiovascular system.

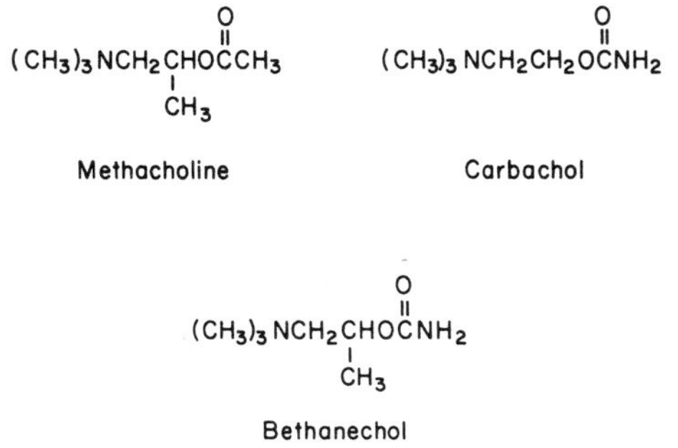

Carbachol and Bethanechol

Carbachol and bethanechol are totally resistant to hydrolysis by acetylcholinesterase or plasma cholinesterase. Bethanechol has mainly muscarinic actions, but both drugs act with some selectivity on the smooth muscle of the gastrointestinal tract and urinary bladder. Carbachol retains a high level of nicotinic activity particularly on autonomic ganglia, which may reflect drug-induced release of endogenous acetylcholine from the terminals of cholinergic fibers. In contrast to methacholine, the cardiovascular effects of carbachol and bethanechol are less prominent than effects on the gastrointestinal and urinary tracts.

Effects on the gastrointestinal tract include increased peristalsis and enhanced secretory activity. Nausea, vomiting, and defecation are manifestations of increased gastrointestinal motility. Selective effects of carbachol and bethanechol include stimulation of ureteral peristalsis and contraction of the detrusor muscle of the urinary bladder. In addition, the trigone and external sphincter are relaxed. These effects evoke evacuation of a neurogenic bladder.

Secretions are increased from all glands that receive parasympathetic nervous system innervation including the lacrimal, tracheobronchial, salivary, digestive, and exocrine sweat glands. Effects on the respiratory system include, in addition to increased tracheobronchial secretion, bronchoconstriction and stimulation of the chemoreceptors of the carotid and aortic bodies. Instilled into the eye, these drugs produce miosis.

Bethanechol is used as a stimulant of the smooth muscle of the gastrointestinal tract and the urinary bladder. For example, oral bethanechol may relieve adynamic ileus or gastric atony following bilateral vagotomy. Bethanechol may be useful in combating urinary retention when mechanical obstruction is absent as in the postoperative and postpartum period and in certain cases of neurogenic bladder, thus avoiding the

$$(CH_3)_3\,NCH_2CHOCCH_3$$
$$\overset{|}{CH_3}$$

Methacholine

$$(CH_3)_3\,NCH_2CH_2OCNH_2$$

Carbachol

$$(CH_3)_3\,NCH_2CHOCNH_2$$
$$\overset{|}{CH_3}$$

Bethanechol

FIGURE 9–16. Synthetic acetylcholine derivatives.

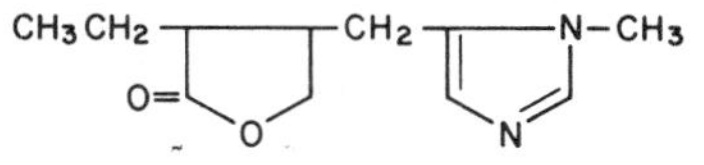

Pilocarpine

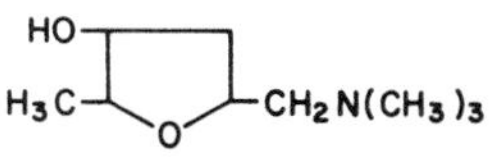

Muscarine

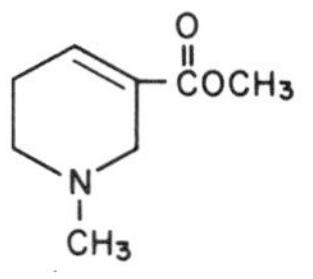

Arecoline

FIGURE 9–17. Cholinomimetic alkaloids.

risk of infection attendant with catheterization. For acute urinary retention, the usual adult dose of bethanechol is 5 mg injected subcutaneously, which can be repeated after 15 to 30 minutes if necessary.

Carbachol is not used for its actions on the gastrointestinal tract and urinary bladder because of its relatively greater nicotinic action at autonomic ganglia. Instead, carbachol is useful as a topical solution in the chronic therapy of narrow-angle glaucoma and to produce miosis during intraocular surgery.

Pilocarpine, Muscarine, and Arecoline

Pilocarpine, muscarine, and arecoline are examples of cholinomimetic alkaloids (Fig. 9-17). The sites of actions of these drugs and pharmacologic actions are the same as for choline agonists. Pilocarpine has a dominant muscarinic action, and sweat glands are particularly sensitive to this drug. Muscarine acts almost exclusively at muscarinic cholinergic receptors. Arecoline acts in addition at nicotinic cholinergic receptors. The clinical use of these drugs is largely limited to the topical administration of pilocarpine as a miotic. Pilocarpine when applied topically to the eye causes miosis, paralysis of accommodation, and a sustained reduction in intraocular pressure. Miosis may persist for several hours, but cycloplegia usually wanes within 2 hours. Pilocarpine is useful for overcoming mydriasis produced by atropine.

REFERENCES

Azar I, Pham AN, Karambelkar DJ, Lear E. The heart rate following edrophonium–atropine and edrophon-ium–glycopyrrolate mixtures. Anesthesiology 1983; 59:139–41.

Balmer HGR, Wyte SR. Antagonism of ketamine or physostigmine (letter). Br J Anaesth 1977;49:510.

Bidwai AV, Stanley TH, Rogers C, Riet EK. Reversal of diazepam-induced postanesthetic somnolence with physostigmine. Anesthesiology 1979;51:256–9.

Bourke DL, Rosenberg M. Allen PD. Physostigmine: Effectiveness as an antagonist of respiratory depression and psychomotor effects caused by morphine or diazepam. Anesthesiology 1984;61:523–8.

Cronnelly R. Muscle relaxant antagonists. Semin Anesth 1985:4:31–40.

Cronnelly R, Miller RD. Onset and duration of edrophonium–pyridostigmine mixtures. Anesthesiology 1984;61:A301.

Cronnelly R, Morris RB. Antagonism of neuromuscular blockade. Br J Anaesth 1982;54:183–93.

Cronnelly R, Morris RB, Miller RD. Edrophonium: Duration of action and atropine requirement in humans during halothane anesthesia. Anesthesiology 1982; 57:261–6.

Cronnelly R, Stanski DR, Miller RD, Sheiner LB. Pyridostigmine kinetics with and without renal function. Clin Pharmacol Ther 1980;28:78–81.

Cronnelly R, Stanski, DR, Miller RD, Sheiner LB, Sohn YJ. Renal function and the pharmacokinetics of neostigmine in anesthetized patients. Anesthesiology 1979;51:222–6.

Donati F, Ferguson A, Bevan DR. Twitch depression and train-of-four ratio after antagonism of pancuronium with edrophonium, neostigmine, or pyridostigmine. Anesth Analg 1983;62:314–6.

Donati F, McCarroll SM, Antzaka C, McCready D, Bevan DR. Dose–response curves for edrophonium, neostigmine, and pyridostigmine after pancuronium and d-tubocurarine. Anesthesiology 1987;66:471–6.

Engbaek J. Ording H, Ostergaard D, Viby-Mogensen J. Edrophonium and neostigmine for reversal of the neuromuscular blocking effect of vecuronium. Acta Anaesthesiol Scand 1985;29:544–6.

Fisher DM, Cronnelly R, Miller RD, Sharma M. The neuromuscular pharmacology of neostigmine in infants and children. Anesthesiology 1983;59:220–5.

Fisher DM, Cronnelly R, Sharma M, Miller RD. Clinical pharmacology of edrophonium in infants and children. Anesthesiology 1984;61:428–33.

Fogdall RP, Miller RD. Antagonism of d-tubocurarine and pancuronium-induced neuromuscular blockades by pyridostigmine in man. Anesthesiology 1973;39:504–9.

Hennis PJ, Cronnelly R, Sharma M, Fisher DM, Miller RD. Metabolites of neostigmine and pyridostigmine do not contribute to antagonism of neuromuscular blockade in the dog. Anesthesiology 1984;61:334–9.

Hill GE, Stanley TH, Sentker CR. Physostigmine reversal of postoperative somnolence. Can Anaesth Soc J 1977;24:707–11.

Jones RM, Pearce AC, Williams JP. Recovery characteristics following antagonism of atracurium with neostigmine or edrophonium. Br J Anaesth 1984;56:453–7.

Karalliedde L, Senanayake N. Organophosphorus insecticide poisoning. Br J Anaesth 1989;63:736–50.

Katz RL. Clinical neuromuscular pharmacology of pancuronium. Anesthesiology 1971;34:550–6.

Kopman A. Recovery times following edrophonium and neostigmine reversal of pancuronium, atracurium, and vecuronium steady-state infusions. Anesthesiology 1986;65:572–8.

Matteo RS, Young WL, Orstein E, Schwartz AE, Silverberg PA, Diaz J. Pharmacokinetics and pharmacodynamics of edrophonium in elderly surgical patients. Anesth Analg 1990;71:334–9.

Miller RD, Booij LDHJ, Agoston S, Crul JF. Aminopyridine potentiates neostigmine and pyridostigmine in man. Anesthesiology 1979;50:416–20.

Miller RD, Larson CP, Way WL. Comparative antagonism of d-tubocurarine-, gallamine-, and pancuronium-induced neuromuscular blockade by neostigmine. Anesthesiology 1972;37:503–9.

Miller RD, Van Nyhius LS, Eger EI, Vitez TS, Way WL. Comparative times to peak effect and duration of action of neostigmine and pyridostigmine. Anesthesiology 1974;41:27–33.

Miller RD, Van Nyhius LS, Eger EI, Way WL. The effect of acid-base balance of neostigmine antagonism of d-tubocurarine–induced neuromuscular blockade. Anesthesiology 1975;42:377–83.

Mirakhur RK. Edrophonium and plasma cholinesterase activity. Can Anaesth Soc J 1986;33:588–90.

Morris RB, Cronnelly R, Miller RD, Stanski DR, Fahey MR. Pharmacokinetics of edrophonium and neostigmine when antagonizing d-tubocurarine neuromuscular blockade in man. Anesthesiology 1981;54:399–402.

Prys-Roberts C. Hemodynamic effects of anesthesia and surgery in renal hypertensive patients receiving large doses of B-receptor antagonists. Anesthesiology 1979;51:S22.

Ramamurthy S, Shaker MH, Winnie AP. Glycopyrrolate as a substitute for atropine in neostigmine reversal of muscle relaxants. Can Anaesth Soc J 1972;19:399–411.

Rothenberg DM, Berns AS, Barkin R, Glantz RH. Bromide intoxication secondary to pyridostigmine bromide therapy. JAMA 1990;263:1121–2.

Roy RC, Stullken EH. Electroencephalographic evidence of arousal in dogs from halothane after doxapram, physostigmine, or naloxone. Anesthesiology 1981;55:392–7.

Rupp SM, McChristian JW, Miller RD, Taboada JA, Cronnelly R. Neostigmine and edrophonium antagonism of varying neuromuscular blockade induced by atracurium, pancuronium, or vecuronium. Anesthesiology 1986;64:711–7.

Smith CE, Donati F, Bevan DR. Dose–response relationships for edrophonium and neostigmine as antagonists of atracurium and vecuronium neuromuscular blockade. Anesthesiology 1989;71:37–43.

Snir-Mor I, Weinstock M, Davidson JT, Bahar M. Physostigmine antagonizes morphine-induced respiratory depression in human subjects. Anesthesiology 1983;59:6–9.

Sprague DH, Severe bradycardia after neostigmine in a patient taking propranolol to control paroxysmal atrial tachycardia. Anesthesiology 1975;42:208–10.

Summers WK, Majovski LV, Marsh GM, Tachiki K, Kling A. Oral tetrahydroaminoacridine in long-term treatment of senile dementia, Alzheimer type. N Engl J Med 1986;315:1241–5.

Wagner DL, Moorthy SS, Stoelting RK. Administration of anticholinesterase drugs in the presence of beta-adrenergic blockade. Anesth Analg 1982;61:153–4.

Weinstock M, Davidson JT, Rosin AJ, Schnieden H. Effect of physostigmine on morphine-induced postoperative pain and somnolence. Br J Anaesth 1982;54:429–34.

Young WL, Matteo RS, Ornstein E. Duration of action of neostigmine and pyridostigmine in the elderly. Anesth Analg 1988;67:775–8.

10

Anticholinergic Drugs

Anticholinergic drugs competitively antagonize the effects of the neurotransmitter acetylcholine at cholinergic postganglionic sites designated as muscarinic receptors. Muscarinic cholinergic receptors are present in the heart, salivary glands, and smooth muscle of the gastrointestinal tract and genitourinary tract. Acetylcholine is also the neurotransmitter at postganglionic nicotinic receptors located at the neuromuscular junction and autonomic ganglia. In contrast to muscarinic receptors, usual doses of anticholinergic drugs exert little or no effect at nicotinic cholinergic receptors. As such, anticholinergic drugs may be considered to be selectively antimuscarinic.

Naturally occurring tertiary amine anticholinergic drugs such as atropine and scopolamine are alkaloids of belladonna plants. Semisynthetic congeners of the belladonna alkaloids represented by glycopyrrolate are usually quaternary ammonium derivatives. These quaternary ammonium derivatives are often more potent than their parent compounds with respect to peripheral anticholinergic effects, but they lack central nervous system activity because of poor penetration into the brain.

STRUCTURE ACTIVITY RELATIONSHIPS

Naturally occurring anticholinergic drugs (atropine and scopolamine) are esters formed by the combination of tropic acid and a complex organic base of either tropine or scopine (Fig. 10-1). Structurally, these drugs resemble cocaine,

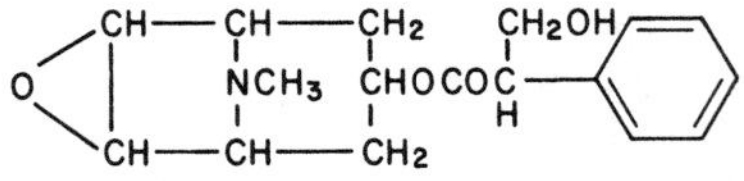

and atropine, in fact, has weak analgesic actions. Atropine and scopolamine comprise mixtures of equal parts of dextrorotatory and levorotatory isomers, but the anticholinergic effect is almost entirely due to the levorotatory form. Synthetic anticholinergic drugs such as glycopyrrolate contain mandelic acid rather than tropic acid (Fig. 10-1). Like acetylcholine, anticholinergic drugs

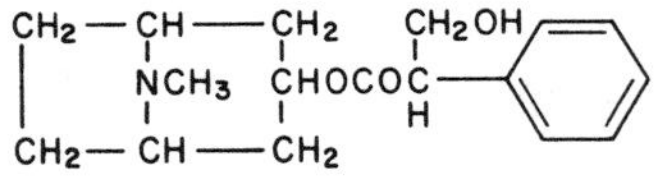

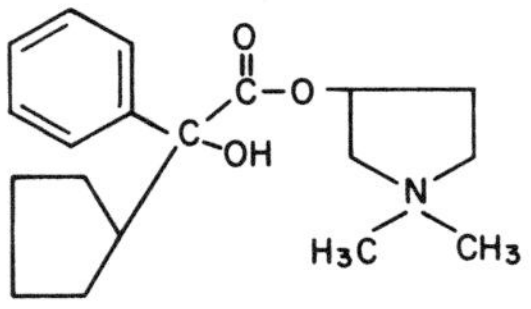

FIGURE 10–1. Naturally occurring and synthetic anticholinergic drugs.

contain a cationic portion that can fit into the muscarinic cholinergic receptor.

MECHANISM OF ACTION

Anticholinergic drugs combine reversibly with muscarinic cholinergic receptors and thus prevent access of the neurotransmitter acetylcholine to these sites. In contrast to acetylcholine, the combination of an anticholinergic drug with the muscarinic receptor does not result in cell membrane changes (inhibition of adenylate cyclase or alteration in calcium permeability) that lead to a cholinergic response. Anticholinergic drugs do not prevent the liberation of acetylcholine nor do they react with acetylcholine. As competitive antagonists, the effect of anticholinergic drugs can be overcome by increasing the concentration of acetylcholine in the area of the muscarinic receptors.

Evidence for subclasses of muscarinic cholinergic receptors (M-1, M-2, and M-3) is the variation in sensitivity among different cholinergic receptors as well as differences in potency among the anticholinergic drugs (Table 10-1) (Goyal, 1989). For example, muscarinic cholinergic receptors that control salivary and bronchial secretions are inhibited by lower doses of anticholinergic drugs than are necessary to inhibit receptors that regulate acetylcholine effects on the heart and eye. Even larger doses of anticholinergic drugs inhibit cholinergic control of the gastrointestinal tract and genitourinary tract, thus decreasing the tone and motility of the intestine and inhibiting micturition. Still larger doses of anticholinergic drugs are required to inhibit gastric secretion of hydrogen ions. As a result, a dose of anticholinergic drug that inhibits gastric secretion of hydrogen ions invariably affects salivary secretion, heart rate, ocular accommodation, and micturition.

Examples of differences in anticholinergic potency between drugs are the greater antisialagogue and ocular effects of scopolamine compared with atropine (Table 10-2) (Eger, 1962). Conversely, atropine has greater anticholinergic effects at the heart, bronchial smooth muscle, and gastrointestinal tract than does scopolamine (Table 10-2) (Eger, 1962).

Atropine, scopolamine, and glycopyrrolate do not discriminate among M-1, M-2, and M-3 receptors; instead, they act as highly selective competitive antagonists of acetylcholine at all muscarinic receptors. Nevertheless, future research may produce anticholinergic drugs that act as selective antagonists on specific muscarinic receptors that mediate unique physiologic responses such as secretion of hydrogen ions by gastric parietal cells. Indeed, pirenzepine seems to be selective in blocking the M-3 receptors responsible for gastric hydrogen ion secretion.

Evidence that anticholinergic drugs are not pure muscarinic cholinergic receptor antagonists is the observation that small doses of atropine, scopolamine, and glycopyrrolate can produce heart rate slowing even when the drug is administered in the presence of bilateral vagotomy. This heart rate slowing reflects a weak, peripheral muscarinic cholinergic receptor agonist effect of the anticholinergic drug. Previous speculation that heart rate slowing following administration of atropine reflected central vagal action before the peripheral blocking effects could occur is not supported by similar heart rate changes following administration of glycopyrrolate, which cannot easily cross the blood-brain barrier.

An additional indirect effect of anticholinergic drugs can result from interference by these drugs with the normal inhibition of the release of endogenous norepinephrine. This indirect effect may manifest as a sympathomimetic effect of atropine.

Table 10–1
Muscarinic-Receptor Subtypes

M-1	M-2	M-3
Neurons and nerve endings	Heart	Exocrine glands
	Neurons and nerve endings	Smooth muscle
	Smooth muscle	Neurons and nerve endings

Table 10–2
Comparative Effects of Anticholinergic Drugs

	Sedation	Antisialagogue	Increase Heart Rate	Relax Smooth Muscle	Mydriasis Cycloplegia	Prevent Motion Sickness	Decrease Gastric Hydrogen Ion Secretion	Alter Fetal Heart Rate
Atropine	+	+	+++	++	+	+	∓	0
Scopolamine	+++	+++	+	+	+++	+++	±	?
Glycopyrrolate	0	++	++	++	0	0	±	0

0 none
  +, mild
 ++, moderate
+++, marked

PHARMACOKINETICS

Oral absorption of even the tertiary amine anticholinergic drugs is not sufficiently predictable for a recommendation of oral administration in the perioperative period. Intramuscular or intravenous administration is used most often for anticholinergic drugs. Despite attempts to develop anticholinergic drugs with greater specificity for certain functions, the sequence of muscarinic cholinergic blockade is similar for all drugs.

Atropine and scopolamine are lipid-soluble tertiary amines that easily penetrate the blood-brain barrier (Fig. 10-2) (Proakis and Harris, 1978). In contrast, glycopyrrolate is a poorly lipid-soluble quaternary ammonium compound with minimal ability to cross the blood-brain barrier and produce central nervous system effects (Fig. 10-2) (Ali-Melkkila et al, 1990; Proakis and Harris, 1978). Absorption of glycopyrrolate after intramuscular injection is rapid (maximum plasma concentration in 16 minutes) and comparable with atropine (Ali-Melkkila et al, 1990). Clearance of glycopyrrolate from the plasma is more rapid than atropine (elimination half-time is 1.25 hours vs 2.3 hours) and nearly 60% of glycopyrrolate is excreted unchanged or as active

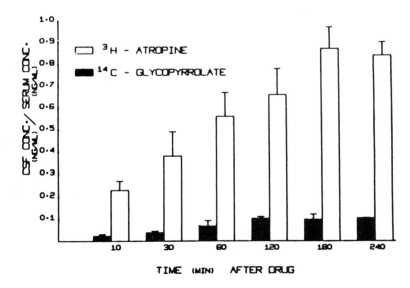

FIGURE 10–2. Cerebrospinal fluid (*CSF*)–to–serum (*S*) concentration ratios (mean ± SE) following intravenous administration of ^{14}C-glycopyrrolate (n=3) or ^{3}H-atropine (n=4) to anesthetized dogs. ^{3}H-atropine produced significantly ($P <0.05$) higher CSF:S concentration ratios over the 4-hour post-drug (0.1 mg·kg^{-1} of each agent) period than did ^{14}C-glycopyrrolate. (From Proakis AG, Harris GB. Comparative penetration of glycopyrrolate and atropine across the blood brain and placental barriers in anesthetized dogs. Anesthesiology 1978; 48: 339–44; with permission.)

metabolites into the urine within 6 hours. The corresponding value for atropine is 18%. Appearance of tropine and tropic acid reflect hydrolysis of atropine to inactive metabolites. Minimal amounts of atropine are destroyed in human plasma, whereas certain animals, such as the rabbit, possess a specific plasma enzyme, atropine esterase, which is capable of hydrolyzing atropine. Conversely, scopolamine is broken down almost entirely in the body with only approximately 1% appearing unchanged in the urine.

CLINICAL USES

Anticholinergic drugs are used in a wide variety of clinical conditions and situations (Mirakhur, 1988). However, the lack of selectivity of these drugs makes it difficult to obtain desired therapeutic responses without concomitant side effects (Table 10-1). The most important uses of anticholinergic drugs in the perioperative period are (1) preoperative medication, (2) treatment of reflex-mediated bradycardia, and (3) protection against the muscarinic effects of anticholinesterase drugs as used to antagonize nondepolarizing neuromuscular blocking drugs (see Chapter 9). Less frequent uses of anticholinergic drugs are (1) bronchodilation, (2) biliary and ureteral smooth muscle relaxation, (3) production of mydriasis and cycloplegia, (4) antagonism of gastric hydrogen ion secretion, (5) prevention of motion-induced nausea, and (6) constitutents in nonprescription cold remedies.

Preoperative Medication

Historically, intramuscular atropine was administered before the induction of anesthesia to protect the heart from vagal reflexes and to prevent excessive secretions. Currently available inhaled or injected anesthetic drugs are not predictably associated with these effects, and it is not mandatory to include an anticholinergic drug in the preoperative medication. When an anticholinergic drug is included in the preoperative medication, the therapeutic goals are to produce sedation or an antisialagogue effect. Anticholinergic drugs in traditional doses used for preoperative medication in adults do not alter gastric fluid pH or volume (Table 10-3) (Stoelting, 1978).

Patients with glaucoma and parturients present special considerations in using anticholinergic drugs for preoperative medication. For example, the mydriatic effects of scopolamine are greater than those of atropine, suggesting caution in the use of scopolamine in patients with glaucoma (Garde et al, 1978). Atropine, 0.4 mg IM or 1 mg IV, as administered with an anticholinesterase drug seems safe because little or no change in pupil size occurs (Balamoutsos et al, 1980). Glycopyrrolate has the least effect on pupil size of all the anticholinergic drugs used for preoperative medication. Both atropine and scopolamine can cross the placenta, but fetal heart rate is not significantly changed following intravenous administration of either atropine or glycopyrrolate (Fig. 10-3) (Abboud et al, 1983; Murad et al, 1981).

Table 10–3

Gastric Fluid pH and Volume Without or With Inclusion of an Anticholinergic Drug in the Perioperative Medication

	Gastric Fluid pH < 2.5 (percent of patients)	*Gastric Fluid Volume >20 ml (percent of patients)*
Morphine (n=75)	65	27
Morphine–atropine (n=75)	57	27
Morphine–glycopyrrolate (n=75)	49	23

n, number of patients.
(Data from Stoelting RK. Responses to atropine, glycopyrrolate, and Riopan of gastric fluid pH and volume in adult patients. Anesthesiology 1978; 48:367–9, with permission.)

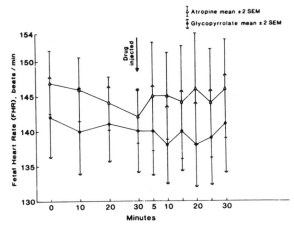

FIGURE 10–3.   Atropine or glycopyrrolate do not alter fetal heart rate following intravenous administration to the mother. Mean ± 2 SEM. (From Abboud T, Raya J, Sadri S, Grobler N, Stine L, Miller F. Fetal and maternal cardiovascular effects of atropine and glycopyrrolate. Anesth Analg 1983; 62: 426–30; with permission.)

Sedation

Scopolamine is selected when sedation is the reason for including an anticholinergic drug in the preoperative medication. Indeed, scopolamine is approximately 100 times more potent than atropine in depressing the reticular activating system. Scopolamine, in addition to depressing the cerebral cortex, also affects other areas of the brain, causing amnesia. Small doses of scopolamine, 0.3 to 0.5 mg IM, usually cause sedation whereas similar doses of atropine produce minimal central nervous system effects. Glycopyrrolate, which does not cross the blood-brain barrier easily, is devoid of sedative effects. Scopolamine also greatly enhances sedative effects of concomitantly administered drugs, especially opioids and benzodiazepines (Frumin et al, 1976). Indeed, the combination of morphine and scopolamine is favored by many anesthesiologists when a reliable sedative effect from the preoperative medication is desired.

Occasionally, central nervous system effects of anticholinergic drugs, especially scopolamine, cause symptoms ranging from restlessness to somnolence. These symptoms are likely to occur in elderly patients and should be considered as a possible explanation for delayed awakening from anesthesia or agitation in the early postoperative period. Inhaled anesthetics can potentiate the effects of anticholinergic drugs on the central nervous system, leading to an increased incidence of postoperative restlessness or somnolence (Holzgrafe et al, 1973). Physostigmine is effective in reversing restlessness or somnolence owing to central nervous system effects of tertiary amine anticholinergic drugs.

Antisialagogue Effect

Scopolamine is approximately three times more potent as an antisialagogue than atropine. For this reason, scopolamine is often selected when both an antisialagogue effect and sedation are desired results of preoperative medication. In equivalent antisialagogue doses, scopolamine, 0.3 to 0.5 mg IM, is less likely than atropine, 0.4 to 0.6 mg IM, to produce heart rate changes. Glycopyrrolate is selected when an antisialagogue effect, in the absence of sedation, is desired. As an antisialagogue, glycopyrrolate is approximately twice as potent as atropine and its duration of action is longer (Murad et al, 1981).

Treatment of Reflex-Mediated Bradycardia

Anticholinergic drugs are the drugs of choice for treating intraoperative bradycardia, particularly that resulting from increased parasympathetic nervous system activity. Administration of atropine, 15 to 70 µg·kg^{-1} IV, and, to a lesser extent, scopolamine and glycopyrrolate, increase the heart rate by blocking the effects of acetylcholine on the sinoatrial node (Gravenstein et al, 1964; Meyers and Tomeldan 1979). Indeed, the maximum increase in heart rate produced by atropine indicates the degree of control normally exerted by the vagus nerve on the sinoatrial node. Equivalent doses of glycopyrrolate produce similar increases in heart rate, but the onset of effect is slower than following the administration of atropine. On the electrocardiogram, the effect of anticholinergic drugs is to shorten the PR interval.

In young adults, in whom vagal tone is greatest, the influence of atropine on heart rate is most marked, whereas in infants or elderly patients even large doses may fail to increase heart rate. During anesthesia that includes a volatile drug, the dose of atropine required to increase heart rate may be decreased compared with awake patients, perhaps reflecting depression of vagal centers during anesthesia. Halothane, like opioids, may increase central vagal tone, accounting for the greater heart rate response following the administration of atropine to patients anesthetized with halothane compared with enflurane (Mirakhur, 1988). Intramuscular administration, in contrast to intravenous injection, is occasionally associated with heart rate slowing, reflecting a peripheral agonist effect of the anticholinergic drug (see the section entitled "Mechanism of Action").

Bronchodilation

The effectiveness of anticholinergic drugs as bronchodilators reflects antagonism of acetylcholine effects on airway smooth muscle via muscarinic receptors, present predominantly in large and medium-sized airways, that respond to vagal nerve activation. The resulting relaxation of bronchial smooth muscle lowers airway resistance and increases dead space, particularly in patients with bronchial asthma or chronic bronchitis. For example, clinical doses of scopolamine decrease airway resistance and increase dead space by approximately one third, but this effect depends largely on the degree of preexisting bronchomotor tone. Glycopyrrolate is equally effective as a bronchodilator and is devoid of effects on the central nervous system, and heart rate effects are minimal (Fig. 10-4) (Gal and Suratt, 1981).

Administration of anticholinergic drugs for preanesthetic medication could result in inspissation of secretions, possibly leading to airway obstruction rather than decreases in airway resistance. Nevertheless, it seems unlikely that a single dose of anticholinergic drug would predictably produce these adverse effects.

Bronchodilation is more likely to occur when anticholinergic drugs are administered by inhalation as aerosols. An advantage of aerosol administration is the absence of adverse cardiovascular side effects that are more likely to accompany systemic administration. Atropine, 1 to 2 mg diluted in 3 to 5 ml of normal saline, can be administered via a nebulizer to treat reflex bronchoconstriction due to parasympathetic nervous system stimulation. Ipratropium is the anticholinergic most often selected for inhalation (Gross, 1988).

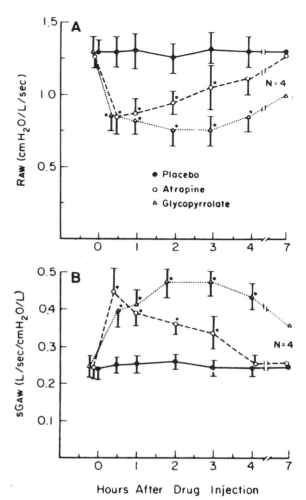

FIGURE 10–4. Atropine and glycopyrrolate are equally effective in lowering airway resistance (R_{AW}) and increasing airway conductance (sGaw). (From Gal TJ, Suratt PM. Atropine and glycopyrrolate effects on lung mechanics in normal man. Anesth Analg 1981;60:85–90; with permission.)

Ipratropium

Ipratropium is a synthetic quaternary ammonium congener of atropine that is administered by metered dose inhaler (40 to 80 μg delivered by two to four actuations of the inhaler). This drug is most effective in preventing and treating bronchospasm that is due to beta-adrenergic antagonists or psychogenic stimuli. In patients with bronchial asthma, ipratropium has a slower onset

(30 to 90 minutes) and is less effective than beta-agonists. Patients with asthma may respond better to beta-agonists because these drugs inhibit the release and the airway smooth muscle contraction caused by mediators such as histamine and leukotrienes. Ipratropium does not influence the release or response to these mediators but is likewise more effective than beta-agonists in producing bronchodilation in patients with chronic bronchitis or emphysema, emphasizing the role of cholinergic tone in the latter patients.

Although not considered the initial bronchodilator of choice for treatment of asthma-induced bronchospasm, ipratropium may be used to augment bronchodilation produced by beta-agonists. Perhaps the strongest argument in favor of the coadministration of beta-agonists and ipratropium is that ipratropium facilitates the rapid onset of beta-agonist effects (5 minutes to 15 minutes) and provides its own sustained activity.

Effects of inhaled ipratropium on the heart rate and intraocular pressure, in contrast to atropine, do not occur, reflecting the minimal systemic absorption (less than 1% of the inhaled dose) of this quaternary ammonium drug. This limited absorption from the airways also accounts for a prolonged effect at the desired site of action. After inhalation of ipratropium, much of the dose is in fact swallowed, but absorption of unchanged drug from the gastrointestinal tract is insignificant. Effects of this drug on mucociliary activity and mucus secretion in the airways are minimal. Ipratropium, like atropine, is not selective for subtypes of muscarinic receptors present in the airways. Tolerance to the bronchodilator effect of ipratropium has not been observed. This is consistent with the concept that antagonists, in contrast to agonists, do not down-regulate but rather may up-regulate the target receptor.

Biliary and Ureteral Smooth Muscle Relaxation

Atropine decreases the tone of the smooth muscle of the biliary tract and ureter. This modest antispasmodic action, however, is unlikely to overcome opioid-induced spasm of the sphincter of Oddi. Conversely, atropine may prevent spasm of the ureter produced by morphine, supporting the custom of administering atropine with an opioid to manage pain due to a renal stone (renal colic).

Therapeutic doses of atropine are thought to diminish the tone of the fundus of the bladder and to increase the tone of the vesical sphincter, possibly contributing to urinary retention.

Mydriasis and Cycloplegia

Circular muscles of the iris that constrict the pupil are innervated by cholinergic fibers from the third cranial nerve, whereas fibers from the same nerve cause contraction of the ciliary muscles allowing the lens to become more convex. Anticholinergic drugs placed topically on the cornea block the action of acetylcholine at both these sites, resulting in mydriasis and cycloplegia. Complete recovery from mydriasis and cycloplegia produced by topical atropine requires 7 to 14 days. In patients with glaucoma, relaxation of the ciliary muscle produced by an anticholinergic drug occludes the angular space, whereas mydriasis obstructs passage of fluid into the venous circulation, resulting in potentially hazardous elevations of intraocular pressure.

Doses of atropine used for preoperative medication are probably inadequate to elevate intraocular pressure even in susceptible patients, assuming medications being used to treat glaucoma are continued. Indeed, mydriasis produced by any anticholinergic drug is completely offset by topical corneal placement of an anticholinesterase drug such as pilocarpine. Nevertheless, intramuscular scopolamine is a more potent mydriatic than either atropine or glycopyrrolate, suggesting the need for caution in using this anticholinergic drug for preoperative medication of a patient with glaucoma.

Antagonists of Gastric Hydrogen Ion Secretion

Anticholinergic drugs have been used to manage peptic ulcer disease. Indeed, glycopyrrolate was originally introduced as an anticholinergic drug to control gastric acidity. Nevertheless, none of the anticholinergic drugs are selective for this effect, and the high doses required to inhibit gastric hydrogen ion secretion are often associated with unacceptable secretory, ocular, and cardiac side effects. Furthermore, the efficacy of H-2 receptor antagonists for reducing gastric hydrogen ion secretion has largely negated the use of anticholinergic drugs for this purpose.

Anticholinergic drugs have predictable effects on the tone and motility of the gastrointestinal tract because the parasympathetic nervous system provides almost exclusive motor innervation to this organ. As with suppression of gastric hydrogen ion secretion, however, large doses of anticholinergic drugs are necessary to alter gastrointestinal motility, often introducing unacceptable side effects. Nevertheless, high doses of anticholinergic drugs do prevent excess peristalsis of the gastrointestinal tract that would otherwise be associated with antagonism of nondepolarizing neuromuscular blocking drugs using anticholinesterase drugs.

Prevention of Motion-Induced Sickness

Transdermal absorption of scopolamine provides sustained therapeutic plasma concentrations that protect against motion-induced nausea without introducing prohibitive side effects such as sedation, cycloplegia, or drying of secretions. For example, a postauricular application of scopolamine delivers the drug at 5 $\mu g \cdot h^{-1}$ for 72 hours (the total absorbed dose is less than 0.5 mg). Protection against motion-induced nausea is greatest if the transdermal application of scopolamine is initiated at least 4 hours before the noxious stimulus. Administration of transdermal scopolamine after the onset of symptoms is less effective than prophylactic administration. Similar protection against motion-induced nausea by oral or intravenous administration of scopolamine would require large doses, resulting in undesirable side effects and subsequent poor patient acceptance. It is presumed that scopolamine blocks transmission to the medulla of impulses arising from overstimulation of the vestibular apparatus of the inner ear. A prophylactic transdermal scopolamine patch applied before induction of anesthesia for gynecologic surgery or cesarean section provides protection against nausea in patients receiving postoperative analgesia with epidural morphine (Kotelko et al, 1989; Loper et al, 1989). Likewise, transdermal scopolamine applied the evening before surgery decreases but does not abolish the occurence of nausea and vomiting after outpatient laparoscopy using general anesthesia (Bailey et al, 1990). Conversely, not all re-

ports describe an antiemetic effect in patients treated with transdermal scopolamine who are undergoing general anesthesia (Koski et al, 1990).

Anisocoria has been attributed to contamination of the eye following digital manipulation of the transdermal scopolamine patch (Price, 1985). More than 90% of unilateral dilated pupils occur on the same side as the patch. The diagnosis is confirmed by history and failure of the mydriasis to respond to topical installation of pilocarpine.

Constituents of Nonprescription Cold Remedies

Anticholinergic drugs are common constituents of nonprescription cold remedies. The apparent efficacy of these drugs is most likely due to inhibition of the production of upper airway secretions. With the exception of allergic mechanisms, it is also likely that contributions of antihistamines in cold remedies are primarily due to their anticholinergic effects.

CENTRAL ANTICHOLINERGIC SYNDROME

Scopolamine, and to a lesser extent atropine, can enter the central nervous system and produce symptoms characterized as the central anticholinergic syndrome. Symptoms range from restlessness and hallucinations to somnolence and unconsciousness (Duvoisin and Katz, 1968). Presumably, these responses reflect blockade of muscarinic cholinergic receptors in the central nervous system. Glycopyrrolate does not easily cross the blood-brain barrier and, thus, is not likely to cause a central anticholinergic syndrome. Indeed, arousal in the first 30 minutes following cessation of anesthesia is delayed following administration of atropine–neostigmine (but not glycopyrrolate–neostigmine) mixtures, which are used to antagonize the effects of nondepolarizing neuromuscular blocking drugs (Baraka et al, 1980). Furthermore, patients premedicated with atropine are more likely than patients who have received glycopyrrolate to demonstrate significant postoperative short-term memory deficit (Simpson et al, 1987).

Physostigmine, a tertiary amine anticholinesterase drug, administered in doses of 15 to 60 $\mu g \cdot kg^{-1}$ IV, is a specific treatment for the central anticholinergic syndrome. Neostigmine and pyridostigmine are not effective antidotes because the quaternary ammonium structure prevents these drugs from easily entering the central nervous system.

OVERDOSE

Deliberate or accidental overdose with an anticholinergic drug produces a rapid onset of symptoms characteristic of muscarinic cholinergic receptor blockade. The mouth becomes dry, swallowing and talking are difficult, vision is blurred, photophobia is present, and tachycardia is prominent. The skin is dry and flushed, and a rash may appear especially over the face, neck, and upper chest (blush area). Even therapeutic doses of anticholinergic drugs sometimes may selectively dilate cutaneous vessels in the blush area. Body temperature is likely to be elevated by anticholinergic drugs, especially when the environmental temperature is also increased. This increase in body temperature largely reflects inhibition of sweating by anticholinergic drugs, emphasizing that innervation of sweat glands is by sympathetic nervous system nerves that release acetylcholine as the neurotransmitter. Small children are particularly vulnerable to drug-induced elevations in body temperature with "atropine fever," occasionally occurring in this age group following administration of even a therapeutic dose of anticholinergic drug. Minute ventilation may be slightly increased due to central nervous system stimulation and the impact of an enlarged physiologic dead space due to bronchodilation. Blood gases are usually unchanged (Nunn and Bergman, 1964). Skeletal muscle weakness and orthostatic hypotension, when present, reflect nicotinic cholinergic receptor blockade. Fatal events owing to an overdose of anticholinergic drug include seizures, coma, and medullary ventilatory center paralysis.

Small children and infants seem particularly vulnerable to developing life-threatening symptoms following an overdose of anticholinergic drug. Physostigmine, administered in doses of 15 to 60 $\mu g \cdot kg^{-1}$ IV, is the specific treatment for reversal of symptoms. Because physostigmine is metabolized rapidly, repeated doses of this anticholinesterase drug may be necessary to prevent a recurrence of symptoms.

DECREASED BARRIER PRESSURE

Barrier pressure is the difference between gastric pressure and lower esophageal sphincter pressure. Administration of atropine (0.6 mg IV) or glycopyrrolate (0.2 to 0.3 mg IV) reduces lower esophageal sphincter pressure a similar amount and thus reduces barrier pressure and the inherent resistance to reflux of acidic fluid into the esophagus (Cotton and Smith, 1981). This effect may persist longer with glycopyrrolate (60 minutes) than following administration of atropine (40 minutes). It is presumed but not documented that intramuscular administration of anticholinergic drugs produces similar effects on lower esophageal sphincter pressure. The clinical significance, if any, of drug-induced decreases in lower esophageal sphincter pressure remains undocumented.

REFERENCES

Abboud T, Raya J, Sadri S, Grobler N, Stine L, Miller F. Fetal and maternal cardiovascular effects of atropine and glycopyrrolate. Anesth Analg 1983;62:426–30.

Ali-Melkkila TM, Kaila T, Kanto J, Iisalo E. Pharmacokinetics of IM glycopyrronium. Br J Anaesth 1990;64:667–9.

Bailey PL, Streisland JB, Pace NL, et al. Transdermal scopolamine reduces nausea and vomiting after outpatient laparoscopy. Anesthesiology 1990;72:922–8.

Balamoutsos NG, Drossou FR, Alevizou FR, Tjvairi E, Papastephanou C, Marios A. Pupil size during reversal of muscle relaxants. Anesth Analg 1980;59:615–6.

Baraka A, Yared J-P, Karam A-M, Winnie A. Glycopyrrolate–neostigmine and atropine–neostigmine mixtures affect postanesthetic times differently. Anesth Analg 1980;59:431–4.

Cotton BR, Smith G. Comparison of the effects of atropine and glycopyrrolate on lower oesophageal sphincter pressure. Br J Anaesth 1981;53:875–79.

Duvoisin RC, Katz RL. Reversal of central anticholinergic syndrome in man by physostigmine. JAMA 1968;206:1963–5.

Eger EI. Atropine, scopolamine and related compounds. Anesthesiology 1962;23:365–83.

Frumin MJ, Herekar VR, Jarvik ME. Amnesic actions of diazepam and scopolamine in man. Anesthesiology 1976;45:406–12.

Gal TJ, Suratt PM. Atropine and glycopyrrolate effects on lung mechanics in normal man. Anesth Analg 1981;60:85–90.

Garde JF, Aston R, Endler GC, Sison OS. Racial mydriatic response to belladonna premedication. Anesth Analg 1978;57:572–6.

Goyal RK. Muscarinic receptor subtypes. Physiology and clinical implications. N Engl J Med 1989; 321:1022–8.

Gravenstein JS, Andersen TW, DePadua CB. Effects of atropine and scopolamine on the cardiovascular system in man. Anesthesiology 1964;25:123–30.

Gross NJ. Ipratropium bromide. Engl J Med 1988; 319:486–94.

Holzgrafe RE, Vondrell JJ, Mintz SM. Reversal of postoperative reactions to scopolamine with physostigmine. Anesth Analg 1973;52:921–5.

Koski EMJ, Mattila MAK, Knapik D, et al. Double blind comparison of transdermal hyoscine and placebo for the prevention of postoperative nausea. Br J Anaesth 1990;64:16–20.

Kotelko DM, Rottman RL, Wright WC, Stone JJ, Yamashir AY, Rosenblatt RM. Transdermal scopolamine decreases nausea and vomiting following cesarean section in patients receiving epidural morphine. Anesthesiology 1989;71:675–78.

Loper KA, Ready LB, Dorman BH. Prophylactic transdermal scopolamine patches reduce nausea in postoperative patients receiving epidural morphine. Anesth Analg 1989;68:144–6.

Meyers EF, Tomeldan SA. Glycopyrrolate compared with atropine in prevention of the oculocardiac reflex during eye muscle surgery. Anesthesiology 1979;51:350–2.

Mirakhur RK. Anticholinergic drugs and anesthesia. Can J Anaesth 1988;35:443–7.

Murad SHN, Conklin KA, Tabsh KMA, Brinkman CR, Erkkola R, Nuwayhid B. Atropine and glycopyrrolate: Hemodynamic effects and placental transfer in the pregnant ewe. Anesth Analg 1981;60:710–4.

Nunn JF, Bergman NA. The effect of atropine on pulmonary gas exchange. Br J Anaesth 1964;36:68–73.

Price JA. Anisocoria from scopolamine patches. JAMA 1985;253:1561.

Proakis AG, Harris GB. Comparative penetration of glycopyrrolate and atropine across the blood brain and placental barriers in anesthetized dogs. Anesthesiology 1978;48:339–4.

Simpson KH, Smith RJ, Davies LF. Comparison of the effects of atropine and glycopyrrolate on cognitive function following general anesthesia. Br J Anaesth 1987;59:966–9.

Stoelting RK. Responses to atropine, glycopyrrolate, and Riopan of gastric fluid *p*H and volume in adult patients. Anesthesiology 1978;48:367–9.

Nonopioid and Nonsteroidal Analgesic, Antipyretic, and Antiinflammatory Drugs

Aspirin (acetylsalicylic acid) is the prototype of the nonopioid analgesic, antipyretic, and antiinflammatory drugs (Fig. 11-1). Despite great variations in chemical structure, these drugs often share therapeutic activities, side effects, and mechanisms of action.

MECHANISM OF ACTION

Aspirin-like drugs produce analgesia through their ability to inhibit activity of cyclooxygenase (prostaglandin synthetase) enzyme, leading to a decrease in the synthesis and release of prostaglandins from cells (see Fig. 20-2). The leukotriene pathway remains intact in the presence of aspirin. Inhibition of cyclooxygenase reflects the ability of aspirin to irreversibly acetylate this enzyme. For example, a 650 mg dose of aspirin will irreversibly inhibit cyclooxygenase enzyme in platelets for the life span of the platelet, which is 8 to 11 days. Aspirin is rapidly hydrolyzed to salicylic acid (orthohydroxybenzoic acid), which lacks acetylating capacity but inhibits prostaglandin synthesis by a nonacetylation mechanism.

Aspirin does not interact with opioid receptors and has little or no effect on release of histamine or serotonin. Unlike opioids, aspirin-like drugs do not produce cardiovascular effects or lead to tolerance or physical dependence.

CLINICAL USES

Aspirin and aspirin-like drugs are most often administered as (1) analgesics for the symptomatic relief of low-intensity pain associated with headache and with musculocutaneous disorders, such

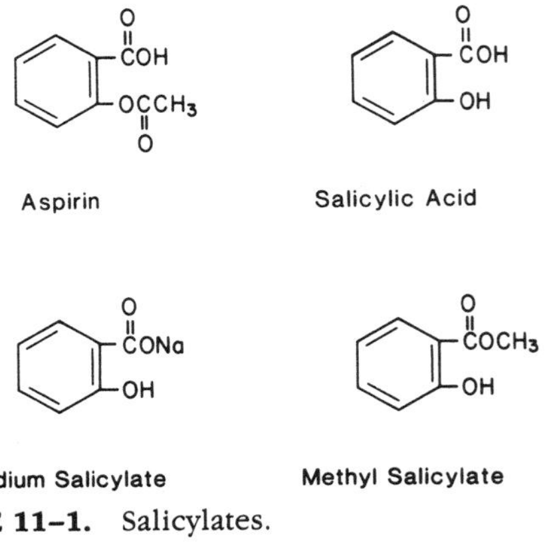

FIGURE 11–1. Salicylates.

252

as osteoarthritis and rheumatoid arthritis; (2) antipyretics; and (3) inhibitors of platelet aggregation in patients vulnerable to vascular obstruction from emboli. There is increasing interest in the use of these drugs as adjunctive therapy for acute pain states, reflecting the presumed role for soft tissue inflammation (prostaglandin release) in the etiology of postoperative pain. Indeed, aspirin seems to be effective as an analgesic only when prostaglandins are produced locally around sensitive nerve endings. Aspirin is not effective against sharp, stabbing (visceral) pain. The analgesic action of aspirin and aspirin-like drugs is confined to a small dose range, below which there is little effect and above which an increase in dose produces toxic effects with little increase in analgesia.

Aspirin, by acetylating cyclooxygenase, decreases the formation of both *thromboxane* (a potent vasoconstrictor and stimulant of platelet aggregation) and *prostacyclin* (a potent vasodilator and inhibitor of platelet aggregation) (see Chapter 20). Low doses of aspirin, 60 to 100 mg daily, selectively suppress the synthesis of platelet thromboxane without inhibiting the production of vascular prostacyclin. This selective suppression may explain the favorable effect of low doses of aspirin in women at risk for pregnancy-induced hypertension and for preventing coronary thrombosis (Benigni et al, 1989; Schiff et al, 1989).

Prostaglandins may play a role in the maintenance of a patent ductus arteriosus, and drugs that inhibit synthesis of prostaglandins, such as indomethacin, have been used with limited success in neonates to evoke closure of the ductus arteriosus (Heymann et al, 1976). Excessive production of prostaglandins is present in Bartter's syndrome and aspirin-like drugs have been used successfully in treatment (Norby, 1976).

Aspirin is effective as an antipyretic by virtue of its ability to prevent pyrogen-induced release of prostaglandins in the central nervous system including the hypothalamus. This is consistent with the known pyrogenic effect of most prostaglandins.

SALICYLATES

The two most frequently used preparations of salicylates are aspirin and salicylic acid (Fig. 11-1).

Aspirin is approximately 50% more effective and toxic than salicylic acid. Among the nonopioid analgesics, aspirin serves as the standard of comparison for analgesic, antipyretic, and antiinflammatory effects. There is often a great deal of individual variation in the response to different aspirin-like drugs, and choice of drug may be largely empirical, especially in the treatment of patients with arthritis.

Pharmacokinetics

Orally administered salicylates are rapidly absorbed from the small intestine and to a lesser extent from the stomach. Rate of absorption is influenced by dissolution rates of the administered tablets and gastric emptying time. If gastric pH is increased, salicylates are more ionized and the rate of absorption is decreased. The presence of food also delays gastric absorption of salicylates. There is no conclusive evidence that sodium bicarbonate given with aspirin (buffered aspirin) has a faster onset of action, greater peak intensity, or longer analgesic effect. In fact, alkalinization of the urine may increase urinary excretion of salicylates requiring administration of a larger dose of aspirin to achieve the same plasma concentration. Aspirin available in buffered effervescent preparations, however, undergoes more rapid systemic absorption and achieves higher plasma concentrations than the corresponding tablet formulations. These effervescent preparations also cause less gastrointestinal irritation.

Salicylates cross the blood-brain barrier slowly, reflecting the highly ionized nature of these drugs at physiologic pH. Conversely, salicylates seem to readily cross the placenta (Turner and Collins, 1975).

Protein Binding

Salicylic acid is highly bound to albumin (80% to 90%). Conversely, aspirin is less avidly bound by albumin. Salicylic acid and protein binding sites compete for thyroxine, triiodothyronine, penicillin, phenytoin, and thiopental. Aspirin-like drugs may displace other drugs such as warfarin, oral hypoglycemics, and methotrexate from protein binding sites. The interaction with warfarin is accentuated because most of the aspirin-like drugs also disturb normal platelet function.

Clearance

Aspirin absorbed into the systemic circulation is rapidly hydrolyzed in the liver to salicylic acid. As a result of this rapid hydrolysis, plasma concentrations of aspirin rarely are more than 20 $\mu g \cdot ml^{-1}$. Nevertheless, aspirin is pharmacologically active and does not require hydrolysis to salicylic acid for its effects. Metabolism of salicylic acid also occurs in the liver where the acid is conjugated with glycine to form salicyluric acid. Salicyluric acid is excreted in the urine along with free salicylic acid. Renal excretion of free salicylic acid is highly variable—from up to 85% of the ingested drug when the urine is alkaline to as low as 5% in acidic urine. Plasma concentrations of salicylic acid are increased in the presence of renal dysfunction that is characterized by decreased glomerular filtration rate or decreased secretory activity of proximal renal tubules. The elimination half-time for aspirin is approximately 15 minutes and for salicylic acid, 2 to 3 hours.

Side Effects

The numerous side effects associated with administration of salicylates include (1) gastric irritation and ulceration, (2) prolongation of bleeding time, (3) central nervous system stimulation, (4) hepatic dysfunction, (5) renal dysfunction, (6) metabolic alterations, (7) uterine effects, and (8) allergic reactions (Settipane, 1981). Epidemiologic evidence has suggested the possibility of an association between the use of aspirin in the treatment of fever in children and the development of Reye's syndrome.

Gastric Irritation and Ulceration

Salicylates may cause gastric irritation and ulceration. Reduction in prostaglandin synthesis, which normally inhibits gastric acid secretion, contributes to gastric mucosa ulceration. Resulting hemorrhage manifests as hematest positive stools and iron deficiency anemia. For example, plasma salicylate concentrations in the usual range for antiinflammatory therapy (12 to 35 $mg \cdot dl^{-1}$ produced by 4 to 5 g of aspirin daily) result in an average daily fecal blood loss of 3 to 8 ml (Leonards and Levy, 1973).

Prolongation of Bleeding Time

Aspirin-induced platelet dysfunction reflects prevention of the formation of thromboxane, which is a potent platelet aggregant. Bleeding time nearly doubles in response to 650 mg of aspirin, presumably reflecting acetylation of platelet cyclooxygenase. This inhibition lasts for the normal life span of platelets, which is 8 to 11 days. Furthermore, large doses of aspirin chronically decrease production of prothrombin, leading to prolonged prothrombin time. Aspirin should be avoided in patients with severe hepatic dysfunction, vitamin K deficiency, hypoprothrombinemia, or hemophilia because inhibition of platelet aggregation in these patients can result in hemorrhage.

Central Nervous System Stimulation

Excessive doses of salicylates (plasma concentration more than 50 $mg \cdot dl^{-1}$) produce stimulation of the central nervous system manifesting as hyperventilation and seizures. Hyperventilation is due to direct stimulation of the medullary ventilatory center. Initially, these changes result in respiratory alkalosis, which is promptly compensated for by renal excretion of bicarbonate, sodium (Na^+), and potassium ions (K^+) with return of the pH toward normal. Ultimately, however, salicylate overdose is likely to progress to metabolic and respiratory acidosis. Metabolic acidosis reflects depression of renal function with accumulation of strong metabolic acids in addition to derangement of carbohydrate metabolism, leading to an increased formation of pyruvic, lactic, and acetoacetic acids. Adults, in contrast to children, however, rarely develop metabolic acidosis regardless of the severity of the overdose. Hyperthermia and dehydration may be life-threatening results of salicylate overdose.

Tinnitus associated with elevated plasma concentrations of salicylates reflects drug-induced increases in labyrinthine pressure or an effect on hair cells of the cochlea. This side effect is the earliest sign of salicylate overdose. Nausea and vomiting are due to irritation of gastric mucosa at low doses and stimulation of the medullary chemoreceptor trigger zone by large doses.

Correction of metabolic acidosis is crucial in the treatment of salicylate overdose because a decrease in pH causes a shift of salicylic acid from plasma into the central nervous system. Metabolic alkalosis produced by the intravenous administration of sodium bicarbonate reverses the direction of transfer of salicylic acid and increases renal excretion. Diuretic-induced diuresis combined with intravenous administration of sodium bicarbonate is effective in speeding renal excretion of salicylic acid.

Hepatic Dysfunction

Salicylates can be associated with elevated plasma concentrations of transaminase enzymes indicating hepatic damage. This drug-induced hepatic dysfunction is reversible and will most likely occur when the plasma concentration of salicylates are more than 25 mg·dl^{-1}. Patients with preexisting liver disease are more likely to develop changes in hepatic function in response to salicylates. In severe salicylate intoxication, fatty infiltration of the liver and kidneys may occur.

Renal Dysfunction

Chronic use of large doses of salicylates may lead to renal papillary necrosis and chronic interstitial nephritis, often initially manifesting as reduced urine concentrating ability (Robinson, 1983). This renal effect may reflect loss of the normal function of prostaglandins in the control of renal circulation. Even small doses of salicylates negate the effects of probenecid and other uricosuric drugs.

Metabolic Alterations

Large doses of salicylates may cause hyperglycemia, glycosuria, and may deplete liver and skeletal muscle glycogen. Salicylates reduce lipogenesis by partially blocking incorporation of free fatty acids.

Uterine Effects

Prolongation of labor by salicylates may reflect loss of the normal uterotropic effects of prostaglandins. Certainly, aspirin should be discontinued before the anticipated time of parturition to avoid prolonging labor or increasing postpartum hemorrhage.

Allergic Reactions

Allergic reactions to aspirin, although rare, can be life threatening. Clinical manifestations may appear within minutes of ingestion and can include vasomotor rhinitis, laryngeal edema, bronchoconstriction, and cardiovascular collapse. Aspirin is more likely than salicylic acid to be associated with an allergic reaction. Despite the resemblance of the response to anaphylaxis, there is no evidence of an immunologic mechanism (Abrishami and Thomas, 1977). Nasal polyps develop in approximately 10% of patients who exhibit asthmatic-like allergic reactions to aspirin. Patients who are allergic to aspirin cross-react to all inhibitors of prostaglandin synthesis.

DIFLUNISAL

Diflunisal is a fluorinated salicylic acid derivative that differs chemically from salicylates but possesses analgesic, antipyretic, and antiinflammatory effects (Fig. 11-2). Like salicylates, this drug inhibits the synthesis of prostaglandins. Diflunisal, 500 to 1000 mg, is useful as an analgesic for the treatment of mild to moderate pain. Antiarthritic effects are prominent, and antipyretic actions, although present, are not clinically useful. Diflunisal also has a uricosuric effect.

Pharmacokinetics

Oral absorption of diflunisal is rapid. Like salicylic acid, diflunisal exhibits nonlinear pharmacokinetics characterized by more than a doubling of the plasma concentration when the dose is doubled. Metabolism of diflunisal is to glucuronide conjugates, which are excreted in the urine.

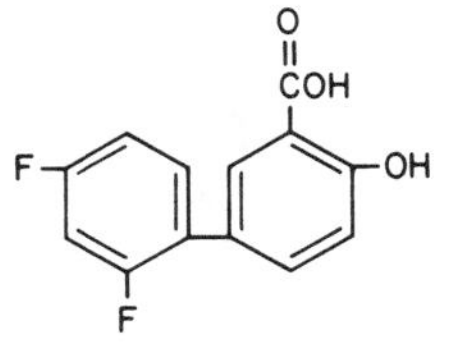

FIGURE 11–2. Diflunisal.

Side Effects

The most frequent side effects of diflunisal are nausea, vomiting, and gastrointestinal irritation. The effect of diflunisal on platelet function and bleeding time is dose-related but is reversible. Acute interstitial nephritis, perhaps due to inhibition of prostaglandin synthesis, may occur. Elevations in plasma concentrations of transaminase enzymes occur in approximately 15% of patients, but severe hepatic dysfunction associated with jaundice is rare. Drowsiness is the most common symptom observed with an overdose of diflunisal.

PHENYLBUTAZONE

Phenylbutazone is an effective antiinflammatory drug that is useful in the therapy of acute gout and treatment of rheumatoid arthritis (Fig. 11-3). Acute exacerbations of these conditions respond well to this drug, and its use should be reserved for such episodes. Phenylbutazone is an effective alternative to colchicine in acute gout, providing control in 85% of patients within 24 to 36 hours. Because of its toxicity, this drug should be given for short periods not exceeding 7 days. Certainly, phenylbutazone should not be used routinely as an analgesic or antipyretic.

Pharmacokinetics

Phenylbutazone is absorbed rapidly and completely from the gastrointestinal tract. Plasma protein binding approaches 98%. Metabolism of phenylbutazone is extensive, involving glucuronidation and hydroxylation of the phenyl rings on the butyl side chain. Oxyphenbutazone is a metabolite of phenylbutazone with antiinflammatory activity similar to the parent drug. Phenylbutazone and oxyphenbutazone are excreted

slowly in the urine because extensive plasma protein binding limits glomerular filtration. The elimination half-time of phenylbutazone is 50 to 100 hours, and significant plasma concentrations may persist in synovial spaces of joints for up to 3 weeks after treatment is discontinued.

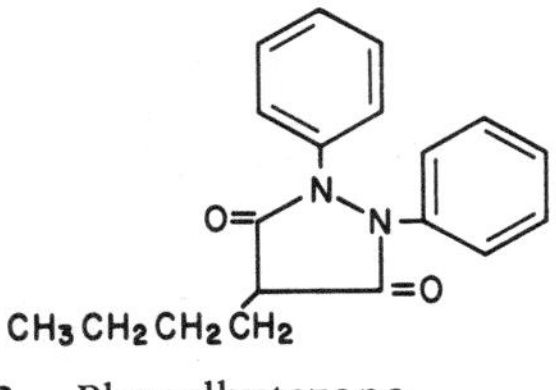

Side Effects

Serious side effects of phenylbutazone therapy are frequent and include anemia and granulocytosis, which limit the usefulness of this drug. Nausea, vomiting, epigastric discomfort, and skin rashes are frequent. Phenylbutazone causes significant Na^+ retention owing to a reversible direct effect on renal tubules. This renal tubular effect is accompanied by decreased urine output. Plasma volume increases as much as 50%, and pulmonary edema may occur in patients with poor cardiac function. Weight gain and the appearance of dilutional anemia reflect drug-induced fluid retention.

Phenylbutazone displaces drugs including warfarin, oral hypoglycemics, and sulfonamides from protein binding sites. Displacement of thyroid hormone from protein binding sites complicates interpretation of thyroid function tests. Phenylbutazone reduces uptake of iodine by the thyroid gland presumably by inhibiting synthesis of organic iodine compounds.

PARA-AMINOPHENOL DERIVATIVES

Phenacetin and its active metabolite, acetaminophen, are useful alternatives to aspirin as analgesics and antipyretics especially in patients in whom salicylates are contraindicated (those with peptic ulcer disease) or when prolongation of bleeding time would be a disadvantage (Fig. 11-4). Indeed, para-aminophenol derivatives, unlike salicylates, do not produce gastric irritation or alter aggregation characteristics of platelets. Furthermore, unlike salicylates, these drugs do not antagonize the effects of uricosuric drugs, thus permitting their administration to patients with gouty arthritis who are taking a uricosuric. Acetaminophen (325 to 650 mg orally every 4 hours in adults) has somewhat less overall toxicity and is usually preferred over phenacetin.

The antiinflammatory effects of phenacetin and acetaminophen are weak (no significant anti-

$CH_3CH_2CH_2CH_2$

FIGURE 11–3. Phenylbutazone.

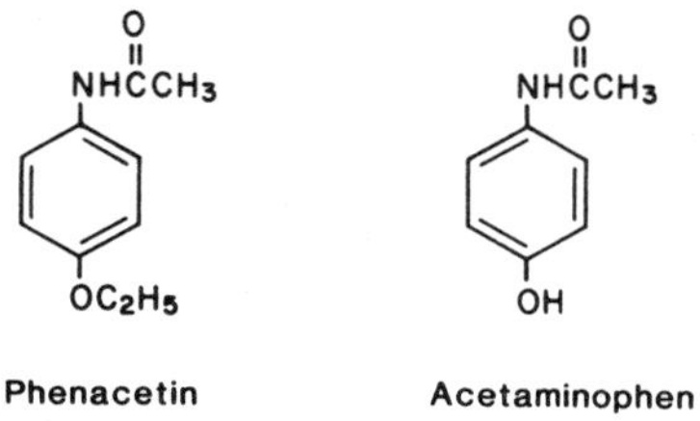

FIGURE 11-4. Para-aminophenol derivatives.

rheumatic effects), presumably reflecting the modest peripheral inhibiting effects on prostaglandin synthesis produced by these drugs. Conversely, strong central inhibition of prostaglandin synthesis confers analgesic and antipyretic effects.

Pharmacokinetics

The systemic absorption of phenacetin and acetaminophen after oral absorption is nearly complete. Significant binding to serum proteins does not occur.

Metabolism

Approximately 75% of phenacetin is dealkylated to acetaminophen in the liver. Acetaminophen is converted by conjugation and hydroxylation in the liver to inactive metabolites with only small amounts of drug being excreted unchanged. High doses of acetaminophen result in formation of *N*-acetyl-p-benzoquinone, which is believed to be responsible for hepatotoxicity. Genetically determined limitations on metabolism of phenacetin to acetaminophen result in formation of other metabolites with the potential to produce methemoglobinemia and hemolysis (see the section entitled "Side Effects").

Side Effects

Methemoglobinemia following administration of phenacetin to susceptible persons and hepatic necrosis after an overdose of acetaminophen are the most serious side effects of para-aminophenol derivatives. Patients who are allergic to salicylates may also exhibit sensitivity to these drugs. Phenacetin may produce a sedative effect. Acid-base changes do not accompany administration of phenacetin or acetaminophen.

Methemoglobinemia

Phenacetin may cause methemoglobinemia and hemolytic anemia in patients with a genetic deficiency of glucose-6-phosphate enzyme in erythrocytes. Hemolysis and subsequent jaundice associated with administration of phenacetin are presumed to be due to metabolites that oxidize glutathione and components of erythrocyte membranes, leading to shortened erythrocyte survival. Anuria may accompany severe intravascular hemolysis.

Hepatic Necrosis

Hepatic necrosis and death may accompany a single dose of acetaminophen of more than 15 g. Renal failure and hypoglycemia may also occur. Clinical manifestations of hepatic damage, including jaundice and coagulation defects, occur 2 to 6 days after the overdose. Liver biopsy reveals centrilobular necrosis. Acetylcysteine administered within the first 8 hours after an acetaminophen overdose may be effective in restoring hepatic stores of glutathione and preventing drug-induced hepatic necrosis (Smilkstein et al., 1988).

INDOMETHACIN

Indomethacin is a methylated indole derivative with analgesic, antipyretic, and antiinflammatory effects comparable with salicylates (Fig. 11-5). This drug is one of the most potent inhibitors of cyclooxygenase enzyme known. Its antiinflammatory effects are useful in the management of patients with arthritis. Indomethacin is the drug of choice in the treatment of ankylosing spondylitis and may be considered for initial therapy of Reiter's syndrome. Indomethacin provides antiinflammatory effects comparable with colchicine in the treatment of acute attacks of gouty arthritis. Conversely, indomethacin does not correct

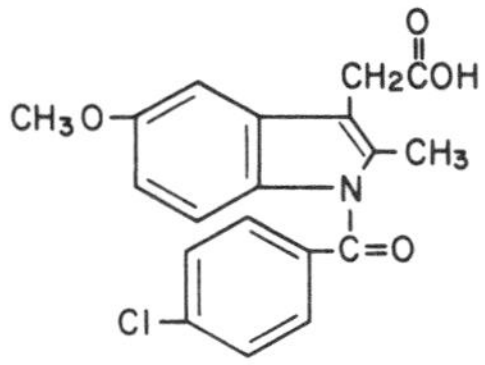

FIGURE 11-5. Indomethacin.

hyperuricemia and therefore is not useful for managing patients with chronic gout. Cardiac failure in neonates caused by patent ductus arteriosus may be controlled with a single dose of indomethacin, emphasizing the ability of this drug to selectively inhibit synthesis of prostaglandins. Indomethacin also appears to be more effective than aspirin in relieving the pain of dysmenorrhea. Finally, patients with Bartter's syndrome have been successfully treated with indomethacin as well as with other inhibitors of prostaglandin synthesis (Norby et al, 1976).

Pharmacokinetics

Indomethacin is absorbed rapidly and almost completely from the gastrointestinal tract following oral administration. Protein binding is extensive, approaching 90%. Hepatic metabolism converts indomethacin to inactive substances.

Side Effects

Severe adverse side effects limit the usefulness of this drug. Gastrointestinal disturbances and severe frontal headaches are common. Liver function tests may become abnormal and patients with preexisting renal disease may experience an exacerbation. Neutropenia, thrombocytopenia, and aplastic anemia are rare. Indomethacin inhibits platelet aggregation. Neutropenia, thrombocytopenia, and aplastic anemia are rare. Allergic reactions may occur, and cross-sensitivity with salicylates is likely.

SULINDAC

Sulindac is a substituted analogue of indomethacin and has similar analgesic, antipyretic, and antiinflammatory effects. The parent drug is inactive but is reduced to the sulfide form, which is responsible for pharmacologic effects. The active metabolite is cleared slowly from the plasma, principally into the bile, with an elimination half-time of approximately 16 hours. Side effects include inhibition of platelet aggregation, gastrointestinal irritation, renal dysfunction, and altered liver function tests.

PROPIONIC ACID DERIVATIVES

Ibuprofen, naproxen, fenoprofen, and ketoprofen are nonsteroidal propionic acid derivatives with prominent analgesic, antipyretic, and antiinflammatory effects, reflecting inhibition of prostaglandin synthesis (Fig. 11-6) (Miller, 1981). Propionic acid derivatives are as useful as salicylates in treating various forms of arthritis including osteoarthritis, rheumatoid arthritis, and acute gouty arthritis. Naproxen is unique in that its longer elimination half-time makes twice daily administration effective.

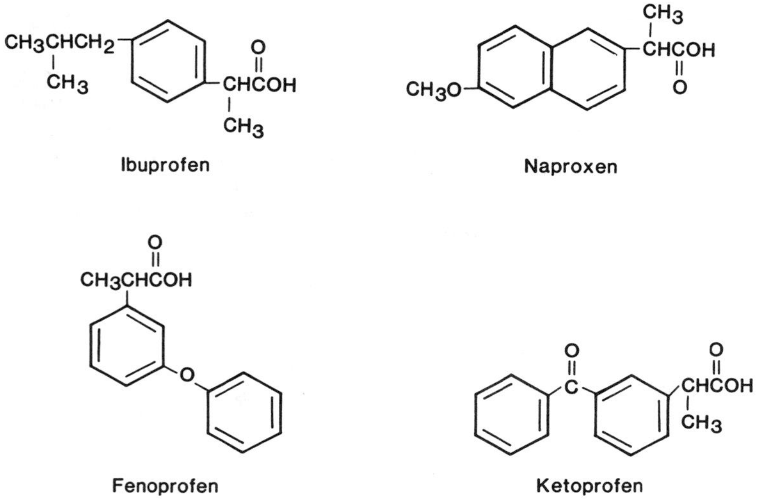

FIGURE 11-6. Propionic acid derivatives.

Gastrointestinal irritation and mucosal ulceration are usually less severe than the irritation and ulceration that may accompany administration of salicylates. Platelet function is altered similarly to that produced by salicylates. Inhibition of prostaglandin synthesis may exacerbate renal dysfunction in patients with preexisting disease in whom prostaglandins are important for maintaining renal blood flow (Robinson, 1983). Fenoprofen is most commonly associated with adverse renal effects. It should be assumed that any patient who is hypersensitive to salicylates may also be allergic to propionic acid derivatives.

Adverse drug interactions often reflect the extensive plasma protein binding to albumin of propionic acid derivatives. For example, the dose of warfarin must be reduced because of its displacement from protein binding sites as well as its alterations in platelet aggregation. Ibuprofen, however, is an exception, presumably because it occupies only a small number of binding sites on albumin. Hematopoietic suppression characterized by agranulocytosis and bone marrow granulocytic aplasia has been associated with chronic administration of ibuprofen (Mamua et al, 1986).

TOLMETIN

Tolmetin is an analgesic, antipyretic, and antiinflammatory drug that, like salicylates, causes gastric irritation and prolongs bleeding time (Fig. 11-7). It is more potent than salicylates and less potent than indomethacin or phenylbutazone. After oral administration, absorption is rapid and binding to plasma proteins is extensive (99%). Most of tolmetin is inactivated by decarboxylation.

ZOMEPIRAC

Zomepirac is a close analogue of tolmetin and possesses similar analgesic, antipyretic, and antiinflammatory properties (Fig. 11-8) (Lewis, 1981). It relieves moderate postoperative pain

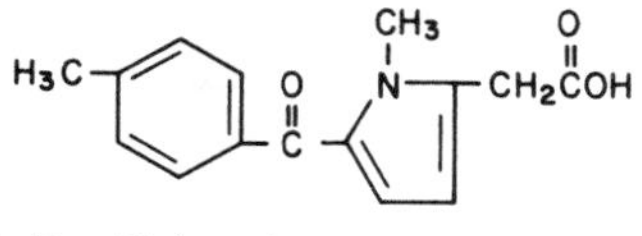

FIGURE 11–7. Tolmetin.

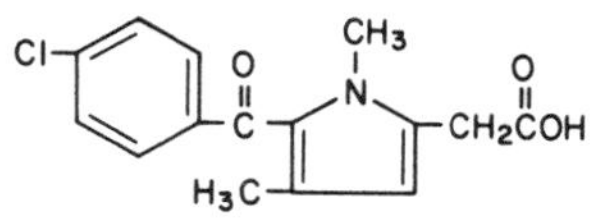

FIGURE 11–8. Zomepirac.

ably by inhibiting prostaglandin synthesis (Dunn et al, 1983). After oral administration of 100 mg, the onset of analgesia is in approximately 30 minutes with a duration of action of 4 to 6 hours. The analgesic effectiveness of zomepirac, 100 mg, is greater than codeine, 60 mg. Zomepirac reduces the need to use opioids in patients with chronic pain.

The incidence of gastrointestinal bleeding with zomepirac is less than with salicylates. Platelet adhesiveness and aggregation are decreased but, in contrast to the irreversible effects of aspirin on platelets, those of zomepirac are transient and normal function returns 24 to 48 hours after the drug is discontinued.

Zomepirac is eliminated primarily by the kidneys, and renal function should be evaluated periodically during long-term use. Allergy to salicylates is likely to manifest as cross-sensitivity with zomepirac. Although zomepirac is highly bound (98.5%) to plasma proteins, it does not interfere with the protein binding of warfarin and does not alter the prothrombin time of patients being treated with warfarin.

PIROXICAM

Piroxicam differs chemically from other nonsteroidal antiinflammatory drugs but produces similar pharmacologic effects (Fig. 11-9). Like salicylates, this drug inhibits prostaglandin synthesis. Administration of 20 mg in a single dose or in divided doses provides prolonged effects. Extensive protein binding (99%) may displace other drugs such as aspirin or oral anticoagulants from albumin binding sites.

KETOROLAC

Ketorolac is a nonsteroidal antiinflammatory drug that exhibits potent analgesic, but only moderate antiinflammatory, activity (Kenny, 1990). This drug is useful for providing postoperative analgesia both as the sole drug and to supplement

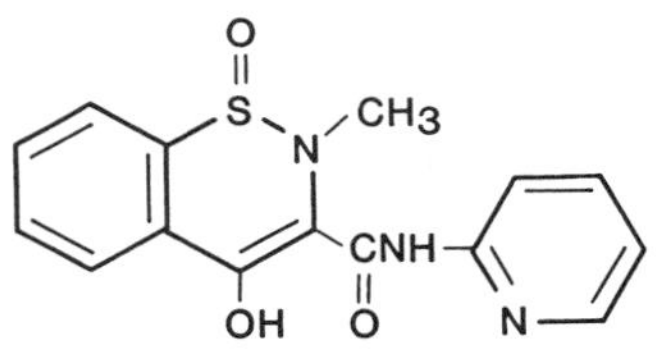

FIGURE 11–9.   Piroxicam.

opioids. Indeed, when postoperative pain is severe, some patients may require no supplementation for adequate pain control; many, however, require supplemental opioids. After intramuscular injection, maximum plasma concentrations are achieved within 45 to 60 minutes, with 30 mg of ketorolac producing analgesia equivalent to 12 mg of morphine or 100 mg of meperidine. The major benefit of ketorolac is that it does not depress ventilation or the cardiovascular system.

In common with other nonsteroidal antiinflammatory drugs, ketorolac inhibits platelet aggregation by reversible inhibition of prostaglandin synthetase. Ketorolac does increase bleeding time, but this apears to have little clinical significance. Likewise, all nonsteroidal antiinflammatory drugs can cause renal insufficiency by decreasing the synthesis of renal prostaglandins. Ketorolac, however, appears to have little potential for renal toxicity when adequate fluid balance is maintained and renal function does not depend on renal prostaglandins. Patients with congestive heart failure, hypovolemia, or hepatic cirrhosis release vasoactive substances; in these circumstances, prostaglandins are important for preventing renal arteriolar constriction, which may decrease renal blood flow. Borderline elevations of liver transaminase enzymes may occur in some patients treated with this drug.

Protein binding exceeds 99%, and clearance of this drug is decreased compared with that of opioids. Clearance is decreased further in elderly patients, and the dose of ketorolac should be less than that given to younger patients. Ketorolac is metabolized principally by glucuronic acid conjugation.

GOLD

Gold may be preferred to glucocorticoids in the treatment of rheumatoid arthritis, producing symptomatic relief most likely by its uptake into macrophages and subsequent inhibition of phagocytosis and the activities of lysosomal enzymes. Gold also reduces immunologic responses. Water-soluble gold salts are rapidly absorbed after intramuscular injection. With chronic use, gold is concentrated in the synovium of affected joints. Renal excretion accounts for 60% to 90% of the administered gold and the remainder is lost via the bile.

Side Effects

Side effects of gold involve the skin and mucous membranes, usually of the mouth. Cutaneous reactions may vary in severity from simple erythema to severe exfoliative dermatitis. Glossitis is common and may extend to the pharynx, trachea, and gastrointestinal tract. A gray to blue pigmentation (chrysiasis) may occur in the skin and mucous membranes, especially in areas exposed to light.

Thrombocytopenia is the most frequent cause of mortality and reflects accelerated degradation of platelets. Leukopenia, agranulocytosis, and aplastic anemia may also occur. Eosinophilia is common during therapy with gold. Proteinuria is frequent, reflecting damage to proximal renal tubules. Nephrosis, characterized by membranous glomerulonephritis, may develop. Rare but other serious complications of gold therapy include encephalitis, peripheral neuritis, hepatitis, and pulmonary infiltrates. Regular examination of the skin and buccal mucosa and performance of platelet counts and renal function tests are indicated to detect early gold-induced toxicity.

COLCHICINE

Colchicine reduces inflammation and thus relieves pain in acute gouty arthritis (Fig. 11-10). This drug is unique in that its beneficial antiinflammatory effects are limited to the treatment of acute attacks of gout as well as prophylaxis against such attacks. Relief of pain and inflammation usually occurs within 24 to 48 hours after oral administration. Colchicine is not an analgesic and does not provide relief of other types of pain or inflammation. Colchicine has been reported to prolong survival in patients with cirrhosis of the liver (Kershenobich et al, 1988).

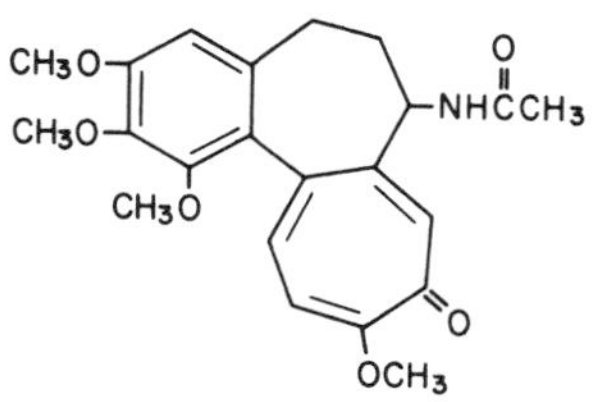

FIGURE 11–10.   Colchicine.

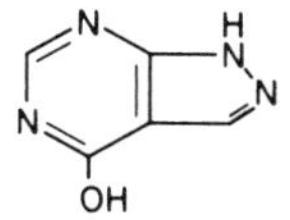

FIGURE 11–11.   Allopurinol.

Mechanism of Action

Colchicine does not influence the renal excretion of uric acid but instead alters fibrillar microtubules in granulocytes, resulting in inhibition of the migration of these cells into inflamed areas. This effect reduces the release of lactic acid and other inflammation-producing enzymes. The result is inhibition of the cycle leading to the inflammatory response evoked by crystals of sodium urate that are deposited in joint tissue. Large amounts of colchicine and its metabolites are excreted in the bile with lesser amounts appearing in the urine.

Side Effects

Nausea, vomiting, diarrhea, and abdominal pain are the most common side effects of colchicine, occurring in approximately 80% of patients. Gastrointestinal intolerance tends to protect the patient from toxic doses of colchicine. Indeed, oral administration of colchicine must be discontinued as soon as gastrointestinal symptoms appear because hemorrhagic gastroenteritis can result in severe fluid and electrolyte losses. Gastrointestinal side effects may be minimized by administering colchicine intravenously. Colchicine enhances effects produced by central nervous system depressants and sympathomimetics. The medullary ventilatory center is depressed. Severe colchicine toxicity may manifest as bone marrow depression with leukopenia and thrombocytopenia.

ALLOPURINOL

Allopurinol is the preferred drug for the therapy of primary hyperuricemia of gout and hyperuricemia that occurs during therapy with chemotherapeutic drugs (Fig. 11-11). In contrast to uricosuric drugs that facilitate renal excretion of urate, allopurinol interferes with the terminal steps of uric acid synthesis by inhibiting xanthine oxidase, the enzyme that converts xanthine to uric acid. Allopurinol is readily absorbed after oral administration and is rapidly converted to oxipurinol with more than 10% of the drug appearing unchanged in the urine. Most of the oxipurinol is excreted unchanged by the kidney. Oxipurinol is also an inhibitor of xanthine oxidase activity and has an elimination half-time of approximately 21 hours compared with 1.3 hours for allopurinol.

The most common side effect of allopurinol is maculopapular rash, frequently preceded by pruritus. Fever and myalgia may occur. These hypersensitivity-like syndromes may be due to allopurinol acting as a hapten to produce immune complex dermatitis. Pruritus is an indication to discontinue therapy with allopurinol. Allopurinol, acting as a hapten, could also result in nephritis and vasculitis. Hepatic dysfunction, ranging from increases in plasma concentrations of transaminase enzymes to hepatitis are common in patients treated with allopurinol.

Allopurinol inhibits the enzymatic inactivation of 6-mercaptopurine and azathioprine such that doses of these drugs must be reduced. Allopurinol also inhibits hepatic drug metabolizing enzymes, which may result in unexpected prolonged effects produced by drugs that are extensively metabolized, including the oral anticoagulants.

URICOSURIC DRUGS

Uricosuric drugs, such as probenecid and sulfinpyrazone, act directly on renal tubules to increase the rate of excretion of uric acid and other organic acids, including penicillin (Fig. 11-12). These drugs are also useful in controlling hyperuricemia resulting from the use of chemotherapeutic drugs or from diseases associated with the accelerated destruction of erythrocytes. Salicylates antagonize the uricosuric action of probenecid but not its capacity to inhibit the renal

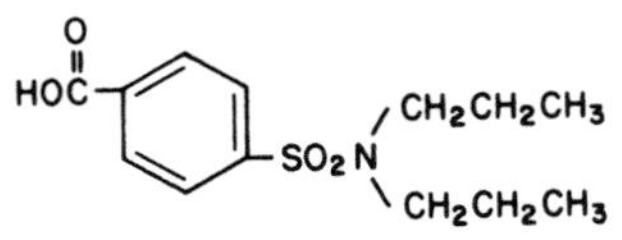

Probenecid

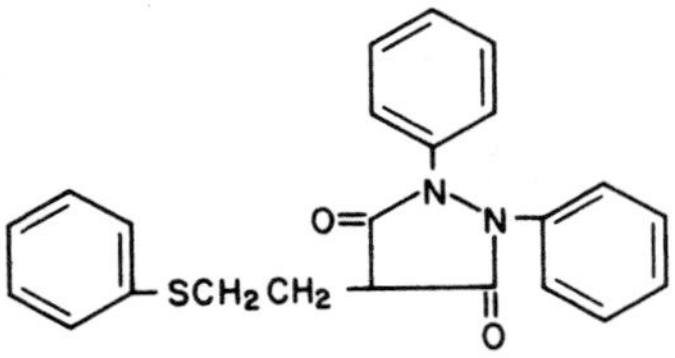

Sulfinpyrazone

FIGURE 11–12. Uricosuric drugs.

tubular excretion of penicillin. Biliary excretion of rifampin is reduced by probenecid, making it possible to achieve higher plasma concentrations of this antituberculosis drug.

Probenecid

Probenecid is completely absorbed after oral administration with peak plasma concentrations occurring in 2 to 4 hours. The elimination half-time is approximately 8 hours. Approximately 90% of probenecid is bound to plasma albumin. A total adult daily dose of 1 g of probenecid in four divided doses is necessary to block effectively the renal excretion of penicillin. Plasma concentrations of penicillin achieved in the presence of probenecid are at least twice the level achieved with the antibiotic alone.

Mild allergic reactions characterized as cutaneous rashes occur in 2% to 4% of patients treated with probenecid. This rash is a diagnostic dilemma when probenecid is administered in conjunction with penicillin. Hepatic dysfunction can occur but is rare.

Sulfinpyrazone

Sulfinpyrazone, an organic congener of phenylbutazone, lacks antiinflammatory effects but instead is a potent inhibitor of the renal tubular reabsorption of uric acid. This uricosuric action

of sulfinpyrazone is antagonized by salicylates. Renal tubular secretion of many drugs is also reduced. For example, sulfinpyrazone may induce hypoglycemia by decreasing the excretion of oral hypoglycemics.

Sulfinpyrazone is well-absorbed after oral administration. Protein binding approaches 98%. The drug undergoes secretion by proximal renal tubules because protein binding limits its glomerular filtration. Approximately 90% of sulfinpyrazone appears unchanged in the urine. The remainder of the drug is metabolized to the para-hydroxyl analogue, which also has uricosuric activity.

Gastrointestinal irritation occurs in 10% to 15% of patients treated with sulfinpyrazone, suggesting caution in the administration of this drug to patients with peptic ulcer disease. Allergic reactions, characterized by rash and fever, occur infrequently. Sulfinpyrazone inhibits platelet function.

REFERENCES

Abrishami MA, Thomas J. Aspirin intolerance—A review. Ann Allergy 1977;39:28–37.

Benigni A, Gregorini G, Frusca T, et al. Effect of low-dose aspirin on fetal and maternal generation of thromboxane by platelets in women at risk for pregnancy-induced hypertension. N Engl J Med 1989;321:357–62.

Dunn GL, Morison DH, Fargas-Babjak AM, Goldsmith CH. A comparison of zomepirac and codeine as analgesic premedicants in short-stay surgery. Anesthesiology 1983;58:265–9.

Heymann MA, Rudolph AM, Silverman NH. Closure of the ductus arteriosus in premature infants by inhibition of prostaglandin synthesis. N Engl J Med 1976;295:530–3.

Kenny GNC. Ketorolac trometamol—a new non-opioid analgesic. Br J Anaesth 1990;65:445–7.

Kershenobich D, Vargas F, Garcia-Tsao G, Tamayo RP, Gent M, Rojkind M. Colchicine in the treatment of cirrhosis of the liver. N Engl J Med 1988;318:1709–13.

Leonards JR, Levy G. Gastrointestinal blood loss during prolonged aspirin administration. N Engl J Med 1973;289:1020–2.

Lewis JR. Zomepirac sodium: New nonaddicting analgesic. JAMA 1981;246:377–9.

Mamua SW, Burton JW, Groat JD, Schulte DA, Lobell M, Zanjani ED. Ibuprofen-associated pure white-cell aplasia. N Engl J Med 1986;314:624–5.

Miller RR. Evaluation of analgesic efficacy of ibuprofen. Pharmacotherapy 1981;1:21–7.

Norby L, Flamenbaum W, Lentz R, Ramwell P. Prostaglandins and aspirin therapy in Bartter's syndrome. Lancet 1976;2:604–6.

Robinson DR. Prostaglandins and mechanism of action of anti-inflammatory drugs. Am J Med 1983;75:26–31.

Schiff E, Peleg E, Goldenberg M, et al. The use of aspirin to prevent pregnancy-induced hypertension and lower the ratio of thromboxane A_2 to prostacyclin in relatively high risk pregnancies. N Engl J Med 1989;321:351–6.

Settipane GA. Adverse reactions to aspirin and related drugs. Arch Intern Med 1981;141:328–32.

Smilkstein MJ, Knapp GL, Kulig KW, Rumack BH. Efficacy of oral *N*-acetylcystene in the treatment of acetaminophen overdose. N Engl J Med 1988;319:1557–62.

Turner G, Collins E. Fetal effects of regular salicylate ingestion in pregnancy. Lancet 1975;2:338–9.

Sympathomimetics include naturally occurring (endogenous) catecholamines, synthetic catecholamines, and synthetic noncatecholamines. Synthetic noncatecholamines are further subdivided into indirect-acting and direct-acting categories (Table 12-1). These drugs evoke physiologic responses similar to those produced by endogenous activity of the sympathetic nervous system. For example, pharmacologic effects of sympathomimetics, although quantitatively different, may include (1) vasoconstriction, especially in the cutaneous and renal circulation; (2) vasodilation in skeletal muscle; (3) bronchodilation; (4) cardiac stimulation characterized by increased heart rate; (4) myocardial contractility, and vulnerability to cardiac dysrhythmias; (5) hepatic glycogenolysis; (6) liberation of free fatty acids from adipose tissue; (7) modulation of insulin, renin, and pituitary hormone secretion; and (8) central nervous system stimulation (Lawson and Wallfisch, 1986; Smith and Corbascio, 1970; Smith and Oldershaw, 1984). The net effect of sympathomimetics on cardiac function is influenced by baroreceptor-mediated reflex responses.

CLINICAL USES

Clinically, sympathomimetics are used most often as positive inotropes to improve myocardial contractility, or as vasopressors to elevate blood pressure from unacceptably low levels that may accompany sympathetic nervous system blockade produced by regional anesthesia. A pulmonary artery catheter permitting measurement of atrial filling pressures and cardiac output as well as calculation of systemic and pulmonary vascular resistances is useful when sympathomimetics are administered as positive inotropes to improve myocardial contractility (Goldberg and Cohn, 1987). Sympathomimetics may also be used as vasopressors to maintain blood pressure during the time needed to eliminate excess inhaled anesthetic or to restore intravascular fluid volume. The prolonged administration of sympathomimetics to support blood pressure in the presence of hypovolemia is not recommended. Indeed, the only time a vasopressor should be administered is when blood pressure must be increased immediately to prevent pressure-dependent reductions in blood flow and resulting organ ischemia. Disadvantages of using sympathomimetics that lack significant beta-1 adrenergic effects to maintain blood pressure include intense vasoconstriction and associated blood pressure elevations that evoke reflex-mediated bradycardia, which lowers cardiac output.

Other uses of selected sympathomimetics include (1) treatment of bronchospasm in patients with asthma, (2) management of life-threatening allergic reactions, and (3) addition to local anesthetic solutions to retard systemic absorption of the local anesthetic (see Chapter 7).

STRUCTURE ACTIVITY RELATIONSHIPS

All sympathomimetics are derived from beta-phenylethylamine (Fig. 12-1). The presence of hydroxyl groups on the 3 and 4 positions of the benzene ring (dihydroxybenzene) of beta-phe-

Table 12-1
Classification and Comparative Pharmacology of Sympathomimetics

	Receptors Stimulated			Mechanism of Action	Cardiac Effects			Peripheral Vascular Resistance	Renal Blood Flow	Mean Arterial Pressure	Airway Resistance	Central Nervous System Stimulation	Single Intravenous Dose (70-kg adult)	Continuous Infusion Dose (70-kg adult)
	Alpha	Beta-1	Beta-2		Cardiac Output	Heart Rate	Dysrhythmias							
Natural Catecholamines														
Epinephrine	+	++	++	Direct	++	++	+++	±	--	+	--	Yes	2–8 µg	1–20 µg·min⁻¹
Norepinephrine	+++	++	0	Direct	-	-	+	+++	---	+++	NC	No	Not used	4–16 µg·min⁻¹
Dopamine	++	++	+	Direct	+++	+	+	+	+++	+	NC	No	Not used	2–20 µg·kg⁻¹ min⁻¹
Synthetic Catecholamines														
Isoproterenol	0	+++	+++	Direct	+++	+++	+++	--	-	±	---	Yes	1–4 µg	1–5 µg·min⁻¹
Dobutamine	0	+++	0	Direct	+++	+	±	NC	++	+	NC		Not used	2–10 µg·kg⁻¹ min⁻¹
Synthetic Noncatecholamines														
Indirect-Acting														
Ephedrine	++	+	+	Indirect, some direct	++	++	++	+	--	++	--	Yes	10–25 mg	Not used
Mephentermine	++	+	+	Indirect	++	++	++	+	--	++	-	Yes	10–25 mg	Not used
Amphetamines	++	+	+	Indirect	+	+	+	++	-	+	NC	Yes	Not used	Not used
Metaraminol	++	+	+	Indirect, direct	-	-	+	+++	---	+++	NC	No	1.5–5 mg	40–500 µg·min⁻¹
Direct-Acting														
Phenylephrine	+++	0	0	Direct	-	-	NC	+++	---	+++	NC	No	50–100 µg	20–50 µg·min⁻¹
Methoxamine	+++	0	0	Direct	-	-	NC	+++	---	+++	NC	No	5–10 mg	

0, none; +, minimal increase; ++, moderate increase; +++, marked increase; —, minimal decrease; ——, moderate decrease; ———, marked decrease. NC, No Change

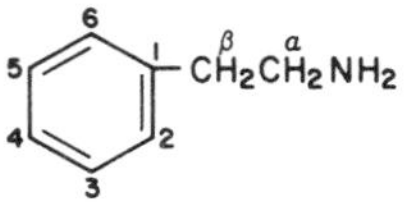

beta-phenylethylamine

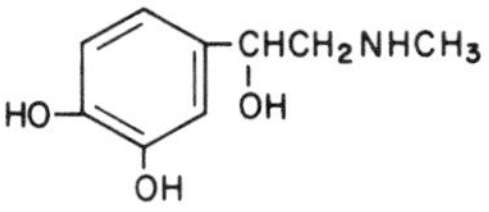

Epinephrine

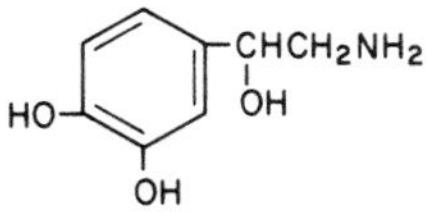

Norepinephrine

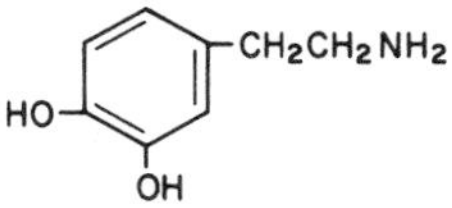

Dopamine

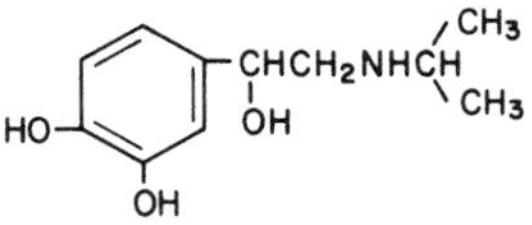

Isoproterenol

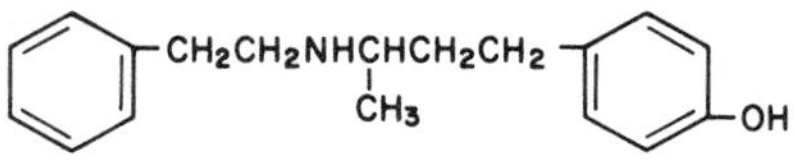

Dobutamine

FIGURE 12–1. Sympathomimetics are derived from beta-phenylethylamine, with a catecholamine being any compound that has hydroxyl groups on the 3 and 4 positions of the benzene ring.

nylethylamine is designated a catechol; drugs with this composition are designated catecholamines. For example, 3,4-dihydroxyphenylethylamine is the endogenous catecholamine dopamine. Hydroxylation of the beta carbon of dopamine results in the endogenous catecholamine and neurotransmitter norepinephrine. The third endogenous catecholamine, epinephrine, results from methylation of the terminal amine of norepinephrine. Addition of an isopropyl group rather than a methyl group to the terminal amine of norepinephrine results in the synthetic catecholamine isoproterenol. The other synthetic catecholamine, dobutamine, possesses a bulky aromatic substituent on the terminal amine. Synthetic noncatecholamines include the beta-phenylethylamine structure but lack hydroxyl groups on the 3 or 4 positions of the benzene ring (Fig. 12-2).

The dextrorotatory forms of norepinephrine and epinephrine are approximately one half as active as the levorotatory isomer. The levorotatory isomer of isoproterenol is more than 1000 times as active as the dextrorotatory isomer.

Receptor Selectivity

The relative selectivity of sympathomimetics for various adrenergic receptors depends on the chemical structure of the drug. Maximal alpha- and beta-adrenergic receptor activity depends on the presence of hydroxyl groups on the 3 and 4 positions of the benzene ring of beta-phenylethylamine (catecholamine). Epinephrine has the optimal structure for producing alpha- and beta-adrenergic effects (Fig. 12-1). Any change in chemical structure compared with epinephrine results in a compound that is less active at alpha- and beta-adrenergic receptors. Indeed, phenylephrine, which lacks the 4-hydroxyl group, is less potent than epinephrine on both alpha- and beta-adrenergic receptors (Fig. 12-2). Despite decreased potency, the removal of this 4-hydroxyl group increases the alpha-1 selectivity of phenylephrine. Substitution on the terminal amine of beta-phenylethylamine increases activity of the drug at beta receptors. For example, norepinephrine possesses minimal beta-2 agonist activity,

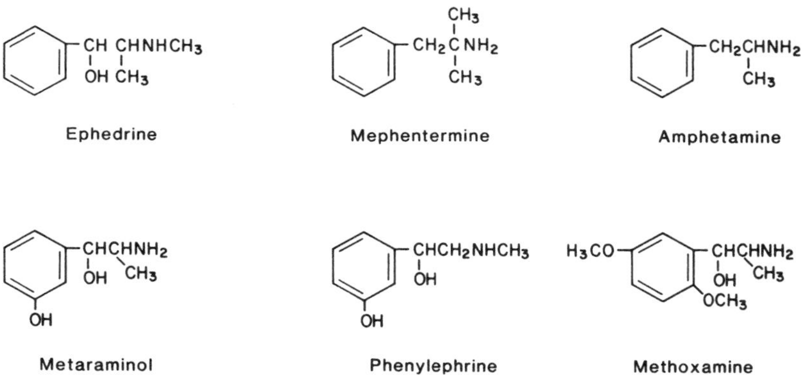

FIGURE 12–2. Indirect-acting and direct-acting synthetic noncatecholamines.

whereas this activity is greatly accentuated in epinephrine with the addition of a methyl group to the terminal amine. Beta-1 and beta-2 receptor activity is maximal in isoproterenol, which contains an isopropyl group on the terminal amine.

Hydroxyl groups in the 3 and 5 positions of the benzene ring confer selective beta-2 agonist activity on compounds with long chain substituents (Fig. 12-3). Thus, metaproterenol, terbutaline, and albuterol relax bronchial smooth muscle without evoking significant beta-1 cardiac effects.

Central Nervous System Stimulation

Central nervous system stimulation is prominent with synthetic noncatecholamines that lack substituents on the benzene ring (methamphetamine) (Fig. 12-2). Substitution of a hydroxyl

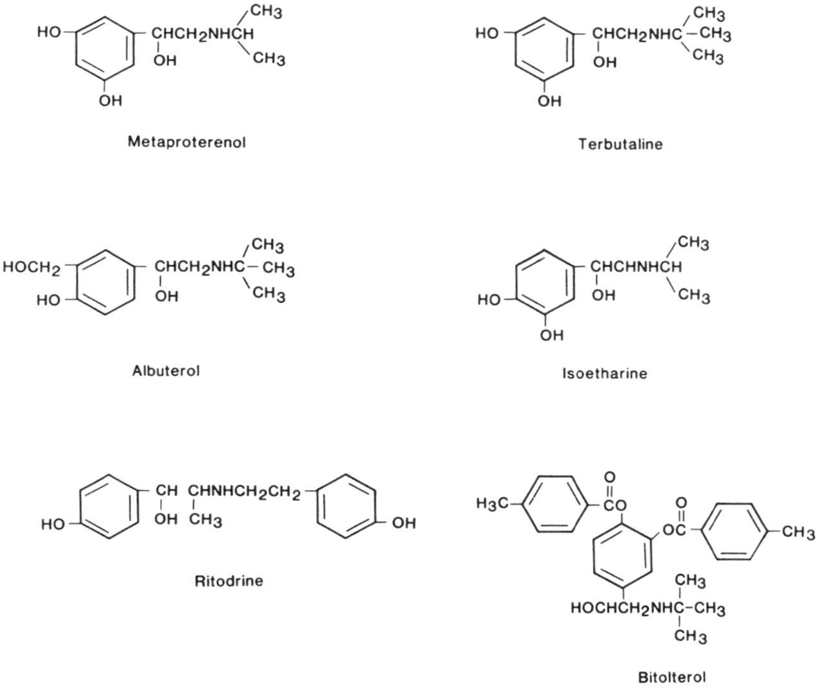

FIGURE 12–3. Selective beta-2 agonists.

group on the beta carbon of the ethylamine side chain (ephedrine) reduces central nervous system stimulant effects presumably by decreasing lipid solubility. Such a substitution, however, enhances alpha- and beta-adrenergic receptor agonist activity. Thus, ephedrine is less potent than methamphetamine as a central nervous system stimulant but is more potent as a bronchodilator and cardiac stimulant. Catecholamines have limited lipid solubility and thus are not likely to cross the blood-brain barrier in sufficient amounts to cause central nervous system stimulation.

MECHANISM OF ACTION

Sympathomimetics exert their pharmacologic effects by activating either directly or indirectly alpha-adrenergic, beta-adrenergic, or dopaminergic receptors. Production of cyclic adenosine monophosphate (cyclic AMP) by stimulating the enzyme adenylate cyclase is the speculated mechanism by which sympathomimetics produce pharmacologic effects considered to reflect beta-adrenergic receptor stimulation (Maze, 1981). For example, increased cyclic AMP stimulates protein kinases, which phosphorylate substrates and enhance inward calcium ion (Ca^{2+}) flux, which increases cytoplasmic Ca^{2+} concentrations. This increased availability of Ca^{2+} enhances the intensity of actin and myosin interaction, manifesting as more forceful myocardial contractions (beta-1 effects). Conversely, beta-2 receptor activation, characterized by relaxation of bronchial and vascular smooth muscle, reflects hyperpolarization of cell membranes and reduced inward Ca^{2+} flux. Alpha-1 receptor stimulation increases inward flux of Ca^{2+} and also probably facilitates the release of bound intracellular Ca^{2+}. Alpha-2 receptor stimulation inhibits adenylate cyclase activity. Dopamine-mediated activation of adenylate cyclase and subsequent increased intracellular concentrations of cyclic AMP is responsible for renal artery dilatation that follows activation of dopamine-1 receptors.

Cyclic AMP is often referred to as the *second messenger,* whereas the water-soluble sympathomimetic that activates adenylate cyclase to catalyze the conversion of adenosine triphosphate to cyclic AMP is referred to as the *first messenger.*

The intracellular level of cyclic AMP also is controlled by phosphodiesterase, which hydrolyzes cyclic AMP to an inactive molecule.

An important factor in the pharmacologic response elicited by a sympathomimetic is the density of alpha- and beta-adrenergic receptors in tissues. There is an inverse relationship between the concentration of available sympathomimetic and the number of receptors. For example, increased plasma concentrations of norepinephrine result in a decrease in the density of beta-adrenergic receptors in cell membranes (down regulation). Likewise, chronic treatment of patients with bronchial asthma, using a beta-2 agonist, results in tachyphylaxis, presumably reflecting decreased receptor density.

The anatomical distribution of alpha- and beta-adrenergic receptors influences the pharmacologic response evoked by sympathomimetics (Table 12-1). For example, norepinephrine has minimal effects on airway resistance because adrenergic receptors in bronchial smooth muscle are principally beta-2 receptors and are not stimulated by this catecholamine. Conversely, epinephrine and isoproterenol are potent bronchodilators as a result of their ability to activate beta-2 receptors. Cutaneous blood vessels possess alpha-adrenergic receptors, resulting almost exclusively in vasoconstriction when activated by norepinephrine or epinephrine. Smooth muscle of blood vessels supplying skeletal muscle contains both beta-2 and alpha-1 receptors such that low doses of epinephrine produce beta-mediated vasodilation and high doses produce alpha-mediated vasoconstriction, which overrides evidence of beta stimulation. Beta-1 receptors are equally responsive to epinephrine and norepinephrine, whereas beta-2 receptors are more sensitive to epinephrine than norepinephrine (Maze, 1981).

Indirect-Acting Sympathomimetics

Indirect-acting sympathomimetics are synthetic noncatecholamines that activate adrenergic receptors by evoking the release of the endogenous neurotransmitter norepinephrine from postganglionic sympathetic nerve endings (Table 12-1) (Fig 12-2). Presumably, these drugs enter postganglionic sympathetic nerve endings from which they displace norepinephrine outward into the synaptic cleft. Denervation or depletion of neurotransmitter, as with repeated doses of sympathomimetics, blunts the pharmacologic responses normally evoked by these drugs. For some synthetic noncatecholamines, such as ephedrine, pharmacologic effects may reflect combinations of direct and indirect actions.

Indirect-acting sympathomimetics are characterized mostly by alpha- and beta-1 agonist effects because norepinephrine is a weak beta-2 agonist (Table 12-1). The blood pressure response to indirect-acting sympathomimetics is reduced by drugs that decrease central sympathetic nervous system activity (Figs. 12-4 and 12-5) (Eger and Hamilton, 1959; Miller et al, 1968).

Direct-Acting Sympathomimetics

Direct-acting sympathomimetics include catecholamines and the synthetic noncatecholamines phenylephrine and methoxamine (Table 12-1) (Fig. 12-2). These sympathomimetics activate adrenergic receptors directly, although the potency of direct-acting synthetic noncatecholamines is less than that of catecholamines. Dener-

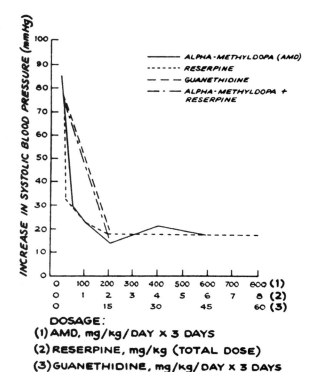

DOSAGE:
(1) AMD, mg/kg/DAY x 3 DAYS
(2) RESERPINE, mg/kg (TOTAL DOSE)
(3) GUANETHIDINE, mg/kg/DAY x 3 DAYS

FIGURE 12-5. Pretreatment with methyldopa (AMD), reserpine, or guanethidine prevents the increase in blood pressure normally evoked by intravenous administration of ephedrine. (From Miller RD, Way WL, Eger EI. The effects of alpha-methyldopa, reserpine, guanethidine, and iproniazid on minimum alveolar anesthetic requirement (MAC). Anesthesiology 1968; 29: 1153–8; with permission.)

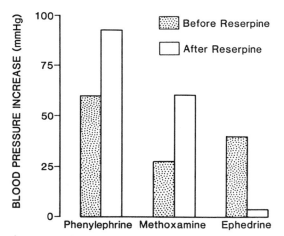

FIGURE 12-4. Reserpine blunts blood pressure elevating effects of an indirect-acting sympathomimetic (ephedrine), whereas blood pressure responses to direct-acting sympathomimetics (phenylephrine and methoxamine) are enhanced. (Data from Eger EI, Hamilton WK. The effect of reserpine on the action of various vasopressors. Anesthesiology 1959;20:641–5; with permission.)

vation or depletion of neurotransmitter does not prevent the activity of these drugs. Most direct-acting sympathomimetics activate both alpha- and beta-adrenergic receptors, but the magnitude of alpha and beta activity varies greatly among drugs from almost pure alpha-agonist activity for phenylephrine to almost pure beta-agonist activity for isoproterenol (Table 12-1).

Sympathetic nervous system blockade, which deprives alpha-adrenergic receptor sites of tonic impulses, results in increased sensitivity of these sites to norepinephrine. As a result, exaggerated blood pressure increases can follow the administration of direct-acting sympathomimetics (Fig. 12-4) (Eger and Hamilton, 1959).

METABOLISM

Catecholamines

All drugs containing the 3,4-dihydroxybenzene (catecholamine) structure are rapidly inactivated by the enzymes monoamine oxidase (MAO) or catechol-O-methyltransferase (COMT). Monoamine oxidase is an enzyme present in the liver, kidneys, and gastrointestinal tract that catalyzes oxidative deamination. Catechol-O-methyltransferase is capable of methylating a hydroxyl group of catecholamines. The resulting inactive methylated metabolites are conjugated with glucuronic acid and appear in the urine as 3-methoxy-4-hydroxymandelic acid; metanephrine (derived from epinephrine); and normetanephrine (derived from norepinephrine).

Despite the importance of enzymatic degradation of catecholamines, the biologic actions of these substances are terminated principally by uptake back into postganglionic sympathetic nerve endings. Inhibition of this uptake mechanism produces a greater potentiation of the effects of epinephrine than does inhibition of either enzyme. The completeness of this uptake mechanism and metabolism is emphasized by the appearance of only minimal amounts of unchanged catecholamines in the urine.

Circulating concentrations of dopamine and epinephrine are not altered in passage across the lungs, whereas norepinephrine is removed to a large extent (Junod, 1977). Because epinephrine traverses the lungs without change, the same concentration exists in arterial and venous blood. In animals, halothane and nitrous oxide decrease removal of norepinephrine from the blood by the lungs (Naito and Gillis, 1973). It is possible that inhaled anesthetics interfere with the amine transport system necessary to deliver norepinephrine into pulmonary cells.

Synthetic Noncatecholamines

Synthetic noncatecholamines lacking a 3-hydroxyl group are not affected by COMT and thus depend on MAO for their metabolism. Metabolism of these sympathomimetics, however, is often slower than that of catecholamines, and inhibition of MAO may even further prolong their duration of action. For this reason, patients treated with MAO inhibitors may manifest exaggerated responses when treated with synthetic noncatecholamines (see Chapter 19).

The presence of an alpha methyl group, as with ephedrine or amphetamine, inhibits deamination by MAO. Ephedrine may be excreted unchanged in the urine. Urinary excretion of unchanged drug is even greater if the urine is acidified, emphasizing the fact that many synthetic noncatecholamines have pK values greater than 9.

ROUTE OF ADMINISTRATION

Oral administration of catecholamines is not effective, presumably reflecting the metabolism of these compounds by enzymes in the gastrointestinal mucosa and liver before reaching the systemic circulation. For this reason, epinephrine is administered subcutaneously or intravenously. Dopamine and norepinephrine are administered only intravenously. Absence of one or both of the 3,4-hydroxyl groups or the presence of an alpha methyl group, as is characteristic of synthetic noncatecholamines, increases oral absorption of these drugs.

NATURALLY OCCURRING CATECHOLAMINES

Naturally occurring catecholamines are epinephrine, norepinephrine, and dopamine (Table 12-1; Fig. 12-1).

Epinephrine

Epinephrine is the prototype drug among the sympathomimetics. Its natural functions on release from the adrenal medulla include regulation of (1) myocardial contractility, (2) heart rate, (3) vascular and bronchial smooth muscle tone, (4) glandular secretions, and (5) metabolic processes such as glycogenolysis and lipolysis. It is the most potent activator of alpha-adrenergic receptors, being two to ten times more active than norepinephrine and more than 100 times more potent that isoproterenol. Epinephrine also activates beta-1 and beta-2 receptors. Oral administration is not effective because epinephrine is rapidly metabolized in the gastrointestinal mucosa and liver. Therefore, epinephrine is administered subcutaneously or intravenously. Absorption after subcutaneous injection is slow because of local vasoconstriction. Epinephrine is poorly lipid soluble, preventing its ready entrance into the central nervous system and accounting for the lack of cortical effects.

Clinical Uses

Clinical uses of epinephrine include (1) addition to local anesthetic solutions to reduce systemic absorption and prolong the duration of action of the anesthetic, (2) treatment of life-threatening allergic reactions, (3) production of course ventricular fibrillation during cardiopulmonary resuscitation, and (4) continuous intravenous infusion to increase myocardial contractility.

Cardiovascular Effects

Cardiovascular effects of epinephrine result from epinephrine-induced stimulation of alpha- and beta-adrenergic receptors (Table 12-1). Small doses of epinephrine (1 to 2 $\mu g \cdot min^{-1}$ IV) administered to adults stimulate principally beta-2 receptors in peripheral vasculature. Stimulation of beta-1 receptors occurs at somewhat greater doses (4 $\mu g \cdot min^{-1}$ IV), whereas large doses of epinephrine (10 to 20 $\mu g \cdot min^{-1}$ IV) stimulate both alpha- and beta-adrenergic receptors with the effects of alpha stimulation predominating in most vascular beds, including the cutaneous and renal circulations. A single rapid injection of epinephrine, 2 to 8 μg IV, produces transient cardiac stimulation lasting 1 to 5 minutes usually without an overshoot of blood pressure or heart rate. During continuous infusion, the concomitant administration of a vasodilator can offset epinephrine-induced vasoconstriction especially in the splanchnic and renal circulations.

Epinephrine stimulates beta-1 receptors to cause an increase in systolic blood pressure, heart rate, and cardiac output. There is a modest reduction in diastolic blood pressure, reflecting vasodilation in skeletal muscles due to activation of beta-2 receptors. The net effect of the blood pressure changes is an increase in pulse pressure and minimal change in mean arterial pressure. Because mean arterial pressure does not change greatly, there is little likelihood that baroreceptor

activation will occur to produce reflex bradycardia. Epinephrine speeds heart rate by accelerating the rate of spontaneous phase 4 depolarization, which also increases the likelihood of cardiac dysrhythmias. Increased cardiac output reflects epinephrine-induced increases in heart rate, myocardial contractility, and venous return. Repeated doses of epinephrine produce similar cardiovascular effects in contrast to tachyphylaxis that accompanies administration of synthetic noncatecholamines that evoke the release of norepinephrine.

Epinephrine predominantly stimulates alpha-1 receptors in the skin, mucosa, and hepatorenal vasculature, producing intense vasoconstriction. In skeletal muscles, epinephrine principally stimulates beta-2 receptors, producing vasodilation. The net effect of these peripheral vascular changes is preferential distribution of cardiac output to skeletal muscles and decreased systemic vascular resistance. Renal blood flow is substantially reduced by epinephrine even in the absence of changes in blood pressure. Indeed, epinephrine is estimated to be two to ten times more potent than norepinephrine for increasing renal vascular resistance. The secretion of renin is increased due to epinephrine-induced stimulation of beta receptors in the kidneys. In usual therapeutic doses, epinephrine has no significant vasoconstrictive effect on cerebral arterioles. Coronary blood flow is enhanced by epinephrine even at doses that do not alter blood pressure.

Chronic elevations in the plasma concentrations of epinephrine, as in patients with pheochromocytoma, result in a decrease of plasma volume owing to loss of protein-free fluid to the extracellular space. Arterial wall damage and local areas of myocardial necrosis may also accompany chronic circulating excesses of epinephrine. Conventional doses of epinephrine, however, do not produce these effects.

Airway Smooth Muscle

Smooth muscles of the bronchi are relaxed by virtue of epinephrine-induced activation of beta-2 receptors. This bronchodilator effect of epinephrine is converted to bronchoconstriction in the presence of beta-adrenergic blockade, reflecting activity of alpha receptors. Beta-2 stimulation, by increasing intracellular concentrations of cyclic AMP, reduces release of vasoactive mediators associated with symptoms of bronchial asthma.

Metabolic Effects

Epinephrine has the most significant effects of all the catecholamines on metabolism. Beta-1 receptor stimulation due to epinephrine increases liver glycogenolysis and adipose tissue lipolysis, whereas alpha-1 receptor stimulation inhibits release of insulin. Liver glycogenolysis results from epinephrine-induced activation of hepatic phosphorylase enzyme. Lipolysis is due to epinephrine-induced activation of triglyceride lipase, which accelerates the breakdown of triglycerides to form free fatty acids and glycerol. Intravenous infusions of epinephrine usually increase plasma concentrations of cholesterol, phospholipids, and low-density lipoproteins.

Release of epinephrine and resulting glycogenolysis and inhibition of insulin secretion is the most likely explanation for the hyperglycemia that commonly occurs during the perioperative period. In addition, epinephrine can produce inhibition of glucose uptake by peripheral tissues, which is also due, in part, to inhibition of insulin secretion. Increased plasma concentrations of lactate presumably reflect glycogenolysis is skeletal muscles due to epinephrine.

Selective beta-2 agonist effects of low-dose infusion of epinephrine ($0.05~\mu g \cdot kg^{-1} \cdot min^{-1}$ IV) are speculated to reflect activation of the sodium–potassium ($Na^+–K^+$) pump in skeletal muscles leading to transfer of K^+ into cells (Fig. 12-6) (Brown et al, 1983). This epinephrine-induced hypokalemia could contribute to cardiac dysrhythmias that occasionally accompany stimulation of the sympathetic nervous system. Conversely, epinephrine may stimulate the release of K^+ from the liver, tending to offset the decrease in extracellular concentrations of this ion produced by entrance into skeletal muscles. Among the exocrine glands, only the salivary glands respond significantly to epinephrine, producing thick, sparse secretions.

Ocular Effects

Epinephrine causes contraction of the radial muscle of the iris, producing mydriasis. Contraction of orbital muscles produces an appearance of exophthalmus considered characteristic of hyperthyroidism. Adrenergic receptors responsible for these ocular effects are probably alpha receptors because norepinephrine is less potent than epinephrine and isoproterenol has practically no ocular effects.

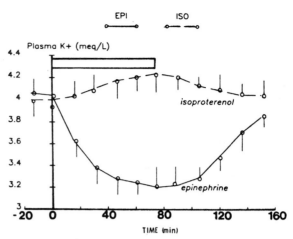

FIGURE 12–6.   Selective beta-2 agonist effects of epinephrine are responsible for stimulating the movement of potassium ions (K^+) into cells with a resulting decrease in the serum concentration of K^+. (From Brown MJ, Brown DC, Murphy MB. Hypokalemia from Beta$_2$-receptor stimulation by circulating epinephrine. N Engl J Med 1983; 309: 1414–9; with permission.)

Gastrointestinal and Genitourinary Effects

Epinephrine, norepinephrine, and isoproterenol produce relaxation of gastrointestinal smooth muscle. Activation of beta-adrenergic receptors relaxes the detrusor muscle of the bladder, whereas activation of alpha-adrenergic receptors contracts the trigone and sphincter muscles.

Coagulation

Epinephrine increases the total leukocyte count but at the same time causes eosinopenia. Blood coagulation is accelerated by epinephrine, presumably owing to increased activity of factor V.

Norepinephrine

Norepinephrine is the endogenous neurotransmitter released from postganglionic sympathetic nerve endings. It is approximately equal in potency to epinephrine for stimulation of beta-1 receptors but, unlike epinephrine, norepinephrine has little agonist effect at beta-2 receptors (Table 12-1). Norepinephrine is a potent alpha-agonist that produces intense arterial and venous vasoconstriction in all vascular beds and lacks bronchodilating effects on airway smooth muscle. Hyperglycemia is unlikely to occur as a result of norepinephrine infusion.

Cardiovascular Effects

A continuous infusion of norepinephrine, 4 to 16 $\mu g \cdot min^{-1}$ IV, may be used to treat refractory hypotension such as may occur in the early period following ligation of the vascular supply to a pheochromocytoma. Placement of norepinephrine in a 5% glucose solution provides sufficient acidity to prevent oxidation of the catecholamine. Extravasation during intravenous infusion can produce severe local vasoconstriction and possible necrosis.

Intravenous administration of norepinephrine results in intense vasoconstriction in skeletal muscles, liver, kidneys, and skin. The resulting increase in systemic vascular resistance reduces venous return to the heart and elevates systolic, diastolic, and mean arterial pressure (Table 12-1). Reduced venous return to the heart combined with baroreceptor-mediated reflex decreases in heart rate due to the marked increase in mean arterial pressure tend to reduce cardiac output despite beta-1 effects of norepinephrine. Peripheral vasoconstriction may reduce tissue blood flow so much that metabolic acidosis occurs. Chronic infusion of norepinephrine or elevated circulating concentrations of this catecholamine, as may be associated with a pheochromocytoma, cause precapillary vasoconstriction and loss of protein-free fluid to the extracellular space.

Dopamine

Dopamine is an important neurotransmitter in the central nervous system and peripheral nervous system. Dopamine-1 receptors are located postsynaptically and mediate vasodilation of renal, mesenteric, coronary, and cerebral blood vessels (Goldberg and Rajfer, 1985). Activation of these receptors is mediated by adenylate cyclase. Dopamine-2 receptors are principally presynaptic and inhibit the release of norepinephrine. Nausea and vomiting produced by dopamine reflect stimulation of dopamine-2 receptors. Dopamine receptors may be associated with the neural mechanism for "reward" that is associated with cocaine or alcohol dependence.

Rapid metabolism of dopamine mandates its use as a continuous infusion of 1 to 20 $\mu g \cdot kg^{-1}$ $\cdot min^{-1}$ IV to maintain therapeutic plasma concentrations. Dopamine should be dissolved in 5% glucose in water for intravenous administration to avoid inactivation of the catecholamine that may occur in alkaline solutions. Depending on the dose, dopamine stimulates principally dopamine-1 receptors (0.5 to 3 $\mu g \cdot kg^{-1} \cdot min^{-1}$ IV) in the renal vasculature to produce renal vasodilation, beta-1 receptors (3 to 10 $\mu g \cdot kg^{-1} \cdot min^{-1}$ IV) in the heart, and alpha receptors (greater than 10 $\mu g \cdot kg^{-1} \cdot min^{-1}$ IV) in the peripheral vasculature. Extravasation of dopamine, like norepinephrine, produces intense local vasoconstriction, which should be treated by the local infiltration of phentolamine. Dopamine is not effective orally and does not cross the blood-brain barrier in sufficient amounts to cause central nervous system effects. The immediate precursor of dopamine, L-dopa, is absorbed from the gastrointestinal tract and readily crosses the blood-brain barrier.

Clinical Uses

Dopamine is used clinically to increase cardiac output in patients with low blood pressure, increased atrial filling pressures, and low urine output. It is unique among the catecholamines in being able to simultaneously increase (1) myocardial contractility, (2) renal blood flow, (3) glomerular filtration rate, (4) excretion of Na^+, and (5) urine output. There is evidence that dopamine inhibits renal tubular solute reabsorption, suggesting that diuresis and natriuresis that frequently accompany dopamine administration may occur independently of the effect on renal blood flow (Hilberman et al, 1984). Inhibition of aldosterone secretion may contribute to increased Na^+ excretion produced by dopamine. No randomized controlled studies have demonstrated a decrease in the incidence of acute renal failure when dopamine is administered to patients considered to be at high risk for developing renal dysfunction (abdominal aorta cross-clamping or cardiopulmonary bypass) (Byrick and Rose, 1990). Hyperglycemia that is commonly present in patients receiving a continuous intravenous infusion of dopamine is likely to reflect drug-induced inhibition of insulin secretion.

Cardiovascular Effects

Dopamine increases cardiac output by stimulation of beta-1 receptors. This increase in cardiac output is usually accompanied by only modest elevations in heart rate, blood pressure, and systemic vascular resistance. A portion of the positive inotropic effect of dopamine is due to stimulation of release of endogenous norepinephrine, which may predispose to the development of cardiac dysrhythmias. Nevertheless, dopamine is less arrhythmogenic than epinephrine. The release of norepinephrine caused by dopamine may be an unreliable mechanism for increasing cardiac output when cardiac catecholamine stores are depleted as in patients in chronic cardiac failure.

Infusion rates of dopamine more than 8 $\mu g \cdot kg^{-1} \cdot min^{-1}$ IV may increase the pulmonary artery occlusion pressure despite concomitant increases in myocardial contractility (Fig. 12-7) (Hess et al, 1979). This paradoxical effect may be a reflection of reduced left ventricular compliance or increased venous return due to venous constriction. Indeed, concomitant intravenous infusion of nitroglycerin prevents the effect of high doses of dopamine on atrial filling pressure. In an animal model, both dopamine and dobutamine (up to 20 $\mu g \cdot kg^{-1} \cdot min^{-1}$ IV) produce similar increases in pulmonary vascular resistance, whereas the response to hypoxic pulmonary vasoconstriction is not altered (Lejeune et al, 1987).

Ventilation Effects

Intravenous infusion of dopamine interferes with the ventilatory response to hypoxemia, reflecting the role of dopamine as an inhibitory neurotransmitter at the carotid bodies (Ward and Belville, 1982). The result is unexpected depression of ventilation in patients who are being treated with dopamine to increase myocardial contractility. Indeed, arterial blood gases have been observed to deteriorate during intravenous infusion of dopamine (Lemaire, 1983).

SYNTHETIC CATECHOLAMINES

The two clinically useful synthetic catecholamines are isoproterenol and dobutamine (Table 12-1) (Fig. 12-1).

Isoproterenol

Isoproterenol is the most potent activator of all the sympathomimetics at beta-1 and beta-2 receptors, being two to ten times more potent than epinephrine and at least 100 times more active than norepinephrine. In clinical doses, isoproterenol is devoid of alpha-agonist effects. Metabolism of isoproterenol in the liver by COMT is rapid, necessitating a continuous intravenous infusion to maintain therapeutic plasma concentrations. Uptake of isoproterenol into postganglionic sympathetic nerve endings is minimal.

Clinical Uses

Clinical uses of isoproterenol include (1) administration intravenously or as an aerosol to produce bronchodilation, (2) continuous infusion of 1 to 5 $\mu g \cdot min^{-1}$ IV to increase heart rate in the presence of complete heart block, and (3) continuous intravenous infusion to decrease pulmonary vascular resistance in patients with pulmonary hypertension. More specific beta-2 agonists, however, have largely replaced isoproterenol as a bronchodilator.

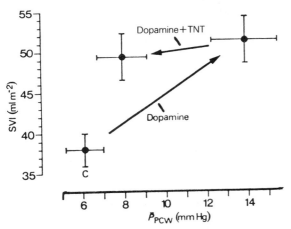

FIGURE 12–7. Plots of left ventricular function (mean ± SE) during the control period (C), during infusion of dopamine, 8 $\mu g \cdot kg^{-1} \cdot min^{-1}$ IV, and during the infusion of the combination of dopamine with nitroglycerin (*TNT*) (mean dose 0.5 $\mu g \cdot kg^{-1} \cdot min^{-1}$ IV). (From Hess W, Klein W, Mueller-Busch C, Tarnow J. Haemodynamic effects of dopamine and dopamine combined with nitroglycerine in patients subjected to coronary bypass surgery. Br J Anaesth 1979; 51: 1063–9; with permission.)

Cardiovascular Effects

Cardiovascular effects of isoproterenol reflect activation of beta-1 receptors in the heart and beta-2 receptors in the vasculature of skeletal muscles. For example, continuous infusion of isoproterenol, 1 to 5 $\mu g \cdot min^{-1}$ IV, greatly increases heart rate, myocardial contractility, and cardiac automaticity, whereas vasodilation in skeletal muscles reduces systemic vascular resistance. The net effect of these changes is an increase in cardiac output that is usually sufficient to increase systolic blood pressure. The mean arterial pressure, however, may decline due to decreases in systemic vascular resistance and associated reductions in diastolic blood pressure. Decreased diastolic blood pressure and cardiac dysrhythmias induced by isoproterenol may decrease coronary blood flow at the same time that myocardial oxygen requirements are elevated by tachycardia and increased myocardial contractility. This combination of events is undesirable in patients with coronary artery disease. Compensatory baroreceptor-mediated reflex slowing of the heart rate does not occur during infusion of isoproterenol because mean arterial pressure is not elevated.

Dobutamine

Dobutamine is a synthetic catecholamine that acts as a selective beta-1 agonist. Rapid metabolism of dobutamine dictates its administration as a continuous infusion at 2 to 10 $\mu g \cdot kg^{-1} \cdot min^{-1}$ IV to maintain therapeutic plasma concentrations. Like dopamine, dobutamine should be dissolved in 5% glucose in water for intravenous infusion to avoid inactivation of the catecholamine that may occur in an alkaline solution.

Clinical Uses

Dobutamine is used to improve cardiac output in patients in cardiac failure, particularly if heart rate and systemic vascular resistance are elevated. Combinations of drugs may be useful to increase the spectrum of activity and improve the distribution of cardiac output. For example, dobutamine may be used to increase cardiac output and a low dose of dopamine may be added to favor renal perfusion. Vasodilators may

be combined with dobutamine or dopamine to reduce afterload to optimize cardiac output in the presence of increased systemic vascular resistance.

Cardiovascular Effects

Dobutamine produces dose-dependent increases in cardiac output and reductions in atrial filling pressures without marked increases in heart rate or blood pressure. The usual small increase in heart rate compared with isoproterenol reflects a lesser effect of dobutamine on the sinoatrial node. Systemic vascular resistance may be decreased but is usually not altered greatly. Indeed, dobutamine may be ineffective in patients who require increased systemic vascular resistance rather than augmentation of cardiac output to increase blood pressure. In an animal model, both dopamine and dobutamine (up to 20 $\mu g \cdot kg^{-1} \cdot min^{-1}$ IV) produce similar increases in pulmonary vascular resistance, whereas the response to hypoxic pulmonary vasoconstriction is not altered (Lejeune et al, 1987). Conversely, in patients with increased pulmonary artery pressure following mitral valve replacement, the infusion of dobutamine (up to 10 $\mu g \cdot kg^{-1} \cdot min^{-1}$ IV) increases cardiac output and decreases systemic and pulmonary vascular resistance (Schwenzer and Miller, 1989). These changes are associated with increases in intrapulmonary shunt flow. Minimal effects on heart rate and blood pressure reduce the likelihood of adverse increases in myocardial oxygen requirements during intravenous infusion of dobutamine. Unlike dopamine, dobutamine does not act indirectly by stimulating the release of endogenous norepinephrine from the heart nor does this catecholamine activate dopaminergic receptors to increase renal blood flow. Renal blood flow, however, improves as a result of increased cardiac output.

High doses of dobutamine (more than 10 $\mu g \cdot kg^{-1} \cdot min^{-1}$ IV) may predispose to tachycardia and cardiac dysrhythmias. Nevertheless, cardiac dysrhythmias are unlikely presumably because of the absence of endogenous catecholamine release. Conduction velocity through the atrioventricular node, however, is increased by dobutamine, raising the possibility that excessive increases in heart rate could occur in patients in atrial fibrillation.

SYNTHETIC NONCATECHOLAMINES

Synthetic noncatecholamines that possess potential clinical usefulness include, but are not limited to, ephedrine, mephentermine, amphetamine, metaraminol, phenylephrine, and methoxamine (Table 12-1; Fig. 12-2) (Smith and Corbascio, 1970).

Ephedrine

Ephedrine is an indirect-acting synthetic noncatecholamine that simulates alpha- and beta-adrenergic receptors. The pharmacological effects of this drug are due in part to endogenous release of norepinephrine (indirect-acting), but the drug also has direct stimulant effects on adrenergic receptors (direct-acting). Ephedrine is resistant to metabolism by MAO in the gastrointestinal tract, thus permitting unchanged drug to be absorbed into the circulation following oral administration. Intramuscular injection of ephedrine is also acceptable because local vasoconstriction is insufficient to greatly delay systemic absorption. Up to 40% of a single dose of ephedrine is excreted unchanged in the urine. Some ephedrine is deaminate by MAO in the liver, and conjugation also occurs. The slow inactivation and excretion of ephedrine are responsible for the prolonged duration of action of this sympathomimetic.

Ephedrine, unlike epinephrine, does not produce marked hyperglycemia. Mydriasis accompanies the administration of ephedrine, and central nervous system stimulation, although less than produced by amphetamine, does occur.

Clinical Uses

Ephedrine, 10 to 25 mg IV administered to adults, is a commonly selected sympathomimetic when drug therapy is used to increase blood pressure in the presence of sympathetic nervous system blockade produced by a regional anesthetic or hypotension due to inhaled or injected anesthetics. Indeed, in an animal model, ephedrine more specifically corrects the noncardiac circulatory changes produced by spinal anesthesia than does either a selective alpha- or beta-agonist drug (Butterworth et al, 1986). Uterine blood flow is not greatly altered when ephedrine is administered to restore maternal blood pressure to normal following production of sympa-

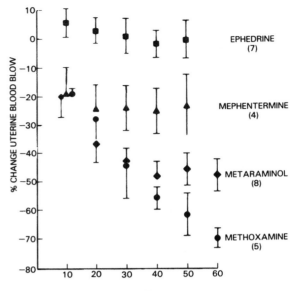

FIGURE 12–8. Ephedrine-induced increases in mean arterial pressure produce the least changes in uterine blood flow. Mephentermine has an intermediate effect, and increases in blood pressure produced by metaraminol and methoxamine result in substantial reductions in uterine blood flow. (From Ralston DH, Shnider SM, deLorimer AA. Effects of equipotent ephedrine, metaraminol, mephentermine and methoxamine on uterine blood flow in the pregnant ewe. Anesthesiology 1974; 40: 354–701; with permission.)

thetic nervous system blockade (Fig 12-8) (Ralston et al, 1974). This contrasts with selective alpha-agonists that restore blood pressure but, at the same time, decrease uterine flow because of vasoconstriction (Fig. 12-8) (Ralston et al, 1974). Ephedrine can be used as chronic oral medication to treat bronchial asthma, reflecting its bronchodilating effects by activation of beta-2 receptors. Compared with epinephrine, the onset of action of ephedrine is slow, becoming complete only 1 hour or more after administration. A decongestant effect accompanying oral administration of ephedrine produces symptomatic relief from acute coryza. Ephedrine 0.5 mg·kg⁻¹ IM has an antiemetic effect similar to droperiodol but with less sedation when administered to patients undergoing out-patient laparoscopy utilizing general anesthesia (Rothenberg et al, 1991).

Cardiovascular Effects

The cardiovascular effects of ephedrine resemble epinephrine, but its blood pressure-elevating response is less intense and lasts approximately 10 times longer. It requires approximately 250 times more ephedrine than epinephrine to produce equivalent blood pressure responses. Intravenous administration of ephedrine results in increases in systolic and diastolic blood pressure, heart rate, and cardiac output. Renal and splanchnic blood flows are decreased, whereas coronary and skeletal muscle blood flows are increased. Systemic vascular resistance may be altered minimally because vasoconstriction in some vascular beds is offset by vasodilation (beta-2 stimulation) in other areas. These cardiovascular effects are due, in part, to alpha receptor-mediated peripheral arterial and venous constriction. The principal mechanism, however, for cardiovascular effects produced by ephedrine is increased myocardial contractility owing to activation of beta-1 receptors. In the presence of preexisting beta blockade, the cardiovascular effects of ephedrine may resemble responses more typical of alpha receptor stimulation.

A second dose of ephedrine produces a less intense blood pressure response than the first dose. This phenomenon, known as tachyphylaxis, occurs with many sympathomimetics and is related to the duration of action of these drugs. Tachyphylaxis probably represents a persistent blockade of adrenergic receptors. For example, ephedrine-induced activation of adrenergic receptors persists even after blood pressure has returned to near predrug levels by virtue of compensatory cardiovascular changes. When ephedrine is administered at this time, the receptors still occupied by ephedrine limit available sites and the blood pressure response is less. Alternatively, tachyphylaxis may be due to depletion of norepinephrine stores.

Mephentermine

Mephentermine is an indirect-acting synthetic noncatecholamine that stimulates alpha- and beta-adrenergic receptors. It is closely related structurally to methylamphetamine but has only modest central nervous system-stimulating qualities. Administered intravenously, mephentermine produces cardiovascular effects that resemble ephedrine. Despite its positive inotropic effect, however, mephentermine exerts a modest antidysrhythmic effect.

Amphetamine

Amphetamine and related sympathomimetics (dextroamphetamine and methamphetamine) resemble ephedrine in evoking alpha- and beta-adrenergic receptor stimulation but differ from ephedrine in producing significant central nervous system stimulation. The central nervous system stimulant effects as well as appetite suppressant actions reflect release of norepinephrine from storage sites in the central nervous system. Tachyphylaxis is prominent, and drug dependence is predictable, considering the ability of these drugs to stimulate the central nervous system.

Acute intravenous administration of dextroamphetamine to dogs increases anesthetic requirements, presumably reflecting the release of norepinephrine into the central nervous system (Johnston et al, 1974). Conversely, chronic administration of dextroamphetamine decreases central nervous system stores of catecholamines, and anesthetic requirements may be reduced (Johnston et al, 1974). Excretion of amphetamine is negligible in alkaline urine (2% to 3%) because the drug exists predominantly in the nonionized fraction that is readily reabsorbed by renal tubules. For this reason, treatment of amphetamine overdose includes acidification of the urine.

Metaraminol

Metaraminol is a synthetic noncatecholamine that stimulates alpha- and beta-adrenergic receptors by indirect and direct effects. This sympathomimetic undergoes uptake into postganglionic sympathetic nerve endings where it substitutes for norepinephrine and acts as a weak false neurotransmitter. Indeed, chronically administered metaraminol (2 to 3 hours by continuous intravenous infusion) lowers blood pressure in hypertensive patients, reflecting the lesser vasoconstrictor potency (estimated to be one tenth) of this sympathomimetic compared with norepinephrine. Sudden withdrawal of a metaraminol infusion can lead to profound hypotension until the nerve ending stores of norepinephrine are replenished. Metaraminol is not a substrate for MAO or COMT.

Cardiovascular Effects

Metaraminol produces more intense peripheral vasoconstriction and less increase in myocardial contractility than ephedrine. Intravenous administration of metaraminol, 1.5 to 5 mg to adults, produces a sustained increase in systolic and diastolic blood pressure that is due almost entirely to peripheral vasoconstriction, emphasizing the predominant alpha-agonist effect of this sympathomimetic. Vasoconstriction decreases renal and cerebral blood flow. Reflex bradycardia often accompanies drug-induced increases in blood pressure, resulting in a decrease in cardiac output. If heart rate slowing is prevented by atropine, then metaraminol can increase cardiac output similar to ephedrine.

Phenylephrine

Phenylephrine is a synthetic noncatecholamine that stimulates principally alpha-1 adrenergic receptors by a direct effect with only a small part of the pharmacologic response being due to its ability to release norepinephrine (indirect acting). There is a minimal effect on beta-adrenergic receptors. The dose of phenylephrine necessary to stimulate alpha-1 receptors is far less than the dose that stimulates alpha-2 receptors. Resulting venoconstriction is greater than arterial constriction. Structurally, phenylephrine is 3-hydroxyphenylethylamine; it differs from epinephrine only in lacking a 4-hydroxyl group on the benzene ring. Clinically, phenylephrine mimics the effects of norepinephrine but is less potent and longer lasting. Central nervous system stimulation is minimal.

Clinical Uses

Phenylephrine, 50 to 200 μg IV, is often administered to adults to treat blood pressure decreases that accompany sympathetic nervous system blockade produced by a regional anesthetic or peripheral vasodilatation, which accompanies administration of injected or inhaled anesthetics. This drug has been used as a continuous intrave-

nous infusion (20–50 μg·min^{-1}) in adults to sustain blood pressure at normal levels during cardiopulmonary bypass or at artificially elevated levels during carotid endarterectomy. The reflex vagal effects produced by phenylephrine can be used to slow heart rate in the presence of hemodynamically significant supraventricular tachydysrhythmias. Topically applied, phenylephrine is a nasal decongestant and produces mydriasis without cycloplegia.

Cardiovascular Effects

Rapid intravenous injection of phenylephrine to patients with coronary artery disease produces dose-dependent peripheral vasoconstriction and elevations in blood pressure that are accompanied by reductions in cardiac output (Fig. 12-9) (Schwinn and Reves, 1989). Reductions in cardiac output may reflect increased afterload but more likely are due to reflex bradycardia in response to drug-induced increases in diastolic blood pressure. It is possible that reductions in cardiac output could limit the associated increases in blood pressure. Stimulation of alpha-1 receptors in the heart by phenylephrine may contribute to the production of cardiac dysrhythmias during halothane anesthesia (Hayashi et al, 1988). Renal, splanchnic, and cutaneous blood flows are reduced but coronary blood flow is increased. Pulmonary arterial pressure is elevated.

Metabolic Effects

Stimulation of alpha receptors by a continuous intravenous infusion of phenylephrine during acute K$^+$ loading interferes with the movement of K$^+$ across cell membranes into cells (Fig. 12-10) (Williams et al, 1984). Administration of phenylephrine in the absence of an acute K$^+$ load does not change the plasma concentration of K$^+$. This effect of alpha stimulation on movement of K$^+$ across cell membranes is the opposite of that produced by beta-2 stimulation (Fig. 12-6) (Brown et al, 1983).

Methoxamine

Methoxamine is a synthetic noncatecholamine that acts directly and selectively on alpha-adrenergic receptors. Beta-adrenergic receptor stimulation is absent. Methoxamine, 5 to 10 mg

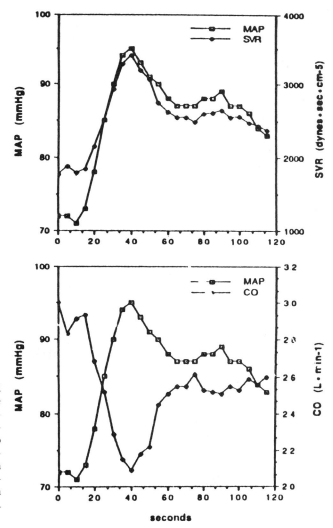

FIGURE 12–9. Hemodynamic response to rapid intravenous injection of phenylephrine in a single patient. Mean arterial pressure (MAP) and systemic vascular resistance (SVR) increase and cardiac output (CO) decreases in response to phenylephrine with peak effects occurring 42 seconds after drug administration. (From Schwinn DA, Reves JG. Time course and hemodynamic effects of alpha-1-adrenergic bolus administration in anesthetized patients with myocardial disease. Anesth Analg 1989; 68: 571–8; with permission.)

IV administered to adults, causes intense arterial vasoconstriction that manifests as increased systolic and diastolic blood pressure and baroreceptor-mediated reflex bradycardia that contributes to a reduction in cardiac output. Venoconstriction is minimal following administration of methoxamine. Renal blood flow is reduced to a greater extent than after equally potent doses of norepinephrine. Conversely, coronary blood flow may increase as a result of increased perfusion pressure and increased time for blood flow owing to reflex bradycardia. Atropine prevents reflex bradycardia and the associated decrease in cardiac

output. Methoxamine exerts a modest antidysrhythmic effect by an unknown mechanism.

SELECTIVE BETA-2 AGONISTS

Selective beta-2 agonists specifically relax bronchiole and uterine smooth muscle, but, in contrast to isoproterenol, generally lack stimulating (beta-1) effects on the heart. The chemical structure of selective beta-2 agonists (placement of hydroxyl groups on the benzene ring at sites different than catecholamines) renders them resis-

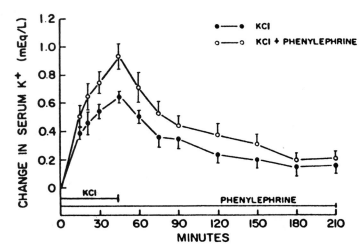

FIGURE 12-10. Plasma potassium (K^+) concentrations during the infusion of KCl increase more in patients also receiving phenylephrine. (From Williams ME, Rosa RM, Silva P, Brown RS, Epstein FH. Impairment of extrarenal potassium disposal by alpha adrenergic stimulation. N Engl J Med 1984; 311: 145–9; with permission.)

tant to methylation by COMT, thus contributing to their sustained duration of action (Figs. 12-1 and 12-3). Metaproterenol, terbutaline, albuterol, and bitolterol are the most selective beta-2 agonists and are preferred to isoetharine because they produce less direct cardiac stimulation and are longer acting (Table 12-2). These drugs are all effective when administered by metered-dose inhaler.

In acute airway obstruction, the traditional approach for rapid relief of bronchospasm has been the subcutaneous injection of epinephrine or terbutaline. It is now accepted that inhalation of beta-2 agonists (metered-dose inhalation or nebulization) is as effective as subcutaneous injection of epinephrine or terbutaline. The presence of a tracheal tube reduces by approximately 50% to 70% the amount of drug delivered by a metered-dose inhaler that reaches the trachea (Crogan and Bishop, 1989). Actuation of the metered-dose inhaler during mechanical inspiration increases the amount of drug that passes beyond the distal end of the tracheal tube. Chronic use of beta-2 agonists to treat elevated airway resistance is often associated with a fine tremor and the development of tolerance. In addition to the

Table 12-2
Comparative Pharmacology of Selective Beta-2 Agonists

	Beta-2 Selectivity	Peak Effect (min)	Duration of Action (h)	Method of Administration
Metaproterenol	+++	30–60	3–4	MDI, Solution, Oral
Terbutaline	++++	60	4	MDI, Solution, Subcutaneous
Albuterol	++++	30–60	4	MDI, Oral
Bitolterol	++++	30–60	5	MDI
Isoetharine	++	15–60	2–3	MDI, Solution
Ritodrine	++++			Intravenous, Oral

++, minimal stimulation; +++, moderate stimulation; ++++, marked stimulation.
MDI, metered-dose inhaler; Solution, solution of nebulization.

treatment of reversible bronchospasm, these drugs have been administered as continuous intravenous infusions to stop uterine contractions in premature labor (tocolytics).

Metaproterenol

Metaproterenol is a selective beta-2 agonist widely used to treat asthma. The drug may be ingested orally, after which it is excreted in the urine principally as conjugates of glucuronic acid. Administered by metered-dose inhaler, the daily dosage should not exceed 16 inhalations with each metered-aerosol actuation delivering approximately 650 μg.

Terbutaline

Terbutaline is a predominantly beta-2 agonist that may be administered orally, subcutaneously, or by inhalation to treat asthma. In general, the subcutaneous injection of terbutaline (0.25 mg) resembles epinephrine but the duration of action may be longer. The subcutaneous dosage of terbutaline may be repeated in 15 to 30 minutes, but no more than 0.5 mg should be administered in any 4-hour period. The subcutaneous dose of terbutaline for children is 0.01 mg·kg^{-1}. Administered by metered-dose inhaler, the daily dose should not exceed 16 to 20 inhalations with each metered-dose actuation delivering approximately 200 μg.

Although not marketed for prevention of premature labor, this drug was used for this purpose before the introduction of ritodrine and is still preferred by some physicians. Indeed, both drugs have equivalent effectiveness and similar potential side effects (tachycardia, pulmonary edema, hyperglycemia, or hypokalemia) when administered intravenously (Hurlbert et al, 1981; Moravec and Hurlbert, 1980; Ravindran et al 1980; Wheeler et al, 1981).

Albuterol

Albuterol is a selective beta-2 agonist that is becoming the standard for the treatment of asthma and other forms of bronchospasm. Because the effects of albuterol and volatile anesthetics such as halothane are additive, this beta-2 agonist is recommended for the treatment of bronchospasm in anesthetized patients (Tobias and Hirshman, 1990). In addition to its peripheral beta-2 agonist effects, albuterol appears to stimulate the ventilatory center. Equally effective doses of albuterol cause fewer cardiovascular side effects than most other beta-2 agonists.

Using a metered-dose inhaler, the drug is delivered by two to three deep inhalations 1 to 5 minutes apart. This may be repeated every 4 to 6 hours. The daily dosage should not exceed 16 to 20 inhalations with each metered-aerosol actuation delivering approximately 90 μg. The duration of action of the inhaled and oral forms is usually approximately 4 hours, but significant relief of symptoms may persist for up to 8 hours after an oral dose. Administered intravenously, beta-1 cardiac effects such as tachycardia begin to manifest and hypokalemia may develop.

Bitolterol

Bitolterol is a selective beta-2 agonist that resembles albuterol but is more potent and lasts longer. When inhaled, bitolterol as a prodrug is converted primarily by pulmonary esterases to the active catecholamine colterol. Cardiovascular side effects are rare. The daily dosage should not exceed 16 to 20 inhalations with each metered-aerosol actuation delivering approximately 370 μg.

Isoetharine

Isoetharine resembles isoproterenol structurally but has less beta-1 activity and produces fewer adverse affects. Used by hand nebulizer, the drug is delivered by one to two inhalations. If the therapeutic response is inadequate after 1 minute, this dose may be repeated once and every 2 to 4 hours thereafter. The metered-dose inhaler delivers approximately 340 μg with each actuation. Overall, this drug is less selective than other beta-2 agonists and its duration of action is brief.

Ritodrine

Ritodrine is the beta-2 agonist most often used to stop uterine contractions of premature labor. This action on uterine activity reflects stimulation of beta-2 receptors through activation of adenylate cyclase. Although ritodrine predominantly stimulates beta-2 receptors, it also has some beta-1 effects manifesting as tachycardia. Ritodrine is administered at doses up to 350 $\mu g \cdot min^{-1}$ IV until uterine contractions are inhibited for at least 12 hours. This is followed by oral ritodrine until delivery of a mature infant is assured. Teratogenic effects have not been shown to accompany the prenatal use of ritodrine after 20 weeks of gestation.

Ritodrine readily crosses the placenta such that cardiovascular and metabolic side effects may occur in the mother and fetus (Benedetti, 1983). Although mean arterial pressure changes little, there is a dose-related tachycardia and increase in cardiac output that most likely results from a reflex response to decreases in diastolic blood pressure combined with direct actions on cardiac beta-1 receptors. Secretion of renin is increased, leading to decreased excretion of Na^+, K^+, and water. Pulmonary edema may occur if hydration is aggressive during therapy, leading to the recommendation that total fluid intake be restricted to less than 2 L in 24 hours and that the electrocardiogram be monitored continuously (Benedetti, 1983). Evidence of cardiac disease limits the use of ritodrine as a tocolytic. Exaggerated blood pressure reductions are possible when ritodrine is given with other drugs that can cause hypotension, such as volatile anesthetics.

Maternal hypokalemia may be associated with intravenous infusion of ritodrine (Hurlbert et al, 1981; Moravec and Hurlbert, 1980). Hypokalemia presumably reflects beta-2 agonist effects that favor translocation of K^+ into the cells. Because total body K^+ stores are unaltered, treatment is not indicated. The possibility of an additive hypokalemic effect with K^+-depleting diuretics should be considered.

Ritodrine, like other beta-2 agonists, can cause marked hyperglycemia. Persistent maternal hyperglycemia may evoke sufficient insulin release to cause reactive hypoglycemia in the fetus. Administration of ritodrine to insulin-dependent diabetics has been followed by ketoacidosis despite prior subcutaneous doses of insulin. (Mordes et al, 1982). Concomitant administration of glucocorticoids to promote fetal lung maturity also is likely to aggravate the diabetic state in these patients and contribute to the beta-agonist actions of ritodrine in promoting glycogenolysis and lipolysis. Nevertheless, abrupt metabolic deterioration is not common in diabetics who receive glucocorticoids without ritodrine. Continuous infusion of insulin may be indicated in the diabetic parturient receiving intravenous ritodrine. Maximum rates of ritodrine infusion may result in at least doubling of previous insulin requirements. Oral ritodrine is not associated with an apparent increase in insulin requirements. Certainly, plasma glucose and K^+ concentrations should be monitored during intravenous administration of ritodrine.

Theophylline

Theophylline (aminophylline is theophylline in complex with ethylenediamine to increase solubility) is the most widely prescribed bronchodilator for maintenance therapy in patients with moderate or severe asthma (Fig. 12-11) (Weinberger, 1984). Administration of aminophylline (loading dose 5 $mg \cdot kg^{-1}$ IV followed by 0.5 to 1 $mg \cdot kg^{-1} \cdot h^{-1}$ IV) often is used for the initial treatment of acute exacerbations of asthma. Nevertheless, the degree of bronchodilation obtained is not different than that produced by selective beta-2 agonists. This has led some to recommend that intravenous administration of aminophylline be considered only when beta-2 agonists and corticosteroids produce an inadequate response (Rees, 1984). In addition to its bronchodilating effect, theophylline has (1) positive cardiac inotropic, (2) vasodilating, (3) diuretic, and (4) central nervous system stimulating effects (see Chapter 33). Theophylline may relax the gastroesophageal sphincter, leading to gastroesophageal reflux. The mechanism of action of theophylline is not defined precisely but may involve increased levels of cyclic AMP, modulation of Ca^{2+} transport, inhibition of adenosine receptors, and antagonism of prostaglandins (Weinberger, 1984). The protective effect of aminophylline on histamine reactivity most likely results from the release of endogenous catecholamines (Tobias et al, 1989).

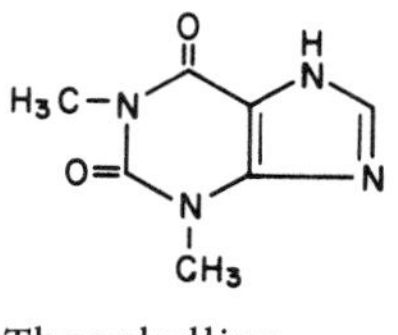

FIGURE 12–11.   Theophylline.

Therapeutic plasma concentrations of theophylline are between 10 and 20 $\mu g \cdot ml^{-1}$, with toxic responses, including cardiac dysrhythmias and seizures, becoming more prevalent at concentrations of more than 20 $\mu g \cdot ml^{-1}$. In the presence of toxic plasma concentrations of aminophylline, the subsequent administration of halothane is more likely than enflurane or isoflurane to be associated with the development of cardiac dysrhythmias. Aminophylline readily crosses the placenta and may produce toxicity in infants of mothers receiving this drug during labor.

Theophylline is metabolized by the liver and excreted by the kidneys. Frequent monitoring of plasma concentrations is indicated because there is great individual variation in rates of metabolism of theophylline. For example, metabolism is slowed in the presence of liver dysfunction due to cardiac failure or alcoholism, treatment with cimetidine, or extremes of age. Conversely, cigarette smoking speeds metabolism of theophylline. The elimination half-time of theophylline is approximately 8.7 hours in nonsmoking adults and 5.5 hours in adults who smoke.

Pentoxifylline

Pentoxifylline is a methylxanthine derivative that increases flexibility of erythrocytes and reduces viscosity of blood, thereby improving capillary blood flow and associated tissue oxygenation. Patients with intermittent claudication owing to chronic occlusive arterial disease of the limbs begin to experience improvement within 2 to 4 weeks after initiation of oral administration of pentoxifylline, 400 mg every 8 hours. This drug is neither a vasodilator nor an anticoagulant and is unrelated to aspirin or dipyridamole.

Side effects are rare but may include hypotension, angina pectoris, and cardiac dysrhythmias. Bleeding or prolonged prothrombin time may occur in the presence of anticoagulants or platelet aggregation inhibitors. Pentoxifylline is compatible with digitalis and beta-adrenergic antagonists.

REFERENCES

Benedetti TJ. Maternal complications of parenteral B-sympathomimetic therapy for premature labor. Am J Obstet Gynecol 1983;145:1–6.

Brown MJ, Brown DC, Murphy MB. Hypokalemia from Beta$_2$-receptor stimulation by circulating epinephrine. N Engl J Med 1983;309:1414–9.

Butterworth JF, Piccione W, Berribeitia LD, Dance G, Shemin RJ, Cohn LH. Augmentation of venous return by adrenergic agonists during spinal anesthesia. Anesth Analg 1986;65:612–6.

Byrick RJ, Rose DK. Pathophysiology and prevention of acute renal failure: The role of the anaesthetist. Can J Anaesth 1990;37:457–67.

Crogan SJ, Bishop MJ. Delivery efficiency of metered dose aerosols given via endotracheal tubes. Anesthesiology 1989;70:1008–10.

Eger EI, Hamilton WK. The effect of reserpine on the action of various vasopressors. Anesthesiology 1959;20:641–5.

Goldberg IF, Cohn JN. New inotropic drugs for heart failure. JAMA 1987;258:493–7.

Goldberg LI, Rajfer SI. Dopamine receptors: Applications in clinical cardiology. Circulation 1985; 72:246–52.

Hayashi Y, Sumikawa K, Tashiro C, Yoshiya I. Synergistic interaction of alpha-1 and beta adrenoreceptor agonists on induction arrhythmias during halothane anesthesia in dogs. Anesthesiology 1988;68:902–7.

Hess W, Klein W, Mueller-Busch. C, Tarnow J. Haemodynamic effects of dopamine and dopamine combined with nitroglycerin in patients subjected to coronary bypass surgery. Br J Anaesth 1979;51:1063–9.

Hilberman M, Maseda J, Stinson EB, et al. The diuretic properties of dopamine in patients following open heart operations. Anesthesiology 1984;61:489–94.

Hurlbert BJ, Edelman JD, David K. Serum potassium levels during and after terbutaline. Anesth Analg 1981;60:723–5.

Johnston PR, Way WL, Miller RD. The effect of central nervous system catecholamine-depleting drugs on dextroamphetamine-induced elevation of halothane MAC. Anesthesiology 1974;41:57–61.

Junod AF. Metabolism of vasoactive agents in lungs. Am Rev Respir Dis 1977;115:51–7.

Lawson NW, Wallfisch HK. Cardiovascular pharmacology: A new look at the pressors. In: Stoelting RK, Barash PG, Gallagher TJ, eds. Advances in Anesthesia. Chicago. Year Book Medical Publishers. 1986:195–270.

Lejeune P, Leeman M, Deloff T, Naeije R. Pulmonary hemodynamic response to dopamine and dobutamine in hyperoxic and in hypoxic dogs. Anesthesiology 1987;66:49–54.

Lemaire F. Effects of catecholamines on pulmonary right-to-left shunt. Int Anesthesiol Clin 1983; 21:43–58.

Maze M. Clinical implications of membrane receptor function in anesthesia. Anesthesiology 1981; 55:160–71.

Miller RD, Way WL, Eger EI. The effects of alpha-methyldopa, reserpine, guanethidine, and iproniazid on minimum alveolar anesthetic requirement (MAC). Anesthesiology 1968;29:1153–8.

Moravec MA, Hurlbert BJ. Hypokalemia associated with terbutaline administration in obstetrical patients. Anesth Analg 1980;59:917–20.

Mordes D, Kreutner K, Metzger W, Colwell JA. Dangers of intravenous ritodrine in diabetic patients. JAMA 1982;248:973–5.

Naito H, Gillis CN. Effects of halothane and nitrous oxide on removal of norepinephrine from the pulmonary circulation. Anesthesiology 1973;39:575–80.

Ralston DH, Shnider SM, deLorimer AA. Effects of equipotent ephedrine, metaraminol, mephentermine and methoxamine on uterine blood flow in the pregnant ewe. Anesthesiology 1974;40:354–70.

Ravindran R, Viegas OJ, Padilla LM, LaBlonde P. Anesthetic considerations in pregnant patients receiving terbutaline therapy. Anesth Analg 1980;59:391–2.

Rees J. Drug treatment in acute asthma. Br Med J 1984;288:1819–21.

Rothenberg DM, Parnass SM, Litwack K, McCarthy RJ, Newman LM. Efficacy of ephedrine in the prevention of postoperative nausea and vomiting. Anesth Analg 1991;72:58–61.

Schwenzer KJ, Miller ED. Hemodynamic effects of dobutamine in patients following mitral valve replacement. Anesth Analg 1989;68:467–72.

Schwinn DA, Reves JG. Time course and hemodynamic effects of alpha-1-adrenergic bolus administration in anesthetized patients with myocardial disease. Anesth Analg 1989;68:571–8.

Smith NT, Corbascio AN. The use and misuse of pressor agents. Anesthesiology 1970;33:58–101.

Smith LDR, Oldershaw PJ. Inotropic and vasopressor agents. Br J Anaesth 1984;56:767–80.

Tobias JD, Hirshman CA. Attenuation of histamine-induced airway constriction by albuterol during halothane anesthesia. Anesthesiology 1990;72:105–10.

Tobias JD, Kubos KL, Hirshman CA. Aminophylline does not attenuate histamine-induced airway constriction during halothane anesthesia. Anesthesiology 1989;71:723–9.

Ward DS, Belville JW. Reduction of hypoxic ventilatory drive by dopamine. Anesth Analg 1982;61:333–7.

Weinberger M. Pharmacology and therapeutic use of theophylline. J Allergy Clin Immunol 1984;73:525–40.

Wheeler AS, Patel KF, Spain J. Pulmonary edema during beta-2-tocolytic therapy. Anesth Analg 1981;60:695–6.

Williams ME, Rosa RM, Silva P, Brown RS, Epstein FH. Impairment of extrarenal potassium disposal by alpha adrenergic stimulation. N Engl J Med 1984;311:145–9.

Digitalis and Related Drugs

Digitalis is the term used for cardiac glycosides that occur naturally in many plants including the foxglove plant. Digoxin, digitoxin, and ouabain are examples of clinically useful cardiac glycosides (Fig. 13-1). Nonglycoside and noncatecholamine drugs that may be administered for similar clinical purposes as cardiac glycosides are calcium (Ca^{2+}), glucagon, amrinone, and milrinone (Fig. 13-2) (Goldenberg and Cohn, 1987).

CLINICAL USES

Cardiac glycosides are used almost exclusively to treat cardiac failure or to slow the ventricular response rate in patients with supraventricular tachydysrhythmias such as paroxysmal atrial tachycardia, atrial fibrillation, or atrial flutter (Smith and Oldershaw, 1984). These drugs are particularly useful in patients with cardiac failure that results from essential hypertension, valvular heart disease, or atherosclerotic heart disease. Digitalis preparations may not be of benefit, however, in high output cardiac failure such as that caused by hyperthyroidism or thiamine deficiency. Before administering a cardiac glycoside to treat a supraventricular dysrhythmia, it is important to confirm that the cardiac dysrhythmia is not due to digitalis toxicity.

Intravenous administration of propranolol or esmolol combined with digoxin may provide more rapid control of supraventricular tachydysrhythmias and minimize the likelihood of toxicity by permitting decreases in the dose of both drugs. Direct current cardioversion in the presence of digitalis may be hazardous because of an alleged increased risk for developing cardiac dysrhythmias including ventricular fibrillation. In approximately 30% of patients with Wolff-Parkinson-White syndrome, digitalis reduces refractoriness in the accessory conduction pathway to the point that rapid atrial impulses can cause ventricular fibrillation. Finally, digitalis may be harmful in patients with hypertrophic subaortic stenosis because increased myocardial contractility intensifies the resistance to ventricular ejection.

STRUCTURE ACTIVITY RELATIONSHIPS

The basic structure of cardiac glycosides is that of a steroid cyclopentenophenanthrene nucleus that consists of a glycone and an aglycone portion (Fig. 13-1). As such, cardiac glycosides are related chemically to bile acids and sex hormones. The glycone portion is a sugar, often glucose, but closely related sugars, such as digitoxose, may also be present. Glycones are pharmacologically inactive but are necessary to assure fixation of cardiac glycosides to cardiac muscle. It is the glycone portion of cardiac glycosides that produces the pharmacologic activity on the heart characterized as "digitalis-like."

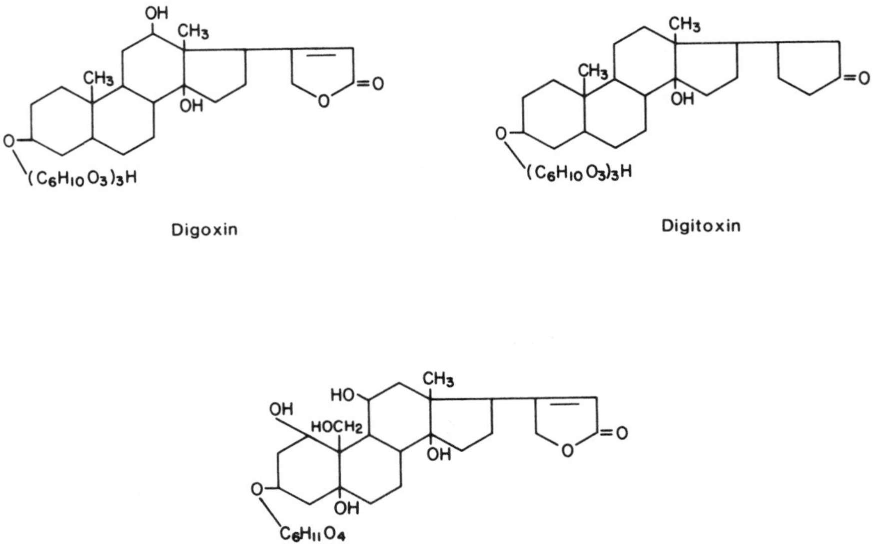

FIGURE 13-1.   Cardiac glycosides.

MECHANISM OF ACTION

The complex mechanism of the positive inotropic effect evoked by cardiac glycosides includes direct effects on the heart, which modify its electrical and mechanical activity, and indirect effects evoked by reflex alterations in autonomic nervous system activity.

Direct Effects on the Heart

The most likely explanation for the direct positive inotropic effect of cardiac glycosides is drug-induced inhibition of the sodium–potassium adenoine triphosphatase (Na^+–K^+ ATPase) ion transport system (Na^+ pump) located in cardiac cell membranes. Cardiac glycosides bind to ATPase enzyme, inducing a conformational change that interferes with outward transport of Na^+ across cardiac cell membranes. The resulting increase in Na^+ concentration in cardiac cells leads to decreased extrusion of Ca^{2+} by the Na^+ pump mechanism. It is presumed that this increased intracellular concentration of Ca^{2+} is responsible for the positive inotropic effects of cardiac glycosides. Conceptually, an increased amount of Ca^{2+} becomes available to react with contractile proteins to generate a greater force to myocardial contraction.

Many of the known effects of cardiac glycosides on the cardiac action potential can be explained on the basis of drug-induced inhibition of the Na^+–K^+ ATPase ion transport system. Indeed, this ion transport system is essential for maintaining normal gradients for Na^+ and K^+ that determine depolarization and excitability characteristics of cardiac cell membranes. For example, cardiac glycosides reduce resting transmembrane potentials and thus increase automaticity (excitability) of cardiac cells by virtue of alterations in K^+ gradients (Fig. 13-3) (Hoffman and Bigger, 1985). Automaticity is also accentuated by drug-induced increases in the slope of phase 4 depolarization. Inhibition of outward transport of Na^+ decreases

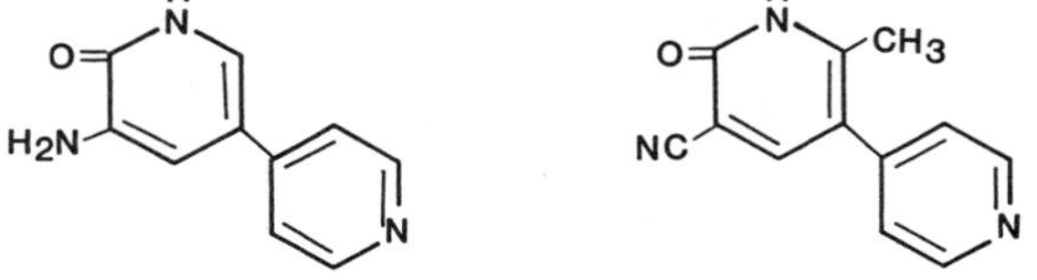

FIGURE 13-2.   Noncardiac glycosides.

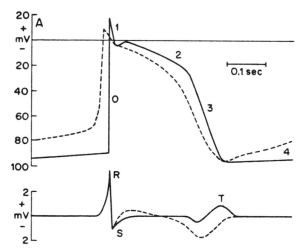

FIGURE 13–3. Schematic depiction of the effects of digitalis (----) on the transmembrane potential and electrocardiogram compared with recordings in the absence of digitalis. In the presence of digitalis, the resting transmembrane potential becomes less negative and the slope of spontaneous phase 4 depolarization is increased (automaticity is enhanced). The change in the slope and duration of phases 2 and 3 of the cardiac action potential change the S-T segment and T wave, and shorten the R-T interval, on the electrocardiogram. (From Hoffman BF, Bigger JT. Digitalis and allied cardiac glycosides. In: Gilman AG, Goodman LS, Rall TW, Murad F, eds. The Pharmacological Basis of Therapeutics, 7th ed. New York. Macmillan Publishing Co., 1987, 716; with permission.)

the slope of phase 0 of the cardiac action potential. The decrease in the duration of the cardiac action potential results largely from shortening of the duration of phase 2. Excessive digitalis-induced increases in intracellular Ca^{2+} concentrations reduce the spread of excitatory current from one myocardial cell to another, manifesting as impaired conduction of cardiac impulses.

Alterations in Autonomic Nervous System Activity

Autonomic nervous system effects of cardiac glycosides include increased parasympathetic nervous system activity owing to sensitization of arterial baroreceptors (carotid sinus) and activation of vagal nuclei and the nodose ganglion in the central nervous system. Enhanced parasympathetic nervous system activity produced by

therapeutic concentrations of digitalis decreases activity of the sinoatrial node and prolongs the effective refractory period, and thus the time for conduction of cardiac impulses through the atrioventricular node. The manifestation of these effects is a slowed heart rate, especially in the presence of atrial fibrillation. Furthermore, the relative predominance of parasympathetic to sympathetic nervous system activity produced by digitalis is consistent with suppression of ectopic cardiac pacemakers. Indirect neurally mediated effects of therapeutic concentrations of digitalis on the specialized ventricular conduction system are less important than effects on the sinoatrial and atrioventricular node.

PHARMACOKINETICS

The assay of plasma concentrations of cardiac glycosides has greatly improved the understanding of the pharmacokinetics of these drugs (Doherty, 1978). At equilibrium, the concentration of cardiac glycosides in the heart is 15 to 30 times greater than those in the plasma. The concentration of cardiac glycosides in skeletal muscle is approximately one half that in the heart.

Digoxin

Absorption of digoxin after oral administration is approximately 75% in the first hour with peak plasma concentrations occurring in 1 to 2 hours (Table 13-1) (Hoffman and Bigger, 1985). Intramuscular administration of digoxin is painful and absorption is often unpredictable. Therapeutic plasma concentrations of digoxin can be achieved rapidly with intravenous administration of the drug (up to 10 µg·kg⁻¹ over approximately 30 minutes), producing an appreciable effect in 5 to 30 minutes. Following achievement of therapeutic plasma concentrations of digoxin by either the oral or intravenous route, the maintenance oral dose is adjusted according to the individual patient's response, the electrocardiogram (ECG), and the plasma concentration of digoxin. The maintenance dose must be equal to the daily loss of drug.

Elimination of digoxin is primarily by the kidneys with approximately 35% of the drug excreted daily. In the presence of renal dysfunction, the elimination half-time of digoxin is depressed in proportion to the reduction in creatinine clearance. For example, elimination half-time of di-

Table 13-1
Comparison of Digoxin and Digitoxin

	Digoxin	Digitoxin
Average Digitalizing Dose		
Oral	0.75–1.5 mg	0.8–1.2 mg
Intravenous	0.5–1 mg	0.8–1.2 mg
Average Daily Maintenance Dose		
Oral	0.125–0.5 mg	0.05–0.2 mg
Intravenous	0.25 mg	0.1 mg
Onset of Effect		
Oral	1.5–6 h	3–6 h
Intravenous	5–30 min	30–120 min
Absorption from Gastrointestinal Tract	75%	90%–100%
Plasma Protein Binding	25%	95%
Route of Elimination	Renal	Hepatic
Enterohepatic Circulation	Minimal	Marked
Elimination Half-Time	31–33 h	5–7 days
Therapeutic Plasma Concentration	0.5–2 ng·ml^{-1}	10–35 ng·ml^{-1}

(Data from Hoffman BF, Bigger JT. Digitalis and allied cardiac glycosides. In: Gilman AG, Goodman LS, Rall TW, Murad F, eds. The Pharmacological Basis of Therapeutics, 7th ed. New York. Macmillan Publishing Co. 1985, 716, with permission.)

goxin is 31 to 33 hours in the presence of normal renal function and up to 4.4 days in the absence of renal function. A practical rule is that the dose of digoxin should be reduced by 50% when the serum creatinine concentration is 3 to 5 mg·dl^{-1} and by 75% in the absence of renal function.

The principal inactive tissue reservoir site for digoxin is skeletal muscle. A decrease in the size of this reservoir, as in elderly patients, results in increased plasma and myocardial levels of the drug. Minimal amounts of digoxin accumulate in fat. Approximately 25% of digoxin is bound to protein. Occasionally, a patient forms antibodies to digoxin, which prevents a therapeutic effect. Metabolism of digoxin is minimal, with a few patients forming the inactive metabolite dihydrogoxin.

Digitoxin

Absorption of digitoxin after oral administration is 90% to 100%, reflecting the greater lipid solubility of this cardiac glycoside compared with digoxin (Table 13-1) (Hoffman and Bigger, 1985). Digitoxin is actively metabolized by hepatic microsomal enzymes; one of these metabolites is digoxin. Approximately 10% of digoxin appears unchanged in the urine. The elimination half-time of digitoxin and its metabolites is 5 to 7 days. Hepatic disease does not appreciably alter the elimination half-time of digitoxin, emphasizing the large reserve capacity of the liver for metabolic degradation of digitoxin. Likewise, impaired renal function does not alter plasma concentrations of digitoxin. The long elimination half-time of digitoxin is an advantage for maintaining therapeutic concentrations should a patient miss several doses.

Ouabain

Ouabain is administered in doses of 1.5 to 3 µg·kg^{-1} IV to provide rapid increases in myocardial contractility or to reduce the heart rate in uncontrolled atrial fibrillation. It is unlikely, however, that ouabain offers any advantages over digoxin administered intravenously for the same reasons. The total adult intravenous dose of ouabain should not exceed 1 mg in 24 hours. Ouabain is rapidly excreted in the urine with approximately 50% of the unchanged drug being recovered in 8 hours. A longer acting digitalis preparation should be substituted for ouabain when maintenance therapy is indicated. Ouabain is not effective when administered orally, reflecting destruction of its glycoside portion in the gastrointestinal tract.

CARDIOVASCULAR EFFECTS

The principal cardiovascular effect of digitalis glycosides administered to patients with cardiac failure is a dose-related increase in myocardial contractility that becomes significant with less than full digitalizing doses. This positive inotropic effect manifests as increased stroke volume, decreased heart size, and reduced left ventricular end-diastolic pressure. Indeed, cardiac glycosides can double stroke volume from a failing and dilated left ventricle. The ventricular function curve (Frank-Starling curve) is shifted to the left (Fig. 13-4). Improved renal perfusion due to the overall increase in cardiac output favors mobilization and excretion of edema fluid, accounting for the diuresis that often accompanies the administration of cardiac glycosides to patients in cardiac failure. Excessive sympathetic nervous system activity that occurs as a compensatory response to cardiac failure is reduced with the improved circulation that accompanies administration of cardiac glycosides. The resulting decrease in systemic vascular resistance further enhances forward left ventricular stroke volume.

In addition to positive inotropic effects, cardiac glycosides enhance parasympathetic nervous system activity, leading to delayed conduction of cardiac impulses through the atrioventricular node and decreases in heart rate. The magnitude of this negative dromotropic effect depends on the preexisting activity of the autonomic nervous system. Increased parasympathetic nervous system activity decreases contractility in the atria, but direct positive inotropic effects of cardiac glycosides more than offset these negative inotropic effects on the ventricles.

Cardiac glycosides also increase myocardial contractility in the absence of cardiac failure. Nevertheless, the resulting tendency for cardiac output to increase may be offset by reductions in heart rate and direct vasoconstricting effects of cardiac glycosides on arterial, and to a lesser extent, on venous smooth muscle. Indeed, cardiac output is often unchanged or even decreased when cardiac glycosides are administered to patients with normal hearts.

ELECTROCARDIOGRAM EFFECTS

The electrophysiologic effects of therapeutic plasma concentrations of cardiac glycosides manifest on the ECG as (1) a prolonged PR interval due to delayed conduction of cardiac impulses through the atrioventricular node; (2) a shortened Q-T interval because of more rapid ventricular repolarization; (3) ST-T segment depression (scaphoid or scooped-out) due to a decreased slope of phase 3 repolarization of cardiac action potentials; and (4) diminished amplitude or inversion of the T wave. The PR interval is rarely prolonged beyond 0.25 second, and the effect on the Q-T interval is independent of parasympathetic nervous system activity. Changes in the ST segment and T wave do not correlate with therapeutic plasma concentrations of cardiac glycosides. Furthermore, ST segment and T wave changes on the ECG may suggest myocardial ischemia. When digitalis is discontinued, the changes on the ECG disappear in approximately 20 days.

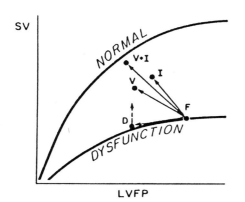

FIGURE 13–4. Cardiac glycosides shift the ventricular function curve of the failing myocardium to the left.

DIGITALIS TOXICITY

Cardiac glycosides have a narrow therapeutic range. Indeed, it is estimated that approximately 20% of patients who are being treated with cardiac glycosides experience some form of digitalis toxicity. Therapeutic effects of cardiac glycosides develop at approximately 35% of the fatal dose, and cardiac dysrhythmias typically manifest at approximately 60% of the fatal dose. The only difference between various cardiac glycosides when toxicity occurs is the duration of adverse effects.

There is general agreement that the toxic effects of cardiac glycosides result from inhibition of the Na^+–K^+ ATPase ion transport system, which leads to an accumulation of intracellular Na^+ and Ca^{2+} and a corresponding reduction in intracellular K^+. The slope of phase 4 depolarization is enhanced by digitalis, especially in the ventricles.

Causes

The most frequent cause of digitalis toxicity in the absence of renal dysfunction is the concurrent administration of diuretics that cause K^+ depletion. During anesthesia, hyperventilation of the lungs can reduce the serum K^+ concentration an average of 0.5 mEq·L^{-1} for every 10 mmHg reduction in $PaCO_2$ (Edwards and Winnie, 1977). Hypokalemia probably increases myocardial binding of cardiac glycosides, resulting in an excess drug effect. Other electrolyte abnormalities that contribute to digitalis toxicity include hypercalcemia and hypomagnesemia. An increase in sympathetic nervous system activity as produced by arterial hypoxemia increases the likelihood of digitalis toxicity. Elderly patients with decreased skeletal muscle mass and reduced renal function are vulnerable to digitalis toxicity if the usual doses of digoxin are administered. Impaired renal function and electrolyte changes (hypokalemia, hypomagnesemia) that may accompany cardiopulmonary bypass could predispose the patient to the development of digitalis toxicity.

Diagnosis

Digitalis is often administered in situations in which the toxic effects of the drug are difficult to distinguish from the effects of the cardiac disease. For this reason, determination of the plasma concentration of the cardiac glycoside may be used to indicate the likely presence of digitalis toxicity (Doherty, 1978). For example, a plasma digoxin concentration of less than 0.5 ng·ml^{-1} eliminates the possibility of digitalis toxicity. Plasma concentrations between 0.5 and 2.5 ng·ml^{-1} are usually considered therapeutic, and levels more than 3 ng·ml^{-1} are definitely in a toxic range. Infants and children have an increased tolerance to cardiac glycosides, and the range of therapeutic concentrations for digoxin is 2.5 to 3.5 ng·ml^{-1}.

It must be appreciated that the relationship between plasma concentrations and observed pharmacologic effects is not always consistent (Doherty, 1978). For example, therapeutic plasma concentrations of digoxin, despite clinical symptoms of digitalis toxicity, are frequently observed in the presence of electrolyte disturbances and recent myocardial infarction. Conversely, high therapeutic plasma concentrations of digoxin, without symptoms of digitalis toxicity, are frequently observed in the treatment of patients with supraventricular tachydysrhythmias, which require large doses to reduce the ventricular response.

Anorexia, nausea, and vomiting are early manifestations of digitalis toxicity. These symptoms, when present preoperatively in patients receiving cardiac glycosides, should arouse suspicion of digitalis toxicity. Excitation of the chemoreceptor trigger zone is the principal mechanism of the production of vomiting. Transitory amblyopia and scotomata have been observed. Pain simulating trigeminal neuralgia may be an early sign of digitalis toxicity. The extremities may also be a site of discomfort.

Electrocardiogram

There are no unequivocal features on the ECG that confirm the presence of digitalis toxicity (Smith and Haber, 1973). Nevertheless, toxic plasma concentrations of digitalis typically cause atrial or ventricular cardiac dysrhythmias (increased automaticity) and delayed conduction of cardiac impulses through the atrioventricular node (prolonged PR interval), culminating in heart block. Activity of the sinoatrial node may also be directly inhibited by high doses of cardiac glycosides. Conduction of cardiac impulses through specialized conducting tissues of the ventricles is not altered, as evidenced by the failure of even toxic plasma concentrations of digoxin to alter the duration of the QRS complex. Ventricular fibrillation is the most frequent cause of death from digitalis toxicity.

Treatment

Treatment of digitalis toxicity includes (1) correction of predisposing causes (hypokalemia or arterial hypoxemia); (2) administration of drugs (phenytoin, lidocaine, or atropine) to treat cardiac dysrhythmias; and (3) insertion of a temporary artificial transvenous cardiac pacemaker if complete heart block is present. Supplemental K^+ decreases the binding of digitalis to cardiac muscle and thus directly antagonizes cardiotoxic effects of cardiac glycosides. Serum K^+ concentrations should be determined before treatment, because supplemental K^+ in the presence of a high preexisting level of K^+ will intensify atrioventricular block and depress the automaticity of ectopic pacemakers in the ventricle, leading to complete heart block. If renal function is normal and atrioventricular conduction block is not present, it is acceptable to administer 0.025 to 0.05 $mEq \cdot kg^{-1}$ IV of K^+ rapidly to treat life-threatening cardiac dysrhythmias associated with digitalis toxicity. Phenytoin (0.5 to 1.5 $mg \cdot kg^{-1}$ IV over 5 minutes) or lidocaine (1 to 2 $mg \cdot kg^{-1}$ IV) is effective in suppressing ventricular cardiac dysrhythmias caused by digitalis; phenytoin is also effective in suppressing atrial dysrhythmias. Atropine, 35 to 70 $\mu g \cdot kg^{-1}$ IV, can be used to increase heart rate by offsetting excessive parasympathetic nervous system activity produced by toxic plasma concentrations of digitalis. Propranolol is effective in suppressing increased automaticity produced by digitalis toxicity, but its tendency to increase atrioventricular node refractoriness limits its usefulness when conduction blockade is present.

Life-threatening digitalis toxicity can be treated by administering antibodies (Fab fragments) to the drug, thus decreasing the plasma concentration of cardiac glycosides available to attach to cardiac cell membranes. The Fab-digitalis complex is eliminated by the kidneys.

PREOPERATIVE PROPHYLACTIC DIGITALIS

Preoperative prophylactic administration of digitalis to patients without signs of cardiac failure is controversial (Deutsch and Dalen, 1969; Selzer and Cohn, 1970). The obvious disadvantage of prophylactic administration of digitalis is the administration of a drug with a narrow therapeutic-to-toxic dose difference to patients with no obvious need for the drug. Furthermore, there may be difficulty in differentiating anesthetic-induced cardiac dysrhythmias from those due to digitalis toxicity (Chung, 1981). Indeed, events such as alterations in renal function, decreases in serum K^+ concentration due to hyperventilation of the lungs, and increases in sympathetic nervous system activity are likely to occur intraoperatively and thus increase the likelihood of an increased pharmacologic effect from circulating digitalis.

Despite these theoretical disadvantages, there is evidence that patients with limited cardiac reserve may benefit from prophylactic digitalis. For example, the preoperative administration of oral digoxin (0.75 mg in divided doses the day before surgery and 0.25 mg before the induction of anesthesia) reduces the occurrence of postoperative supraventricular cardiac dysrhythmias in elderly patients undergoing thoracic or abdominal surgery (Chee et al, 1982). Prophylactic administration of digoxin also reduces evidence of impaired cardiac function in patients with coronary artery disease recovering from anesthesia (Fig. 13-5) (Pinaud et al, 1983). Based on these observations, it may be reasonable to conclude that beneficial effects of prophylactic digitalis administered to appropriately selected patients in the preoperative period outweigh the potential hazards of digitalis toxicity. Certainly, there are no data to support discontinuing digitalis in any patient preoperatively, including those undergoing cardiopulmonary bypass. It is particularly important to continue digitalis therapy throughout the perioperative period in patients who are receiving the drug for heart rate control.

DRUG INTERACTIONS

Quinidine produces a dose-related increase in the plasma concentration of digoxin that be-

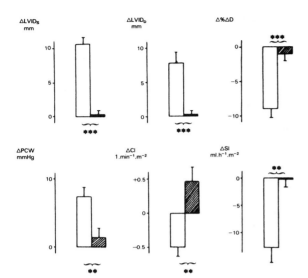

FIGURE 13–5. Preoperative and postoperative measurements (mean ± SE) of cardiac function in patients with coronary artery disease receiving (▨) or not receiving (▢) digitalis. ΔLVID$_S$, end-systolic left ventricular internal dimension; ΔLVID$_D$, end-diastolic left ventricular internal dimension; Δ%D, shortening fraction; ΔPCW, pulmonary capillary occlusion pressure; CI, change in cardiac index; ΔSI, change in stroke index. **P <0.01, ***P <0.001. (From Pinaud MLJ, Blanloeil YAG, Souron RJ. Preoperative prophylactic digitalization of patients with coronary artery disease—A randomized echocardiographic and hemodynamic study. Anesth Analg 1983; 62: 865–9; with permission.)

comes apparent within 24 hours after the first dose of the antidysrhythmic drug. This effect of quinidine may be due to displacement of digoxin from binding sites in tissues.

Succinylcholine, or any other drug that can abruptly increase parasympathetic nervous system activity, could theoretically have an additive effect with cardiac glycosides. Cardiac dysrhythmias also could reflect succinylcholine-induced catecholamine release and resulting cardiac irritability. Despite these theoretical concerns, clinical experience does not support the occurrence of an increased incidence of cardiac dysrhythmias in patients being treated with cardiac glycosides and receiving succinylcholine (Bartolone and Rao, 1983).

Sympathomimetics with beta-adrenergic agonist effects as well as pancuronium may increase the likelihood of cardiac dysrhythmias in the presence of cardiac glycosides (Bartolone and Rao, 1983). Ca^{2+} may precipitate cardiac dysrhythmias in patients receiving cardiac glycosides. Any drug that facilitates renal loss of K$^+$ increases the likelihood of hypokalemia and associated digitalis toxicity. The simultaneous administration of an oral antacid and digitalis decreases the gastrointestinal absorption of cardiac glycosides. Halothane can antagonize digitalis-induced cardiac dysrhythmias (Morrow and Townley, 1964). Fentanyl, enflurane, and, to a lesser extent, isoflurane protect against digitalis-enhanced cardiac automaticity (Ivankovich et al, 1976).

NONCATECHOLAMINE NONGLYCERIDE CARDIAC INOTROPES

Calcium

Ca^{2+}, when injected intravenously, produces an intense positive inotropic effect lasting 10 to 20 minutes and manifesting as increases in stroke volume and decreases in left ventricular end-diastolic pressure (Denlinger et al, 1975). Heart rate and systemic vascular resistance decrease. The inotropic effects of Ca^{2+} are enhanced in the presence of preexisting hypocalcemia. The risk of cardiac dysrhythmias when Ca^{2+} is administered to patients receiving digitalis should be considered, especially if hypokalemia is also present.

Calcium chloride, 5 to 10 mg·kg^{-1} IV to adults, is often used to improve myocardial contractility and stroke volume at the conclusion of cardiopulmonary bypass. Indeed, myocardial contractility at the conclusion of cardiopulmonary bypass may be depressed by hypocalcemia owing to (1) use of K$^+$-containing cardioplegia solutions, (2) administration of citrated stored whole blood, and (3) treatment of metabolic acidosis with sodium bicarbonate. A 10% solution of calcium chloride contains more Ca^{2+} than a 10% calcium gluconate solution does, although the availability of ionized Ca^{2+} is prompt regardless of the preparation administered (see Chapter 35).

Glucagon

Glucagon is a polypeptide hormone produced by alpha cells of the pancreas. Like catecholamines, glucagon enhances formation of cyclic adenosine monophosphate (cyclic AMP), but, unlike catecholamines, does not act via beta-adrenergic receptors. Inhibition of phosphodiesterase enzyme does not occur. Glucagon also evokes the release of catecholamines, but this is not the predominant mechanism of its cardiovascular effects. The principal cardiac indication for glucagon is to increase myocardial contractility and heart rate in the presence of intense drug-induced beta-adrenergic blockade. Because glucagon is a peptide, it must be administered intravenously or intramuscularly.

Cardiovascular Effects

In adults, glucagon, as a rapid injection (1 to 5 mg IV) or as a continuous intravenous infusion (20 mg·h^{-1}) reliably increases stroke volume and heart rate independent of adrenergic receptor activation. Tachycardia, however, may be sufficiently great to interfere with the augmented cardiac output. Abrupt increases in heart rate can occur when glucagon is administered to patients in atrial fibrillation. Mean arterial pressure may increase modestly, whereas systemic vascular resistance is unchanged or reduced. In contrast to other sympathomimetics, glucagon enhances automaticity in the sinoatrial and atrioventricular nodes without increasing automaticity in the ventricle. The renal effect is similar to that of dopamine, but glucagon is less potent. In contrast to these acute cardiovascular effects, the chronic administration of glucagon is not effective in evoking sustained positive inotropic and chronotropic effects.

Side Effects

In awake patients, intravenous administration of glucagon often evokes nausea and vomiting. Hyperglycemia is a predictable effect following intravenous administration of glucagon. Paradoxical hypoglycemia may occur in patients lacking sufficient hepatic glycogen stores to offset the increased insulin release caused by glucagon. Hypokalemia reflects increased secretion of insulin and subsequent intracellular transfer of glucose and K$^+$. Glucagon stimulates release of catecholamines and could evoke hypertension in a patient with an unrecognized pheochromocytoma. In this regard, glucagon, 1 to 2 mg IV,

may be used as a provocative test in the differential diagnosis of pheochromocytoma. This dose of glucagon will evoke a three-fold or greater increase in the plasma concentrations of catecholamines 1 to 3 minutes following administration to a patient with pheochromocytoma. A simultaneous increase in blood pressure of at least 20/15 mmHg is also likely.

Amrinone

Amrinone is a noncatecholamine nonglycoside bipyridine derivative that produces dose-dependent positive inotropic and vasodilator effects manifesting as increased cardiac output and decreased left ventricular end-diastolic pressure (Fig. 13-2) (LeJemtel et al, 1980; Wynn et al, 1980). Heart rate may increase and blood pressure may decline. Controversy exists as to whether the predominant action of amrinone is inotropic or vasodilating (Goldenberg and Cohn, 1987). Amrinone possesses neither antidysrhythmic nor arrhythmogenic properties.

Amrinone-induced inhibition of phosphodiesterase enzyme leads to increased intracellular concentrations of cyclic AMP, which potentiates delivery of Ca^{2+} to the myocardial contractile system (Goldberg and Cohn, 1987). Positive inotropic effects are not prevented by alpha- or beta-adrenergic blockade, depletion of catecholamines, or inhibition of the Na$^+$–K$^+$ ATPase ion transport system. Indeed, amrinone can be used in conjunction with digitalis without provoking digitalis toxicity, suggesting the mechanism of action of these two drugs is different. The elimination half-time of amrinone is approximately 6 hours with the principle route of excretion being that of unchanged drug in the urine.

Amrinone is effective when administered orally as well as intravenously. Administration of a single dose, 0.5 to 1.5 mg·kg^{-1} IV, increases cardiac output within 5 minutes with detectable positive inotropic effects persisting for approximately 2 hours (Wilmshurst et al, 1983). Following the initial injection, continuous intravenous infusion of 2 to 10 µg·kg^{-1}·min^{-1} produces positive inotropic effects that are maintained during the infusion (tachyphylaxis does not occur) and for several hours following discontinuation of the infusion. The recommended maximum daily dose of amrinone is 10 mg·kg^{-1} including the initial loading dose, which may be repeated 30 minutes after the first injection. Patients who have failed to respond to catecholamines may respond to amrinone.

An adverse side effect of amrinone is occasional hypotension due to vasodilation. Thrombocytopenia may occur with chronic therapy. In animals, chronic administration of amrinone has been associated with hepatic dysfunction. Overall, the therapeutic index of amrinone is approximately 100:1 compared with 1.2:1 for cardiac glycosides.

Milrinone

Milrinone is a bypyridine derivative that, like amrinone, produces positive inotropic and vasodilating effects (Fig. 13-2). It can be administered orally or intravenously and acts through nonglycoside and noncatecholamine mechanisms most likely reflecting enhancement of Ca^{2+} entry into cells. This increased Ca^{2+} entry is due in part to drug-induced inhibition of phosphodiesterase, which results in increased myocardial levels of cyclic AMP (Goldberg and Cohn, 1987). Increased cyclic AMP levels result in stimulation of protein kinases that phosphorylate substances responsible for inward Ca^{2+} movement.

Compared with amrinone, milrinone causes a greater decrease in left ventricular pressure and blood pressure probably secondary to its vasodilator properties (Grose et al, 1984). Side effects seem to be fewer with milrinone (Baim et al, 1986). In the treatment of patients with chronic congestive heart failure, milrinone improves exercise tolerance but offers no advantage over digoxin (DiBianco et al, 1989).

REFERENCES

Baim DS, Colucci WS, Monrad ES, et al. Survival of patients with severe congestive heart failure treated with oral milrinone. J Am Coll Cardiol 1986; 7:661–70.

Bartolone RS, Rao TLK. Dysrhythmias following muscle relaxant administration in patients receiving digitalis. Anesthesiology 1983;58:567–9.

Chee TP, Prakash NS, Desser KB, Benchimol A. Postoperative supraventricular arrhythmias and the role of prophylactic digoxin in cardiac surgery. Am Heart J 1982;104:974–7.

Chung DC. Anesthetic problems associated with the treatment of cardiovascular disease: I. Digitalis toxicity. Can Anaesth Soc J 1981;28:6–16.

Denlinger JP, Kaplan JA, Lecky JH, Wollman H. Cardiovascular responses to calcium administered intravenously to man during halothane anesthesia. Anesthesiology 1975;42:390–7.

Deutsch S, Dalen JE. Indications for prophylactic digitalization. Anesthesiology 1969;30:648–56.

DiBianco R, Shabetai R, Kostuk W, et al. A comparison of oral milrinone, digoxin, and their combination in the treatment of patients with chronic heart failure. N Engl J Med 1989;320:677–83.

Doherty JE. How and when to use digitalis serum levels. JAMA 1978;239:2594–6.

Edwards R, Winnie AP, Ramamurphy S. Acute hypocapnic hypokalemia: An iatrogenic complication. Anesth Analg 1977;56:786–92.

Goldenberg IF, Cohn JN. New inotropic drugs for heart failure. JAMA 1987;258:493–6.

Grose RM, Strain JE, Bergman MJ, et al. Milrinone vs. dobutamine. A comparative study. Circulation 1984;70:1–11.

Hoffman BF, Bigger JT. Digitalis and allied cardiac glycosides. In: Gilman AG, Goodman LS, Rall TW, Murad F, eds. The Pharmacological Basis of Therapeutics, 7th ed. New York. Macmillan Publishing Co. 1985, 716–47.

Ivankovich AD, Miletich DJ, Grossman RK, Albrecht RF, El-Etr AA, Cairoli VJ. The effect of enflurane, isoflurane, fluroxene, methoxyflurane and diethyl ether anesthesia on ouabain tolerance in the dog. Anesth Analg 1976;55:360–5.

LeJemtel TH, Keung E, Ribner HS, et al. Sustained beneficial effects of oral amrinone on cardiac and renal function in patients with severe congestive heart failure. Am J Cardiol 1980;45:123–9.

Morrow DH, Townley NT. Anesthesia and digitalis toxicity: An experimental study. Anesth Analg 1964; 43:510–19.

Pinaud MLJ, Blanloeil YAG, Souron RJ. Preoperative prophylactic digitalization of patients with coronary artery disease—A randomized echocardiographic and hemodynamic study. Anesth Analg 1983;62:865–9.

Selzer A, Cohn KE. Some thoughts concerning the prophylactic use of digitalis. Am J Cardiol 1970;26:214–6.

Smith LDR, Oldershaw PF. Inotropic and vasopressor agents. Br J Anaesth 1984;56:767–80.

Smith TW, Haber E. Digitalis. N Engl J Med 1973;289:1063–72;1125–9.

Wilmshurst PT, Thompson DS, Jenkins BS, Coltart DJ, Webb-Peploe M. Haemodynamic effects of intravenous amrinone in patients with impaired left ventricular function. Br Heart J 1983;49:77–82.

Wynn J, Malacoff RF, Benotti JR, et al. Oral amrinone in refractory congestive heart failure. Am J Cardiol 1980;45:1245–9.

Chapter

14

Alpha- and Beta-Adrenergic Receptor Antagonists

INTRODUCTION

Alpha- and beta-adrenergic receptor antagonists prevent the interaction of the endogenous neurotransmitter, norepinephrine, or sympathomimetics with the corresponding adrenergic receptor (Foex, 1984). Interference with normal adrenergic receptor function attenuates sympathetic nervous system homeostatic mechanisms and evokes predictable pharmacologic responses.

ALPHA-ADRENERGIC RECEPTOR ANTAGONISTS

Alpha-adrenergic receptor antagonists bind selectively to alpha-adrenergic receptors and interfere with the ability of catecholamines or other sympathomimetics to provoke alpha-responses. Drug-induced alpha-adrenergic blockade prevents the effects of catecholamines and sympathomimetics on the heart and peripheral vasculature. The inhibitory action of epinephrine on insulin secretion is also prevented. Orthostatic hypotension, baroreceptor-mediated reflex tachycardia, and impotence are invariable side effects of alpha-adrenergic blockade. Furthermore, absence of beta-adrenergic blockade permits maximum expression of cardiac stimulation from norepinephrine. These side effects prevent the

use of nonselective alpha-adrenergic antagonists in the management of ambulatory essential hypertension.

Mechanism of Action

Phentolamine, prazosin, and yohimbine are competitive (reversible binding with receptors) alpha-adrenergic antagonists. In contrast, phenoxybenzamine binds covalently to alpha-adrenergic receptors to produce an irreversible and insurmountable type of blockade. Once alpha-blockade has been established with phenoxybenzamine, even massive doses of sympathomimetics are ineffective until the effect of phenoxybenzamine is terminated by metabolism.

Phentolamine and phenoxybenzamine are nonselective alpha-antagonists acting at postsynaptic alpha-1 receptors as well as presynaptic alpha-2 receptors. Prazosin is selective for alpha-1 receptors, whereas yohimbine is selective for alpha-2 receptors.

Phentolamine

Phentolamine is a substituted imidazoline derivative that produces transient nonselective alpha-adrenergic blockade (Fig. 14-1). Administered

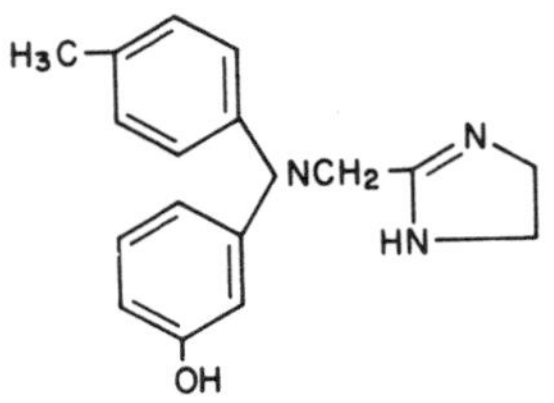

FIGURE 14–1.   Phentolamine.

intravenously, phentolamine produces peripheral vasodilation and a decrease in blood pressure that manifests within 2 minutes and lasts 10 to 15 minutes. This vasodilation reflects alpha-1 receptor blockade and a direct action of phentolamine on vascular smooth muscle. Decreases in blood pressure cause baroreceptor-mediated increases in sympathetic nervous system activity manifesting as cardiac stimulation. In addition to reflex stimulation, phentolamine-induced alpha-2 receptor blockade permits enhanced neural release of norepinephrine manifesting as increased heart rate and cardiac output. Indeed, cardiac dysrhythmias and angina pectoris may accompany the administration of phentolamine. Hyperperistalsis, abdominal pain, and diarrhea may be caused by a predominance of parasympathetic nervous system activity.

Clinical Uses

The principal use of phentolamine is in the treatment of acute hypertensive emergencies, such as may accompany intraoperative manipulation of a pheochromocytoma or autonomic hyperreflexia. Administration of phentolamine, 30 to 70 $\mu g \cdot kg^{-1}$ IV, produces a prompt but transient decrease in blood pressure. A continuous intravenous infusion of phentolamine may be used to maintain normal blood pressure during intraoperative resection of a pheochromocytoma. Local infiltration with a phentolamine-containing solution (2.5 to 5 mg in 10 ml) is appropriate when a sympathomimetic accidentally is administered extravascularly.

Phenoxybenzamine

Phenoxybenzamine is a haloalkylamine derivative that acts as a nonselective alpha-adrenergic antagonist by combining covalently with alpha-

adrenergic receptors (Fig. 14-2). Blockade at postsynaptic alpha-1 receptors is more intense than at alpha-2 receptors.

Pharmacokinetics

Absorption of phenoxybenzamine from the gastrointestinal tract is incomplete. Onset of alpha-adrenergic blockade is slow, taking up to 60 minutes to reach peak effect even following intravenous administration. This delay in onset is due to the time required for structural modification of the phenoxybenzamine molecule, which is necessary to render the drug active. The elimination half-time of phenoxybenzamine is about 24 hours, emphasizing the likelihood of cumulative effects with repeated doses.

Cardiovascular Effects

Phenoxybenzamine administered to a supine, normovolemic patient in the absence of elevated sympathetic nervous system activity produces little change in blood pressure. Orthostatic hypotension, however, is prominent, especially in the presence of preexisting hypertension or hypovolemia. In addition, impairment of compensatory vasoconstriction results in exaggerated blood pressure reductions in response to blood loss or vasodilating drugs such as volatile anesthetics. Despite reductions in blood pressure, cardiac output is often increased and renal blood flow is not greatly altered unless preexisting renal vasoconstriction is present. Cerebral and coronary vascular resistances are not changed.

Noncardiac Effects

Phenoxybenzamine prevents the inhibitory action of epinephrine on the secretion of insulin. Catecholamine-induced glycogenolysis in skeletal muscle or lipolysis is not altered.

Stimulation of the radial fibers of the iris is prevented, and miosis is a prominent component

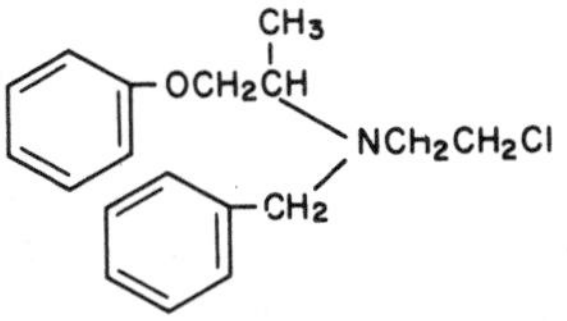

FIGURE 14–2.   Phenoxybenzamine.

of the response to phenoxybenzamine. Sedation may accompany chronic phenoxybenzamine therapy. Nasal stuffiness is due to unopposed vasodilation in mucous membranes in the presence of alpha-adrenergic blockade.

Clinical Uses

Phenoxybenzamine, 0.5 to 1 mg·kg^{-1} orally (or prazosin) is administered preoperatively to control blood pressure in patients with pheochromocytoma. Chronic alpha-adrenergic blockade, by relieving intense peripheral vasoconstriction, permits expansion of intravascular fluid volume as reflected by a decrease in the hematocrit. Excessive vasoconstriction with associated tissue ischemia, such as accompanies hemorrhagic shock, may be reversed by phenoxybenzamine, but only after intravascular fluid volume has been replenished.

Treatment of peripheral vascular disease characterized by intermittent claudication is not favorably influenced by alpha-adrenergic blockade because cutaneous rather than skeletal muscle blood flow is increased. The most beneficial clinical responses to alpha-adrenergic blockade are in diseases with a large component of vasoconstriction, such as Raynaud's syndrome.

Yohimbine

Yohimbine is a selective antagonist at presynaptic alpha-2 receptors leading to enhanced release of norepinephrine from nerve endings. As a result, this drug may be useful in treatment of the rare patient suffering from idiopathic orthostatic hypotension. Observations that alpha-2 agonists can reduce anesthetic requirements by actions on presynaptic alpha-2 receptors in the central nervous system suggests a possible interaction of yohimbine with volatile anesthetics.

Prazosin

Prazosin (see Chapter 15) is a selective postsynaptic alpha-1 receptor antagonist that leaves intact the inhibiting effect of alpha-2 receptor activity on norepinephrine release from nerve endings. As a result, prazosin is less likely than nonselective alpha-adrenergic antagonists to evoke reflex tachycardia. Prazosin dilates both arterioles and veins.

BETA-ADRENERGIC RECEPTOR ANTAGONISTS

Beta-adrenergic receptor antagonists bind selectively to beta-adrenergic receptors and interfere with the ability of catecholamines or other sympathomimetics to provoke beta-responses. Drug-induced beta-adrenergic blockade prevents effects of catecholamines and sympathomimetics on the heart and smooth muscle of the airways and blood vessels. Beta-antagonist drug therapy should be continued throughout the perioperative period to maintain desirable effects and to avoid the risk of sympathetic nervous system hyperactivity associated with abrupt discontinuation of these drugs. Propranolol is the standard beta-antagonist with which all other drugs are compared.

Mechanism of Action

Beta-adrenergic receptor antagonists exhibit selective affinity for beta-adrenergic receptors where they act by competitive inhibition. Binding of antagonist drugs to beta-adrenergic receptors is reversible such that drug can be displaced from receptors if sufficiently large amounts of agonist become available. Competitive antagonism causes a rightward displacement of the dose-response curve for the agonist, but the slope of the curve remains unchanged, emphasizing that sufficiently large doses of the agonist may still exert a full pharmacologic effect. Chronic administration of beta-adrenergic antagonists is associated with an increase in the number of beta-adrenergic receptors.

Structure Activity Relationships

Beta-adrenergic antagonists are derivatives of the beta-agonist drug isoproterenol (Fig. 14-3). Substituents on the benzene ring determine whether the drug acts on beta-adrenergic receptors as an antagonist or agonist. The levorotatory forms of beta-antagonists and agonists are more potent than the dextrorotatory forms. For example, the dextrorotatory isomer of propranolol has

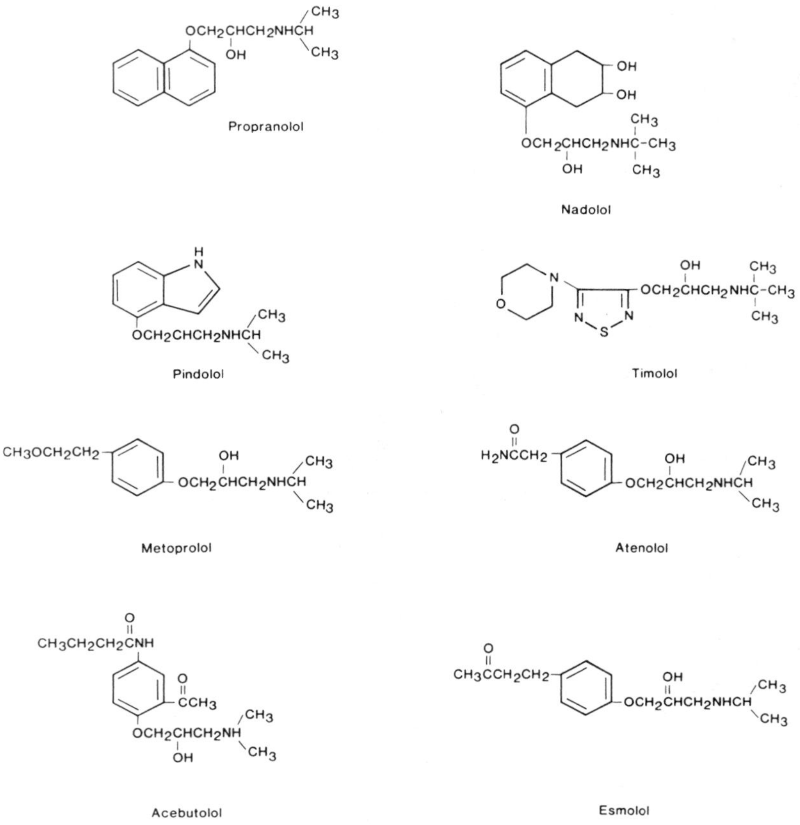

FIGURE 14–3. Beta-adrenergic antagonists.

less than 1% of the potency of the levorotatory isomer for blocking beta-adrenergic receptors.

Classification

Beta-adrenergic receptor antagonists are classified as nonselective and selective for beta-1 and beta-2 receptors (Table 14-1). Beta-antagonists are further classified as partial or pure antagonists on the basis of the presence or absence of intrinsic sympathomimetic activity (Table 14-1). Antagonists with intrinsic sympathomimetic activity cause less direct myocardial depression and heart rate slowing than drugs that lack this intrinsic sympathomimetic activity. As a result, partial antagonists may be better tolerated than pure antagonists by patients with poor left ventricular function.

Selective beta-1 antagonists include metoprolol and atenolol. It is important to recognize that beta-1 selectivity is dose dependent and is lost when large doses of the antagonist are administered. This emphasizes that selectivity should not be interpreted as specificity for a specific type of beta-adrenergic receptor.

Beta-adrenergic antagonists may produce some degree of membrane stabilization in the heart and thus resemble quinidine (Table 14-1). This membrane stabilization effect, however, is detectable only at plasma concentrations that are far greater than needed to produce clinically adequate beta-adrenergic blockade. Indeed, bradycardia and direct myocardial depression produced by beta-adrenergic antagonists are due to removal of sympathetic nervous system innervation to the heart and not membrane stabilization (Foex, 1984).

Table 14-1
Comparative Characteristics of Beta-Adrenergic Receptor Antagonists

	Cardio-Selective Activity	Intrinsic Sympathomimetic Activity	Membrane Stabilizing Activity	Protein Binding (percent)	Clearance	Active Metabolites	Elimination Half-Time (h)	Adult Oral Dose (mg)
Propranolol	No	0	++	90–95	Hepatic	Yes	2–3	40–1000
Nadolol	No	0	0	30	Renal	No	20–24	40–640
Pindolol	No	+	+/–	40–60	Hepatic Renal	No	3–4	5–40
Timolol	No	+/–	0	10	Hepatic	No	3–4	5–45
Metoprolol	Yes	0	+/–	10	Hepatic	No	3–4	50–400
Atenolol	Yes	0	0	5	Renal	No	6–7	50–300
Acebutolol	Yes	+	+	25	Hepatic Renal	Yes	3–4	200–800
Esmolol	Yes				Plasma hydrolysis		0.15	10–80 mg IV 100–300 $\mu g \cdot kg^{-1} \cdot min^{-1}$ IV

Propranolol

Propranolol is a nonselective beta-adrenergic receptor antagonist that lacks intrinsic sympathomimetic activity and thus is a pure antagonist (Table 14-1). Antagonism of beta-1 and beta-2 receptors produced by propranolol is about equal. As the first beta-antagonist introduced clinically, propranolol remains the standard drug with which all other beta-antagonists are compared.

Cardiac Effects

The most important pharmacologic effects of propranolol are on the heart. Propranolol, because of beta-1 receptor blockade, decreases heart rate and cardiac output, especially during exercise or in the presence of increased sympathetic nervous system activity. Heart rate slowing induced by propranolol lasts longer than the negative inotropic effects, suggesting a possible subdivision of beta-1 receptors. Concomitant blockade of beta-2 receptors by propranolol increases peripheral vascular resistance, including coronary vascular resistance. Although prolongation of systolic ejection and dilatation of the cardiac ventricles caused by propranolol increases myocardial oxygen requirements, the oxygen-sparing effects of decreased heart rate and myocardial contractility predominate. As a result, propranolol may relieve myocardial ischemia even though drug-induced increases in coronary vascular resistance oppose coronary blood flow. Sodium ion (Na^+) retention associated with propranolol therapy most likely results from intrarenal hemodynamic changes that accompany drug-induced reductions in cardiac output.

Pharmacokinetics

Propranolol is rapidly and almost completely absorbed from the gastrointestinal tract, but systemic availability of the drug is limited by extensive hepatic first-pass metabolism, which may account for up to 70% of the absorbed dose. Considerable individual variation in the magnitude of hepatic first-pass metabolism exists, accounting for the up to 20-fold differences in plasma concentrations of propranolol in patients after oral administration of comparable doses (Shand, 1975). Hepatic first-pass metabolism is the reason the oral dose of propranolol must be substantially greater than the intravenous dose.

PROTEIN BINDING. Propranolol is extensively bound (90% to 95%) to plasma proteins. Heparin-induced increases in plasma concentrations of free fatty acids owing to elevated lipoprotein lipase activity results in decreased plasma protein binding of propranolol (Fig. 14-4) (Wood et al, 1979). In addition, hemodilution that occurs when cardiopulmonary bypass is initiated may alter protein binding of drugs because of the nonphysiologic protein concentration in the pump prime.

METABOLISM. Clearance of propranolol from the plasma is by hepatic metabolism. An active metabolite, 4-hydroxypropranolol, is detectable in the plasma after administration of propranolol (Nies and Shand, 1975) . Indeed, cardiac beta-blocking activity following equivalent doses of propranolol is greater after oral than after intravenous administration, presumably reflecting the

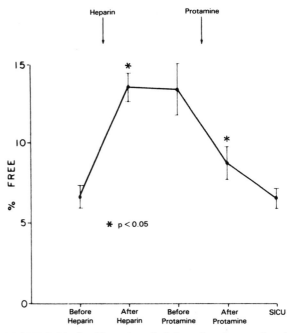

FIGURE 14–4. Heparin administration is associated with decreased plasma protein binding of propranolol manifesting as an increased plasma concentration of free (unbound) drug. Mean ± SE. SICU, surgical intensive care unit. (From Wood M, Shand DG, Wood AJJ. Propranolol binding in plasma during cardiopulmonary bypass. Anesthesiology 1979; 51: 512–6; with permission.)

effects of this metabolite, which is equivalent in activity to the parent compound. The elimination half-time of propranolol is 2 to 3 hours, whereas that of 4-hydroxypropranolol is even shorter. The plasma concentration of propranolol or the total dose administered does not correlate with its therapeutic effects.

Elimination of propranolol is greatly reduced when hepatic blood flow decreases. In this regard, propranolol may decrease its own clearance rate by decreasing cardiac output and hepatic blood flow. Alterations in hepatic enzyme activity may also influence the rate of hepatic metabolism. Renal failure does not alter the elimination half-time of propranolol, but accumulation of metabolites may occur.

CLEARANCE OF LOCAL ANESTHETICS. Propranolol reduces clearance of amide local anesthetics by decreasing hepatic blood flow and inhibiting metabolism in the liver (Bowdle et al, 1987). For example, in humans, propranolol causes clearance to be reduced to a much greater extent (46%) than would be predicted from a maximum 25% reduction in hepatic blood flow, implying that drug metabolism in the liver has also been affected (Conrad et al, 1983). Bupivacaine clearance is relatively insensitive to changes in hepatic blood flow (low extraction drug), suggesting that the 35% decrease in clearance of the local anesthetic reflects propranolol-induced reductions in metabolism (Fig. 14-5) (Bowdle et al, 1987). Because clearance of drugs with low extraction ratios is inversely related to plasma protein binding, an increase in bupivacaine binding to alpha-1 acid glycoprotein (responsible for 90% binding of the local anesthetic) caused by propranolol could explain a decrease in clearance. Nevertheless, propranolol does not alter alpha-1 acid glycoprotein concentrations (Conrad et al, 1983). It is conceivable that systemic toxicity of local anesthetics would be increased by propranolol and presumably other beta-antagonists that interfere with clearance of local anesthetics.

CLEARANCE OF OPIOIDS. Pulmonary first-pass uptake of fentanyl is substantially reduced in patients being treated chronically with propranolol (Roerig et al, 1989). As a result, two to four times as much injected fentanyl enters the systemic circulation in the time period immediately after injection. This response most likely reflects the ability of one basic lipophilic amine (propra-

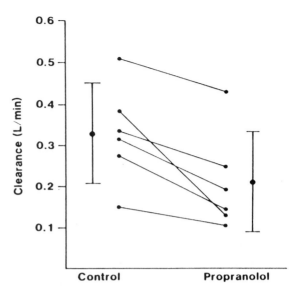

FIGURE 14–5. Bupivacaine clearance is decreased 35% in subjects treated with propranolol compared with control measurements. (From Bowdle TA, Freund PR, Slattery JT. Propranolol reduces bupivacaine clearance. Anesthesiology 1987; 66: 36–8; with permission.)

nolol) to inhibit the pulmonary uptake of a second basic lipophilic amine (fentanyl).

Nadolol

Nadolol is a nonselective beta-adrenergic receptor antagonist that is unique in that its long duration of action permits once-daily administration.

Pharmacokinetics

Nadolol is slowly and incompletely absorbed (an estimated 30%) from the gastrointestinal tract. Metabolism does not occur, with about 75% of the drug being excreted unchanged in the urine and the remainder in the bile. Therefore, wide individual variations in plasma concentrations that occur with nadolol cannot be attributed to differences in metabolism such as occur with propranolol. The elimination half-time is 20 to 40 hours, accounting for the need to administer this drug only once a day. The dosing interval should be extended beyond 14 hours in patients with renal dysfunction. The plasma concentration of nadolol, like propranolol, does not correlate with therapeutic effects of the drug.

Pindolol

Pindolol is a nonselective beta-adrenergic receptor antagonist with intrinsic sympathomimetic activity. Because it possesses intrinsic sympathomimetic activity, this drug causes minimal resting bradycardia. Also, because of this characteristic, large doses of the drug may cause an unexpected increase in blood pressure.

Pharmacokinetics

Pindolol is well absorbed from the gastrointestinal tract, but plasma concentrations of the drug vary greatly. Protein binding of pindolol is 40% to 60%. Approximately 40% to 50% of a single dose of pindolol can be recovered unchanged in the urine. No active metabolites have been identified. The elimination half-time of pindolol is 3 to 4 hours, and this is increased to longer than 11 hours in patients with renal failure.

Timolol

Timolol is a nonselective beta-adrenergic receptor antagonist that is as effective as propranolol for various therapeutic indications. In addition, timolol is effective in the treatment of glaucoma as a result of its ability to decrease intraocular pressure, presumably by reducing the production of aqueous humor. Timolol is administered as eye drops in the treatment of glaucoma, but systemic absorption may be sufficient to cause resting bradycardia and increased airway resistance. Indeed, bradycardia and hypotension that are refractory to treatment with atropine have been observed during anesthesia in pediatric and adult patients receiving topical timolol with or without pilocarpine (Mishra et al, 1983). Timolol may be associated with impaired control of ventilation in neonates, resulting in unexpected postoperative apnea (Bailey, 1984). Immaturity of the neonate's blood-brain barrier may facilitate access of this drug to the central nervous system.

Pharmacokinetics

Timolol is rapidly and almost completely absorbed after oral administration. Nevertheless, extensive hepatic first-pass metabolism limits the amount of drug reaching the systemic circulation to about 50% of that absorbed from the gastrointestinal tract. Protein binding of timolol is not ex-

tensive. The elimination half-time is about 4 hours.

Metoprolol

Metoprolol is a selective beta-1 antagonist that prevents inotropic and chronotropic responses to beta-adrenergic stimulation. Conversely, bronchodilator, vasodilator, and metabolic effects of beta-2 receptors remain intact such that metoprolol is less likely to cause adverse effects in patients with chronic obstructive airway disease, peripheral vascular disease and patients vulnerable to hypoglycemia. It is important to recognize, however, that selectivity is dose related, and large doses of metoprolol are likely to become nonselective, exerting antagonist effects at beta-2 receptors as well as beta-1 receptors. Indeed, airway resistance may increase in asthmatic patients treated with metoprolol, although the magnitude of increase will be less than that evoked by propranolol. Furthermore, metoprolol-induced elevations in airway resistance are more readily reversed with beta-2 agonists such as terbutaline.

Pharmacokinetics

Metoprolol is readily absorbed from the gastrointestinal tract, but this is offset by substantial hepatic first-pass metabolism such that only about 40% of the drug reaches the systemic circulation. Protein binding is low, being estimated to account for about 10% of the drug. None of the hepatic metabolites have been identified as active. A small amount (less than 10%) of the drug appears unchanged in the urine. The elimination half-time of metoprolol is 3 to 4 hours. Plasma concentrations of metoprolol do not correlate with therapeutic effects of the drug.

Atenolol

Atenolol is a selective beta-1 receptor antagonist that may have specific usefulness in patients in whom the continued presence of beta-2 receptor activity is desirable.

Pharmacokinetics

About 50% of an orally administered dose of atenolol is absorbed from the gastrointestinal tract. Atenolol undergoes little or no hepatic metabolism and is eliminated principally by renal excretion. The elimination half-time is 6 to 7 hours, and this may increase to more than 24 hours in patients with renal failure. Plasma concentrations of atenolol do not correlate with therapeutic effects of the drug.

The antihypertensive effect is prolonged, and atenolol can be administered once a day for the treatment of hypertension. Like nadolol, atenolol does not enter the central nervous system in large amounts, but fatigue and mental depression still occur. Unlike nonselective beta-antagonists, atenolol does not appear to potentiate insulin-induced hypoglycemia and can thus be administered with caution to patients with diabetes mellitus whose hypertension is not controlled by other antihypertensives.

Esmolol

Esmolol is a rapid-onset and short-acting selective beta-1 receptor antagonist (Fig. 14-3). These characteristics may make esmolol a useful drug for preventing or treating adverse blood pressure and heart rate increases that occur intraoperatively in response to noxious stimulation, as during intubation of the trachea (Fig. 14-6) (Menkhaus et al, 1985). Administered as a continuous infusion (200 $\mu g \cdot kg^{-1} \cdot min^{-1}$ IV) beginning 5 minutes before induction of anesthesia, esmolol prevents increases in heart rate associated with noxious stimulation in patients undergoing coronary artery–bypass graft opera-

tions (Girard et al. 1986). Alternatively, a bolus of esmolol, 80 mg IV, followed by a continuous infusion (12 $mg \cdot min^{-1}$ IV) lowers heart rate and blood pressure in adult patients undergoing noncardiac surgery (Gold et al, 1989). Other reports describe prevention of perioperative tachycardia and hypertension with esmolol, 100 to 200 mg IV, administered over 15 seconds before the induction of anesthesia (Oxorn et al; 1900; Sheppard et al, 1990). Prior administration of esmolol, 500 $\mu g \cdot kg^{-1} \cdot min^{-1}$ IV, to patients undergoing electroconvulsive therapy with anesthesia induced by methohexital and succinylcholine results in attenuation of the heart rate increase and a decrease in the length of the electrically induced seizures (Howie et al, 1990). Esmolol has been used during resection of pheochromocytoma and may be useful in the perioperative management of thyrotoxicosis, pregnancy-induced hypertension (toxemia of pregnancy), and epinephrine- or cocaine-induced cardiovascular toxicity (Nicholas et al, 1988; Ostman et al, 1988; Pollan and Tadjziechy, 1989; Thorne and Bedford, 1989; Zakowski et al, 1989). The beta-1 selectivity of esmolol may unmask beta-2–stimulated vasodilation by epinephrine-secreting tumors. Administration of esmolol to patients chronically treated with beta-antagonists has not been observed to produce additional negative inotropic effects (deBruijn et al, 1987a). The presumed reason for this observation is that esmolol, in the dose employed, does not occupy sufficient additional beta-receptors to produce detectable increases in beta-blockade.

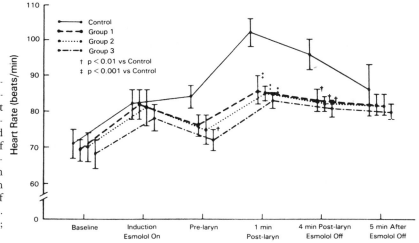

FIGURE 14–6. Esmolol administered as a continuous intravenous infusion attenuates heart rate responses to direct laryngoscopy. Groups 1, 2, and 3 received cumulative esmolol doses of 1100, 2000, and 2700 $\mu g \cdot kg^{-1}$, respectively. Mean ± SE. (From Menkhaus PG, Reves JG, Kisson I, et al. Cardiovascular effects of esmolol in anesthetized humans. Anesth Analg 1985; 64: 327–34; with permission.)

Pharmacokinetics

The short duration of effect of esmolol is due to its rapid metabolism in blood by hydrolysis of the methyl ester, resulting in an inactive acid metabolite and clinically insignificant amounts of methanol. Plasma esterases responsible for hydrolysis of esmolol are distinct from plasma cholinesterase, and the duration of action of succinylcholine is not predictably prolonged in patients treated with esmolol (McCammon et al, 1985). Evidence of the short duration of action is return of the heart rate to predrug levels within 15 minutes of discontinuing esmolol. The elimination half-time is about 10 minutes (deBruijn et al, 1987b). Indeed, plasma concentrations of esmolol are usually not detectable 15 minutes after discontinuing the drug. Poor lipid solubility limits transfer of esmolol into the central nervous system or across the placenta (Ostman et al, 1988).

Side Effects of Beta-Antagonists

Side effects of beta-antagonists are similar for all available drugs, although the magnitude may differ depending on their selectivity and the presence or absence of intrinsic sympathomimetic activity. Beta-antagonists exert their most prominent pharmacologic effects as well as side effects on the cardiovascular system. These drugs may also alter airway resistance, carbohydrate and fat metabolism, and the distribution of extracellular potassium ions (K^+). Additive effects between drugs used for anesthesia and beta-antagonists may occur. Beta-antagonists penetrate the blood-brain barrier and cross the placenta. Gastrointestinal side effects of beta-antagonists include nausea, vomiting, and diarrhea. Fever, rash, myopathy, alopecia, and thrombocytopenia have been associated with chronic beta-antagonist treatment. Beta-antagonists have been reported to reduce plasma concentrations of high-density lipoproteins and to increase triglyceride and uric acid levels.

The principal contraindication to administration of beta-antagonists is preexisting atrioventricular heart block or cardiac failure not caused by tachycardia. Nonselective beta-antagonists or high doses of selective beta-antagonists should not be administered to patients with chronic obstructive airway disease. In patients with diabetes mellitus, there is the risk that beta-adrenergic blockade may mask the signs of hypoglycemia and thus delay its recognition.

Cardiovascular System

Beta-antagonists produce negative inotropic and chronotropic effects. In addition, the conduction speed of cardiac impulses through the atrioventricular node is slowed and the rate of spontaneous phase 4 depolarization is decreased. Preexisting atrioventricular heart block owing to any cause may be accentuated by beta-antagonists.

The cardiovascular effects of beta-adrenergic blockade reflect removal of sympathetic nervous system innervation to the heart (beta-1 blockade) and not membrane stabilization, which occurs only at high plasma concentrations of the antagonist drug. In addition, nonselective beta-adrenergic blockade resulting in beta-2 receptor antagonism may impede left ventricular ejection owing to unopposed alpha-adrenergic receptor-mediated peripheral vasoconstriction. The magnitude of cardiovascular effects produced by beta-antagonists is greatest when preexisting sympathetic nervous system activity is increased, as during exercise or in patients in cardiac failure. Indeed, the tachycardia of exercise is consistently attenuated by beta-antagonists. Furthermore, administration of a beta-antagonist may precipitate cardiac failure in a patient who was previously compensated. Resting bradycardia is minimized, and cardiac failure is less likely to occur when a partial beta-antagonist with intrinsic sympathomimetic activity is administered. Acute cardiac failure is rare with oral administration of beta-antagonists.

Classically, beta-antagonists prevent inotropic and chronotropic effects of isoproterenol as well as baroreceptor-mediated increases in heart rate evoked by decreases in blood pressure in response to vasodilator drugs. Conversely, the cardiac-stimulating effects of calcium, glucagon, and digitalis preparations are not detectably influenced by beta-antagonists. Likewise, beta-antagonists do not alter the response to alpha-adrenergic agonists such as epinephrine or phenylephrine. Indeed, the pressor effect of epinephrine is enhanced because nonselective beta-antagonists prevent the beta-2 vasodilating effect of epinephrine and leave unopposed the alpha-adrenergic effect of this catecholamine. The presence of unopposed alpha-adrenergic–induced vasoconstriction may provoke paradoxical hypertension, and may even precipitate cardiac failure in a diseased myocardium that cannot respond to sympathetic nervous system stimulation because of beta-adrenergic blockade. Unexpected hypertension has occurred in patients receiving clonidine or alpha-methyldopa who subsequently receive a nonselective beta-antagonist (Nies and Shand, 1973). Presumably, blockade of the vasodilating effect normally produced by activity of beta-2 receptors leaves unopposed alpha-adrenergic effects to provoke peripheral vasoconstriction with resulting hypertension.

Patients with peripheral vascular disease do not tolerate well the peripheral vasoconstriction associated with beta-2 receptor blockade produced by nonselective beta-antagonists. Indeed, the development of cold hands and feet is a common side effect of beta-blockade. Vasospasm associated with Raynaud's disease is accentuated by propranolol.

The principal antidysrhythmic effect of beta-adrenergic blockade is to prevent the arrhythmogenic effect of endogenous or exogenous catecholamines or sympathomimetics. This reflects a reduction in sympathetic nervous system activity. Membrane stabilization is probably of little importance in the antidysrhythmic effects produced by usual doses of beta-antagonists.

TREATMENT OF EXCESS MYOCARDIAL DEPRESSION. Excessive bradycardia and/or reductions in cardiac output owing to drug-induced beta-blockade should be treated initially with atropine in incremental doses of 70 $\mu g \cdot kg^{-1}$ IV. Atropine is likely to be effective by blocking vagal effects on the heart and thus unmasking any residual sympathetic nervous system innervation. If atropine is ineffective, the use of drugs to produce direct positive chronotropic and inotropic effects is indicated. For example, continuous intravenous infusion of the nonselective beta-agonist, isoproterenol, in doses sufficient to overcome competitive beta-blockade, is appropriate. The necessary dose of isoproterenol may be 2 to 25 $\mu g \cdot min^{-1}$ IV, which is five to twenty times the necessary dose in the absence of beta-blockade. When a pure beta-antagonist is responsible for excessive cardiovascular depression, a pure beta-1 agonist such as dobutamine is recommended because isoproterenol, with beta-1 and beta-2 agonist effects, can produce vasodilation

before the inotropic effect develops. Dopamine is not recommended because alpha-adrenergic–induced vasoconstriction is likely to occur with the high doses required to overcome beta-blockade. Calcium chloride, 250 to 1000 mg IV, or glucagon, 1 to 5 mg IV, administered to adults, effectively reverses myocardial depression produced by beta-antagonists at normal doses because these drugs do not exert their effect by means of beta-adrenergic receptors. In the presence of life-threatening bradycardia, the placement of a transvenous artificial cardiac pacemaker may be necessary.

Airway Resistance

Nonselective beta-antagonists, such as propranolol, consistently increase airway resistance as a manifestation of bronchoconstriction owing to blockade of beta-2 receptors. These airway resistance effects are exaggerated in patients with pre-existing obstructive airway disease. Because bronchodilation is a beta-2 agonist response, selective beta-1 antagonists, such as metoprolol, are less likely than propranolol to increase airway resistance.

Metabolism

Beta-antagonists alter carbohydrate and fat metabolism. For example, nonselective beta-antagonists, such as propranolol, interfere with glycogenolysis that ordinarily occurs in response to release of epinephrine during hypoglycemia. This emphasizes the need for beta-2 receptor activity in the occurrence of glycogenolysis. Furthermore, tachycardia, which is an important warning sign of hypoglycemia in insulin-treated diabetics, is blunted by beta-antagonists. For this reason, nonselective beta-antagonists are not recommended for administration to patients with diabetes mellitus who may be at risk for developing hypoglycemia because of treatment with insulin or oral hypoglycemics. Altered fat metabolism is evidenced by failure of sympathomimetics or sympathetic nervous system stimulation to increase plasma concentrations of free fatty acids in the presence of beta-adrenergic blockade.

Distribution of Extracellular Potassium

Distribution of K^+ across cell membranes is influenced by sympathetic nervous system activity as well as insulin. Specifically, stimulation of beta-2 adrenergic receptors seems to facilitate movement of K^+ intracellularly. As a result, beta-adrenergic blockade inhibits uptake of K^+ into skeletal muscle and the plasma concentration of K^+ is increased. Indeed, increases in the plasma concentration of K^+ associated with intravenous infusion of this ion are greater in the presence of beta-adrenergic blockade produced by propranolol (Fig. 14-7) (Rosa et al, 1980). In animals, elevations in the plasma concentrations of K^+ following administration of succinylcholine last longer when beta-adrenergic blockade is present (McCammon and Stoelting, 1984). In view of the speculated role of beta-2 receptors in regulating plasma concentrations of K^+, it is likely that selective beta-1 antagonists would impair skeletal muscle uptake of K^+ less than nonselective beta-antagonists.

Interactions with Anesthetics

Myocardial depression produced by inhaled or injected anesthetics could be additive with depression produced by beta-antagonists. Never-

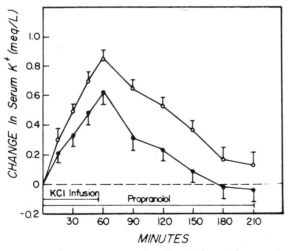

FIGURE 14–7. Increases in plasma (serum) potassium (K^+) concentration in response to infusion of potassium chloride (KCl) are greater in the presence of propranolol (O) than in its absence (●). Mean ± SE (From Rosa RM, Silva P, Young JB, et al. Adrenergic modulation of external potassium disposal. N Engl J Med 1980; 302: 431–4; with permission.)

theless, clinical experience, as well as controlled studies in patients and animals, has confirmed that additive myocardial depression between anesthetics and beta-antagonists is not excessive, and treatment with beta-antagonists may therefore be safely maintained up to the time of anesthesia induction (Foex, 1984). An exception may be patients treated with topical timolol in whom profound bradycardia has been observed in the presence of inhaled anesthetics.

Additive cardiovascular effects between inhaled anesthetics and beta-antagonists seem to be greatest with enflurane, intermediate with halothane, and least with isoflurane (Foex, 1984; Kopriva et al, 1978; Philbin and Lowenstein, 1976; Roberts et al, 1976a). For example, cardiac output and blood pressure are similar with or without beta-adrenergic blockade in the presence of 1 or 2 MAC isoflurane (Philbin and Lowenstein, 1976). Even acute hemorrhage does not alter the interaction between isoflurane or halothane and beta-antagonists (Horan et al, 1977a; Roberts et al, 1976b). In contrast, cardiac depression is more likely to occur in the presence of beta-blockade when acute hemorrhage occurs in animals anesthetized with enflurane (Horan et al, 1977b). Cardiovascular responses to even high doses of opioids such as fentanyl are not altered by preexisting beta-adrenergic blockade. In the presence of anesthetic drugs that increase sympathetic nervous system activity (ketamine) or when excessive sympathetic nervous system activity is present because of hypercarbia, the acute administration of a beta-antagonist may unmask direct negative inotropic effects of concomitantly administered anesthetics with resulting reductions in blood pressure and cardiac output (Foex and Ryder, 1981).

Nervous System

Beta-antagonists may cross the blood-brain barrier to produce side effects. For example, fatigue and lethargy are commonly associated with chronic propranolol therapy. Vivid dreams are frequent, but psychotic reactions are rare. Memory loss and mental depression are not infrequent. Peripheral paresthesias have been described. Atenolol and nadolol are less lipid soluble than other beta-antagonists and thus may be associated with a lower incidence of central nervous system effects.

Fetus

Beta-antagonists can cross the placenta and cause bradycardia, hypotension, and hypoglycemia in newborn infants of mothers who are receiving the drug. Breast milk is also likely to contain beta-antagonists administered to the mother.

Withdrawal Hypersensitivity

Acute discontinuation of beta-antagonist therapy can result in excess sympathetic nervous system activity that manifests in 24 to 48 hours. Presumably, this enhanced activity reflects an increase in the number of beta-adrenergic receptors (up-regulation) during chronic therapy with beta-antagonists. Continuous infusion of propranolol, 3 mg·h^{-1} IV, is effective in maintaining therapeutic plasma concentrations in adult patients who cannot take drugs orally during the perioperative period (Smulyan et al, 1982).

Clinical Uses of Beta-Antagonists

Clinical uses of beta-adrenergic antagonists are multiple but most often include (1) treatment of essential hypertension, (2) management of angina pectoris, (3) treatment of postmyocardial infarction patients, (4) preoperative preparation of hyperthyroid patients, (5) suppression of cardiac dysrhythmias, and (6) prevention of excess sympathetic nervous system activity. In equivalent doses, all beta-antagonists seem to be equally effective in producing desired therapeutic effects.

Treatment of Essential Hypertension

Chronic therapy with beta-antagonists results in gradual reductions in blood pressure. The antihypertensive effect of beta-adrenergic blockade is largely dependent on reductions in cardiac output owing to decreased heart rate. Large doses of beta-antagonists may depress myocardial contractility as well. In many patients, systemic vascular resistance remains unchanged. An important advantage in use of beta-antagonists for the treatment of essential hypertension is the absence of orthostatic hypotension. Often a beta-antagonist is used in combination with a vasodilator to minimize reflex baroreceptor-mediated increases in heart rate and cardiac output produced by the vasodilator. All beta-antagonists appear to be equally effective antihypertensive drugs.

Release of renin from the juxtaglomerular apparatus that occurs in response to stimulation of beta-2 receptors is prevented by nonselective beta-antagonists such as propranolol. This may account for a portion of the antihypertensive effect of propranolol, especially in patients with high circulating plasma concentrations of renin. Because drug-induced reductions in secretion of renin will lead to decreased release of aldosterone, beta-antagonists will also prevent the compensatory Na$^+$ and water retention that accompanies treatment with a vasodilator.

Management of Angina Pectoris

Beta-antagonists are equally effective in reducing the likelihood of myocardial ischemia manifesting as angina pectoris. This desirable response reflects drug-induced reductions in myocardial oxygen requirements secondary to decreased heart rate and cardiac output.

The concept that beta-antagonists and calcium entry blockers act on different determinants of the myocardial oxygen supply-demand ratio suggests combined use of these drugs would be beneficial in the management of patients with coronary artery disease. Nevertheless, the evidence from clinical studies suggests that patients managed with combined therapy do not experience greater therapeutic effects but may experience more adverse effects than if they had received optimal treatment with a single drug (Packer, 1989).

Treatment of Postmyocardial Infarction Patients

Chronic therapy with a beta-antagonist may reduce the mortality after acute myocardial infarction, although which patients are most likely to benefit, when to institute treatment, and how long the protective effect lasts are still unresolved questions (Ruskin, 1989; Yusuf et al, 1985). Treatment should probably be instituted 5 days to 4 weeks after myocardial infarction and continued for at least 1 to 3 years. Whether beta-antagonists can reduce mortality in patients with angina pectoris who have not yet had a myocardial infarction is unknown. Intravenous administration of beta-blockers within 12 hours of the onset of myocardial infarction pain may reduce infarct size and the frequency of ventricular dysrhythmias (Yusuf et al, 1985).

The cardioprotective effect of beta-antagonists is present with both cardioselective and nonselective drugs and does not depend on membrane-stabilizing properties (Table 14-1). The mechanism of the cardioprotective effect is uncertain, but antidysrhythmic actions may be particularly important. A nonselective beta-antagonist that prevents epinephrine-induced reductions in plasma K^+ concentrations (a beta-2–mediated response) may be useful in decreasing the incidence of ventricular dysrhythmias.

Preoperative Preparation of Hyperthyroid Patients

Thyrotoxic patients can be prepared for surgery, in an emergency, by intravenous injection of esmolol or propranolol or, electively, by oral administration of propranolol (40 to 320 mg·day^{-1}) (Lee et al, 1982; Lennquits et al, 1985). Advantages of beta-antagonists include rapid control of autonomic nervous system hyperreactivity and elimination of the need to administer iodine or antithyroid drugs.

Suppression of Cardiac Dysrhythmias

Beta-antagonists reduce sympathetic nervous system activity to the heart with a resulting decrease in the rate of spontaneous phase 4 depolarization of ectopic cardiac pacemakers. In addition, decreased sympathetic nervous system activity owing to beta-blockade decreases activity of the sinoatrial node and slows conduction of the cardiac impulse through the atrioventricular node. Resting transmembrane potentials and repolarization are not altered by beta-antagonists.

The cardiac effects of beta-blockade are responsible for the efficacy of beta-antagonists in suppressing intraoperative supraventricular tachydysrhythmias as well as ventricular cardiac dysrhythmias (Foex, 1984). For example, supraventricular and ventricular cardiac dysrhythmias are suppressed by the administration of propranolol, 5 to 15 μg·kg^{-1} IV, especially if digitalis overdose is responsible for the abnormal rhythm. Seldom is a total dose of propranolol greater than 70 μg·kg^{-1} required.

Prevention of Excess Sympathetic Nervous System Activity

Beta-adrenergic blockade is associated with attenuated heart rate and blood pressure changes in response to direct laryngoscopy and intubation of the trachea (Foex, 1984; Prys-Roberts et al, 1973). Hypertrophic obstructive cardiomyopathies are often treated with beta-antagonists. Tachycardia and cardiac dysrhythmias associated with pheochromocytoma and hyperthyroidism are effectively suppressed by propranolol. The likelihood of cyanotic episodes in patients with tetralogy of Fallot is minimized by beta-blockade. Propranolol has been used intraoperatively to prevent reflex baroreceptor-mediated increases in heart rate evoked by vasodilators administered to produce controlled hypotension. Even anxiety states as associated with public speaking have been treated with propranolol.

COMBINED ALPHA- AND BETA-ADRENERGIC RECEPTOR ANTAGONISTS

Labetalol

Labetalol exhibits selective alpha-1 and nonselective beta-1 and beta-2 antagonist effects (Fig. 14-8) (MacCarthy and Bloomfield, 1983; Wallin and O'Neill, 1983). Presynaptic alpha-2 receptors are spared by labetalol. The drug is one fifth to one tenth as potent as phentolamine in its ability to block alpha-receptors and is approximately one fourth to one third as potent as propranolol in blocking beta-receptors. In humans, the ratio of alpha- to beta-receptor blockade is estimated to be 1:3 after oral ingestion and 1:7 after intravenous administration.

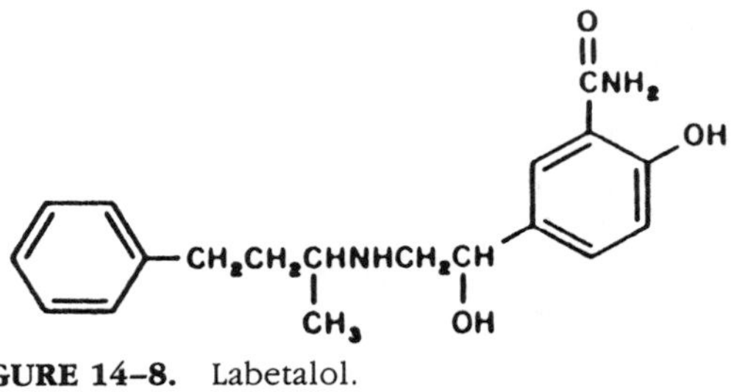

FIGURE 14–8. Labetalol.

Pharmacokinetics

Metabolism or labetalol is by conjugation to glucuronic acid, with less than 5% of the drug recovered unchanged in the urine. The elimination half-time is 5 to 8 hours, being prolonged in the presence of liver disease and unchanged by renal dysfunction.

Cardiovascular Effects

Administration of labetalol, 0.1 to 0.5 mg·kg^{-1} IV, over 2 minutes acutely lowers blood pressure by decreasing systemic vascular resistance (alpha-1 blockade), whereas reflex tachycardia triggered by vasodilation is attenuated by simultaneous beta-blockade. Cardiac output may also be decreased. The maximum blood pressure–lowering effect of an intravenous dose of labetalol is present in 5 to 10 minutes. If necessary, additional doses may be injected every 10 minutes or, alternatively, a continuous infusion, 0.5 to 2 mg·min^{-1} IV, may be initiated.

Clinical Uses

Labetalol can be administered to attenuate increases in blood pressure and heart rate that occur during and following surgery (Leslie et al, 1987). Rebound hypertension following withdrawal of clonidine therapy and hypertensive responses in patients with pheochromocytoma can be effectively treated with labetalol. In contrast to nitroprusside, controlled hypotension produced with intermittent injections of labetalol, 10 mg IV, is not associated with increases in heart rate, intrapulmonary shunt, or cardiac output (Goldberg et al, 1990). Availability of both an oral and an intravenous preparation is useful for converting a patient with a hypertensive crisis to oral therapy after initial control with intravenous therapy.

Side Effects

All the precautions and risks relating to use of beta-antagonists (bronchospasm, congestive heart failure, heart block, fatigue, mental depression) are also present for labetalol, although the incidence and severity are probably less. Orthostatic hypotension is the most common side effect. Fluid retention is the reason for combining labetalol with a diuretic during chronic therapy.

REFERENCES

Bailey PL. Timolol and postoperative apnea in neonates and young infants. Anesthesiology 1984; 61:622.

Bowdle TA, Freund PR, Slattery JT. Propranolol reduces bupivacaine clearance. Anesthesiology 1987;66:36–8.

Conrad KA, Beyers JM, Finley PR, Burnham L. Lidocaine elimination: Effects of metoprolol and of propranolol. Clin Pharmacol Ther 1983;33:133–8.

deBruijn NP, Croughwell N, Reves JG. Hemodynamic effects of esmolol in chronically B-blocked patients undergoing aortocoronary bypass surgery. Anesth Analg 1987a;66:137–41.

deBruijn NP, Reves JG, Croughwell N. Clements F, Drissel DA. Pharmacokinetics of esmolol in anesthetized patients receiving chronic beta blocker therapy. Anesthesiology 1987b;66:323–6.

Foex P. Alpha- and beta-adrenoceptor antagonists. Br J Anaesth 1984;56:751–65.

Foex P, Ryder WA. Interactions of adrenergic beta-receptor blockade (oxprenolol) and PCO$_2$ in the anesthetized dog: Influence of intrinsic sympathomimetic activity. Br J Anaesth 1981;53:19–26.

Girard D, Shulman BJ, Thys DM, Mindich BP, Mikula SK, Kaplan JA. The safety and efficacy of esmolol during myocardial revascularization. Anesthesiology 1968;65:157–64.

Gold MI, Sacks DJ, Grosnoff DB, Herrington C, Skillman CA. Use of esmolol during anesthesia to treat tachycardia and hypertension. Anesth Analg 1989;68:101–4.

Goldberg ME, McNulty SE, Azad SS, et al. A comparison of labetalol and nitroprusside for inducing hypotension during major surgery. Anesth Analg 1990;70:537–42.

Horan BF, Prys-Roberts C, Roberts JG, Bennett MJ, Foex P. Haemodynamic responses to isoflurane anaesthesia and hypovolaemia in the dog, and their modification by propranolol. Br J Anaesth 1977a;49:1179–87.

Horan BF, Prys-Roberts C, Hamilton WK, Roberts JG. Haemodynamic responses to enflurane anaesthesia and hypovolaemia in the dog, and their modification by propranolol. Br J Anaesth 1977b;49:1189–97.

Howie MB, Black HA, Zvara D, McSweeney TD, Martin DJ, Coffman EA. Esmolol reduces autonomic hypersensitivity and length of seizures induced by electroconvulsive therapy. Anesth Analg 1990;71:384–8.

Kopriva CJ, Brown ACD, Pappas G. Hemodynamics during general anesthesia in patients receiving propranolol. Anesthesiology 1978;48:28–33.

Lee TC, Coffey RJ, Currier BM, Ca X-P, Canary JJ. Propranolol and thyroidectomy in the treatment of thyrotoxicosis. Ann Surg 1982;195:766–72.

Lennquits S, Jortso E, Anderberg B, Smeds S. Beta blockers compared with antithyroid drug as preoperative treatment in hyperthyroidism: Drug tolerance, complications, and postoperative thyroid function. Surgery 1985;98:1141–6.

Leslie JB, Kalayjian RW, Sirgo MA, Plachetka JR, Watkins WD. Intravenous labetalol for treatment of postoperative hypertension. Anesthesiology 1987; 67:413–6.

MacCarthy EP, Bloomfield SS. Labetalol: A review of its pharmacology, pharmacokinetics, clinical uses and adverse effects. Pharmacotherapy 1983;3:193–219.

McCammon RL, Hilgenberg JC, Sandage BW, Stoelting RK. The effect of esmolol on the onset and duration of succinylcholine-induced neuromuscular blockade. Anesthesiology 1985;63:A317.

McCammon RL, Stoelting RK. Exaggerated increase in serum potassium following succinylcholine in dogs with beta blockade. Anesthesiology 1984;61:723–5.

Menkhaus PG, Reves JG, Kisson I, et al. Cardiovascular effects of esmolol in anesthetized humans. Anesth Analg 1985;64:327–34.

Mishra P, Calvey TN, Williams NE, Murray GR. Intraoperative bradycardia and hypotension associated with timolol and pilocarpine eye drops. Br J Anaesth 1983;55:897–9.

Nicholas E, Deutschman CS, Allo M, Rock P. Use of esmolol in the intraoperative management of pheochromocytoma. Anesth Analg 1988;67:1114–7.

Nies AS, Shand DG. Hypertensive response to propranolol in a patient treated with methyldopa—a proposed mechanism. Clin Pharmacol Ther 1973; 14:823–6.

Nies AS, Shand DG. Clinical pharmacology of propranolol. Circulation 1975;52:6–15.

Ostman PL, Chestnut DH, Robillard JE, Weiner CP, Hdez MJ. Transplacental passage and hemodynamic effects of esmolol in the gravid ewe. Anesthesiology 1988;69:738–41.

Oxorn D, Knox JWD, Hill J. Bolus doses of esmolol for the prevention of perioperative hypertension and tachycardia. Can J Anaesth 1990;37:206–9.

Packer M. Combined beta-adrenergic and calcium-entry blockade in angina pectoris. N Engl J Med 1989;320:709–17.

Philbin DM, Lowenstein E. Lack of beta-adrenergic activity of isoflurane in the dog: A comparison of circulatory effects of halothane and isoflurane after propranolol administration. Br J Anaesth 1976; 48:1165–70.

Pollan S, Tadjziechy M. Esmolol in the management of epinephrine-and cocaine-induced cardiovascular toxicity. Anesth Analg 1989;69:663–4.

Prys-Roberts C, Foex P, Biro GP, Roberts JG. Studies of anaesthesia in relation to hypertension. V. Adrenergic beta-receptor blockade. Br J Anaesth 1973;45:671–81.

Roberts JG, Foex P, Clarke TNS, Bennett MJ. Haemodynamic interactions of high-dose propranolol pretreatment and anaesthesia in the dog. I. Halothane dose-response studies. Br J Anaesth 1976a;48:315–25.

Roberts JG, Foex P, Clarke TNS, Bennett MJ, Saner CA. Haemodynamic interactions of high-dose propranolol pretreatment and anaesthesia in the dog. III. The effects of haemorrhage during halothane and trichlorethylene anaesthesia. Br J Anaesth 1976b; 48:411–8.

Roerig DL, Kotrly KJ, Ahlf SB, Dawson CA, Kampine JP. Effect of propranolol on the first pass uptake of fentanyl in the human and rat lung. Anesthesiology 1989;71:62–8.

Rosa RM, Silva P, Young JB, et al. Adrenergic modulation of extrarenal potassium disposal. N Engl J Med 1980;302:431–4.

Ruskin JN. The cardiac arrhythmia suppression trial (CAST). N Engl J Med 1989;321:386–8.

Shand DG. Drug therapy—propranolol. N Engl J Med 1975;293:280–5.

Sheppard S, Eagle CJ, Strunin L. A bolus dose of esmolol attenuates tachycardia and hypertension after tracheal intubation. Can J Anaesth 1990 37:202–5.

Smulyan H, Weinberg SE, Howanitz PJ. Continuous propranolol infusion following abdominal surgery. JAMA 1982;247:2539–42.

Thorne AC, Bedford RF. Esmolol for perioperative management of thyrotoxic goiter. Anesthesiology 1989;71:291–4.

Wallin JD, O'Neill WM. Labetalolol: Current research and therapeutic status. Arch Intern Med 1983; 143:485–90.

Wood M, Shand DG, Wood AJJ. Propranolol binding in plasma during cardiopulmonary bypass. Anesthesiology 1979;51:512–6.

Yusuf S, Peto R, Lewis J, Collins R, Sheight P. Beta blockade during and after myocardial infarction: An overview of the randomized trails. Prog Cardiovasc Dis 1985;27:335–71.

Zakowski M, Kaufman B, Berguson P, Tissot M, Yarmush L, Turndorf H. Esmolol use during resection of pheochromocytoma: Report of three cases. Anesthesiology 1989;20:875–7.

Chapter
15
Antihypertensive Drugs

INTRODUCTION

All available antihypertensive drugs act to some extent by interfering with normal homeostatic mechanisms. Efficacy, toxicity, and suitable combinations of antihypertensive drugs can often be predicted by consideration of both the sites and mechanisms of action of the drugs. The effectiveness of a given drug, however, cannot necessarily be taken as evidence that its mechanisms of action relate to the pathogenesis of the elevated blood pressure.

The potential adverse interaction between antihypertensive drugs and anesthetics has been exaggerated. When interactions are likely, they are usually predictable and can thus be avoided or their significance minimized. Specific concerns during administration of anesthesia to patients being treated with antihypertensive drugs include (1) attenuation of sympathetic nervous system activity, (2) modification of the response to sympathomimetic drugs, and (3) sedation. Attenuation of sympathetic nervous system activity is reflected by orthostatic hypotension and exaggerated blood pressure decreases during anesthesia in response to (1) blood loss, (2) body position change, or (3) decreased venous return owing to positive-pressure ventilation of the lungs. Antihypertensive drugs that deplete norepinephrine or that act on peripheral vascular smooth muscle decrease the sensitivity to predominantly indirect-acting sympathomimetic drugs (Eger and Hamilton, 1959). Conversely, sympathetic nervous system blockade, which deprives the alpha-adrenergic receptors of tonic impulses, results in exaggerated responses to catecholamines and direct-acting sympathomimetic drugs.

Patients remaining on antihypertensive therapy show less extreme swings in blood pressure and heart rate during anesthesia and are less likely to exhibit cardiac dysrhythmias (Prys-Roberts et al, 1971). It is an inescapable conclusion that antihypertensive drugs should be continued throughout the perioperative period. In this regard, the usual dose and unique pharmacology of each antihypertensive drug as well as the physiologic reflexes that occur in response to drug-induced blood pressure changes must be considered when planning the management of anesthesia (Table 15-1).

METHYLDOPA

Methyldopa is an effective antihypertensive drug that acts in the central nervous system (Fig. 15-1). The average daily adult dose of methyldopa is 1 g, with little additional effect with doses greater than 2 g. Methyldopa is given in divided doses, usually three times daily. Intravenous doses of methyldopa are 0.5 to 1 g.

Mechanism of Action

Methyldopa enters the central nervous system where it serves as an alternative substrate to dopa, being decarboxylated to methyldopamine and beta-hydroxylated to alpha-methylnorepinephrine in central adrenergic neurons. When released, alpha-methylnorepinephrine intensely stimu-

Table 15–1
Principal Site of Action of Antihypertensive Drugs

Central Nervous System
  Methyldopa
  Clonidine
  Reserpine
  Guanabenz

Peripheral Vascular Smooth Muscle
  Hydralazine
  Prazosin
  Minoxidil
  Trimazosin
  Terazosin

Peripheral Sympathetic Nervous System
  Guanethidine
  Guanadrel

Peripheral Alpha- and Beta-Adrenergic Receptors
  Labetalol

Angiotensin Converting Enzyme
  Captopril
  Enalapril

Angiotensin II Receptors
  Saralasin

Tyrosine Hydroxylase Enzyme
  Metyrosine

lates inhibitory alpha-2 adrenergic receptors in the hypothalamus, which inhibits sympathetic nervous system outflow from the vasomotor center to the periphery. As a result, decreases in systemic vascular resistance and blood pressure occur. Evidence that the centrally active substance is alpha-methylnorepinephrine is inhibition of antihypertensive effects by prevention of central nervous system decarboxylation or beta-hydroxylation of methyldopa.

Although the major mechanism of the antihypertensive effect of methyldopa seems to be via the central nervous system, some impact of peripheral mechanisms cannot be ruled out. For example, a reduction in renal vascular resistance may be related to the fact that alpha-methylnore-

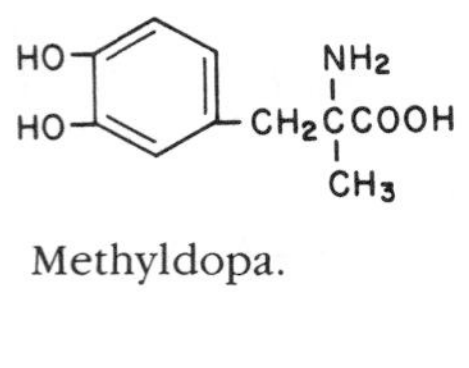

FIGURE 15–1. Methyldopa.

pinephrine is a much weaker vasoconstrictor in this vascular bed than is norepinephrine.

Pharmacokinetics

The extent of absorption of methyldopa after oral administration is only about 25%. Renal excretion of methyldopa or its conjugates accounts for about two thirds of the clearance of drug from the circulation. Nevertheless, there is no evidence that the dose should be substantially altered in the presence of hepatic or renal disease.

Cardiovascular Effects

Methyldopa produces significant decreases in blood pressure and systemic vascular resistance, whereas cardiac output and renal, cerebral, and myocardial blood flow are maintained. Predominance of parasympathetic nervous system activity may be manifested as bradycardia. The decrease in blood pressure is maximal within 4 to 6 hours after an oral dose and persists for as long as 24 hours. Secretion of renin is modestly decreased but is not necessary for the antihypertensive effect of the drug. Because methyldopa does not work solely by its effects on the sympathetic nervous system, a moderate decrease in supine blood pressure is usually not accompanied by orthostatic hypotension, emphasizing the fact that compensatory sympathetic nervous system reflexes remain intact.

Decreased sympathomimetic responses following the administration of ephedrine have been documented in animals pretreated with methyldopa (Miller et al, 1969). Nevertheless, the clinical observation is that patients receiving methyldopa respond appropriately to ephedrine. Methyldopa is a logical choice in patients with renal disease, because this drug maintains or increases renal blood flow.

Side Effects

Side effects of methyldopa treatment include (1) sedation, (2) hepatic dysfunction, (3) development of a positive Coombs' test, (4) interactions with concomitantly administered drugs, and (5) rebound hypertension (Husserl and Messerli,

1981). In addition, methyldopa and its metabolites can interfere with some of the chemical tests for catecholamines, producing false-positive tests for pheochromocytoma. Depending on the chemical method used for analysis, methyldopa may also interfere with the measurement of serum creatinine, uric acid, and transaminase enzymes. Retention of sodium ions (Na^+) and water with weight gain and edema may occur during treatment with methyldopa. Methyldopa does not cause bradycardia or decreased salivary flow to the same extent as clonidine. Sexual dysfunction, primarily impotence, can occur. Orthostatic hypotension is possible but not frequent.

Sedation

Methyldopa predictably causes sedation, but this effect tends to decrease with chronic therapy. In animals, anesthetic requirements (MAC) for volatile drugs are decreased 20% to 40% by methyldopa (Fig. 15-2) (Miller et al, 1969).

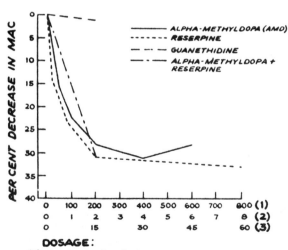

DOSAGE:
(1) AMD, mg/kg/DAY x 3 DAYS
(2) RESERPINE, mg/kg (TOTAL DOSE)
(3) GUANETHIDINE, mg/kg/DAY x 3 DAYS

FIGURE 15-2. Methyldopa (AMD) and reserpine, but not guanethidine, produce dose-related reductions in anesthetic requirements (MAC). (From Miller RD, Way WL, Eger EI. The effects of alpha-methyldopa, reserpine, guanethidine and iproniazid on minimum alveolar anesthetic requirement (MAC). Anesthesiology 1969; 29: 1153–8; with permission.)

Hepatic Dysfunction

Methyldopa may be associated with elevations of plasma concentrations of transaminase enzymes and alkaline phosphatase, especially during the first 6 to 12 weeks of treatment (Husserl and Messerli, 1981). Fever, malaise, and, rarely, jaundice may accompany this drug-induced hepatic dysfunction. Fatal hepatic necrosis has occurred with reexposure to the drug. Liver function tests should probably be performed at monthly intervals during the early period of treatment with methyldopa.

Positive Coombs' Test

A positive Coombs' test develops in 10% to 20% of patients taking 1 g of methyldopa daily for longer than 6 months. Hemolytic anemia occurs in fewer than 5% of these patients and is generally reversible when the drug is discontinued. Nevertheless, the Coombs' test may remain positive for several months. Because most patients developing a positive Coombs' test do not also develop hemolytic anemia, a positive Coombs' test is not a contraindication to continued use of the drug. The principal problem presented by a positive Coombs' test is the difficulty in crossmatching blood. The antibody responsible for the positive Coombs' test is an immunoglobulin G directed at the erythrocyte membrane.

Drug Interactions

Dementia has been observed in patients treated with methyldopa who subsequently receive a butyrophenone drug, such as haloperidol (Thornton, 1976). This dementia may be caused by the ability of both drugs to prevent dopamine from acting at specific receptors in the central nervous system.

Propranolol may elicit paradoxical hypertensive responses when administered to animals pretreated with methyldopa (Niles and Shand, 1973). This hypertensive response presumably reflects the ability of propranolol to block the beta-2 vasodilating component of alpha-methylnorepinephrine. As a result, only the alpha-vasoconstricting effect of this metabolite is apparent.

Rebound Hypertension

Sudden withdrawal of methyldopa therapy can cause rebound hypertension. The incidence of this complication, however, seems to be less than that observed after discontinuation of other centrally acting antihypertensive drugs (see the section entitled "Clonidine").

CLONIDINE

Clonidine is a centrally acting alpha-2 agonist that acts as an antihypertensive drug (Fig. 15-3). The usual daily adult dose is 0.2 to 0.3 mg orally. A parenteral form of clonidine is not available. Transdermal clonidine administered once every 7 days lowers blood pressure in patients with mild to moderate hypertension (White and Gilbert, 1985).

In addition to treatment of patients with essential hypertension, clonidine has been used to aid in the diagnosis of pheochromocytoma (Bravo et al, 1981). For example, clonidine, 0.3 mg orally, will decrease the plasma concentration of catecholamines in normal patients but not in the presence of a pheochromocytoma. This reflects the ability of clonidine to suppress the endogenous release of catecholamines from nerve endings but not the diffusion of excess catecholamines into the circulation from a pheochromocytoma. Clonidine is also effective in suppressing the signs and symptoms of withdrawal from opioids. It is speculated that clonidine replaces opioid-mediated inhibition with alpha-2–mediated inhibition of central nervous system sympathetic activity (Gold et al, 1980).

Clonidine administered into the epidural or subarachnoid space produces intense analgesia and, unlike opioids, does not produce depression of ventilation, pruritus, or nausea and vomiting (Bonnet et al, 1989a; Eisenach et al, 1989; Glynn et al, 1988). Activation of alpha-2 receptors in the substantia gelatinosa is the presumed mechanism by which clonidine produces analgesia. As such, clonidine and morphine, when used as neuraxial analgesics, do not show cross-tolerance (Milne et al, 1985). Pretreatment of patients with a single oral dose of clonidine, 5 $\mu g \cdot kg^{-1}$, administered with the preoperative med-

ication (1) blunts reflex tachycardia associated with direct laryngoscopy for intubation of the trachea; (2) reduces intraoperative lability of blood pressure and heart rate; (3) decreases plasma catecholamine concentrations; and (4) substantially reduces anesthetic requirements (MAC) (Engelman et al, 1989; Flacke et al, 1987; Ghignone et al, 1987). Clonidine does not significantly potentiate morphine-induced depression of ventilation (Bailey et al, 1991). Addition of clonidine, 75 to 150 μg, to a solution containing tetracaine or bupivacaine, placed in the subarachnoid space, prolongs the duration of sensory and motor blockade produced by the local anesthetic (Bonnet et al, 1989b; Racle et al, 1987). The need for intravenous infusion of fluids and the decline in diastolic blood pressure may be greater in patients receiving clonidine containing local anesthetic solutions. Fetal bradycardia may limit the usefulness of subarachnoid clonidine in large doses (greater than 10 $\mu g \cdot kg^{-1}$) in obstetrics (Eisenach and Dewan, 1990).

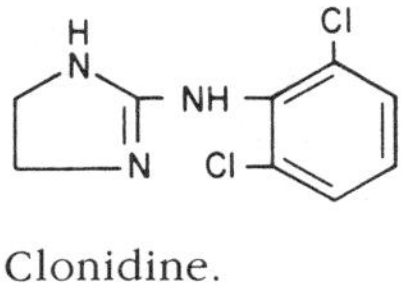

Mechanism of Action

Clonidine stimulates alpha-2 inhibitory neurons in the medullary vasomotor center. As a result, there is a reduction of sympathetic nervous system outflow from the central nervous system to peripheral tissues. Reduced peripheral sympathetic nervous system activity is manifested as decreases in blood pressure, heart rate, and cardiac output. A selective agonist action on postsynaptic alpha-2 receptors in the central nervous system (cell membranes becomes hyperpolarized) may be the mechanism for profound reductions in anesthetic requirements produced by clonidine and other even more selective alpha-2 agonists such as dexmedetomidine. Neuraxial placement of clonidine inhibits spinal substance P release and nociceptive neuron firing produced by noxious stimulation.

Pharmacokinetics

Clonidine is well absorbed after oral administration, and about 60% of the drug appears unchanged in the urine. The duration of hypotensive effect after a single oral dose is about 8 hours. The elimination half-time averages 8.5 hours.

FIGURE 15–3. Clonidine.

Cardiovascular Effects

The decrease in systolic blood pressure produced by clonidine is more prominent than the decrease in diastolic blood pressure. In patients treated chronically, systemic vascular resistance is little affected, and cardiac output, which is initially reduced, returns toward predrug levels. Homeostatic cardiovascular reflexes are maintained, thus avoiding the problems of orthostatic hypotension or hypotension during exercise. The ability of clonidine to decrease blood pressure without paralysis of compensatory homeostatic reflexes is highly desirable. Renal blood flow and glomerular filtration rate are maintained.

Side Effects

The most frequent side effects produced by treatment with clonidine are sedation and xerostomia. Consistent with sedation and, perhaps more specifically, an agonist effect on postsynaptic alpha-2 receptors in the central nervous system are nearly 50% reductions in anesthetic requirements for inhaled anesthetics (MAC) and injected opioids in patients pretreated with clonidine, 5 to 20 $\mu g \cdot kg^{-1}$ (Engelman et al, 1989; Flacke et al, 1987; Ghignone et al, 1987). Patients pretreated with clonidine often manifest lower plasma concentrations of catecholamines in response to surgical stimulation and occasionally require treatment of bradycardia with atropine. As with other antihypertensive drugs, retention of Na^+ and water often occurs such that combination of clonidine with a diuretic is often necessary. Skin rashes and constipation are frequent. Impotence occurs occasionally and orthostatic hypotension rarely.

Rebound Hypertension

Abrupt discontinuation of clonidine therapy can result in rebound hypertension as soon as 8 hours and as late as 36 hours after the last dose (Brodsky and Bravo, 1976; Bruce et al, 1979; Husserl and Messerli, 1981). Rebound hypertension is most likely to occur in patients who are receiving more than 1.2 mg of clonidine daily. The increase in blood pressure is associated with more than a 100% increase in circulating concentra-tions of catecholamines and intense peripheral vasoconstriction. Symptoms of nervousness, diaphoresis, headache, abdominal pain, and tachycardia precede the actual rise in blood pressure. Beta-adrenergic blockade may exaggerate the magnitude of rebound hypertension by blocking the beta-2 vasodilating effects of catecholamines and leaving unopposed their alpha-vasoconstricting actions. Likewise, tricyclic antidepressant therapy may exaggerate rebound hypertension associated with discontinuation of clonidine therapy (Stiff and Harris, 1983). Indeed, tricyclic antidepressants can potentiate the pressor effects of norepinephrine. Naloxone has also been observed to reverse the antihypertensive effects of clonidine in animals (Farsang and Kunos, 1979).

Rebound hypertension can usually be controlled by reinstituting clonidine therapy or by administering a vasodilating drug such as hydralazine or nitroprusside. Beta-adrenergic blocking drugs are useful but probably should be administered only in the presence of alpha-adrenergic blockade so as to avoid unopposed alpha-vasoconstricting actions. In this regard, labetalol with alpha- and beta-antagonist effects may be useful in management of patients experiencing rebound hypertension. If clonidine therapy is interrupted because of surgery, the prior substitution of alternative drugs such as hydralazine or methyldopa, alone or in conjunction with nitroprusside as necessary, is effective (Stiff and Harris, 1983). Alternatively, transdermal clonidine may provide continued drug effect for 7 days, including the time oral administration is interrupted (White and Gilbert, 1985). For a planned withdrawal, clonidine dosage should be decreased gradually over 7 days or more.

Rebound hypertension following abrupt discontinuation of antihypertensive drugs is not unique to clonidine. Indeed, rebound hypertension similar to that observed after abrupt discontinuation of clonidine has also been observed following sudden cessation of treatment with methyldopa, reserpine, guanethidine, guanabenz, and beta-adrenergic receptor antagonists (Husserl and Messerli, 1981). Antihypertensive drugs that act independently of central and peripheral sympathetic nervous system mechanisms (direct vasodilators, converting enzyme inhibitors) do not seem to be associated with rebound hypertension following sudden discontinuation of therapy.

RESERPINE

Reserpine depletes stores of catecholamines and serotonin in the central nervous system. Reduced concentrations of catecholamines can be measured within an hour after administration of reserpine, and depletion is maximal by 24 hours. The norepinephrine content of the heart is also reduced by reserpine. Despite rapid depletion of catecholamines, the antihypertensive effect of reserpine may not become maximal for up to 21 days. This antihypertensive effect is usually associated with decreased cardiac output and bradycardia. Orthostatic hypotension is prominent.

Side Effects

Dose-related side effects of reserpine manifest principally in the central nervous system and gastrointestinal tract. For example, sedation and decreased requirements for volatile anesthetics presumably reflect central nervous system depletion of vital neurotransmitters (Miller et al, 1969). Mental depression also is most likely due to depletion of neurotransmitters. Signs of parasympathetic nervous system predominance include bradycardia, nasal stuffiness, xerostomia, increased gastric hydrogen ion secretion, and exaggerated gastrointestinal motility manifesting as abdominal cramps and diarrhea. Nasal congestion is usually of minor importance but may occasionally cause signs of airway obstruction in neonates born of mothers treated with reserpine.

Increased sensitivity to catecholamines and direct-acting sympathomimetics may occur in patients treated with reserpine. This response resembles denervation hypersensitivity. Conversely, the response to indirect-acting sympathomimetics is reduced in the presence of reserpine therapy.

GUANABENZ

Guanabenz is a guanidine derivative that lowers blood pressure by inhibiting sympathetic nervous system outflow from the central nervous system by activation of central alpha-adrenergic receptors (Fig. 15-4). Oral absorption is rapid with a single dose, producing a peak plasma concentration in 4 hours. The duration of action of a single dose is 12 to 24 hours. Approximately 80%

FIGURE 15–4. Guanabenz.

of an oral dose is excreted in the urine as metabolites.

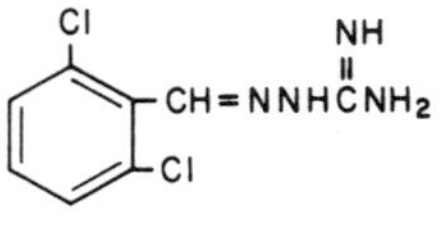

Sedation and dryness of the mouth are the most common side effects of guanabenz therapy. Orthostatic hypotension is possible but less frequent than with guanethidine.

HYDRALAZINE

Hydralazine is a phthalazine derivative that decreases blood pressure by a direct relaxant effect on vascular smooth muscle, the dilatation effect on arterioles being greater than on veins (Fig. 15-5). Vasodilatory effects are more pronounced on the coronary, cerebral, renal, and splanchnic circulations. Vasodilatation probably reflects hydralazine-related interference with calcium ion transport in vascular smooth muscle.

The usual adult oral dose of hydralazine is 20 to 40 mg administered four times daily. Concomitant administration with a beta-adrenergic antagonist to limit the reflex increase in sympathetic nervous system activity induced by hydralazine is common. Beta-adrenergic blockade effectively prevents cardiac stimulation and increased secretion of renin. Treatment of a hypertensive crisis can be accomplished with hydralazine, 2.5 to 10 mg IV. The antihypertensive effect begins within 15 minutes after intravenous administration and lasts 3 to 4 hours.

Pharmacokinetics

Extensive hepatic first-pass metabolism limits availability of hydralazine following oral administration. Acetylation seems to be the major route of metabolism of hydralazine. Rapid acetylators

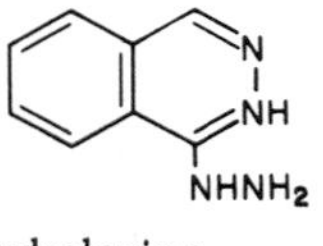

FIGURE 15–5. Hydralazine.

have lower bioavailability (about 30%) than do slow acetylators (about 50%) following oral administration of hydralazine. During multiple oral dosing, slow acetylators attain higher concentrations of hydralazine in plasma than do those who acetylate the drug rapidly. The elimination half-time averages 3 hours. Following intravenous administration, less than 15% of the drug appears unchanged in the urine.

Cardiovascular Effects

Hydralazine often decreases diastolic blood pressure more than systolic blood pressure. Systemic vascular resistance is reduced. Heart rate, stroke volume, and cardiac output increase, reflecting reflex baroreceptor-mediated increases in sympathetic nervous system activity owing to decreases in blood pressure. Nevertheless, tachycardia induced by hydralazine is greater than would be expected solely on a reflex basis and is poorly correlated with changes in blood pressure. This exaggerated heart rate increase may reflect a direct effect of hydralazine on the heart and in the central nervous system in addition to baroreceptor-mediated responses.

The preferential dilatation of arterioles compared with veins minimizes orthostatic hypotension and promotes an increase in cardiac output. The effect of hydralazine develops gradually over about 15 minutes even after intravenous administration. Splanchnic, coronary, cerebral, and renal blood flow usually increase. Glomerular filtration rate, renal tubular function, and urine volume are not consistently affected. Renin activity is often increased, presumably reflecting hydralazine-induced reflex increases in sympathetic nervous system activity leading to increased secretion of renin by the renal juxtaglomerular cells.

Side Effects

Like other vasodilators, hydralazine causes Na$^+$ and water retention if a diuretic is not given concomitantly. Other common side effects of hydralazine therapy include vertigo, diaphoresis, nausea, and tachycardia. Myocardial stimulation associated with hydralazine therapy can evoke angina pectoris and produces changes on the electrocardiogram (ECG) that are characteristic of myocardial ischemia. Side effects are less frequent and less severe when the dose of hydralazine is increased slowly, and tolerance may develop with continued administration. Drug fever, urticaria, polyneuritis, anemia, and pancytopenia are rare but require termination of hydralazine therapy. Peripheral neuropathies have been successfully treated with pyridoxine. Hydrazine-containing compounds, such as hydralazine, may lead to enhanced defluorination of enflurane (Mazze et al, 1982).

A lupus erythematosus–like syndrome occurs in 10% to 20% of patients treated chronically (longer than 6 months) with hydralazine, especially if the dose is greater than 400 mg. The syndrome occurs predominantly in patients who are slow acetylators. Symptoms disappear when the drug is discontinued, differentiating it from the true disease.

PRAZOSIN

Prazosin is a quinazoline derivative that produces peripheral vasodilation via selective and competitive postsynaptic alpha-1 receptor blockade (Fig. 15-6). Absence of a presynaptic alpha-2 effect leaves the normal inhibition of norepinephrine release intact.

In addition to treating essential hypertension, prazosin may be of value for reducing afterload in patients with cardiac failure. Effectiveness of prazosin as a cardiac antidysrhythmic is evidenced by an increased dose of epinephrine necessary to evoke cardiac dysrhythmias during halothane anesthesia in animals (see Fig. 2-15) (Maze and Smith, 1983). This suggests a role for postsynaptic alpha-adrenergic receptors in the myocardium for halothane-induced sensitization of the heart. Prazosin is often combined with a beta-adrenergic antagonist, a diuretic, or both to maximize its antihypertensive effects at the lowest possible dose. In addition, prazosin is useful in the preoperative preparation of patients with a pheochromocytoma.

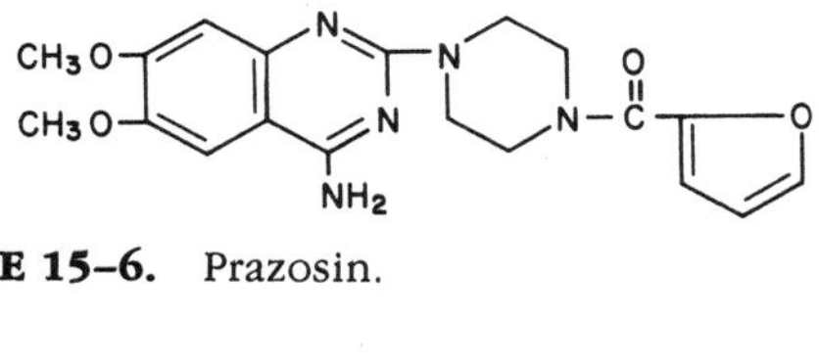

FIGURE 15–6. Prazosin.

Pharmacokinetics

Prazosin is nearly completely metabolized, and less than a 60% bioavailability after oral administration suggests the occurrence of substantial hepatic first-pass metabolism. The elimination half-time is about 3 hours, being prolonged by cardiac failure but not by renal dysfunction. The fact that this drug is metabolized in the liver permits its use in patients with renal failure without altering the dose.

Cardiovascular Effects

Prazosin reduces systemic vascular resistance without causing reflex-induced tachycardia or increases in renin activity as occur with hydralazine or minoxidil. Failure to alter plasma renin activity reflects continued activity of alpha-2 receptors that normally inhibit release of renin. Vascular tone in both resistance and capacitance vessels is reduced, resulting in decreased venous return and cardiac output. Because of its greater affinity for alpha-receptors in veins than in arteries, prazosin produces hemodynamic changes (orthostatic hypotension) that resemble nitroglycerin more than hydralazine.

Side Effects

Side effects of prazosin include vertigo, fluid retention, and orthostatic hypotension. Fluid retention requires the concomitant administration of a diuretic. Syncope may occur early in treatment with prazosin, especially if the initial dose is greater than 1 mg every 8 hours and the patient is volume depleted. In most instances, this syncopal response is due to orthostatic hypotension, presumably reflecting abrupt peripheral vasodilation. Eventually, patients may tolerate up to 20 mg of prazosin daily. The antihypertensive effect of prazosin can be abolished by the prostaglandin synthesis inhibitor indomethacin. Dryness of the mouth, nasal congestion, nightmares, urinary frequency, lethargy, and sexual dysfunction may accompany treatment with this drug.

MINOXIDIL

Minoxidil is an orally active antihypertensive drug that reduces blood pressure by direct relax-

FIGURE 15–7. Minoxidil.

ation of arteriolar smooth muscle (Fig. 15-7) (Campese, 1981). There is little effect on venous capacitance vessels. Minoxidil is particularly effective in patients with renal disease complicated by accelerated hypertension. Minoxidil should be used in combination with a beta-adrenergic antagonist and diuretic to minimize the dose (10 to 40 mg daily) and thus reduce the magnitude of cardiovascular stimulation and fluid retention that may accompany therapy with this drug.

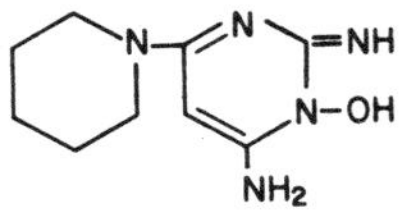

Pharmacokinetics

About 90% of an oral dose of minoxidil is absorbed from the gastrointestinal tract, and peak plasma levels are attained within 1 hour. Metabolism to inactive minoxidil glucuronide is extensive, and only 10% of the drug is recovered unchanged in the urine. The elimination half-time is about 4 hours.

Cardiovascular Effects

The hypotensive effect of minoxidil is accompanied by marked increases in heart rate and cardiac output. This same reflex stimulation of the sympathetic nervous system is also accompanied by increases in the plasma concentrations of norepinephrine and renin with associated Na^+ and water retention. Orthostatic hypotension is not prominent in patients treated with minoxidil.

Side Effects

Fluid retention, manifesting as weight gain and edema, is a common side effect of minoxidil therapy. Furosemide or even dialysis may be necessary if fluid retention is unresponsive to less potent diuretics. Pulmonary hypertension associated with minoxidil is more likely due to fluid retention than a unique effect of this drug on pulmonary vasculature.

A potentially serious side effect of minoxidil therapy is the development of pericardial effusion and cardiac tamponade in about 3% of patients, especially if severe renal dysfunction is present (Husserl and Messerli, 1981). Echocardiographic studies should be performed if pericardial effusion is suspected. Abnormalities on the ECG are characterized by flattening or inversion of the T wave and increased voltage of the QRS complex. During long-term therapy, T-wave abnormalities generally disappear and the QRS voltage is reduced. Hypertrichosis, most notable around the face and arms, is an unpleasant but harmless side effect that appears, to some degree, in nearly all patients treated for longer than 1 month (Husserl and Messerli, 1981). This side effect cannot be attributed to any definite endocrine abnormality.

TRIMAZOSIN

Trimazosin is related to prazosin, but its effect on alpha-1 receptors is less pronounced. There is dilation of both arterioles and venules. Metabolism is in the liver, and the elimination half-time is about 2.7 hours.

TERAZOSIN

Terazosin is a long-acting selective alpha-1 antagonist that decreases blood pressure by dilation of both arterioles and venules.

GUANETHIDINE

Guanethidine acts exclusively on the peripheral sympathetic nervous system and produces its antihypertensive effect by inhibiting the presynaptic release of the neurotransmitter, norepinephrine, in response to sympathetic nervous system stimulation (Fig. 15-8). With time, there is a depletion of tissue concentrations of norepinephrine that persists for several days after the drug is discontinued. Uptake of guanethidine into adrenergic neurons by the same mechanism

responsible for reentry of norepinephrine into the neurons is essential for the antihypertensive action of guanethidine.

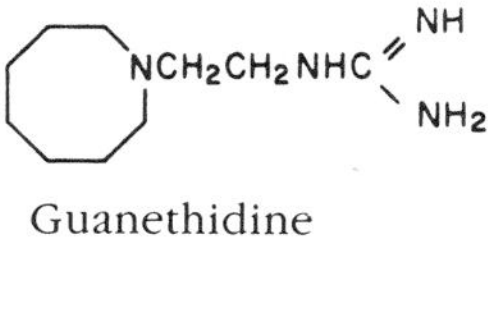

Guanethidine is used in the treatment of essential hypertension that is resistant to less potent drugs. Another rare use of guanethidine is its intravenous injection into an extremity isolated from the circulation for the treatment of reflex sympathetic dystrophy (Hannington-Kiff, 1974).

Pharmacokinetics

Absorption of guanethidine after oral administration (25 to 50 mg daily) is variable, ranging from 3% to 30% of the administered dose. Almost all of the guanethidine that enters the circulation in humans is eliminated in the urine as unchanged drug or inactive metabolites. Elimination half-time is prolonged, averaging about 5 days, allowing for a once-daily dosing interval. The effect of guanethidine may not occur for 7 to 14 days after therapy is initiated. Furthermore, antihypertensive effects may persist for several days after guanethidine is discontinued reflecting the drug's prolonged elimination half-time.

Cardiovascular Effects

Orthostatic hypotension is the most prominent side effect of treatment with guanethidine. Decreased sympathetic nervous system activity at the heart may precipitate cardiac failure, particularly in the presence of fluid retention and preexisting cardiac disease. Fluid retention can lead to resistance to the antihypertensive effect if a diuretic is not administered concurrently. Diarrhea occurs in a high percentage of patients, reflecting a predominance of parasympathetic nervous system activity in the presence of sympathetic nervous system blockade. The antihypertensive effect of guanethidine is prevented by drugs (tricyclic antidepressants, phenothiazines, amphetamines, cocaine) that prevent passage of norepinephrine as well as this drug into postganglionic sympathetic nerve endings.

Chronic administration of guanethidine produces a denervation hypersensitivity phenomena. Indeed, hypertensive crisis can occur if direct-acting sympathomimetics are administered or if a patient with a pheochromocytoma receives guanethidine. Conversely, the response to indirect-acting sympathomimetics is attenuated.

FIGURE 15–8. Guanethidine

Concentrations of catecholamines in the central nervous system are not altered by guanethidine, reflecting the limited ability of this poorly lipid-soluble drug to cross the blood-brain barrier. Indeed, sedation and associated reductions in anesthetic requirements (MAC) are not produced by guanethidine (Fig. 15-2) (Miller et al, 1969). Further evidence of lack of guanethidine entrance into the central nervous system is the absence of mental depression when this drug is administered.

GUANADREL

Guanadrel has a mechanism of action and hemodynamic effects similar to those of guanethidine, but it has a more rapid onset and shorter duration of action (Fig. 15-9). In contrast to guanethidine, guanadrel causes less orthostatic hypotension, diarrhea, and impotence.

Following oral administration, the maximal hypotensive effect occurs in 4 to 6 hours. Protein binding is estimated to be 20%. Unchanged drug and metabolites excreted in the urine account for 85% of an administered dose. The elimination half-time ranges from 5 to 45 hours.

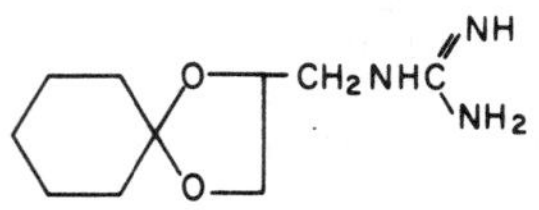

CAPTOPRIL

Captopril is an orally effective antihypertensive drug that acts by competitive inhibition of angiotensin I-converting enzyme (peptidyl dipeptidase) (Fig. 15-10) (Williams, 1988). This is the enzyme that converts inactive angiotensin I to active angiotensin II. Angiotensin II is responsible for stimulating secretion of aldosterone by the adrenal cortex. As a result of inhibition of this enzyme by captopril, there is a predictable decrease in circulating plasma concentrations of angiotensin II and aldosterone accompanied by compensatory increases in angiotensin I and renin levels. The increase in plasma concentrations of renin reflects the loss of negative feedback control normally provided by angiotensin II. The de-

FIGURE 15-10.   Captopril.

crease in aldosterone secretion results in a slight increase in serum potassium (K^+) levels.

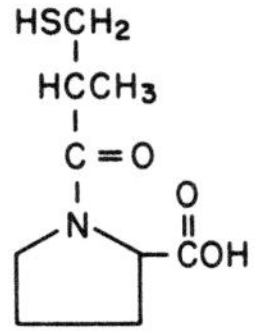

Patients with renovascular hypertension are particularly likely to respond to captopril. Nevertheless, this drug is often efficacious in treating hypertension even in patients who exhibit normal plasma renin activity. In particular, captopril may be useful in the treatment of hypertension in patients with diabetes mellitus (Williams, 1988). Part of the broad efficacy of captopril and other drugs classified as converting enzyme inhibitors may reflect effects on a number of different hormonal systems. For example, there may be increased synthesis of vasodilating prostaglandins, and the effects of plasma kinins may be exaggerated because the same converting enzyme inhibited by captopril is also responsible for the metabolism of bradykinin. Measures of general well-being (cognitive function, work performance, physical symptoms, sexual function) are better maintained in patients treated with captopril than in those treated with drugs acting on the central nervous system, leading to improved patient compliance with drug therapy (Croog et al, 1986).

Pharmacokinetics

Captopril is well absorbed after oral administration, with 25% to 30% of the drug reversibly bound to protein in the circulation. Inhibition of converting enzyme occurs within 15 minutes following oral administration. Excretion of unchanged drug in the urine accounts for about 50% of captopril. Indeed, renal dysfunction leads to drug retention.

Cardiovascular Effects

The antihypertensive effect of captopril is due to a decrease in systemic vascular resistance as a re-

FIGURE 15-9.   Guanadrel.

sult of decreased Na$^+$ and water retention. Decreased systemic vascular resistance is particularly prominent in the kidneys, whereas cerebral blood flow and coronary blood flow appear to remain autoregulated. Nevertheless, decreases in cerebral blood flow with or without captopril-induced reductions in blood pressure have been described (Jensen et al, 1989). Besides evoking arteriolar dilation, captopril increases compliance of large arteries, which also contributes to reductions in blood pressure.

Typically, captopril reduces blood pressure without concomitant alterations in cardiac output or heart rate. Orthostatic hypotension is unlikely because this drug does not interfere with sympathetic nervous system activity. The absence of a compensatory reflex-mediated increase in heart rate when blood pressure is decreased suggests that captopril may cause changes in baroreceptor sensitivity (Williams, 1988). Unlike beta-adrenergic antagonists, this antihypertensive drug lacks metabolic effects and is useful in patients with diabetes mellitus. Simultaneous administration of captopril with a diuretic or beta-adrenergic antagonist is often used to increase antihypertensive effects. Captopril may improve the efficacy of vasodilators in treating cardiac failure, presumably by blocking vasodilator-induced increases in renin output. Dramatic reversal of vascular and renal effects of scleroderma may follow the administration of captopril.

Side Effects

The most common side effect of captopril therapy, occurring in about 10% of patients, is a skin rash sometimes accompanied by fever and joint discomfort (Husserl and Messerli, 1981). Pruritus may accompany the rash. Loss of taste sensation occurs in 1% to 2% of treated patients. Proteinuria has been observed in patients with preexisting renal disease treated for prolonged periods with high doses of captopril. Captopril may cause elevations in the serum concentrations of creatinine when administered to volume-depleted patients or those with renal disease. Elevated transaminase enzymes have been noted, but a cause-and-effect relationship has not been established. Neutropenia has occurred in about 0.3% of patients, being most frequent in patients with severe renal disease or those receiving immuno-

suppressive therapy. For this reason, white blood cell counts should be performed frequently during the first few months of captopril treatment. The gravest but rarest. side effect of captopril is angioedema, which may be due to a drug-induced inhibition of the metabolism of bradykinin.

Captopril may increase serum K$^+$ levels and cause hyperkalemia, especially in patients with impaired renal function. The risk of hyperkalemia is increased if a K$^+$-sparing diuretic is given with captopril (Williams, 1988).

Appearance of cough and, in patients with chronic obstructive airway disease, an exacerbation of dyspnea and wheezing, may accompany the administration of captopril (Semple and Herd, 1986). It is speculated that these responses reflect potentiation of the effects of kinins owing to captopril-induced inhibition of peptidyl dipeptidase activity. This cough is not associated with an increase in airway resistance (Boulet et al, 1989).

The initial dose of captopril may cause an abrupt fall in blood pressure, particularly in patients who are volume depleted by prior diuretic therapy. Neurologic disturbances have been observed in patients receiving captopril and cimetidine concurrently. Nonsteroidal anti-inflammatory drugs may antagonize the antihypertensive effects of captopril, suggesting the possible role of prostaglandin synthesis in the blood pressure–lowering effects of this drug.

ENALAPRIL

Enalapril is a converting enzyme inhibitor that resembles captopril with respect to pharmacologic effects (Fig. 15-11). This drug binds tightly to the enzyme such that a single daily oral dose may be effective. Enalapril is a prodrug that is metabolized in the liver to its active dicarboxylic acid form, enalaprilat. This active form lacks the sulfhydryl group thought to be responsible for

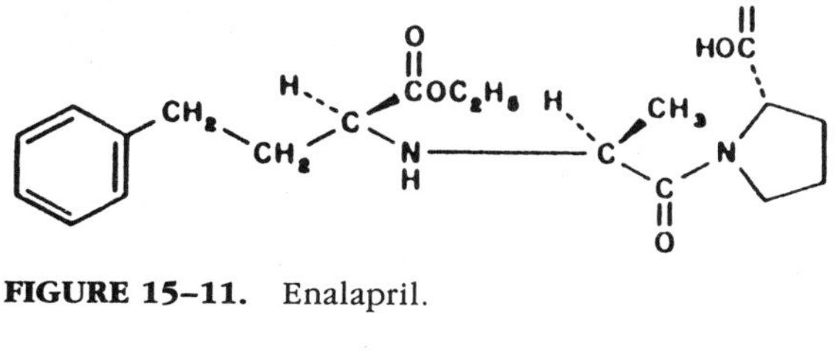

FIGURE 15–11. Enalapril.

some of the adverse effects of captopril. Indeed, rash and taste disturbances are less common with enalapril than with captopril.

SARALASIN

Saralasin and related drugs preferentially compete with angiotensin II for receptors on vascular smooth muscle that mediate angiotensin II-induced vasoconstriction. Because the agonist activity of saralasin is only about 1% of that of angiotensin II, this drug acts as a competitive inhibitor, resulting in a decrease in systemic vascular resistance and a decrease in blood pressure in patients with renin-dependent hypertension. Conversely, administration of this drug to hypertensive patients with subnormal plasma renin activity may evoke a pressor response, reflecting the intrinsic agonist activity of saralasin. Another important agonist action of saralasin in the absence of elevated plasma renin activity is stimulation of aldosterone secretion. The elimination half-time of saralasin is brief (about 4 minutes), necessitating a continuous intravenous infusion to achieve a sustained effect.

METYROSINE

Metyrosine, 2 to 4 g daily, administered orally to adults, blocks catecholamine synthesis by inhibiting tyrosine hydroxylase, the enzyme that catalyzes the conversion of tyrosine to dopa (Fig. 15-12; see Fig. 42-5). This is the first step in catecholamine synthesis and is also the rate-limiting step. When administered to patients with pheochromocytoma, metyrosine reduces catecholamine production and usually decreases the frequency and severity of hypertensive attacks. This drug may be useful for the preoperative treatment of patients with pheochromocytoma and for long-term therapy when surgery is not feasible. Metyrosine has not been compared to the traditional treatment regimen of alpha-adrenergic blockade with or without concomitant beta-adrenergic blockade in the preoperative preparation of patients with a pheochromocytoma. This drug is not consistently effective in the treatment of essential hypertension.

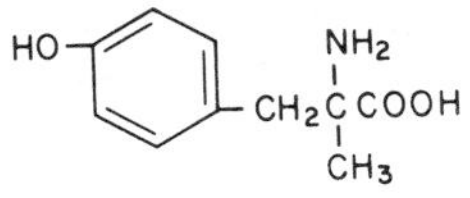

Pharmacokinetics

Metyrosine is well absorbed from the gastrointestinal tract, with maximal biochemical effects occurring within 1 to 3 days after the initiation of therapy. The urinary concentration of catecholamines usually returns to pretreatment levels within 3 to 4 days after discontinuing the drug. Excretion of metyrosine is principally in the urine as unchanged drug.

Side Effects

Sedation is the most common side effect of metyrosine. Insomnia and psychic stimulation may occur when the drug is discontinued. Extrapyramidal reactions occur in about 10% of treated patients, and these effects may be potentiated by butyrophenones. Diarrhea may be severe in about 10% of patients. The risk of nephrolithiasis is reduced by increased water intake to achieve a daily urine output of at least 2 L. Metyrosine should be discontinued if crystalluria persists despite an increase in water intake. Increased transaminase levels and eosinophilia have been observed rarely.

REFERENCES

Bailey PL, Sperry RJ, Johnson GK et al. Respiratory effects of clonidine alone and combined with morphine, in humans. Anesthesiology 1991;74:43–48.

Bonnet F, Boico O, Rostaing S, et al. Postoperative analgesia with extradural clonidine. Br J Anaesth 1989a;63:465–9.

Bonnet F, Brun-Buisson V, Saada M, Boico O, Rostaing S, Touboul C. Dose-related prolongation of hyperbaric tetracaine spinal anesthesia by clonidine in humans. Anesth Analg 1989b;68:619–22.

Boulet L-P, Milot J, Lampron N, Lacouciere Y. Pulmonary function and airway responsiveness during long-term therapy with captopril. JAMA 1989;261:413–6.

Bravo EL, Taraji RC, Fouad FM, Vidt DG, Gifford RW. Clonidine suppression: A useful aid in the diagnosis of pheochromotycoma. N Engl J Med 1981;305:623–6.

Brodsky JB, Bravo JJ. Acute postoperative clonidine

FIGURE 15–12. Metyrosine.

withdrawal syndrome. Anesthesiology 1976; 44:519–20.

Bruce DL, Croley TF, Lee JS. Preoperative clonidine withdrawal syndrome. Anesthesiology 1979;51:90–2.

Campese VM. Minoxidil: A review of its pharmacological properties and therapeutic use. Drugs 1981;22:257–78.

Croog SH, Levine S, Testa MA, et al. The effects of antihypertensive therapy on the quality of life. N Engl J Med 1986;314:1657–64.

Eger EI, Hamilton WK. The effect of reserpine on the action of various vasopressors. Anesthesiology 1959;20:641–5.

Eisenach JC, Dewan DM. Intrathecal clonidine in obstetrics: Sheep studies. Anesthesiology 1990; 72:663–8.

Eisenach JC, Dewan DM, Rose JC, Angelo JM. Epidural clonidine produces antinociception, but not hypotension, in sheep. Anesthesiology 1987;66:496–501.

Engelman E, Lipszyc M, Gilbart E, et al. Effects of clonidine on anesthetic drug requirements and hemodynamic response during aortic surgery. Anesthesiology 1989;71:178–87.

Farsang C, Kunos G. Naloxone reverses the antihypertensive effect of clonidine. Br J Pharmacol 1979;67:161–4.

Flacke JW, Bloor BC, Flacke WE, et al. Reduced narcotic requirement by clonidine with improved hemodynamic and adrenergic stability in patients undergoing coronary bypass surgery. Anesthesiology 1987;67:11–9.

Ghignone M. Calvillo O, Quintin L. Anesthesia and hypertension: The effect of clonidine on perioperative hemodynamics and isoflurane requirements. Anesthesiology 1987;67:3–10.

Glynn C, Dawson D, Sanders R. A double-blind comparison between epidural morphine and epidural clonidine in patients with chronic non-cancer pain. Pain 1988;34:123–8.

Gold MS, Pottash AC, Sweeney DR, Kleber HD. Opiate withdrawal using clonidine: A safe, effective and rapid nonopiate treatment. JAMA 1980;242:343–6.

Hannington-Kiff G. Intravenous regional sympathetic block with guanethidine. Lancet 1974;1:1019–20.

Husserl FE, Messerli FH. Adverse effects of antihypertensive drugs. Drugs 1981;22:188–210.

Jensen K, Bunemann L, Riisager S, Thomsen LJ. Cerebral blood flow during anaesthesia: Influence of pretreatment with metoprolol or captopril. Br J Anaesth 1989;62:321–3.

Maze M, Smith CM. Identification of receptor mechanism mediating epinephrine-induced arrhythmias during halothane anesthesia in the dog. Anesthesiology 1983;59:322–6.

Mazze RI, Woodruff RE, Heerdt ME. Isoniazid-induced enflurane defluorination in humans. Anesthesiology 1982;57:5–8.

Miller RD, Way WL, Eger EI. The effects of alpha-methyldopa, reserpine, guanethidine and iproniazid on minimum alveolar anesthetic requirement (MAC). Anesthesiology 1969;29:1153–8.

Milne B, Cervenko FW, Jhamandas K, Sutak M. Local clonidine: Analgesia and effect on opiate withdrawal in the rat. Anesthesiology 1985;62:34–8.

Niles AS, Shand DG. Hypertensive response to propranolol in a patient treated with methyldopa: A proposed mechanism. Clin Pharmacol Ther 1973;14:823–6.

Prys-Roberts C, Meloche R, Foex P. Studies of anaesthesia in relation to hypertension. I: Cardiovascular responses to treated and untreated patients. Br J Anaesth 1971;43:122–37.

Racle JP, Benkhadra A, Poy JY, Gleizal B. Prolongation of isobaric bupivacaine spinal anesthesia with epinephrine and clonidine for hip surgery in the elderly. Anesth Analg 1987;66:442–6.

Semple PF, Herd GW. Cough and wheeze caused by inhibitors of angiotensin-converting enzyme. N Engl J Med 1986;314:61.

Stiff JL, Harris DB. Clonidine withdrawal complicated by amitriptyline therapy. Anesthesiology 1983;59:73–4.

Thornton WE. Dementia induced by methyldopa with haloperidol. N Engl J Med 1976;194:1222.

White WB, Gilbert JC. Transdermal clonidine in a patient with resistant hypertension and malabsorption. N Engl J Med 1985;313:1418.

Williams GH. Converting-enzyme inhibitors in the treatment of hypertension. N Engl J Med 1988; 319:1517–25.

16

Peripheral Vasodilators

INTRODUCTION

Peripheral vasodilators are most frequently used clinically to (1) treat hypertensive crises, (2) produce controlled hypotension, and (3) facilitate left ventricular forward stroke volume, as in patients with regurgitant valvular heart lesions or acute cardiac failure (Fyman et al, 1986). Peripheral vasodilators that are administered intravenously, often as a continuous infusion, include nitroprusside, nitroglycerin, trimethaphan, and diazoxide (Fig. 16-1). Conceptually, vasodilators lower blood pressure by decreasing systemic vascular resistance (arterial vasodilators) or by decreasing venous return and cardiac output (venous vasodilators). Decreased systemic vascular resistance also reduces the impedance to left ventricular ejection and allows for an increased forward left ventricular stroke volume, decreased left ventricular chamber size, and reduced myocardial oxygen requirements. Indeed, the present trend in treatment of cardiac failure is to optimize cardiac output by manipulating the peripheral circulation (Fyman et al, 1986).

NITROPRUSSIDE

Nitroprusside is a direct-acting, nonselective peripheral vasodilator that causes relaxation of arterial and venous vascular smooth muscle (Fig. 16-1) (Kaplan et al, 1980; Tinker and Michenfelder, 1976). This drug lacks significant effects on other smooth muscle and on cardiac muscle.

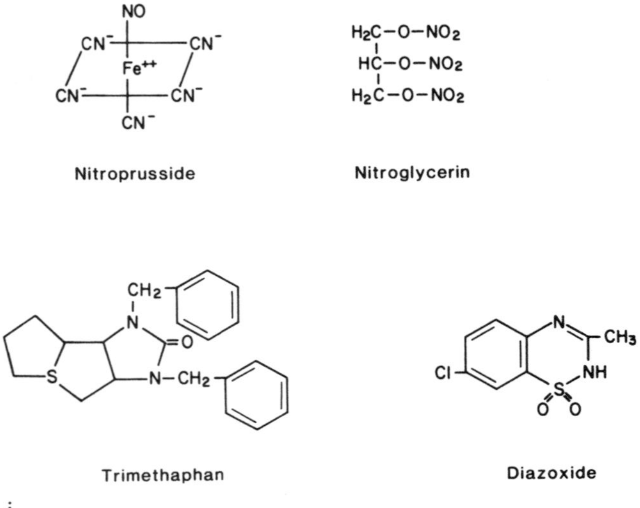

FIGURE 16-1. Peripheral vasodilators.

Nitroprusside

Nitroglycerin

Trimethaphan

Diazoxide

Its onset of action is almost immediate, and its duration of action is transient, requiring continuous intravenous infusion to maintain a therapeutic effect. The extreme potency of nitroprusside necessitates careful titration of dosage as provided by continuous infusion devices and frequent monitoring of blood pressure, often by an intraarterial catheter attached to a transducer.

Clinical Uses

Nitroprusside is used when prompt and reliable reduction in blood pressure is mandatory, as in treatment of hypertensive crises or production of controlled hypotension (Thompson et al, 1978). In addition, nitroprusside-induced decreases in left ventricular impedance, even in the absence of changes in blood pressure, can improve cardiac output in patients with acute cardiac failure due to myocardial ischemia or regurgitant valvular heart lesions.

Nitroprusside, 1 to 2 $\mu g \cdot kg^{-1}$ IV as a rapid injection, is useful to offset blood pressure elevations produced by direct laryngoscopy for intubation of the trachea (Fig. 16-2) (Stoelting,

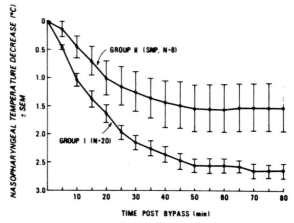

FIGURE 16-3. Nitroprusside (SNP)-induced vasodilation during the rewarming phase of cardiopulmonary bypass minimizes the subsequent decline in nasopharyngeal temperature (group II) compared with untreated patients (group I). (From Noback CR, Tinker JR. Hypothermia after cardiopulmonary bypass in man: Amelioration by nitroprusside-induced vasodilation during rewarming. Anesthesiology 1980; 53: 277–80; with permission.)

1979). Administration of nitroprusside, and presumably other vasodilators such as nitroglycerin, during the rewarming phase of cardiopulmonary bypass results in vasodilation that permits increased flow rates and, thus, improved heat delivery to peripheral tissues. As a result, the decline in nasopharyngeal temperature following cessation of cardiopulmonary bypass is minimized (Fig. 16-3) (Noback and Tinker, 1980).

Mechanism of Action

Organic nitrates, such as nitroprusside, nitroglycerin, and hydralazine, can produce nitric oxide, which activates the enzyme guanylate cyclase (Parker, 1987). Guanylate cyclase results in increased concentrations of cyclic guanosine monophosphate in smooth muscle, leading to vasodilation in veins and arteries. The mechanism of vasodilation induced by cyclic guanosine monophosphate is not completely understood, but it may be secondary to decreased calcium ion (Ca^{2+}) entry into muscle cells or increased Ca^{2+} uptake by the sarcoplasmic reticulum (Parker, 1987).

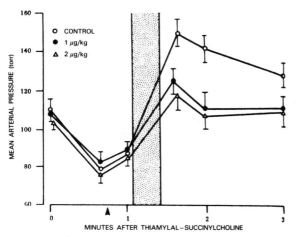

FIGURE 16-2. Intravenous administration of nitroprusside attenuates the blood pressure response evoked by direct laryngoscopy (shaded area) and intubation of the trachea. Arrow denotes the injection of nitroprusside. (From Stoelting RK. Attenuation of blood pressure response to laryngoscopy and tracheal intubation with sodium nitroprusside. Anesth Analg 1979; 58: 116–9; with permission.)

Metabolism

Metabolism of nitroprusside begins with the transfer of an electron from the iron of oxyhemoglobin to nitroprusside, yielding methemoglobin and an unstable nitroprusside radical (Fig. 16-4) (Tinker and Michenfelder, 1976; Vesey et al, 1976). This electron transfer is independent of enzyme activity. The unstable nitroprusside radical promptly breaks down, releasing all five cyanide ions, one of which reacts with methemoglobin to form cyanmethemoglobin. The remaining free cyanide ions are available to rhodanase enzyme in the liver and kidney for conversion to thiocyanate. Any free cyanide that is not rapidly converted to thiocyanate can bind to cytochrome oxidase, impairing aerobic respiration. Anaerobic respiration occurs, yielding lactic acid and metabolic acidosis (see the section entitled "Cyanide Toxicity"). The breakdown of nitroprusside to cyanide by plasma glutathione or tissue

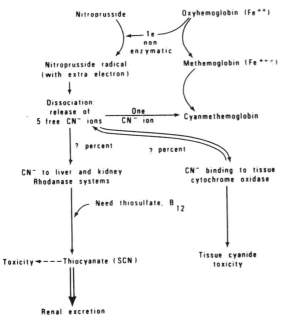

FIGURE 16-4. Metabolism of nitroprusside begins with the transfer of an electron from the iron of oxyhemoglobin to nitroprusside, yielding methemoglobin and an unstable nitroprusside radical. (From Tinker JH, Michenfelder JD. Sodium nitroprusside: Pharmacology, toxicity and therapeutics. Anesthesiology 1976; 45: 340–54; with permission.)

sulfhydryl groups is too slow to be of any significance. The nonenzymatic release of cyanide from nitroprusside is not inhibited by hypothermia as may be present during cardiopulmonary bypass, whereas enzymatic conversion of cyanide to thiocyanate may be delayed (Moore et al, 1985).

Because the conversion of nitroprusside to cyanide is independent of enzyme activity, the amount of cyanide release from nitroprusside depends entirely on the total dose of drug that is administered. The subsequent rate at which cyanide is converted to thiocyanate by rhodanase enzyme is dependent on the availability of a sulfur donor for the enzyme. Usually, endogenous thiosulfate is the sulfur donor, being derived from the amino acid cysteine.

Thiocyanate is cleared slowly by the kidney, with an elimination half-time of 4 to 7 days. Thus, thiocyanate accumulates with prolonged therapy or in the presence of renal failure. If the plasma concentration of thiocyanate is greater than 10 $mg \cdot dl^{-1}$, there may be skeletal muscle weakness, nausea, and mental confusion. Prolonged elevations of plasma thiocyanate concentrations can result in hypothyroidism because thiocyanate inhibits uptake of iodide ions by the thyroid gland. Oxyhemoglobin can slowly oxidize thiocyanate back to sulfate and cyanide, but this is insufficient to cause cyanide toxicity.

Solutions of nitroprusside exposed to light may release cyanide *in vitro*. For this reason, the container and tubing used to deliver nitroprusside to patients are commonly covered with aluminum foil. Nevertheless, differences in cyanide concentrations do not occur in light-exposed compared with light-protected solutions during the first 8 hours (Ikeda et al, 1987). When protected from light, *in vitro* breakdown to cyanide is not excessive in the first 24 hours after the solution of nitroprusside is prepared.

Cyanide Toxicity

There is a linear relationship between the plasma concentration of cyanide and the total dose of nitroprusside administered (Vesey et al, 1976). Cyanide toxicity from spontaneous breakdown of nitroprusside should be suspected in any patient who is resistant to the hypotensive effects of the drug despite adequate infusion rates (up to 8 $\mu g \cdot kg^{-1} \cdot min^{-1}$ IV), or in a previously responsive patient who becomes unresponsive to the blood pressure–lowering effects of the drug despite increasing doses (tachyphylaxis). Mixed venous PO_2 is elevated in the presence of cyanide toxicity, indicating paralysis of cytochrome oxidase and inability of the tissues to use oxygen. At the same time, metabolic acidosis develops as a reflection of anaerobic metabolism in the tissues. Decreased cerebral oxygen use is evidenced by the increased cerebral venous oxygen content.

Blood cyanide levels are increased while thiocyanate levels are unchanged in patients who develop cyanide toxicity following short-term administration of nitroprusside (Vesey et al, 1976). Indeed, measurement of blood thiocyanate levels is of no value in the recognition of cyanide toxicity (Michenfelder and Tinker, 1977). Even measurement of plasma cyanide concentrations may be of limited value because circulating cyanide rapidly binds to tissue cytochrome oxidase.

The phenomenon of resistance to the therapeutic effects of nitroprusside may be related to an abnormality in the cyanide-thiocyanate pathway that allows cyanide to accumulate (Davies et al, 1975). For example, patients who have Leber's optic atrophy or tobacco amblyopia manifest elevated blood concentrations of cyanide. The mechanism by which cyanide results in resistance or tachyphylaxis to the blood pressure–lowering effects of nitroprusside is not confirmed but could reflect cyanide-induced stimulation of cardiac output, which would tend to offset the hypotensive effects of the vasodilator. Furthermore, most patients who are resistant or develop tachyphylaxis to the hypotensive effects of nitroprusside are children or young adults. It is speculated that active baroreceptor reflexes in this age group evoke increases in sympathetic nervous system activity in response to drug-induced reductions in blood pressure. As a result, a larger initial dose or the subsequent need to increase the dose of nitroprusside is required to produce a decrease in blood pressure, leading to the likelihood of dose-dependent cyanide toxicity. Propranolol can be administered to blunt these baroreceptor-mediated responses and thus minimize the total dose of nitroprusside required to produce the desired blood pressure effect. Likewise, volatile anesthetics blunt baroreceptor reflex activity, thus contributing to decreased dose requirements for nitroprusside.

There is no evidence that preexisting hepatic or renal disease increases the likelihood of cyanide toxicity. In fact, renal failure may prevent sulfate excretion, which allows production of more thiosulfate to act as a sulfur donor and thus convert cyanide to thiocyanate (Fig.16-5) (Tinker and Michenfelder, 1980).

Treatment of Cyanide Toxicity

Appearance of tachyphylaxis in a previously sensitive patient in association with metabolic acidosis and elevated mixed venous PO_2 mandates immediate discontinuation of nitroprusside administration. Sodium thiosulfate, 150 mg·kg^{-1} IV, administered over 15 minutes, is a recommended therapy for cyanide toxicity (Michenfelder and Tinker, 1977). Thiosulfate acts as a sulfur donor to convert cyanide to thiocyanate. If cyanide toxicity is severe, with deteriorating hemodynamics and metabolic acidosis, the treatment is the slow administration of sodium nitrate, 5 mg·kg^{-1} IV, to convert hemoglobin to methemoglobin (Tinker and Michenfelder, 1976). Methemoglobin acts as an antidote to cyanide toxicity by converting cyanide to cyanmethemoglobin. Alternatively, administration of hydroxocobalamin, which reacts with cyanide to form cyanocobalamin, has been recommended (Cottrell et al, 1979).

Dose

Nitroprusside should be administered on the basis of total dose and not the blood pressure effect that is achieved. The maximum acceptable

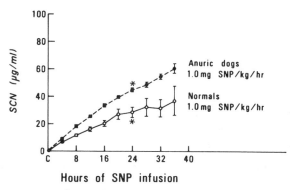

FIGURE 16–5. Plasma thiocyanate (SCN) concentrations are greater in anuric than normal dogs. (From Tinker JH, Michenfelder JD. Increased resistance to nitroprusside-induced cyanide toxicity in anuric dogs. Anesthesiology 1980; 52: 40–7; with permission.)

continuous infusion rate of nitroprusside is 8 $\mu g \cdot kg^{-1} \cdot min^{-1}$ IV for a 1- to 3-hour administration or 0.5 $mg \cdot kg^{-1} \cdot h^{-1}$ IV for chronic infusion (Michenfelder and Tinker, 1977). Nevertheless, the vast majority of anesthetized patients do not require a dose near this maximum amount, with the usual continuous intraoperative infusion rate being 0.5 to 2 $\mu g \cdot kg^{-1} \cdot min^{-1}$ IV. Volatile anesthetics, which decrease baroreceptor sensitivity, are associated with greatly reduced dose requirements for nitroprusside (Chen et al, 1982). Like volatile anesthetics, propranolol can also be used to blunt baroreceptor reflex responses and renin release, thus minimizing the dose of nitroprusside required to produce desirable degrees of blood pressure reduction (Marshall et al, 1981). Conversely, hypotension produced by nitroprusside is followed by increased baroreceptor sensitivity (baroreceptors are reset), which could contribute to subsequent increased dose requirements for nitroprusside to maintain blood pressure at a reduced level (Fig.16-6) (Chen et al, 1982). Whenever the dose of nitroprusside approaches the maximum infusion rate, it is important to monitor pH for evidence of metabolic acidosis as a manifestation of cyanide toxicity.

Effects on Organ Systems

The principal pharmacologic effects of nitroprusside are manifest on the (1) cardiovascular system, (2) blood flow to the central nervous system, (3) hypoxic pulmonary vasoconstriction, and (4) platelet aggregation. Nitroprusside lacks direct effects on the central or autonomic nervous system. In animals, nitroprusside-induced decreases in blood pressure do not result in hepatic hypoxia or changes in hepatic blood flow (Sivarajan et al, 1985). Furthermore, hepatic blood flow does not change when cardiac output is maintained in anesthetized patients despite 20% to 60% reductions in blood pressure produced by nitroprusside (Chauvin et al, 1985).

Cardiovascular System

Nitroprusside produces prompt decreases in blood pressure as a result of arterial and venous vasodilation (Tinker and Michenfelder, 1976). Peripheral vascular resistance is decreased as evidence of arterial vasodilation, whereas venous return is decreased because of vasodilation of venous capacitance vessels. It is likely that reductions in right atrial pressure reflect pooling of blood in veins. Baroreceptor-mediated reflex responses to nitroprusside-induced decreases in blood pressure manifest as tachycardia and increased myocardial contractility. Indeed, these reflex-mediated responses may offset the blood pressure–lowering effects of nitroprusside. Although decreased venous return would tend to reduce cardiac output, the net effect is often an increase in cardiac output owing to reflex-mediated increases in peripheral sympathetic nervous system activity combined with decreased impedance to left ventricular ejection. There is no evidence that nitroprusside exerts direct inotropic or chronotropic effects on the heart.

Nitroprusside-induced reductions in blood pressure often result in decreases in renal function (Tinker and Michenfelder, 1976). Release of renin may accompany blood pressure decreases produced by nitroprusside and contribute to blood pressure overshoots when the drug is discontinued (Khambatta et al, 1979; Miller et al,

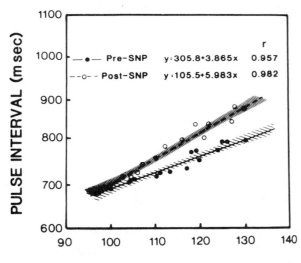

FIGURE 16–6. Baroreceptor sensitivity increases following nitroprusside-induced hypotension (post-SNP) compared with pre-SNP. (From Chen RYZ, Matteo RS, Fan F-C, Schuessler GB, Chien S. Resetting of baroreceptor sensitivity after induced hypotension. Anesthesiology 1982; 56: 29–35; with permission.)

1977). Indeed, infusion of saralasin, a competitive inhibitor of angiotensin II, prevents blood pressure overshoot following discontinuation of nitroprusside, thus confirming the participation of the renin-angiotensin system in this response (Delaney and Miller, 1980). Increased plasma concentrations of catecholamines also accompany hypotension produced by nitroprusside but not by trimethaphan (Fig. 16-7) (Knight et al, 1983).

Nitroprusside may increase the area of damage associated with a myocardial infarction. It is speculated that nitroprusside causes an intracoronary steal of blood flow away from ischemic areas by arteriolar vasodilation (Becker, 1978). Coronary steal occurs because nitroprusside dilates resistance vessels in nonischemic myocardium, resulting in diversion of blood flow from ischemic areas where vessels are already maximally dilated. Clinical evidence of a coronary steal phenomenon is the appearance of ischemic changes on the electrocardiogram (ECG). Reductions in diastolic blood pressure produced by nitroprusside may also contribute to myocardial ischemia by decreasing coronary blood flow (Sivarajan et al, 1985).

Cerebral Blood Flow

Nitroprusside is a direct cerebral vasodilator, leading to increased cerebral blood flow and cerebral blood volume. These changes, when they occur in patients with reduced intracranial compliance, may cause undesirable elevations of intracranial pressure (Turner et al, 1977). It is speculated that the rapidity of blood pressure decrease produced by nitroprusside exceeds the capacity of the cerebral circulation to autoregulate its blood flow such that intracranial pressure and blood pressure change simultaneously but in opposite directions (Rogers et al, 1979). Nevertheless, increases in intracranial pressure produced by nitroprusside are maximal during modest reductions (less than 30%) in mean arterial pressure. When nitroprusside-induced reductions in mean arterial pressure exceed 30% of the awake level, the intracranial pressure decreases to less than the awake value (Turner et al, 1977). Furthermore, decreasing blood pressure over 5 minutes with nitroprusside in the presence of hypocarbia and hyperoxia negates the increase in intracranial pressure that accompanies the rapid infusion of nitroprusside (Fig. 16-8) (Marsh et al, 1979). Clearly, the potential adverse effects of nitroprusside on intracranial pressure are not present if this drug is administered after the dura is opened.

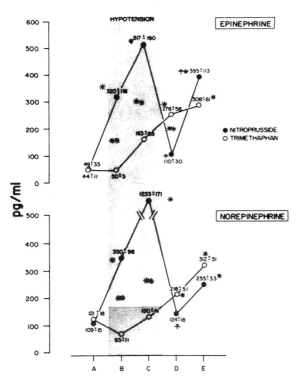

FIGURE 16–7. Increased plasma concentrations of epinephrine and norepinephrine accompany hypotension induced by nitroprusside but not by trimethaphan. (From Knight PR, Lane GA, Hensinger RN, Bolles RS, Bjoraker DJ. Catecholamine and renin-angiotensin response during hypotensive anesthesia induced by sodium nitroprusside or trimethaphan camsylate. Anesthesiology 1983; 59: 248–53; with permission.)

Hypoxic Pulmonary Vasoconstriction

Reductions in the PaO_2 may accompany the infusion of nitroprusside and other peripheral vasodilators as used to produce controlled hypotension. Attenuation of hypoxic pulmonary vasoconstriction by peripheral vasodilators is the presumed mechanism for this effect on arterial oxygenation (Colley et al, 1979). Addition of propranolol to the vasodilator regimen does not alter

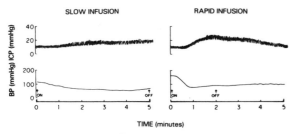

FIGURE 16–8. Compared with rapid infusion, the slow intravenous administration of nitroprusside does not increase the intracranial pressure. (From Marsh ML, Aidinis SJ, Naughton KVH, Marshall LF, Shapiro HM. The technique of nitroprusside administration modifies the intracranial pressure response. Anesthesiology 1979; 51: 538–41; with permission.)

the magnitude of reduction in PaO_2 (Miller et al, 1982). Furthermore, peripheral vasodilator–induced reductions in blood pressure may be more likely to increase the shunt fraction in patients with normal lungs than in those with chronic obstructive airway disease (Casthely et al, 1982). It is speculated that hypotension in normal patients leads to decreased pulmonary artery pressure such that preferential perfusion of dependent but poorly ventilated alveoli occurs. In contrast, patients with chronic obstructive airway disease may develop destructive vascular changes that prevent alterations in distribution of pulmonary blood flow in response to vasodilation. The addition of positive end-expiratory pressure may reverse vasodilator-induced reductions in the PaO_2 (Berthelsen et al, 1986).

Platelet Aggregation

Infusion rates of nitroprusside greater than 3 $\mu g \cdot kg^{-1} \cdot min^{-1}$ IV (or a total dose of more than 16 mg) may result in dose-related decreases in platelet aggregation (Fig. 16-9) (Hines and Barash, 1989). This reduction in platelet aggregation is accompanied by an increase in bleeding time, which could result in excessive operative and postoperative blood loss. It is speculated that impaired platelet aggregation reflects nitroprusside-induced inhibition of thrombosthenin, a smooth muscle-like protein. Conversely, the increase in bleeding time may be independent of an alteration in platelet function and rather a result of vasodilation secondary to a direct effect of nitroprusside on vascular tone.

NITROGLYCERIN

Nitroglycerin is an organic nitrate that acts principally on venous capacitance vessels to produce peripheral pooling of blood, reduction of heart size, and decreased cardiac ventricular wall tension (Fig. 16-1) (Kaplan et al, 1980; Parker, 1987). As the dose of nitroglycerin is increased, there is also relaxation of arterial vascular smooth muscle. The most common clinical use of nitroglycerin is sublingual or intravenous administration for the treatment of angina pectoris owing either to atherosclerosis of the coronary arteries or intermittent vasospasm of these vessels. Production of controlled hypotension has also been achieved with the continuous intravenous infusion of nitroglycerin.

Route of Administration

Nitroglycerin is most frequently administered by the sublingual route, but it is also available as an oral tablet, a buccal or transmucosal tablet, a lingual spray, and a transdermal ointment or patch. Sublingual administration of nitroglycerin results in peak plasma concentrations within 4 minutes. Only about 15% of the blood flow from the sublingual area passes through the liver, which limits the initial first-pass hepatic metabolism of nitroglycerin.

Transdermal absorption of nitroglycerin, 5 to 10 mg over 24 hours, provides sustained protection against myocardial ischemia. The plasma

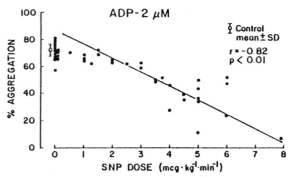

FIGURE 16–9. Platelet aggregation (%) at varying intravenous infusion rates of nitroprusside (SNP). (From Hines R, Barash PG. Infusion of sodium nitroprusside induces platelet dysfunction *in vitro.* Anesthesiology 1989; 70: 611–5; with permission.)

concentration resulting from transdermal absorption of nitroglycerin is low, but tolerance to the drug effect occurs when the patches are left in place longer than 24 hours (Parker, 1987). It is likely that removing the patches after 14 to 16 hours will prevent the development of tolerance.

Continuous intravenous infusion of nitroglycerin, via special delivery tubing to reduce absorption of the drug into plastic, is a useful approach to maintain a constant plasma concentration of nitroglycerin.

Mechanism of Action

(See also the section entitled "Nitroprusside.")

The ability of nitroglycerin to reduce myocardial oxygen requirements is the most likely mechanism by which this drug relieves angina pectoris in patients with atherosclerotic disease of the coronary arteries. For example, nitroglycerin-induced venodilatation and increased venous capacitance decreases venous return (preload) to the heart, resulting in reduced ventricular end-diastolic pressure and volume and, therefore, decreased myocardial oxygen requirements. In addition, any drug-induced reduction in systemic vascular resistance decreases afterload and myocardial oxygen requirements. Nitroglycerin does not increase total coronary blood flow in patients with angina pectoris owing to atherosclerosis.

The ability of nitroglycerin to dilate selectively large conductive coronary arteries may be an important mechanism in the relief of angina pectoris owing to vasospasm. Specifically, nitroglycerin appears to cause redistribution of coronary blood flow to ischemic areas of subendocardium by selective dilatation of large epicardial vessels. Indeed, nitroglycerin increases the washout rate of radioactive xenon from ischemic areas of the ventricle, indicating that blood flow to this region has increased. Nitroglycerin, in contrast to nitroprusside, may decrease the area of damage associated with a myocardial infarction, presumably by preferentially diverting blood flow to the ischemic area.

Pharmacokinetics

Nitroglycerin has an elimination half-time of about 1.5 minutes (Parker, 1987). There is a large volume of distribution, reflecting tissue uptake, and it has been estimated that only 1% of total body nitroglycerin is present in plasma. For this reason, plasma nitroglycerin concentrations may vary widely as a result of minor changes in tissue binding.

Metabolism

Nitroglycerin is metabolized in the liver by nitrate reductase (glutathione dependent) to glycerol dinitrate and nitrite, which are excreted in the urine (Kaplan et al, 1980). Resulting denitrated metabolites of nitroglycerin are about ten times less potent as vasodilators. The nitrite metabolite of nitroglycerin is capable of oxidizing the ferrous ion in hemoglobin to the ferric state with the production of methemoglobin. Although significant methemoglobin formation is unlikely when total nitroglycerin doses are less than 5 mg·kg^{-1}, there are reports of methemoglobinemia in patients receiving lesser doses of nitroglycerin (Fibuch et al, 1979; Zurick et al, 1984). Treatment is with methylene blue, 1 to 2 mg·kg^{-1} IV, administered over 5 minutes, to facilitate the conversion of methemoglobin to hemoglobin.

Clinical Uses

Angina Pectoris

Sublingual nitroglycerin, 0.3 mg, is the most useful of the organic nitrates for the acute and chronic treatment and prevention of angina pectoris owing to atherosclerotic coronary artery disease or coronary artery vasospasm. Failure of three sublingual tablets in a 15-minute period to relieve angina pectoris may reflect myocardial infarction. Other, more expensive, sublingual nitrates do not appear to be more effective than nitroglycerin. (See the section entitled "Isosorbide Dinitrate"). Application of 2% nitroglycerin ointment over a skin area of 2.5 by 5 cm produces sustained protection from angina pectoris for up to 4 hours.

Continuous intravenous infusion of nitroglycerin, 0.25 to 1 µg·kg^{-1}·min^{-1}, has been used intraoperatively as prophylaxis against myocardial ischemia in anesthetized patients with known coronary artery disease (Kaplan et al, 1976). Nevertheless, nitroglycerin, 0.5 to 1 µg·kg^{-1}·min^{-1}

IV, cannot be demonstrated to prevent changes of myocardial ischemia on the ECG of patients anesthetized with nitrous oxide-fentanyl and paralyzed with pancuronium (Gallagher et al, 1986; Thomson et al, 1984). Nitroglycerin does, however, reduce the incidence of hypertension as may occur during direct laryngoscopy and intubation of the trachea.

Headache is common and may be severe following administration of sublingual nitroglycerin. Presumably, headache reflects dilatation of meningeal vessels. Arterial dilatation in the face and neck manifests as facial flushing. Tolerance, which occurs with frequent exposure to high doses of organic nitrates, does not develop with the intermittent sublingual administration of nitroglycerin as used to treat angina pectoris.

Cardiac Failure

Nitroglycerin primarily reduces preload and relieves pulmonary edema. Intravenous infusion of nitroglycerin to patients with acute myocardial infarction can improve cardiac output, relieve pulmonary congestion, and decrease myocardial oxygen requirements, thus potentially limiting the size of the myocardial infarction.

Controlled Hypotension

Nitroglycerin can be used to produce controlled hypotension, but it is less potent than nitroprusside. For example, equivalent reductions in blood pressure are achieved by the continuous intravenous infusion of nitroglycerin, 4.7 $\mu g \cdot kg^{-1} \cdot min^{-1}$, and nitroprusside, 2.5 $\mu g \cdot kg^{-1} \cdot min^{-1}$ (Fahmy, 1978). At comparable systolic blood pressures, the mean and diastolic blood pressures are higher with nitroglycerin than with nitroprusside. Evidence of myocardial ischemia may appear on the ECG during infusion of nitroprusside, presumably reflecting the impact of decreased diastolic blood pressure on coronary blood flow (Fahmy, 1978). Because nitroglycerin acts predominantly on venous capacitance vessels, the production of controlled hypotension using this drug may be more dependent on intravascular fluid volume as compared with nitroprusside.

Acute Hypertension

Nitroglycerin may be effective in controling acute increases in blood pressure that may ac-

company noxious stimulation in the parturient, as during cesarean section (Snyder et al, 1979). This drug crosses the placenta because of its low molecular weight (227) and nonionized state, but should not produce adverse metabolic or central nervous system effects in the fetus. Conversely, a theoretical concern exists as to the possible adverse effects of cyanide that is detectable in fetal blood following administration of nitroprusside to the mother. Trimethaphan effectively controls maternal blood pressure but may produce undesirable autonomic nervous system effects in the neonate, including paralytic ileus.

Effects on Organ Systems

The principal pharmacologic actions of nitroglycerin manifest as cardiovascular effects. Nitroglycerin also acts on smooth muscle in the airways and gastrointestinal tract. For example, bronchial smooth muscle is relaxed regardless of the preexisting tone (Byrick et al, 1983). Smooth muscle of the biliary tract, including the sphincter of Oddi, is relaxed. Indeed, pain that mimics angina pectoris but is due to opioid-induced biliary tract spasm will often be relieved by nitroglycerin. Relief of this pain by nitroglycerin may lead to the incorrect conclusion that myocardial ischemia had been present. Esophageal muscle tone is reduced, as is ureteral and uterine smooth muscle tone, although these latter effects are somewhat unpredictable. Like nitroprusside, nitroglycerin is a cerebral vasodilator and may increase intracranial pressure in patients with decreased intracranial compliance (Gagnon et al, 1979).

Cardiovascular Effects

Nitroglycerin doses up to 2 $\mu g \cdot kg^{-1} \cdot min^{-1}$ IV produce dilatation of veins that predominates over that produced in arterioles (Gerson et al, 1982). Venodilatation results in decreased venous return as well as reduced left and right ventricular end-diastolic pressures. In normal individuals and patients with coronary artery disease, but in the absence of cardiac failure, nitroglycerin decreases cardiac output. This decreased cardiac output reflects reduced venous return as nitroglycerin is devoid of any direct inotropic effect on the heart. Heart rate is often not changed or only slightly increased during administration of nitroglycerin.

Nitroglycerin-induced decreases in blood pressure are more dependent on blood volume that are blood pressure changes produced by nitroprusside. Indeed, marked hypotension may occasionally follow sublingual administration of nitroglycerin, especially if the patient is standing, as this position augments venous pooling and further decreases cardiac output. Excessive decreases in diastolic blood pressure may decrease coronary blood flow. These decreases in diastolic blood pressure may also evoke baroreceptor-mediated reflex increases in sympathetic nervous system activity manifesting as tachycardia and increased myocardial contractility. The combination of decreased coronary blood flow and changes that increase myocardial oxygen requirements may provoke angina pectoris in susceptible patients.

Calculated systemic vascular resistance is usually relatively unaffected by nitroglycerin. Pulmonary vascular resistance, is, however, consistently decreased, presumably reflecting a direct relaxant effect of nitroglycerin on pulmonary vasculature (Tinker and Michenfelder, 1976). Indeed, in an animal model for pulmonary hypertension, nitroglycerin, but not nitroprusside, was effective in decreasing pulmonary artery pressures and pulmonary vascular resistance (Pearl et al, 1983).

Nitroglycerin primarily dilates larger conductance vessels of the coronary circulation, often leading to an increase in coronary blood flow for ischemic subendocardial areas. In contrast, nitroprusside may produce a coronary steal phenomenon. Indeed, the frequency of S-T segment elevation on the ECG during acute coronary artery occlusion in dogs is reduced by nitroglycerin but increased by nitroprusside (Chiariello et al, 1976). For these reasons, nitroglycerin has been recommended in favor of nitroprusside for the treatment of hypertension in patients with coronary artery disease (Kaplan et al, 1976).

Nitroglycerin produces a dose-related prolongation of bleeding time that parallels the decrease in blood pressure (Fig. 16-10) (Lichtenthal et al, 1985). Platelet aggregation is not altered, suggesting that prolonged bleeding time is due to vasodilation and increased venous capacitance.

TRIMETHAPHAN

Trimethaphan is a peripheral vasodilator and ganglionic blocker that acts rapidly but so briefly that it must be given by continuous intravenous infusion (Fig. 16-1). Because trimethaphan directly relaxes capacitance vessels and blocks autonomic nervous system reflexes, it lowers blood pressure both by decreasing cardiac output and by reducing systemic vascular resistance (Harioka et al, 1984; Wang et al, 1977). Histamine release does not contribute to decreases in blood pressure produced by trimethaphan (Fahmy and Soter, 1985). In contrast to nitroprusside, trimethaphan-induced decreases in blood pressure are not associated with increases in plasma concentrations of catecholamines and renin, reflecting the effect of ganglionic blockade (Fig. 16-7) (Knight et al, 1983). Increases in heart rate secondary to administration of trimethaphan most likely reflect parasympathetic nervous system ganglionic blockade.

Ganglionic blockade produced by trimethaphan reflects occupation of receptors normally responsive to acetylcholine as well as stabilization of postsynaptic membranes against the actions of acetylcholine liberated from presynaptic nerve endings. The route of metabolism of trimethaphan is unclear, although hydrolysis by plasma cholinesterase has been implicated. As a quaternary ammonium drug, trimethaphan has a limited passage across the blood-brain barrier and central nervous system effects are unlikely.

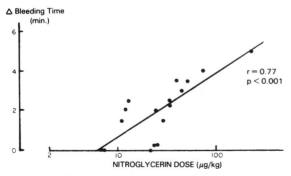

FIGURE 16–10. Nitroglycerin produces dose-related increases in bleeding time. (From Lichtenthal PR, Rossi EC, Louis G, et al. Dose-related prolongation of the bleeding time by intravenous nitroglycerin. Anesth Analg 1985; 64: 30–3; with permission.)

Clinical Uses

Trimethaphan is most often used as a continuous intravenous infusion (10 to 200 $\mu g \cdot kg^{-1} \cdot min^{-1}$) to produce controlled hypotension. Tachycardia may accompany drug-induced decreases in blood pressure, and cardiac output is likely to be reduced as a manifestation of decreased venous return (Harioka et al, 1984). Furthermore, tachycardia may offset the blood pressure–lowering effects of trimethaphan, requiring the administration of propranolol.

Side Effects

A number of side effects may accompany the use of trimethaphan for production of controlled hypotension. Mydriasis, reduced gastrointestinal activity culminating in ileus, and urinary retention accompany ganglionic blockade produced by this drug. Mydriasis produced by trimethaphan may interfere with neurologic evaluation of patients following intracranial surgery. Deleterious cerebral metabolic disturbances in dogs characterized by decreased brain oxygen availability have occurred following production of controlled hypotension with trimethaphan but not with nitroprusside (Michenfelder and Theye, 1977). In monkeys anesthetized with halothane-nitrous oxide, production of controlled hypotension by the administration of trimethaphan, but not nitroprusside, reduces cerebral blood flow, whereas cerebral metabolic rate for oxygen remains unchanged (Fig. 16-11) (Sivarajan et al, 1985). There is evidence that blood pressure decreases produced by trimethaphan evoke smaller increases in intracranial pressure than those associated with comparable degrees of hypotension produced by nitroprusside or nitroglycerin (Turner et al, 1977). This may reflect a slower onset of action of trimethaphan, allowing autoregulation of cerebral blood flow to occur.

Trimethaphan-induced controlled hypotension in animals is associated with decreased coronary blood flow but unchanged renal and hepatic blood flow (Sivarajan et al, 1985). Trimethaphan is a potent inhibitor of plasma cholinesterase such that the duration of action of succinylcholine is likely to be prolonged (Sklar and Lanks, 1977). Histamine release that may accompany the administration of trimethaphan makes

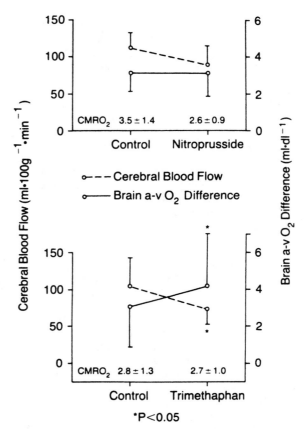

FIGURE 16–11. Hypotension produced by trimethaphan, but not by nitroprusside, reduces cerebral blood flow, whereas cerebral metabolic oxygen requirements, as reflected by an increased brain a-V oxygen difference, remain unchanged (From Sivarajan M, Amory DW, McKenzie SM. Regional blood flows during induced hypotension produced by nitroprusside or trimethaphan in the rhesus monkey. Anesth Analg 1985; 64: 759–66; with permission.)

administration of this drug to patients with pheochromocytoma questionable.

DIAZOXIDE

Diazoxide, a benzothiadiazene derivative, is related chemically to the thiazide diuretics (Fig. 16-1). This drug is used to treat acute blood pressure increases as in patients with accelerated and severe hypertension associated with glomerulonephritis. For example, diazoxide, 1 to 3 mg·kg^{-1} IV, (30-mg miniboluses up to 150 mg in a single injection) administered to a hypertensive patient produces a decrease in systolic and diastolic blood pressure within 1 to 2 minutes that lasts 6 or 7 hours. The drug can be repeated at intervals of 5 to 15 minutes. Diazoxide is highly protein bound, and it was previously thought that the drug had to be given as a bolus to exceed the binding capacity of albumin. Subsequent experience has shown that an adequate therapeutic response can be obtained with a slower infusion (Garrett and Kaplan, 1982). Diazoxide is eliminated principally as unchanged drug by the kidneys, with an elimination half-time of 28 hours. Although excessive blood pressure reductions are unlikely, a disadvantage of diazoxide, compared with nitroprusside, is the inability to titrate the dose of this drug in accordance with the patient's response.

Cardiovascular Effects

Diazoxide-induced decreases in blood pressure are associated with significant increases in cardiac output and often an elevation in heart rate. Systemic vascular resistance is decreased. Because diazoxide increases cardiac output and left ventricular ejection velocity, this drug is unsuitable for the treatment of hypertension associated with a dissecting aortic aneurysm. Indeed, excessive hypotension that evokes reflex sympathetic nervous system stimulation leading to myocardial ischemia may occur unpredictably in such patients. Conversely, the hypotensive effect of diazoxide may be accentuated in patients receiving beta-adrenergic antagonists because baroreceptor-mediated reflex increases in sympathetic nervous system activity (increased heart rate and cardiac output) are prevented. The principal site of action of diazoxide is on arteriolar resistance rather than venous capacitance vessels.

Side Effects

Unlike thiazide diuretics, diazoxide causes sodium ion (Na$^+$) and water retention, which may result in cardiac failure in susceptible patients. This effect may necessitate concomitant administration of a thiazide diuretic. Retention of Na$^+$ oc-

curs independently of reductions in glomerular filtration rate and renal blood flow that predictably accompany diazoxide-induced decreases in blood pressure. Diazoxide is a powerful uterine relaxant, being capable of stopping labor. Hyperglycemia can occur 4 to 5 hours after a single intravenous injection, reflecting a drug-induced alpha-adrenergic agonist–like inhibition of insulin release from the pancreas. Thiazide diuretics may enhance the hyperglycemic effects of diazoxide. Blood glucose concentrations should be monitored daily during chronic use of diazoxide, as hyperglycemic, hyperosmolar, nonketoacidotic coma has occurred. Stimulation of catecholamine release prohibits the use of diazoxide in patients with pheochromocytoma.

ISOSORBIDE DINITRATE

Isosorbide dinitrate is the most commonly administered oral nitrate for the prophylaxis of angina pectoris. This direct-acting vasodilator has predominant effects on the venous circulation and also improves regional distribution of myocardial blood flow in patients with coronary artery disease. During oral administration, the elimination half-time may be as long as 15 hours (Parker, 1987). The metabolite of isosorbide dinitrate, isosorbide-5-mononitrate, is more active than the parent compound. Orthostatic hypotension accompanies acute administration of isosorbide dinitrate, but tolerance to this and other pharmacologic effects seems to develop with chronic therapy.

Despite its common use, isosorbide dinitrate, 5 to 10 mg orally, is not more effective than placebo in decreasing the frequency of angina pectoris or increasing the patient's exercise tolerance. Higher doses of isosorbide dinitrate, 20 to 40 mg orally every 4 hours, are effective but are also associated with an increased incidence of side effects.

DIPYRIDAMOLE

Dipyridamole is administered orally as prophylaxis against angina pectoris, although convincing evidence of efficacy is not available (Fig. 16-12). In combination with warfarin, dipyridamole is administered to patients with prosthetic heart

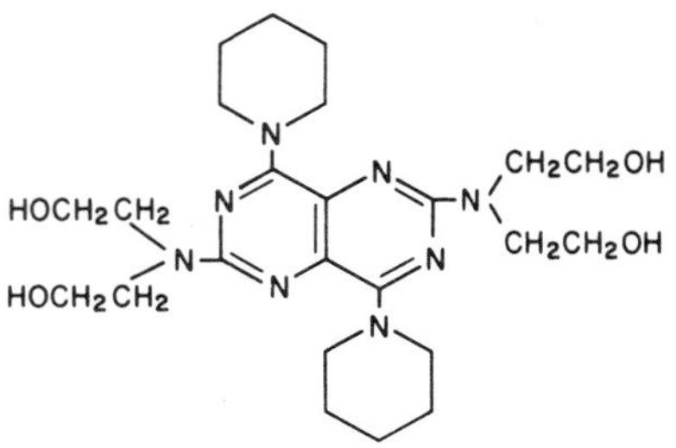

FIGURE 16–12.   Dipyridamole.

valves as prophylaxis against thromboemboli. This clinical use reflects the ability of dipyridamole, like aspirin, to inhibit platelet aggregation. Dipyridamole may interfere with platelet function by potentiating the effect of prostacyclin or by inhibiting phosphodiesterase enzyme activity, thus increasing intracellular concentrations of cyclic adenosine monophosphate.

Coronary vascular resistance is decreased, whereas coronary blood flow and oxygen tension in coronary sinus blood are increased by dipyridamole. The drug appears to act principally on small resistance vessels in the coronary circulation with little effect on resistance to flow in ischemic areas of the myocardium where vessels are already maximally dilated. These actions of dipyridamole are linked to the metabolism and transport of adenosine and adenine nucleotides. Adenosine is released from ischemic myocardium, acting as a vasodilator and an important signal for the autoregulation of coronary artery blood flow. Indeed, dipyridamole inhibits cellular uptake of adenosine.

PAPAVERINE

Papaverine is a nonspecific smooth muscle relaxant present in opium but unrelated chemically or pharmacologically to the opioid alkaloids (Fig. 16-13). It is possible that papaverine-induced vas-

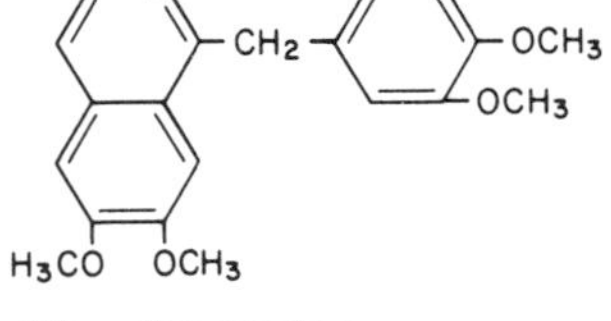

FIGURE 16–13.   Papaverine

odilatation is related to its ability to inhibit phosphodiesterase, leading to increased intracellular concentrations of cyclic adenosine monophosphate. Papaverine has not been demonstrated to be efficacious in any condition.

PURINES

Purines are represented by adenosine and adenine nucleotides.

Adenosine

Adenosine is an endogenous nucleotide occurring in all cells of the body (Fig. 16-14). This nucleotide in high doses has inhibitory effects on conduction of cardiac impulses through the atrioventricular node, whereas its potent vasodilator effects are important in the regulation of local blood flow in vascular beds, including the heart and brain. Clinical uses of adenosine include administration as an antidysrhythmic or to produce controlled hypotension.

Antidysrhythmic Action

Adenosine slows conduction of cardiac impulses through the atrioventricular node, can interrupt reentry pathways through the atrioventricular node, and can restore normal sinus rhythm in patients with paroxysmal supraventricular tachycardia, including that associated with Wolff-Parkinson-White syndrome. Administration of adenosine, 6 to 12 mg IV, as a rapid injection usually

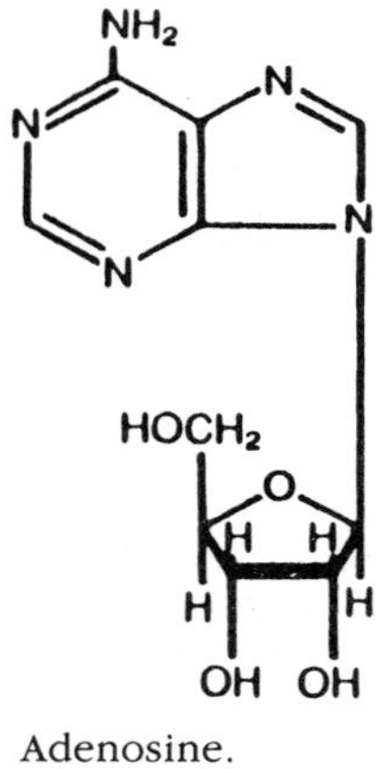

FIGURE 16–14.   Adenosine.

converts paroxysmal supraventricular tachycardia to normal sinus rhythm within 1 minute. This dose has no hemodynamic effects, and its rapid metabolism precludes any influence of hepatic or renal dysfunction. The elimination half-time is less than 10 seconds owing to rapid metabolism to inosine and adenosine monophosphate. Adenosine is antagonized competitively by methylxanthines, such as caffeine and theophylline, and potentiated by blockers of nucleoside transport, such as dipyridamole. Adenosine is not effective in the treatment of atrial flutter, atrial fibrillation, and ventricular tachycardia. In the absence of a functioning artificial cardiac pacemaker, adenosine should not be administered in the presence of second- or third-degree atrioventricular heart block or in the presence of sick sinus syndrome.

Controlled Hypotension

Adenosine-induced controlled hypotension is characterized by rapid onset and a stable level of hypotension that is promptly reversed when the infusion is discontinued (Sollevi et al, 1984). Rapid recovery of blood pressure reflects the brief elimination half-time of adenosine. During controlled hypotension produced by adenosine, there is a marked reduction in systemic vascular resistance and a modest increase in heart rate. Cardiac output is enhanced, coronary sinus blood flow is increased, and cardiac filling pressures are maintained, suggesting the absence of negative inotropic effects and minimal alterations in venous capacitance and venous return to the heart (Bloor et al, 1985). The rate of adenosine infusion required to produce controlled hypotension (approximately 220 $\mu g \cdot kg^{-1} \cdot min^{-1}$ IV) is unlikely to result in plasma concentrations that alter cardiac automaticity or conduction of cardiac impulses (Owall et al, 1987). Furthermore, the necessary infusion rate of adenosine can be reduced by about one third when patients are pretreated with an adenosine uptake inhibitor, such as dipyridamole (Sollevi et al, 1984).

The unchanging adenosine infusion requirements to maintain constant decreases in blood pressure for as long as 120 minutes confirm the absence of tachyphylaxis. Likewise, plasma concentrations of renin and catecholamines do not increase, which is again consistent with unchanging adenosine dose requirements and the ab-

sence of rebound hypertension when the infusion is discontinued (Bloor et al, 1985; Owall et al, 1987). Acid-base disturbances do not accompany adenosine-induced hypotension. Uric acid levels may increase 10% to 20% when adenosine is used for controlled hypotension, suggesting caution in selecting this drug for patients with a purine metabolic disturbance such as gout (Owall et al, 1987).

REFERENCES

Becker LC. Conditions for vasodilator-induced coronary steal in experimental myocardial ischemia. Circulation 1978;57:1103–10.

Berthelsen P, St Haxholdt O, Husum R, Rasmussen JP. PEEP reverses nitroglycerin-induced hypoxemia following coronary artery bypass surgery. Acta Anaesthesiol Scand 1986;30:243–6.

Bloor BC, Fukunaga AF, Ma C, et al. Myocardial hemodynamics during induced hypotension: A comparison between sodium nitroprusside and adenosine triphosphate. Anesthesiology 1985;63:517–25.

Byrick RJ, Hobbs EG, Martineau R, Noble WH. Nitroglycerin relaxes large airways. Anesth Analg 1983;62:421–5.

Casthely PA, Lear S, Cottrell JE, Lear E. Intrapulmonary shunting during induced hypotension. Anesth Analg 1982;61:231–5.

Chauvin M, Bonnet F, Montembault C, Lafay M, Curet P, Viars P. Hepatic plasma flow during sodium nitroprusside-induced hypotension in humans. Anesthesiology 1985;63:287–93.

Chen RYZ, Matteo RS, Fan F-C, Schuessler GB, Chien S. Resetting of baroreceptor sensitivity after induced hypotension. Anesthesiology 1982;56:29–35.

Chiariello M, Gold HK, Leinbach RC, Davis MA, Maroko PR. Comparison between the effects of nitroprusside and nitroglycerin on ischemic injury during acute myocardial infarction. Circulation 1976;54:766–73.

Colley PS, Cheney FW, Hlastala MP. Ventilation-perfusion and gas exchange effects of sodium nitroprusside in dogs with normal and edematous lungs. Anesthesiology 1979;50:489–95.

Cottrell JE, Casthely P, Brodie JD, Patel K, Klein A, Turndorf H. Prevention of nitroprusside-induced cyanide toxicity with hydroxocobalamin. N Engl J Med 1979;298:809–11.

Davies DW, Greiss L, Steward DJ. Sodium nitroprusside in children: Observations on metabolism during normal and abnormal responses. Can Anaesth Soc J 1975;22:553–60.

Delaney TJ, Miller ED. Rebound hypertension after sodium nitroprusside prevented by saralism in rats. Anesthesiology 1980;52:154–6.

Fahmy NR. Nitroglycerin as a hypotensive drug during general anesthesia. Anesthesiology 1978;49:17–20.

Fahmy NR, Soter NA. Effects of trimethaphan on arterial blood histamine and systemic hemodynamics in humans. Anesthesiology 1985;62:562–6.

Fibuch EE, Cecil WT, Reed WA. Methemoglobinemia associated with organic nitrate therapy. Anesth Analg 1979;58:521–3.

Fyman PN, Cottrell JR, Kushing L, Casthely PA. Vasodilator therapy in the perioperative period. Can Anaesth Soc J 1986;33:629–43.

Gagnon RL, Marsh ML, Smith RW, Shapiro HM. Intracranial hypertension caused by nitroglycerin. Anesthesiology 1979;51:86–7.

Gallagher JD, Moore RA, Jose AB, Botros SB, Clark DL. Prophylactic nitroglycerin infusions during coronary artery bypass surgery. Anesthesiology 1986;64:785–9.

Garrett BN, Kaplan NM. Efficacy of slow infusion of diazoxide in treatment of severe hypertension without organ hypoperfusion. Am Heart J 1982;103:390–4.

Gerson JI, Allen FB, Seltzer JL, Parker FB, Markowitz AH. Arterial and venous dilation by nitroprusside and nitroglycerin—is there a difference? Anesth Analg 1982;61:256–60.

Harioka T, Hatano Y, Mori K, Toda N. Trimethaphan is a direct arterial vasodilator and an alpha-adrenoceptor antagonist. Anesth Analg 1984;63:290–6.

Hines R, Barash PG. Infusion of sodium nitroprusside induces platelet dysfunction *in vitro*. Anesthesiology 1989;70:611–5.

Ikeda S, Schweiss JF, Frank PA, Homan SM. *In vitro* cyanide release from sodium nitroprusside. Anesthesiology 1987;66:381–5.

Kaplan JA, Dunbar RW, Jones EL. Nitroglycerin infusion during coronary artery surgery. Anesthesiology 1976;45:14–21.

Kaplan JA, Finlayson DC, Woodward S. Vasodilator therapy after cardiac surgery: A review of the efficacy and toxicity of nitroglycerin and nitroprusside. Can Anaesth Soc J 1980;27:154–8.

Khambatta HJ, Stone G, Khan E. Hypertension during anesthesia on discontinuation of sodium nitroprusside-induced hypotension. Anesthesiology 1979; 51:127–30.

Knight PR, Lane GA, Hensinger RN, Bolles RS, Bjoraker DJ. Catecholamine and renin-angiotensin response during hypotensive anesthesia induced by sodium nitroprusside or trimethaphan camsylate. Anesthesiology 1983;59:248–53.

Lichtenthal PR, Rossi EC, Louis G, et al. Dose-related prolongation of the bleeding time by intravenous nitroglycerin. Anesth Analg 1985;64:30–3.

Marsh ML, Aidinis SJ, Naughton KVH, Marshall LF, Shapiro HM. The technique of nitroprusside administration modifies the intracranial pressure response. Anesthesiology 1979;51:538–41.

Marshall WK, Bedford RF, Arnold WP, et al. Effects of propranolol on the cardiovascular and renin-angiotensin systems during hypotension produced by sodium nitroprusside in humans. Anesthesiology 1981;55:277–80.

Michenfelder JD, Theye RA. Canine systemic and cerebral effects of hypotension induced by hemorrhage, trimethaphan, halothane, or nitroprusside. Anesthesiology 1977;46:188–95.

Michenfelder JD, Tinker JH. Cyanide toxicity and thiosulfate protection during chronic administration of sodium nitroprusside in the dog: Correlation with a human case. Anesthesiology 1977;47:441–8.

Miller ED, Ackerly JA, Vaughn ED, Peach MJ, Epstein RM. The renin-angiotensin system during controlled hypotension with sodium nitroprusside. Anesthesiology 1977;47:257–62.

Miller JR, Benumof JL, Trousdale FR. Combined effects of sodium nitroprusside and propranolol on hypoxic pulmonary vasoconstriction. Anesthesiology 1982; 57:267–71.

Moore RA, Geller EA, Gallagher JD, Clark DL. Effect of hypothermic cardiopulmonary bypass on nitroprusside metabolism. Clin Pharmacol Ther 1985; 37:680–3.

Noback CR, Tinker JR. Hypothermia after cardiopulmonary bypass in man: Amelioration by nitroprusside-induced vasodilation during rewarming. Anesthesiology 1980;53:277–80.

Owall A, Gordon E, Lagerkranser M, Lindquist C, Rudehill A, Sollevi A. Clinical experience with adenosine for controlled hypotension during cerebral aneurysm surgery. Anesth Analg 1987;66:229–34.

Parker JO. Nitrate therapy in stable angina pectoris. N Engl J Med 1987;316:1635–42.

Pearl RG, Rosenthal MH, Ashton JPA. Pulmonary vasodilator effects of nitroglycerin and sodium nitroprusside in canine oleic acid–induced pulmonary hypertension. Anesthesiology 1983;58:514–8.

Rogers MC, Hamburger C, Owen K, Epstein MH. Intracranial pressure in the cat during nitroglycerin-induced hypotension. Anesthesiology 1979;51:227–9.

Sivarajan M, Amory DW, McKenzie SM. Regional blood flows during induced hypotension produced by nitroprusside or trimethaphan in the rhesus monkey. Anesth Analg 1985;64:759–66.

Sklar GS, Lanks KW. Effects of trimethaphan and sodium nitroprusside on hydrolysis of succinylcholine *in vitro*. Anesthesiology 1977;47:31–3.

Snyder SW, Wheeler AS, James FM. The use of nitroglycerin to control severe hypertension of pregnancy during cesarean section. Anesthesiology 1979;51:563–4.

Sollevi A, Lagerkranser M, Irestedt L, Gordon E, Lindquist C. Controlled hypotension with adenosine in cerebral aneurysm surgery. Anesthesiology 1984;61:400–5.

Stoelting RK. Attenuation of blood pressure response to laryngoscopy and tracheal intubation with sodium nitroprusside. Anesth Analg 1979;58:116–9.

Thompson GE, Miller RD, Stevens WC, Murray WR.

Hypotensive anesthesia for total hip arthroplasty: A study of blood loss and organ function (brain, heart, liver, and kidney). Anesthesiology 1978;48:91–6.

Thomson IR, Mutch WAC, Culligan JD. Failure of intravenous nitroglycerin to prevent intraoperative myocardial ischemia during fentanyl-pancuronium anesthesia. Anesthesiology 1984;61:385–93.

Tinker JH, Michenfelder JD. Sodium nitroprusside: Pharmacology, toxicity and therapeutics. Anesthesiology 1976;45:340–54.

Tinker JH, Michenfelder JD. Increased resistance to nitroprusside-induced cyanide toxicity in anuric dogs. Anesthesiology 1980;52:40–7.

Turner JM, Powell D, Gibson RM, McDowell DG. Intracranial pressure changes in neurosurgical patients during hypotension induced with sodium nitroprusside or trimethaphan. Br J Anaesth 1977;49:419–24.

Vesey CJ, Cole PV, Simpson PJ. Cyanide and thiocyanate concentrations following sodium nitroprusside infusion in man. Br J Anaesth 1976;48:651–60.

Wang HH, Liu LMP, Katz RL. A comparison of the cardiovascular effects of sodium nitroprusside and trimethaphan. Anesthesiology 1977;46:40–8.

Zurick AM, Wagner RH, Starr NJ, Lytle B, Estafanous FG. Intravenous nitroglycerin, methemoglobinemia, and respiratory distress in a postoperative cardiac surgical patient. Anesthesiology 1984;61:464–6.

Chapter

17

Cardiac Antidysrhythmic Drugs

INTRODUCTION

Treatment of cardiac dysrhythmias and disturbances in conduction of cardiac impulses with antidysrhythmic drugs is based on an understanding of the electrophysiologic basis of the abnormality and the mechanism of action of the therapeutic drug to be employed. Even when information is incomplete and the diagnosis uncertain, it is possible to treat most cardiac dysrhythmias and conduction disturbances by applying knowledge gained from prior clinical experience. Indeed, the selection of an antidysrhythmic drug may be empirical, with the ultimate choice being determined by which drug proves to be effective with minimal side effects (Lucas et al, 1990).

Patients may be taking antidysrhythmic drugs for chronic suppression of cardiac rhythm disturbances. These drugs pose little threat to the uneventful course of anesthesia and should be continued up to the time of induction of anesthesia. Surprisingly, chronic treatment of asymptomatic to minimally symptomatic ventricular dysrhythmias with flecainide or encainide following myocardial infarction is associated with a substantial increase in the sudden death rate (The Cardiac Arrhythmia Suppression Trial [CAST] Investigators, 1989).

The majority of cardiac dysrhythmias that occur during anesthesia do not require therapy. Cardiac dysrhythmias, however, do require treat-

ment when (1) they cannot be corrected by removing the precipitating cause, (2) hemodynamic function is compromised, and (3) the disturbance predisposes to more serious cardiac rhythm changes. During the perioperative period, antidysrhythmic drugs are most often administered by the intravenous route.

The mechanism of cardiac dysrhythmias may be different with or without anesthesia. For example, anesthetic-related cardiac dysrhythmias have been ascribed to abnormal pacemaker activity characterized by suppression of the sinoatrial node, with the emergence of latent pacemakers within or below the atrioventricular tissues (Atlee and Bosnjak, 1990). Furthermore, development of reentry circuits is likely to be important in the mechanism of cardiac dysrhythmias that occur during anesthesia. Certainly anesthetics, particularly inhaled drugs, have effects on the specialized conduction system for cardiac impulses.

CLASSIFICATION

Antidysrhythmic drugs are classified into four groups based on their mechanism of action (Table 17-1). Available drugs differ in their pharmacokinetics and efficacy in treating specific types of cardiac dysrhythmias (Tables 17-2 and 17-3) (Lucas et al, 1990).

Membrane Stabilizers

Membrane stabilizers are divided into three subgroups. The dominant electrophysiologic properties of group Ia drugs (quinidine, procainamide, disopyramide) are related to their ability to block the rapid inward flux of sodium ions (Na^+) during phase 0 depolarization. This effect causes a reduced level of membrane responsiveness and slowed conduction of cardiac impulses. In addition to slowed conduction of cardiac impulses, these drugs decrease the rate of spontaneous phase 4 depolarization, resulting in reduced automaticity. Group Ia drugs induce a bidirectional block and thus interrupt reentry.

Group Ib drugs (lidocaine, tocainide, mexiletine, phenytoin) decrease automaticity by reducing the rate of spontaneous phase 4 depolarization. Unlike group Ia drugs, however, there is little effect on membrane responsiveness produced by these drugs. As a result, antegrade conduction can take place and thus interrupt reentry.

Group Ic drugs (flecainide, encainide, lorcainide) exhibit fairly selective depressant effects on fast Na^+ channels. Thus, they decrease V_{max} and overshoot of action potentials in atrial and ventricular fibers and markedly slow conduction of cardiac impulses.

Quinidine

Quinidine is effective in the treatment of acute and chronic supraventricular dysrhythmias (Fig. 17-1). A frequent indication for quinidine is to prevent recurrence of supraventricular tachydysrhythmias or to suppress ventricular premature contractions. For example, quinidine is often administered to slow the atrial rate in the presence of atrial fibrillation. Indeed, about 25% of patients with atrial fibrillation will convert to normal sinus rhythm when treated with quinidine. Supraventricular tachydysrhythmias associated with Wolff-Parkinson-White syndrome are effectively suppressed by quinidine.

It is common to administer prior digitalis when treating atrial fibrillation with quinidine because an occasional patient will manifest a paradoxical increase in the rate of ventricular response when quinidine is administered. Of interest is an occasional patient in whom a previously stable plasma concentration of digoxin increases dramatically when quinidine is acutely added to the treatment regimen (Leahey et al, 1978). Apparently, quinidine causes displacement of digoxin from myocardial and peripheral tissue stores. An associated reduction in renal excretion of digoxin is due to a decrease in the renal tubular secretion of digoxin.

Table 17–1
Classification of Antidysrhythmic Drugs

Class	Mechanism	Examples
I	Membrane stabilizers (sodium channel blockade)	
IA	Slow conduction—moderate	Quinidine
		Procainamide
		Disopyramide
IB	Slow conduction—mild	Lidocaine
		Tocainide
		Mexiletine
		Phenytoin
IC	Slow conduction—marked	Flecainide
		Encainide
		Lorcainide
II	Beta-adrenergic antagonists	Propranolol
III	Prolonged repolarization	Bretylium
		Amiodarone
IV	Calcium entry blockers	Verapamil
		Diltiazem

Table 17-2
Pharmacokinetics of Cardiac Antidysrhythmic Drugs

	Principal Clearance Mechanism	Protein Binding (percent)	Elimination Half-Time (h)	Therapeutic Plasma Concentration
Quinidine	Hepatic	80–90	5–12	2–8 $\mu g \cdot ml^{-1}$
Procainamide	Renal/hepatic	15	2.5–5	4–10 $\mu g \cdot ml^{-1}$
Disopyramide	Renal/hepatic	15	8–12	2–4 $\mu g \cdot ml^{-1}$
Lidocaine	Hepatic	55	1.4–1.8	1–5 $\mu g \cdot ml^{-1}$
Tocainide	Hepatic/renal	10–30	12–15	4–10 $\mu g \cdot ml^{-1}$
Mexiletine	Hepatic	60–75	6–12	0.75–2 $\mu g \cdot ml^{-1}$
Phenytoin	Hepatic	93	8–60	10–20 $\mu g \cdot ml^{-1}$
Flecainide	Hepatic	35–45	13–30	0.3–1.5 $\mu g \cdot ml^{-1}$
Encainide	Hepatic/renal	70	1–3	0.3–0.6 $\mu g \cdot ml^{-1}$
Propranolol	Hepatic	90–95	2–4	10–30 $ng \cdot ml^{-1}$
Bretylium	Renal	<10	8–12	75–100 $ng \cdot ml^{-1}$
Amiodarone	Hepatic	96	8–107 days	1.5–2 $\mu g \cdot ml^{-1}$
Verapamil	Hepatic	90	4.5–12	100–300 $ng \cdot ml^{-1}$

Quinidine is most often administered orally in a dose of 300 to 500 mg four times daily. Oral absorption of quinidine is rapid, with peak concentrations in the plasma attained in 60 to 90 minutes and an elimination half-time of 5 to 12 hours. The therapeutic blood level of quinidine is 2 to 8 $\mu g \cdot ml^{-1}$. Intramuscular injection is not recommended because of associated pain at the injection site. The intravenous administration of quinidine is limited because peripheral vasodilation and myocardial depression can occur.

MECHANISM OF ACTION. Quinidine is the dextro isomer of quinine and, like quinine, has antimalarial and antipyretic effects. Unlike quinine, however, quinidine has intense effects on the heart. For example, quinidine decreases the slope of phase 4 depolarization, explaining its effectiveness in suppressing cardiac dysrhythmias caused by enhanced automaticity. Quinidine increases the fibrillation threshold in the atria and ventricles. Quinidine-induced slowing of the conduction of cardiac impulses through normal and abnormal fibers may be responsible for the ability of quinidine to occasionally convert atrial flutter or fibrillation to normal sinus rhythm. This drug can abolish reentry dysrhythmias by prolonging conduction of cardiac impulses in an area of injury, thus converting one-way conduction blockade to two-way conduction blockade.

Reduction of atrial rate during atrial flutter or fibrillation may reflect slowed conduction velocity, a prolonged effective refractory period in the atria, or both.

METABOLISM AND EXCRETION. Quinidine is hydroxylated in the liver to inactive metabolites, which are excreted in the urine (Table 17-2). About 20% of quinidine is excreted unchanged in the urine. Enzyme induction significantly shortens the duration of action of quinidine. As a result of its dependence on renal excretion and hepatic metabolism for clearance from the body, accumulation of quinidine or its metabolites may occur in the presence of impaired function of these organs. About 80% to 90% of quinidine in plasma is bound to albumin. Quinidine accumulates rapidly in most tissues except the brain.

SIDE EFFECTS. Quinidine has a low therapeutic ratio, and side effects are predictable if the plasma concentration becomes excessive. As the plasma concentration increases above 2 $\mu g \cdot ml^{-1}$, the P-R interval, QRS complex, and Q-T interval on the electrocardiogram (ECG) are prolonged, emphasizing the importance of the ECG for monitoring patients being treated with quinidine. A 50% increase in the duration of the QRS complex requires a reduction in dosage of quinidine or heart blockade will likely ensue. Occasionally,

Table 17–3
Efficacy of Antidysrhythmic Drugs for Treatment of
Specific Cardiac Dysrhythmias

	Conversion of Atrial Fibrillation	Paroxysmal Supraventricular Tachycardia	Premature Ventricular Contractions	Ventricular Tachycardia
Quinidine	+	++	++	+
Procainamide	+	++	++	++
Disopyramide	+	++	++	++
Lidocaine	0	0	++	++
Tocainide	0	0	++	++
Mexiletine	0	0	++	++
Phenytoin	0	0	++	++
Flecainide	0	+	++	++
Encainide	0	+	++	++
Propranolol	+	++	+	+
Bretylium	0	0	+	++
Amiodarone	+	++	++	++
Verapamil	+	++	0	0

0, no effect; +, effective; ++, highly effective

uniquely susceptible patients being treated with quinidine experience syncope or sudden death despite low plasma concentrations of drug. Quinidine syncope may reflect the occurrence of ventricular dysrhythmias owing to delayed intraventricular conduction of cardiac impulses. Persons with a preexisting prolongation of the Q-T interval or evidence of atrioventricular heart block on the ECG should not be treated with quinidine.

Quinidine can cause significant hypotension, particularly if administered intravenously. This response most likely reflects peripheral vasodilation from alpha-adrenergic blockade. High plasma concentrations depress myocardial contractility, and this is further accentuated by hyperkalemia.

Patients in normal sinus rhythm treated with quinidine may show an increase in heart rate which, presumably, is due either to an anticholinergic action and/or a reflex increase in sympathetic nervous system activity. This atropine-like action of quinidine opposes its direct depressant actions on the sinoatrial and atrioventricular nodes.

Fever may accompany administration of quinidine and disappears when the drug is withdrawn. Thrombocytopenia is a rare occurrence that is due to drug-platelet complexes that evoke production of antibodies. Discontinuation of quinidine results in return of the platelet count to normal in 2 to 7 days. Nausea, vomiting, and diarrhea occur in about one third of treated patients.

Like other cinchona alkaloids and salicylates, quinidine can cause cinchonism. Symptoms of cinchonism include tinnitus, decreased hearing acuity, blurring of vision, and gastrointestinal upset. In severe cases, there may be abdominal pain and mental confusion.

Because quinidine is an alpha-adrenergic blocking drug, it can interact in an additive manner with drugs that cause vasodilation. For example, nitroglycerin can cause exaggerated orthostatic hypotension in patients being treated with quinidine.

Quinidine interferes with normal neuromuscular transmission and may accentuate the effect of neuromuscular blocking drugs (Harrah et al, 1970). Recurrence of skeletal muscle paralysis in

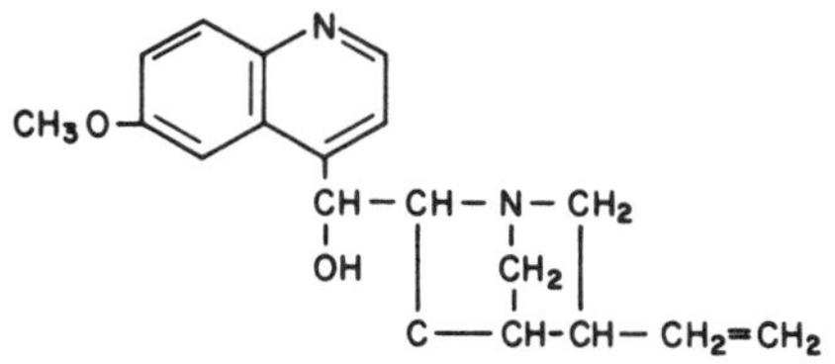

FIGURE 17–1. Quinidine.

the immediate postoperative period has been observed in association with the administration of quinidine (Way et al, 1967).

Procainamide

Procainamide has similar therapeutic uses as quinidine (Table 17-3; Fig. 17-2). Premature ventricular contractions and paroxysmal ventricular tachycardia are suppressed in most patients within a few minutes after intravenous administration. The effectiveness of procainamide against atrial dysrhythmias is comparable to that of quinidine.

Procainamide, 3 to 6 g, is effectively absorbed following oral administration, reaching peak concentrations in 45 to 75 minutes. The plasma concentration of procainamide associated with antidysrhythmic effects is 4 to 10 $\mu g \cdot ml^{-1}$. The probability of toxicity becomes greater when the plasma concentration of procainamide increases to more than 8 $\mu g \cdot ml^{-1}$. Intramuscular and intravenous routes of administration of procainamide are acceptable. For example, procainamide can be administered in doses of 1.5 $mg \cdot kg^{-1}$ IV over 1 minute and repeated every 5 minutes until the cardiac dysrhythmia is controlled or the total dose reaches about 15 $mg \cdot kg^{-1}$. The total loading dose is never given as a single intravenous injection because it can cause hypotension. When the cardiac dysrhythmia is controlled, a constant rate of intravenous infusion is used to maintain a therapeutic plasma concentration of procainamide. Although procainamide and quinidine have a broader spectrum of antidysrhythmic effects than lidocaine (useful in treatment of supraventricular and ventricular cardiac dysrhythmias), they are rarely used during anesthesia because of their propensity to produce hypotension.

MECHANISM OF ACTION. Procainamide is eliminated by renal excretion and hepatic metabolism (Table 17-2). In humans, 40% to 60% of procainamide is excreted unchanged by the kidneys. In the liver, the remaining procainamide is acetylated to N-acetyl procainamide (NAPA), which is also eliminated by the kidneys. This metabolite is cardioactive and probably contributes to the antidysrhythmic effects of procainamide. In the presence of renal failure, plasma concentrations of NAPA may reach dangerous levels. Eventually, 90% of an administered dose of procainamide is recovered as unchanged drug or its metabolites.

The activity of the N-acetyltransferase enzyme responsible for the acetylation of procainamide is genetically determined. In fast acetylators, the elimination half-time of procainamide is 2.5 hours, compared with 5 hours in slow acetylators. The blood level of NAPA exceeds that of procainamide in rapid but not slow acetylators.

Unlike its analogue, procaine, procainamide is highly resistant to hydrolysis by plasma cholinesterase. Indeed, only 2% to 10% of an administered dose of procainamide is recovered unchanged in the urine as para-aminobenzoic acid.

Only about 15% of procainamide is bound to plasma proteins. Despite this limited binding in plasma, procainamide is avidly bound to tissue proteins with the exception of brain.

SIDE EFFECTS. The incidence of side effects is high when procainamide is used as an antidysrhythmic drug. Rapid intravenous injection of procainamide can cause hypotension, whereas higher plasma concentrations slow conduction of cardiac impulses through the atrioventricular node and intraventricular conduction system. Indeed, ventricular asystole or fibrillation may occur when procainamide is administered in the presence of heart block as associated with digitalis toxicity. Direct myocardial depression that occurs at high plasma concentrations of procainamide is exaggerated by hyperkalemia. As with quinidine, ventricular dysrhythmias may accompany excessive plasma concentrations of procainamide.

A syndrome resembling systemic lupus erythematosus, most often manifesting as arthralgia and hepatomegaly, may accompany chronic but not acute therapy with procainamide. Antinuclear antibodies are present, and the LE cell preparation is often positive. Slow acetylators are more prone than rapid acetylators to develop these antinuclear antibodies. Symptoms disappear when procainamide is discontinued.

Fever may force the discontinuation of procainamide therapy. Agranulocytosis may occur in

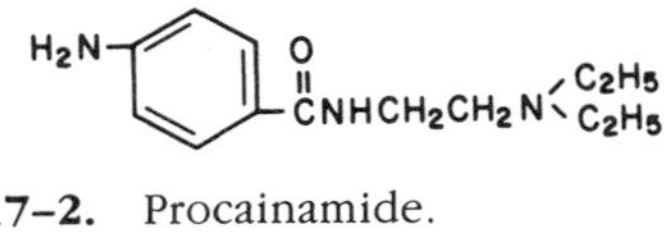

FIGURE 17–2. Procainamide.

the early weeks of therapy, emphasizing the need for monitoring complete blood counts periodically. Gastrointestinal irritation is less frequent than observed during administration of quinidine. Central nervous system symptoms can occur but are less likely than when patients are treated with lidocaine.

Disopyramide

Disopyramide is effective in the control of atrial and ventricular cardiac dysrhythmias (Table 17-3; Fig. 17-3). The oral dose is 100 to 200 mg administered four times daily. About 90% of an oral dose is absorbed, with peak plasma concentrations occurring in 1 to 2 hours. The elimination half-time is 8 to 12 hours.

Disopyramide resembles quinidine with respect to effects on the duration of the cardiac action potential and membrane responsiveness. There is little change in heart rate, and changes in the P-R interval, QRS complex, and Q-T interval on the ECG are less than observed with quinidine.

About 50% of disopyramide is excreted unchanged by the kidney. As a result, the elimination half-time is greatly prolonged in the presence of renal disease. A dealkylated metabolite with less antidysrhythmic and atropine-line activity than the parent compound accounts for about 20% of the drug.

The anticholinergic action of disopyramide produces a substantial incidence of dry mouth, blurred vision, and, occasionally, urinary retention. The potential for direct myocardial depression, especially in patients with preexisting left ventricular dysfunction, seems to be greater with this drug than with quinidine and procainamide.

Lidocaine

Lidocaine is used principally for suppression of ventricular dysrhythmias, having minimal effects on supraventricular dysrhythmias (Table 17-3; see Fig. 7-2). This drug is particularly effective in suppressing reentry dysrhythmias, such as premature ventricular contractions and ventricular tachycardia. The value of prophylactic lidocaine therapy for preventing early ventricular fibrillation following acute myocardial infarction has not been documented (MacMahon et al, 1988).

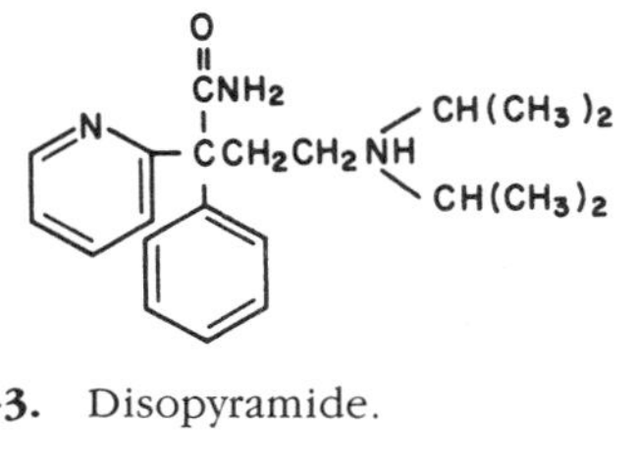

Rapid intravenous administration of lidocaine, 1 to 1.5 mg·kg^{-1}, provides antidysrhythmic effects lasting 15 to 60 minutes. This short duration of action is related to rapid tissue redistribution and metabolism of lidocaine. Maintenance of a therapeutic plasma lidocaine concentration of 1 to 5 µg·ml^{-1} following a single initial intravenous injection is most often achieved by the continuous intravenous infusion of 15 to 60 µg·kg^{-1}·min^{-1}. Decreased hepatic blood flow, as produced by anesthetics, shock, or congestive heart failure, may decrease by 50% the rate of intravenous lidocaine infusion necessary to maintain therapeutic plasma levels.

Advantages of lidocaine compared with quinidine and procainamide include a more rapid onset and prompt disappearance of effects when the continuous intravenous infusion is terminated. This permits moment-to-moment titration of the infusion rate, which is necessary to produce an antidysrhythmic effect. Lidocaine for intravenous injection differs from that used for local anesthesia by not containing a preservative.

Lidocaine is well absorbed after oral administration but is subject to extensive hepatic first-pass metabolism. Indeed, only about one third of the drug reaches the circulation, resulting in low and often unpredictable plasma concentrations.

Intramuscular absorption of lidocaine is nearly complete. In an emergency situation, lidocaine, 4 to 5 mg·kg^{-1} IM, will produce a therapeutic plasma concentration in about 15 minutes, and this level is maintained for about 90 minutes.

MECHANISM OF ACTION. Lidocaine delays the rate of spontaneous phase 4 depolarization by preventing or diminishing the gradual decrease in potassium ion permeability that normally occurs during this phase (Table 17-1). Higher doses of lidocaine result in slowing of phase 0 depolarization (the rapid spike phase). This effect is presumably due to inhibition of inward movement of Na$^+$ across membranes of cardiac cells. This is similar to the effect that produces conduction

FIGURE 17–3. Disopyramide.

blockade (local anesthesia) in peripheral nerves. Lidocaine reduces the disparity in the duration of action potentials in normal (shortens refractory period) and ischemic (prolongs refractory period) myocardial cells and thus improves the chances of a uniform spread of depolarization through the myocardium. Retrograde conduction is inhibited, and reentry fails to occur.

Effectiveness of lidocaine in suppressing premature ventricular contractions reflects its ability to decrease the rate of spontaneous phase 4 depolarization. Ineffectiveness of lidocaine against supraventricular dysrhythmias presumably reflects its inability to alter the rate of spontaneous phase 4 depolarization in atrial cardiac cells.

METABOLISM AND EXCRETION. Metabolites of lidocaine may possess antidysrhythmic activity (see Chapter 7).

SIDE EFFECTS. Lidocaine is essentially devoid of effects on the ECG or cardiovascular system when the plasma concentration remains less than 5 μg$\cdot$ml^{-1} (Table 17-2). For example, in contrast to quinidine and procainamide, lidocaine does not alter the duration of the QRS complex on the ECG and activity of the sympathetic nervous system is not changed. Toxic plasma concentrations of lidocaine (greater than 5 to 10 μg$\cdot$ml^{-1}) produce peripheral vasodilation and direct myocardial depression with resulting hypotension. In addition, slowing of conduction of cardiac impulses manifests as bradycardia, a prolonged P-R interval, and widened QRS complex on the ECG.

The principal side effects of lidocaine are on the central nervous system. Stimulation of the central nervous system occurs in a dose-related manner, with symptoms appearing when plasma concentrations of lidocaine are greater than 5 μg$\cdot$ml^{-1}. Seizures are possible at plasma concentrations of lidocaine of 5 to 10 μg$\cdot$ml^{-1}. Central nervous system depression, apnea, and cardiac arrest are possible when plasma concentrations of lidocaine are greater than 10 μg$\cdot$ml^{-1}. The convulsive threshold for lidocaine is reduced during arterial hypoxemia, hyperkalemia, or acidosis, emphasizing the importance of monitoring these parameters during continuous intravenous infusion of lidocaine to patients for suppression of cardiac dysrhythmias.

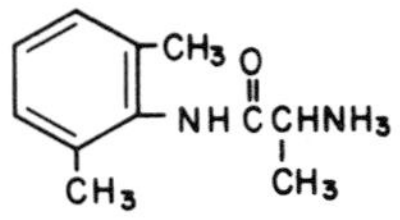

FIGURE 17-4. Tocainide.

Tocainide

Tocainide is an orally effective amine analogue of lidocaine that is used for the suppression of symptomatic ventricular dysrhythmias (Fig. 17-4) (Roden and Woosley, 1986b). The addition of the amine side group enables tocainide to avoid significant hepatic first-pass metabolism that limits the effectiveness of orally administered lidocaine. The usual daily adult maintenance dose of tocainide is 800 to 2200 mg in three divided oral doses.

MECHANISM OF ACTION. Electrophysiologically, tocainide is similar to lidocaine, producing decreases in the effective refractory period and duration of the action potential with an unchanged QRS complex on the ECG.

METABOLISM AND EXCRETION. Absorption of tocainide from the gastrointestinal tract is rapid and complete. About 40% of the drug is excreted unchanged in the urine, and the remainder undergoes hepatic metabolism to inactive metabolites. Therapeutic plasma concentrations are 4 to 10 μg$\cdot$ml^{-1}, and the elimination half-time is about 15 hours.

SIDE EFFECTS. A modest negative inotropic effect accompanies use of tocainide, and there is a potential for aggravating cardiac failure. Headache, tremor, paresthesia, dizziness, and gastrointestinal irritation are not infrequent and may become intolerable to the patient. It is possible that lidocaine, as administered intravenously in the perioperative period to treat cardiac dysrhythmias or provide additional protection against noxious stimulation, would have an additive effect with circulating tocainide.

Mexiletine

Mexiletine, like tocainide, is an orally effective amine analogue of lidocaine that is used for the treatment of symptomatic ventricular dysrhythmias.

Phenytoin

Phenytoin is particularly effective in suppression of ventricular dysrhythmias associated with digitalis toxicity (Table 17-3; see Fig. 30-1). This drug is not effective in suppression of atrial tachycardia or fibrillation. Phenytoin should be administered orally or by intermittent intravenous injection. Intramuscular absorption is too unreliable to treat cardiac dysrhythmias. The intravenous dose is 1.5 mg^{-1}·kg^{-1} every 5 minutes until the cardiac dysrhythmia is controlled or 10 to 15 mg·kg^{-1} (maximum 1000 mg) has been administered.

MECHANISM OF ACTION. The effects of phenytoin on automaticity and velocity of conduction of cardiac impulses resemble those of lidocaine. Like lidocaine, phenytoin has little effect on the ECG. Conduction of cardiac impulses through the atrioventricular node is improved, but activity of the sinus node may be depressed. The possible interaction with volatile anesthetics that may also depress the sinoatrial node should be remembered if consideration is given to administering phenytoin during general anesthesia.

METABOLISM AND EXCRETION. Phenytoin is hydroxylated and then conjugated with glucuronic acid for excretion in the urine. The elimination half-time is about 24 hours.

SIDE EFFECTS. The most prominent effects of phenytoin during acute treatment of cardiac dysrhythmias are on the central nervous system. Symptoms of central nervous system toxicity include nystagmus, sedation, and ataxia. Neurologic symptoms are usually indicative of plasma concentrations of phenytoin greater than 20 μg·ml^{-1}. Cardiac dysrhythmias that have not been suppressed at this concentration are unlikely to respond favorably to further increases in the dosage of phenytoin.

Flecainide

Flecainide is a fluorinated local anesthetic analogue of procainamide that is effective in suppression of nonsustained ventricular dysrhythmias in patients with normal or nearly normal left ventricular function (Roden and Woosley, 1986a). Conversely, patients with recurrent sustained ventricular tachycardia or ventricular fibrillation may experience an exacerbation of their dysrhythmia when treated with this drug. Chronic treatment of ventricular dysrhythmias with flecainide following myocardial infarction is not recommended owing to an increased incidence of sudden death in treated patients. In contrast to procainamide, flecainide prolongs the duration of the P-R and QRS intervals on the ECG. These changes suggest the possibility of atrioventricular or infranodal conduction block of cardiac impulses. Furthermore, flecainide may depress sinus node function in a manner similar to that of calcium entry blockers. Pacing threshold is increased, emphasizing caution in the use of this drug in patients with artificial cardiac pacemakers.

Oral absorption of flecainide is excellent, and prolonged elimination half-time makes a twice daily dose of 100 to 200 mg acceptable. About 25% of flecainide is excreted unchanged by the kidney, and the remainder appears as weakly active metabolites. Vertigo and difficulty in visual accommodation are common dose-related side effects of flecainide therapy.

Encainide

Encainide is a unique antidysrhythmic drug that combines the electrophysiologic effects of quinidine and lidocaine to suppress ventricular cardiac dysrhythmias (Fig. 17-5) (Woosley et al, 1988). A distinctive feature of encainide therapy is widening of the QRS on the ECG that usually occurs at concentrations required for pharmacologic effects and most likely reflects Na$^+$ channel blockade that slows the conduction of cardiac impulses. In contrast to quinidine, this drug lacks peripheral-vasodilating or direct negative inotropic effects such that alterations in blood pressure are uncommon after oral or intravenous administration. Chronic treatment of ventricular dysrhythmias with encainide following myocardial infarction is not recommended owing to an

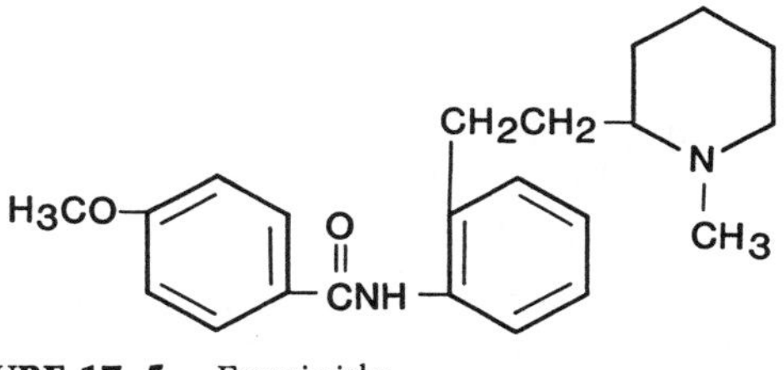

FIGURE 17–5. Encainide.

increased incidence of sudden death in treated patients.

Encainide undergoes extensive hepatic metabolism, forming active metabolites that contribute to the sustained antidysrhythmic effect of this drug. About 7% of the population have a genetically determined inability to efficiently metabolize encainide. The elimination half-time of encainide in these patients is 8 to 12 hours compared with 0.5 to 4 hours in those who metabolize the drug at a normal rate. Plasma concentrations of unchanged drug do not correlate closely with efficacy because of the contribution of active metabolites.

Beta-Adrenergic Antagonists

Beta-adrenergic antagonists depress both automaticity and conduction of cardiac impulses, with the latter effect being highly dependent on the degree of underlying sympathetic nervous system activity. At very high doses, certain beta-adrenergic antagonists, such as propranolol, also exhibit membrane-depressant actions.

Propranolol

Propranolol is used principally to slow the ventricular response to atrial fibrillation or paroxysmal supraventricular tachycardia (Table 17-3; see Fig. 14-3). Premature ventricular contractions are also suppressed by propranolol. It is a useful drug for suppression in the prolonged Q-T interval syndrome. Propranolol abolishes ventricular dysrhythmias induced by digitalis, but it is associated with a greater incidence of side effects than are lidocaine or phenytoin.

Propranolol is given orally for long-term treatment of cardiac dysrhythmias. For emergency use, propranolol can be given intravenously during monitoring of the ECG and blood pressure. The usual dose of propranolol is 5 to 15 $\mu g \cdot kg^{-1}$ IV to a total dose of 1 to 3 mg. The therapeutic plasma concentration of propranolol may vary from 10 to 30 $ng \cdot ml^{-1}$. The elimination half-time of propranolol is 2 to 4 hours, although the duration of antidysrhythmic activity usually persists for 6 to 8 hours.

MECHANISM OF ACTION. Antidysrhythmic effects of beta-adrenergic antagonists most likely reflect blockade of responses of beta-receptors in the heart to sympathetic nervous system stimulation and circulating catecholamines. As a result, the rate of spontaneous phase 4 depolarization is decreased and the rate of sinoatrial discharge is reduced. The electrical threshold of the atria and ventricles is minimally altered by propranolol. There is a substantial increase in the effective refractory period of the atrioventricular node owing to beta-adrenergic receptor blockade. Reentry dysrhythmias are prevented by an increase in the refractoriness of the atrioventricular node.

In addition to beta-adrenergic blockade, propranolol causes alterations in the electrical activity of myocardial cells. This cell membrane effect is probably responsible for some of the antidysrhythmic effects of propranolol. Indeed, dextropropranolol, which lacks beta-adrenergic antagonist activity, is an effective antidysrhythmic.

METABOLISM AND EXCRETION. Orally administered propranolol is extensively metabolized in the liver, and a hepatic first-pass effect is responsible for the variation in plasma concentration of propranolol. The primary metabolite of propranolol is 4-hydroxypropranolol, which possesses beta-adrenergic antagonist activity. This active metabolite most likely contributes to the antidysrhythmic activity following oral administration of propranolol.

SIDE EFFECTS. Propranolol often prolongs the P-R interval, with a minimal effect on the QRS complex and Q-T interval recorded on the ECG. In patients with chronic cardiac failure, a high level of sympathetic nervous system activity is essential for cardiac support. Treatment of cardiac dysrhythmias in these patients with propranolol reduces this vital compensatory mechanism and can result in accentuation of cardiac failure. The use of propranolol in the presence of preexisting atrioventricular blockade is not recommended.

Drugs That Prolong Repolarization

Antiadrenergic drugs that prolong repolarization by increasing the duration of action potentials in ventricular and Purkinje fibers are effective in treating ventricular cardiac dysrhythmias. Absence of this effect on the duration of action potentials of atrial muscle is consistent with the ineffectiveness of these drugs in treating supraventricular cardiac dysrhythmias.

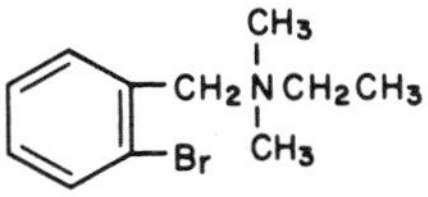

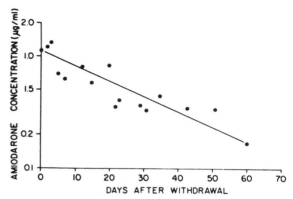

FIGURE 17-6. Bretylium.

Bretylium

Bretylium is uniquely effective in the treatment of ventricular tachycardia and ventricular fibrillation (Table 17-3; Fig. 17-6). The usual dose is 5 to 10 $mg^{-1} \cdot kg^{-1}$ IV, and the duration of action is 8 to 24 hours. The most striking electrophysiologic effect of bretylium is prolongation of the ventricular action potential and refractory period, explaining the effectiveness of this drug in suppressing ventricular dysrhythmias. Bretylium initially causes the release of norepinephrine from postganglionic sympathetic nerve endings, which can transiently lead to hypertension. Ultimately, the presence of bretylium in nerve endings prevents the release of norepinephrine and may lead to orthostatic hypotension and bradycardia.

The elimination half-time of bretylium is 8 to 12 hours, which is directly related to renal clearance (Table 17-3). About 70% of the drug is excreted unchanged in the urine in the first 24 hours, and by 48 hours, 98% of the initially injected drug is recovered. Hepatic metabolism has not been demonstrated for bretylium. Prolonged and/or cumulative effects are predictable when bretylium is administered to patients with impaired renal function.

Amiodarone

Amiodarone is administered for the prevention of (1) recurrent paroxysmal supraventricular tachydysrhythmias such as atrial fibrillation that may accompany Wolff-Parkinson-White syndrome and (2) recurrent ventricular tachycardia or ventricular fibrillation (Table 17-3) (Mason, 1987). The usual daily adult oral dose is 3 to 5 $mg \cdot kg^{-1}$. The onset of action after an oral dose is slow, and full antidysrhythmic effects may not occur for several days. Administered over 2 to 5 minutes, a dose of 5 $mg \cdot kg^{-1}$ IV produces a prompt antidysrhythmic effect that lasts up to 4 hours.

On discontinuation, the therapeutic effects of amiodarone may persist for prolonged periods. Indeed, chronic oral administration of amiodarone results in an elimination half-time of 29 days (Fig. 17-7) (Kannan et al, 1982). This is the

FIGURE 17-7. Following discontinuation of amiodarone, the plasma concentration declines slowly, resulting in an elimination half-time of 29 days. (From Kannan R, Nademannee K, Hendrickson JA, Rostami HJ, Singh BN. Amiodarone kinetics after oral doses. Clin Pharmacol Ther 1982; 31: 438–44; with permission.)

longest elimination half-time of any antidysrhythmic drug. A pharmacologic effect of amiodarone lasts more than 45 days after its discontinuation. Because of potentially serious side effects, amiodarone is recommended only when other drugs have been deemed ineffective or contraindicated in the treatment of life-threatening tachydysrhythmias.

MECHANISM OF ACTION. Amiodarone is a benzofurane derivative with a chemical structure that resembles thyroxine (Fig. 17-8). Like bretylium, amiodarone prolongs the duration of action potentials in atrial and ventricular muscle without altering the resting membrane potential, in effect delaying repolarization. The effective refractory period is increased. Amiodarone depresses sinoatrial and atrioventricular nodal function and slows conduction of cardiac impulses through the atrioventricular node. In most patients with the Wolff-Parkinson-White syndrome, amiodarone increases the refractory period of the accessory pathway, accounting for the efficacy of

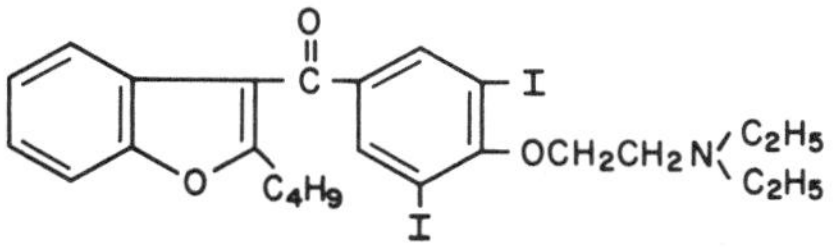

FIGURE 17-8. Amiodarone.

this drug in the management of patients with this disorder.

Amiodarone produces Na$^+$ channel blockade as estimated by the rate of rise of the action potential. This Na$^+$ channel blockade occurs principally during phase 2 and part of phase 3 of the cardiac action potential. As a result, amiodarone has a more marked effect on depolarized tissue (as in myocardial ischemia), tissue with a brief phase 4 (as during tachycardia), and tissue with prolonged repolarization (Mason, 1987).

Amiodarone acts as an effective antianginal drug by dilating coronary arteries and increasing coronary blood flow. Antiadrenergic effects of amiodarone most likely reflect noncompetitive blockade of alpha- and beta-adrenergic receptors.

METABOLISM AND EXCRETION. Amiodarone is minimally dependent on renal excretion as reflected by an unchanged elimination half-time in the absence of renal function (Kannan et al, 1982). The principal metabolite, desmethylamiodarone, has a longer elimination half-time than the parent drug, but it is not known whether this metabolite is pharmacologically active. Protein binding is extensive, and the drug is not removed by hemodialysis. There is an inconsistent relationship between the plasma concentration of amiodarone and its pharmacologic effects. Indeed, the ultimate concentration of drug in the myocardium is 10 to 50 times that in the plasma.

SIDE EFFECTS. Side effects of amiodarone are dose dependent, becoming most likely when the total daily dose is greater than 200 mg (Heger et al, 1981). Depressant effects on the heart are alleged to be minimal, although an animal study suggests amiodarone is a direct myocardial depressant (MacKinnon et al, 1983). The heart rate often slows, and the Q-T interval on the ECG is prolonged. Heart rate slowing is resistant to the effects of atropine, and responsiveness to catecholamine and sympathetic nervous system stimulation is reduced as a result of drug-induced inhibition of alpha- and beta-adrenergic receptors. Antiadrenergic effects of amiodarone may be enhanced in the presence of general anesthesia manifesting as sinus arrest, atrioventricular heart block, low cardiac output, or hypotension (Teasdale and Downar, 1990). Drugs that inhibit automaticity of the sinoatrial node, such as halothane and lidocaine, could accentuate the effects of amiodarone and increase the likelihood of

sinus arrest. The potential need for a temporary artificial cardiac (ventricular) pacemaker and administration of sympathomimetics such as isoproterenol should be considered in patients being treated with this drug and scheduled to undergo surgery (Navalgund et al, 1986). Amiodarone may act as a coronary artery and peripheral vascular vasodilator. Indeed, intravenous administration of amiodarone may result in hypotension and atrioventricular heart block. Neurologic abnormalities, including proximal skeletal muscle weakness, gait abnormalities, tremor, and peripheral neuropathies, have been reported (Heger et al, 1981).

Pulmonary toxicity manifestisting as pulmonary fibrosis and decreased diffusing capacity for carbon monoxide occurs in as many as 13% of patients treated with amiodarone (Mason, 1987). There is increasing evidence that patients with preexisting evidence of amiodarone-induced pulmonary toxicity are at increased risk for developing adult respiratory distress syndrome following surgery that requires cardiopulmonary bypass (Kupferschmid et al, 1989; Nalos et al, 1987). The mechanism for this response is unknown but may reflect a form of oxygen toxicity. Overall, patients with preexisting pulmonary disease may be unlikely candidates for amiodarone therapy, and those receiving the drug are often monitored with periodic chest radiographs and, perhaps, determination of diffusion capacity.

Chronic amiodarone therapy is associated with an alteration in thyroid function, causing either hypothyroidism or hyperthyroidism in 2% to 4% of patients. Hyperthyroidism has occurred up to 5 months after discontinuation of amiodarone. Patients with preexisting thyroid dysfunction seem more likely to develop amiodarone-related alterations in thyroid function. Despite the rarity of clinically significant drug-induced thyroid dysfunction, amiodarone invariably alters results of blood tests (increased thyroxine concentrations) used to measure thyroid function.

Corneal microdeposits occur after several weeks in many patients, but visual impairment is unlikely. Photosensitivity and rash develop in up to 10% of patients. Rarely, there may be a cyanotic discoloration of the face that persists even after the drug is discontinued. Transient, mild elevations in plasma transaminase enzyme concentrations are common, and fatty liver infiltration has been observed (Heger et al, 1981). Amiodarone displaces digoxin from protein binding sites and may increase its plasma concentration as much as 70%. The digoxin dose should be reduced at least 50% when administered in the presence of amiodarone. Amiodarone may directly depress vitamin K–dependent clotting factors.

Calcium Entry Blockers

Group 4 drugs are the calcium entry blockers that specifically inhibit inward passage of calcium ions (Ca^{2+}) across cardiac cell membranes (see Chapter 18).

Verapamil

Verapamil is uniquely effective in the suppression of reentrant supraventricular tachydysrhythmias (Table 17-3; see Fig. 18-1). The usual dose of verapamil is 75 to 150 $\mu g \cdot kg^{-1}$ IV infused over 1 to 3 minutes followed by a continuous infusion of about 5 $\mu g \cdot kg^{-1} \cdot min^{-1}$ IV to maintain a sustained effect.

The oral dose of verapamil required for antidysrhythmic activity is about ten times the intravenous dose, emphasizing the extensive hepatic first-pass effect that occurs. The duration of action is 4 to 6 hours, which correlates with the elimination half-time of 4.5 to 12 hours (Table 17-2).

MECHANISM OF ACTION. Verapamil slows the rate of spontaneous phase 4 depolarization in sinoatrial and atrioventricular nodal tissue. The action of verapamil on phase 4 depolarization is related to inhibition of the inward flux of Ca^{2+}. In addition, the duration of the cardiac action potential and repolarization are shortened by verapamil. Calcium entry blockers are relatively ineffective in suppressing ectopic pacemaker activity of ventricular automatic cells.

METABOLISM AND EXCRETION. An estimated 70% of an injected dose of verapamil is eliminated by the kidneys, whereas up to 15% may be present in the bile. A metabolite, norverapamil, may contribute to the parent drug's antidysrhythmic effects.

SIDE EFFECTS. Side effects of verapamil as used to treat cardiac dysrhythmias reflect extensions of the drug's atrioventricular pharmacologic effects (see Chapter 18). Atrioventricular heart block is more likely in patients with preexisting defects in the conduction of cardiac impulses. Direct myocardial depression and reduced cardiac output are likely to be exaggerated in patients with poor left ventricular function. Peripheral vasodilation may contribute to hypotension. There may be potentiation of anesthetic-produced myocardial depression, and effects of neuromuscular blocking drugs may be exaggerated (see Chapter 18).

REFERENCES

Atlee JL, Bosnjak ZJ. Mechanisms for cardiac dysrhythmias during anesthesia. Anesthesiology 1990;72:347–74.

Harrah MD, Way WL, Katzung BG. The interaction of d-tubocurarine with antiarrhythmic drugs. Anesthesiology 1970;33:406–10.

Heger JJ, Prystowsky EN, Jackman WM, et al. Amiodarone: Clinical efficacy and electrophysiology during long-term therapy for recurrent ventricular tachycardia or ventricular fibrillation. N Engl J Med 1981;305:539–45.

Kannan R, Nademannee K, Hendrickson JA, Rostami HJ, Singh BN. Amiodarone kinetics after oral doses. Clin Pharmacol Ther 1982;31:438–44.

Kupferschmid JP, Rosengart TK, McIntosh CL, Leon MB, Clark RE. Amiodarone-induced complications after cardiac operation for obstructive hypertrophic cardiomyopathy. Ann Thorac Surg 1989;48:359–64.

Leahey EB, Reiffel JA, Drusin RE, Hissenbuttel RH, Lovejoy WP, Bigger JT. Interaction between quinidine and digoxin. JAMA 1978;240:533–4.

Lucas WJ, Maccioli GA, Mueller RA. Advances in oral antiarrhythmic therapy: Implications for the anaesthetist. Can J Anaesth 1990;37:94–101.

MacKinnon G, Landymore R, Marble A. Should oral amiodarone be used for sustained ventricular tachycardia in patients requiring open-heart surgery? Can J Surg 1983;26:355–7.

MacMahon S, Collins R, Peto R, Koster PW, Yusuf S. Effects of prophylactic lidocaine in suspected acute myocardial infarction: An overview of results from the randomized, controlled trials. JAMA 1988;260:1910–6.

Mason JW. Amiodarone. N Engl J Med 1987;316:455–63.

Navalgund AA, Alifimoff JK, Jakymec AJ, Bleyaert AL. Amidarone-induced sinus arrest successfully treated with ephedrine and isoproterenol. Anesth Analg 1986;65:414–6.

Nalos PC, Kass RM, Gang ES, Fishbein MC, Mandel WJ, Peter T. Life-threatening postoperative pulmonary complications in patients with previous amiodarone pulmonary toxicity undergoing cardiothoracic operations. J Thorac Cardiovase Surg 1987;93:904–12.

Roden DM, Woosley RL. Flecainide. N Engl J Med 1986a;315:36–41.

Roden DM, Woosley RL. Tocainide. N Engl J Med 1986b;315:41–5.

Teasdale S, Downar E. Amiodarone and anaesthesia. Can J Anaesth 1990;37:151–5.

The Cardiac Arrhythmia Suppression Trial (CAST) Investigators. Preliminary report: Effect of encanide and flecainide on mortality in a randomized trial of arrhythmia suppression after myocardial infarction. N Engl J Med 1989;321:406–12.

Way WL, Katzung BG, Larson CP. Recurarization with quinidine. JAMA 1967;200:163–4.

Woosley RL, Wood AJJ, Roden DM. Encainide. N Engl J Med 1988;318:1107–15.

Chapter
18

Calcium Entry Blockers

INTRODUCTION

Calcium entry blockers (also known as calcium antagonists and calcium channel blockers) are a diverse group of structurally unrelated compounds that selectively interfere with inward calcium ion (Ca^{2+}) movement across cell membranes (Durand et al, 1991; Kaplan, 1989). Commonly used calcium entry blockers are verapamil, nifedipine, diltiazem, and nicardipine (Fig. 18-1).

MECHANISM OF ACTION

Channels with a system of gates exist in membranes of excitable cells for the inward transfer of Ca^{2+}, sodium (Na^+), and potassium ions (K^+). Conceptually, a slow Ca^{2+} channel and a fast Na^+ channel are present. Slow channels are 100 times more selective for Ca^{2+} than for Na^+ or K^+. Two different gates are postulated to be present on slow Ca^{2+} channels (Fig. 18-2) (Antman et al, 1980). The gate on the extracellular membrane (outer gate) is voltage dependent, opening with depolarization and closing with repolarization. A second gate on the intracellular surface (inner gate) modulates Ca^{2+} ion flux. Cyclic adenosine monophosphate allows widening of this gate, which facilitates inward movement of Ca^{2+}. Cyclic guanosine monophosphate causes narrowing of this gate.

Calcium entry blockers selectively interfere with inward transfer of Ca^{2+} through slow Ca^{2+} channels. Verapamil may act principally at the inner gate, whereas nifedipine probably blocks the outer gate. Verapamil and diltiazem also have some blocking activity at fast Na^+ channels.

PHARMACOLOGIC EFFECTS

The pharmacologic effects of calcium entry blockers can be predicted from a consideration of the normal role of Ca^{2+} in production of the cardiac action potential. For example, the slow plateau portion of the cardiac action potential (phase 2) is thought to be due to inward Ca^{2+} flux. This phase of the action potential is particularly important in the excitation-contraction of cardiac muscle and vascular smooth muscle and, to a lesser extent, skeletal muscle. In addition, Ca^{2+} movement during phase 2 of the cardiac action potential is responsible for depolarization in sinoatrial and atrioventricular nodal tissue. Based on these known effects of Ca^{2+} transport on the action potential, it is predictable that calcium entry blockers will produce (1) decreased myocardial contractility, (2) decreased heart rate, (3) decreased rate of conduction of cardiac impulses through the atrioventricular node, and (4) vascular smooth muscle relaxation with associated vasodilation and reductions in blood pressure (Reves et al, 1982). The predominant hemodynamic effect of calcium entry blockers is a decrease in blood pressure owing to a decline in systemic vascular resistance. Although all vascular beds are dilated, these drugs appear to affect primarily arterial rather than venous vascular tone.

The relative abilities of calcium entry blockers to evoke these pharmacologic effects

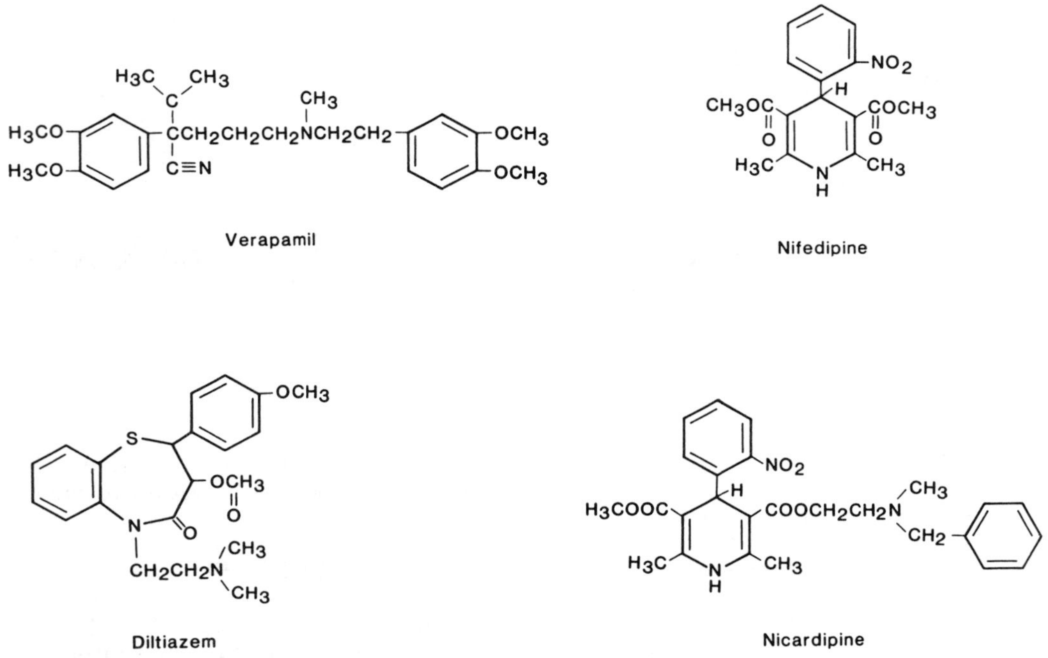

Verapamil

Nifedipine

Diltiazem

Nicardipine

FIGURE 18–1. Calcium entry blockers.

differs among the drugs (Table 18-1). In addition, verapamil and diltiazem also have some blocking activity at fast Na^+ channels responsible for rapid phase 0 and phase 1 portions of the cardiac action potential. This effect on the fast Na^+ channels is consistent with the local anesthetic activity of these two drugs.

CLINICAL USES

Differences in cardiovascular effects produced by the various calcium entry blockers may influence the specific drug selected for individual patients (Table 18-1). With this in mind, calcium entry blockers are particularly useful in the treatment of essential hypertension and management of supraventricular tachydysrhythmias. Other uses of calcium entry blockers may include (1) management of angina pectoris owing to coronary artery vasospasm or atherosclerosis, (2) management of cerebral vasospasm, (3) cerebral protection after global ischemia, (4) myocardial protection during cardiopulmonary bypass, (5) production of controlled hypotension, (6) pre-

vention of bronchospasm associated with exercise-induced asthma, and (7) treatment of esophageal spasms (Reves et al, 1982). Antihypertensive effects reflect principally decreases in systemic vascular resistance, although reductions in left ventricular contractility may accompany administration of calcium entry blockers such as verapamil.

Essential Hypertension

As a reflection of their efficacy and relatively mild side effects, calcium entry blockers have been recommended for initial monotherapy for hypertension (Kaplan, 1989). These drugs are similar in antihypertensive efficacy but differ in their effects on the atrioventricular node and degree of peripheral vasodilation (Table 18-1). Drugs with more specific vasodilating actions and less negative inotropic effects may be preferable in patients with congestive heart failure related to chronic essential hypertension. A mild natriuretic action of calcium entry blockers may reduce the need for concomitant dietary Na^+ re-

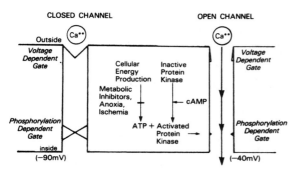

FIGURE 18-2. Schematic depiction of the slow calcium channel demonstrating a voltage-dependent gate on the extracellular membrane and a phosphorylation-dependent gate on the intracellular surface. (From Antman EM, Stone PH, Muller JE, Braunwald E. Calcium channel blocking agents in the treatment of cardiovascular disorders. I: Basic and clinical electrophysiologic effects. Ann Intern Med 1980; 93: 875–85; with permission.)

striction or administration of diuretics. The antihypertensive efficacy of calcium entry blockers directly parallels the pretreatment blood pressure with little or no effect in normotensive subjects.

Calcium entry blockers are useful choices for treating many subsets of patients with essential hypertension. These include patients with preexisting disease (diabetes mellitus, asthma, gout, peripheral vascular disease) that limits or precludes use of other antihypertensives. Furthermore, patients with preexisting diseases (coronary artery disease, cerebrovascular disease, esophageal spasm) may secondarily benefit from treatment of essential hypertension with calcium entry blockers.

Supraventricular Tachydysrhythmias

Verapamil, but not nifedipine, is effective in terminating paroxysmal supraventricular tachycardia by delaying conduction of cardiac impulses through the atrioventricular node (Waxman et al, 1981). The recommended dose of verapamil for treatment of supraventricular tachydysrhythmias is 75 to 150 $\mu g \cdot kg^{-1}$ IV (5 to 10 mg IV for an adult) infused over 3 to 5 minutes. Diltiazem, 0.1 $mg \cdot kg^{-1}$ IV, slows heart rate in patients with atrial fibrillation who develop supraventricular tachydysrhythmias intraoperatively (Iwatsuki et al, 1985).

Verapamil may be useful in the treatment of maternal and fetal tachydysrhythmias as well as premature labor (Murad et al, 1985a). Indeed, verapamil administered intravenously to the mother prolongs atrioventricular conduction in the fetus despite limited placental transport of the drug (the ratio of umbilical vein to uterine artery verapamil concentrations is 0.35 to 0.45). Fetal hepatic extraction of verapamil is substantial, as evidenced by a plasma concentration in the fetal carotid artery less than in the umbilical vein. Verapamil may decrease uterine blood flow, suggesting caution in the administration of this drug to parturients with impaired uteroplacental perfusion (Murad et al, 1985b).

Verapamil is as effective and more rapid in onset than digitalis in slowing the ventricular response in the presence of atrial flutter or fibrillation (Waxman et al, 1981). Reversion to sinus rhythm, however, is uncommon. In patients with mitral valve disease and rapid atrial fibrillation, verapamil may abruptly slow heart rate and relieve pulmonary congestion. The administration of verapamil orally to prevent recurrences of

Table 18-1
Comparative Effects of Calcium Entry Blockers

	Verapamil	Nifedipine	Diltiazem	Nicardipine
Blood pressure	−	−	−	−
Heart rate	−	+/NC	−	+/NC
Nodal conduction	− −	NC	−	NC
Myocardial contractility	− −	NC	−	NC
Peripheral vasodilation	−	− −	−	− −

− indicates decrease, + indicates increase, NC indicates no change.

tachydysrhythmias appears to be safer than digitalis for use before electrical cardioversion. Depending on conduction through the accessory pathway, verapamil may or may not be beneficial in the management of patients with preexcitation syndromes such as the Wolff-Parkinson-White syndrome. In some of these patients, verapamil may actually increase the ventricular response during atrial fibrillation (Rinkenberger et al, 1980). Indeed, the rate of retrograde conduction of cardiac impulses through accessory pathways is not altered by verapamil. Verapamil should probably be avoided in patients with sick sinus syndrome and in the presence of any degree of preexisting atrioventricular heart block.

Ventricular cardiac dysrhythmias are not predictably responsive to treatment with calcium entry blockers. A possible exception is ventricular tachycardia and fibrillation in patients with coronary artery vasospasm (Kapur et al, 1984b). In addition, diltiazem administered to dogs increases the dose of epinephrine necessary to produce ventricular cardiac dysrhythmias during halothane anesthesia and abolishes premature ventricular contractions that appear spontaneously in patients anesthetized with halothane (Iwatsuki et al, 1985).

Coronary Artery Vasospasm

Coronary artery vasospasm is characterized by angina pectoris that occurs at rest in association with S-T changes on the electrocardiogram (ECG). Verapamil administered intravenously or nifedipine administered orally or sublingually are equally effective treatment for coronary artery vasospasm (Johnson et al, 1981). The incidence of perioperative myocardial ischemia is not altered by chronic treatment with calcium entry blockers (Chung et al, 1988; Slogoff and Keats, 1988.)

Exercise-Induced Angina Pectoris

Improvement in the balance of oxygen supply and demand is the presumed mechanism for the effectiveness of calcium entry blockers in the treatment of angina owing to coronary atherosclerosis. For example, the beneficial effect of nifedipine in the treatment of exercise-induced angina pectoris appears to be due principally to its peripheral vasodilator action rather than to an effect on the coronary arteries.

Cerebral Artery Vasospasm

Cerebral artery vasospasm is focal or diffuse narrowing of one or more of the large arteries at the base of the brain. Vasospasm occurs frequently between 4 and 14 days after subarachnoid hemorrhage and is thought to cause neurologic deficits. The initial event in the development of vasospasm may be an intracellular influx of Ca^{2+} that causes contraction of smooth muscle cells in large cerebral arteries.

Nimodipine is a lipid-soluble analogue of nifedipine that gains entrance to the central nervous system and selectively blocks the influx of extracellular Ca^{2+}. In animals, the effect of nimodipine is greater on the basilar artery than the femoral artery. Administration of nimodipine within 96 hours of subarachnoid hemorrhage reduces the severity of ischemic neurologic deficits from vasospasm (Allen et al, 1983). Likewise, patients experiencing acute ischemic stroke may benefit from early treatment with nimodipine (Gelmers et al, 1988). Side effects have not been reported to accompany the administration of nimodipine, although drug-induced cerebral vasodilation could evoke increases in intracranial pressure, particularly in patients with preexisting reductions in intracranial compliance.

Cerebral Protection

The theoretical basis for considering calcium entry blockers is the observation that lack of oxygen interferes with maintenance of the normal Ca^{2+} gradient across cells membranes, leading to massive increases (at least 200-fold) in the intraneuronal concentrations of this ion. Calcium entry blockers may be effective in ameliorating ischemic brain injury (White et al, 1984). Indeed, nimodipine, a calcium entry blocker that rapidly enters the central nervous system, is associated with improved neurologic outcome when administered within 5 minutes to primates previously experiencing 17 minutes of cerebral ischemia (Steen et al, 1985). Nevertheless, administration of nimodipine following cardiac arrest does not seem to influence ultimate neurologic outcome in humans (Forsman et al, 1989; Roine et al, 1991).

Myocardial Protection

Calcium entry blockers may exert a protective effect during global myocardial ischemia associated with cardiopulmonary bypass by suppressing energy-dependent Ca^{2+}-mediated myocardial activity. The combination of blockade of slow channels with a calcium entry blocker and fast channels with K^+ may result in even a greater reduction in myocardial oxygen consumption than either intervention alone. High doses of calcium entry blockers as used for this myocardial protection, however, could depress myocardial contractility in the period following cessation of cardiopulmonary bypass. Calcium entry blockers have not been found to be cardioprotective either during or after myocardial infarction.

DRUG INTERACTIONS

The known pharmacologic effects of calcium entry blockers on cardiac, skeletal, and vascular smooth muscle as well as on the conduction velocity of cardiac impulses make drug interactions possible. For example, myocardial depression and peripheral vasodilation produced by volatile anesthetics could be exaggerated by similar actions of calcium entry blockers. Indeed, volatile anesthetics may interfere with Ca^{2+} movement across cell membranes. Furthermore, delayed conduction of cardiac impulses through the atrioventricular node produced by halothane may be, in part, due to Ca^{2+} channel blockade (Chapter 2). The likelihood of adverse circulatory changes owing to interactions between calcium entry blockers and anesthetic drugs would seem to be greater in patients with preexisting atrioventricular heart block or left ventricular dysfunction. In addition to the possibility of drug interaction effects on the cardiovascular system, calcium entry blockers may potentiate neuromuscular blocking drugs (van Poorten et al, 1984). Nevertheless, therapy with calcium entry blockers can be continued until the time of surgery without risk of significant drug interactions, especially with respect to conduction of cardiac impulses (Henling et al, 1984).

Anesthetic Drugs

Calcium entry blockers are vasodilators and myocardial depressants. In fact, negative inotropic effects, depressant effects on sinus node function, and peripheral vasodilating effects of calcium entry blockers and inhaled anesthetics are similar, and there is evidence that inhaled anesthetics have blocking effects on Ca^{2+} channels (Merin, 1987). For these reasons, calcium entry blockers must be administered with caution during anesthesia, especially to patients with impaired left ventricular function or hypovolemia. Nevertheless, administration of verapamil, 150 $\mu g \cdot kg^{-1}$ IV over 10 minutes, to patients with normal left ventricular function anesthetized with halothane does not produce adverse circulatory changes other than modest further reductions in blood pressure, even in the presence of chronic low-dose beta-adrenergic antagonist therapy (Figs. 18-3 and 18-4) (Schulte-Sasse et al, 1984). Patients treated with a combination of beta-blockers and nifedipine tolerate high-dose fentanyl anesthesia and show no undue depression of cardiac function when verapamil is infused (Kapur et al, 1986b). Conversely, in anesthetized patients with preexisting left ventricular dysfunction, administration of verapamil is associated with myocardial depression and decreased cardiac output (Chew et al, 1981). Furthermore, intravenous administration of verapamil or diltiazem during open-chest surgery in patients with depressed ventricular function and anesthetized with volatile anesthetics may be associated with further decreases in ventricular function (Merin, 1987). Treatment of cardiac dysrhythmias with calcium entry blockers in patients anesthetized with halothane produces only transient decreases in blood pressure and infrequent prolongation of the P-R interval on the ECG. Because of the tendency to produce atrioventricular heart block, verapamil should be used cautiously in patients taking digitalis or beta-adrenergic antagonists. Nevertheless, in patients without preoperative evidence of cardiac conduction abnormalities, the chronic combined administration of calcium entry blockers and beta-adrenergic antagonists is not associated with cardiac conduction abnormalities in the perioperative period (Table 18-2) (Henling et al, 1984). Beta-agonists increase the number of functioning slow Ca^{2+} channels in myocardial cell membranes through a cyclic adenosine monophosphate mechanism and readily counter the effects of calcium entry blockers. Nevertheless, there is no evidence that patients being treated chronically with calcium entry blockers are at increased risk for anesthesia.

In animals, continuous intravenous infusion of verapamil in the presence of anesthetic doses of halothane, enflurane, or isoflurane produces dose-dependent reductions in mean arterial pres-

sure, heart rate, and cardiac index, whereas the P-R interval on the ECG is increased (Fig. 18-5) (Kapur et al, 1984a). Reductions in blood pressure and the occurrence of conduction abnormalities are more prominent in animals anesthetized with enflurane than in those anesthetized with halothane or isoflurane (Kapur et al, 1984a). Dogs given nifedipine during halothane anesthesia develop exaggerated reductions in blood pressure, whereas increasing concentrations of

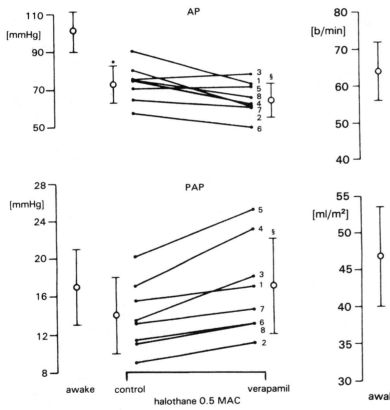

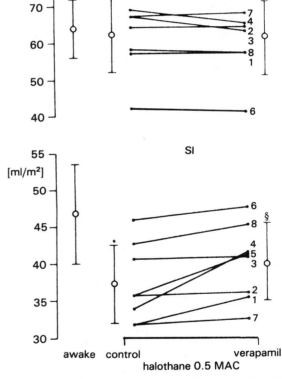

FIGURE 18–3. Administration of verapamil, 150 $\mu g \cdot kg^{-1}$ IV, over 10 minutes to patients receiving chronic beta-adrenergic antagonist drug therapy anesthetized with halothane produces modest decreases in arterial pressure (AP), whereas pulmonary arterial pressure (PAP) increases. Mean ± SD. (From Schulte-Sasse U, Hess W, Markschies-Harnung A, Tarnow J. Combined effects of halothane anesthesia and verapamil on systemic hemodynamics and left ventricular myocardial contractility in patients with ischemic heart disease. Anesth Analg 1984; 63: 791–8; with permission.)

FIGURE 18–4. Administration of verapamil, 150 $\mu g \cdot kg^{-1}$ IV, over 10 minutes, to patients receiving chronic beta-adrenergic antagonist drug therapy and anesthetized with halothane does not alter heart rate (HR) or stroke index (SI). Mean ± SD. (From Schulte-Sasse U, Hess W, Markschies-Harnung A, Tarnow J. Combined effects of halothane anesthesia and verapamil on systemic hemodynamics and left ventricular myocardial contractility in patients with ischemic heart disease. Anesth Analg 1984; 63: 791–8; with permission.)

Table 18–2

Effect of Chronic Antianginal Therapy on Perioperative Heart Rate
(beats· min⁻¹) and P-R Interval (msec)

	Before Induction	After Induction	Ten Minutes After Cardiopulmonary Bypass
Control			
Heart rate	72	71	87
P-R interval	160	156	164
Calcium Entry Blockers			
Heart rate	69	70	86
P-R interval	168	169	175
Beta-Adrenergic Antagonists			
Heart rate	59	65	78
P-R interval	168	171	183
Nifedipine and Beta-Adrenergic Antagonists			
Heart rate	67	69	86
P-R interval	175	177	186

(Data from Henling CE, Slogoff S, Kodali SV, Arlund C. Heart block after coronary artery bypass: Effect of chronic administration of calcium-entry blockers and beta-blockers. Anesth Analg 1984; 63: 515–20; with permission.)

halothane attenuate the usual reflex increases in heart rate produced by this drug.

Cardiovascular depression is accentuated in halothane-anesthetized dogs rendered acutely hyperkalemic (Nugent et al, 1984). Administration of intravenous Ca^{2+} is only partially effective in reversing this cardiovascular depression and of no value in antagonizing prolongation of the P-R interval on the ECG. Acute intravenous administration of verapamil to dogs in doses sufficient to prolong the P-R interval on the ECG lowers halothane MAC from 0.97% to 0.72% (Maze and Mason, 1983).

Neuromuscular Blocking Drugs

Calcium entry blockers alone do not produce a skeletal muscle relaxant effect as evidenced by failure to alter twitch height (Fig. 18-6) (Durant et al, 1984). Conversely, these drugs potentiate the effects of depolarizing and nondepolarizing neuromuscular blocking drugs (Fig. 18-6) (Durant et al, 1984). This potentiation resembles

that produced by mycin antibiotics in the presence of neuromuscular blocking drugs (see Chapter 28). The local anesthetic effect of verapamil, reflecting inhibition of Na^+ flux via fast Na^+ channels, may also contribute to the potentiation of neuromuscular blocking drugs. Observations of skeletal muscle weakness following administration of verapamil to a patient with muscular dystrophy is consistent with diminished release of neurotransmitter (Zalman et al, 1983). Therefore, the neuromuscular effects of verapamil may be more likely to manifest in patients with a compromised margin of safety of neuromuscular transmission.

Antagonism of neuromuscular blockade may be impaired because of diminished presynaptic release of acetylcholine in the presence of a calcium entry blocker (Lawson et al, 1983). Indeed, Ca^{2+} is essential for the release of acetylcholine at the neuromuscular junction. In one report, edrophonium, but not neostigmine, was effective in antagonizing nondepolarizing neuromuscular blockade that was potentiated by verapamil (Jones et al, 1985).

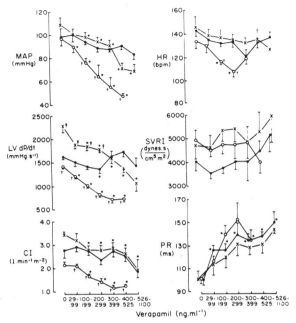

FIGURE 18-5. In animals, the continuous intravenous infusion of verapamil during halothane (●), enflurane (O), or isoflurane (x—x) produces dose-dependent decreases in mean arterial pressure (MAP), heart rate (HR), left ventricular (LV) dp/dt, and cardiac index (CI). Systemic vascular resistance is unchanged, and the P-R interval on the electrocardiogram is prolonged. *P <0.05 compared with control. †P <0.05 compared with both halothane and isoflurane. ‡P <0.05 compared with halothane. Mean ± SE. (From Kapur PA, Bloor BC, Flacke WE, Olewine SK. Comparison of cardiovascular response to verapamil during enflurane, isoflurane, or halothane anesthesia in the dog. Anesthesiology 1984; 61: 156–60; with permission.)

Local Anesthetics

Verapamil has potent local anesthetic activity, which may increase the risk of local anesthetic toxicity when regional anesthesia is administered to patients being treated with this drug (Rosenblatt et al, 1984).

Potassium-Containing Solutions

Calcium entry blockers slow the inward movement of K^+. For this reason, hyperkalemia in patients treated with verapamil may occur after much smaller amounts of exogenous K^+ infusion as associated with use of potassium chloride to treat hypokalemia or administration of stored whole blood (Nugent et al, 1984). In animals, however, pretreatment with verapamil does not alter increases in plasma K^+ concentration following the administration of succinylcholine (Roth et al, 1985).

Dantrolene

The ability of both verapamil and dantrolene to inhibit intracellular Ca^{2+} flux and excitation-contraction coupling would suggest this combination might be useful in the treatment of malignant hyperthermia. In swine, however, the administration of dantrolene in the presence of verapamil or diltiazem results in hyperkalemia and cardiovascular collapse (Fig. 18-7) (Saltzman et al, 1984a; Saltzman et al, 1984b). A patient being treated with verapamil developed hyperkalemia and myocardial depression within 1.5 hours of being treated with dantrolene administered intravenously (Rubin and Zablocki, 1987). The same patient did not experience

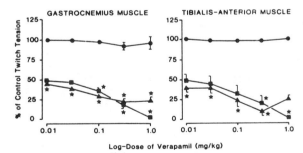

Log-Dose of Verapamil (mg/kg)

FIGURE 18-6. Infusion of verapamil in the absence of neuromuscular blocking drugs (●) does not alter twitch height response (*twitch tension*) of indirectly stimulated rabbit skeletal muscle. When twitch tension is reduced to about 50% of control by the continuous infusion of pancuronium (■) or succinylcholine (▲), the addition of verapamil further reduces twitch tension. *P <0.05 compared with the twitch tension before verapamil. Mean ± SE. (From Durant NN, Nguyen N, Katz R. Potentiation of neuromuscular blockade by verapamil. Anesthesiology 1984; 60: 298–303; with permission.)

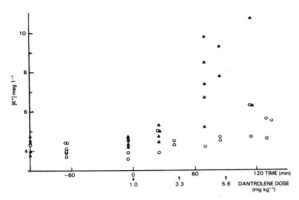

FIGURE 18–7. Administration of dantrolene to swine pretreated with verapamil (▲) results in hyperkalemia (*K*⁺) compared with animals receiving only dantrolene (O) (From Saltzman LS, Kates RA, Corke BC, Norfleet EA, Heath KR. Hyperkalemia and cardiovascular collapse after verapamil and dantrolene administration in swine. Anesth Analg 1984; 63: 473–8; with permission.)

hyperkalemia when nifedipine was substituted for verapamil prior to pretreatment with dantrolene. Whenever calcium entry blockers, especially verapamil or diltiazem, and dantrolene must be administered concurrently, invasive hemodynamic monitoring and frequent measurement of plasma K⁺ concentrations are recommended. It is speculated that verapamil alters normal homeostatic mechanisms for regulation of plasma K⁺ potassium concentrations and results in hyperkalemia from dantrolene-induced K⁺ release. Furthermore, there is evidence that verapamil does not influence the ability of known triggering agents to evoke malignant hyperthermia in susceptible animals (Gallant et al, 1985).

Platelet Function

Calcium entry blockers interfere with Ca²⁺-mediated platelet functions.

Digoxin

Calcium entry blockers may increase the plasma concentration of digoxin, presumably by reducing plasma clearance.

VERAPAMIL

Verapamil is a synthetic derivative of papaverine that is supplied as a racemic mixture (Fig. 18-1). The dextro isomer is devoid of activity at slow Ca²⁺ channels but instead acts on fast Na⁺ channels, accounting for the local anesthetic effects of verapamil (1.6 times as potent as procaine) (Kraynack et al, 1982). The levo isomer, however, is specific for slow Ca²⁺ channels, and the predominance of this action accounts for the classification of verapamil as a calcium entry blocker. Furthermore, it has been demonstrated that the parent drug of verapamil, papaverine, also possesses slow Ca²⁺ channel blocking effects.

Verapamil produces direct depressant effects on the sinoatrial node and delays antegrade transmission of cardiac impulses through the atrioventricular node (Table 18-1) (Reves, 1984). Retrograde transmission of cardiac impulses through the atrioventricular node or in accessory pathways is not significantly altered by verapamil. Negative inotropic effects of verapamil are not prominent except in patients with preexisting left ventricular dysfunction and possibly in those being treated with beta-adrenergic antagonists.

Verapamil, administered intravenously, is effective in the treatment of acute supraventricular tachydysrhythmias. Although the principal pharmacologic effect of verapamil is on the sinoatrial and atrioventricular nodes, it also possesses mild vasodilating properties, making this drug useful in the treatment of angina pectoris and essential hypertension. Verapamil is not as active as nifedipine in its effects on vascular smooth muscle and, therefore, causes a less pronounced decrease in blood pressure and less reflex peripheral sympathetic nervous system activity (Table 18-1) (Reves, 1984). Isoproterenol may be useful to increase heart rate acutely in the presence of drug-induced heart block when life-threatening situations require temporary artificial cardiac pacing. Intravenous administration of verapamil can produce hypotension, especially when administered to patients with preexisting left ventricular dysfunction. Although verapamil is highly effective in some patients with hypertrophic cardiomyopathy, there have also been instances of drug-induced cardiovascular depression. Elevated plasma transaminase and alkaline phosphatase concentrations accompanied by hepatitis develop rarely.

Pharmacokinetics

Oral verapamil is almost completely absorbed, but extensive hepatic first-pass metabolism limits bioavailability to 10% to 20% (Table 18-3) (Reves et al, 1982). As a result, the oral dose (80 to 160 mg three times daily) is about ten times the intravenous dose. The therapeutic plasma concentration of verapamil is 100 to 300 ng·ml^{-1}.

Demethylated metabolites of verapamil predominate, with norverapamil possessing sufficient activity to contribute to the antidysrhythmic properties of the parent drug. In view of the nearly complete hepatic metabolism of verapamil, almost none of the drug appears unchanged in the urine. Conversely, an estimated 70% of an injected dose of verapamil is recovered in the urine as metabolites and about 15% is excreted via the bile. Chronic oral administration of verapamil or renal dysfunction leads to the accumulation of norverapamil.

The elimination half-time of verapamil is 2 to 7 hours but may be prolonged to over 13 hours in patients with liver disease. Like nifedipine, verapamil is highly protein bound (90%), and the presence of other drugs (lidocaine, diazepam, propranolol) can increase the pharmacologically active, unbound portion of the drug.

NIFEDIPINE

Nifedipine is a dihydropyridine derivative with greater coronary and peripheral arterial vasodilator properties than verapamil (Table 18-1 and Fig. 18-1) (Reves, 1984). There is minimal effect on venous capacitance vessels. Unlike verapamil, nifedipine has little or no direct depressant effect on sinoatrial or atrioventricular nodal activity. Peripheral vasodilation and the resulting decrease in blood pressure produced by nifedipine activate baroreceptors, leading to increased peripheral sympathetic nervous system activity most often manifesting as an elevated heart rate. This increased sympathetic nervous system activity counters the direct negative inotropic, chrono-

Table 18–3
Characteristics of Calcium Entry Blockers

	Verapamil	*Nifedipine*	*Diltiazem*
Dosage			
Oral	80–160 mg every 8 hours	10–20 mg every 8 hours	60–90 mg every 8 hours
Intravenous	75–150 µg·kg^{-1}	5– 15 µg·kg^{-1}	75–150 µg·kg^{-1}
Absorption (percent)			
Oral	>90	>90	>90
Bioavailability	10–20	65–70	40
Onset of Effect (min)			
Oral	<30	<20	30
Sublingual		3	
Intravenous	1–3	1–3	1–3
Protein Binding (percent)	90	90	70–80
Clearance Mechanisms			
Renal (percent)	70	80	35
Fecal (percent)	15	<15	60
Active Metabolites	Yes	No	Yes
Elimination Half-Time (h)	6–12	2–5	3–5

(Data from Reves JG, Kissin I, Lell WA, Tosone S. Calcium entry blockers: Uses and implications for anesthesiologists. Anesthesiology 1982; 57:504–18.)

tropic, and dromotropic effects of nifedipine. Nevertheless, nifedipine may produce excessive myocardial depression, especially in patients with (1) aortic stenosis, (2) preexisting left ventricular dysfunction, or (3) beta-adrenergic antagonist therapy.

Nifedipine, 10 to 20 mg, administered orally three times daily, is used to treat patients with angina pectoris, especially that due to coronary artery vasospasm. The drug is oxidized by light and must, therefore, be protected during storage. This extreme light sensitivity makes availability of an intravenous preparation unlikely.

Pharmacokinetics

Absorption of an oral or sublingual dose of nifedipine is about 90%, with onset of an effect being detectable within about 20 minutes after administration (Table 18-3) (Reves et al, 1982). Protein binding approaches 90%. Hepatic metabolism is nearly complete, with elimination of inactive metabolites principally in the urine (about 80%) and, to a lesser extent, in the bile. The elimination half-time of nifedipine is 4 to 6 hours. Glucose intolerance and hepatic dysfunction occur rarely. Abrupt discontinuation of nifedipine has been associated with coronary artery vasospasm.

DILTIAZEM

Diltiazem is a calcium entry blocker derived from benzothiazapine (Fig. 18-1). Its cardiovascular effects are similar to those of verapamil (Table 18-1) (Reves, 1984). Resting heart rate is often decreased by diltiazem. Coronary and peripheral arteries are dilated. Diltiazem exerts minimal cardiodepressant effects and is unlikely to interact with beta-antagonists to decrease contractility (Packer, 1989). Intravenous infusion of diltiazem produces dose-related prolongation of the P-R interval on the ECG and decreases in blood pressure in dogs anesthetized with enflurane (Kapur et al, 1986a).

Diltiazem is administered orally or intravenously for the management of patients with angina pectoris (see Table 18-3). Oral absorption is excellent. Diltiazem is 80% bound to protein and is excreted as inactive metabolites principally in the bile (about 60%) and, to a lesser extent, in the urine (about 35%). The elimination half-time is 4

to 6 hours. The clinical uses and drug interactions for diltiazem are similar to verapamil.

REFERENCES

Allen GS, Ahn HS, Preziosi TJ, et al. Cerebral arterial spasm: A controlled trial of nimodipine in patients with subarachnoid hemorrhage. N Engl J Med 1983;308:619–24.

Antman EM, Stone PH, Muller JE, Braunwald E. Calcium channel blocking agents in the treatment of cardiovascular disorders. I: Basic and clinical electrophysiologic effects. Ann Intern Med 1980;93:875–85.

Chew CYC, Hecht HS, Collett JT, McAllister RG, Singh BN. Influence of severity of ventricular dysfunction on hemodynamic responses to intravenously administered verapamil in ischemic heart disease. Am J Cardiol 1981;47:917–22.

Chung F, Houston PL, Cheng DCH, et al. Calcium channel blockade does not offer adequate protection from perioperative myocardial ischemia. Anesthesiology 1988;69:343–7.

Durand P-G, Lehot J-J, Foex P. Calcium-channel blockers and anaesthesia. Can J Anaesth 1991; 38:75-89.

Durant NN, Nguyen N, Katz R. Potentiation of neuromuscular blockade by verapamil. Anesthesiology 1984;60:298–303.

Forsman M, Aarseth HP, Nordby H, Skulberg A, Steen PA. Effects of nimodipine on cerebral blood flow and cerebrospinal fluid pressure after cardiac arrest: Correlation with neurologic outcome. Anesth Analg 1989;68:436–43.

Gallant EM, Foldes FF, Rempel WE, Gronert GA. Verapamil is not a therapeutic adjunct to dantrolene in porcine malignant hyperthermia. Anesth Analg 1985;64:601–6.

Gelmers HJ, Gorter K, deWeerdt CJ, Wiezer HJA. A controlled trial of nimodipine in acute ischemic stroke. N Engl J Med 1988;318:303–7.

Henling CE, Slogoff S, Kodali SV, Arlund C. Heart block after coronary artery bypass: Effect of chronic administration of calcium-entry blockers and beta-blockers. Anesth Analg 1984;63:515–20.

Iwatsuki N, Katoh M, Ono K, Amaha K. Antiarrhythmic effect of diltiazem during halothane anesthesia in dogs and in humans. Anesth Analg 1985;64:964–70.

Johnson SM, Mauritson DR, Willerson JT, Hillis LD. Controlled trial of verapamil for Prinzmetal's variant angina. N Engl J Med 1981;304:862–6.

Jones RM, Cashman JN, Casson WR, Broadbent MP. Verapamil potentiation of neuromuscular blockade: Failure of reversal with neostigmine but prompt reversal with edrophonium. Anesth Analg 1985;64:1021–5.

Kaplan NM. Calcium entry blockers in the treatment of hypertension: Current status and future prospects. N Engl J Med 1989;262:817–23.

Kapur PA, Bloor BC, Flacke WE, Olewine SK. Comparison of cardiovascular response to verapamil during enflurane, isoflurane, or halothane anesthesia in the dog. Anesthesiology 1984a;61:156–60.

Kapur PA, Campos JH, Buchea OC. Plasma diltiazem levels, cardiovascular function, and coronary hemodynamics during enflurane anesthesia in the dog. Anesth Analg 1986a;65:918–24.

Kapur PA, Norel E, Dajee H, Cimochowski G. Verapamil treatment of intractable ventricular arrhythmias after cardiopulmonary bypass. Anesthesiology 1984b;63:460–3.

Kapur PA, Norel EJ, Dajee H, Cohen G, Flacke W. Hemodynamic effects of verapamil administration after large doses of fentanyl in man. Can Anaesth Soc J 1986b;33:138–44.

Kraynack BJ, Lawson NW, Gintautas J. Local anesthetic effect of verapamil *in vitro*. Reg Anesth 1982;7:114–7.

Lawson NW, Kraynack BJ, Gintautas J. Neuromuscular and electrocardiographic responses to verapamil in dogs. Anesth Analg 1983;62:50–4.

Maze M, Mason DM. Verpamil decreases the MAC for halothane in dogs. Anesth Analg 1983;62:274.

Merin RG. Calcium channel blocking drugs and anesthetics: Is the drug interaction beneficial or detrimental? Anesthesiology 1987;66:111–3.

Murad SHN, Tabsh KMA, Conklin KA, et al. Verapamil: Placental transfer and effects on maternal and fetal hemodynamics and atrioventricular conduction in the pregnant ewe. Anesthesiology 1985a;62:49–53.

Murad SHN, Tabsh KMA, Shilyanski G, et al. Effects of verapamil on uterine blood flow and maternal cardiovascular function in the awake pregnant ewe. Anesth Analg 1985b;64:7–10.

Nugent M, Tinker JH, Moyer TP. Verapamil worsens rate of development and hemodynamic effects of acute hyperkalemia in halothane-anesthetized dogs: Effects of calcium therapy. Anesthesiology 1984;60:435–9.

Packer M. Combined beta-adrenergic and calcium-entry blockade in angina pectoris. N Engl J Med 1989;320:709–17.

Reves JG. The relative hemodynamic effects of CA^{++} entry blockers. Anesthesiology 1984;61:3–5.

Reves JG, Kissin I, Lell WA, Tosone S. Calcium entry blockers: Uses and implications for anesthesiologists. Anesthesiology 1982;57:504–18.

Rinkenberger RL, Prystowsky EN, Heger JJ, Troup PJ, Jackman WM, Zipes DP. Effects of intravenous and chronic oral verapamil administration in patients with supraventricular tachyarrhythmias. Circulation 1980;62:996–1010.

Roine RO, Kaste M. Kinnunen A, Nikki P. Seppo S, Kajaste S. Nimodipine after resuscitation from out-of-hospital ventricular fibrillation. A placebo-controlled, double-blind, randomized trial. JAMA 1990;264:3171–77.

Rosenblatt RM, Weaver JM, Want Y, Tallman RD. Verapamil potentiates the toxicity of local anesthetics. Anesth Analg 1984;63:269.

Roth JL, Nugent M, Gronert GA. Verapamil does not alter succinylcholine-induced increases in serum potassium during halothane anesthesia in normal dogs. Anesth Analg 1985;64:1202–4.

Rubin AS, Zablocki AD. Hyperkalemia, verapamil, and dantrolene. Anesthesiology 1987;66:246–9.

Saltzman LS, Kates RA, Corke BC, Norfleet EA, Heath KR. Hyperkalemia and cardiovascular collapse after verapamil and dantrolene administration in swine. Anesth Analg 1984a;63:473–8.

Saltzman LS, Kates RA, Norfleet EA, Corke BC, Heath KS. Hemodynamic interactions of diltiazem-dantrolene and nifedipine-dantrolene. Anesthesiology 1984b;61:A11.

Schulte-Sasse U, Hess W, Markschies-Harnung A, Tarnow J. Combined effects of halothane anesthesia and verapamil on systemic hemodynamics and left ventricular myocardial contractility in patients with ischemic heart disease. Anesth Analg 1984;63:791–8.

Slogoff S, Keats AS. Does chronic treatment with calcium entry blocking drugs reduce perioperative myocardial ischemia? Anesthesiology 1988;68:676–80.

Steen PA, Gisvold SE, Milde JH, et al. Nimodipine improves outcome when given after complete cerebral ischemia in primates. Anesthesiology 1985;62:406–14.

van Poorten JF, Chasmana KM, Kuypers SM, Erdmann W. Verapamil and reversal of vecuronium neuromuscular blockade. Anesth Analg 1984;63:155–7.

Waxman HL, Myerberg RJ, Appel R, Sung RJ. Verapamil for control of ventricular rate in paroxysmal supraventricular tachycardia and atrial fibrillation of flutter. Ann Intern Med 1981;94:1–6.

White BC, Wiegenstein JG, Winegar CD. Brain ischemic anoxia: Mechanism of injury. JAMA 1984;251:1586–90.

Zalman F, Perloff JK, Durant NW, Campion DS. Acute respiratory failure following intravenous verapamil in Duchenne's muscular dystrophy. Am Heart J 1983;105:510–1.

19

Drugs Used in Treatment of Psychiatric Disease

INTRODUCTION

About 20% of prescriptions written in the United States are for drugs intended to alter mood or behavior. Classes of drugs effective in the symptomatic treatment of psychiatric disease include (1) phenothiazines and structurally similar thioxanthenes, (2) butyphenones, (3) lithium, (4) tricyclic antidepressants, (5) tetracyclic antidepressants, (6) serotonin uptake inhibitors, and (7) monoamine oxidase inhibitors (MAOI) (Table 19-1). Phenothiazines, thioxanthenes, and butyrophenones are most often administered for the treatment of schizophrenia, which accounts for their frequent designation as antipsychotics. Treatment of mania is with antipsychotics or lithium. Tricyclic antidepressants, tetracyclic antidepressants, and MAOI are most often used in the treatment of depression.

PHENOTHIAZINES AND THIOXANTHENES

Phenothiazines and thioxanthenes have a high therapeutic index and a relatively flat dose-response curve, accounting for the remarkable safety of these drugs over a wide dose range. Even large overdoses are unlikely to cause life-threatening depression of ventilation. These

drugs do not produce physical dependence, although abrupt discontinuation may be accompanied by skeletal muscle discomfort. In addition to their use in the treatment of psychiatric disease, phenothiazines and thioxanthenes possess other clinically useful properties, including antiemetic and antihistaminic effects and potentiation of analgesics.

Structure Activity Relationships

Phenothiazines have a three-ring structure in which two benzene rings are linked by a sulfur and a nitrogen atom (Fig. 19-1). If the nitrogen atom at position 10 is replaced by a carbon atom with a double bond to the side chain, the compound becomes a thioxanthene (Fig. 19-1). Phenothiazines and thioxanthenes used to treat psychiatric disease have three carbon atoms interposed between position 10 of the central ring and the first amino nitrogen atom of the side chain at this position. In addition, the amine is always tertiary. This structure contrasts with that of phenothiazines with significant antihistamine activity (promethazine) or phenothiazines with significant anticholinergic activity (ethopropazine, diethazine), which have only two carbon atoms separating the amino

Table 19–1
Classification of Drugs Useful in the Treatment of Psychiatric Disease

Phenothiazines
Chlorpromazine
Thioridazine
Fluphenazine
Perphenazine
Trifluoperazine

Thioxanthenes
Chlorprothixene
Thiothixene

Butyrophenones
Droperidol
Haloperidol

Lithium

Tricyclic Antidepressants
Imipramine
Desipramine
Amitriptyline
Nortriptyline
Doxepin
Protriptyline
Trimipramine
Amoxamine

Tetracyclic Antidepressants
Malprotiline

Serotonin Uptake Inhibitors
Fluoxetine
Trazodone

Monoamine Oxidase Inhibitors
Phenelzine
Isocarboxazid
Tranylcypromine
Selegiline

group from position 10 of the central ring. Loss of a methyl group or other substituents on the tertiary amino group, as can occur during metabolism, results in a loss of pharmacologic activity.

Mechanism of Action

Phenothiazines and thioxanthenes most likely produce their antipsychotic actions by antagonism of dopamine as a neurotransmitter in the basal ganglia and limbic portions of the fore-brain. Indeed, most phenothiazines and thioxanthenes are potentially associated with extrapyramidal side effects, indicating interference with the normal actions of dopamine. Antiemetic effects of these drugs likely reflect interference with the action of dopamine at the chemoreceptor trigger zone in the medulla.

Pharmacokinetics

Phenothiazines and thioxanthenes often display erratic and unpredictable patterns of absorption following oral administration. These drugs are highly lipid soluble and accumulate in well-perfused tissues such as the brain. Passage across the placenta and accumulation of drug in the fetus are possible. Avid binding to protein in plasma and tissues limits effectiveness of hemodialysis in removing these drugs.

Metabolism

Metabolism of phenothiazines and thioxanthenes is principally by oxidation in the liver followed by conjugation. Most oxidative metabolites are pharmacologically inactive, with a notable exception being 7-hydroxychlorpromazine. Metabolites appear primarily in the urine and to a lesser extent in the bile. Typical elimination half-times of these drugs are 10 to 20 hours, permitting once-daily dosing intervals. The elimination half-time may be prolonged in the fetus and in the elderly, who have decreased capacity to metabolize these drugs.

Side Effects

Side effects produced by treatment with phenothiazine or thioxanthenes are common and include (1) cardiovascular effects, (2) extrapyramidal symptoms, (3) endocrine changes, (4) neuroleptic malignant syndrome, (5) obstructive jaundice, (6) antiemetic effects, (7) anticholinergic effects, (8) sedation, (9) hypothermia, (10) altered seizure threshold, (11) skeletal muscle relaxation, (12) cutaneous reactions, and (13) drug interactions. Many of these side effects also accompany administration of butyrophenones. Despite the common occurrence of side effects, these drugs have a large margin of safety and overdoses are seldom fatal.

Cardiovascular Effects

Intravenous administration of chlorpromazine causes a decrease in blood pressure resulting from (1) depression of vasomotor reflexes mediated by the hypothalamus or brain stem, (2) peripheral alpha-adrenergic blockade, (3) direct relaxant effects on vascular smooth muscle, and (4) direct cardiac depression. Alpha-adrenergic blockade produced by chlorpromazine is sufficient to blunt or prevent the pressor effects of epinephrine. Miosis that occurs predictably may also be due to alpha-adrenergic blockade. A cardiac antidysrhythmic effect of chlorpromazine may reflect the potent local anesthetic activity of this drug. Changes in the electrocardiogram (ECG) include prolongation of the P-R and Q-T intervals and depression of the S-T segment.

Oral administration of these drugs is associated with less pronounced blood pressure–lowering effects. Indeed, tolerance to the hypotensive effect develops so that after several weeks of therapy, the blood pressure returns toward normal. Nevertheless, some element of orthostatic hypotension may persist for the duration of therapy.

Extrapyramidal Effects

Acute dystonic reactions characterized as facial grimacing and torticollis may be seen with the initiation of phenothiazine or thioxanthene therapy. Tardive dyskinesia, characterized by involuntary skeletal muscle movements, develops in 5% to 10% of patients treated with antipsychotics longer than 1 year. Compensatory increases in the function of dopamine activity in the basal ganglia may be responsible for the development of tardive dyskinesia.

Endocrine Changes

Prolactin secretion is stimulated by phenothiazines, presumably reflecting inhibition of the action of dopamine at the hypothalamus and pituitary. Galactorrhea and gynecomastia may accompany excess prolactin secretion. Amenorrhea is a possible but rare complication of therapy. Decreased secretion of corticosteroids may be due to diminished corticotropin release from the anterior pituitary. Chlorpromazine may impair glucose tolerance and the release of insulin in some patients.

Neuroleptic Malignant Syndrome

Neuroleptic malignant syndrome occurs in 0.5% to 1% of all patients treated with antipsychotic drugs. Abrupt withdrawal of levodopa therapy in patients with Parkinson's disease has also been associated with this syndrome. The syndrome typically develops over 24 to 72 hours in young males and is characterized by (1) hyperthermia; (2) generalized hypertonicity of skeletal muscles; (3) instability of the autonomic nervous system manifesting as alterations in blood pressure, tachycardia, and cardiac dysrhythmias; and (4) fluctuating levels of consciousness (Guze and Baxter, 1985). Autonomic nervous system dysfunction may precede the onset of other symptoms. Increased skeletal muscle tone may so reduce chest-wall compliance that it becomes necessary to provide mechanical support of ventilation. Creatine phosphokinase is often elevated, and liver transaminase enzymes are increased. Mortality is 20% to 30%, with common causes of death being ventilatory failure, cardiac failure and/or dysrhythmias, renal failure, and thromboembolism.

Malignant hyperthermia associated with anesthesia and the central anticholinergic syndrome may mimic the neuroleptic malignant syndrome (Guze and Baxter, 1985). A distinguishing feature is the ability of nondepolarizing neuromuscular blocking drugs, such as pancuronium, to produce flaccid paralysis in patients with neuroleptic malignant syndrome but not in

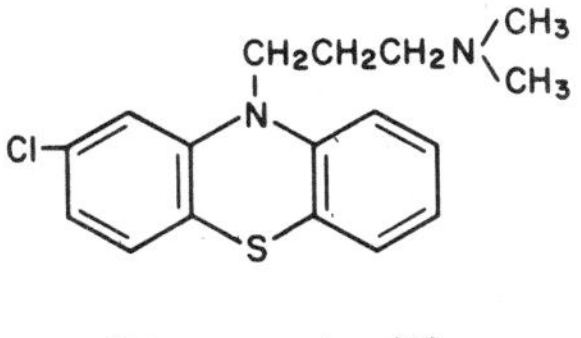

FIGURE 19–1. Phenothiazines (A) and thioxanthenes (B).

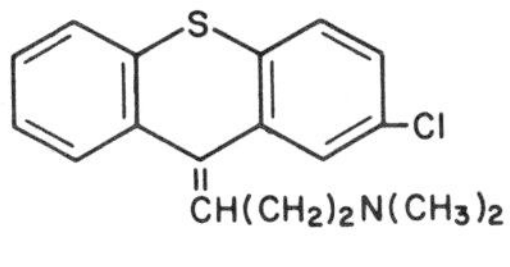

Chlorpromazine (A)

Chlorprothixene (B)

those persons experiencing malignant hyperthermia (Sangal and Dimitrijevic, 1985). The cause of neuroleptic malignant syndrome is not known and, as a result, its treatment is empirical and includes symptomatic measures and the administration of dantrolene. The reported efficacy of dopamine agonists, such as bromocriptine and amantadine, in treatment of the associated skeletal muscle rigidity as well as the prevention of the onset of the syndrome with abrupt withdrawal of levodopa therapy suggests a role of dopamine receptor blockade in the development of this syndrome (Granato et al, 1983).

Obstructive Jaundice

Obstructive jaundice that is considered to be an allergic reaction occurs rarely 2 to 4 weeks after the administration of phenothiazines or thioxanthenes. Indeed, there is prompt recurrence of jaundice if the offending drug, usually chlorpromazine, is again administered. If jaundice is not observed in the first month of therapy, it is unlikely to occur at a later date.

Antiemetic Effects

Antiemetic effects of antipsychotic drugs reflect their interaction with dopaminergic receptors in the chemoreceptor trigger zone of the medulla. Motion sickness is not controlled. A high incidence of extrapyramidal side effects limits the usefulness of these drugs as antiemetics.

Anticholinergic Effects

Chlorpromazine has moderate anticholinergic effects manifesting as blurring of vision, decreased gastric hydrogen ion secretion, and reduced gastrointestinal motility. Decreased sweating and salivation are additional manifestations of anticholinergic effects.

Sedation

Phenothiazines and thioxanthenes, particularly chlorpromazine, produce sedative effects that are often most intense early in the treatment phase. With chronic therapy, tolerance develops to the sedative effects produced by these drugs.

Hypothermia

An effect of chlorpromazine on the hypothalamus is most likely responsible for the poikilothermic effect of this drug. In the past, this effect was used to facilitate the production of surgical hypothermia.

Seizure Threshold

Many antipsychotic drugs lower the seizure threshold and produce a pattern on the electroencephalogram (EEG) similar to that associated with seizure disorders. Chlorpromazine causes a slowing of the EEG pattern, with some increase in burst activity and spiking. Sensory evoked potentials are often decreased in amplitude, and there is an increase in latency.

Skeletal Muscle Relaxation

Chlorpromazine causes skeletal muscle relaxation in some types of spastic conditions, presumably by actions on the central nervous system, as the drug is devoid of actions at the neuromuscular junction.

Cutaneous Reactions

Cutaneous reactions manifesting as urticaria or photosensitivity occur in about 5% of patients treated with chlorpromazine. Contact dermatitis may occur in personnel who handle chlorpromazine.

Drug Interactions

Ventilatory depressant effects of opioids are likely to be exaggerated by antipsychotic drugs. Likewise, the miotic and sedative effects of opioids are increased, and the analgesic actions are likely to be potentiated. These drugs may interfere with the actions of exogenously administered dopamine, and the effects of alcohol are enhanced.

BUTYROPHENONES

Butyrophenones, such as droperidol and haloperidol, structurally resemble and evoke pharmacologic effects similar to phenothiazines and thioxanthenes (Fig. 19-2). Like these drugs, butyrophenones can reduce the anxiety accompanying psychoses. Conversely, butyrophenones are less effective against acute situational anxiety such as that present in the preoperative period.

Droperidol is the butyrophenone most often administered in the perioperative period. Haloperidol has a longer duration of action than droperidol and lacks significant alpha-adrenergic antagonist effects such that reductions in blood pressure are unlikely. The principal use of haloperidol is as a long-acting antipsychotic drug.

Mechanism of Action

Butyrophenones act at postsynaptic receptor sites to decrease the neurotransmitter function of dopamine. Conceptually, there are two distinct binding sites on a single postsynaptic receptor (Richter, 1981). Dopamine binds to one site, and dopamine antagonists, such as droperidol, bind to the other site. Presumably, antipsychotic effects of butyrophenones reflect antagonism of dopaminergic receptors in various areas of the central nervous system. Droperidol is metabolized in the liver, with maximal excretion of metabolites occurring during the first 24 hours.

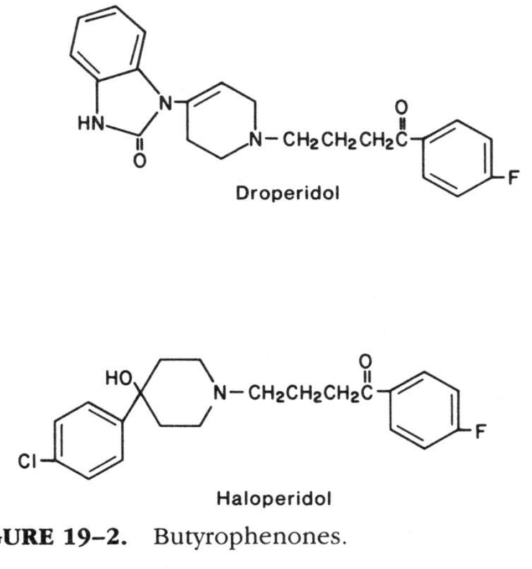

Droperidol

Haloperidol

FIGURE 19-2. Butyrophenones.

Pharmacokinetics

In patients anesthetized with nitrous oxide–fentanyl, the elimination half-time of droperidol is 104 minutes, clearance 14.1 ml·kg^{-1}·min^{-1}, and the volume of distribution 2.04 L·kg^{-1} (Fischler et al, 1986). The total body clearance of droperidol is similar to hepatic blood flow, emphasizing the importance of hepatic metabolism. In this regard, potential accumulation of droperidol is more likely to occur when the hepatic blood flow is decreased rather than with an alteration in hepatic enzyme activity. The short elimination half-time is not consistent with the prolonged central nervous system effects of droperidol, which may reflect slow dissociation of the drug from receptors or retention of droperidol in the brain.

Clinical Uses

Clinical uses of droperidol are principally limited to production of neuroleptanalgesia and use as an antiemetic.

Neuroleptanalgesia

Droperidol combined with fentanyl is administered for the production of neuroleptanalgesia. A commercially available 50:1 combination of droperidol with fentanyl is known as *Innovar.* This fixed combination of drugs is not associated with enhanced depression of ventilation as compared with either drug alone (Harper et al, 1976). Droperidol does not enhance analgesia produced by fentanyl but rather prolongs its duration of action. Orthostatic hypotension and dysphoria are more likely to occur following the administration of Innovar compared with fentanyl alone.

Neuroleptanalgesia is characterized by trance-like (cataleptic) immobility in an outwardly tranquil patient who is dissociated and indifferent to the surroundings. Analgesia is intense, allowing performance of a variety of diagnostic and minor surgical procedures such as bronchoscopy and cystoscopy. Disadvantages of neuroleptanalgesia are prolonged central nervous system depression and failure to depress sympathetic nervous system responses predictably to painful stimulation.

Antiemetic

Droperidol is a powerful antiemetic as a result of inhibition of dopaminergic receptors in the chemoreceptor trigger zone of the medulla. For example, droperidol, 1.2 to 2.5 mg, administered intravenously before the conclusion of elective cesarean section surgery, decreases the incidence of postoperative nausea and vomiting (Fig. 19-3) (Santos and Datta, 1984). Droperidol, 20 $\mu g \cdot kg^{-1}$ IV, administered 2 minutes before the induction of general anesthesia, is an effective antiemetic for female outpatients undergoing laparoscopy (Pandit et al, 1989). In unpremedicated children undergoing elective strabismus surgery, the administration of droperidol, 7.5 $\mu g \cdot kg^{-1}$ IV, at the induction of anesthesia greatly reduces the incidence of postoperative nausea and vomiting and does not delay awakening from anesthesia (Christensen et al, 1989). Sedation and delayed discharge time are likely only after the use of doses of droperidol greater than 2.5 mg (Cohen

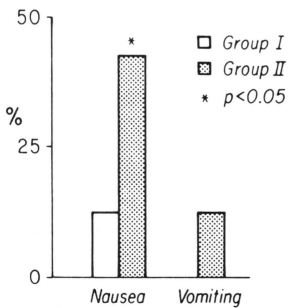

FIGURE 19–3. Droperidol, 1.2 to 2.5 mg IV, administered to group I patients before the conclusion of surgery, decreases the incidence of nausea and vomiting. Group II patients did not receive droperidol but underwent similar surgery. (From Santos A, Datta S. Prophylactic use of droperidol for control of nausea and vomiting during spinal anesthesia for cesarean section. Anesth Analg 1984; 63: 85–7; with permission.)

et al, 1984). Labyrinthine-induced vomiting (motion sickness) is not influenced by droperidol.

Side Effects

(See also the section entitled "Phenothiazines and Thioxanthenes.") As a dopamine antagonist, droperidol evokes extrapyramidal reactions in about 1% of patients (Rivera et al, 1975; Wiklund and Ngai, 1971). For this reason, droperidol should not be administered to patients being treated for Parkinson's disease. Diphenhydramine administered intravenously is an effective treatment for droperidol-induced extrapyramidal reactions.

The outwardly calming effect of droperidol may mask an overwhelming fear of surgery. This possible dysphoric reaction detracts from the use of droperidol in preoperative medication (Lee and Yeakel, 1975). Akathisia (most often a feeling of restlessness in the legs) may accompany administration of droperidol as preoperative medication (Ward, 1989). Droperidol may be of value in reducing shivering associated with deliberate hypothermia.

Central Nervous System Effects

Droperidol is a cerebral vasoconstrictor leading to a reduction in cerebral blood flow, whereas cerebral metabolic rate for oxygen is not greatly altered. Failure to lower metabolic rate despite reduced cerebral blood flow could be undesirable in patients with cerebral vascular disease. The reticular activating system is not depressed, and alpha rhythm persists on the EEG. Droperidol does not produce amnesia, nor does it have an anticonvulsant action.

Cardiovascular Effects

Droperidol can decrease blood pressure as a result of actions in the central nervous system and by peripheral alpha-adrenergic blockade (Whitwam and Russell, 1971). The decrease in blood pressure is usually minimal, although occasionally a patient may experience marked hypotension. Systemic and pulmonary vascular resistances are only modestly and transiently reduced. Myocardial contractility is not altered by droperidol.

Hypertension has been reported following administration of droperidol to patients with pheochromocytoma (Bittar, 1979; Sumikawa and Amakata, 1977). This blood pressure response reflects droperidol-induced release of catecholamines from the adrenal medulla as well as inhibition of catecholamine uptake into chromaffin granules (Fig. 19-4) (Sumikawa et al, 1985).

Droperidol is a cardiac antidysrhythmic and protects against epinephrine-induced dysrhythmias (Bertolo et al, 1972). The mechanism for this cardiac antidysrhythmic effect has not been established but may reflect blockade of alpha-adrenergic receptors in the myocardium, stabilization of excitable membranes of myocardial cells by local anesthetic effects, and decreases in blood pressure that reduce the likelihood of pressure-dependent cardiac dysrhythmias. Large doses of droperidol, 0.2 to 0.6 mg·kg^{-1} IV, depress conduction of the cardiac impulse along ac-

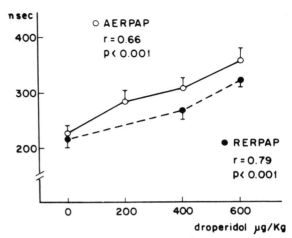

FIGURE 19–5. Droperidol produces dose-dependent prolongation of the antegrade and retrograde effective refractory period of accessory pathways. (From Gomez-Arnau J, Marquez-Montes J, Avello F. Fentanyl and droperidol effects on the refractoriness of the accessory pathway in the Wolff-Parkinson-White syndrome. Anesthesiology 1983; 58: 307–13; with permission.)

cessory pathways responsible for tachydysrhythmias that occur in patients with Wolff-Parkinson-White syndrome (Fig. 19-5) (Gomez-Arnau et al, 1983).

Ventilation

Resting ventilation and the ventilatory response to carbon dioxide are not altered by droperidol (Soroker et al, 1978). Furthermore, droperidol administered intravenously augments the ventilatory response evoked by arterial hypoxemia, presumably by blocking the action of the inhibitory neurotransmitter, dopamine, at the carotid body (Fig. 19-6) (Ward, 1984). For this reason droperidol may be an acceptable preoperative medication in patients with chronic obstructive airway disease who are dependent on carotid body drive to prevent hypoventilation.

LITHIUM

Lithium is used for the treatment of mania and for the prevention of recurrent attacks of manic-depressive illness (Havdala et al, 1979). When given to manic patients who characteristically

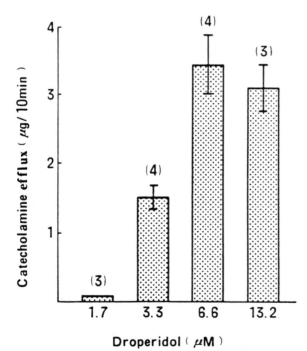

FIGURE 19–4. Catecholamine efflux (mean ± SE) from the perfused dog adrenal medulla is increased by droperidol. The number of experiments is indicated by the figure in parentheses. (From Sumikawa K, Hirano H, Amakata Y, Kashimoto T, Wada A, Isumi F. Mechanism of the effect of droperidol to induce catecholamine efflux from the adrenal medulla. Anesthesiology 1985; 62: 17–22; with permission.)

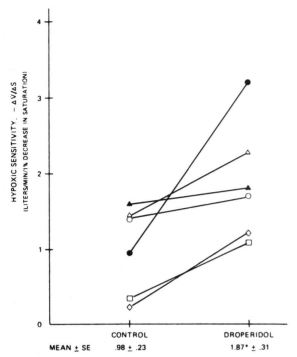

FIGURE 19-6. The ventilatory response to arterial hypoxemia (hypoxic sensitivity) is enhanced by droperidol. Solid symbols represent repeated experiments on the same subjects as those represented by the open symbols. (From Ward DS. Stimulation of hypoxic ventilatory drive by droperidol. Anesth Analg 1984; 63: 106-10; with permission.)

sleep very little, lithium corrects the sleep disorder as the mania abates. These changes are associated with diffuse slowing on the EEG. Plasma lithium concentrations should not exceed 2 $mEq \cdot L^{-1}$ (ideally 0.75 to 1.5 $mEq \cdot L^{-1}$) during initial treatment and should be maintained within a range of 0.4 to 1 $mEq \cdot L^{-1}$ during chronic therapy. Monitoring of plasma concentrations of lithium is indicated, as the therapeutic and toxic concentrations do not differ greatly.

Mechanism of Action

At the cellular level, lithium ions act as imperfect substitutes for sodium ions (Na^+). For example, lithium ions can replace Na^+ in supporting a single action potential, but they are not an adequate substrate for the Na^+–K^+ pump and cannot, therefore, maintain transmembrane potentials. Furthermore, once in the cell, lithium ions can be extruded at a rate only 10% that of Na^+. The resulting intracellular accumulation of lithium ions appears to interfere with the ability of several hormones to activate adenylate cyclase and produce cyclic adenosine monophosphate. Reduced availability of cyclic adenosine monophosphate would be associated with decreased responses of receptors to neurotransmitters and reduced cellular activity.

Pharmacokinetics

Lithium is almost completely absorbed from the gastrointestinal tract, with peak concentrations in plasma occurring 2 to 4 hours after an oral dose. Initial distribution is in the extracellular fluid, with subsequent accumulation in various tissues. Passage across the blood-brain barrier is slow, but ultimately the concentration of lithium in the cerebrospinal fluid is about 40% of the concentration in plasma. There is no evidence of lithium binding to plasma proteins.

Approximately 95% of a single dose of lithium is eliminated in the urine. About one third to two thirds of an acute dose is excreted during a 6- to 12-hour initial phase of excretion followed by a slow excretion over the next 10 to 14 days. Because 80% of the filtered lithium is reabsorbed by renal tubules, lithium clearance by the kidney is about 20% of that for creatinine. Most of the renal tubular reabsorption of lithium seems to occur in proximal convoluted tubules. Na^+ loading produces a small enhancement of lithium excretion, but Na^+ depletion promotes a clinically important degree of retention of the ion. Indeed, reabsorption of lithium back into the circulation can be produced by any diuretic (thiazides, furosemide) that causes increased renal elimination of Na^+. Triamterene may increase excretion of lithium, suggesting that some reabsorption of the ion may occur in distal renal tubules. Conversely, spironolactone does not increase the excretion of lithium.

Side Effects

Na^+ is retained, and, in some cases, peripheral edema manifests in the initial phases of lithium therapy. An occasional lithium-treated patient develops benign diffuse thyroid enlargement. Rarely, lithium inhibits the release of thyroid hormones to the extent that hypothyroidism develops.

Polydipsia and polyuria may occur in patients treated with lithium. Indeed, nephrogenic diabetes insipidus has occurred in patients maintained chronically with therapeutic plasma concentrations of lithium (Burroughs et al, 1978). The mechanism of polyuria may involve inhibition of the action of antidiuretic hormone on renal adenylate cyclase, resulting in reduced stimulation for reabsorption of water across the renal tubules.

Prolonged use of lithium causes a benign and reversible depression of T waves on the ECG. This effect is not related to depletion of Na^+ or potassium ions. An increase in the circulating concentration of leukocytes occurs during chronic treatment with lithium.

The association of sedation with lithium therapy suggests that anesthetic requirements for injected and inhaled drugs could be reduced. High plasma concentrations of lithium may delay recovery from central nervous system depressant effects of barbiturates (Mannisto and Saarnivaara, 1976). Responses to depolarizing and nondepolarizing neuromuscular blocking drugs may be prolonged in the presence of lithium (Hill et al, 1977).

Toxicity

The therapeutic range for lithium is narrow, with plasma concentrations less than 0.8 mEq·L^{-1} often being ineffective, whereas levels greater than 1.5 mEq·L^{-1} may produce toxicity. Mild lithium toxicity is reflected by sedation, nausea, skeletal muscle weakness, and changes on the ECG characterized by widening of the QRS complex. Atrioventricular heart block, hypotension, cardiac dysrhythmias, and seizures may occur when plasma concentrations of lithium are greater than 2 mEq·L^{-1}. It is not uncommon for elderly patients who excrete lithium slowly to become confused even in the presence of therapeutic plasma concentrations of this ion.

Diuretics that stimulate renal loss of Na^+ cause retention of lithium ions. Indeed, even short-term administration of thiazide diuretics or furosemide can quickly cause lithium toxicity. In parturients, concomitant use of diuretics and low Na^+ diets contribute to maternal and neonatal lithium intoxication.

Treatment of lithium intoxication is supportive. If renal function is adequate, excretion of lithium ions can be modestly accelerated by osmotic diuresis and intravenous administration of sodium bicarbonate. Hemodialysis is also effective in removing excess lithium ions from the body.

TRICYCLIC ANTIDEPRESSANTS AND RELATED DRUGS

The efficacy of tricyclic antidepressants in alleviating mental depression is well established. These drugs may also be used in the treatment of chronic pain, presumably reflecting a link between serotonin and nociception and the ability of tricyclic antidepressants to block the uptake of this neurotransmitter (Rosenblatt et al, 1984).

Structure Activity Relationships

The structure of tricyclic antidepressants resembles that of phenothiazines (Fig. 19-7). *Tricyclic* denotes the three-ring chemical structure of the central portion of the molecule (Fig. 19-7). Imipramine, which is the prototype of the tricyclic antidepressants, differs from the phenothiazines only in the replacement of the sulfur atom with an ethylene linkage to produce a seven-membered central ring. Desipramine is the principal metabolite of imipramine, and nortriptyline is the demethylated metabolite of amitriptyline. Malprotiline is a tetracyclic antidepressant with a clinical profile that resembles imipramine.

Fluoxetine and trazodone are effective antidepressants that inhibit central nervous system neuronal uptake of serotonin. Structurally, they are unrelated to tricyclic or tetracyclic antidepressants. Depressant effects of these drugs on conduction of cardiac impulses are weak, and anticholinergic responses are slight.

Mechanism of Action

Tricyclic antidepressants potentiate the actions of biogenic amines (especially norepinephrine and/or serotonin) in the central nervous system

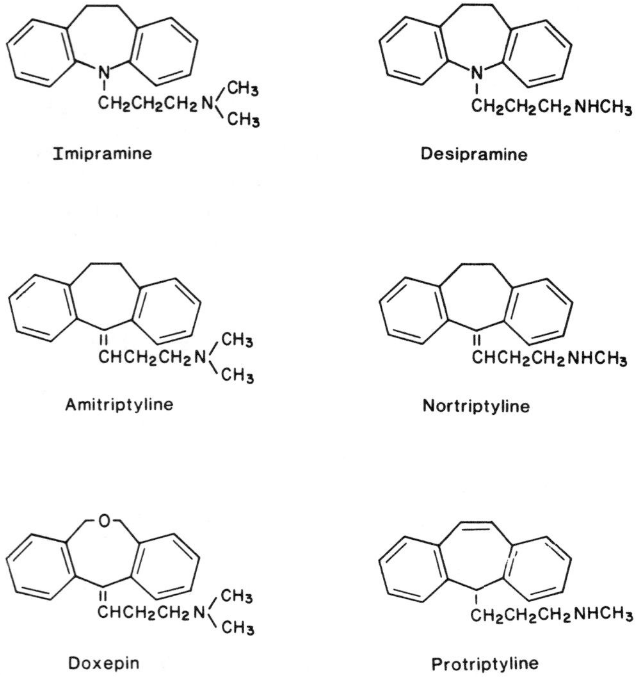

Imipramine

Desipramine

Amitriptyline

Nortriptyline

Doxepin

Protriptyline

FIGURE 19-7.   Tricyclic antidepressants.

by interfering with the uptake (reuptake) of these amines into postganglionic sympathetic nerve endings. Despite the prompt onset of this effect, the development of a therapeutic antidepressant effect is inexplicably delayed for 2 to 3 weeks. For this reason, there is doubt that antidepressant effects are totally due to an accumulation of biogenic amines in the brain. Furthermore, some drugs without effects on uptake of biogenic amines are effective antidepressants. It seems likely that potentiation of monoaminergic neurotransmission in the brain is only an early event in a complex cascade of events that eventually results in an antidepressant effect. Indeed, chronic administration of these drugs is associated with (1) decreased sensitivity of postsynaptic beta-1 and serotonin-2 receptors and of presynaptic alpha-2 receptors; and (2) increased sensitivity of postsynaptic alpha-1 receptors.

Pharmacokinetics

Tricyclic antidepressants are efficiently absorbed from the gastrointestinal tract after oral administration, reflecting their high lipid solubility. Peak plasma concentrations occur within 2 to 8 hours after oral administration. Therapeutic plasma concentrations (parent compound plus the pharmacologically active demethylated metabolites) are 100 to 300 ng·ml^{-1}, whereas toxicity is likely at levels higher than 500 ng·ml^{-1}. Tricyclic antidepressants are strongly bound to plasma and tissue proteins, which, in combination with high lipid solubility, results in a large volume of distribution (up to 50 L·kg^{-1}) for these drugs. The long elimination half-time (17 to 30 hours) and wide range of therapeutic plasma concentrations make once-daily dosing intervals effective.

Metabolism

Tricyclic antidepressants are oxidized by microsomal enzymes in the liver with subsequent conjugation with glucuronic acid. The individual variation in rate of metabolism between patients is 10- to 30-fold. This inactivation and elimination of tricyclic antidepressants occurs over several days, with 1 week or longer required for excretion.

Imipramine is metabolized to the active compound, desipramine. Both these active compounds are inactivated by oxidation of hydroxy metabolites and by conjugation with glucuronic acid. Nortriptyline, which is the pharmacologically active demethylated metabolite of imipramine and amitriptyline, can accumulate to levels that exceed the precursors. Doxepin also appears to be converted to an active metabolite, nordoxepin, by demethylation.

Side Effects

Side effects of tricyclic antidepressants are frequent, most commonly manifesting as (1) anticholinergic effects, (2) cardiovascular effects, (3) central nervous system effects, and (4) drug interactions (Table 19-2). Marked individual variation in the incidence and type of side effects may be related to the plasma concentrations of tricyclic antidepressant and its active metabolites. Weakness and fatigue are attributable to central nervous system effects and may resemble those seen with phenothiazines. Extrapyramidal reactions are rare, although a fine tremor develops in about 10% of patients, especially the elderly. These drugs produce insignificant effects on ventilation. Side effects are less with fluoxetine and trazodone, accounting for the increasing popularity of these drugs as antidepressants.

Anticholinergic Effects

Anticholinergic effects of tricyclic antidepressants, in contrast to the antipsychotic drugs, are prominent, especially at high doses. Amitriptyline causes the highest incidence of anticholinergic effects (dry mouth, blurred vision, tachycardia, urinary retention, slowed gastric

Table 19-2
Comparative Pharmacology of Tricyclic Antidepressants

	Anticholinergic Effect	Sedative Effect
Imipramine	Moderate	Minimal
Desipramine	Minimal	Minimal
Amitriptyline	Marked	Marked
Nortriptyline	Moderate	Moderate
Doxepin	Moderate	Marked

emptying), whereas desipramine produces the fewest such effects (Table 19-2). For this reason, desipramine is often selected when tachycardia would be undesirable.

Cardiovascular Effects

Orthostatic hypotension and modest increases in heart rate are the most common side effects of treatment with tricyclic antidepressants. Previous suggestions that tricyclic antidepressants increase the risks of cardiac dysrhythmias and sudden death have not been substantiated in the absence of drug overdose (Thompson et al, 1983). Furthermore, in the absence of severe preexisting cardiac dysfunction, tricyclic antidepressants lack adverse effects on left ventricular function and may even possess cardiac antidysrhythmic properties (Veith et al, 1982). In particular, nortriptyline has minimal effects on myocardial contractility and may be a useful drug to select when left ventricular dysfunction accompanies mental depression (Roose et al, 1986). Previous reports that doxepin is less cardiotoxic than other tricyclic antidressants have not been confirmed. Tricyclic antidepressants produce depression of conduction of cardiac impulses through the atria and ventricles, manifesting on the ECG as prolongation of the P-R interval, widening of the QRS complex, and flattening or inversion of the T wave. Nevertheless, these electrocardiographic changes are probably benign and may gradually disappear with continued therapy (Thompson et al, 1983). Atropine is useful when tricyclic antidepressants dangerously slow atrioventricular or interventricular conduction of cardiac impulses.

Direct cardiac depressant effects may reflect quinidine-like actions on the heart. Conceivably, there could also be enhancement of depressant cardiac effects of anesthetics by tricyclic antidepressants. Quinidine-like properties of tricyclic antidepressants are thought to reflect slowing of Na^+ flux into cells, resulting in altered repolarization and conduction of cardiac impulses.

Central Nervous System Effects

Sedation associated with tricyclic antidepressant therapy may be desirable for management of agitated patients. For this purpose, amitriptyline and doxepin produce the greatest degree of sedation (Table 19-2). Tricyclic antidepressants produce evidence of seizure activity on the EEG, introducing the question as to the safety of administering these drugs to patients with seizure disorders or to those receiving drugs that may produce seizures. Children seem to be especially vulnerable to the seizure-inducing effects of tricyclic antidepressants.

Drug Interactions

The anticholinergic and catecholamine uptake blocking properties of the tricyclic antidepressants are most likely to be responsible for drug interactions. Drug interactions may be prominent with (1) sympathomimetics, (2) inhaled anesthetics, (3) anticholinergics, (4) antihypertensives, and (5) opioids. Binding of tricyclic antidepressants to plasma albumin can be reduced by competition from other drugs, including phenytoin, aspirin, and scopolamine.

SYMPATHOMIMETICS. Tricyclic antidepressants, by inhibiting uptake of norepinephrine into postganglionic sympathetic nerve endings, make more neurotransmitter available to act at postsynaptic adrenergic receptors. As a result, the pressor response evoked by an indirect-acting sympathomimetic, such as ephedrine, is increased two- to tenfold in the presence of tricyclic antidepressants. Even epinephrine present in a local anesthetic solution could evoke hypertension if administered to a patient being treated with a tricyclic antidepressant (Boakes et al, 1973). If a sympathomimetic is required, a direct-acting drug, such as phenylephrine in a reduced dose, would be an acceptable choice.

INHALED ANESTHETICS. An increased incidence of cardiac dysrhythmias, including sinus tachycardia, ventricular tachycardia, and ventricular fibrillation, has been observed in halothane-anesthetized dogs pretreated with imipramine and receiving pancuronium (Fig. 19-8) (Edwards et al, 1979). Presumably, there is an interaction between the tricyclic antidepressant and the anticholinergic and/or sympathetic nervous system stimulating effect of pancuronium (Fig. 19-9) (Edwards et al, 1979). Theoretically, ketamine might produce a similar adverse response as pancuronium when administered in the presence of tricyclic antidepressants.

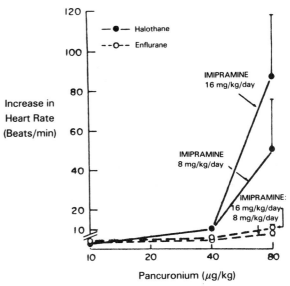

FIGURE 19–8. Correlation between dose of pancuronium and maximum increase in heart rate in dogs during halothane or enflurane anesthesia. Dogs were pretreated with 8 or 16 $mg \cdot kg^{-1} \cdot day^{-1}$ of imipramine for 15 days. (From Edwards RP, Miller RD, Roizen RF, et al. Cardiac responses to imipramine and pancuronium during anesthesia with halothane or enflurane. Anesthesiology 1979; 50:421–5; with permission.)

Induction of anesthesia may be associated with an increased incidence of cardiac dysrhythmias in patients being treated with tricyclic antidepressants. Likewise, the dose of exogenous epinephrine necessary to produce cardiac dysrhythmias during anesthesia with a volatile anesthetic, such as halothane, is reduced by tricyclic antidepressants (Wong et al, 1980). Theoretically, increased availability of norepinephrine in the central nervous system could result in increased anesthetic requirements for inhaled drugs. Treatment with tricyclic antidepressants may enhance the central nervous system stimulating effects of enflurane (Sprague and Wolf, 1982).

ANTICHOLINERGICS. Because anticholinergic side effects of drugs may be additive, the use of centrally active anticholinergic drugs for preoperative medication of patients being treated with tricyclic antidepressants could increase the likelihood of postoperative delirium and confu-

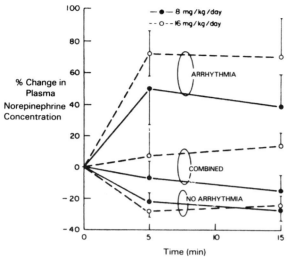

— ● — 8 mg/kg/day
-- O-- 16 mg/kg/day

100

80

60   ARRHYTHMIA

% Change in
Plasma
Norepinephrine 40
Concentration

20

0   COMBINED

-20   NO ARRHYTHMIA

-40

0   5   10   15

Time (min)

FIGURE 19–9.   Dogs pretreated with imipramine that developed cardiac dysrhythmias following administration of pancuronium during halothane anesthesia also manifested increased plasma concentrations of norepinephrine. (From Edwards RP, Miller RD, Roizen RF, et al. Cardiac responses to imipramine and pancuronium during anesthesia with halothane and enflurane. Anesthesiology 1979; 50: 421–5; with permission.)

sion (central anticholinergic syndrome) (see Chapter 10). Glycopyrrolate would be less likely to evoke this drug interaction in patients being treated with tricyclic antidepressants.

ANTIHYPERTENSIVES. Tricyclic antidepressants prevent the antihypertensive effect of guanethidine, presumably by interfering with uptake of guanethidine into postganglionic sympathetic nerve endings. These drugs can also block the centrally mediated antihypertensive action of alpha-methyldopa and clonidine. Rebound hypertension following abrupt discontinuation of clonidine may be accentuated and prolonged by concomitant tricyclic antidepressant therapy (Stiff and Harris, 1983). Conceivably, increased plasma concentrations of catecholamines can persist for longer periods in the presence of tricyclic antidepressants that prevent uptake of norepinephrine back into the postganglionic sympathetic nerve endings. The combination of a tricyclic antidepressant and an MAOI has been associated with central nervous system

toxicity manifesting as hyperthermia, seizures, and coma.

OPIOIDS. In animals, tricyclic antidepressants augment the analgesic and ventilatory depressant effects of opioids. Likewise, the sedative and depressant effects of barbiturates are increased in animals. If these responses also occur in patients, it is predictable that doses of these drugs should be reduced so as to avoid exaggerated and/or prolonged depressant effects.

Tolerance

Tolerance to anticholinergic effects (dry mouth, blurred vision, tachycardia) and orthostatic hypotension develops during chronic therapy with tricyclic antidepressants. Conversely, tolerance to desirable effects often fails to develop. Abrupt discontinuation of high doses of tricyclic antidepressants may be associated with a mild withdrawal syndrome characterized by malaise, chills, coryza, and skeletal muscle aching.

Overdose

Tricyclic antidepressant overdose probably represents the most common life-threatening form of drug ingestion (Frommer et al, 1987). Progression from alert to life-threatening symptoms may be rapid. Intractable myocardial depression or ventricular cardiac dysrhythmias are the most frequent terminal event.

Presenting features of a tricyclic antidepressant overdose include agitation and seizures followed by coma; depression of ventilation; hypotension; hypothermia; and striking signs of anticholinergic effects, including mydriasis, flushed dry skin, urinary retention, and tachycardia. The QRS complex on the ECG may be prolonged to more than 100 msec. Indeed, the likelihood of seizures and ventricular dysrhythmias is increased when the duration of the QRS complex is greater than 100 msec (Boehnert and Lovejoy, 1985). Conversely, plasma concentrations of tricyclic antidepressants do not allow prediction of the likely occurrence of seizures or cardiac dysrhythmias (Boehnert and Lovejoy, 1985).

The comatose phase of tricyclic antidepressant overdose lasts 24 to 72 hours. Even after this phase passes, the risk of life-threatening cardiac dysrhythmias persists for up to 10 days, necessitating continued monitoring of the ECG in these patients.

Treatment

Treatment of a life-threatening overdose of a tricyclic antidepressant is directed toward management of central nervous system and cardiac toxicity (Table 19-3) (Frommer et al, 1987). Coma usually resolves within 24 hours but is frequently severe enough to require active airway support. Extrapyramidal effects and organic brain syndrome usually require supportive care only, although judicious use of physostigmine, 0.5 to 2 mg IV, for obvious anticholinergic psychosis may be indicated.

Seizures may precede cardiac arrest and should be treated aggressively with diazepam. After initial suppression of seizure activity with diazepam, it may be necessary to provide sustained effects with a longer-acting drug, such as phenytoin. Acidosis associated with seizure activity may abruptly increase unbound tricyclic antidepressants in the circulation and predispose to cardiac dysrhythmias. In this regard, alkalinization of the plasma (pH greater than 7.45) either

Table 19-3
Pharmacologic Treatment of Tricyclic Antidepressant Overdose

Symptom	Treatment
Seizures	Diazepam
	Sodium bicarbonate
	Phenytoin
Ventricular cardiac dysrhythmias	Sodium bicarbonate
	Lidocaine
	Phenytoin
Heart block	Isoproterenol
Hypotension	Crystalloid or colloid solution
	Sodium bicarbonate
	Sympathomimetics
	Inotropes

(Data from Frommer DA, Kulig KW, Marx JA, Rumack B: Tricyclic antidepressant overdose. JAMA 1987; 257: 521–6; with permission.)

by intravenous administration of sodium bicarbonate or deliberate hyperventilation of the lungs can temporarily reverse drug-induced cardiotoxicity. Lidocaine and phenytoin may be used subsequently to provide sustained suppression of cardiac ventricular dysrhythmias.

Hypotension may be the result of direct tricyclic antidepressant–induced vasodilation, alpha-blockade, or myocardial depression. Patients remaining hypotensive despite intravascular fluid replacement and alkalinization of the plasma may require support with sympathomimetics, inotropes, or both.

Gastric lavage may be useful early in treatment, but this is most safely performed with a cuffed tracheal tube already in place. Activated charcoal significantly absorbs drug throughout the gastrointestinal tract ("intestinal dialysis"). Conversely, avid protein binding of tricyclic antidepressants negates any therapeutic value of hemodialysis or drug-induced diuresis.

MONOAMINE OXIDASE INHIBITORS

Monoamine oxidase inhibitors constitute a heterogenous group of drugs that have in common the ability to prevent oxidative deamination of naturally occurring monoamines in the central and peripheral autonomic nervous systems (Fig. 19-10). Clinically used MAOI are classified as hydrazine or nonhydrazine derivatives, with a further subdivision based on the presence or absence of selectivity for the A or B form of the enzyme (Table 19-3) (Michaels et al, 1984). These drugs are administered only by the oral route, being readily absorbed from the gastrointestinal tract.

Clinical Uses

The use of MAOI is limited by serious drug interactions and hepatotoxicity. The development of tricyclic antidepressants with few perceived side effects led to decreased clinical usage of MAOI. There now seems to be a resurgence of interest in the use of MAOI not only for treatment of mental depression but also obsessive-compulsive disorders, eating disorders, essential hypertension (pargyline), chronic pain syndromes, and migraine headache (Stack et al, 1988; Wells and Bjorksten, 1989). Tranylcypromine and phenal-

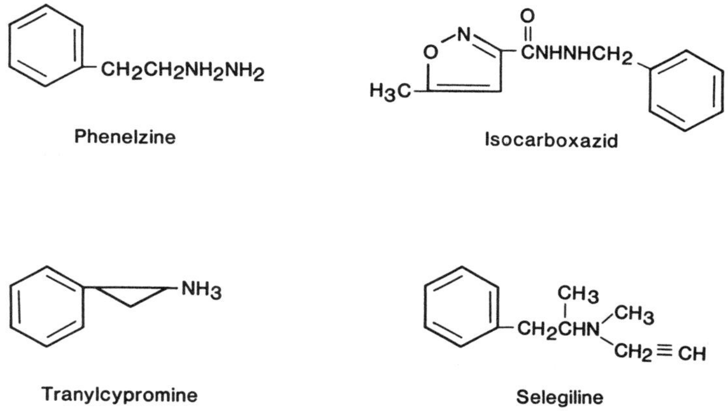

FIGURE 19-10. Monoamine oxidase inhibitors.

zine account for over 90% of all MAOI currently prescribed.

Mechanism of Action

Monoamine oxidase inhibitors form a stable and irreversible complex with monoamine oxidase enzyme. Monoamine oxidase is the principal intraneuronal enzyme responsible for the oxidative deamination of amine neurotransmitters, including dopamine, norepinephrine, epinephrine, and serotonin. Synthesis of new monoamine oxidase is a slow process, accounting for the prolonged effect of MAOI following their discontinuation.

Inhibition of monoamine oxidase by MAOI results in accumulation of amine neurotransmitters in the brain within a few hours. Although the therapeutic action was originally believed to reflect this amine accumulation, recent evidence has cast considerable doubt on this view (Wells and Bjorksten, 1989). Indeed, as with tricyclic antidepressants, the therapeutic effects of MAOI are delayed several days beyond the early increase in brain neurotransmitters. It seems likely that the initial increase in brain neurotransmitters produced by MAOI activates a feedback loop that leads to decreased synthesis of these amines and delayed antidepressant effects. With chronic MAOI therapy, there is a reduction in the responsiveness of alpha-, beta-, and serotonergic receptors manifesting as a general reduction in sympathetic nervous system activity.

Two forms of monoamine oxidase (MAO-A and MAO-B) have been defined on the basis of differences in substrate preferences (Table 19-4) (Michaels et al, 1984; Wells and Bjorksten, 1989). Type A enzyme preferentially deaminates serotonin, dopamine, and norepinephrine (Fig. 19-11) (Michaels et al, 1984). Inhibition of MAO-A is clinically relevant, because serotonin and norepinephrine are important neurotransmitters in psychiatric disorders. Type B enzyme preferentially deaminates phenethylamine and tyramine (Fig. 19-11) (Michaels et al, 1984). Human brain contains approximately 60% MAO-A. Theoretically, use of selective MAOI could reduce the incidence of side effects that accompany the administration of nonselective MAOI. It must be recognized, however, that substrate specificity is

Table 19-4
Drug Selectivity for Monoamine Oxidase (MAO) Enzymes

	MAO-A	MAO-B
Hydrazine Compound		
Phenelzine	+	+
Isocarboxazid	+	+
Iproniazid	+	+
Nonhydrazine Compound		
Tranylcypromine	+	+
Pargyline	?	+
Clorgyline	+	0
Selegiline	?	+

(Data from Michaels I, Sevrins M, Shier NQ, Barash PG. Anesthesia for cardiac surgery in patients receiving monoamine oxidase inhibitors. Anesth Analg 1984; 63: 1041–4; with permission.)

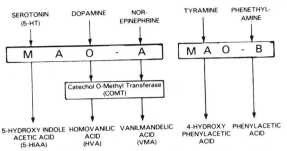

FIGURE 19–11 The two forms of monoamine oxidase enzyme (MAO-A and MAO-B) exhibit substrate selectivity. (From Michaels I, Serrins M, Shier NQ, Barash PG. Anesthesia for cardiac surgery in patients receiving monoamine oxidase inhibitors. Anesth Analg 1984; 63;1041–4; with permission.)

concentration dependent, and both subtypes of monoamine oxidase are capable of metabolizing all substrates if presented in appropriate concentrations.

Hypotensive effects of MAOI are attributed to accumulation of a false neurotransmitter, octopamine, in postganglionic sympathetic nerve endings. Release of this false neurotransmitter in response to a neural stimulus produces less vasoconstriction than does norepinephrine. As a result, blood pressure declines as a manifestation of a decrease in systemic vascular resistance. This is the presumed mechanism of action of pargyline in the treatment of essential hypertension.

Side Effects

The most common side effects produced by MAOI are sedation, blurred vision, dryness of the mouth, and orthostatic hypotension. Hepatotoxicity associated with hydrazine-containing compounds has led to discontinuation of the use of several MAOI. Peripheral neuropathy following the use of MAOI may be related to pyridoxine deficiency. Effects of MAOI on the EEG are slight and not seizure-like, which contrasts with tricyclic antidepressants. Also in contrast with tricyclic antidepressants is the failure of MAOI to produce cardiac dysrhythmias (Wong et al, 1980).

A common recommendation is to discontinue MAOI for a period of 14 to 21 days before elective surgery. This recommendation is based on isolated and anecdotal reports rather than controlled scientific studies. Adherence to this approach may place patients at risk for psychiatric complications, including suicide. There is now growing appreciation that anesthesia can be safely administered to most patients in the presence of chronic use of these drugs (El-Ganzouri et al, 1985; Michaels et al, 1984; Wells and Bjorkstein, 1989). Caution is still indicated, however, as adverse responses may occur in rare patients (Sides, 1987).

Overdose

Overdose with MAOI is reflected by signs of excessive sympathetic nervous system activity (tachycardia, hyperthermia, mydriasis), seizures, and coma. Treatment is supportive plus gastric lavage, because MAOI delay gastric emptying. Dantrolene has been advocated for treatment of skeletal muscle rigidity and associated symptoms of hypermetabolism following an overdose of MAOI (Kaplan et al, 1986).

Sympathomimetics

The actions of indirect-acting and, to a lesser extent, direct-acting sympathomimetics, including those in cold or asthma remedies, may be exaggerated by MAOI. This reflects the fact that MAOI act primarily intraneuronally such that more neurotransmitter becomes available for release by indirect-acting sympathomimetics. If hypotension occurs in a patient receiving an MAOI, direct-acting sympathomimetics such as phenylephrine, in reduced doses, are recommended. Monoamine oxidase inhibitors may have less potentiating effects on exogenously administered catecholamines because metabolism by catechol-O-methyltransferase and neuronal uptake partially offset the reduced activity of monoamine oxidase (Boakes et al, 1973). Even the incidence of hypertension in response to indirect-acting sympathomimetics seems to be lower than previously suggested (Wells and Bjorksten, 1989).

Tyramine in Food

Monoamine oxidase is widely distributed in the body, with high concentrations of the enzyme being present in the liver and gastrointestinal tract. Ingestion of tyramine-containing foods (cheese, chicken liver, chocolate, beer, wine) by patients being treated with MAOI may evoke hyperthermia and a hypertensive crisis, since tyramine is no longer inactivated in the gastrointestinal tract or liver. This allows tyramine to evoke the release of endogenous catecholamines that are present in excess amounts. Headache may be the first sign of life-threatening hypertension owing to this food-drug interaction. The precipitous hypertension resembles that which occurs with release of catecholamines from a pheochromocytoma. Treatment of hypertension is with a peripheral vasodilator (nitroprusside) or an alpha-adrenergic antagonist (phentolamine). Cardiac dysrhythmias that persist after control of blood pressure are treated with lidocaine or a beta-antagonist.

Orthostatic Hypotension

Orthostatic hypotension occurs with all MAOI, possibly reflecting the accumulation of the false neurotransmitter octopamine in the cytoplasm of postganglionic sympathetic nerve endings. Release of this less potent vasoconstrictor in response to neural impulses is the most likely explanation for orthostatic hypotension as well as the antihypertensive effects associated with chronic administration of MAOI.

Hyperthermia

Hyperthermia may accompany the administration of meperidine to patients receiving an MAOI. The most likely mechanism for hyperthermia is the ability of meperidine to impair the neuronal uptake of serotonin (Wells and Bjorksten, 1989). This response occurs in about 20% of patients receiving an MAOI, suggesting that a critical cerebral concentration of serotonin must be reached to trigger the response (Stack et al, 1988). In addition to hyperthermia, there may be hypertension, hypotension, depression of ventilation, skeletal muscle rigidity, seizures, and coma. Morphine does not interfere with serotonin uptake and, therefore, hyperthermic reactions in patients taking MAOI are less likely, although the ventilatory depressant effects of morphine may be exaggerated (Wells and Bjorksten, 1989). Fentanyl has also been administered without incidence to patients being treated with MAOI (El-Ganzouri et al, 1985; Wong 1980).

Inhibition of Hepatic Enzymes

Inhibition of hepatic enzymes other than monoamine oxidase by MAOI has been proposed as an explanation for exaggerated depressant effects produced by opioids and barbiturates. For this reason, the dose of opioid should be decreased to one fourth the usual amount (Janowsky et al, 1981). Exaggerated effects of antihistamines, anticholinergics, and tricyclic antidepressants may also reflect slow metabolism resulting from MAOI-induced decreases in enzyme activity. There is one documented case of prolonged apnea following administration of succinylcholine to a patient being treated with phenelzine (Bodley et al, 1969). It was subsequently demonstrated that plasma cholinesterase levels were reduced in 40% of patients treated with phenelzine but in no patient receiving other MAOI. As with opioids and sympathomimetics, the dangers of barbiturate usage in patients being treated with MAOI seems to have been exaggerated.

Anesthetic Requirements

In animals, anesthetic requirements for volatile drugs are increased, presumably reflecting accumulation of norepinephrine in the central nervous system (Miller et al, 1968).

DISULFIRAM

Disulfiram is a thiuram derivative that inhibits acetaldehyde dehydrogenase activity necessary for the oxidation of acetaldehyde, which results from breakdown of alcohol by alcohol dehydrogenase. As a result, ingestion of alcohol in the presence of disulfiram leads to accumulation of acetaldehyde in the plasma, manifesting as flushing, vertigo, nausea, hyperventilation, tachycardia, and diaphoresis. Symptoms usually last 30 to 60 minutes but in some patients may persist for several hours. Sedation is predictable following waning of symptoms. Severe reactions occur less frequently and include hypoventilation, hypotension, cardiac dysrhythmias, cardiac failure, syncope, and seizures. Hypotension may reflect the ability of disulfiram to inhibit dopamine beta-hydroxylase activity necessary for the synthesis of norepinephrine from dopamine. The unpleasantness of symptoms that accompany ingestion of alcohol in the presence of inhibition of acetaldehyde dehydrogenase activity is the basis for the use of disulfiram as an adjunctive drug with psychiatric counseling to decrease consumption of alcohol. Compliance with long-term oral disulfiram therapy is often poor.

Management of anesthesia in patients being treated with disulfiram should consider the potential presence of disulfiram-induced sedation and hepatotoxicity. Preoperative determination of liver function tests seems prudent. Decreased drug requirements could reflect an additive effect with preexisting sedation or the ability of disulfiram to inhibit metabolism of drugs other than alcohol. For example, disulfiram may result in potentiation of the effects of benzodiazepines. Acute and otherwise unexplained hypotension during general anesthesia could reflect inadequate stores of norepinephrine owing to disulfiram-induced inhibition of dopamine beta-hydroxylase (Diaz and Hill, 1979). This hypotension responds to ephedrine, although a direct-acting sympathomimetic such as phenylephrine would seem more logical for treatment of hypotension owing to depletion of norepinephrine. Use of regional anesthesia may be influenced by the occasional patient treated with disulfiram who develops polyneuropathy. Alcohol-containing solutions as used for skin cleansing should be avoided in these patients.

REFERENCES

Bertolo L, Novakovic L, Penna M. Antiarrhythmic effects of droperidol. Anesthesiology 1972;37:529–35.

Bittar DA. Innovar-induced hypertensive crisis in patients with pheochromocytoma. Anesthesiology 1979;50:366–9.

Boakes AJ, Laurence DR, Teoh PC, Barar FSK, Benedikter LT, Prichard BNC. Interactions between sympathomimetic amines and antidepressant agents in man. Br Med J 1973;1:311–5.

Bodley PO, Halwax K, Potts L. Low serum pseudocholinesterase levels complicating treatment with phenelzine. Br Med J 1969;3:510–2.

Boehnert MT, Lovejoy FH. Value of the QRS duration versus the serum drug level in predicting seizures and ventricular arrhythmias after an acute overdose of tricyclic antidepressants. N Engl J Med 1985;313:474–9.

Burroughs GD, Davies B, Kincaid-Smith P. Unique tubular lesion after lithium (letter). Lancet 1978;1:1310.

Christensen S, Farrow-Gillespie A, Lerman J. Incidence of emesis and postanesthetic recovery after strabismus surgery in children: A comparison of droperidol and lidocaine. Anesthesiology 1989;70:251–4.

Cohen SE, Woods WA, Wyner J. Antiemetic efficacy of droperidol and metoclopramide. Anesthesiology 1984;60:67–9.

Diaz JH, Hill GE. Hypotension with anesthesia in disulfiram-treated patients. Anesthesiology 1979;51:366–8.

Edwards RP, Miller RD, Roizen RF, et al. Cardiac responses to imipramine and pancuronium during anesthesia with halothane or enflurane. Anesthesiology 1979;50:421–5.

El-Ganzouri AR, Ivankovich AD, Braverman B, McCarthy R. Monoamine oxidase inhibitors: Should they be discontinued preoperatively? Anesth Analg 1985;64:592–6.

Fischler M, Bonnet F, Trang H et al. The pharmacokinetics of droperidol in anesthetized patients. Anesthesiology 1986;64:486–9.

Frommer DA, Kulig KW, Marx JA, Rumack B. Tricyclic antidepressant overdose. JAMA 1987;257:521–6.

Gomez-Arnau J, Marquez-Montes J, Avello F. Fentanyl and droperidol effects on the refractoriness of the accessory pathway in the Wolff-Parkinson-White syndrome. Anesthesiology 1983;58:307–13.

Granato JE, Stern, Ringel A, et al. Neuroleptic malignant syndrome: Successful treatment with dantrolene and bromocriptine. Ann Neurol 1983;14:89–90.

Guze BH, Baxter LR. Neuroleptic malignant syndrome. N Engl J Med 1985;313:163–6.

Harper MH, Hickey RF, Cromwell TH, Linwood S. The magnitude and duration of respiratory depression produced by fentanyl and fentanyl plus droperidol in man. J Pharmacol Exp Ther 1976;199;464–8.

Havdala HS, Borison RL, Diamond BI. Potential hazards and applications of lithium in anesthesiology. Anesthesiology 1979;50:534–7.

Hill GE, Wong KC, Hodges MR. Lithium carbonate and neuromuscular blocking agents. Anesthesiology 1977;46:122–6.

Janowsky EC, Risch C, Janowsky DS. Effect of anesthesia on patients taking psychotropic drugs. J Clin Psychopharmacol 1981;1:14–20.

Kaplan RF, Feinglass NG, Webster W, Mudra S. Phenelzine overdose treated with dantrolene sodium. JAMA 1986;255:642–4.

Lee CM, Yeakel AE. Patients refusal of surgery following Innovar premedication. Anesth Analg 1975;54:224–6.

Mannisto PT, Saarnivaara L. Effect of lithium and rubidium on the sleeping time caused by various anaesthetics in the mouse. Br J Anaesth 1976;48:185–9.

Michaels I, Serrins M, Shier NQ, Barash PG. Anesthesia for cardiac surgery in patients receiving monoamine oxidase inhibitors. Anesth Analg 1984;63:1041–4.

Miller RD, Way WL, Eger EI. The effects of alpha-methyldopa, reserpine, guanethidine, and iproniazid on minimum alveolar anesthetic requirement (MAC). Anesthesiology 1968;29:1153–8.

Pandit SK, Kothary SP, Pandit UA, Randel G, Levy L. Dose-response study of droperidol and metoclopramide as antiemetics for outpatient anesthesia. Anesth Analg 1989;68:798–802.

Richter JJ. Current theories about the mechanisms of benzodiazepines and neuroleptic drugs. Anesthesiology 1981;54:66–72.

Rivera VM, Keichian AH, Oliver RE. Persistent parkinsonism following neuroleptanalgesia. Anesthesiology 1975;42:635–7.

Roose SP, Glassman AH, Giardina E-GV, et al. Nortriptyline in depressed patients with left ventricular impairment. JAMA 1986;256:3523–7.

Rosenblatt RM, Reich J, Dehring D. Tricyclic antidepressants in treatment of depression and chronic pain. Anesth Analg 1984;63:1025–32.

Sangal R, Dimitrijevic R. Neuroleptic malignant syndrome: Successful treatment with pancuronium. JAMA 1985;254:2795–6.

Santos A, Datta S. Prophylactic use of droperidol for control of nausea and vomiting during spinal anesthesia for cesarean section. Anesth Analg 1984; 63:85–7.

Sides CA. Hypertension during anaesthesia with monoamine oxidase inhibitors. Anaesthesia 1987;46:633–5.

Soroker D, Barjilay E, Konichezky S, Bruderman I. Respiratory function following premedication with droperidol or diazepam. Anesth Analg 1978;57:695–9.

Sprague DH, Wolf S. Enflurane seizures in patients taking amitriptyline. Anesth Analg 1982;61:67–8.

Stack CG, Rogers P, Linter SPK. Monoamine oxidase inhibitors and anaesthesia. Br J Anaesth 1988;60:222–7.

Stiff JL, Harris DB. Clonidine withdrawal complicated by amitriptyline therapy. Anesthesiology 1983;59:73–4.

Sumikawa K, Amakata Y. The pressor effect of droperidol on a patient with pheochromocytoma. Anesthesiology 1977;46:359–61.

Sumikawa K, Hirano H, Amakata Y, Kashimoto T, Wada A, Izumi F. Mechanism of the effect of droperidol to induce catecholamine efflux from the adrenal medulla. Anesthesiology 1985;62:17–22.

Thompson TL, Moran MG, Nies AS. Psychotropic drug use in the elderly. N Engl J Med 1983;308:194–8.

Veith RC, Raskind MA, Caldwell JH, Barnes RF, Gumbrecht G, Ritchie JL. Cardiovascular effects of tricyclic antidepressants in depressed patients with chronic heart disease. N Engl J Med 1982;306:954–9.

Ward DS. Stimulation of hypoxic ventilatory drive by droperidol. Anesth Analg 1984;63:106–10.

Ward NG. Akathisia associated with droperidol during epidural anesthesia. Anesthesiology 1989;71:786–7.

Wells DG, Bjorksten AR. Monoamine oxidase inhibitors revisited. Can J Anaesth 1989;36:64–74.

Whitwam JG, Russell WJ. The acute cardiovascular changes and adrenergic blockade by droperidol in man. Br J Anaesth 1971;581–90.

Wiklund RA, Ngai SH. Rigidity and pulmonary edema after Innovar in a patient on levodopa therapy: Report of a case. Anesthesiology 1971;35:545–7.

Wong KC, Puerto AX, Puerto BA, Blatnick RA. Influence of imipramine and pargyline on the arrythmogenicity of epinephrine during halothane, enflurane or methoxyflurane anesthesia in dogs. Anesthesiology 1980;53:S25.

20

Prostaglandins

INTRODUCTION

Prostaglandins are among the most prevalent of the naturally occurring, physiologically active endogenous substances (autacoids), having been detected in almost every tissue and body fluid. No other autacoids (histamine, serotonin, angiotensin II, plasma kinins) show more numerous and diverse effects than do prostaglandins.

NOMENCLATURE AND STRUCTURE ACTIVITY RELATIONSHIPS

The designation of a substance as a prostaglandin reflects the initial observation that human semen contained a lipid-soluble acid that caused the uterus to relax. The generic term *eicosanoids* refers to the 20-carbon, hairpin-shaped fatty acid chain that includes a cyclopentane ring, characteristic of prostaglandins (Fig. 20-1).

The letters PG denote the word *prostaglandin*. A third letter indicates the structure of the cyclopentane ring, such that PGE has a different ring structure than PGF. A subscript that follows the third letter denotes the number of double bonds in the structure as well as the fatty acid precursor of the prostaglandin. For example, PGE_1 has one double bond, whereas PGE_2 has two double bonds. The subscript 2 also designates arachidonic acid as the fatty acid precursor. Indeed, arachidonic acid is the most common fatty acid precursor of prostaglandins in humans. Alpha or beta following the subscript indicates the orientation of the hydroxyl group at the number 9 carbon atom in relation to the plane of the cyclopentane ring.

SYNTHESIS

Prostaglandins are derived principally from the polyunsaturated 20-carbon essential fatty acid, arachidonic acid. Arachidonic acid is a ubiquitous component of cell membranes and is released by the action of phospholipase enzyme. This enzyme is activated by various physical and chemical stimuli and inhibited by corticosteroids. Histamine is known to activate phospholipase, leading to the formation of prostaglandins, including prostacyclin. Inhaled anesthetics, as a result of their solubility in lipid cell membranes, may increase availability of arachidonic acid as a substrate (Shayevitz et al, 1985). Once released, arachidonic acid becomes available to serve as a substrate for production of prostaglandins via either the cyclooxygenase or the lipoxygenase pathway (Fig. 20-2).

Cyclooxygenase

Cyclooxygenase is a widely distributed complex of microsomal enzymes necessary for the initial synthesis of prostaglandins (PGG_2 and PGH_2) known as *endoperoxides* (Fig. 20-2). Subsequent

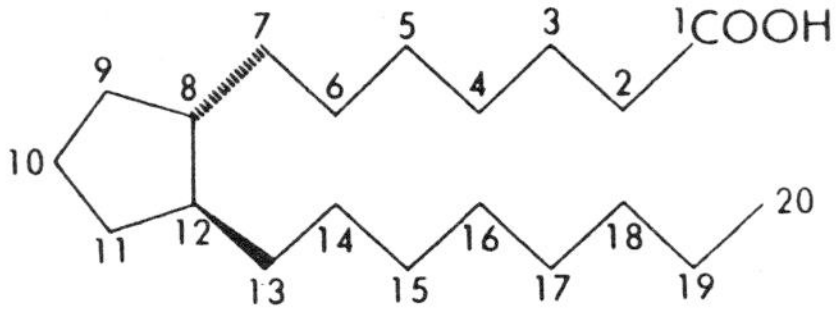

FIGURE 20-1. A 20-carbon hairpin-shaped fatty acid chain is characteristic of prostaglandins.

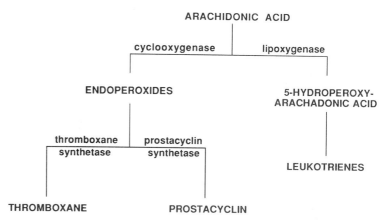

FIGURE 20–2. Synthesis of prostaglandins from arachidonic acid occurs via a cyclooxygenase pathway and a lipoxygenase pathway.

conversion of PGH_2 to thromboxane (TXA_2) and prostacyclin (PGI_2) requires the activity of tissue specific enzymes, thromboxane synthetase and prostacyclin synthetase (Fig. 20-2). In contrast to the wide tissue distribution of cyclooxygenase, thromboxane synthetase is principally present in platelets and the lungs, whereas prostacyclin synthetase is principally present in vascular endothelium.

Lipoxygenase

Lipoxygenase enzymes are localized principally in platelets, vascular endothelium, the lungs, and leukocytes. Compounds formed by these enzymes from arachidonic acid include 5-hydroperoxyarachidonic acid (HPETE) and its degradation product, 12-hydroxyarachidonic acid (HETE) (Fig. 20-2). Leukotrienes result from lipoxygenation of arachidonic acid and further addition of water-soluble substituents. The term *leukotriene* denotes the initial discovery of these substances in leukocytes and their conjugated structure. Elevated concentrations of leukotrienes have been measured in several disease states, including bronchial asthma, neonatal hypoxemia with pulmonary hypertension, and the adult respiratory distress syndrome (Matthay et al, 1984). Leukotriene D (formerly designated a slow-reacting substance of anaphylaxis) has preferential effects on peripheral airways and is a more potent bronchoconstrictor than histamine. Furthermore, leukotriene-induced increases in vascular permeability occur at lower concentrations than histamine. Leukotriene B released from alveolar macrophages and other leukocytes stimulates neutrophil adhesion to endothelial cells, with subsequent degranulation, enzyme release, and superoxide generation (Samuelsson, 1983).

MECHANISM OF ACTION

In many tissues, prostaglandins act on specific receptors to stimulate synthesis of cyclic adenosine monophosphate (cyclic AMP) by activation of adenylate cyclase. The acidic lipid nature of prostaglandins is unique among the autacoids and other substances that react with specific cell membrane receptors. Stimulation of smooth muscle by prostaglandins appears to be associated with the depolarization of cellular membranes and the release of calcium ions (Ca^{2+}).

METABOLISM

Initial metabolism of prostaglandins to inactive substances is rapid, being catalyzed by specific enzymes that are widely distributed in the body, in such organs as the lungs, kidneys, liver, and the gastrointestinal tract. For example, 95% of infused PGE_2 is inactivated during one passage through the lungs. The unique position of the pulmonary circulation between the venous and arterial circulations allows the lungs to act as a filter for many of the prostaglandins, thus protecting the cardiovascular system and other organs from prolonged effects due to recirculation of these substances. Thromboxane is hydrolyzed rapidly (elimination half-time 30 seconds) to an inactive product, thus largely limiting its actions to the microenvironment of its release. Prostacyclin, with an elimination half-time of about 3 minutes, is nonenzymatically converted to 6-keto-prostaglandin (PGF_{1a}). Measurement of plasma concentrations 6-keto-PGF_{1a} serves as an indicator of prostacyclin release or lack of release as in the presence of known inhibitors (aspirin, ibuprofen) or H_1 receptor antagonists (diphenhydramine).

The initial rapid metabolism of prostaglandins is followed by a slower breakdown, during which the existing inactive metabolites are oxidized by enzymes responsible for oxidation of most fatty acids. The liver is the major site for this oxidation, and the resulting metabolites appear in the urine often as dicarboxylic acid.

EFFECTS ON ORGAN SYSTEMS

The possible role of prostaglandins as mediators of effects on organ systems depend on the system under consideration (Table 20-1) (Oates et al, 1988). For example, inhibitors of prostaglandin synthesis usually have little effect on the cardiovascular system or lungs, suggesting a negligible role of prostaglandins in the basal regulation of these systems. Conversely, normal platelet function and hemostasis are likely to be under strict regulation of prostaglandins, as emphasized by the ability of nonsteroidal anti-inflammatory drugs to interfere with normal platelet aggregation. Renal blood flow may be influenced by the presence or absence of prostaglandins in the kidneys (see the section entitled "Kidneys").

Hematologic System

Thromboxane, the principal cyclooxygenase product of arachidonic acid in platelets, acts as an intense stimulus for platelet aggregation, presumably reflecting inhibition of adenylate cyclase and subsequent reduced cyclic AMP synthesis in platelets. Conversely, release of prostacyclin from vascular endothelium opposes platelet aggregation. Prostacyclin stimulates platelet production of cyclic AMP, leading to decreased platelet adhesiveness and prolonged platelet survival.

A normal thromboxane-to-prostacyclin ratio is important in maintaining platelet activity and coagulation. An increase in this ratio, as may occur when atherosclerotic plaques release substances that inhibit synthesis of prostacyclin, results in a predominance of thromboxane activity manifesting as platelet aggregation and vasoconstriction. This sequence of events could lead to reduced blood flow in the area of an atherosclerotic plaque manifesting as ischemia or infarction in organs such as the heart, brain, and kidneys. A similar imbalance in the ratio of thromboxane to prostacyclin in the venous circulation could lead to venous thromboembolism.

Table 20-1
Comparative Effects of Prostaglandins

	Platelet Aggregation	*Systemic Vascular Resistance*	*Airway Resistance*	*Uterine Muscle Tone*
Thromboxane	I	I	I	
Prostacyclin	D	D	D	
Iloprost	D	D	D	
Alprostadil (PGE_2)	D	D	I	I
Carboprost				I
Dinoprost (PGF_{2a})		I/D	I	I
Dinoprostone (PGE_2)				I

I, increased; D, decreased.

Bleeding disorders are likely in the presence of thromboxane depletion or excess prostacyclin. The speculated role for platelet aggregation in myocardial ischemia suggests a potentially useful role for prostacyclin in both dilating coronary arteries and preventing aggregation of platelets. These same effects of prostacyclin could be useful in treating acute ischemic pain in extremities and in promoting healing of ischemic ulcerations.

Prostacyclin present in low concentrations in the plasma may be responsible for preventing aggregation of normal platelets. A break in the vascular endothelium releases thromboxane, causing intense local vasoconstriction and platelet aggregation leading to formation of a hemostatic plug. It seems likely that cyclooxygenase enzyme in the platelets that synthesizes thromboxane is more sensitive to inhibition by aspirin than is the same enzyme in vascular endothelium that synthesizes prostacyclin. As a result, thromboxane production in platelets is stopped by small doses of aspirin, whereas large doses of aspirin inhibit both thromboxane and prostacyclin production. If a patient is taking low doses of aspirin, thromboxane is no longer present to oppose prostacyclin, and platelet aggregation does not occur.

Platelets are activated and consumed when blood passes over the surfaces of materials used for extracorporeal circulation. Continuous intravenous infusion of prostacyclin during extracorporeal circulation minimizes the degree of thrombocytopenia, and maintenance of platelet function is suggested by reduced postoperative bleeding (Fig. 20-3) (Longmore et al, 1981). Prostacyclin use is limited by its instability at physiologic pH and intense vasodilating activity that results in severe hypotension.

Iloprost

Iloprost is a prostacyclin analogue that is a potent inhibitor of platelet aggregation. This drug produces its platelet effect immediately and has an elimination half-time of 15 to 30 minutes such that platelet reactivity returns usually within 3 hours after cessation of administration. It has no effect on the activity of coagulation factors other than platelets. Iloprost causes vasodilation, but it is associated with less hypotension than prostacyclin. Nevertheless, iloprost may produce hypotension that is resistant to relatively large doses of phenylephrine (Kraenzler and Starr, 1988).

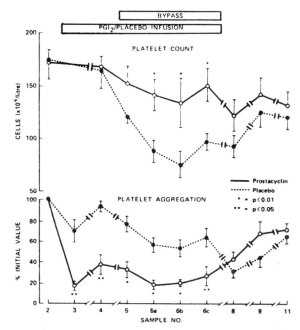

FIGURE 20–3. Variations in platelet count and platelet aggregation with prostacyclin (PGI$_2$) (—) and without prostacyclin (-----). (From Longmore DB, Bennett JG, Hoyle PM, et al. Prostacyclin administration during cardiopulmonary bypass in man. Lancet 1981; 1: 800–4; with permission.)

Iloprost added to the cardiopulmonary bypass circuit preserves circulating platelet count and prevents platelet granule release during simulated extracorporeal circulation (Addonizio et al, 1985). This drug may be useful during cardiac surgery to prevent interaction of platelets with antigens such as heparin in patients with heparin-induced thrombocytopenia.

Cardiovascular System

The effects of prostaglandins on cardiac function are complex, being dependent on direct inotropic effects, the activity of the sympathetic nervous system relative to the parasympathetic nervous system, and the metabolic status of the heart. For example, PGE$_2$ produces an increase in heart rate and contractility by direct inotropic effects as well as by increasing reflex sympathetic nervous system activity. The intravenous administration of prostacyclin causes a decrease in blood pressure resulting from a decline in systemic vascular resistance, reflecting vasodilation in several vascular beds, including coronary, renal, mesenteric, and skeletal muscle circulations. Prostacyclin is not inactivated in the lungs and is thus an effective vasodilator when administered intravenously. The effects of prostacyclin on heart rate are variable, apparently depending on the basal level of autonomic nervous system activity.

Mesenteric traction during aortic surgery may produce facial flushing, decreased blood pressure and systemic vascular resistance, and increased heart rate and cardiac output (Hudson et al, 1990). These changes are associated with increased plasma concentrations of 6-keto-PGF_{1a}, suggesting prostacyclin as a mediator. Indeed, ibuprofen, a cyclooxygenase inhibitor, prevents facial flushing and cardiovascular changes associated with mesenteric traction (Hudson et al, 1990). Likewise, d-tubocurarine–induced hypotension is associated with similar evidence for prostacyclin release and prevention of hypotension by pretreatment with aspirin (Hatano et al, 1990).

The activity of vascular smooth muscle in various vascular beds may be modulated by the relative magnitude of vasoconstriction and vasodilation produced by thromboxane and prostacyclin, respectively. For example, events leading to coronary artery spasm and thrombosis may arise from a deficiency of prostacyclin-induced vasodilation relative to thromboxane-induced vasoconstriction.

Local generation of PGE_2 and prostacyclin may participate in the transition of the fetal circulation to that of a normal neonate. Indeed, prostaglandin synthesis inhibitors may contribute to the closure of the ductus arteriosus (Olley and Coceani, 1981).

Alprostadil

Alprostadil (PGE_1) has a variety of pharmacologic effects, among which the most important are vasodilation, inhibition of platelet aggregation, and stimulation of gastrointestinal and uterine smooth muscle (Fig. 20-4). This drug is a potent relaxant of the smooth muscle of the ductus arteriosus and, when infused intravenously, preserves ductal patency in neonates (Cole et al, 1981). For this reason, alprostadil is used in neonates with ductal-dependent congen-

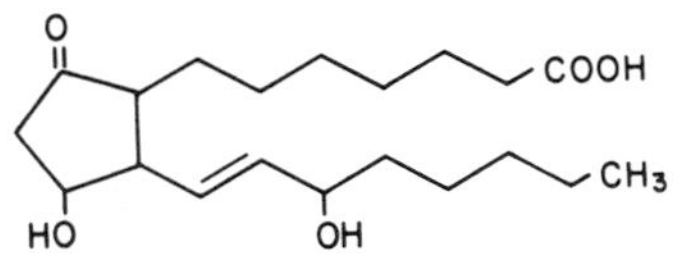

FIGURE 20–4.   Aprostadil (prostaglandin E_2 [PGE_2]).

ital heart disease (pulmonary atresia, tetralogy of Fallot) to maintain patency of the ductus arteriosus until surgery can be performed.

Alprostadil is metabolized so rapidly that it must be administered as a continuous intravenous infusion ($0.1 \ \mu g \cdot kg^{-1} \cdot min^{-1}$ or less). Nearly 70% of circulating alprostadil is metabolized in one passage through the lungs, and the metabolites are excreted by the kidneys. Depression of ventilation, bronchoconstriction, flushing, bradycardia, and hyperthermia may be evoked by continuous intravenous infusion of this drug (Lewis et al, 1981). Alprostadil should not be administered to infants with respiratory distress syndrome.

Misoprostol

Misoprostol is a prostaglandin E_1 analogue with oral bioavailability that improves renal function and reduces the incidence of acute rejection in renal-transplant patients treated concurrently with cyclosporine and prednisone (Fig. 20-5) (Moran et al, 1990). Indeed, cyclosporine-induced nephrotoxicity may reflect inhibition of the synthesis of renal prostaglandins.

Pulmonary Circulation

Pulmonary vasoconstriction may be related to increased circulating concentrations of thromboxane, PGE_2, and PGE_{2a}. Pulmonary vasoconstriction, pulmonary hypertension, and bronchoconstriction that, on rare occasions, are associated with the administration of protamine may reflect protamine-induced production of the prostaglandin vasoconstrictor, thromboxane (Nuttal et al, 1991). Short-term intravenous infusions of prostacyclin, 12.5 to 35 $ng \cdot kg^{-1} \cdot min^{-1}$, decrease pulmonary artery pressure in patients with pulmonary hypertension during the adult respiratory distress syndrome (Radermacher et al, 1990). In this regard, prostacyclin may become useful in the management of acute respiratory

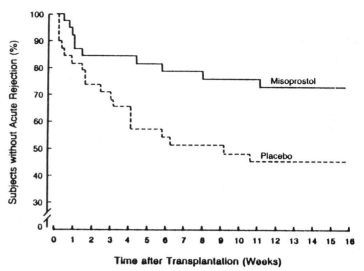

FIGURE 20–5. Treatment with misoprostal is associated with a significant decrease in acute rejection in renal-transplant recipients. (From Moran M, Mozes MF, Maddux MS, et al. Prevention of acute graft rejection by the prostaglandin E, analogue of misoprostol in renal-transplant recipients treated with cyclosporin and prednisone. N Engl J Med 1990; 322: 1183–8; with permission.)

failure. Release of prostacyclin from the lungs into the pulmonary circulation could prevent aggregation of platelets. This effect would provide a physiologic mechanism for dispersing clumps of platelets trapped in small pulmonary blood vessels.

As a potent pulmonary vasoconstrictor, PGF_{2a} has been shown to enhance vasoconstriction in an atelectatic lung, diverting pulmonary blood flow to ventilated alveoli and increasing the PaO_2 (Scherer et al, 1985). In essence, PGF_{2a} is capable of potentiating hypoxic pulmonary vasoconstriction and thus improving arterial oxygenation. Because 70% to 98% of this prostaglandin is inactivated in one passage across the lung, it is possible, with the proper infusion rate, to selectively produce effects on the pulmonary vasculature to the exclusion of the systemic circulation.

Lungs

The lungs are a major site of prostaglandin synthesis. Prostaglandins may produce bronchoconstriction or bronchodilation. Indeed, an imbalance between production of thromboxane and prostacyclin in the lungs might contribute to symptoms of bronchial asthma. Asthmatic patients experience increased airway resistance with far lower inhaled amounts of PGF_{2a} than do normal patients. Both PGE_1 and PGE_2 produce bronchodilatation when given by aerosol, but the

associated irritant effect of this inhalation offsets their clinical usefulness.

Leukotrienes are several thousand times more potent as constrictors of bronchial smooth muscle than is histamine. A predominant role of leukotrienes in asthma-induced bronchoconstriction in individual patients is suggested by the ineffectiveness of antihistamines. Furthermore, the relatively slow metabolism of leukotrienes in the lungs contributes to long-lasting bronchoconstriction. Aspirin-induced asthma may reflect inhibition of the cyclooxygenase pathway by the drug, leading to increased availability of arachidonic acid to the lipoxygenase pathway to form leukotrienes (Fig. 20-2).

Kidneys

Intrarenal release of prostaglandins may be an important mechanism for modulating renal blood flow and regulating urine formation. Indeed, the kidneys are a major site of prostaglandin synthesis. The antihypertensive effect of normally functioning kidneys may be related to their capacity to synthesize and release into the circulation PGE_2 or prostacyclin, which causes diuresis, natriuresis, and a decrease in blood pressure. These effects of prostaglandins may be due to a direct action on renal tubular transport processes or a change in the distribution of renal blood flow. Renal vasodilation produced by PGE_2

may offset renal vasoconstriction produced by events such as drug-induced increases in sympathetic nervous system activity. Prostacyclin and PGE_2 influence angiotensin-induced vasoconstriction as a result of their ability to increase the release of renin from the kidney. Indeed, drugs such as aspirin and indomethacin that inhibit synthesis of prostaglandins by way of the cyclooxygenase enzyme pathway are effective in the treatment of primary hyperreninemia (Bartter's syndrome). Conversely, inhibition of cyclooxygenase enzyme by aspirin or nonsteroidal anti-inflammatory drugs may interfere with normal renal prostaglandin protective mechanisms and accentuate catecholamine-induced renal vasoconstriction (Byrick and Rose, 1990). Certain prostaglandins may induce erythropoiesis by stimulating the release of erythropoietin from the renal cortex.

Gastrointestinal Tract

Certain prostaglandins inhibit gastric acid secretion evoked by histamine or gastrin. Methylated analogues of prostaglandins have been shown to decrease the volume of gastric fluid and its acidity after oral or intravenous administration. Nausea, vomiting, and diarrhea associated with the use of PGE_2 to induce abortion reflect stimulation of smooth muscle of the gastrointestinal tract as well as the uterus.

Uterus

The nongravid and gravid uterus are predictably contracted by PGE_2 and PGF_{2a}, leading to the speculation that these prostaglandins are important in the initiation and maintenance of labor. Intravenous infusion of these prostaglandins results in prompt and dose-dependent elevations in uterine muscle tone. In contrast to oxytocin, this effect of prostaglandins is observed at all stages of pregnancy, accounting for the usefulness of PGE_2 or PGF_{2a} for inducing abortion as well as labor. Prompt depression of progesterone output and reabsorption of the corpus luteum follow parenteral injection of PGF_{2a} to animals. This effect interrupts early pregnancy, which is dependent on luteal rather than placental progesterone.

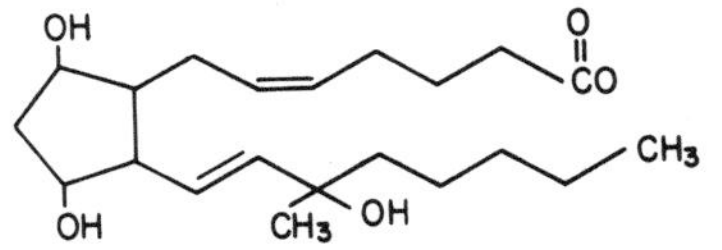

FIGURE 20–6. Carboprost.

Increased synthesis of prostaglandins in the endometrium is speculated to be a possible cause of dysmenorrhea. Indeed, inhibitors of prostaglandin synthesis such as aspirin or indomethacin reduce pain associated with dysmenorrhea. Chronic use of aspirin increases the average length of gestation and the duration of spontaneous labor. Likewise, these inhibitors of prostaglandin synthesis reduce contractions of the uterus in premature labor and could increase the likelihood of postpartum uterine atony.

Prostaglandins may be important in the control of uteroplacental circulation. Changes in the production of prostaglandins have been implicated in the pathophysiology of preeclampsia.

Carboprost

Carboprost is a synthetic analogue of naturally occurring PGF_{2a} (Fig. 20-6). The addition of a methyl group at carbon 15 results in a longer duration of action. Drug-induced uterine contractions are similar to those that accompany labor. Induction of elective abortion with carboprost is successful in more than 90% of patients between 12 and 20 weeks of gestation. Mean time to abortion is 16 hours following intramuscular injection of carboprost, 2.6 mg. Adverse effects are common but usually are not serious. Vomiting and diarrhea occur in more than 60% of patients. Body temperature elevation of 1° to 2°C occurs in nearly 10% of patients and must be differentiated from that resulting from endometritis. Delivery of a live fetus with carboprost-induced abortion is possible.

Dinoprost

Dinoprost (PGF_{2a}) is administered intra-amniotically to induce uterine contractions (Fig. 20-7). The mean abortion time is about 20 hours. Nausea and vomiting occur in most patients and can often be ameliorated by antiemetics. Bronchospasm may occur in asthmatic patients. Grand mal sei-

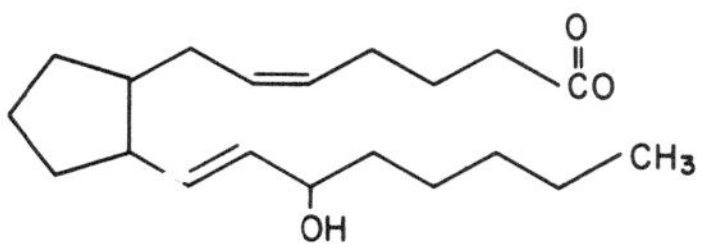

FIGURE 20–7. Dinoprost.

zures are possible in patients prone to epilepsy. Inadvertent intravenous administration produces immediate bronchospasm, tetanic uterine contraction, and hypotension or hypertension.

Dinoprostone

Dinoprostone (PGE_2) produces physiologic-like uterine contractions by activating adenylate cyclase and thus increasing intracellular concentrations of Ca^{2+} (Fig. 20-8). Therapeutically, this prostaglandin is most often administered as a vaginal suppository to induce elective abortion. Side effects of PGE_2 include increases in heart rate and cardiac output as well as tachypnea and hyperthermia that may mimic the onset of sepsis (Hughes and Hughes, 1989). Diuresis is speculated to reflect increased renal blood flow secondary to renal artery dilation. In addition, PGE_2 stimulates steroid formation in the adrenal cortex by activating adenylate cyclase while suppressing epinephrine-induced lipolysis.

Immune System

Prostaglandins such as prostacyclin contribute to the signs and symptoms of inflammation, accentuating the pain and edema produced by bradykinin. Conversely, other prostaglandins suppress the release of chemical mediators from mast cells of patients experiencing allergic reactions.

Antibody responses may be decreased by PGE_1, possibly allowing greater acceptance of tissue transplants. Indeed, immunosuppressant ef-

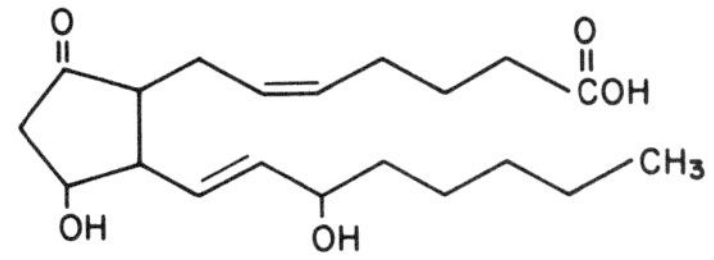

FIGURE 20–8. Dinoprostone.

fects of certain tumors may reflect their ability to produce prostaglandins. Hypercalcemia associated with a tumor may reflect osteolytic activity of certain prostaglandins. Overproduction of PGD_2 is principally responsible for the systemic (flushing, tachycardia, hypotension) and pulmonary (bronchoconstriction) manifestations of mastocytosis (Oates et al, 1988).

REFERENCES

Addonizio VP, Fisher CA, Jenkin BK, Strauss JF, Musial JF, Edmunds LH. Iloprost (ZK36374), a stable analogue of prostacyclin, preserves platelets during simulated extracorporeal circulation. J Thorac Cardiovasc Surg 1985;89:926–33.

Byrick RJ, Rose DK. Pathophysiology and prevention of acute renal failure: The role of the anaesthetist. Can J Anaesth 1990;37:457–67.

Cole RB, Abman S, Azis KU, Bharati S, Lev M. Prolonged prostaglandin E infusion: Histologic effects on patent ductus arteriosus. Pediatrics 1981; 67:816–9.

Hatano Y, Arai T, Noda J, et al. Contribution of prostacyclin to d-tubocurarine-induced hypotension in humans. Anesthesiology 1990;72:28–32.

Hudson JC, Wurm WH, O'Donnell TF, et al. Ibuprofen pretreatment inhibits prostacyclin release during abdominal exploration in aortic surgery. Anesthesiology 1990;72:443–9.

Hughes WA, Hughes SC. Hemodynamic effects of prostaglandin E2. Anesthesiology 1989;70:713–6.

Kraenzler EJ, Starr NJ. Heparin-associated thrombocytopenia: Management of patients for open heart surgery. Case reports describing the use of Iloprost. Anesthesiology 1988;69:964–7.

Lewis AB, Scheinman MM, Gonzalez R, Hess D. Side-effects of therapy with prostaglandin E in infants with critical congenital heart disease. Circulation 1981;64:893–8.

Longmore DB, Bennett JG, Hoyle PM, et al. Prostacyclin administration during cardiopulmonary bypass in man. Lancet 1981;1:800–4.

Matthay M, Eschenbacher W, Goetzl E. Elevated concentrations of leukotriene D4 in pulmonary edema fluid of patients with adult respiratory distress syndrome. J Clin Immunol 1984;4:479–83.

Moran M, Mozes MF, Maddux MS, et al. Prevention of acute graft rejection by the prostaglandin E, analogue of misoprostol in renal-transplant recipients treated with cyclosporin and prednisone. N Engl J Med 1990;322:1183–8.

Nuttall GA, Murray MJ, Bowie EJW. Protamine-herparine induced pulmonary hypertension in pigs: Effects of treatment with a thromboxane receptor agtogonist on hemodynamics and coagulation. Anesthesiology 1991;74:138–45.

Oates JA, Fitzgerald GA, Branch RA, Jackson EK, Knapp HK, Roberts LJ. Clinical implications of prostaglandin and thromboxane A_2 formation. N Engl J Med 1988;319:689–98.

Olley PM, Coceani F. Prostaglandins and ductus arteriosus. Annu Rev Med 1981;32:375–85.

Radermacher P, Santak B, Wust HJ, Tarnow J, Falke KJ. Prostacyclin for the treatment of pulmonary hypertension in adult respiratory distress syndrome: Effects on pulmonary capillary pressure and ventilation-perfusion distributions. Anesthesiology 1990; 72:238–44.

Samuelsson B. Leukotrienes: Mediators of immediate hypersensitivity reactions and inflammation. Science 1983;220:568–75.

Scherer RW, Vigfusson G, Hultsch E, Van Aken H, Lawin P. Prostaglandin F_2 alpha improves oxygen tension and reduces ventilation admixture during one-lung ventilation in anesthetized paralyzed dogs. Anesthesiology 1985;62:23–8.

Shayevitz JR, Traystman RJ, Adkinson NF, Sciuto AM, Gurtner GH. Inhalation anesthetics augment oxidant-induced pulmonary vasoconstriction: Evidence for a membrane effect. Anesthesiology 1985; 63:624–32.

Chapter

21

Histamine and Histamine Receptor Antagonists

HISTAMINE

Histamine is a low–molecular-weight amine that is one of several naturally occurring endogenous substances (autacoids) which produce intense physiologic effects when released locally or into the circulation (Fig. 21-1). Other autacoids include prostaglandins, serotonin, angiotensin II, and plasma kinins (see Chapters 20 and 22). Histamine is present in mast cells located in the skin, lungs, and gastrointestinal tract. Circulating basophils also contain large amounts of histamine. Histamine does not easily cross the blood-brain barrier, and central nervous system effects are usually not evident.

Synthesis

Synthesis of histamine in tissues is by decarboxylation of histidine. Histamine is stored in vesicles in a complex with heparin. Stored histamine is subsequently released in response to antigen-antibody reactions or stimuli such as drugs. Histamine ingested with food is largely destroyed in the liver or lungs or excreted in the urine.

Metabolism

There are two pathways of histamine metabolism in humans. The most important pathway involves methylation catalyzed by histamine-N-methyltransferase, resulting in N-methylhistamine, which is further degraded by monoamine oxidase. In the other pathway, histamine undergoes oxidative deamination catalyzed by diamine oxidase (histaminase), which is a nonspecific enzyme widely distributed in body tissues. Resulting metabolites from both pathways are pharmacologically inactive and are excreted in the urine.

Receptors

Effects of histamine are mediated via histamine receptors that are classified as H-1, H-2, and H-3 (Table 21-1). These receptors are presumed to be components of cell membranes (Maze, 1981).

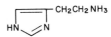

FIGURE 21–1. Histamine.

393

Table 21–1

Effects Mediated by Activation of Histamine Receptors

	Receptor Subtype Activated
Increased intracellular cyclic guanosine monophosphate	H-1
Mediate release of prostacyclin	H-1
Slowed conduction of cardiac impulses through the atrioventricular node	H-1
Coronary artery vasoconstriction	H-1
Bronchostriction	H-1
Increased intracellular cyclic adenosine monophosphate	H-2
Central nervous system stimulation	H-2
Cardiac dysrhythmias	H-2
Increased myocardial contractility	H-2
Increased heart rate	H-2
Coronary artery vasodilation	H-2
Bronchodilation	H-2
Increased secretion of acidic gastric fluid	H-2
Increased capillary permeability	H-1, H-2
Peripheral vascular vasodilation	H-1, H-2
Inhibited synthesis and release of histamine	H-3

H-1 Receptors

H-1 receptors mediate histamine-induced contraction of smooth muscle in the gastrointestinal tract and bronchi (Maze, 1981). The only cardiac effect mediated by these receptors is a delay in the conduction of cardiac impulses through the atrioventricular node. Increased capillary permeability and relaxation of vascular smooth muscle are a reflection of histamine activation of both H-1 and H-2 receptors. The release of prostacyclin from vascular endothelium is mediated via H-1 receptors. Indeed, histamine activates the enzyme phospholipase, which leads to the release of prostacyclin. Elevated intracellular concentrations of cyclic guanosine monophosphate (cyclic GMP) may accompany activation of H-1 receptors. In many respects, the responses evoked by stimulation of H-1 receptors are analogous to those associated with activation of alpha-adrenergic receptors. Histamine-induced effects mediated by activation of H-1 receptors are suppressed by specific H-1 receptor antagonists (Table 21-2).

H-2 Receptors

H-2 receptors mediate histamine-induced secretion of gastric hydrogen ions (H^+) (Maze, 1981). Increased myocardial contractility and heart rate reflect histamine activation of these receptors in

Table 21–2

Classification of Histamine Receptor Antagonists

	Sedative Effects	Anticholinergic Activity	Antiemetic Effects	Duration of Action (h)	Adult Dose (mg)
H-1 Antagonists					
Diphenhydramine	Marked	Marked	Moderate	3–6	50
Pyrilamine	Mild	None	None	3–6	25–50
Chlorpheniramine	Mild	Mild	None	4–12	2–4
Brompheniramine	Mild	Mild	None	4–12	4–8
Cyclizine	Moderate	Minimal	Mild	4–6	50
Promethazine	Moderate	Marked	Marked	4–24	25–50
Terfenadine	Absent			6–12	60
H-2 Antagonists					
Cimetidine	Mild*	None	None	5–7	300
Ranitidine	None	None	None	8–12	150
Famotidine	None	None	None	12	20–40
Nizatidine	None	None	None	8–12	150

*Manifests as confusion and agitation.

the heart. H-2 receptors are also present in the central nervous system. Increased capillary permeability and relaxation of vascular smooth muscle reflect histamine activation of both H-1 and H-2 receptors. Occupation of H-2 receptors by histamine activates adenylate cyclase, thus increasing intracellular concentrations of cyclic adenosine monophosphate (cyclic AMP). The increased levels of cyclic AMP activate the proton pump of the parietal cell to secrete H^+. In many respects, the responses evoked by stimulation of H-2 receptors are analogous to those associated with activation of beta-adrenergic receptors.

Histamine-induced effects mediated by activation of H-2 receptors are suppressed by specific H-2 receptor antagonists (Table 21-2). H-2 receptors in the central nervous system are blocked by lysergic acid diethylamide. Similar central nervous system actions of cimetidine, an H-2 receptor antagonist, would be consistent with confusional states noted in patients with renal dysfunction and in those receiving high doses of cimetidine.

H-3 Receptors

H-3 receptors that function as autoreceptors to inhibit the synthesis and release of histamine have been described (Arrang et al, 1987). Activity of these receptors may be impaired by H-2 antagonists. This could result in enhancement of histamine release when histamine-releasing drugs are administered to patients pretreated with H-2 antagonists. For this reason, it may be prudent to avoid rapid intravenous injection of drugs known to be capable of evoking the release of histamine in patients receiving concomitant treatment with H-2 antagonists. Indeed, atracurium-induced blood pressure decreases are greater in patients pretreated only with an H-2 antagonist compared with an H-1 antagonist or a combination of an H-1 and an H-2 antagonist (Hosking et al, 1988).

Effects on Organ Systems

Histamine exerts profound effects on the cardiovascular system, airways, and gastric H^+ ion secretion. Histamine in large doses stimulates ganglion cells and chromaffin cells in the adrenal medulla, evoking the release of catecholamines. Central nervous system effects do not accompany peripheral release of histamine because this compound cannot easily cross the blood-brain barrier.

Cardiovascular System

The predominant cardiovascular effects of histamine are due to dilatation of arterioles and capillaries, leading to (1) flushing, (2) decreased peripheral vascular resistance, (3) decreases in blood pressure, and (4) increased capillary permeability. Vascular dilatation results from a direct effect of histamine on the blood vessels, mediated by both H-1 and H-2 receptors independently of autonomic nervous system innervation. Activation of either type of receptor can evoke maximal vasodilation, but H-1 receptors are activated at lower concentrations of histamine, producing a rapid onset and transient vasodilatation compared with a slower onset and more sustained vasodilation in response to H-2 receptor activation. Although peripheral vasodilation is generalized, flushing is most obvious in the skin of the face and upper part of the body (the blush area). Increased capillary permeability is characterized as outward passage of plasma proteins and fluid into the extracellular fluid space, manifesting as edema. This increased capillary permeability is due to histamine-induced contraction of capillary endothelial cells, thus exposing the freely permeable basement membranes of capillaries to protein-containing intravascular fluid.

In addition to peripheral vasodilatation, histamine can produce inotropic, chronotropic, and antidromic effects. Positive inotropic effects are due to histamine-mediated stimulation of H-2 receptors as well as the ability of histamine to evoke the release of catecholamines from the adrenal medulla. Positive chronotropic effects and the development of cardiac dysrhythmias reflect direct activation of H-2 receptors by histamine as well as an indirect effect due to histamine-induced catecholamine release. Slowed conduction of cardiac impulses through the atrioventricular node is due to histamine activation of H-1 receptors. Changes in the threshold for ventricular fibrillation may be caused by the liberation of small amounts of histamine that are not detectable as changes in the plasma concentration. It is conceivable that regional tissue release of histamine could contribute to cardiac dysrhythmias. Coronary artery vasoconstriction is mediated by

H-1 receptors, whereas coronary artery vasodilation is mediated by H-2 receptors (Ginsberg et al, 1980).

The triple response elicited by histamine in the skin consists of (1) dilatation of capillaries in the injured area, (2) edema due to increased permeability of the capillaries, and (3) a flare consisting of dilated arteries surrounding the edema. The flare component of the triple response is an example of the ability of histamine to stimulate nerve endings. Histamine also causes pruritus when injected into superficial layers of the skin.

Decreases in blood pressure induced by histamine are prevented by the prior administration of the combination of H-1 and H-2 receptor antagonists (Philbin et al, 1981). Blockade of either receptor alone does not completely prevent the subsequent blood pressure–lowering effects of histamine.

Airways

Histamine activates H-1 receptors to constrict bronchial smooth muscle, whereas stimulation of H-2 receptors relaxes bronchial smooth muscle. In normal patients, the bronchoconstrictor action of histamine is negligible. Conversely, patients with obstructive airway disease, such as asthma or bronchitis, are more likely to develop increases in airway resistance in response to histamine.

Gastric Hydrogen Ion Secretion

Histamine evokes copious secretion of gastric fluid containing high concentrations of H^+. This response occurs in the presence of plasma concentrations of histamine that do not alter blood pressure. A doubling of the plasma histamine concentration is usually considered necessary to evoke changes in blood pressure (Rosow et al, 1980).

Increased gastric H^+ secretion is believed to result from a direct stimulant effect of histamine on parietal cells where, acting on H-2 receptors that are linked to adenylate cyclase, histamine activates a membrane pump (H^+-K^+-ATPase) that extrudes protons. The presence of vagal activity results in even a higher rate of H^+ secretion. For example, after vagotomy in humans, the maximal secretory response to histamine decreases to about one third of its usual value. Cholinergic blockade, such as is produced by high doses of

atropine, also decreases the gastric secretory response to histamine.

Allergic Reactions

During allergic reactions, histamine is only one of several chemical mediators released, and its relative importance in producing symptoms is greatly dependent on the species studied. Likewise, protection afforded by histamine receptor antagonists is highly variable and species dependent. In humans, histamine receptor antagonists (antihistamines) are effective in preventing edema formation and pruritus. Hypotension is attenuated but not totally blocked, whereas bronchoconstriction is often not prevented, emphasizing the predominant role of leukotrienes in this response in humans.

Responses to histamine-releasing drugs are better controlled by histamine receptor antagonists than are allergic responses (Moss and Rosow, 1983; Philbin et al, 1981). Fewer chemical mediators are presumably involved in drug-induced responses, and histamine and possibly prostacyclin are relatively more important.

Clinical Uses

Histamine has been used to assess the ability of the stomach to secrete H^+ and to determine parietal cell mass. Anacidity or hyposecretion of H^+ in response to histamine may reflect pernicious anemia, atrophic gastritis, or gastric carcinoma. Hypersecretion of H^+ in response to histamine is present with Zollinger-Ellison syndrome and may be found in the presence of duodenal ulcer. Distressing side effects produced by histamine alone can be reduced by prior administration of an H-1 receptor antagonist that does not oppose histamine-induced gastric secretion. An alternative to histamine for gastric function tests is pentagastrin, a synthetic pentapeptide derivative of gastrin. Side effects from pentagastrin are minimal.

The fact that intradermal histamine causes a flare that is mediated by axon reflexes allows a test for the integrity of sensory nerves that may be of value in the diagnosis of certain neurologic conditions. The stimulant effect of histamine on chromaffin cells has been used in the past as a provocative test in patients with pheochromocytoma.

HISTAMINE RECEPTOR ANTAGONISTS

Depending on what responses to histamine are inhibited, drugs are classified as H-1 or H-2 receptor antagonists (Table 21-2). This classification is similar to terminology applied to drugs that act as antagonists at alpha- or beta-receptors. H-1 and H-2 receptor antagonists are presumed to act by occupying receptors on effector cell membranes, to the exclusion of agonist molecules, without themselves initiating a response. For histamine receptor antagonists, this is a competitive and reversible interaction (Maze, 1981). It is important to recognize that H-1 and H-2 receptor antagonists do not inhibit release of histamine, but rather, attach to receptors and prevent responses mediated by histamine.

H-1 Receptor Antagonists

Several H-1 receptor antagonists (ethanolamines, ethylenediamines, alkylamines, piperazines, and phenothiazines) are available, but individual variability in responses makes it difficult to document unique effects or advantages of a single drug (Table 21-2). H-1 receptor antagonists resemble histamine in that they contain a substituted ethylamine (Fig. 21-2). Unlike histamine, the H-1 receptor antagonists contain a tertiary amino group linked to two aromatic substituents (Fig. 21-2). In addition to acting as antagonists at the H-1 receptor, those drugs that are classified as ethanolamines also possess some blocking activity at serotonin receptors.

Pharmacokinetics

H-1 receptor antagonists are readily absorbed from the gastrointestinal tract following oral administration, reaching maximal plasma concentrations in 1 to 2 hours. Plasma concentrations parallel the pharmacologic effects of these drugs. The elimination half-time of most H-1 receptor antagonists is about 3.5 hours, with extensive metabolism occurring in the liver such that little if any drug is excreted unchanged in the urine.

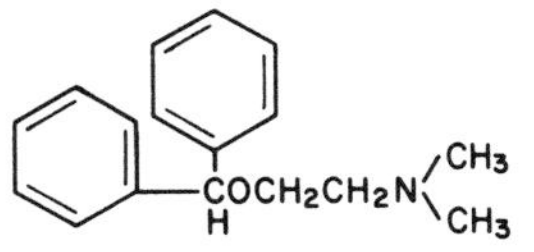

Diphenhydramine

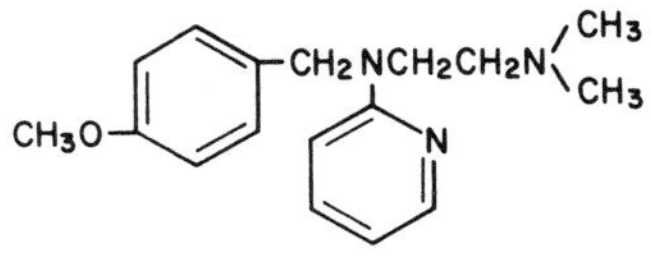

Pyrilamine

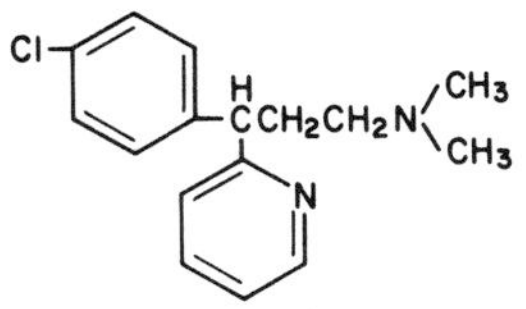

Chlorpheniramine

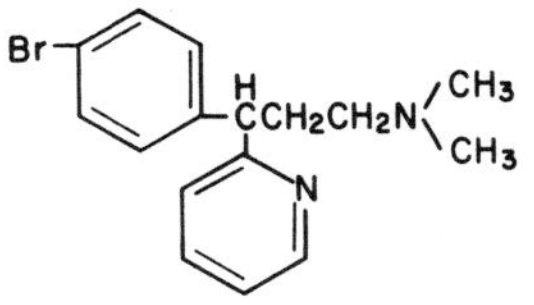

Brompheniramine

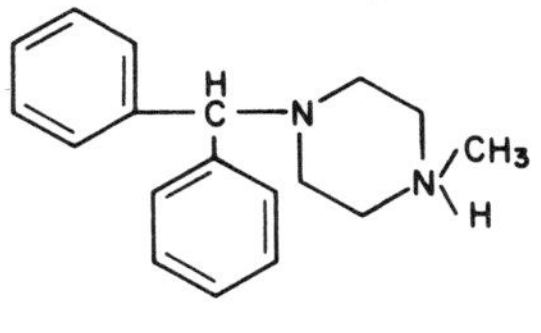

Cyclizine

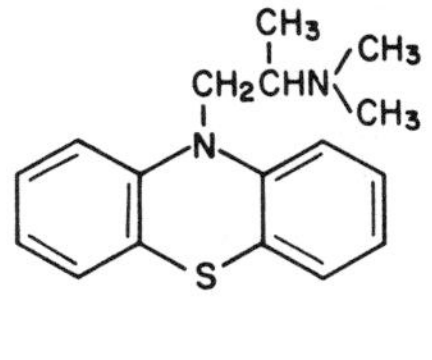

Promethazine

FIGURE 21–2. H-1 receptor antagonists.

Side Effects

The most common side effect of H-1 receptor antagonists is sedation, although the magnitude of this response varies with the specific drug being most prominent, with ethanolamines represented by diphenhydramine (Table 21-2). Central nervous system sedation is less with ethylenediamines, such as pyrilamine, and the alkylamines, represented by chlorpheniramine and absent with terfenadine. Less commonly, small doses of H-1 receptor antagonists may evoke activation of the electroencephalogram and epileptiform seizures in patients with disease of the central nervous system.

Anticholinergic effects of H-1 receptor antagonists manifesting as dry mouth and increased heart rate may be prominent, with the exception of the ethylenediamine, pyrilamine (Table 21-2). Despite these anticholinergic effects, gastric secretion of H^+ is not altered by H-1 receptor antagonists.

H-1 receptor antagonists possess local anesthetic activity but only at concentrations far greater than that necessary to antagonize the effects of histamine. Rapid intravenous injection of an H-1 receptor antagonist can transiently decrease blood pressure, possibly reflecting this local anesthetic (quinidine-like) effect. Oral administration of an H-1 receptor antagonist, however, does not usually alter blood pressure.

Smooth muscle responses in bronchi and peripheral vasculature are inhibited by H-1 receptor antagonists. In guinea pigs, protection is provided against bronchospasm that accompanies an allergic reaction, but this is not so in humans, in whom allergic bronchoconstriction is mediated less by histamine and more by leukotrienes. On peripheral vascular smooth muscle, H-1 receptor antagonists inhibit both vasoconstrictor and vasodilator effects (Table 21-1). Residual vasodilation reflects the role of H-2 receptors, emphasizing the need to block both H-1 and H-2 receptors so as to prevent the decrease in blood pressure produced by histamine. Allergic dermatitis is not uncommon with topical application of H-1 receptor antagonists such as those used to treat pruritus.

Acute overdose with an H-1 receptor antagonist, particularly if it occurs in small children, can produce central nervous system excitation culminating in seizures. Fixed, dilated pupils with flushed face and fever are common in children but not in adults. These latter symptoms are similar to atropine overdose. Ultimately, H-1 receptor antagonist overdose may progress to cardiopulmonary depression and coma. Treatment is symptomatic, with support of vital organ function.

Clinical Uses

H-1 receptor antagonists such as terfenadine are effective in the symptomatic treatment of rhinitis because of their ability to antagonize the effects of histamine released from the nasal mucosa in response to irritants such as pollens. Sneezing, rhinorrhea, and conjunctivitis are predictably suppressed. These drugs are not effective in the treatment of bronchial asthma, allergic reactions, or angioedema in which chemical mediators other than histamine are responsible for the symptoms.

H-1 receptor antagonists may be used for the prophylaxis and treatment of motion sickness. Diphenhydramine and promethazine are effective in this regard, but scopolamine is even more efficacious (Table 21-2). A possible explanation for the efficacy of these drugs in the management of motion sickness is central nervous system antagonism of acetylcholine similar to scopolamine.

Allergic dermatitis usually responds to H-1 receptor antagonists. These drugs prevent the action of histamine that results in increased capillary permeability and formation of edema as well as pruritus.

Sedative effects of H-1 receptor antagonists are present in nonprescription drugs used to treat insomnia. Even pyrilamine, which is considered to have minimal sedative effects on the central nervous system, is a frequent component of these preparations.

H-2 Receptor Antagonists

The relationship between gastric hypersecretion of fluid containing high concentrations of H^+ and peptic ulcer disease emphasizes the potential value of a drug that selectively blocks H-2 receptor-mediated secretion of acidic gastric fluid (Feldman and Burton, 1990). Cimetidine, ranitidine, famotidine and nizatidine are reversible and selective competitive antagonists of the actions of histamine on H-2 receptors (Fig. 21-3). Despite the presence of H-2 receptors throughout the body, inhibition of

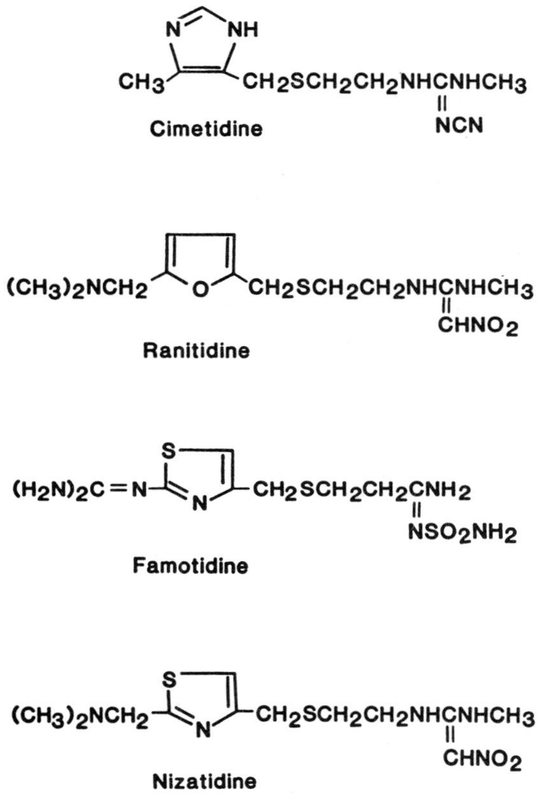

FIGURE 21-3. H-2 receptor antagonists.

histamine binding to the receptors on gastric parietal cells is the major beneficial clinical effect of H-2 receptor antagonists.

Cimetidine

Cimetidine is a selective and competitive H-2 receptor antagonist that blocks histamine-induced secretion of H^+ by gastric parietal cells. The magnitude of this effect is dose related and parallels the plasma concentration of cimetidine. There is no significant effect of cimetidine on gastric emptying time, lower esophageal sphincter tone, or pancreatic secretions.

In addition to blockade of H-2 receptors, cimetidine also prevents the increase in gastric fluid secretion normally produced by gastrin and acetylcholine. The mechanism of this blockade is not clear but may reflect a final common-mediator phenomenon in which gastrin or acetyl-

choline renders histamine more available to parietal cell H-2 receptors.

PHARMACOKINETICS. Cimetidine is readily absorbed from the small intestine following oral administration, with peak plasma concentrations occurring in 60 to 90 minutes. After an oral dose of 300 mg, therapeutic plasma concentrations of cimetidine are maintained for at least 4 hours, whereas 90% or greater suppression of gastric H^+ secretion persists for 5 to 7 hours. Cimetidine can also be administered intramuscularly or intravenously. This drug easily crosses lipid barriers such as the blood-brain barrier or placenta.

Cimetidine is rapidly filtered and excreted by the kidneys, with 50% to 70% of the drug being excreted unchanged within 24 hours. Some reabsorption of cimetidine occurs in proximal renal tubules in addition to a small amount of tubular secretion. Hepatic inactivation occurs primarily by conversion of the side chain of cimetidine to a thioether or sulfoxide. These metabolites appear in the urine as 5-hydroxymethyl and/or sulfoxide metabolites. Bacteria in the gastrointestinal tract, however, can convert some sulfoxide back to cimetidine. Only about 10% of cimetidine is excreted in the bile. The elimination half-time of cimetidine is 1.5 to 2 hours in the presence of normal renal function and is doubled in anephric patients.

CLINICAL USES. Cimetidine is of value in the treatment of duodenal ulcer disease associated with hypersecretion of gastric H^+. The recommended dose is 300 mg orally four times a day. Zollinger-Ellison syndrome, characterized by hypersecretion of large amounts of acidic gastric fluid, is an indication for treatment with an H-2 receptor antagonist.

A number of investigators have confirmed the ability of cimetidine administered orally, intramuscularly, or intravenously to increase gastric fluid pH prior to the induction of anesthesia (Table 21-3) (Coombs et al, 1979; Stoelting, 1978; Weber and Hirschman, 1979). For this reason, cimetidine has been advocated as a useful drug in preoperative medication to reduce the risk of acid pneumonitis if inhalation of acidic gastric fluid occurs in the perioperative period. A frequent approach is administration of cimetidine, 300 mg orally (3 to 4 mg·kg^{-1}), 1.5 to 2 hours before the induction of anesthesia, with or with-

Table 21-3

Influence of Cimetidine on Gastric Fluid pH

	Gastric Fluid pH (percent of patients)		
	<2.5	2.5-5	>5
No cimetidine	60	34	6
Cimetidine 300 mg orally evening before operation	22	38	40
Cimetidine 300 mg orally with preanesthetic medication	16	24	60

(Data from Stoelting RK. Gastric fluid pH in patients receiving cimetidine. Anesth Analg 1978; 57:675–7; with permission.)

out a similar dose the preceding evening. This dose may need to be increased to about 7.5 mg·kg^{-1} in pediatric patients and in obese adults (Goudsouzian et al, 1981). When a more rapid onset of effect is needed, the intramuscular or intravenous route is preferable to oral administration. The effects of cimetidine on gastric fluid volume are not consistent. Furthermore, cimetidine, in contrast to antacids, has no influence on the pH of the gastric fluid that is already in the stomach. Cimetidine crosses the placenta but does not adversely affect the fetus when administered prior to cesarean section (Hodgkinson et al, 1983; Johnston et al, 1983).

Preoperative preparation of patients with allergic histories or patients undergoing procedures associated with an increased likelihood of allergic reactions (chymopapain injection, radiographic dye injection) may include prophylactic oral administration of an H-1 receptor antagonist (diphenhydramine, 0.5 to 1 mg·kg^{-1}) and H-2 antagonist (cimetidine, 4 mg·kg^{-1}) every 6 hours in the 24 hours preceding the possible triggering event (Stoelting, 1983). A corticosteroid, such as prednisone, 50 mg orally every 6 hours, may also be added to this regimen. An implied goal of histamine antagonist pretreatment is to occupy receptors normally responsive to histamine such that subsequent release of this chemical mediator will be less likely to evoke life-threatening symptoms. Despite the logic of this approach, symptomatic allergic reactions to chymopapain, and presumably to other triggering events, may still occur (Bruno et al, 1984).

Administration of cimetidine intravenously to treat life-threatening allergic reactions must be

tempered with the realization that such treatment could exacerbate bronchospasm owing to sudden unmasking of unopposed H-1 activity on bronchial smooth muscle. The risk of further hypotension as may accompany intravenous administration of cimetidine is also a consideration. Furthermore, H-2 activity could have desirable effects during allergic reactions including increased myocardial contractility and coronary artery vasodilation. It is possible that descriptions of dramatic reversals of life-threatening allergic reactions following the intravenous administration of cimetidine may reflect the cumulative effect of prior epinephrine administration in the presence of a prolonged circulation time (DeSoto and Turk, 1989; Kelly and Prielipp, 1990).

Drug-induced histamine release that may follow rapid intravenous administration of morphine, d-tubocurarine, or atracurium is not altered by pretreatment with an H-1 receptor antagonist (diphenhydramine or chlorpheniramine) plus cimetidine (Moss et al, 1981; Philbin et al, 1981). The magnitude of the blood pressure reduction evoked by these drugs is, however, reduced, confirming that prior occupation of histamine receptors with an antagonist attenuates the cardiovascular effects of subsequently released histamine (Philbin et al, 1981). Treatment with diphenhydramine or cimetidine alone is not effective in preventing cardiovascular effects of released histamine, emphasizing the role of both H-1 and H-2 receptors in these responses. In fact, drug-induced histamine release may be exaggerated in patients pretreated only with H-2 antagonists (see the section entitled "H-3 Receptors").

SIDE EFFECTS. Side effects of cimetidine are frequent but predictable, considering the widespread distribution of H-2 receptors. Administration of cimetidine, 300 mg IV over 2 minutes, to postoperative adult patients often produces transient reductions in blood pressure that are maximal 2 minutes following the infusion (Iberti et al, 1986). The mechanism for this blood pressure decline appears to be a direct drug-induced peripheral vasodilation. Bradycardia, heart block, and even cardiac arrest have been observed following rapid intravenous administration of cimetidine to critically ill or elderly patients (Cohen et al, 1979; Shaw et al, 1980). Cardiovascular changes following intravenous administration of cimetidine are not surprising, considering that cardiac effects of histamine are mediated principally by H-2 receptors (Table 21-1.) Cimetidine may increase airway resistance in patients with bronchial asthma, reflecting loss of H-2 receptor–mediated bronchodilation and leaving unopposed H-1 receptor–mediated bronchoconstriction (Table 21-1).

Since histamine is likely to be a neurotransmitter in the central nervous system, it is predictable that cimetidine, because of its ability to cross the blood-brain barrier, could produce significant neurologic side effects. Indeed, central nervous system dysfunction characterized by confusion, agitation, hallucinations, seizures, and coma have been observed, especially in elderly patients treated with cimetidine (Schentag et al, 1979). Central nervous system dysfunction is more likely to occur in the presence of high plasma concentrations of cimetidine associated with renal dysfunction. Delayed awakening from anesthesia has been attributed to lingering central nervous system effects of cimetidine (Viegas et al, 1982). Physostigmine may reverse cimetidine-induced central nervous system dysfunction (Mogelnicki et al, 1979).

Prolonged H-2 receptor blockade and associated gastric achlorhydria may weaken the gastric barrier to bacteria and predispose to systemic infection (Cristiano and Paradisi, 1982). Likewise, pulmonary infections from inhaled secretions may be more likely if the acid-killing effect on bacteria in the stomach is altered. Sustained elevations of gastric fluid pH may lead to an overgrowth of other organisms such as *Candida albicans.* This may account for the occasional case of Candida peritonitis observed after peptic ulcer perforation in patients treated with cimetidine. Prolonged elevation of gastric fluid pH also results in the production of nitroso compounds as a result of an increase in the nitrate-reducing bacteria (Milton-Thompson et al, 1982). Nitroso derivatives are potent mutagens *in vitro,* but there is no evidence that this occurs *in vivo* in association with chronic cimetidine therapy.

Cimetidine has occasionally been associated with mild increases in serum transaminase enzymes, alkaline phosphatase, or both. Transient elevations in serum creatinine occur in about 3% of chronically treated patients, presumably reflecting a reversible interstitial nephritis. Cimetidine-induced neutropenia and thrombocytopenia are rare and usually reversible. Nevertheless, white blood cell counts should be monitored during chronic cimetidine therapy. A weak antiandrogen effect manifesting as gynecomastia in males has been observed during chronic therapy with high doses of cimetidine.

Cimetidine retards metabolism of drugs, such as propranolol and diazepam, that normally undergo high hepatic extraction (Donovan et al, 1981; Klotz and Reimann, 1980). This reduced rate of metabolism may reflect cimetidine-induced reductions in hepatic blood flow as well as inhibition of the hepatic mixed function P-450 oxidase system by means of binding to microsomal cytochrome enzymes (Feely et al, 1981). Indeed, benzodiazepines, such as oxazepam and lorazepam, that are eliminated almost entirely by glucuronidation are not altered by cimetidine-induced effects on P-450 enzyme activity (Klotz and Reimann, 1980). Slowed metabolism and prolonged elimination half-time with associated exaggerated pharmacologic effects of propranolol and diazepam have been documented with only 24 hours of treatment with cimetidine (Figs. 21-4 and 21-5) (Feely et al, 1981; Klotz and Reimann, 1980).

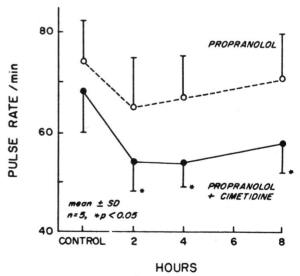

FIGURE 21–4. The effect of propranolol on resting heart rate is accentuated by the concomitant administration of cimetidine. (From Feely J, Wilkinson GR, Wood AJJ. Reduction of liver blood flow and propranolol metabolism by cimetidine. N Engl J Med 1981; 304: 692–5; with permission.)

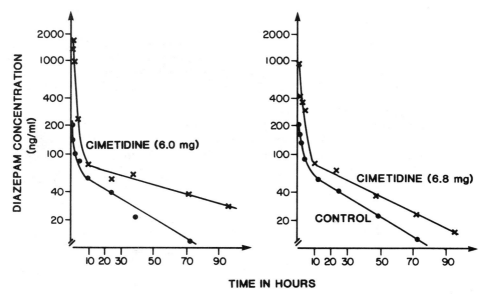

FIGURE 21–5.   The rate of decline in the plasma concentration of diazepam, 0.1 mg·kg^{-1} IV, is slowed by the prior administration of cimetidine, 6 to 6.8 mg·kg^{-1}. (From Klotz U, Reimann I. Delayed clearance of diazepam due to cimetidine. N Engl J Med 1980; 302: 1012–4; redrawn with permission.)

Cimetidine may slow metabolism of lidocaine and thus increase the possibility of systemic toxicity (Feely et al, 1982). In contrast, plasma concentrations of bupivacaine after epidural anesthesia for cesarean section are not influenced by a single dose of cimetidine administered before induction of anesthesia (Fig. 21-6) (Flynn et al, 1989; Kuhnert et al, 1987). This is important since bupivacaine has a narrow therapeutic range because of its cardiotoxicity, and cimetidine is likely to be used for aspiration pneumonitis prophylaxis before cesarean section performed under epidural anesthesia with this local anesthetic.

A previous suggestion, that the duration of action of succinylcholine is significantly prolonged in patients receiving cimetidine, has not been reproducible (Woodworth et al, 1989). Indeed, plasma cholinesterase activity is not altered by cimetidine (Kambam and Franks, 1988). Cimetidine modestly reduces defluorination of methoxyflurane and inhibits oxidative metabolism of halothane (Wood et al, 1986).

Ranitidine

Ranitidine is a selective and competitive H-2 receptor antagonist which, unlike cimetidine, has a furan rather than an imidazole structure (Fig. 21-3) (Zeldis et al, 1983). The imidazole ring present in histamine and cimetidine had previously been considered to be essential for antagonism of H-2 receptors. Ranitidine has the same clinical uses as cimetidine but is five to eight times more potent than cimetidine in antagonizing H$^+$ secretion by gastric parietal cells (Fig. 21-7) (Francis and Kwik, 1982). Like cimetidine, ranitidine has no significant effect on gastric emptying time, lower esophageal sphincter tone, or pancreatic secretions.

PHARMACOKINETICS.   Ranitidine is rapidly absorbed from the gastrointestinal tract, with an oral dose of 150 mg producing a peak plasma concentration in 30 to 60 minutes (Zeldis et al, 1983). Bioavailability of ranitidine is about 50% compared with 70% for cimetidine, reflecting a more significant hepatic first-pass effect for

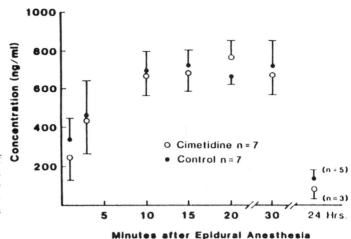

FIGURE 21-6. Maternal plasma levels of bupivacaine after epidural anesthesia. (From Kuhnert BR, Zuspan KJ, Kuhnert PM, Syracuse CD, Brashear WT, Brown DE. Lack of influence of cimetidine on bupivacaine levels during parturition. Anesth Analg 1987; 66: 986–90; with permission.)

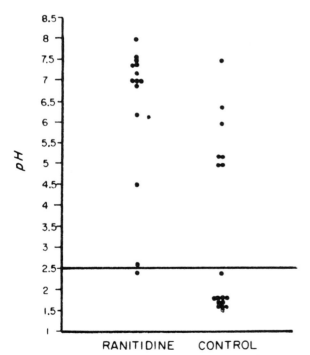

FIGURE 21-7. Distribution of pH values of gastric fluid in patients receiving ranitidine, 150 mg orally the evening before the morning of surgery, compared with untreated patients. (From Francis RN, Kwik RSH. Oral ranitidine for prophylaxis against Mendelson's syndrome. Anesth Analg 1982; 61:130–2; with permission.)

ranitidine. The duration of inhibition of gastric H^+ secretion is prolonged, lasting 8 to 12 hours.

About 50% of ranitidine is excreted by the kidney as unchanged drug. Up to 30% is metabolized in the liver to nitrogen oxide, sulfuric oxide, and desmethyl derivatives. The elimination half-time of ranitidine is 2 to 3 hours, and this is prolonged in the presence of renal dysfunction. For example, the elimination half-time of ranitidine is prolonged about 50% in elderly patients, presumably reflecting an age-related decline in glomerular filtration rate. Likewise, hepatic dysfunction increases the bioavailability and elimination half-time of ranitidine. In patients with renal disease, therapeutic plasma concentrations of ranitidine can be achieved with one half the usual dose.

SIDE EFFECTS. Side effects may be less likely to follow administration of ranitidine than of cimetidine (Zeldis et al, 1983). For example, elderly patients and patients with renal or hepatic dysfunction may be less likely to develop central nervous system dysfunction during treatment with ranitidine. Presumably, this reflects minimal entrance of ranitidine into the central nervous system. In contrast to cimetidine, ranitidine does not bind to androgen receptors; thus, gynecomastia does not occur. Neutropenia and thrombocytopenia, which occur rarely during therapy with cimetidine, have not occurred with ranitidine treatment. Indeed, human lymphocytes have receptors for cimetidine but not ranitidine. Elevations in serum creatinine and development of interstitial nephritis seem to be less likely with ranitidine than with cimetidine therapy. As with cimetidine, transient increases in serum transaminase concentrations have been reported in patients treated with ranitidine (Barr and Piper, 1981). Adverse cardiac effects seem infrequent, but bradycardia has been observed after intravenous infusion of ranitidine (Camarri et al, 1982).

Ranitidine binds less avidly than cimetidine to hepatic microsomal P-450 enzymes. For this reason, ranitidine, in contrast to cimetidine, does not alter the rate of metabolism of drugs with a high hepatic extraction ratio. Both ranitidine and cimetidine, however, decrease hepatic blood flow.

Famotidine

Famotidine is a potent (40 mg equally potent to ranitidine 150 mg) and highly selective H-2 receptor antagonist (Campoli-Richards and Clissold, 1986). After oral administration of famotidine, peak plasma levels occur in 1 to 3 hours, and suppression of gastric H$^+$ secretion is considered to last 12 hours, reflecting the slow dissociation of this drug from receptors. Its effects on hepatic blood flow and enzyme induction are negligible in comparison with other H-2 antagonists. Also, unlike cimetidine or ranitidine, this drug has almost no adverse hemodynamic effects, with blood pressure, heart rate, and cardiac rhythm remaining unchanged after oral or intravenous administration. Famotidine, 20 to 40 mg, administered orally the evening before surgery and/or the morning of surgery before induction of anesthesia, increases gastric fluid pH and decreases gastric fluid volume without adverse side effects (Abe et al, 1989; Dubin et al, 1989).

Nizatidine

Nizatidine is a highly selective H-2 receptor antagonist that resembles ranitidine in potency and famotidine in structure (Feldman and Burton, 1990). In contrast to the other H-2 receptor antagonists, there is little first pass metabolism and bioavailability approaches 100%. Hepatic metabolism is the principal pathway for elimination of cimetidine, ranitidine, and famotidine, whereas renal excretion is the principal pathway for elimination of nizatidine. Only nizatidine appears to have an active metabolite with 60% of the activity of the parent drug. Nizatidine does not bind significantly to the cytochrome P-450 system and is unlikely to inhibit the oxidative metabolism of other drugs.

Omeprazole

Omeprazole is a substituted benzimidazole that blocks gastric acid secretion by selective inhibition of the H$^+$-K$^+$-ATPase proton pump in the parietal cell membrane (Fig. 21-8). Virtual anacidity can be achieved for sustained periods following oral or intravenous administration. In the treatment of gastric ulcer disease, omeprazole is superior to H-2 antagonists (Walan et al, 1989).

CROMOLYN

Cromolyn inhibits antigen-induced release of histamine and other autacoids, including leukotrienes from pulmonary mast cells as well as from mast cells at other sites during antibody-mediated allergic responses (Fig. 21-9). Cromolyn does not prevent the interaction between cell-bound immunoglobulin E and specific antigens, but rather suppresses the secretory response elicited by the reaction. Release of histamine from basophils is not altered by cromolyn. Cromolyn does not relax bronchial or vascular smooth muscle.

The mechanism of action of cromolyn is not known but has been attributed to a membrane-stabilizing action that may reflect blockade of calcium channels. Oral absorption is poor, and the drug is therefore administered by inhalation. After inhalation, 8% to 10% of the drug enters the circulation where it has an elimination half-time of about 80 minutes. Cromolyn is not metabo-

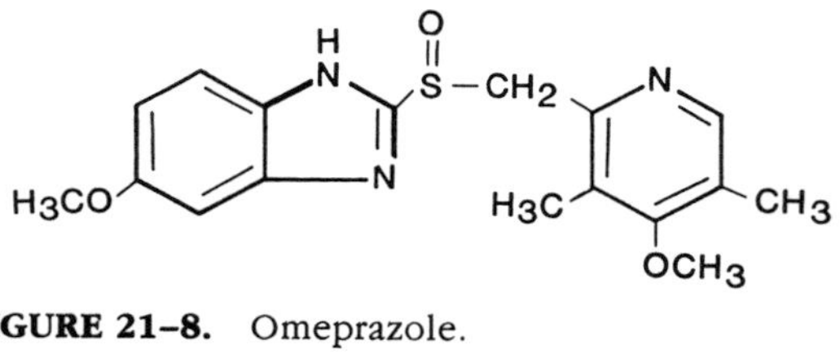

FIGURE 21–8.   Omeprazole.

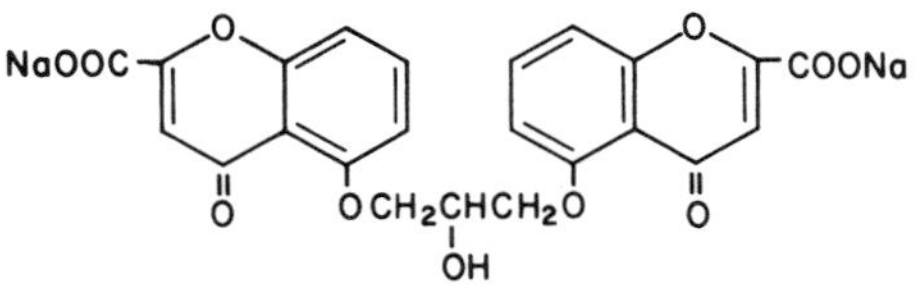

FIGURE 21–9. Cromolyn.

lized, being excreted unchanged in the urine and bile in approximately equal amounts.

Side effects of cromolyn are rare and usually minor. Infrequent but more serious side effects, probably attributable to allergic reactions to the drug, include laryngeal edema, angioedema, urticaria, and anaphylaxis.

The principal use of cromolyn is in the prophylactic treatment of bronchial asthma. Given before an antigenic challenge, cromolyn will inhibit bronchoconstriction and prevent signs and symptoms of an acute asthmatic attack. This protective effect can last for hours. Evidence that cromolyn has no role in the treatment of established bronchoconstriction is the observation that its administration as early as 1 minute after an antigen challenge is ineffective in altering the response.

REFERENCES

Abe K, Shibata M, Demizu A, et al. Effect of oral and intramuscular famotidine on pH and volume of gastric contents. Anesth Analg 1989;68:541–4.

Arrang JM, Garbarg M, Lancelot JC, et al. Highly potent and selective ligands for H_3 receptors. Nature 1987;327:117–23.

Barr GD, Piper DW. Possible ranitidine hepatitis. Med J Aust 1981;2:421.

Bruno LA, Smith DS, Bloom MJ, et al. Sudden hypotension with a test dose of chymopapain. Anesth Analg 1984;63:533–5.

Camarri E, Chirone E, Fanteria G, Zocchi M. Ranitidine induced bradycardia. Lancet 1982;2:160.

Campoli-Richards DM, Clissold SF. Famotidine: Pharmacodynamic and pharmacokinetic properties and a preliminary review of its therapeutic use in peptic ulcer disease and Zollinger-Ellison syndrome. Drugs 1986;32:197–221.

Cohen J, Weetman AP, Dargie HJ, Krikler DM. Life-threatening arrhythmias and intravenous injection of cimetidine. Br Med J 1979;2:768.

Coombs DW, Hooper D, Colton T. Acid aspiration prophylaxis by use of preoperative oral administration of cimetidine. Anesthesiology 1979;51:352–6.

Cristiano P, Paradisi F. Can cimetidine facilitate infections by the oral route? Lancet 1982;2:45.

DeSoto H, Turk P. Cimetidine in anaphylactic shock refractory to standard therapy. Anesth Analg 1989; 69:264–5.

Donovan M, Hagerty A, Pael L, Castleden M, Pohl JEF. Cimetidine and bioavailability of propranolol. Lancet 1981;1:164.

Dubin SA, Silverstein PI, Wakefield ML, Jense HG. Comparison of the effects of oral famotidine and ranitidine on gastric volume and pH. Anesth Analg 1989;69:680–3.

Feely J, Wilkinson GR, McCallister CB, et al. Increased toxicity and reduced clearance of lidocaine by cimetidine. Ann Intern Med 1982;96:592–4.

Feely J, Wilkinson GR, Wood AJJ. Reduction of liver blood flow and propranolol metabolism by cimetidine. N Engl J Med 1981;304:692–5.

Feldman M, Burton ME. Histamine$_2$-receptor antagonists. N Engl J Med 1990;323:1672–80.

Flynn RJ, Moore J, Collier PS, McClean E. Does pretreatment with cimetidine and ranitidine affect the disposition of bupivacaine? Br J Anaesth 1989;62:87–91.

Francis RN, Kwik RSH. Oral ranitidine for prophylaxis against Mendelson's syndrome. Anesth Analg 1982;61:130–2.

Ginsberg R, Bristow MR, Stinson EB, Harrison DC. Histamine receptors in the human heart. Life Sci 1980;26:2245–9.

Goudsouzian N, Cote CJ, Liu LMP, Dedrick DF. The dose-response effects of oral cimetidine on gastric pH and volume in children. Anesthesiology 1981;55:533–6.

Hodgkinson R, Glassenberg R, Joyce TH, Coombs DW, Ostheimer GW, Gibbs CP. Comparison of cimetidine (Tagamet) with antacid for safety and effectiveness in reducing gastric acidity before elective cesarean section. Anesthesiology 1983;59:86–90.

Hosking MP, Lennon RL, Gronert GA. Combined H_1 and H_2 receptor blockade attenuates the cardiovascular effects of high-dose atracurium for rapid sequence endotracheal intubation. Anesth Analg 1988;67:1089–92.

Iberti TJ, Paluch TA, Helmer L, Murgolo VA, Benjamin E. The hemodynamic effects of intravenous cimetidine in intensive care patients: A double-blind, prospective study. Anesthesiology 1986;64:87–9.

Johnston JR, Moore J, McCaughey W, et al. Use of cimetidine as an oral antacid in obstetric anesthesia. Anesth Analg 1983;62:720–6.

Kambam JR, Franks JJ. Cimetidine does not affect plasma cholinesterase activity. Anesth Analg 1988;67:69–70.

Kelly JS, Prielipp RC. Is cimetidine indicated in the treatment of acute anaphylactic shock? Anesth Analg 1990;71:104–5.

Klotz U, Reimann I. Delayed clearance of diazepam

due to cimetidine. N Engl J Med 1980;302:1012–4.

Kuhnert BR, Zuspan KJ, Kuhnert PM, Syracuse CD, Brashear WT, Brown DE. Lack of influence of cimetidine on bupivacaine levels during parturition. Anesth Analg 1987;66:986–90.

Maze M. Clinical implications of membrane receptor function in anesthesia. Anesthesiology 1981; 55:160–71.

Milton-Thompson GJ, Lightfoot NF, Ahmet Z, et al. Intragastric acidity, bacteria, nitrite, and N-nitroso compounds before, during and after cimetidine treatment. Lancet 1982;1:1091–5.

Mogelnicki S, Walle J, Finalyson D. Physostigmine reversal of cimetidine-induced mental confusion. JAMA 1979;241:826–7.

Moss J, Rosow CE. Histamine release by narcotics and muscle relaxants in humans. Anesthesiology 1983; 59:330–9.

Moss J, Roscow CE, Savarose JJ, Philbin DM, Kniffen KJ. Role of histamine in the hypotensive action of d-tubocurarine in man. Anesthesiology 1981;55:19–25.

Philbin DM, Moss J, Akins CW, et al. The use of H_1 and H_2 histamine blockers with high dose morphine anesthesia: A double-blind study. Anesthesiology 1981;55:292–6.

Rosow CE, Basta SJ, Savarese JJ, Ali HH, Kniffen KJ, Moss J. Correlation of cardiovascular effects with increases in plasma histamine. Anesthesiology 1980;53:S270.

Schentag JJ, Cerra FB, Calleri G, DeGlopper E, Ross JQ, Bernard H. Pharmacokinetic and clinical studies in patients with cimetidine associated mental confusion. Lancet 1979;1:177–81.

Shaw RG, Mashford ML, Desmond PV. Cardiac arrest after intravenous injection of cimetidine. Med J Aust 1980;2:629–30.

Stoelting RK. Gastric fluid pH in patients receiving cimetidine. Anesth Analg 1978;57:675–7.

Stoelting RK. Allergic reactions during anesthesia. Anesth Analg 1983;62:341–56.

Viegas OJ, Stoops CA, Ravindran RS. Reversal of cimetidine-induced postoperative somnolence. Anesthesiol Rev 1982;9:30–1.

Walan A, Bader J-P, Classen M, et al. Effect of omeprazole and ranitidine on ulcer healing and relapse rates in patients with benign gastric ulcer. N Engl J Med 1989;320:69–75.

Weber L, Hirshman CA. Cimetidine for prophylaxis of aspiration pneumonitis: Comparison of intramuscular and oral dose schedules. Anesth Analg 1979;58:426–7.

Wood M, Vetrecht J, Pythyon JM, et al. The effect of cimetidine on anesthetic metabolism and toxicity. Anesth Analg 1986;65:481–8.

Woodworth GE, Sears DH, Grove TM, Ruff RH, Kosek, Katz RC. The effect of cimetidine and ranitidine on the duration of action of succinylcholine. Anesth Analg 1989;68:295–7.

Zeldis JB, Friedman LS, Isselbacher KJ. Ranitidine: A new H_2 receptor antagonist. N Engl J Med 1983; 309:1368–73.

Chapter

22

Renin, Plasma Kinins, and Serotonin

RENIN

Renin is a proteolytic enzyme that is synthesized and stored by juxtaglomerular cells present in the walls of renal afferent arterioles as they enter the glomeruli. The most important stimulus for the release of renin is a decrease in renal perfusion pressure associated with hemorrhage, dehydration, chronic sodium ion (Na^+) depletion, or renal artery stenosis. The secretion of renin is also increased by sympathetic nervous system stimulation caused by activation of beta-adrenergic receptors.

Formation of Angiotensins

Release of renin initiates the formation of active hormones known as *angiotensins*. The first step is the reaction of renin with circulating angiotensinogen, a substrate synthesized in the liver, to form a decapeptide prohormone known as *angiotensin I* (Fig. 22-1). This prohormone is promptly hydrolyzed to the octapeptide, angiotensin II, by converting enzyme (peptidyl dipeptidase) that is present in highest concentrations in the lungs. Indeed, the lungs convert 20% to 40% of angiotensin I to angiotensin II in a single circulation. This same converting enzyme is also responsible for the breakdown of plasma kinins, creating the situation in which the most potent endogenous vasoconstrictor (angiotensin II) and vasodilator (bradykinin) are cleared by the same enzyme. Angiotensin II is metabolized to the heptapeptide angiotensin III by aminopeptidase enzyme (Fig. 22-1).

The renin-angiotensin-aldosterone system does not play an active role in the Na^+-repleted patient but is of major importance in maintaining blood pressure and intravascular fluid volume during Na^+ deprivation or in the presence of hypovolemia. Furthermore, plasma renin activity is elevated in only about 15% of patients with essential hypertension. Nevertheless, the frequent efficacy of renin-angiotensin antagonists in treating essential hypertension suggests a much wider involvement than would be indicated solely by elevations in plasma renin activity.

Effects on Organ Systems

Vasoconstriction and stimulation of the synthesis and secretion of aldosterone by the adrenal cortex are the principal pharmacologic effects of angiotensin II. Aldosterone causes renal conservation of Na^+ with retention of water and loss of potassium (K^+) and hydrogen ions (H^+). Other less intense effects include stimulation of the heart and sympathetic nervous system and increased release of antidiuretic hormone. Angiotensin III produces similar but less marked physiologic effects compared with angiotensin II. For example, its pressor effect is less than 50% of that of angiotensin II. Angiotensin III, however, is as potent or more so for evoking output of aldosterone when compared with angiotensin II. Angiotensin I has less than 1% of the activity of

407

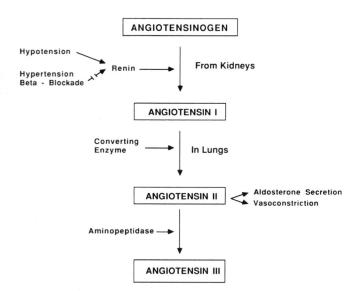

FIGURE 22–1. Schematic diagram of the renin-angiotensin-aldosterone system.

angiotensin II on vascular smooth muscle, the heart, or the adrenal cortex. Effects of angiotensin are most likely mediated through specific receptors on cell membranes.

Cardiovascular Effects

Angiotensin II produces vasoconstriction of precapillary arterioles and, to a lesser extent, postcapillary venules. Angiotensin II is the most powerful endogenous vasoconstrictor, being 40 times more potent than norepinephrine. This intense vasoconstriction reflects a direct action of angiotensin II on vascular smooth muscle and indirect activation of the sympathetic nervous system. The vasoconstrictive effect is greatest in skin, splanchnic vasculature, and kidneys, with blood flow being greatly reduced to these areas. Coronary artery vasoconstriction may jeopardize the adequacy of coronary blood flow. Vasoconstriction is less in cerebral vessels and even weaker in skeletal muscles. In fact, total blood flow in these two regions may increase as the increased perfusion pressure more than offsets a modest increase in systemic vascular resistance. Likewise, changes in pulmonary vascular pressures are usually modest.

Angiotensin II acts directly on cardiac cells to prolong the plateau phase of the cardiac action potential, which increases inward calcium ion (Ca^{2+}) movement that drives the contractile ele-ments. Central and peripheral stimulant effects on the sympathetic nervous system may increase heart rate and myocardial contractility. Nevertheless, increased blood pressure may activate baroreceptors, which reflexively slow heart rate and decrease myocardial contractility. Changes in central venous pressure are modest, since angiotensin II has weak vasoconstrictor effects on large veins and thus reduces venous capacitance less than norepinephrine. The net result of all these changes is often a reduction in cardiac output.

Angiotensin II reduces intravascular fluid volume through loss of extracellular fluid in response to constriction of postcapillary venules, which increases capillary filtration pressure. In addition, angiotensin II increases vascular permeability in large arterioles by causing separation of the endothelial cells.

Central Nervous System

Central nervous system effects of angiotensin II occur despite the fact that peptides are generally regarded as being incapable of crossing the blood-brain barrier. Sustained hypertension reflects enhanced central outflow of sympathetic nervous system impulses caused by effects of angiotensin II on the medullary vasomotor center. Angiotensin II can also enhance release of adrenocorticotrophic hormone, presumably via a central nervous system action.

Peripheral Autonomic Nervous System

Peripheral autonomic nervous system effects of angiotensin II include stimulation of sympathetic nervous system ganglion cells and facilitation of ganglionic transmission. This may result in enhanced responsiveness of the innervated organ to norepinephrine as well as increased output of norepinephrine from postganglionic sympathetic nerve endings. Angiotensin-induced prolongation of the nerve action potential with influx of Ca^{2+} contributes to facilitation of norepinephrine release in response to each nerve impulse.

Angiotensin II stimulates release of catecholamines from the adrenal medulla by directly depolarizing the chromaffin cells. Resulting hypertension may be particularly marked in patients with pheochromocytoma.

Adrenal Cortex

Angiotensin II directly stimulates the synthesis and secretion of aldosterone from the adrenal cortex by facilitating the Ca^{2+}-dependent mechanism necessary for the conversion of cholesterol to pregnenolone. This effect occurs with low concentrations of angiotensin II that lack effects on the blood pressure. Aldosterone subsequently acts on the kidneys to cause retention of Na^+ and excretion of K^+ and H^+. The stimulant effects of angiotensin II on aldosterone secretion are enhanced when the plasma concentration of Na^+ is reduced or when the plasma K^+ concentration is elevated. These changes in responsiveness presumably reflect alterations in the number of receptors for angiotensin II on the zona glomerulosa cells.

In addition to angiotensin II, hyponatremia, hyperkalemia, and adrenocorticotrophic hormone can stimulate the zona glomerulosa of the adrenal cortex to release aldosterone. Indeed, control of aldosterone secretion is not lost following bilateral nephrectomies, although responsiveness is blunted.

Factors that Alter Plasma Renin Activity

Institution of positive end-expiratory pressure results in significant increases in plasma renin activity, plasma aldosterone concentration, and circulating levels of antidiuretic hormone (Annat et al, 1983). Nitroprusside-induced hypotension

is associated with modest increases in plasma renin activity and marked elevations in the plasma concentrations of antidiuretic hormone (Fig. 22-2) (Knight et al, 1983; Zubrow et al, 1983). Propranolol administered during nitroprusside-induced hypotension prevents the usual rise in plasma renin activity (Marshall et al, 1981). Plasma renin activity increases may contribute to tachyphylaxis during infusion of nitroprusside as well as overshoot of blood pressure above predrug levels when nitroprusside is discontinued. In contrast to nitroprusside, blood pressure reductions produced by trimethaphan do not increase plasma renin activity, presumably because blockade of sympathetic nervous system ganglia by this vasodilator inhibits the release of renin (Fig. 22-2) (Knight et al, 1983).

In Na^+-repleted animals, plasma renin activity does not change during anesthesia with halothane, enflurane, or ketamine (Miller et al, 1978b). Conversely, in Na^+-depleted animals, plasma renin activity increases during adminis-

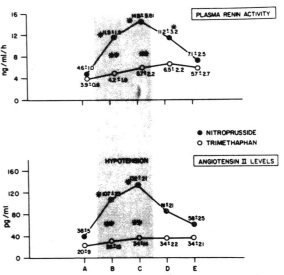

FIGURE 22–2. Plasma renin activity and angiotensin II concentrations are increased during nitroprusside-induced hypotension (O) but not during decreases in blood pressure produced by trimethaphan (●). (From Knight PR, Lane GA, Hensinger RN, Bolles RS, Bjoraker DG. Catecholamine and renin-angiotensin response during hypotensive anesthesia induced by sodium nitroprusside or trimethaphan camsylate. Anesthesiology 1983; 59: 248–53; with permission.)

tration of these anesthetics (Miller et al, 1978a). Furthermore, subsequent infusion of saralasin to these animals accentuates blood pressure decreases, suggesting that the renin-angiotensin-aldosterone system is important in maintaining blood pressure in Na^+-depleted and anesthetized animals. There is no evidence that anesthetics influence the rate of conversion of angiotensin I to angiotensin II (Miller et al, 1979).

Activation of the sympathetic nervous system may contribute to the release of renin via stimulation of beta-adrenergic receptors in the kidneys (Pettinger, 1978). Indeed, plasma renin activity and plasma concentrations of aldosterone increase dramatically during cardiopulmonary bypass (Fig. 22-3) (Bailey et al, 1975). Therefore, the renin-angiotensin-aldosterone system may play a role in blood pressure regulation during cardiopulmonary bypass, which could manifest as urinary excretion of K^+ with associated hypokalemia.

Exogenous Infusion of Angiotensin II

Intravenous infusion of commercially available angiotensin II produces intense vasoconstriction and increases in blood pressure. Too rapid infusion can increase blood pressure to dangerous levels and produce myocardial ischemia. Compared with norepinephrine, angiotensin II has the following effects: (1) it is a more potent vasoconstrictor, (2) it produces a more sustained effect, (3) cardiac dysrhythmias are infrequent, and (4) hypotension is less likely to occur when a

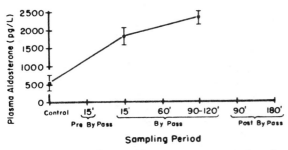

FIGURE 22–3. Plasma aldosterone concentrations increase dramatically during cardiopulmonary bypass. (From Bailey DR, Miller ED, Kaplan JA, Rogers PW. The renin-angiotensin-aldosterone system during cardiac surgery with morphine–nitrous oxide anesthesia. Anesthesiology 1975; 42:538–44; with permission.)

chronic infusion is abruptly discontinued. Spasm of the vein used for intravenous infusion does not occur, and tissue necrosis has not manifested, even with extravasation of angiotensin II. Like norepinephrine, angiotensin II diminishes intravascular fluid volume by promoting the loss of fluid from the circulation to tissues. As a constrictor of capacitance vessels, angiotensin II is less potent than norepinephrine. The lack of a positive inotropic effect on the heart may be a disadvantage of angiotensin II compared with norepinephrine.

Antagonists of the Renin-Angiotensin-Aldosterone System

Antagonists of the renin-angiotensin-aldosterone system act by blocking receptors responsive to angiotensin II (saralasin) and by inhibiting activity of the converting enzyme necessary for conversion of angiotensin I to angiotensin II (captopril). In addition, beta-adrenergic blockade impairs secretion of renin by sympathetic nervous system stimulation of juxtaglomerular cells. Furthermore, clonidine may decrease renin secretion by an action within the central nervous system.

PLASMA KININS

Plasma kinins are polypeptides that include kallidin and bradykinin. These two kinins are the result of enzyme-induced cleavage of kininogens that exist in the plasma as alpha-2 globulins. These alpha-2 globulin enzymes are collectively referred to as *kininogenases* and include kallikreins, trypsin, and plasmin.

Plasma kinins are the most potent endogenous vasodilators known. Furthermore, in low plasma concentrations, kinins (1) increase capillary permeability, (2) produce edema, and (3) evoke intense burning pain by acting on nerve endings. Plasma kinins are about ten times more potent than histamine in causing vasodilation. Injected intravenously, plasma kinins cause flushing in the blush area and dilatation in renal, coronary, and cerebral arterioles. Vasodilation results in marked decreases in systolic and diastolic blood pressure. In contrast to effects on arterioles, plasma kinins tend to constrict large veins, leading to increased venous return. Increased venous return combined with reflexly increased baroreceptor reflex activity owing to diastolic hypotension results in increased cardiac output and heart rate. Increased capillary permeability produced by plasma kinins resembles that occurring in response to histamine and serotonin. Indeed, intradermal injections of plasma kinins produce a "wheal and flare" response. Finally, plasma kinins may increase airway resistance in patients with reactive airway disease, such as bronchial asthma.

Mechanism of Action

Specific plasma kinin receptors are postulated, whereas some responses to kinins may be mediated by production of prostaglandins. Certain of the direct effects on blood vessels may reflect the ability of plasma kinins to evoke the release of histamine from mast cells.

Pharmacokinetics

The elimination half-time of plasma kinins is less than 15 seconds, with more than 90% being metabolized during a single passage through the lungs. Other tissues are also capable of rapidly metabolizing the plasma kinins. The enzyme responsible for this rapid metabolism is known as *converting enzyme* (peptidyl dipeptidase) and is identical to the enzyme necessary for the conversion of angiotensin I to angiotensin II.

Bradykinin

Bradykinin (so named because it produces slow contraction of the gastrointestinal tract) is formed from a high–molecular-weight kininogen by the action of the enzyme kallikrein. Typically, minimal amounts of bradykinin are present because plasma kallikrein circulates in an inactive form known as *prekallikrein*. Changes that activate prekallikrein and lead to the formation of bradykinin include alteration in pH or temperature and contact with negatively charged surfaces such as collagen when exposed by tissue damage. Indeed, many of the factors that activate prekallikrein are involved in factor XII-initiated coagulation and fibrinolysis.

Hereditary angioedema is associated with the absence of the C_1 esterase inhibitor of the complement system, which is also an inhibitor of kallikrein. For this reason, it is speculated that episodes of edema that are characteristic of this disease may be in part due to excess formation of bradykinin. Other diseases that may be associated with excess formation of plasma kinins such as bradykinin include (1) septic shock, (2) allergic reactions, and (3) carcinoid syndrome. Conversely, inadequate amounts of bradykinin may be associated with essential hypertension. Indeed, accumulation of plasma kinins resulting from inhibition of the converting enzyme by captopril may contribute to the blood pressure–lowering effects of this drug.

Aprotinin

Aprotinin is a polypeptide inhibitor of kallikrein that may be useful in the treatment of acute pancreatitis and carcinoid syndrome.

SEROTONIN

Serotonin (5-hydroxytryptamine [5-HT]) is a widely distributed endogenous vasoactive substance (autacoid) that also serves as an inhibitory neurotransmitter in the central nervous system. About 90% of endogenous serotonin is present in enterochromaffin cells of the gastrointestinal tract. The remaining serotonin is present primarily in the central nervous system and in platelets. Mast cells of some species, but not of humans, contain serotonin. The function of serotonin in platelets is unknown but may reflect an inactive storage site for serotonin that escapes from cells, particularly in the gastrointestinal tract. Indeed, the potentiating effect of serotonin on platelet aggregation is small, and platelets depleted of serotonin function normally.

Mechanism of Action

Receptors specific for serotonin are confirmed by the effectiveness of serotonin antagonist drugs. It is likely that subtypes of receptors (5-HT_1; 5-HT_2) that respond to serotonin exist, as emphasized by different responses evoked by various antagonist drugs. For example, methysergide and cyproheptadine antagonize effects of serotonin on peripheral tissues but do not act as antagonists in the central nervous system. Changes in cell membrane permeability to inorganic ions, including Ca^{2+}, seem to be important in the function of serotonin receptors. Likewise, intracellular accumulation of cyclic adenosine monophosphate may be important in serotonin-induced responses.

Serotonin receptors and alpha-receptors have many overlapping functions and may share common binding sites. For example, large doses of serotonin antagonists or alpha-antagonists exert blocking effects at alpha- and serotonin receptors, respectively (Marwood and Stokes, 1984). In animals, pretreatment with ketanserin attenuates opioid-induced skeletal muscle rigidity, suggesting a possible role of central 5-HT_2 receptors in this response (Weinger et al, 1987).

Synthesis and Metabolism

Serotonin is synthesized in cells from tryptophan (Fig. 22-4). In cells, tryptophan is first hydroxylated to 5-hydroxytryptophan, which is then decarboxylated to serotonin by the same nonspecific decarboxylase enzyme that is involved in the synthesis of catecholamines. Tryptophan ingested in food is not available for this endogenous synthesis of serotonin, because it is metabolized in the liver or lungs before it reaches tissue sites. An exception is platelets, which acquire tryptophan derived from exogenous sources during their passage through the gastrointestinal tract. In cells, serotonin is stored in vesicles located in the cytoplasm for subsequent release.

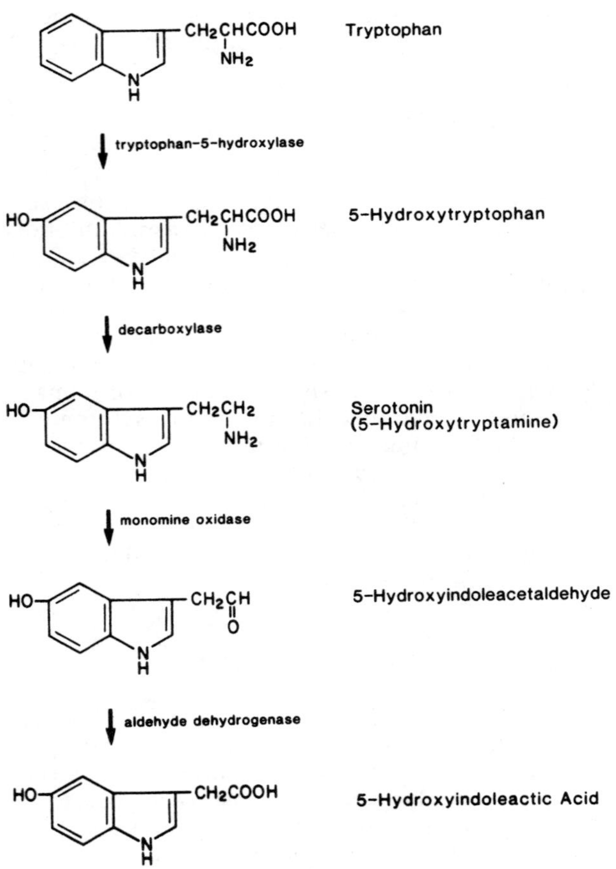

FIGURE 22–4. Synthesis and metabolism of serotonin.

Turnover rates of serotonin in the brain and gastrointestinal tract are about 1 and 17 hours, respectively. Carcinoid tumors that synthesize serotonin may divert so much tryptophan from protein synthesis to production of serotonin that hypoalbuminemia and pellagra result. Serotonin undergoes oxidative deamination by monoamine oxidase, ultimately resulting in the formation of 5-hydroxyindolacetic acid (Fig. 22-4). Patients with carcinoid tumors or those who have just ingested certain foods, such as bananas, manifest an elevated urinary excretion of this metabolite. Oral administration of serotonin followed by measurement of urinary excretion of 5-hydroxyindolacetic acid provides a method for testing the degree of inhibition of monoamine oxidase activity.

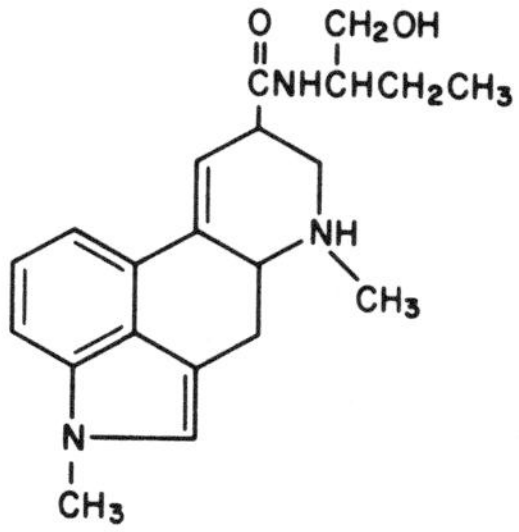

FIGURE 22–5. Methysergide.

Effects on Organ Systems

Serotonin produces vasoconstriction of vascular smooth muscle, particularly in the splanchnic and renal circulations. Cerebral vasoconstriction may be marked. Pulmonary vasoconstriction induced by serotonin is less prominent in humans than in other species. Vasodilation occurs in skeletal muscles and skin, producing an intense flush response followed by cyanosis, presumably indicating stasis owing to venoconstriction. Indeed, serotonin acts as a potent constrictor of veins. Positive inotropic and chronotropic actions of serotonin are masked by reflex-mediated baroreceptor responses.

Bronchoconstriction is a prominent response to serotonin in animals but rarely in humans, except perhaps in patients with bronchial asthma. Motility of the gastrointestinal tract is greatly increased by circulating serotonin. Serotonin present in the peripheral circulation penetrates the blood-brain barrier poorly, producing minimal central nervous system effects.

Antagonists

Tricyclic antidepressants inhibit the uptake of serotonin back into tryptaminergic nerve endings similar to the effect exerted on catecholamines. A long-lasting depletion of serotonin is produced by the anorexiant drug fenfluramine. Lysergic acid derivatives are specific competitive antagonists at receptors normally responsive to serotonin. Other drugs that act as serotonin antagonists include H-1 receptor blockers of the ethylenediamine type; phenothiazines, especially chlorpromazine; and beta-haloalkylamines, such as phenoxybenzamine.

Methysergide

Methysergide is a congener of lysergic acid but lacks significant central nervous system effects (Fig. 22-5). It inhibits peripheral vasoconstriction evoked by serotonin. Clinical uses include prophylaxis against development of migraine and other vascular headaches. This drug is not effective after a headache has developed. Methysergide is useful in treating malabsorption and diarrhea in patients with carcinoid syndrome. It may also alleviate similar symptoms in patients with postgastrectomy dumping syndrome. Methysergide depresses prolactin secretion, perhaps by dopamine-like actions. An infrequent but serious side effect of treatment with methysergide is an inflammatory reaction that may manifest as retroperitoneal, pleuropulmonary, coronary, or endocardial fibrosis.

Cyproheptadine

Cyproheptadine resembles the structure of H-1 receptor antagonists and is able to block receptors for both histamine and serotonin (Fig. 22-6). In addition, this drug possesses weak anticholinergic activity and mild central nervous system depressant properties. The actions of cyproheptadine as an antagonist during allergic reactions are not relevant, because serotonin is not involved in human allergic responses. Uses of this drug are in the treatment of intestinal hypermo-

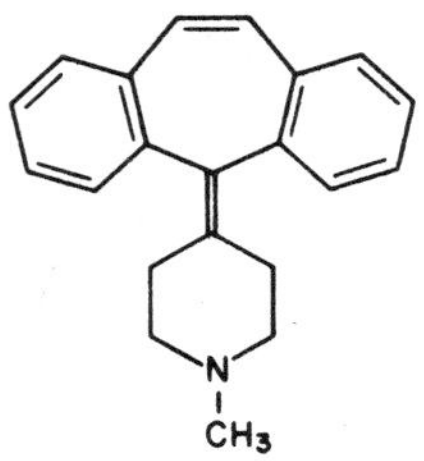

FIGURE 22–6. Cyproheptadine.

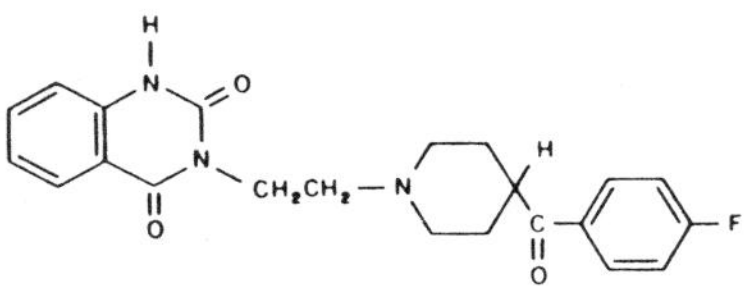

FIGURE 22–7. Ketaneserin.

tility associated with carcinoid syndrome and in the postgastrectomy dumping syndrome. Side effects of cyproheptadine include sedation and dry mouth, as a reflection of H-1 receptor antagonism. Increased growth in children has been observed, perhaps as a result of altered secretion of insulin and growth hormone.

Ketanserin

Ketanserin is a quinazoline derivative that selectively antagonizes the effects of serotonin at peripheral $5\text{-}HT_2$ receptors, thus attenuating serotonin-induced vasoconstriction, bronchoconstriction, and platelet aggregation (Fig. 22-7) (Marwood and Stokes, 1984). This drug, however, is nonspecific in that it has substantial affinity for alpha-1 receptors, H-1 receptors, and, to a lesser degree, dopamine receptors. In addition, ketanserin appears to inhibit sympathetic nervous system outflow from the central nervous system.

Uses of ketanserin include treatment of patients with carcinoid (5 to 30 mg IV infused over 3 minutes) and management of hypertension. It is possible that the antihypertensive effects of this drug reflect alpha-1 antagonist effects unrelated to actions at serotonin receptors.

REFERENCES

Annat G, Viale JP, Xuan BB, et al. Effect of PEEP ventilation on renal function, plasma renin, aldosterone, neurophysins and urinary ADH, and prostaglandins. Anesthesiology 1983;58:136–141.

Bailey DR, Miller ED, Kaplan JA, Rogers PW. The renin-angiotensin-aldosterone system during cardiac surgery with morphine-nitrous oxide anesthesia. Anesthesiology 1975;42:538–44.

Knight PR, Lane GA, Hensinger RN, Bolles RS, Bjoraker DG. Catecholamine and renin-angiotensin response during hypotensive anesthesia induced by sodium nitroprusside or trimethaphan camsylate. Anesthesiology 1983;59:248–53.

Marshall WK, Bedford RF, Arnold WP, et al. Effects of propranolol on the cardiovascular and renin-angiotensin systems during hypotension produced by sodium nitroprusside in humans. Anesthesiology 1981;55:277–80.

Marwood JF, Stokes GS. Serotonin (5HT) and its antagonists: Involvement in cardiovascular system. Clin Exp Pharmacol Physiol 1984;11:439–56.

Miller ED, Ackerly JA, Peach MJ. Blood pressure support during general anesthesia in a renin-dependent state in the rat. Anesthesiology 1978a;48:404–8.

Miller ED, Gianfagna W, Ackerly JA, Peach MJ. Converting-enzyme activity and pressure responses to angiotensin I and II in the rat awake and during anesthesia. Anesthesiology 1979;50:88–92.

Miller ED, Longnecker DE, Peach MJ. The regulatory function of the renin-angiotensin system during general anesthesia. Anesthesiology 1978b;48:399–403.

Pettinger WA. Anesthetics and the renin-angiotensin-aldosterone axis (editorial). Anesthesiology 1978; 48:393–6.

Weinger MB, Cline EJ, Smith NT, Koob GF. Ketanserin pretreatment reverses alfentanil-induced muscle rigidity. Anesthesiology 1987;67:348–54.

Zubrow AB, Daniel SS, Startk RI, Husain MK, James LS. Plasma renin, catecholamine, and vasopressin during nitroprusside-induced hypotension in ewes. Anesthesiology 1983;58:245–9.

Chapter

23

Hormones as Drugs

INTRODUCTION

Preparations that contain active hormones secreted endogenously by endocrine glands may be administered as drugs. These synthetic hormones resemble the endogenous substances in structure and activity. Typically, the clinical application of these drugs is for hormone replacement to provide a physiologic effect. In certain patients, however, large doses of the synthetic hormone are used to exert a pharmacologic effect. Recombinant deoxyribonucleic acid (DNA) technology permits the incorporation of synthetic genes that code for the synthesis of specific human hormones by bacteria, thus permitting production of pure hormones devoid of allergenic properties.

ANTERIOR PITUITARY HORMONES

Anterior pituitary hormones include (1) growth hormone, (2) prolactin, (3) gonadotropins, including luteinizing hormone and follicle stimulating hormone, (4) adrenocorticotrophic hormone (ACTH), and (5) thyroid stimulating hormone (TSH). Growth hormone, gonadotropins, and ACTH can be administered in the form of synthetic drugs.

Perioperative replacement of anterior pituitary hormones may be necessary for patients receiving exogenous hormones because of prior hypophysectomy. For example, cortisol must be provided continuously. Conversely, thyroid hormone has such a long elimination half-time that it can be omitted for several days without adverse effects. Likewise, the loss of other anterior pituitary hormones has no immediate implications.

Growth Hormone

Growth hormone is used to treat hypopituitary dwarfism, based on documentation that the plasma concentration of the hormone is inadequate. In this regard, radioimmunoassays for growth hormone are used to measure plasma concentrations of the hormone. Treatment must be maintained for several months or years, corresponding to childhood. Injection of hormone at weekly intervals is usually adequate for treatment, despite an elimination half-time of about 20 minutes.

Gonadotropins

Gonadotropins are used most often for the treatment of infertility and cryptorchism. Induction of ovulation can be stimulated in females who are infertile because of pituitary insufficiency. Excessive ovarian enlargement and maturation of many follicles leading to multiple births is a possibility. Gonadotropins are effective only by parenteral injection. Radioimmunoassays are useful in measuring the plasma and urine concentrations of gonadotropins.

Adrenocorticotrophic Hormone

The physiologic and pharmacologic effects of ACTH result from this hormone's stimulation of secretion of corticosteroids from the adrenal cortex, principally cortisol. An important clinical use of ACTH is as a diagnostic aid in patients with suspected adrenal insufficiency. For example, a normal increase in the plasma concentration of cortisol in response to administration of ACTH rules out primary adrenocortical insufficiency. Furthermore, ACTH may be administered therapeutically to evoke the release of cortisol. Treatment of disease states with ACTH is not physiologically equivalent to administration of a specific hormone, because ACTH exposes the tissues to a mixture of glucocorticoids, mineralocorticoids, and androgens. Indeed, there may be associated retention of sodium ions (Na^+), development of hypokalemic metabolic alkalosis, and appearance of acne, which are unlikely to accompany selective acting corticosteroids.

Absorption of ACTH after intramuscular injection is prompt. Following intravenous injection, ACTH disappears rapidly from the plasma, with an elimination half-time of about 15 minutes. Maximal stimulation of the adrenal cortex is produced by ACTH, 25 units, absorbed over 8 hours. Allergic reactions ranging from mild fever to life-threatening anaphylaxis may be associated with administration of ACTH.

THYROID GLAND HORMONES

The thyroid gland is the source of triiodothyronine (T_3), thyroxine (T_4), and calcitonin (Fig. 23-1). Commercial preparations of T_3 and T_4 are available for treatment of hypothyroidism, as may be encountered in patients with a simple goiter. The effectiveness of treatment is judged by the return of the plasma concentration of TSH to normal and a decrease in the size of the goiter. Certain carcinomas of the thyroid gland, particularly papillary tumors, may remain sensitive to TSH. Indeed, administration of thyroid hormones may suppress this responsiveness and cause regression of the malignant lesion. Thyroid hormones enhance the effects of coumarin anticoagulants by increasing catabolism of vitamin K–dependent clotting factors. Cholestyramine binds orally administered thyroid hormone in the gastrointestinal tract.

Levothyroxine

Levothyroxine is the most frequently administered drug for treatment of diseases requiring thyroid hormone replacement. Oral administration is preferred, but intravenous injection is acceptable in emergency situations. Most patients can be maintained in a euthyroid state with 100 to 200 mg daily.

Liothyronine

Liothyronine is the levorotatory isomer of T_3, being 2.5 to 3 times as potent as levothyroxine. Its rapid onset and short duration of action preclude use of liothyronine for long-term thyroid replacement.

DRUGS THAT INHIBIT THYROID HORMONE SYNTHESIS

A large number of substances are capable of interfering with the synthesis of thyroid hormones. These compounds include (1) antithyroid drugs, (2) inhibitors of the iodide transport mechanism, (3) iodide, and (4) radioactive iodine.

Antithyroid Drugs

Propylthiouracil and methimazole are antithyroid drugs that inhibit the formation of thyroid hormone by interfering with the incorporation of iodine into tyrosine residues of thyroglobulin (Fig. 23-2) (Cooper, 1984). In addition to blocking hormone synthesis, these drugs also inhibit the peripheral deiodination of T_4 to T_3. These drug-induced effects on thyroid hormone synthesis render antithyroid drugs useful in the treat-

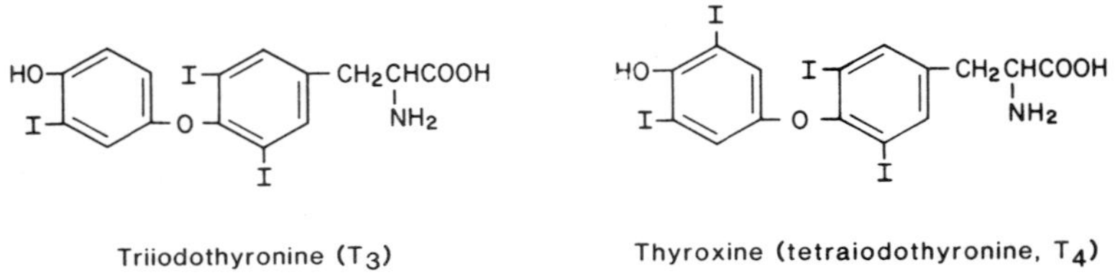

Triiodothyronine (T_3)

Thyroxine (tetraiodothyronine, T_4)

FIGURE 23–1. Thyroid gland hormones.

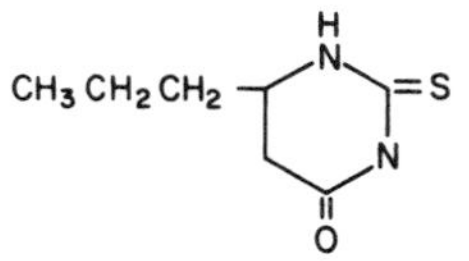

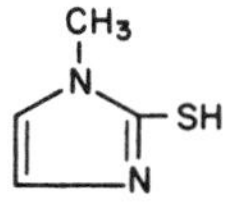

FIGURE 23-2. Antithyroid drugs.

ment of hyperthyroidism prior to elective thyroidectomy.

Antithyroid drugs are not available as parenteral preparations, necessitating their administration by way of a gastric tube if drugs cannot be administered orally, such as during thyroid storm. Drug-induced reductions in excessive thyroid activity usually require several days, because preformed hormone must be depleted before symptoms begin to wane. In a few patients, especially those with severe hyperthyroidism, definite improvement is evident in 1 to 2 days.

Side Effects

The incidence of side effects produced by propylthiouracil and methiamazole are similar. The most common reaction is an urticarial or papular skin rash often associated with pruritus that occurs in about 3% of patients. This rash may disappear spontaneously without interrupting treatment. In others, this side effect necessitates changing to the other drug, since cross-sensitivity is not likely.

Granulocytopenia and agranulocytosis are serious but rare side effects that are most likely to occur in the first 2 months of therapy with an antithyroid drug. Periodic white blood cell counts, although helpful for detecting gradual reductions in the leukocyte count, should not be relied on to detect agranulocytosis because of the rapidity with which this complication can develop. Fever or pharyngitis may be the earliest manifestation of the development of agranulocytosis. Recovery is likely if the antithyroid drug is discontinued at the first sign of this side effect.

Antithyroid drugs cross the placenta and appear in breast milk. Placental passage, however, is limited for propylthiouracil, making it the preferred drug for use in the parturient.

Inhibitors of Iodine Transport Mechanisms

Inhibitors of iodide transport mechanisms are thiocyanate and perchlorate. These ions are similar in size to iodide and, in some way, interfere with the uptake of iodide ions by the thyroid gland. Thiocyanate can result from the metabolism of nitroprusside or ingestion of cabbage, neither of which is likely to be clinically significant. Perchlorate is capable of producing aplastic anemia and is thus rarely used.

Iodide

Iodide is the oldest available therapy for hyperthyroidism, providing a paradoxical treatment that is effective for reasons that are not fully understood. The response of the patient with hyperthyroidism to iodide is often discernible within 24 hours, emphasizing that release of hormone into the circulation is quickly interrupted. Indeed, the most important clinical effect of high doses of iodide is inhibition of the release of thyroid hormone. This may reflect the ability of iodide to antagonize the ability of both TSH and cyclic adenosine monophosphate to stimulate hormone release.

Iodide is particularly useful in the treatment of hyperthyroidism prior to elective thyroidectomy. Indeed, the combination of oral potassium iodide and propranolol is a recommended approach (Feek et al, 1980). Vascularity of the thyroid gland is also reduced by iodide therapy. Chronic treatment with iodide, however, is often associated with a recurrence of previously suppressed excessive thyroid gland activity.

Allergic reactions may accompany treatment with iodide or administration of organic preparations that contain iodine. Angioedema and laryngeal edema may become life-threatening.

Radioactive Iodine

Among the radioactive isotopes of iodine, ^{131}I is the most frequently administered. This isotope is rapidly and efficiently trapped by thyroid gland cells, and the subsequent emission of destructive beta rays acts almost exclusively on these cells with little or no damage to surrounding tissue. It is possible to completely destroy the thyroid gland with [131]I. Indeed, hypothyroidism occurs in about 10% of treated patients in the first year following ^{131}I administration and increases about 2% to 3% each year thereafter. For this reason, iatrogenic hypothyroidism must be considered preoperatively in any patient who has previously been treated with [131]I.

Hyperthyroidism is treated with orally administered ^{131}I, with symptoms of excessive thyroid gland activity gradually abating over a period of 2 to 3 months. One half to two thirds of patients are cured by a single dose of isotope, and the remainder require an additional one to two doses. Despite the safety and effectiveness of ^{131}I, surgery is often selected for patients younger than 30 years of age because of the concern about potential carcinogenic effects of radiation. Nevertheless, there is no evidence that ^{131}I has ever caused cancer in adults.

The principal indication for ^{131}I treatment is hyperthyroidism in elderly patients and in those with heart disease. Indeed, hypothyroidism is not a common sequela following treatment with ^{131}I for toxic nodular goiter, the usual cause of hyperthyroidism in elderly patients. The use of ^{131}I is contraindicated during pregnancy, because the fetal thyroid gland would concentrate the isotope.

Most thyroid carcinomas except for follicular carcinoma accumulate little radioactive iodine. As a result, the therapeutic usefulness of ^{131}I for treatment of thyroid carcinoma is limited.

OVARIAN HORMONES

An understanding of the synthesis and action of ovarian hormones, including estrogens and progesterone, permits therapeutic interventions in certain disease states. Equally important is the therapeutic use of drugs that can mimic effects of these hormones and act as contraceptives.

Estrogens

Estrogens are effective in treating unpleasant side effects of menopause (Fig. 23-3). Senile or atrophic vaginitis responds to topical estrogen. There is no evidence that administration of estrogen delays the progression of atherosclerosis in postmenopausal women. Treatment of postmenopausal osteoporosis is as effective with calcium ions (Ca^{2+}) as with estrogens. Estrogens are administered to decrease milk production in the postpartum period. The presence of receptors for estrogen increases the likelihood of a palliative response to estrogen therapy in women with metastatic breast cancer. An important use of estrogens is in combination with progestins as oral contraceptives.

Route of Administration

The absorption of most estrogens and their derivatives from the gastrointestinal tract is prompt and nearly complete. Metabolism in the liver,

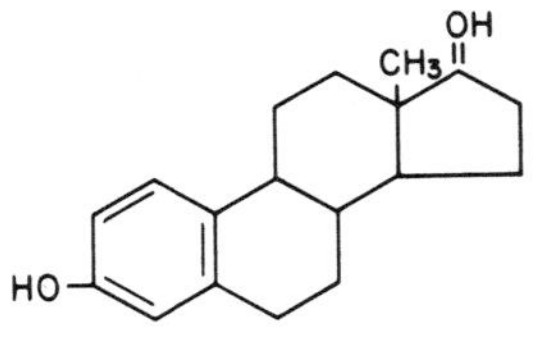

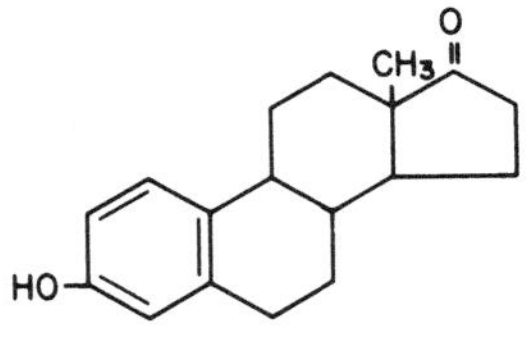

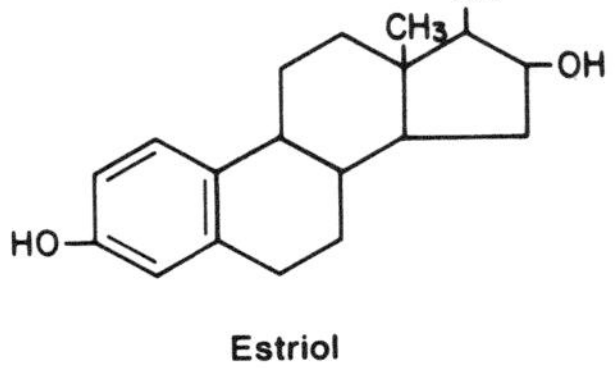

FIGURE 23–3.   Estrogens.

however, limits the effectiveness of orally administered estrogens. Topical and intramuscular administration of estrogens is also effective. Radioimmunoassay methods are highly specific and sensitive for measuring the plasma concentrations of estrogens.

Side Effects

The most frequent unpleasant symptom associated with the use of estrogens is nausea. Large doses of estrogens may cause retention of Na^+ and water, which is particularly undesirable in patients with cardiac or renal disease. There is an increased incidence of vaginal and cervical adenocarcinoma in daughters of mothers treated with diethylstilbestrol or other synthetic estrogens during the first trimester of pregnancy. Most of the affected women have been 20 to 25 years of age when diagnosed. Use of estrogen by postmenopausal women increases the risk of developing endometrial carcinoma.

Antiestrogens

Clomiphene and tamoxifen act as antiestrogens by binding to estrogen receptors (Fig. 23-4). The subsequent loss of normal feedback inhibition of estrogen synthesis causes an increased secretion of gonadotropins. The most prominent effect of increased plasma concentrations of gonadotropins is enlargement of the ovaries and enhancement of fertility in otherwise infertile women.

Progesterone

Orally active derivatives of progesterone are designated progestins (Fig. 23-5). Progestins are often combined with estrogens as oral contraceptives. Dysfunctional uterine bleeding can be treated with small doses of a progestin for a few days, with the goal being induction of progesterone-withdrawal bleeding. Progestins, like estrogens, are effective in suppressing lactation in the immediate postpartum period. Palliative treatment of metastatic endometrial carcinoma is achieved with progestins. Absorption of progestins from the gastrointestinal tract is rapid, but hepatic first pass metabolism is extensive.

Oral Contraceptives

Oral contraceptives are most often a combination of an estrogen and a progestin. This combination inhibits ovulation, presumably by preventing release of follicle-stimulating hormone by estrogen and luteinizing hormone by progesterone.

Side Effects

Estrogens in combined preparations are believed to be responsible for most, if not all, the side effects of oral contraceptives. For example, estrogens seem to be responsible for the increased incidence of thrombophlebitis and thromboembolism. Indeed, patients taking estrogens manifest increased blood concentrations of some clotting factors as well as increased platelet aggregation. Nausea, vomiting, weight gain, and discomfort in the breasts resemble early pregnancy and are attributable to the estrogen component of oral contraceptives. The incidence of myocardial infarction and stroke is increased in patients who chronically take oral contraceptives (Kaplan, 1978). Hypertension occurs in about 5% of females taking oral contraceptives chronically (Laragh, 1976). This response probably reflects estrogen-induced increases in circulating plasma concentrations of renin and angiotensin, with associated retention of Na^+ and water.

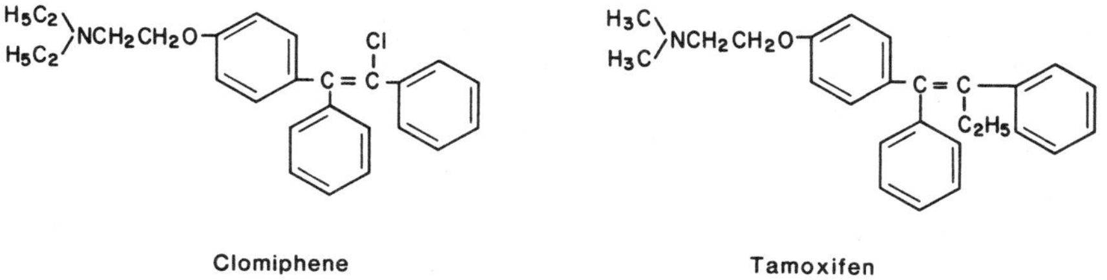

Clomiphene

Tamoxifen

FIGURE 23–4. Antiestrogens.

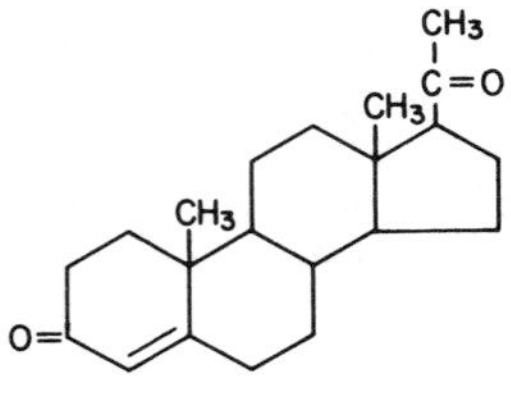

Progesterone

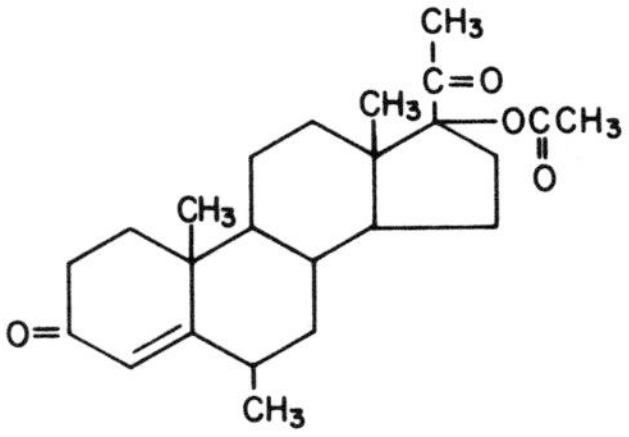

Medroxyprogesterone Acetate

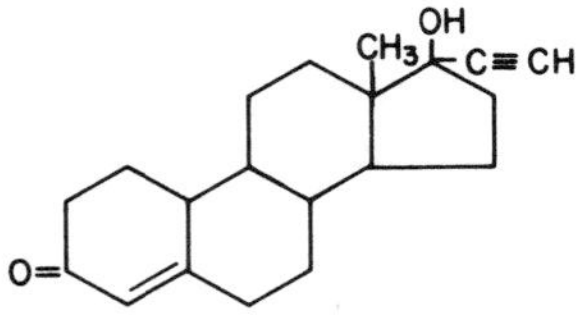

Norethindrone

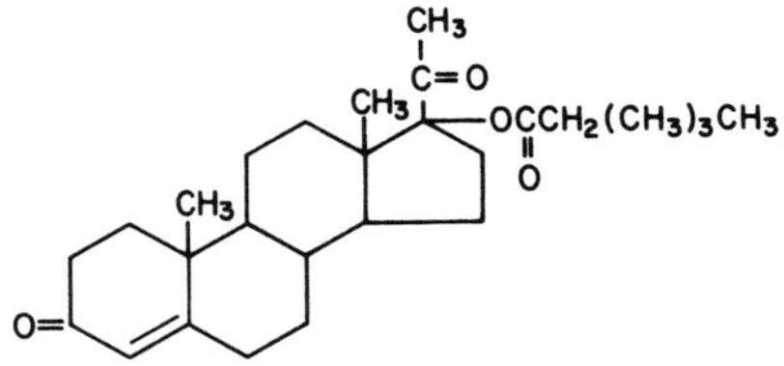

Hydroxyprogesterone Caproate

FIGURE 23–5. Progestins.

Oral contraceptives containing high doses of estrogen may produce alterations in the glucose tolerance curve of patients with preclinical diabetes mellitus. These drugs increase the concentration of cholesterol in bile, which is consistent with an increased incidence of cholelithiasis. Benign hepatomas have been associated with the use of oral contraceptives. An increased incidence of breast tumors in patients taking estrogen-containing oral contraceptives has not been demonstrated. Depression of mood and fatigue have been attributed to the progestin component of oral contraceptives.

ANDROGENS

Androgens are most often administered to males to stimulate the development and maintenance of secondary sexual characteristics (Fig. 23-6). The most common indication for androgen therapy in females is palliative management of metastatic carcinoma of the breast. Androgens enhance erythropoiesis by stimulation of renal production of erythropoietin as well as by a direct dose-related stimulation of erythropoietin-sensitive elements in bone marrow. In addition, there is a drug-induced increase in 2,3-diphosphoglycerate levels, which decreases hemoglobin affinity for oxygen, thus enhancing the availability of oxygen to tissues. For these reasons, androgen therapy is often instituted in the patient with aplastic anemia, hemolytic anemia, and anemia associated with chronic renal failure. Androgen-anabolic steroids have been used in the treatment of chronic debilitating diseases. These drugs promote a feeling of well-being and may improve appetite when administered to patients with terminal illnesses. The efficacy of anabolic steroids to improve athletic performance is not documented and is condemned on ethical grounds. Finally, androgens are useful in the treatment of hereditary angioedema (see the section entitled "Danazol").

Route of Administration

Testosterone administered orally is readily absorbed but is metabolized so extensively by the liver that therapeutic effects do not occur. Alkylation of androgens at the 17 position retards their hepatic metabolism and permits such derivatives to be effective orally (Fig. 23-6). About 99% of

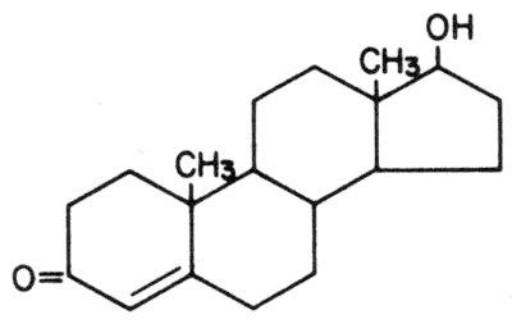

FIGURE 23–6. Androgens.

testosterone circulating in the plasma is bound to sex hormone–binding globulin. As a result, this globulin determines the concentration of free testosterone in the plasma and thus its elimination half-time, which is 10 to 20 minutes.

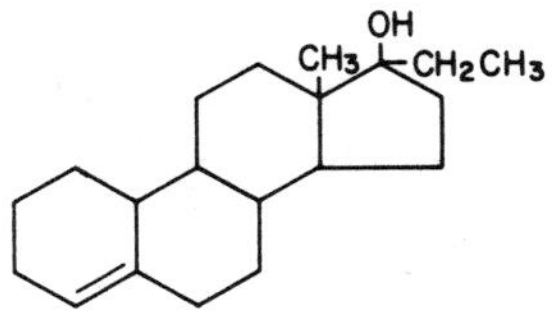

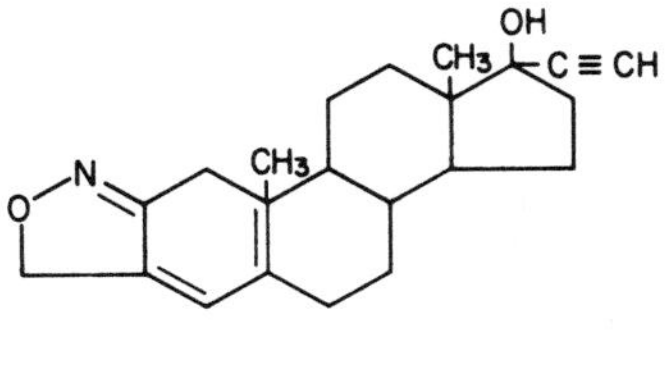

Side Effects

Dose-related cholestatic hepatitis and jaundice are particularly likely to accompany androgen therapy for palliation in neoplastic disease. Elevations in plasma alkaline phosphatase and transaminase enzymes are also likely. Prolonged therapy (longer than 1 year) with androgens, as for management of anemia, is associated with an increased incidence of hepatic adenocarcinoma. Retention of Na^+ and water is also likely to accompany palliative treatment of cancer with high doses of androgens. Androgens increase the potency of coumarin anticoagulants and the likelihood of spontaneous hemorrhage. Androgens can decrease the concentration of thyroid-binding globulin in plasma and thus influence thyroid function tests.

Danazol

The low androgenic activity of danazol makes it the preferred androgen for treatment of hereditary angioedema (Fig. 23-6). There is a remission of symptoms as well as increased production of previously deficient plasma protein factors. As with other androgens, danazol therapy has been associated with abnormal liver function tests and jaundice. Danazol also reduces breast pain and nodularity in many women with fibrocystic breast disease. Symptoms of endometriosis are reduced, and fertility is often restored by danazol. In patients with hemophilia A, danazol increases factor VIII activity and reduces the incidence of hemorrhage (Gralnick et al, 1985).

CORTICOSTEROIDS

The actions of corticosteroids are classified according to the potencies of these compounds to (1) evoke distal renal tubular reabsorption of Na^+ in exchange for potassium ions (K^+) (mineralocorticoid effect), or (2) produce an anti-inflammatory response (glucocorticoid effect). Naturally occurring corticosteroids are cortisol (hydrocortisone), cortisone, corticosterone, desoxycorticosterone, and aldosterone (Fig. 23-7). Several synthetic corticosteroids are available, principally for use to produce anti-inflammatory effects. Although it is possible to separate mineralocorticoid and glucocorticoid effects using synthetic drugs, it has not been possible to separate the various components of the glucocorticoid effects. Consequently, all synthetic corticosteroids, when used in pharmacologic doses for their anti-inflammatory effects, also produce less desirable effects, such as suppression of the hypothalamic-pituitary-adrenal axis, weight gain, and skeletal muscle wasting.

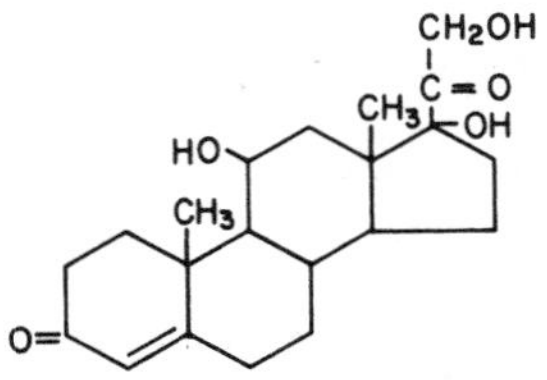

Cortisol

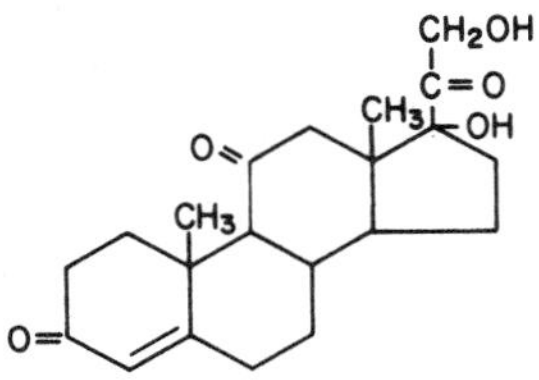

Cortisone

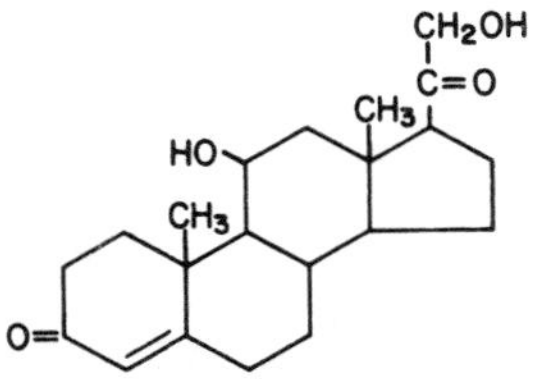

Corticosterone

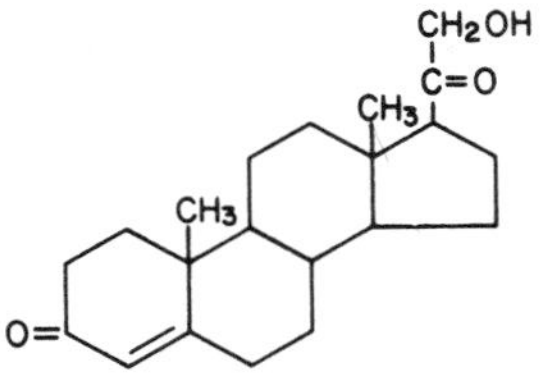

Desoxycorticosterone

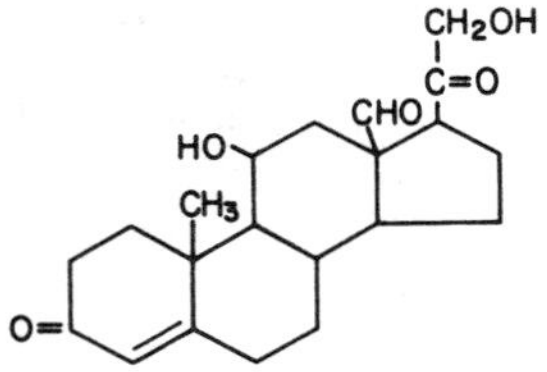

Aldosterone

FIGURE 23–7. Endogenous corticosteroids.

Structure Activity Relationships

All corticosteroids are constructed on the same primary molecular framework, designated as the steroid nucleus (Fig. 23-7). Changes in molecular structure may result in altered biologic responses owing to changes in absorption, protein binding, rate of metabolism, and intrinsic effectiveness of the drug at receptors. Modifications of structure, such as the introduction of a double bond in prednisolone and prednisone, have resulted in synthetic corticosteroids with more potent glucocorticoid effects than the two closely related natural hormones, cortisol and cortisone, respectively (Table 23-1). At the same time, mineralocorticoid effects and the rate of hepatic metabolism of these synthetic drugs are less than those of the natural hormones. Despite increased anti-inflammatory effects, it has not been possible to separate this response from alterations in carbohydrate and protein metabolism. This suggests that the multiple manifestations of drug-induced glucocorticoid effects are mediated by the same receptor.

Pharmacokinetics

Synthetic cortisol and its derivatives are effective orally (Table 23-1). Antacids, but not food, interfere with the oral absorption of corticosteroids. Water-soluble cortisol succinate can be administered intravenously to achieve prompt elevations in plasma concentrations. More prolonged effects are possible with intramuscular injection. Cortisone acetate may be given orally or intramuscularly but cannot be given intravenously. The acetate preparation is a slow-release preparation lasting 8 to 12 hours. After release, cortisone is converted into cortisol in the liver. Cortico-

Table 23-1

Comparative Pharmacology of Endogenous and Synthetic Corticosteroids

	Anti-inflammatory Potency	Sodium Retaining Potency	Equivalent Dose (mg)	Elimination Half-Time (h)	Duration of Action	Route of Administration
Cortisol	1	1	20	1.5–3	8–12	Oral, IV, IM, IA
Cortisone	0.8	0.8	25	0.5	8–36	Oral, IM
Prednisolone	4	0.8	5	2–4	12–36	Oral, IV, IM, IA
Prednisone	4	0.8	5	3–4	18–36	Oral
Methylprednisolone	5	05	4	2–4	12–36	Oral, IV, IM, IA
Betamethasone	25	0	0.75	5	36–54	Oral, IV, IM, IA
Dexamethasone	25	0	0.75	3.5–5	36–54	Oral, IV, IM, IA
Triamcinolone	5	0	4	3.5	12–36	Oral, IM, IA
Fludrocortisone	10	125	—	—	24	Oral

IV, intravenous; IM, intramuscular; IA, intraarticular.

steroids are also promptly absorbed after topical application or aerosol administration.

Cortisol is highly bound (90% or more) in the plasma to corticosteroid-binding globulin. Nevertheless, cortisol and related compounds readily cross the placenta. Small amounts of cortisol appear unchanged in the urine, but at least 70% is conjugated in the liver to inactive or poorly active metabolites. These water-soluble conjugated metabolites appear in the urine. The elimination half-time of cortisol is 1.5 to 3 hours (Table 23-1).

Synthetic Corticosteroids

Synthetic corticosteroids administered for their glucocorticoid effects include prednisolone, prednisone, methylprednisolone, betamethasone, dexamethasone, and triamcinolone (Table 23-1, Fig. 23-8). Fludrocortisone is a synthetic halogenated derivative of cortisol, administered for its mineralocorticoid effect (Table 23-1, Fig. 23-8). Naturally occurring corticosteroids, such as cortisol and cortisone, are also available as synthetic drugs (Table 23-1; Fig. 23-7.)

Prednisolone

Prednisolone is an analogue of cortisol that is available as an oral or parenteral preparation. The anti-inflammatory effect of 5 mg of prednisolone is equivalent to that of 20 mg of cortisol. This drug and prednisolone are suitable for sole re-

placement therapy in adrenocortical insufficiency because of the presence of glucocorticoid and mineralocorticoid effects.

Prednisone

Prednisone is an analogue of cortisone that is available as an oral or parenteral preparation. It is rapidly converted to prednisolone after its absorption from the gastrointestinal tract. Its anti-inflammatory effect and clinical uses are similar to those of prednisolone.

Methylprednisolone

Methylprednisolone is the methyl derivative of prednisolone. The anti-inflammatory effect of 4 mg of methylprednisolone is equivalent to that of 20 mg of cortisol. The acetate preparation administered intraarticularly has a prolonged effect. Methylprednisolone succinate is highly soluble in water and is used intravenously to produce an intense glucocorticoid effect.

Betamethasone

Betamethasone is a fluorinated derivative of prednisolone. The anti-inflammatory effect of 0.75 mg is equivalent to that of 20 mg of cortisol. Betamethasone lacks the mineralocorticoid properties of cortisol and thus is not acceptable for sole replacement therapy in adrenocortical insufficiency. Oral or parenteral administration is acceptable.

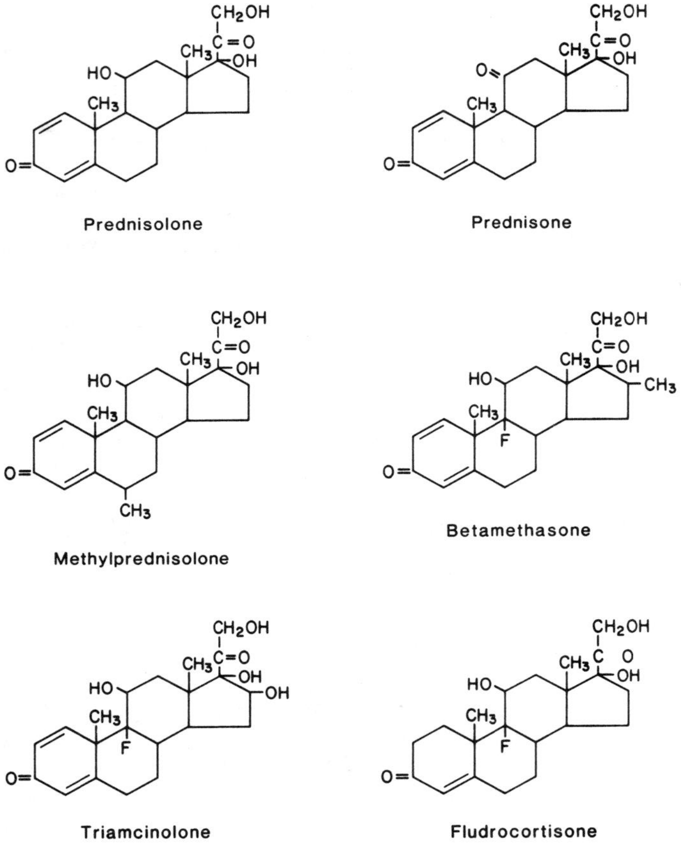

FIGURE 23–8. Synthetic corticosteroids.

Dexamethasone

Dexamethasone is a fluorinated derivative of prednisolone and an isomer of betamethasone. The anti-inflammatory effect of 0.75 mg is equivalent to that of 20 mg of cortisol. Oral and parenteral preparations are available. The acetate preparation is used as a long-acting repository suspension. Dexamethasone sodium phosphate is water soluble, rendering it appropriate for parenteral use. This corticosteroid is commonly chosen to treat certain types of cerebral edema.

Triamcinolone

Triamcinolone is a fluorinated derivative of prednisolone. The anti-inflammatory effect of 4 mg is equivalent to that of 20 mg of cortisol.

Triamcinolone has less mineralocorticoid effect than does prednisolone. Oral and parenteral preparations are available. The hexacetonide preparation injected intraarticularly may provide therapeutic effects for 3 months or longer. This drug is often used for epidural injections in the treatment of lumbar disc disease.

During the first days of treatment with triamcinolone, mild diuresis with Na^+ loss may occur. Conversely, edema may occur in patients with decreased glomerular filtration rates. Triamcinolone does not increase K^+ loss except when administered in large doses.

An unusual adverse side effect of triamcinolone is an increased incidence of skeletal muscle weakness. Likewise, anorexia rather than appetite stimulation, and sedation rather than euphoria, may accompany administration of triamcinolone.

Clinical Uses

The only universally accepted clinical use of corticosteroids and their synthetic derivatives is as replacement therapy for deficiency states. With this exception, the use of corticosteroids in disease states is empirical and not curative, although anti-inflammatory responses exert an intense palliative effect. The safety of corticosteroids is such that it is acceptable to administer a single large dose in a life-threatening situation on the presumption that unrecognized adrenal or pituitary insufficiency may be present.

Prednisolone or prednisone are recommended when an anti-inflammatory effect is desired. The low mineralocorticoid potency of these drugs limits Na$^+$ and water retention when large doses are administered to produce the desired glucocorticoid effect. It must be recognized, however, that the anti-inflammatory effect of corticosteroids is palliative, because the underlying cause of the response remains. Nevertheless, suppression of the inflammatory response may be lifesaving in some situations. Conversely, masking of the symptoms of inflammation may delay diagnosis of life-threatening illnesses such as peritonitis owing to perforation of a peptic ulcer.

Deficiency States

Acute adrenal insufficiency requires electrolyte and fluid replacement as well as supplemental corticosteroids. Cortisol is administered at a rate of 100 mg IV every 8 hours following an initial injection of 100 mg. Management of chronic adrenal insufficiency in adults is with the daily oral administration of cortisone, 25 to 37.5 mg. A typical regimen is 25 mg in the morning and 12.5 mg in the late afternoon. This schedule mimics the normal diurnal cycle of adrenal secretion. An orally effective mineralocorticoid such as fludrocortisone, 0.1 to 0.3 mg daily, is required by most patients.

Cerebral Edema

Corticosteroids in large doses are of value in the reduction or prevention of cerebral edema and the resulting increases in intracranial pressure that may accompany intracranial tumors and metastatic lesions. There is no doubt about the benefit of corticosteroids in the treatment of cerebral edema resulting from global ischemic injury. Conversely, cerebral edema owing to closed head injury is not predictably responsive to corticosteroids. Dexamethasone, with minimal mineralocorticoid activity, is frequently selected to reduce cerebral edema and associated increases in intracranial pressure.

Aspiration Pneumonitis

The use of corticosteroids in the treatment of aspiration pneumonitis is controversial. There is evidence in animals that corticosteroids administered immediately after inhalation of acidic gastric fluid may be effective in reducing pulmonary damage (Dudley and Marshall, 1974). Conversely, other data show no beneficial effect or suggest that the use of corticosteroids may enhance the likelihood of gram-negative pneumonia (Downs et al, 1974; Wynne et al, 1981). Despite the absence of confirmatory evidence that corticosteroids are beneficial, it is not uncommon for the treatment of aspiration pneumonitis to include the empiric use of pharmacologic doses of these drugs.

Lumbar Disc Disease

An alternative to surgical treatment of lumbar disc disease is the epidural or subarachnoid placement of corticosteroids (Abram, 1978; Bullard and Houghton, 1977; Winnie et al, 1972). Corticosteroids may reduce inflammation and edema of the nerve root that has resulted from compression. A common regimen is epidural injection of 25 to 50 mg of triamcinolone or 40 to 80 mg of methylprednisolone, with 5 ml of lidocaine at the interspace corresponding to the distribution of pain. In animals, the epidural injection of triamcinolone, 2 mg·kg^{-1}, interferes with the ability of the adrenal cortex to release cortisol in response to hypoglycemia for 4 weeks (Table 23-2) (Gorski et al, 1982). If this also occurs in patients receiving a single epidural injection of corticosteroid, it is conceivable that tolerance to stress would be reduced.

Organ Transplantation

In organ transplantation, high doses of corticosteroids are often administered at the time of sur-

Table 23-2
Epidural Triamcinolone and Plasma Cortisol Response to Stress (Plasma Cortisol [μg·dl⁻¹] Before and After Hypoglycemia)

| Control | | Days After Administration of Epidural Triamcinolone (2 mg·kg⁻¹) | | | | | | | | | |
| | | 1 | | 7 | | 21 | | 28 | | 35 | |
Before	After	Before	After	Before	After	Before	After	Before	After	Before	After
5.1	7.4	2.3	2.2	2.7	2.3	2.5	2.1	2.5	2.9	4.8	8.3*

*$P < 0.05$ compared with "Before."
(Data from Gorski DW, Rao TLK, Glisson SN, Chinthagada M, El-Etr AA. Epidural triamcinolone and adrenal response to hypoglycemic stress in dogs. Anesthesiology 1982; 57: 364–6; with permission.)

gery. Smaller maintenance doses of corticosteroids are continued indefinitely, and the dosage is increased if rejection of the transplanted organ is threatened

CYCLOSPORINE. Cyclosporine is a metabolite produced by the fungus, *Tolypocladium inflatum gams.* The drug selectively inhibits helper T-lymphocyte–mediated immune responses while not effecting B lymphocytes. Cyclosporine binds and inhibits calmodulin, an intracytoplasmic protein, that is involved in Ca^{2+}-mediated activities and is required for activation of T cells. Use of this immunosuppressant drug in combination with corticosteroids has greatly increased the success of organ transplantation. Cyclosporine must be administered before T-lymphocyte cells undergo proliferation as a result of exposure to specific antigens presented by organ transplantation. There is some evidence that insulin-dependent diabetes mellitus may be prevented or alleviated if treatment with cyclosporine is initiated promptly after diagnosis (Assan et al, 1985). Cyclosporine has beneficial therapeutic effects in patients with active Crohn's disease that is unresponsive to corticosteroids (Brynskov et al, 1989). Uveitis, psoriasis, and rheumatoid arthritis may respond to cyclosporine therapy. Cyclosporine is extensively metabolized, with less than 1% excreted unchanged in the urine.

Serious side effects may accompany administration of cyclosporine, emphasizing the need to monitor blood concentrations and reduce the dose accordingly to minimize adverse effects (Kahan, 1989). Nephrotoxicity is the most important adverse effect, occurring in 25% to 38% of patients. For this reason, it is recommended that

renal function tests be performed regularly during therapy. In renal transplant patients, it may be difficult to differentiate cyclosporine nephrotoxicity from acute rejection reactions (Ptachcinski et al, 1985). Cyclosporine-induced hypertension assoicated with activation of the sympathetic nervous system often requires medical therapy especially in heart transplant patients (Scherrer et al, 1990). Limb paresthesias occur in about 50% of patients. Even though cyclosporine is not believed to cross the blood-brain barrier, there is a significant incidence of headache, confusion, and somnolence. Seizures of new onset may be triggered by cyclosporine therapy. The use of cyclosporine almost doubles the incidence of cholestasis with hyperbilirubinemia and elevation of liver transaminases in renal transplant recipients. Rarely, patients have experienced allergic reactions to cyclosporine. Other side effects include gum hyperplasia, hirsutism, and hyperglycemia. To avoid interactions with plasticizers in intravenous solution bags, cyclosporine is dispensed from glass bottles.

Asthma

Corticosteroids are useful in the long-term treatment and suppression of asthma. The efficacy of corticosteroids in treatment of the acute phase of asthma is less well defined. Nevertheless, a controlled clinical study demonstrated that methylprednisolone, 125 mg IV, administered to adults with acute bronchial asthma, reduces the need for subsequent hospitalization compared with placebo-treated patients (Littenberg and Gluck, 1986).

Oral administration of methylprednisolone, 160 or 320 mg daily, is as effective as an intravenous injection, 500 or 1000 mg daily, in the treatment of status asthmaticus (Ratto et al, 1988). Status asthmaticus has also been treated with administration of cortisol, 50 to 1000 mg IV every 8 hours, until the acute episode is suppressed. Subsequently, prednisolone may be required for about 10 days, but the goal remains to gradually decrease the dose and ultimately discontinue the corticosteroid.

Severe chronic bronchial asthma that is uncontrolled by other measures may respond to aerosol administration of a corticosteroid. Aerosol therapy is predictably ineffective, however, in acute asthmatic attacks when airways may be plugged with mucus. Systemic effects are minimal with aerosol administration of corticosteroids, but pharyngeal candidiasis develops in a high percentage of patients.

Manifestations of allergic diseases that are of limited duration, such as hay fever, contact dermatitis, drug reactions, angioneurotic edema, and anaphylaxis, can be suppressed by adequate doses of corticosteroids. Life-threatening allergic reactions, however, must be treated with epinephrine, since the onset of the anti-inflammatory effect produced by corticosteroids is delayed. Indeed, any beneficial effect of corticosteroids in the management of severe allergic reactions is probably related to suppression of the inflammatory response rather than to inhibition of production of immunoglobulins.

Arthritis

The criterion for initiating corticosteroid therapy in patients with rheumatoid arthritis is progressive disability despite maximal medical therapy. Corticosteroids are administered in the smallest dose possible that provides significant but not complete symptomatic relief. The usual initial dose is prednisolone, 10 mg (or its equivalent), in divided doses. Intraarticular injection of corticosteroids is recommended for treatment of episodic manifestations of acute joint inflammation associated with osteoarthritis. However, painless destruction of the joint is a risk of this treatment.

Collagen Diseases

Manifestations of collagen diseases, such as polymyositis, polyarteritis nodosa, and Wegener's granulomatosis, but not scleroderma, are re-

duced, and longevity is improved by chronic corticosteroid therapy. Fulminating systemic lupus erythematosus is a life-threatening illness that is aggressively treated initially with large doses of prednisone, 1 mg·kg^{-1}, or its equivalent. Large doses of corticosteroids are effective for inducing a remission of sarcoidosis. In temporal arteritis, corticosteroid therapy is necessary to prevent blindness, which occurs in about 20% of untreated patients. Some forms of nephrotic syndrome respond favorably to corticosteroids. Rheumatic carditis may be suppressed by large doses of corticosteroids.

Ocular Inflammation

Corticosteroids are used to suppress ocular inflammation (uveitis and iritis) and thus preserve sight. Instillation of corticosteroids into the conjunctival sac results in therapeutic concentrations in the aqueous humor. Topical corticosteroid therapy often increases intraocular pressure. For this reason, it is recommended that intraocular pressure be monitored when topical ocular corticosteroids are used for more than 2 weeks. Corticosteroids are contraindicated in herpes simplex (dendritic keratitis) of the eye. Topical corticosteroids should not be used for treatment of ocular abrasions, because delayed healing and infection may occur.

Cutaneous Disorders

Topical administration of corticosteroids is frequently effective in the treatment of skin diseases. Effectiveness is increased by application of the corticosteroid as an ointment under an occlusive dressing. Systemic absorption is also occasionally enhanced to the degree that suppression of the pituitary-adrenal axis occurs or manifestations of Cushing's syndrome appear. Corticosteroids may also be administered systemically for treatment of severe episodes of acute skin disorders and exacerbations of chronic disorders.

Postintubation Laryngeal Edema

Treatment of postintubation laryngeal edema may include administration of corticosteroids, such as dexamethasone, 0.1 to 0.2 mg·kg^{-1} IV. Nevertheless, the efficacy of corticosteroids for treatment of this condition has not been proved.

Ulcerative Colitis

Corticosteroid therapy is indicated in selected patients with chronic ulcerative colitis. A disadvantage of this therapy is that signs and symptoms of intestinal perforation and peritonitis may be masked.

Myasthenia Gravis

Corticosteroids are usually reserved for patients with severe myasthenia gravis who are unresponsive to medical or surgical therapy. These drugs seem to be most effective after thymectomy. The mechanism of beneficial effects produced by corticosteroids is not known but may reflect drug-induced suppression of the production of an immunoglobulin that normally binds to the neuromuscular junction.

Respiratory Distress Syndrome

Administration of corticosteroids at least 24 hours before delivery reduces the incidence and severity of respiratory distress syndrome in neonates born between 26 and 34 weeks' gestation. Dexamethasone administered for prolonged periods (42 days) improves pulmonary and neurodevelopmental outcome in low-birth-weight infants at risk for bronchopulmonary dysplasia (Cummings et al, 1989).

Hypercalcemia

Pharmacologic doses of corticosteroids, by antagonizing the effects of vitamin D, are often effective in treating hypercalcemia caused by increased intestinal absorption of Ca^{2+}. Corticosteroids also prevent hypercalcemia in patients with multiple myeloma by decreasing reabsorption of Ca^{2+} from bone. These drugs are usually ineffective, however, when hypercalcemia is due to increased levels of parathyroid hormone, either from hyperparathyroidism or from a neoplasm that secretes a parathyroid hormone–like substance.

Leukemia

The antilymphocytic effects of glucocorticoids are used to advantage in combination chemotherapy of acute lymphocytic leukemia and lymphomas, including Hodgkin's disease and multiple myeloma. For example, prednisone and vincristine produce remissions in about 90% of children with lymphoblastic leukemia.

Septic Shock

Corticosteroids have been recommended as part of the therapeutic regimen, along with antibiotics and volume replacement in the treatment of septic shock (Schumer, 1976). Nevertheless, controlled studies in humans fail to confirm any value of high-dose corticosteroid therapy in the prevention of shock, the reversal of shock, or overall mortality (Bone et al, 1987; Sprung et al, 1984; Bone et al, 1987; The Veterans Administration Systemic Sepsis Cooperative Study Group, 1987). Mortality related to infection may be increased in corticosteroid-treated patients. The overwhelming evidence is that corticosteroids provide no benefit in the treatment of sepsis and septic shock and are not indicated as adjunctive therapy.

Cardiac Arrest

Glucocorticoids have been given to patients following global brain ischemia. This practice is based on the well-established benefit of these drugs in the treatment of perifocal vasogenic edema around an intrinsic mass. Nevertheless, the value of glucocorticoids in treatment of intracellular cytotoxic edema, as is thought to occur after global ischemia, is unproven. Indeed, glucocorticoids have not been shown to improve survival or neurologic recovery rate following cardiac arrest, and their administration to these patients is not recommended (Jastremski et al, 1989).

Side Effects

Side effects of chronic corticosteroid therapy include (1) suppression of the hypothalamic-pituitary-adrenal axis, (2) electrolyte and metabolic changes, (3) osteoporosis, (4) peptic ulcer disease, (5) skeletal muscle myopathy, (6) central nervous system dysfunction, (7) peripheral blood changes, and (8) inhibition of normal growth. Increased susceptibility to bacterial or fungal infection accompanies treatment with corticosteroids. Corticosteroid administration is associated with greater clearance of salicylates and reduced effectiveness of anticoagulants.

Suppression of the Hypothalamic-Pituitary-Adrenal Axis

Corticosteroid therapy may result in suppression of the hypothalamic-pituitary-adrenal axis with the result that release of cortisol in response to stress, such as that produced by surgery, is blunted or does not occur. It is not possible to define the precise dose of corticosteroid or duration of therapy that will produce pituitary and adrenocortical suppression in a given patient, because there is marked variation among patients. Typically, however, the larger the dose and the more prolonged the therapy, the greater is the likelihood of suppression. When appropriate, a dose of a corticosteroid administered every other day is less likely to suppress the anterior pituitary release of ACTH than is the daily administration of the drug.

CORTICOSTEROID SUPPLEMENTATION. Corticosteroid supplementation should be increased whenever the patient being treated for chronic hypoadrenocorticism undergoes a surgical procedure. This recommendation is based on the concern that these patients are susceptible to cardiovascular collapse because they cannot release additional endogenous cortisol in response to the stress of surgery. More controversial is the management of the patient who may manifest suppression of the hypothalamic-pituitary-adrenal axis because of current or previous administration of corticosteroids for treatment of a disease unrelated to pituitary or adrenocortical dysfunction.

A rational regimen for corticosteroid supplementation in the perioperative period is the administration of cortisol, 25 mg IV, at the induction of anesthesia followed by a continuous intravenous infusion of cortisol, 100 mg, during the following 24 hours (Symreng et al, 1981). This approach maintains the plasma concentration of cortisol above normal during major surgery in patients receiving chronic treatment with corticosteroids and manifesting a subnormal response to the preoperative infusion of ACTH (Fig. 23-9) (Symreng et al, 1981). It is likely that patients undergoing minor operations will need minimal to no additional corticosteroid coverage during the perioperative period.

In addition to intravenous supplementation with cortisol, patients receiving daily maintenance doses of a corticosteroid should also re-

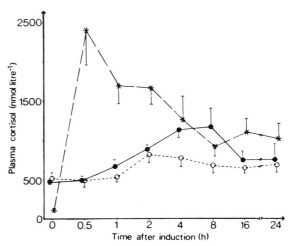

FIGURE 23–9. Administration of cortisol, 25 mg IV, plus a continuous intravenous infusion of 100 mg over 24 hours, maintains the plasma cortisol concentration above normal in patients (*) receiving chronic treatment with corticosteroids and manifesting a subnormal response to the preoperative infusion of adrenocorticotropic hormone. (From Symreng T, Karlberg BE, Kagedal B, Schildt B. Physiological cortisol substitution of long-term steroid-treated patients undergoing major surgery. Br J Anaesth 1981; 53: 949–53; with permission.)

ceive this dose with the preoperative medication on the day of surgery. There is no objective evidence to support increasing the maintenance dose of corticosteroid preoperatively. In those instances in which events such as burns or sepsis could exaggerate the need for exogenous corticosteroid supplementation, the continuous intravenous infusion of cortisol, 100 mg, every 12 hours should be sufficient. Indeed, endogenous cortisol production during stress introduced by major surgery or extensive burns is not greater than 150 mg daily (Hardy and Turner, 1957; Hume et al, 1962).

Electrolyte and Metabolic Changes

Hypokalemic metabolic alkalosis reflects mineralocorticoid effects of corticosteroids on distal renal tubules, leading to enhanced reabsorption of Na^+ and loss of K^+. Edema and weight gain accompany this corticosteroid effect.

Corticosteroids inhibit use of glucose in peripheral tissues and promote hepatic gluconeogenesis. The resulting corticosteroid-induced hyperglycemia can usually be managed with diet, insulin, or both. The dose requirement for oral hypoglycemics may be increased by corticosteroids.

There is a redistribution of body fat characterized by deposition of fat in the back of the neck (buffalo hump), supraclavicular area, and face (moon facies) and loss of fat from the extremities. The mechanism by which corticosteroids elicit this redistribution of body fat is not known.

Peripherally, corticosteroids mobilize amino acids from tissues. This catabolic effect manifests as reduced skeletal muscle mass, osteoporosis, thinning of the skin, and a negative nitrogen balance.

Osteoporosis

Osteoporosis, vertebral compression fractures, and rib fractures are frequent and serious complications of corticosteroid therapy in patients of all ages. Corticosteroids appear to inhibit the activities of osteoblasts and stimulate osteoclasts by inhibition of Ca^{2+} absorption from the gastrointestinal tract, which causes an increased secretion of parathyroid hormone. Osteoporosis is an indication for withdrawal of corticosteroid therapy. Evidence of osteoporosis should be sought on radiographs of the spines of patients being treated chronically with corticosteroids. The presence of osteoporosis could predispose patients to fractures during positioning in the operating room.

Peptic Ulcer Disease

Although a cause-and-effect relationship has not been proved, the incidence of peptic ulcer disease seems to be increased by chronic corticosteroid therapy. Indeed, corticosteroids may decrease the normal protective barrier provided by gastric mucus.

Skeletal Muscle Myopathy

Skeletal muscle myopathy characterized by weakness of the proximal musculature is occasionally observed in patients taking large doses of corticosteroids. In some patients, this skeletal muscle weakness is so severe that ambulation is not possible and corticosteroid therapy must be discontinued.

Central Nervous System Dysfunction

Corticosteroid therapy is associated with an increased incidence of neuroses and psychoses. Behavioral changes include manic depression and suicidal tendencies. Cataracts develop in almost all patients who receive prednisone, 20 mg daily, or its equivalent for at least 4 years.

Peripheral Blood Changes

Corticosteroids tend to increase the hematocrit and number of circulating leukocytes. Conversely, a single dose of cortisol reduces, by almost 70%, the number of circulating lymphocytes and, by over 90%, the number of circulating monocytes in 4 to 6 hours. This acute lymphocytopenia most likely reflects sequestration from the blood rather than destruction of cells.

Inhibition of Normal Growth

Inhibition or arrest of growth can result from the administration of relatively small doses of glucocorticoids to children. This cannot be overcome with exogenous human growth hormone. The mechanism for this effect is presumed to be the generalized inhibitory effect of glucocorticoids on DNA synthesis and cell division.

Inhibitors of Corticosteroid Synthesis

Metyrapone

Metyrapone reduces cortisol secretion by inhibition of the 11-beta-hydroxylation reaction, resulting in accumulation of 11-desoxycortisol. Metyrapone may induce acute adrenal insufficiency in patients with reduced adrenocortical function. A deficiency of mineralocorticoids does not occur, because metyrapone-induced inhibition of 11-beta-hydroxylation results in increased production of the mineralocorticoid 11-desoxycorticosterone. Metyrapone has been used to treat excessive adrenocortical function that results from adrenal neoplasms that function autonomously or as a result of ectopic production of ACTH by tumors.

Aminoglutethimide

Aminoglutethimide inhibits the conversion of cholesterol to 20-alpha-hydroxycholesterol. This inhibition interrupts production of both cortisol and aldosterone. As such, this drug is effective in decreasing the excessive secretion of cortisol in autonomously functioning adrenal tumors and in hypersecretion resulting from ectopic production of ACTH.

POSTERIOR PITUITARY HORMONES

Antidiuretic hormone (ADH) and oxytocin are the two principal hormones secreted by the posterior pituitary. The target sites for ADH are renal collecting ducts, where this hormone acts to increase permeability of cell membranes to water. As a result, water is passively reabsorbed from renal collecting ducts into extracellular fluid. Nonrenal actions of ADH include intense vasoconstriction, accounting for its alternative designation as vasopressin. Oxytocin elicits contractions of the uterus, which are indistinguishable from those that occur in spontaneous labor.

Antidiuretic Hormone

Antidiuretic hormone and its congeners (desmopressin, lypressin) are used in the treatment of diabetes insipidus that results from inadequate secretion of the hormone by the posterior pituitary. Failure to secrete adequate amounts of ADH results in polyuria and hypernatremia. Trauma and surgery in the region of the pituitary and hypothalamus are recognized causes of diabetes insipidus. Nephrogenic diabetes insipidus resulting from an inability of the renal tubules to respond to adequate amounts of centrally produced ADH does not respond to exogenous administration of the hormone or its congeners.

The oral hypoglycemic chlorpropamide sensitizes renal tubules to the effects of low circulating concentrations of ADH, accounting for its beneficial effects in patients with diabetes insipidus. Inhibition of prostaglandin production produced by chlorpropamide may be responsible for increased sensitivity of the renal tubules to ADH. This drug is not effective in the treatment of nephrogenic diabetes insipidus. A high incidence of hypoglycemic reactions detracts from the therapeutic value of chlorpropamide in the treatment of diabetes insipidus. Acetaminophen and indomethacin probably enhance the effects of ADH by a similar inhibitory effect on the synthesis of prostaglandins. Clofibrate may directly stimulate secretion of ADH by the posterior pituitary, leading to a significant antidiuretic action in patients with diabetes insipidus. The combination of clofibrate with chlorpropamide may produce an additive effect, emphasizing the speculated differences in mechanism of action of these drugs. Thiazide diuretics exert a paradoxical antidiuretic action in patients with nephrogenic diabetes insipidus and serve as the only drugs effective in the treatment of this disorder.

Inappropriate and excessive secretion of ADH with subsequent retention of water and dilutional hyponatremia may occur in patients with head injuries, intracranial tumors, meningitis, and pulmonary infections. Aberrant production of ADH is observed most commonly in patients with cancer, especially oat cell carcinoma, in which the tumor itself produces ADH. In these patients, the antibiotic demeclocycline promotes diuresis by antagonizing the effects of ADH on renal tubules.

Vasopressin

Vasopressin is the exogenous preparation of ADH used for the (1) treatment of ADH-sensitive diabetes insipidus, (2) evaluation of the urine-concentrating abilities of the kidneys as following administration of a fluorinated volatile anesthetic, and (3) management of uncontrolled hemorrhage from esophageal varices. This drug is not effective in the management of the patient with nephrogenic diabetes insipidus.

Vasopressin administered intravenously is used for the initial evaluation of patients with suspected diabetes insipidus, which may follow head trauma or hypophysectomy. Under these circumstances, polyuria may be transient, and a longer antidiuretic effect (1 to 3 days) as produced by intramuscular vasopressin tannate in oil could produce water intoxication. Oral administration of vasopressin is followed by rapid inactivation by trypsin, which cleaves a peptide linkage. Likewise, intravenous administration of vasopressin results in a brief effect because of rapid enzymatic breakdown by peptides in the tissues, especially the kidneys.

Vasopressin may serve as an adjunct in the control of bleeding esophageal varices and during abdominal surgery in patients with cirrhosis and portal hypertension. Infusion of 20 units over 5 minutes results in marked reductions in hepatic blood flow and pressure lasting about 30 minutes. Only a moderate rise in blood pressure occurs. This effect on portal circulation is attributable to marked splanchnic vasoconstriction. An alternative to systemic administration is infusion of vasopressin directly into the superior mesenteric artery. It has not been established whether selective arterial administration is safer than systemic administration with respect to cardiac and vascular side effects.

SIDE EFFECTS. Vasoconstriction and increased blood pressure occur only with doses of vasopressin that are much larger than those administered for the treatment of diabetes insipidus. This response is due to a direct and generalized effect on vascular smooth muscle that is not antagonized by denervation or adrenergic blocking drugs. Facial pallor owing to cutaneous vasoconstriction may also accompany large doses of vasopressin. The magnitude of elevation in blood pressure caused by vasopressin depends, to some extent, on the reactivity of the baroreceptor reflexes. For example, when baroreceptor reflexes are depressed by anesthesia, smaller amounts of vasopressin are capable of evoking a pressor response. Pulmonary artery pressures are also increased by vasopressin.

Vasopressin, even in small doses, may produce selective vasoconstriction of the coronary arteries, with reductions in coronary blood flow manifesting as angina pectoris, electrocardiographic evidence of myocardial ischemia, and, in some instances, myocardial infarction. Ventricular cardiac dysrhythmias may accompany these cardiac effects.

Large doses of vasopressin stimulate gastrointestinal smooth muscle, and the resulting increased peristalsis may manifest as abdominal pain, nausea, and vomiting. Smooth muscle of the uterus is also stimulated by large doses of vasopressin.

The circulating plasma concentrations of factor VIII are increased by vasopressin (Mannucci et al, 1977; Sutor et al, 1978). As a result, these drugs may be beneficial in the management of moderately severe hemophilia, particularly to reduce bleeding associated with surgery. The mechanisms of this effect are not known.

Allergic reactions ranging from urticaria to anaphylaxis may occasionally follow the administration of vasopressin. Prolonged use of vasopressin may result in antibody formation and a shortened duration of action of the drug.

Desmopressin

Desmopressin is a synthetic analogue of ADH possessing intense antidiuretic effects that last 6 to 20 hours as well as hemostatic responses (see chapter 36). Administered intranasally, twice daily, using a calibrated catheter (rhinyle), desmopressin is the drug of choice in the treatment of diabetes insipidus owing to inadequate ADH production by the posterior pituitary. Desmopressin, like all the ADH analogues, is not effective in the treatment of nephrogenic diabetes insipidus. There are fewer side effects produced by desmopressin than are associated with vasopressin, although nausea and increases in blood pressure can occur.

Lypressin

Lypressin is a synthetic analogue of ADH that produces antidiuresis for about 4 hours following intranasal administration. Its short duration of action limits its usefulness in the treatment of diabetes insipidus.

Oxytocin

Oxytocin, along with ergot derivatives and certain prostaglandins, is sufficiently selective in its stimulation of uterine smooth muscle to be clinically useful.

Clinical Uses

The principal clinical uses of oxytocin are to induce labor at term and to counter uterine hypotonicity and reduce hemorrhage in the postpartum or postabortion period.

For induction of labor, a continuous intravenous infusion is preferred, because the low dose of oxytocin needed can be precisely controlled. Indeed, the sensitivity of the uterus to oxytocin increases as pregnancy progresses. To induce labor, a dilute solution (10 milliunits·ml^{-1}) is administered intravenously by a constant infusion pump beginning at 1 to 2 milliunits·min^{-1}. This infusion rate is increased 1 to 2 milliunits·min^{-1} every 15 to 30 minutes until an optimal response (one uterine contraction every 2 to 3 minutes) is obtained. The average dose of oxytocin to induce labor is 8 to 10 milliunits·min^{-1}. Infusion rates up to 40 milliunits·min^{-1} of oxytocin may be necessary to treat uterine atony initially following delivery. Intramuscular injections of oxytocin are commonly used to provide sustained uterine contraction in the postpartum period.

All preparations of oxytocin used clinically are synthetic, and their potency is described in units. These synthetic preparations are identical to the hormone normally released from the posterior pituitary but devoid of contamination by other polypeptide hormones and proteins found in natural preparations.

Side Effects

High doses of oxytocin produce a direct relaxant effect on vascular smooth muscle that manifests as a decrease in systolic and diastolic blood pressure and flushing. Reflex tachycardia and increased cardiac output accompany this transient reduction in blood pressure. When high doses are infused continuously, the brief reduction in blood pressure is followed by a modest but sustained increase in blood pressure. The amounts of oxytocin administered for most obstetric purposes are inadequate to produce marked alterations in blood pressure. A marked fall in blood pressure, however, may occur if oxytocin is administered to patients with blunted compensatory reflex responses, as may be produced by anesthesia. Likewise, hypovolemic patients would be particularly susceptible to oxytocin-induced hypotension.

In the past, oxytocin preparations were often contaminated with ergot alkaloids, resulting in exaggerated blood pressure elevations when administered to patients previously treated with a sympathomimetic. Modern synthetic commercial preparations are pure oxytocin and do not introduce the risk of exaggerated vasoconstriction when administered in the presence of a sympathomimetic drug.

Oxytocin exhibits a slight ADH-like activity when administered in high doses, introducing the possibility of water intoxication if an excessive volume of fluid is administered. The risk of this complication can be minimized by infusion of oxytocin in an electrolyte-containing solution rather than in dextrose in water.

Ergot Derivatives

Ergot is the product of a fungus that grows on grain. Ingestion of contaminated grain results in generalized and intense vasoconstriction, reflecting the peripheral vascular effects of ergot alkaloids. The ergot alkaloids, ergotamine and ergonovine, are derivatives of 6-methylergoline. Hydrolysis of ergonovine yields lysergic acid and an amine. Semisynthetic derivatives of the ergot alkaloids include lysergic acid diethylamide and methylergonovine. Methysergide is formed by the addition of a methyl group to the indole nitrogen of methylergonovine.

Clinical Uses

All the natural alkaloids of ergot produce dose-related increases in the motor activity of the uterus. The sustained elevation of resting uterine tone produced by high doses of ergot precludes its use for induction of labor but increases its value in the postpartum or postabortion period to control bleeding and maintain uterine contraction. Ergonovine is less toxic and produces a more rapid uterine response than ergotamine. For these reasons, ergonovine and its semisynthetic derivatives methylergonovine have replaced other ergot derivatives. Ergonovine and methylergonovine are rapidly absorbed after oral or intramuscular (0.2 mg) administration, producing a uterotonic action within about 10 minutes that lasts 3 to 6 hours. Administered intravenously (0.2 mg), uterine contraction occurs within 30 to 45 seconds. The uterine-stimulating effects of these drugs most likely reflect interactions with specific receptors.

Ergotamine may be effective in relieving migraine headaches. This beneficial effect may be due to ergotamine-induced constriction of dilated cerebral blood vessels, particularly in the meningeal branches of the external carotid artery. In addition to reducing extracranial blood flow, ergotamine reduces hyperperfusion of regions supplied by the basilar artery and decreases shunting of blood via arteriovenous anastomoses. Caffeine increases approximately twofold the absorption of ergotamine following oral administration. Metabolism is almost complete, as emphasized by minimal recovery of unchanged drug in the urine. Storage in the tissues probably accounts for prolonged therapeutic and toxic effects, despite an elimination half-time of about 2 hours. Other types of headache are not improved and may even be aggravated by ergotamine.

Ergoloid is the combination of three ergot alkaloids (dihydroergocristine, dihydroergocornine, and dihydroergocryptine [as the mesylates]) that may provide symptomatic relief in some elderly patients who are manifesting changes of idiopathic mental decline (Alzheimer's disease). Improvement in cognitive and emotional symptoms is presumed to reflect a drug-induced effect on cerebral metabolism and not a direct cerebrovascular action. Following oral administration, the elimination half-time of ergoloid is about 4 hours. Side effects of treatment with ergoloid include nausea, vomiting, and gastric irrigation. Sinus bradycardia occasionally occurs. A sublingual preparation of ergoloid may produce local tissue irritation.

Side Effects

Ergonovine and methylergonovine are weak peripheral vasoconstrictors but produce additive effects with sympathomimetics, such as ephedrine and phenylephrine (Munson, 1965). Intravenous injection of these drugs has been associated with intense vasoconstriction leading to acute hypertension, seizures, cerebrovascular accidents, and retinal detachment (Abouleish, 1976). For this reason, these drugs should be used cautiously, if at all, in patients with preeclampsia, essential hypertension, or cardiac disease. Both drugs should be avoided in patients with atherosclerotic peripheral vascular disease. Nausea and vomiting most likely reflect a direct central nervous system effect.

CHYMOPAPAIN

Chymopapain is a proteolytic enzyme used in the treatment of herniated lumbar intervertebral disc disease that has not responded to conservative therapy. Injected into the intervertebral disc, chymopapain dissolves the proteoglycan portion of the nucleus pulposus but does not affect collagenous components. Evidence of dissolution of the nucleus pulposus is the appearance in the urine of glycosaminoglycans of the type known to occur in human intervertebral discs. Dissolution of the nucleus pulposus of the herniated intervertebral disc by chymopapain is known as *chemonucleolysis*. The recommended dose is 2000 to 5000 units per disc in a volume of 1 to 2 ml. The maximal dose in a patient with multiple disc herniations is 10,000 units.

Injection of chymopapain into the intervertebral space has been associated with allergic reactions of varying severity, including cardiovascular collapse and death (Rajagopalan et al, 1974). Almost all allergic reactions occur immediately but, on occasion, the symptoms do not appear for up to 2 hours, emphasizing the need for close observation after the injection. The allergic potential of chymopapain appears to be greatest in females and in those with preexisting allergies. Known allergy to papaya is a contraindication to injection of chymopapain, because this enzyme is derived from the crude latex of *Carica papaya*. Preoperative administration of a corticosteroid (prednisone, 50 mg) plus H-1 (diphenhydramine, 50 to 100 mg) and H-2 (cimetidine 300 to 600 mg) receptor antagonists as a single dose with the preoperative medication or up to four doses every 6 hours in the 24 hours preceding the induction of anesthesia may decrease the incidence and severity of allergic reactions (Bruno et al, 1984). Using preoperative histamine receptor antagonists and avoiding chemonucleolysis in patients with known allergies have reduced the incidence of allergic reactions following injection of chymopapain to 0.44% (Moss et al, 1985). Chymopapain is extremely toxic if injected into the subarachnoid space.

REFERENCES

Abouleish E. Postpartum hypertension and convulsion after oxytocic drugs. Anesth Analg 1976;55:813–5.

Abram SE. Subarachnoid corticosteroid injection following inadequate response to epidural steroids for sciatica. Anesth Analg 1978;57:313–5.

Assan R, Debray-Sachs M, Laborie C, et al. Metabolic and immunological effects of cyclosporine in recently diagnosed type 1 diabetes mellitus. Lancet 1985;1:67–71.

Bone RC, Fisher CJ, Clemmer TP et al. A controlled clinical trial of high-dose methylprednisolone in the treatment of severe sepsis and septic shock. N Engl J Med 1987;317:653–8.

Bruno LA, Smith DS, Bloom MJ, et al. Sudden hypotension with a test dose of chymopapain. Anesth Analg 1984;63:533–5.

Bullard JR, Houghton FM. Epidural steroid treatment of acute herniated nucleus pulposus. Anesth Analg 1977;56:862–3.

Brynskov J, Freund L, Rasmussen ST, et al. A placebo-controlled double-blind, randomized trial of cyclosporine therapy in active chronic Crohn's disease. N Engl J Med 1989;321:845–50.

Cooper DS. Antithyroid drugs. N Engl J Med 1984;311:1353–62.

Cummings JJ, D'Eugenio DB, Gross SJ. A controlled trial of dexamethasone in preterm infants at high risk for bronchopulmonary dysplasia. N Engl J Med 1989;320:1505–10.

Downs JB, Chapman RL, Modell JH, Hood CI. An evaluation of steroid therapy in aspiration pneumonitis. Anesthesiology 1974;40:129–35.

Dudley WR, Marshall BE. Steroid treatment for acid-aspiration pneumonia. Anesthesiology 1974;40:136–41.

Feek CM, Stewart J, Sawers A, et al. Combination of potassium iodide and propranolol in preparation of patients with Graves' disease for thyroid surgery. N Engl J Med 1980;302:883–5.

Gorski DW, Rao TLK, Glisson SN, Chinthagada M, El-Etr AA. Epidural triamcinolone and adrenal response to hypoglycemic stress in dogs. Anesthesiology 1982;57:364–6.

Gralnick HR, Maisonneuve P, Sultan Y, Rick ME. Benefits of danazol treatment in patients with hemophilia A (classic hemophilia). JAMA 1985;253:1151–3.

Hardy JD, Turner MD. Hydrocortisone secretion in man: Studies of adrenal vein blood. Surgery 1957;42:194–201.

Hume DM, Bell CC, Bartter FC. Direct measurement of adrenal secretion during operative trauma and convalescence. Surgery 1962;52:174–87.

Jastremski M, Sutton-Tyrrell K, PerVaagenes PH, et al. Glucocorticoid treatment does not improve neurologic recovery following cardiac arrest. JAMA 1989;262:3427–30.

Kahan BD. Cyclosporine. N Engl J Med 1989;321:1725–8.

Kaplan NM. Cardiovascular complications of oral contraceptives. Annu Rev Med 1978;29:31–40.

Laragh JH. Oral contraceptive—induced hypertension: Nine years later. Am J Obstet Gynecol 1976;126:141–7.

Littenberg B, Gluck EH. A controlled trial of methylprednisolone in the emergency treatment of acute asthma. N Engl J Med 1986;314:150–2.

Mannucci PM, Pareti H, Ruggeri ZM, Capitano A. I-desamino-8-arginine vasopressin: A new pharmacological approach to the management of haemophilia and vonWillebrand's disease. Lancet 1977;1:869–72.

Moss J, Roizen MF, Norbdy ET, et al. Decreased incidence and mortality of anaphylaxis to chymopapain. Anesth Analg 1985;64:1197–201.

Munson WM. The pressor effect of various vasopressor-oxytocic combinations: A laboratory study and review. Anesth Analg 1965;44:114–9.

Ptachcinski RJ, Burckarl GJ, Venkataramanan R. Cyclosporine. Drug Intell Clin Pharm 1985;19:90–100.

Rajagopalan R, Tindal S, MacNab LT, et al. Anaphylactic reactions to chymopapain during general anesthesia: A case report. Anesth Analg 1974;53;191–3.

Ratto D, Alfaro C, Sipsey J, Glovsky MM, Sharma OP. Are intravenous corticosteroids required in status asthmaticus? JAMA 1988;260:527–9.

Scherrer U, Vissing SF, Morgan BJ, et al. Cyclosporine-induced sympathetic activation and hypertension after heart transplantation. N Engl J Med 1990;323:693–9.

Schumer W. Steroids in the treatment of clinical peptic shock. Ann Surg 1976;184:333–9.

Sprung CV, Caralis PV, Marcial EH, et al. The effects of high-dose corticosteroids in patients with peptic shock: A prospective, controlled study. N Engl J Med 1984;311:1137–43.

Sutor AH, Uollman H, Arends P. Intrasanal application of DDAVP in severe haemophilia (letter). Lancet 1978;1:446.

Symreng T, Karlberg BE, Kagedal B, Schildt B. Physiological cortisol substitution of long-term steroid-treated patients undergoing major surgery. Br J Anaesth 1981;53:949–53.

The Veterans Administration Systemic Sepsis Cooperative Study Group. Effect of high-dose glucocorticoid therapy on mortality in patients with clinical signs of systemic sepsis. N Engl J Med 1987;317:659–65.

Winnie AP, Hartman JT, Meyers HL, Ramamurthy S, Barangan V. Pain clinic. II: Intradural and extradural corticosteroids for sciatica. Anesth Analg 1972;51:990–1003.

Wynne JW, DeMarco FJ, Hood CI. Physiological effects of corticosteroids in foodstuff aspiration. Arch Surg 1981;116:46–9.

24

Insulin and Oral Hypoglycemics

Insulin administered exogenously is the only effective treatment for Type I diabetes mellitus. Oral hypoglycemic drugs may serve as alternatives to exogenous administration of insulin to patients with Type II diabetes mellitus.

INSULIN

Insulin is synthesized in the beta cells of the islets of Langerhans as a single polypeptide precursor, preproinsulin, which is subsequently converted to proinsulin. Proinsulin forms equimolar amounts of insulin and C peptide (also referred to as "connecting peptide"). The two most important effects of insulin are to facilitate transport of glucose across cell membranes and to enhance phosphorylation of glucose within cells. For example, insulin can increase the rate of carrier-mediated diffusion of glucose seven- to tenfold. It is not known whether insulin increases the amount of carrier in cell membranes or whether it increases the rate at which chemical reactions take place between glucose and the carrier.

Structure Activity Relationships

Insulin comprises two chains (A and B) of amino acids joined by three disulfide bonds (Fig. 24-1) (Larner, 1985). Porcine insulin most closely resembles human insulin, differing only by substitution of an alanine residue on the B chain. The activity of various mammalian insulins is similar,

ranging from 22 to 26 units·mg^{-1}. Proinsulin has only slight biologic activity, whereas the separated A and B amino acid chains are inactive.

Pharmacokinetics

The elimination half-time of insulin injected intravenously is 5 to 10 minutes in normal patients or in the presence of diabetes mellitus. Insulin is metabolized in the kidneys and liver by a proteolytic enzyme. Approximately 50% of the insulin that reaches the liver by way of the portal vein is destroyed in a single passage through the liver. Nevertheless, renal dysfunction alters the disappearance rate of circulating insulin to a greater extent than does hepatic disease. Indeed, unexpected prolonged effects of insulin may occur in patients with renal disease, reflecting impairment of both metabolism and excretion of this hormone by the kidneys. Peripheral tissues such as skeletal muscles and fat can bind and inactivate insulin, but this is of minor quantitative significance.

Despite rapid clearance from the plasma following intravenous injection of insulin, there is a sustained pharmacologic effect for 30 to 60 minutes, because insulin is tightly bound to tissue receptors. Insulin administered subcutaneously is released slowly into the circulation to produce a sustained biologic effect.

Insulin is secreted into the portal venous system in the basal state at a rate of approximately 1 unit·h^{-1}. Food intake results in a prompt five- to

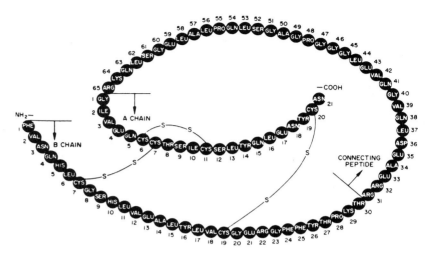

FIGURE 24–1. Proinsulin, which is converted to insulin by proteolytic cleavage of amino acids 31, 32, 64, 65, and the connecting peptide. (From Larner J. Insulin and oral hypoglycemic drugs; glucagon. In Gilman AG, Goodman LS, Rall TW, Murad F, eds. The Pharmacological Basis of Therapeutics, 7th ed. New York: Macmillan Publishing Co., 1985;1490–1516; with permission.)

tenfold increase in the rate of insulin secretion. The total daily secretion of insulin is approximately 40 units. The sympathetic and parasympathetic nervous systems innervate the insulin-producing islet cells and thus influence the basal rate of hormone secretion as well as the response to stress. For example, alpha-adrenergic stimulation reduces, and beta-adrenergic or parasympathetic nervous system stimulation increases, the basal secretion of insulin.

Receptors

Receptors for insulin in cell membrane surfaces are characterized as insulin-binding proteins. The receptor contains two alpha and two beta subunits joined together by disulfide bonds (Ullrich et al, 1985). The addition of insulin and adenosine triphosphate *in vitro* causes the receptor to become phosphorylated on tyrosine residues of the beta subunit. It has not, however, been proved that insulin activates adenylate cyclase to increase the intracellular concentrations of cyclic adenosine monophosphate. In fact, it is possible that insulin actually inhibits adenylate cyclase, leading to an increase in glycogen synthesis.

Insulin receptors become fully saturated with low circulating concentrations of insulin. For example, continuous intravenous infusion of insulin, 1 to 2 units·h^{-1}, has the same or even greater pharmacologic effect than a single larger

intravenous dose that is cleared rapidly from the circulation. Large doses of insulin, however, will last longer and exert a greater net effect than small doses.

The number of insulin receptors seems to be inversely related to the plasma concentration of insulin. This relationship may reflect the ability of insulin to regulate the population of its receptors. Obesity and insulin-dependent diabetes mellitus appear to be associated with a decrease in the number of insulin receptors.

Preparations

Insulin preparations differ in their concentration, time to onset, duration of action, purity, and species of origin. Commercially prepared insulin is bioassayed, and its physiologic activity (potency), based on the ability to lower the blood glucose concentration, is expressed in units. The potency of insulin is 22 to 26 units·mg^{-1}. Insulin U-100 (100 units·ml^{-1}) is the most commonly used commercial preparation. A total daily exogenous dose of insulin for treatment of diabetes mellitus is usually in the range of 20 to 60 units. This insulin requirement, however, may be acutely increased by stress associated with sepsis or trauma.

Human Insulins

The goal of producing the purest insulins possible has resulted in development of semisynthetic and biosynthetic methods for synthesizing insulin identical to that produced by the human pancreas (Zinman, 1989). The semisynthetic method is to begin with porcine insulin and, by an enzymatic process, substitute threonine for the terminal alanine on the B chain, making the structure identical to human insulin. Alternatively, a biosynthetic method that applies recombinant deoxyribonucleic acid technology can be used to splice synthetic genes for insulin A and B chains to *Escherichia coli* genes for beta-galactosidase. The insulin chains are cleaved from the beta-galactosidase and joined with sulfide bonds to form the insulin molecule. The proinsulin gene can also be introduced into *E. coli* and the resulting proinsulin then converted to insulin.

Classification

Insulin preparations are classified as fast acting, intermediate acting, and long acting, based on the time to onset, duration of action, and intensity of action following subcutaneous administration (Table 24-1). These classifications are, however, artificial; a particular insulin preparation can show wide variations of activity in a group of patients and even within an individual patient, especially one with labile diabetes mellitus.

REGULAR INSULIN. Regular insulin is a fast-acting preparation and is the only one that can be administered intravenously as well as subcutaneously. This form of insulin can be mixed in the same syringe with other insulin preparations, assuming that the pH of the solutions is similar. Zinc, present in longer-acting insulin preparations, may retard full activity of regular insulin when the two are mixed in the same syringe.

Administration of regular insulin is the preparation of choice for treating the abrupt onset of hyperglycemia or the appearance of ketoacidosis. In the perioperative period, regular insulin is administered as single injections (1 to 5 units IV) or as a continuous infusion (0.5 to 2 units·h^{-1} IV) to treat metabolic derangements associated with diabetes mellitus.

SEMILENTE INSULIN. Semilente insulin is a rapid-acting insulin preparation that is most often used to supplement intermediate- and long-acting insulin preparations. The rapid onset and short duration of action of semilente insulin reflect its small size and amorphous structure.

Lente insulin preparations (semilente insulin, lente insulin, and ultralente insulin) contain methylparaben as a preservative, whereas all other insulin preparations use phenol or cresol for this purpose. Methylparaben resembles para-

Table 24-1
Classification of Insulin Preparations

	Hours After Subcutaneous Administration*				
	Onset	*Peak*	*Duration*	*Modifier*	*Source*
Fast-acting					
Regular	0.5–1	2–4	6–8	None	B,P,H
Semilente	1–3	5–10	16	Zinc	B,P
Intermediate-acting					
Isophane (NPH)	2–4	6–12	18–26	Protamine	B,P,H
Lente	2–4	6–12	18–26	Zinc	B,P,H
Long-acting					
Protamine zinc	4–8	14–24	28–36	Protamine	B,P
Ultralente	4–8	14–24	28–36	Zinc	B,P

*Approximate.
B, bovine; P, porcine; H, human (Humulin).
NPH, neutral (N) solution, protamine (P), with origin in Hagedorn's laboratory (H).

aminobenzoic acid and has been incriminated as a cause of allergic reactions, especially when combined with local anesthetics.

ISOPHANE INSULIN. Isophane insulin (NPH) is an intermediate-acting preparation whose absorption from its subcutaneous injection site is delayed because the insulin is conjugated with protamine. The acronym NPH designates a neutral solution (N), protamine (P), and origin in Hagedorn's laboratory (Hagedorn et al, 1936). This insulin preparation contains 0.005 mg·unit^{-1}) of protamine.

LENTE INSULIN. Lente insulin is a mixture of 30% semilente (prompt onset) and 70% ultralente (extended duration) insulin. Lente insulin is used interchangeably with NPH insulin in the initial treatment of diabetes mellitus. Zinc is present in lente insulin to provide stability, but proteins such as protamine are lacking.

PROTAMINE ZINC INSULIN. Protamine zinc insulin (PZI) results from letting insulin and zinc react with the basic protein protamine. Each unit of PZI is combined with 0.028 mg of protamine. Injected subcutaneously, this insulin preparation has a delayed onset and prolonged duration of action. These characteristics have led to the infrequent clinical use of this preparation.

ULTRALENTE INSULIN. Ultralente insulin is long acting, reflecting the large particle size and crystalline form of this insulin preparation. This insulin preparation lacks protamine but, like PZI, has limited clinical usefulness because of its slow onset and prolonged duration of action.

Side Effects

Side effects of treatment with insulin may manifest as (1) hypoglycemia, (2) allergic reactions, (3) lipodystrophy, (4) insulin resistance, and (5) drug interactions.

Hypoglycemia

The most serious side effect of insulin therapy is hypoglycemia. Patients vulnerable to hypoglycemia are those who continue to receive exogenous insulin in the absence of carbohydrate intake, as may occur in the perioperative period, especially prior to surgery. Initial symptoms of hypoglycemia reflect the compensatory effects of increased epinephrine secretion manifesting as diaphoresis, tachycardia, and hypertension. Rebound hyperglycemia caused by sympathetic nervous system activity in response to hypoglycemia (the Somogyi effect) may mask the correct diagnosis. Symptoms of hypoglycemia involving the central nervous system include mental confusion progressing to seizures and coma. The intensity of central nervous system effects reflects the dependence of the brain on glucose as a selective substrate for oxidative metabolism. A prolonged period of hypoglycemia may result in irreversible brain damage.

The diagnosis of hypoglycemia during general anesthesia is made difficult because classic signs of sympathetic nervous system stimulation are likely to be masked by the anesthetic drugs. If signs of sympathetic nervous system stimulation owing to hypoglycemia occur, they are likely to be confused with responses evoked by painful stimulation in a lightly anesthetized patient. Furthermore, autonomic nervous system neuropathy associated with diabetes mellitus could alter the usual heart rate and blood pressure changes caused by hypoglycemia (Burgos et al, 1989). Finally, nonselective beta antagonists may also mask signs and symptoms of hypoglycemia.

Severe hypoglycemia is treated with 50 to 100 ml of 50% glucose solution administered intravenously. Alternatively, glucagon 0.5 to 1 mg IV or administered subcutaneously may be used. Nausea and vomiting are frequent side effects of glucagon treatment. In the absence of central nervous system depression, carbohydrates may be given orally.

Allergic Reactions

Local or systemic allergic reactions to insulin may occur. Local allergic reactions are approximately 10 times more frequent than systemic allergic reactions. These local allergic reactions are characterized by an erythematous indurated area that develops at the site of insulin injection. The cause of local allergic reactions is likely to be noninsulin materials in the insulin preparation.

Systemic allergic reactions to insulin range from urticaria to life-threatening cardiovascular collapse. These allergic reactions have been ascribed to sensitivity to the insulin molecule, as reflected by high circulating concentrations of antibodies to insulin. Commonly, there is a history of allergy to other drugs such as penicillin. A systemic allergic reaction to insulin requires changing to insulin derived from a different species or source. In this regard, porcine insulin is less antigenic than the bovine product.

Chronic exposure to low doses of protamine in certain insulin preparations (NPH insulin or PZI) may serve as an antigenic stimulus for the production of antibodies against protamine. These patients remain asymptomatic until a relatively large dose of protamine is administered intravenously to antagonize the anticoagulant effects of heparin. Indeed, patients with diabetes mellitus being treated with NPH insulin have a 50-fold increase in the likelihood of experiencing an allergic reaction to protamine (Stewart et al, 1984).

Lipodystrophy

Lipodystrophy reflects atrophy of fat at the sites of subcutaneous injection of insulin. This side effect is minimized by frequently changing the site used for injection of insulin.

Insulin Resistance

Patients requiring more than 100 units of exogenous insulin daily are considered to be manifesting insulin resistance. Even this value is high, since insulin requirements for pancreatectomized adults are often as low as 30 units.

Insulin resistance may be acute or chronic. Acute insulin resistance is associated with trauma, as produced by surgery and infection. It is likely that increased circulating plasma cortisol concentrations contribute to this acute resistance. Chronic insulin resistance is often associated with circulating antibodies against insulin. Sulfonylureas can reduce insulin requirements in some resistant patients, presumably by causing the release of endogenous insulin, which has less affinity for circulating antibodies than does exogenous porcine or bovine insulin.

Drug Interactions

Hormones administered as drugs that counter the hypoglycemic effect of insulin include adrenocorticotrophic hormone, estrogens, and glucagon. Epinephrine inhibits the secretion of insulin and stimulates glycogenolysis. Guanethidine decreases blood glucose concentrations and may reduce exogenous insulin requirements. Certain antibiotics (tetracycline or chloramphenicol), salicylates, and phenylbutazone increase the duration of action of insulin and may also have a direct hypoglycemic effect. The hypoglycemic effect on insulin may be potentiated by monoamine oxidase inhibitors.

ORAL HYPOGLYCEMICS

Sulfonylurea compounds that function as oral hypoglycemics account for approximately 1% of

Table 24–2
Classification and Pharmacokinetics of Sulfonylurea Oral Hypoglycemics

	Relative Potency	Average Dose (mg)	Doses per Day	Duration of Action* (h)	Elimination Half-Time* (h)
First Generation					
Tolbutamide	1	1500	2–3	6–10	4–8
Acetohexamide	2.5	1000	2	12–18	1.3–6
Tolazamide	5	250	1–2	16–24	4.7–8
Chlorpropamide	6	250	1	24–72	30–36
Second Generation					
Glyburide	150	7.5	1–2	18–24	4.6–12
Glipizide	100	10	1–2	16–24	4–7

*Approximate.

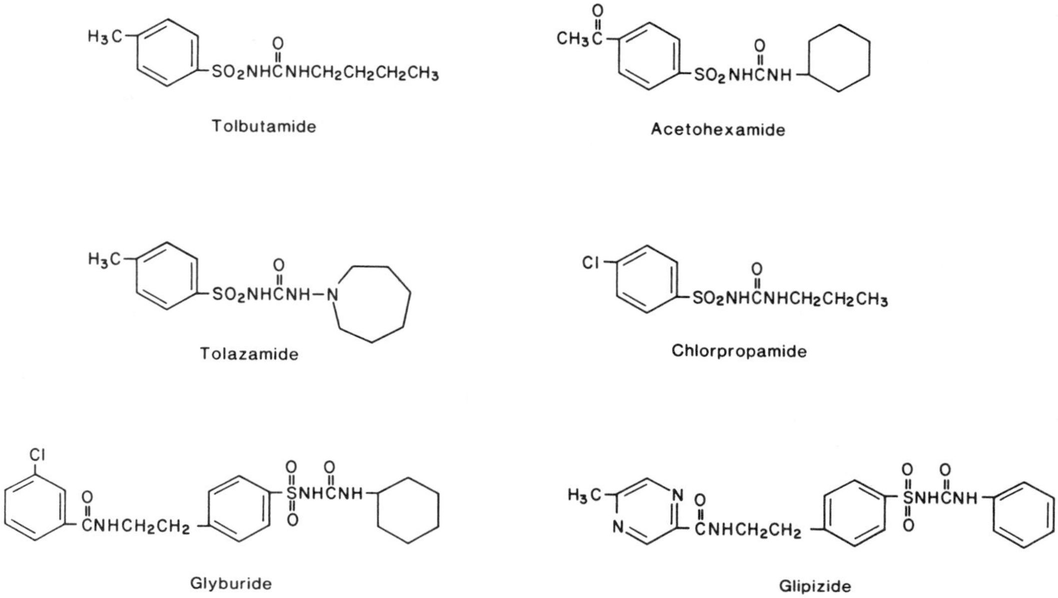

FIGURE 24–2. Oral hypoglycemics derived from sulfonylurea.

all prescriptions written in the United States (Table 24-2; Fig. 24-2) (Gerich, 1989). Three drugs, chlorpropamide, glyburide, and glipizide, account for approximately 70% of these prescriptions. The biguanide oral hypoglycemic drug phenformin causes lactic acidosis in some patients and for this reason is no longer commercially available.

Approximately one third of unselected patients with noninsulin-dependent diabetes mellitus do not achieve satisfactory glycemic control with sulfonylurea treatment. Conversely, many patients with noninsulin-dependent diabetes mellitus who are treated with insulin may achieve equally good control with sulfonylureas. Certain characteristics identify patients whose initial response is likely to be satisfactory (Table 24-3). Of patients who at first achieve satisfactory glycemic control, 5% to 10% experience secondary failure each year. Secondary failure results from poor patient selection; dietary noncompliance; islet beta cell exhaustion; concomitant drug therapy (thiazide diuretics or beta antagonists); or the development of another disorder. It is important to distinguish between true secondary failure and a temporary loss of effectiveness owing to intercurrent illness (sepsis, trauma, or myocardial infraction) because satisfactory glycemic control may again be achieved with a sulfonylurea after temporary insulin therapy and recovery from the illness. The use of sulfonylureas is contraindicated in patients allergic to sulfa drugs and in patients with insulin-dependent diabetes mellitus.

Mechanism of Action

Sulfonylureas increase islet beta cell sensitivity to glucose so more insulin is released. These drugs do not increase the synthesis of insulin and are ineffective in the absence of endogenous insulin. Sulfonylurea receptors are present on pancreatic beta cells, and their activation results in

Table 24–3

Characteristics of Patients with Noninsulin Diabetes Mellitus (NIDDM) Likely to Respond to Sulfonylureas

---

Over 40 years of age

Duration of NIDDM <5 years

Body weight 110% to 160% of ideal

Fasting blood glucose <180 mg·dl^{-1}

Satisfactory glycemic control with <40 units of insulin daily

---

inhibition of the efflux of potassium ions, which leads to depolarization of pancreatic beta cell membrane. Oral hypoglycemics may also reduce the release of glucagon and improve tissue sensitivity to insulin. Although sulfonylureas are derivatives of sulfonamides, they have no antibacterial action.

Pharmacokinetics

Oral hypoglycemics are readily absorbed from the gastrointestinal tract, with the most important distinguishing features being differences in duration of action and elimination half-time (Table 24-2). These drugs are weakly acidic and circulate bound to protein (90% to 98%), principally to albumin. Metabolism in the liver is extensive, and resulting active and inactive metabolites are eliminated by renal tubular secretion. Approximately 50% of glyburide is excreted in the feces.

Side Effects

Sulfonylureas are generally well tolerated, with the most common severe complication of these drugs being hypoglycemia (Table 24-4) (Gerich, 1989). The frequency of hypoglycemia is related to the potency and duration of action of the drug with the highest incidence occurring with chlorpropamide and glipizide. Hypoglycemia may be prolonged and require intravenous glucose infusion for several days. Risk factors for sulfonylurea-induced hypoglycemia include impaired nutrition as in the perioperative period; age greater than 60 years; impaired renal function; and concomitant drug therapy that can potentiate sulfonylureas (phenylbutazone, sulfonamide antibiotics, or warfarin) or in itself produce hypoglycemia (alcohol or salicylates). Renal disease decreases elimination of sulfonylureas and their active metabolites, thus increasing the likelihood of hypoglycemia. In this regard, only small amounts of tolbutamide and glipizide are excreted unchanged in the urine, making these drugs preferable for patients with renal disease. Sulfonylureas cross the placenta and may produce fetal hypoglycemia.

Approximately 1% to 3% of patients treated with oral hypoglycemics experience gastrointestinal disturbances that include nausea, vomiting, abnormal liver function tests, and cholestasis. Liver disease may prolong the elimination half-time and enhance the hypoglycemic action of all the sulfonylureas except acetohexamide. Disulfiram-like reactions and inappropriate secretion of antidiuretic hormone (ADH) with resulting hyponatremia are unique side effects of chlorpropamide.

Tolbutamide

Tolbutamide is the shortest-acting and least potent sulfonylurea (Table 24-2). It is extensively metabolized in the liver to much less potent compounds that are excreted in the urine. Of all the sulfonylureas, tolbutamide probably causes the fewest side effects, although it can produce hypoglycemia and hyponatremia.

Acetohexamide

Acetohexamide differs from other sulfonylureas in that most of its hypoglycemic action is due to its principal metabolite hydroxyhexamide, which is 2.5 times as potent as the parent compound. After oral ingestion, peak plasma concentrations of acetohexamide and its active metabolite occur after 1.5 and 3.5 hours, respectively. This drug is not recommended for patients with renal disease because the active metabolite is excreted by the kidneys. This is the only sulfonylurea with uricosuric properties, making it an appropriate drug for the diabetic patient with gout.

Tolazamide

Tolazamide is slowly absorbed after oral administration with an onset of hypoglycemic action after 4 to 6 hours that persists for 16 to 24 hours (Table 24-2). Metabolism in the liver produces several different products, some of which possess weak hypoglycemic activity. These active as well as inactive metabolites are excreted by the kidneys.

Chlorpropamide

Chlorpropamide is the longest-acting sulfonylurea, with a duration of action that may approach 72 hours (Table 24-2). Because of the long elimi-

Table 24-4
Side Effects of Sulfonylurea Oral Hypoglycemics

	Overall Incidence of Side Effects (%)	Incidence of Hypoglycemia (%)	Antidiuretic	Diuretic
Tolbutamide	3	<1	Yes	Yes
Acetohexamide	4	1	No	Yes
Tolazamide	4	1	No	Yes
Chlorpropamide	9	4–6	Yes	No
Glyburide	7	4–6	No	Yes
Glipizide	6	2–4	No	Yes

nation half-time (average 33 hours), the maximal effect of chlorpropamide may not be apparent for 7 to 14 days, and several weeks may be required for complete elimination of the drug. Because 20% of a dose is excreted unchanged, impaired renal function can lead to chlorpropamide accumulation and an enhanced hypoglycemic effect. Chlorpropamide is unique in being associated with reactions similar to those produced by disulfiram (facial flushing after ingestion of alcohol) and with the inappropriate secretion of ADH, which can cause severe hyponatremia. Approximately 5% of patients treated with chlorpropamide have serum sodium concentrations of less than 129 $mEq \cdot L^{-1}$, but they are usually asymptomatic. Risk factors include age greater than 60 years, female sex, and the concomitant use of thiazide diuretics. If all are present, the frequency of hyponatremia increases threefold.

Glyburide

Glyburide stimulates insulin secretion over a 24-hour period after a morning oral dose (Feldman, 1985). Peak plasma levels occur approximately 3 hours after oral administration. Peripheral effects include increased sensitivity to insulin and inhibition of hepatic glucose production. Metabolism is in the liver with metabolites excreted equally in the urine and feces. One of the hepatic metabolites of glyburide has approximately 15% of the activity of the parent compound. A mild diuretic effect accompanies use of this drug. When administration is discontinued, the drug is cleared from the plasma in approximately 36 hours.

Glipizide

Glipizide stimulates insulin secretion over a 12-hour period after a morning oral dose. Peak plasma levels occur in approximately 1 hour after oral administration. Peripheral effects include increased glucose uptake and suppression of hepatic glucose output (Lebovitz, 1985). These effects on insulin secretion persist for prolonged periods (at least 3 years) without evidence of tolerance. Metabolism in the liver produces inactive substances (in contrast to glyburide), which are excreted in the urine. A mild diuretic effect accompanies use of this drug. Relatively rapid clearance from the plasma should minimize the potential for glipizide to produce long-lasting hypoglycemia.

Metformin

Metformin is a biguanide oral hypoglycemic drug that rarely produces lactic acidosis (Fig. 24-3) (Gerich 1989). This drug produces satisfactory results in approximately 50% of cases in which sulfonylureas have failed. In contrast to sulfonylureas, metformin rarely causes hypoglycemia, is not bound to plasma proteins, and does not undergo metabolism. It is eliminated by the kidneys with 90% of an oral dose being excreted in ap-

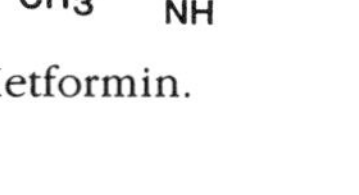

FIGURE 24–3. Metformin.

proximately 12 hours. Peak plasma levels of metformin occur approximately 2 hours after oral administration. The drug has an elimination half-time of 2 to 4 hours, requiring its administration up to 3 times a day (500 to 1000 mg with meals). The most common side effects are anorexia, nausea, and diarrhea, occurring initially in 5% to 20% of patients. Fewer than 5% of patients experience side effects sufficient to warrant withdrawal of the drug. The mechanism of action of metformin does not involve stimulation of insulin secretion but rather an effect on the liver to reduce basal hepatic glucose production.

Intestinal Glycosidase Inhibitors

Acarbose is an intestinal glycosidase inhibitor that delays systemic absorption of glucose and is devoid of dangerous side effects (Gerich, 1989). This drug improves the effectiveness of injected insulin in patients with insulin-dependent diabetes mellitus and partially compensates for delayed insulin secretion in patients with noninsulin-dependent diabetes mellitus who are being treated with diet or sulfonylureas. Because the principal effect of acarbose is on postprandial hyperglycemia, it is probably suitable for most patients only as adjunctive therapy.

REFERENCES

Burgos LG, Ebert TJ, Asiddao C, et al. Increased intraoperative cardiovascular morbidity in diabetics with autonomic neuropathy. Anesthesiology 1989; 70:591–7.

Feldman JM. Glyburide: Second generation sulfonylurea hypoglycemic agent; History, chemistry, metabolism, pharmacokinetics, clinical use and adverse effects. Pharmacotherapy 1985;5:43–62.

Gerich JE. Oral hypoglycemic agents. N Engl J Med 1989;321:1231–43.

Hagedorn HC, Jensen BN, Krarup NB, Woodstrup I. Protamine insulinate. JAMA 1936;106:179–80.

Larner J. Insulin and oral hypoglycemic drugs; glucagon. In: Gilman AG, Goodman LS, Rall TW, Murad F, eds. The Pharmacological Basis of Therapeutics, 7th ed. New York. Macmillan Publishing Co. 1985;1:1490–1516.

Lebovitz HE. Glipizide: Second-generation sulfonylurea hypoglycemic agent. Pharmacology, pharmacokinetics and clinical use. Pharmacotherapy 1985;5:63–77.

Stewart WJ, McSweeney SM, Kellett MA, Faxon DP, Ryan TJ. Increased risk of severe protamine reactions in NPH–insulin-dependent diabetics undergoing cardiac catheterization. Circulation 1984;70:788–92.

Ullrich A, Bell JR, Chen EY, et al. Human insulin receptor and its relationship to the tyrosine kinase family of oncogenes. Nature 1985;313:756–61.

Zinman B. The physiologic replacement of insulin. An elusive goal. N Engl J Med 1989;321:363–70.

Chapter
25
Diuretics

Diuretics are among the most frequently prescribed drugs, with the classic pharmacologic response being diuresis. These drugs are classified according to their site of action on renal tubules and the mechanism by which they alter the excretion of solute as (1) thiazide diuretics, (2) loop diuretics, (3) osmotic diuretics, (4) potassium-sparing diuretics, (5) aldosterone antagonists, and (6) carbonic anhydrase inhibitors (Tables 25-1 and 25-2) (Merin and Bastron, 1986).

THIAZIDE DIURETICS

Thiazide diuretics are administered orally in divided daily doses to treat essential hypertension and mobilize edema fluid associated with renal, hepatic, or cardiac dysfunction (Fig. 25-1). Most often, a thiazide diuretic is selected as the initial treatment of essential hypertension, either as the sole drug or in combination with an antihypertensive drug. In combination with thiazide diuretics, the dose of more potent antihypertensive drugs can be reduced 25% to 50%, thus minimizing drug-induced side effects. Less common uses of thiazide diuretics include management of diabetes insipidus and treatment of hypercalcemia.

Mechanism of Action

Thiazide diuretics produce diuresis by inhibiting reabsorption of sodium (Na^+) and chloride (Cl^-) ions, principally in the cortical portion of the ascending loops of Henle and, to a lesser extent, in the proximal renal tubules and distal renal tubules (Table 25-2) (Merin and Bastron, 1986).

The result is a marked increase in the urinary excretion of Na^+, Cl^-, and bicarbonate ions (HCO_3^-) (Table 25-3) (Tonnesen, 1983.). An associated increased secretion of potassium ions (K^+) into the renal tubules occurs whenever there is enhanced distal delivery of Na^+ and water. This emphasizes that the normal driving force for K^+ secretion by distal renal tubules is the transtubular electrical potential difference created by Na^+ reabsorption. Thiazide diuretics, by inhibiting Na^+ reabsorption, lead to the delivery of higher concentrations of Na^+ to the distal

Table 25–1
Classification of Diuretics

Thiazide Diuretics
Chlorothiazide
Hydrochlorothiazide
Benzthiazide
Cyclothiazide

Loop Diuretics
Ethacrynic Acid
Furosemide

Osmotic Diuretics
Mannitol
Urea

Potassium-sparing Diuretics
Triamterene
Amiloride

Aldosterone Antagonists
Spironolactone

Carbonic Anhydrase Inhibitors
Acetazolamide

Table 25–2
Sites of Action of Diuretics

	Thiazide Diuretics	Loop Diuretics	Osmotic Diuretics	Potassium-Sparing Diuretics	Aldosterone Antagonists	Carbonic Anhydrase Inhibitors
Early proximal convoluted tubule		+	+			
Proximal convoluted tubule	+	+				+++
Medullary portion of ascending loop of Henle		+++	+++			
Cortical portion of ascending loop of Henle	+++	+	+			
Distal convoluted tubule	+	+	+	+++		+
Collecting duct					+++	

+, minor site of action; +++, major site of action
(Adapted from Merin RG, Bastron RD. Diuretics. In: Smith NT, Miller RD, Corbascio AN, eds. Drug Interactions in Anesthesia. Philadelphia: Lea and Febiger 1986; 206–24; with permission.)

renal tubules and the subsequent enhancement of secretion of K^+ into the renal tubules. The diuretic effect of thiazide diuretics is independent of acid-base balance.

Antibypertensive Effect

The antihypertensive effect of thiazide diuretics is due initially to a reduction in extracellular fluid volume, often with a reduction in cardiac output. The sustained antihypertensive effect of thiazide diuretics, however, is due to peripheral vasodilation, which takes several weeks to develop. This peripheral vasodilation may reflect a diminished effect of sympathetic nervous system activity at peripheral vascular smooth muscle, which correlates roughly with the reduction in total body stores of Na^+. This diuretic-induced reduction in systemic vascular resistance is accompanied by at least partial correction of the decreased extracellular fluid volume. The importance of diuretic-induced Na^+ excretion is sug-

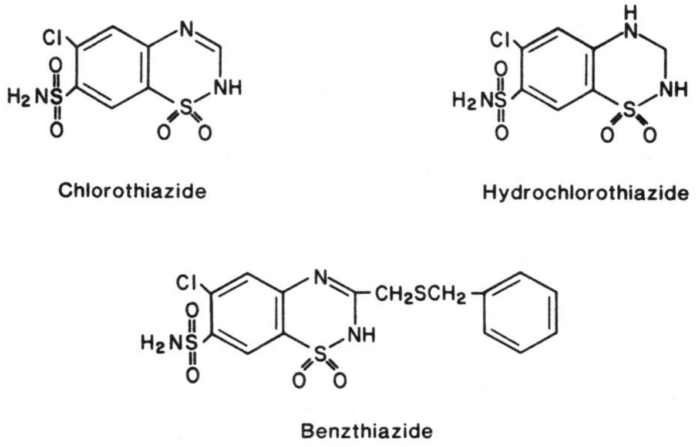

Chlorothiazide

Hydrochlorothiazide

Benzthiazide

FIGURE 25–1. Thiazide diuretics.

Table 25-3
Effects of Diuretics on Urine Composition

	Volume (ml·min^{-1})	pH	Sodium (mEq·L^{-1})	Potassium (mEq·L^{-1})	Chloride (mEq·L^{-1})	Bicarbonate (mEq·L^{-1})
No drug	1	6.4	50	15	60	1
Thiazide diuretics	13	7.4	150	25	150	25
Loop diuretics	8	6.0	140	25	155	1
Osmotic diuretics	10	6.5	90	15	110	4
Potassium-sparing diuretics	3	7.2	130	10	120	15
Carbonic anhydrase inhibitors	3	8.2	70	60	15	120

(Adapted from Tonnesen AS. Clinical pharmacology and use of diuretics. In: Hershey SG, Bamforth BJ, Zander H, eds. Review Courses in Anesthesiology. Philadelphia: JB Lippincott Co. 1983; 217–26; with permission.)

gested by the absence of an antihypertensive effect when thiazide diuretics are administered to anephric animals (Freis, 1976).

Side Effects

Thiazide diuretic-induced hypokalemic, hypochloremic, metabolic alkalosis is a common side effect when these drugs are administered chronically, as in the treatment of essential hypertension (Table 25-4). Depletion of Na$^+$ and magnesium ions may accompany kaliuresis. Cardiac dysrhythmias may occur as the result of diuretic-induced hypokalemia or hypomagnesemia. Other important side effects of hypokalemia that may occur include (1) skeletal muscle weakness, (2) gastrointestinal ileus, (3) nephropathy characterized by polyuria and azotemia, (4) increased likeli-

hood of developing digitalis toxicity, and (5) potentiation of nondepolarizing neuromuscular blocking drugs.

Intravascular fluid volume should be evaluated in all patients being treated with thiazide diuretics and scheduled for surgery. The presence of orthostatic hypotension in such patients should arouse suspicion that intravascular fluid volume is reduced. Laboratory evidence of hemoconcentration (increased hematocrit and elevated blood urea nitrogen concentration) and decreased right or left atrial filling pressures are further evidence of hypovolemia.

Thiazide diuretics may cause hyperglycemia and aggravate diabetes mellitus. The mechanism of hyperglycemia is unknown but may reflect drug-induced inhibition of insulin release from the pancreas and blockade of peripheral glucose utilization.

Table 25-4
Side Effects of Diuretics

	Hypokalemic, Hypochloremic, Metabolic Alkalosis	Hyperkalemia	Hyperglycemia	Hyperuricemia	Hyponatremia
Thiazide diuretics	Yes	No	Yes	Yes	Yes
Loop diuretics	Yes	No	Minimal	Minimal	Yes
Potassium-sparing diuretics	No	Yes	Minimal		Minimal
Aldosterone antagonists	No	Yes	No	No	Yes

Inhibition of renal tubular secretion of urate by thiazide diuretics can result in hyperuricemia. This thiazide-induced retention of uric acid can exacerbate gouty arthritis, even in patients being treated with probenecid.

Borderline renal or hepatic function may deteriorate further during treatment with thiazide diuretics, presumably reflecting drug-induced reductions in blood flow to these organs. A maculopapular rash occurs in 1% or more of patients treated with chlorothiazide.

LOOP DIURETICS

Ethacrynic acid and furosemide are examples of diuretics that inhibit reabsorption of Na^+ and Cl^- primarily in the medullary portion of the ascending limb of Henle's loop (Table 25-2; Fig. 25-2) (Merin and Bastron, 1986). This site of action accounts for the designation of these drugs as loop diuretics. Intravenous administration of either ethacrynic acid or furosemide produces within 2 to 10 minutes a diuretic response that is independent of acid-base changes (Table 25-3) (Tonnesen, 1983). Indeed, responsiveness to furosemide is directly related to the glomerular filtration rate over a wide range. Conversely, responses to thiazide diuretics follow this relationship only when glomerular filtration rates are greatly reduced to less than 20 ml·min^{-1}.

Pharmacokinetics

Ethacrynic Acid

Ethacrynic acid is effective when administered orally (0.75 to 3 mg·kg^{-1}) or intravenously (0.5 to 1 mg·kg^{-1}). A high incidence of gastrointestinal reactions follows oral administration of this diuretic. Protein binding is extensive. Ethacrynic acid is excreted by the kidneys as unchanged drug and an unstable metabolite.

Furosemide

Furosemide is effective when administered orally (0.75 to 3 mg·kg^{-1}) or intravenously (0.1 to 1 mg·kg^{-1}). Protein binding to albumin is extensive, accounting for approximately 90% of the drug. Glomerular filtration and renal tubular secretion account for approximately 50% of furosemide excretion. Approximately one third of a dose of furosemide is metabolized or excreted unchanged in the bile. The elimination half-time is less than 1 hour, accounting for the short duration of action of furosemide.

Clinical Uses

Clinically, furosemide is used far more often than ethacrynic acid. Common clinical uses of furosemide include (1) mobilization of edema fluid owing to renal, hepatic, or cardiac dysfunction; (2) treatment of increased intracranial pressure; and (3) differential diagnosis of acute oliguria. Loop diuretics have little use in the chronic treatment of essential hypertension. Indeed, the antihypertensive effect of furosemide is due entirely to its ability to reduce intravascular fluid volume, which, if it occurs rapidly, may evoke baroreceptor reflex–mediated increases in sympathetic nervous system activity. Acceleration of excretion of other drugs, such as long-acting nondepolarizing neuromuscular blocking drugs, by furosemide-induced diuresis is limited because this diuretic does not increase glomerular filtration rate or renal tubular secretion.

Mobilization of Edema Fluid

Furosemide, administered in doses of 0.1 to 1 mg·kg^{-1} IV, produces prompt diuresis of edema fluid owing to renal, hepatic, or cardiac dysfunction. Peripheral vasodilation precedes the onset of diuresis, and the associated reduction in ve-

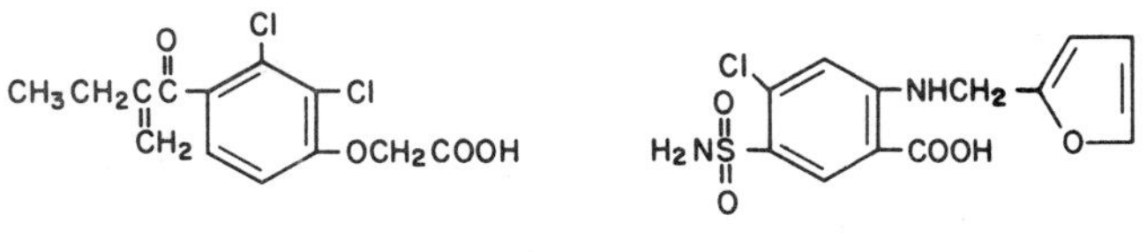

Ethacrynic Acid   Furosemide   **FIGURE 25–2.** Loop diuretics.

nous return is consistent with the prompt and efficacious effects of furosemide in the management of acute pulmonary edema. Furosemide also increases thoracic duct lymph flow (Fig. 25-3) (Szwed et al, 1972).

Treatment of Increased Intracranial Pressure

Administration of furosemide, 0.1 to 1 mg·kg^{-1} IV, decreases intracranial pressure without producing alterations in plasma osmolarity (Cottrell et al, 1977). This reflects mobilization of edema fluid and intracellular dehydration. Furthermore, furosemide may decrease production of cerebrospinal fluid by interfering with Na$^+$ transport in glial tissue.

In addition, alterations in the blood-brain barrier do not influence the immediate or subsequent effects of furosemide on intracranial pressure. This contrasts with mannitol, which may produce rebound intracranial hypertension if a disrupted blood-brain barrier allows mannitol to enter the central nervous system.

Differential Diagnosis of Acute Oliguria

Furosemide administered in small doses (0.1 mg·kg^{-1} IV) will stimulate diuresis in the presence of excessive antidiuretic hormone effect.

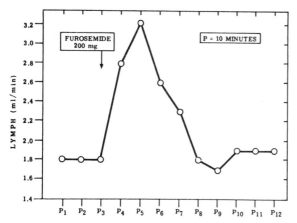

FIGURE 25–3. Furosemide increases flow of lymph through the thoracic duct. (From Szwed JJ, Kleit SA, Hamburger RJ. Effect of furosemide and chlorothiazide on the thoracic duct lymph flow in the dog. J Lab Clin Med 1972;79:693–700; with permission.)

This drug must not be used, however, to treat acute oliguria owing to decreased intravascular fluid volume because furosemide-induced diuresis could further exaggerate hypovolemia and aggravate renal ischemic changes that result from poor renal blood flow. Furthermore, continued urine output in the presence of furosemide can no longer be considered evidence of adequate intravascular fluid volume, cardiac output, and renal blood flow.

The use of furosemide to treat acute renal failure is controversial. Attempts to convert oliguric renal failure into the nonoliguric form, which is associated with a lower mortality, has not proven beneficial when compared with untreated controls (Byrick and Rose, 1990). Nevertheless, furosemide has been used to decrease metabolic activity by inhibiting active cellular transport of solutes with the speculation that this change would be protective if a subsequent renal tubular ischemic event should occur.

Large doses of furosemide (up to 10 mg·kg^{-1} IV) can increase renal blood flow principally to the renal cortex (Koechel, 1981). This increase in renal blood flow, however, occurs only when intravascular fluid volume is maintained. Redistribution of renal blood flow may reflect furosemide-induced release of prostaglandins and renin. Indeed, indomethacin in doses adequate to block the synthesis of prostaglandins prevents an increase in renal blood flow following the administration of furosemide (Patak et al, 1975). In an animal model, furosemide, 1 to 10 mg·kg^{-1} IV, administered during or immediately following an acute ischemic insult (unilateral renal artery infusion of norepinephrine for 40 minutes), limits the extent of experimental renal failure (Cronin et al, 1978).

Side Effects

Side effects of loop diuretics are most often manifested as abnormalities of fluid and electrolyte balance. Loss of K$^+$ and Cl$^-$ is prominent, and hypokalemia is a constant threat in patients treated with furosemide (Table 25-4).

In animals, loop diuretics deplete myocardial K$^+$ stores and increase the likelihood of digitalis toxicity. Hypokalemia has been associated with enhancement of the effects of nondepolarizing neuromuscular blocking drugs. Furosemide may also act on presynaptic nerve terminals to inhibit production of cyclic adenosine monophosphate and the subsequent release of acetylcholine, which would also potentiate nondepolarizing neuromuscular blocking drugs (Miller et al, 1976). As with thiazide diuretics, loop diuretics may cause hyperuricemia, but this is rarely clinically significant. Likewise, hyperglycemia, although possible, is less likely to occur than with thiazide diuretics.

Furosemide elevates renal tissue concentrations of aminoglycosides and enhances the possible nephrotoxic effect of these antibiotics. Cephalosporin nephrotoxicity may also be increased by furosemide. Furosemide has been associated with allergic interstitial nephritis similar to that occasionally produced by penicillin. Cross-sensitivity may exist between furosemide and patients allergic to other sulfonamides. The renal clearance of lithium is decreased in the presence of diuretic-induced reductions in Na^+ reabsorption. Consequently, plasma concentrations in lithium may be acutely increased by the intravenous administration of furosemide in the perioperative period (Havdala et al, 1979). In symptomatic hypercalcemia, furosemide may lower the plasma concentration of calcium by stimulating urine output.

High doses of furosemide, such as may be used to treat acute renal failure, can result in the accumulation of reactive intermediary metabolites. These reactive intermediary metabolites can produce hepatic necrosis in animals (Mitchell et al, 1974). At the usual clinical doses, however, hepatotoxicity is not observed, but this theoretical possibility should be kept in mind when large doses of furosemide are administered to patients with renal failure.

Development of deafness, either transient or permanent, is a rare and unique complication produced by furosemide and ethacrynic acid. This side effect is most likely to occur with prolonged elevations of the plasma concentrations of these drugs. Drug-induced changes in the electrolyte composition of the endolymph is a possible mechanism. Patients who are allergic to sulfonamide-containing drugs (sulfonamide antibiotics or thiazide diuretics) may be at increased risk for developing allergic reactions when treated with furosemide (Hansbrough et al, 1987). A similar cross-sensitivity with ethacrynic acid is less likely because this diuretic lacks a sulfonamide nucleus (Figs. 25-1 and 25-2).

OSMOTIC DIURETICS

Osmotic diuretics such as mannitol and urea are freely filterable at the glomerulus, undergo limited reabsorption from renal tubules, resist metabolism, and are pharmacologically inert. These characteristics permit administration of osmotic diuretics in sufficiently large quantities to alter the osmolarity of the plasma, glomerular filtrate, and renal tubular fluid, resulting in osmotic diuresis.

Mannitol

Mannitol is the most frequently used osmotic diuretic. Structurally, mannitol is a six-carbon sugar that does not undergo metabolism (Fig. 25-4). It is not absorbed from the gastrointestinal tract, which necessitates its exclusive use by intravenous injection to achieve a diuretic effect. Mannitol does not enter cells, and its only means of clearance from the plasma is by way of the glomerular filtrate.

Mechanism of Action

Following intravenous administration, mannitol is completely filtered at the glomeruli, and none of the filtered drug is subsequently reabsorbed from the renal tubules (Table 25-2) (Merin and Bastron, 1986). As a result, mannitol raises the osmolarity of renal tubular fluid and prevents reabsorption of water. Na^+ is diluted in this retained water in the renal tubules, leading to less reabsorption of this ion. As a result of this osmotic effect in the renal tubular fluid, there is an osmotic diuretic effect, with urinary excretion of water, Na^+, Cl^-, and HCO_3^- (Table 25-3) (Tonnesen, 1983). Urinary pH is not altered by mannitol-induced osmotic diuresis (Table 25-3) (Tonnesen, 1983).

$$
\begin{array}{c}
CH_2OH \\
| \\
HOCH \\
| \\
HOCH \\
| \\
HCOH \\
| \\
HCOH \\
| \\
CH_2OH
\end{array}
$$

FIGURE 25-4. Mannitol.

In addition to renal tubular effects, intravenous administration of mannitol also increases plasma osmolarity, thus drawing fluid from intracellular to extracellular spaces. This increased plasma osmolarity may result in an acute expansion of the intravascular fluid volume. Redistribution of fluid from intracellular to extracellular sites decreases brain size and may increase renal blood flow. Likewise, the acute increase in intravascular fluid volume may have detrimental effects in patients with poor myocardial function.

Clinical Uses

Mannitol is administered for prophylaxis against (1) acute renal failure, (2) differential diagnosis of acute oliguria, (3) treatment of increases in intracranial pressure, and (4) reduction of intraocular pressure.

PROPHYLAXIS AGAINST ACUTE RENAL FAILURE.
Mannitol is used as prophylaxis against acute renal failure, which may occur after (1) cardiovascular surgery, (2) extensive trauma, (3) surgery in the presence of jaundice, and (4) hemolytic transfusion reactions.

Experimental data suggest that the administration of hypertonic mannitol prior to an ischemic insult will reduce renal damage (Byrick and Rose, 1990). There are several proposed mechanisms for this protective effect. For example, mannitol, by remaining in the renal tubules, increases distal renal tubular delivery of Na^+, thus providing a flushing effect for any necrotic cellular debris that might enter the renal tubules following ischemic injury. Furthermore, the concentration of any nephrotoxin in the renal tubular fluid does not reach the excessively high levels that would occur in the presence of more complete reabsorption of water. Another possible mechanism for the protective effect of mannitol may be the ability of the hyperosmotic state induced by this drug to reduce endothelial cell swelling, thus decreasing vascular congestion that would limit blood flow to inner medullary regions of the kidneys. Prophylactic administration of mannitol and low-dose dopamine during and following infrarenal cross-clamping of the abdominal aorta has not been shown to prevent transient deteriorations in renal function in patients whose hemodynamic stability is maintained (Byrick and Rose, 1990). Likewise, the protective effect of mannitol administration after the development of oliguria is not well established. The protective effect of mannitol as used for prevention of acute renal failure following a transfusion reaction has not been proven (Goldfinger, 1977). The rationale for its use, which is relief of renal tubular obstruction by precipitated hemoglobin, has been largely discounted.

TREATMENT OF INCREASED INTRACRANIAL PRESSURE.
Mannitol, $0.25-1$ g·kg^{-1} IV, acts to decrease intracranial pressure by increasing plasma osmolarity, which draws water from tissues, including the brain, along an osmotic gradient. There is little difference in the effect of this dose range on intracranial pressure, but the larger dose may last longer (Marsh et al, 1977). Importantly, mannitol is not associated with a high incidence of rebound increases in intracranial pressure. An intact blood-brain barrier is necessary to prevent entrance of mannitol into the central nervous system. If the blood-brain barrier is not intact, mannitol may enter the brain, drawing fluid with it and producing rebound cerebral edema. Regardless, the brain eventually adapts to sustained elevations in plasma osmolarity such that chronic use of mannitol is likely to become less effective for lowering intracranial pressure.

DIFFERENTIAL DIAGNOSIS OF ACUTE OLIGURIA.
Mannitol, 0.25 g·kg^{-1} IV, is useful in the differential diagnosis of acute oliguria. For example, urine output is increased by mannitol when the cause of acute oliguria is decreased intravascular fluid volume. Conversely, when glomerular or renal tubular function are severely compromised, mannitol will not increase urine flow.

REDUCTION OF INTRAOCULAR PRESSURE.
Mannitol, glycerin, and isosorbide are occasionally used for the short-term reduction of intraocular pressure in patients undergoing ophthalmologic surgery. By increasing plasma osmolarity, fluid leaves the intraocular space along an osmotic gradient. Glycerin and isosorbide are administered orally and may contribute to an increased gastric fluid volume at the time of anesthesia induction. A maximal reduction in intraocular pressure and vitreous volume occurs approximately 1 hour after oral administration of glycerin, with a return to pretreatment levels in approximately 5 hours. Metabolism of glycerin to glucose can cause hy-

perglycemia and glycosuria, emphasizing the need for caution in administering this substance to patients with diabetes mellitus. Because it is rapidly metabolized, glycerin produces minimal diuresis, and routine urinary bladder catheterization for surgery is not required. Isosorbide does not adversely affect blood glucose levels and is preferred in patients with diabetes mellitus.

Side Effects

In patients with oliguria secondary to cardiac failure, acute mannitol-induced increases in intravascular fluid volume may precipitate pulmonary edema. Conversely, hypovolemia may follow excessive excretion of water and Na^+. Nephrotoxins and prolonged renal ischemia may damage the renal tubular epithelium so that renal tubules are no longer impermeable to mannitol and the osmotic effect of the diuretic is lost.

Diuresis secondary to mannitol does not alter the elimination rate of long-acting nondepolarizing neuromuscular blocking drugs. This is predictable because these neuromuscular blocking drugs depend on glomerular filtration, which is not altered by mannitol. Venous thrombosis is not likely to occur after the intravenous administration of mannitol and tissue necrosis is unlikely if extravasation occurs.

Urea

Urea, 1 to 1.5 $g \cdot kg^{-1}$ IV, is an effective osmotic diuretic, but, unlike mannitol, its small molecular size results in reabsorption of more than 60% of urea filtered at the glomerulus (Fig. 25-5). This drug eventually penetrates cells and crosses the blood-brain barrier, resulting in a greater degree of rebound increase in intracranial pressure than occurs after administration of mannitol. Another disadvantage of urea is a high incidence of venous thrombosis and the possibility of tissue necrosis if extravasation of urea-containing solutions occurs. Elevated blood urea nitrogen concentrations following administration of urea should not be confused with acute renal failure.

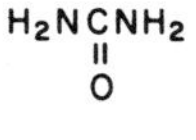

$$H_2NCNH_2$$
$$\overset{\|}{O}$$

FIGURE 25–5.   Urea.

POTASSIUM-SPARING DIURETICS

Potassium-sparing diuretics such as triamterene and amiloride act directly on renal tubular transport mechanisms in the distal convoluted tubule independent of aldosterone to produce diuresis (Table 25-2; Fig. 25-6) (Merin and Bastron, 1986). This diuresis is characterized by an increase in the urinary excretion of Na^+, Cl^-, and HCO_3^- and an elevation of the urine pH (Table 25-3) (Tonnesen, 1983). Diuresis is accompanied either by no increase or a decrease in K^+ excretion in the urine (Table 25-3) (Tonnesen, 1983). The lack of diuretic-induced K^+ excretion results from inhibition of K^+ secretion into distal renal tubules.

Clinical Uses

The greatest value of potassium-sparing diuretics is in combination with hydrochlorothiazide. This combination maximizes diuretic efficiency of both drugs while offsetting their opposite effects on urinary excretion of K^+. Aerosolized amiloride administered to patients with cystic fibrosis improves sputum viscosity presumably by inhibiting excessive absorption of Na^+ across the airway epithelium (Knowles et al, 1990).

Side Effects

Hyperkalemia is the principal side effect of therapy with potassium-sparing diuretics (Table 25-4). Unlike other diuretics, these drugs do not produce hyperuricemia.

ALDOSTERONE ANTAGONISTS

Spironolactone is the prototype of drugs that act as competitive antagonists at receptor sites on collecting ducts that otherwise respond to aldosterone (Table 25-2; Fig. 25-7) (Merin and Bastron, 1986). This drug is effective only when aldosterone is present. Normally, aldosterone augments the renal tubular reabsorption of Na^+ and Cl^- and increases the excretion of K^+. Spironolactone blocks these renal tubular effects of aldosterone, as reflected by inhibition of the reabsorption of Na^+ and Cl^-.

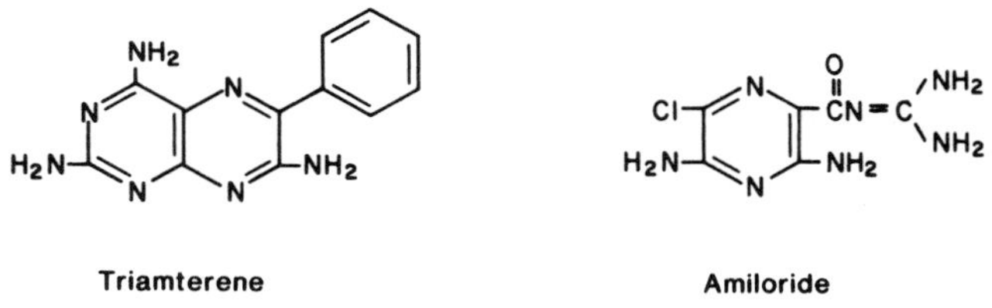

FIGURE 25–6. Potassium-sparing diuretics.

Triamterene   Amiloride

Clinical Uses

Spironolactone is often prescribed for fluid overload owing to cirrhosis of the liver on the assumption that reduced hepatic function and metabolism lead to increased plasma concentrations of aldosterone. The antihypertensive effect of this diuretic is similar to that of thiazide diuretics, but side effects are different. The combination of spironolactone and hydrochlorothiazide (Aldactazide) is an attempt to maximize diuretic efficiency of both drugs while offsetting their opposite effects of K^+ secretion.

Side Effects

Hyperkalemia, especially in the presence of renal dysfunction, is the most serious side effect of treatment with spironolactone (Table 25-4). In contrast to thiazide diuretics, spironolactone does not cause hypokalemia, hyperglycemia, or hyperuricemia (Table 25-4).

CARBONIC ANHYDRASE INHIBITORS

Acetazolamide is the prototype of a class of sulfonamide drugs that bind tightly to the carbonic anhydrase enzyme, producing noncompetitive inhibition of enzyme activity, principally in the proximal renal tubules (Table 25-2; Fig. 25-8) (Merin and Bastron, 1986). As a result of this enzyme inhibition, the excretion of hydrogen ions

(H^+) is diminished and loss of HCO_3^- is increased (Table 25-3) (Tonnesen, 1983). Cl^- is retained by the kidney to offset the loss of HCO_3^- and thus maintain an ionic balance. Decreased availability of H^+ in the distal renal tubules results in excretion of K^+ in exchange for Na^+. The net effect of all these changes is excretion of an alkaline urine in the presence of hyperchloremic metabolic acidosis. The diuretic action of acetazolamide is not altered by metabolic or respiratory acidosis. Following oral administration, acetazolamide is excreted unchanged by the kidneys in 24 hours.

Clinical Uses

The most common clinical uses of acetazolamide, 250 to 500 mg administered orally, are to reduce intraocular pressure in the treatment of glaucoma and as an adjuvant for management of petit mal and grand mal epilepsy. Decreased intraocular pressure reflects the presence of high concentrations of carbonic anhydrase enzyme in the ocular structures, and a resulting decrease in formation of aqueous humor when enzyme activity is inhibited by acetazolamide. Formation of cerebrospinal fluid is also inhibited by acetazolamide. Acetazolamide inhibits seizure activity, presumably by producing metabolic acidosis.

Beneficial effects of acetazolamide in the management of familial periodic paralysis may reflect drug-induced metabolic acidosis, which raises the local concentration of K^+ in skeletal

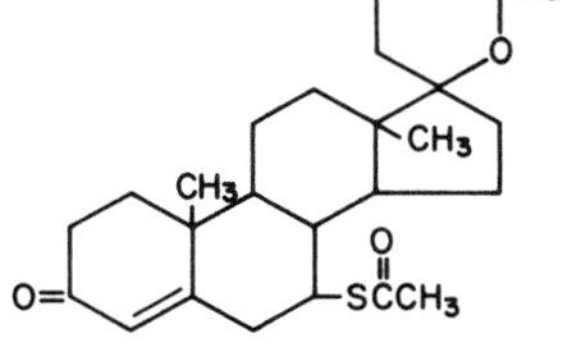

FIGURE 25–7. Spironolactone.

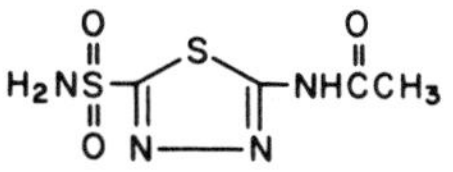

FIGURE 25–8. Acetazolamide.

muscle. Acetazolamide, by producing metabolic acidosis, may stimulate ventilation in patients who are hypoventilating as a compensatory response to metabolic alkalosis. Conversely, the loss of HCO_3^- necessary to buffer carbon dioxide may result in exacerbation of hypercarbia in patients with chronic obstructive airway disease, leading to central nervous system depression.

REFERENCES

Byrick RJ, Rose DK. Pathophysiology and prevention of acute renal failure: The role of the anaesthetist. Can J Anaesth 1990;37:457–67.

Cottrell JE, Robustelli A, Post K, Turndorf H. Furosemide and mannitol-induced changes in intracranial pressure and serum osmolality and electrolytes. Anesthesiology 1977;47:28–30.

Cronin RE, McColl AL, DeTorrente A, McDonald KM, Schrier RW. Norepinephrine-induced acute renal failure. Kidney Int 1978;14:73–6.

Freis ED. Salt, volume, and the prevention of hypertension. Circulation 1976;53:589–95.

Goldfinger D. Acute hemolytic transfusion reactions—A fresh look at pathogenesis and considerations regarding therapy. Transfusion 1977;17:985–98.

Hansbrough JR, Wedner J, Chaplin DD. Anaphylaxis to intravenous furosemide. J Allergy Clin Immunol 1987;80:538–41.

Havdala HS, Borison RL, Diamond BI. Potential hazards and applications of lithium in anesthesiology. Anesthesiology 1979;50:534–7.

Knowles MR, Church NL, Waltner WE, et al. A pilot study of aerosolized amiloride for the treatment of lung disease in cystic fibrosis. N Engl J Med 1990;322:1189–94.

Koechel DA. Ethacrynic acid and related diuretics: Relationship of structure to beneficial and detrimental actions. Ann Rev Pharmacol Toxicol 1981;21:265–93.

Marsh ML, Marshall LF, Shapiro HM. Neurosurgical intensive care. Anesthesiology 1977;47:149–63.

Merin RG, Bastron RD. Diuretics. In: Smith NT, Miller RD, Corbascio AN, eds. Drug Interactions in Anesthesia. Philadelphia. Lea and Febiger. 1986;206–24.

Miller RD, Sohn YJ, Matteo RS. Enhancement of d-tubocurarine neuromuscular blockade by diuretics in man. Anesthesiology 1976;45:442–5.

Mitchell JR, Potter WZ, Hinson JA, Jollow DJ. Hepatic necrosis caused by furosemide. Nature 1974;251:508–11.

Patak R, Mookerjee BK, Bentzel CJ, Hysert PE, Babej M, Lee JB. Antagonism of the effects of furosemide by indomethacin in normal and hypertensive man. Prostaglandins 1975;10:649–53.

Szwed JJ, Kleit SA, Hamburger RJ. Effect of furosemide and chlorothiazide on the thoracic duct lymph flow in the dog. J Lab Clin Med 1972;79:693–700.

Tonnesen AS. Clinical pharmacology and use of diuretics. In: Hershey SG, Bamforth BJ, Zauder H, eds. Review Courses in Anesthesiology, Philadelphia. JB Lippincott Co. 1983:217–26.

26

Chapter 76

Gastric Antacids, Stimulants, and Antiemetics

GASTRIC ANTACIDS

Gastric antacids are drugs that neutralize or remove acid from the gastric contents. Clinically useful antacids are aluminum, calcium, and magnesium salts that react with hydrochloric acid to form neutral, less acidic, or poorly soluble salts. Doses of antacids that increase gastric fluid pH above 5 inactivate pepsin and facilitate healing of a peptic ulcer. Neutralization of gastric fluid pH increases gastric motility via the action of gastrin (with the exception of aluminum hydroxide) and increases lower esophageal sphincter tone by a mechanism that is independent of gastrin. Liquid preparations are generally more effective than tablets for neutralizing acids *in vivo*. When antacids are appropriately used, they are as effective as cimetidine in the treatment of peptic ulcer, reflux esophagitis, and prophylaxis against stress-induced ulceration and hemorrhage.

Side Effects

The only adverse effects shared by all antacids are those resulting from changes in gastric and urinary pH and alterations in acid-base status. Gastric alkalinization has been suggested as a cause of increased susceptibility to various acid-sensitive microbial pathogens. In the presence of renal failure, all antacids except aluminum compounds can cause metabolic alkalosis. Elevation of the urinary pH may persist for longer than 24 hours following administration of an antacid, leading to alterations in the renal elimination of drugs. Alkalinization of the urine may predispose to urinary tract infections; if it is chronic, urolithiasis is possible.

Drug Interactions

Because gastric alkalinization hastens gastric emptying, antacids other than aluminum compounds will hasten delivery of drugs into the small intestine. This may speed absorption of drugs that are poorly absorbed or it may shorten the time available for absorption. The rate of absorption of salicylates, indomethacin, and naproxen is increased when gastric fluid pH is elevated. Aluminum hydroxide accelerates absorption and increases bioavailability of diazepam by an unknown mechanism. Conversely, bioavailability of drugs may be decreased because of their capacity to form complexes with antacids. For example, antacids reduce bioavailability of orally administered cimetidine by approximately 15% (Gulger et al, 1981). One hour should elapse between the ingestion of an antacid and oral cimetidine to minimize this interaction. Antacids containing aluminum, and to a lesser extent calcium and magnesium, interfere with the absorption of tetracyclines and possibly digoxin from the gastrointestinal tract.

Commercial Preparations

Aluminum Hydroxide

Aluminum hydroxide is actually a mixture of aluminum hydroxide, aluminum oxide, and some fixed carbon dioxide as carbonate. Systemic absorption of aluminum is minimal, but in patients with renal disease, the plasma and tissue concentrations of aluminum may become excessive (Berlyne et al, 1970). Encephalopathy in patients undergoing hemodialysis has been attributed to intoxication with aluminum (Alfrey et al, 1976). Among the compounds formed in the intestine from aluminum hydroxide are insoluble aluminum phosphates, which pass through the intestinal tract unabsorbed. Hypophosphatemia can occur and is the basis for the occasional therapeutic use of aluminum hydroxide in the treatment of phosphate nephrolithiasis. Decreased phosphate absorption is accompanied by increased calcium ion (Ca^{2+}) absorption, which sometimes causes hypercalciuria and nephrolithiasis. Hypomagnesemia can also occur. Aluminum compounds, in contrast to other antacids, cause slowing of gastric emptying and marked constipation. These effects, in addition to an unpleasant taste, contribute to poor patient acceptance.

SUCRALFATE. Sucralfate is a complex of sulfated sucrose and aluminum hydroxide that is used for the short-term (up to 8 weeks) treatment of duodenal ulcer. This compound lacks antacid action but instead adheres to the ulcer to form a protective barrier against pepsin penetration. The efficacy of sucralfate in facilitating healing of duodenal ulcers appears to be comparable with that of cimetidine. The most common side effect of sucralfate is constipation. Simultaneous administration of antacids may interfere with the action of sucralfate.

Calcium Carbonate

Calcium carbonate produces rapid and effective neutralization of gastric acidity. Although systemic absorption is slight, sufficient absorption occurs with chronic therapy to produce a detectable metabolic alkalosis. The plasma concentration of Ca^{2+} is increased transiently. Clinically, dangerous hypercalcemia may occur in patients with renal disease. The administration of calcium carbonate-containing antacids may be accompanied by hyperphosphatemia. Even small amounts of calcium carbonate-containing antacids evoke hypersecretion of hydrogen ions (H^+); (acid rebound) (Clayman, 1980). The chalky taste of calcium carbonate is a disadvantage. The release of carbon dioxide in the stomach may cause eructation and flatulence. Constipation is minimized by including magnesium oxide with calcium carbonate. Acute appendicitis has been produced by impacted calcium carbonate fecaliths.

MILK-ALKALI SYNDROME. The milk-alkali syndrome may occur after prolonged administration of calcium carbonate with sodium bicarbonate or homogenized milk containing vitamin D. This rare syndrome is characterized by hypercalcemic alkalosis, nausea, and occasionally renal failure. Conjunctival and episcleral suffusion accompanies the alkalosis. Ca^{2+} deposits manifest as band keratopathy. Symptoms are reversible with discontinuation of the antacid or milk. Magnesium and aluminum salts have not been implicated in this syndrome.

Magnesium Oxide

Magnesium hydroxide (milk of magnesia) produces prompt neutralization of gastric acid and is not associated with significant acid rebound. In contrast to aluminum hydroxide, a prominent laxative effect is characteristic of magnesium hydroxide. Systemic absorption of magnesium may be sufficient to cause neurologic, neuromuscular, and cardiovascular impairment in patients with renal dysfunction. In normal patients, absorption of magnesium is associated with little danger of systemic alkalosis. Magnesium is often combined with aluminum hydroxide.

Sodium Bicarbonate

The high solubility of sodium bicarbonate results in an immediate and rapid antacid action in the stomach. The effect, however, is short-lived, and systemic alkalosis is possible. Weight gain may be prominent with chronic therapy. Sodium bicarbonate is useful when the goal is to alkalinize the urine.

Table 26-1
Contents (mg per 5 ml) of Particulate Antacids

	Aluminum Hydroxide	Magnesium Hydroxide	Calcium Carbonate	Sodium
Aludrox	307	103		1.1
Amphojel	320			6.9
Di-Gel	282	85		10.6
Gelusil	200	200		0.7
Maalox	225	200		1.35
Mylanta	200	200		0.68
Riopan	480			0.3
Tums			500	<3
WinGel	180	160		<2.5

Antacid Selection

There is considerable variation in the acid-neutralizing effects of different antacids (Table 26-1). Poorly absorbed antacids are preferred in the treatment of peptic ulcer. Mixtures of aluminum hydroxide and magnesium hydroxide are used most frequently. Calcium carbonate has a greater neutralizing capacity, but it is infrequently used because of concern about systemic Ca^{2+} absorption and Ca^{2+}-induced acid rebound. There is no convincing evidence that mixtures of antacids have greater beneficial effects than those provided by the individual antacid.

Preoperative Administration of Antacids

Preoperative administration of antacids to increase gastric fluid pH prior to the induction of general anesthesia would theoretically reduce the risk of acid pneumonitis if inhalation (aspiration) of gastric fluid occurs. Indeed, approximately 17% of patients scheduled for elective surgery have a gastric fluid pH less than 2.5 and a gastric fluid volume more than 20 ml (Table 26-2) (Stoelting, 1978). Despite the predictability of antacids to increase gastric fluid pH and theoretically reduce the risk associated with aspiration, it has not been documented that routine

Table 26-2
Percentages of Patients with Gastric Fluid pH <2.5 and/or Volume >20 ml

	pH <2.5 (%)	Volume >20 ml (%)	pH <2.5, Volume >20 ml (%)
Morphine (n = 75)	63	27	16
Morphine-atropine (n = 75)	58	27	17
Morphine-glycopyrrolate (n = 75)	52	23	16
Morphine–atropine–Riopan (n = 25)	0*	60*	0

*P < 0.05 compared with morphine.
n, number of patients.
(Data from Stoelting RK. Responses to atropine, glycopyrrolate, and Riopan of gastric fluid pH and volume in adult patients. Anesthesiology 1978; 48: 367–9; with permission.)

use of antacids in a high-risk patient population (parturients) decreases mortality (Taylor, 1975; Tompkinson et al, 1982). Furthermore, antacids or other prophylactic drugs (H-2 receptor antagonists or metoclopramide) do not reduce the possibility of regurgitation and aspiration.

The duration of antacid action is highly dependent on gastric emptying time. For example, opioid-induced slowing of gastric motility prolongs the pH-elevating effects of antacids in these patients compared with the effects in patients not receiving opioids (O'Sullivan and Bullingham, 1985). Repeated administration of antacids, such as to the parturient who has also received opioids, can result in a greatly increased gastric fluid volume and can predispose the parturient to regurgitation if general anesthesia is induced. In this regard, it is logical to administer an antacid as a single dose approximately 30 minutes before the induction of anesthesia.

Even a single dose of antacid may increase the gastric fluid volume, and it has been speculated that this effect could offset desirable effects on pH if aspiration occurs. Nevertheless, in an animal model, mortality was 90% following inhalation of 0.3 ml·kg^{-1} of gastric fluid with a pH of 1 compared with 14% mortality following inhalation of 1 to 2 ml·kg^{-1} of gastric fluid with a pH of more than 1.8 (Table 26-3) (James et al, 1984). These data suggest that an increased gastric fluid volume produced by administration of an antacid will not increase the likelihood of aspiration

Table 26–3
Mortality Rate (%) for Rats After Aspiration of Solutions of Various pH and Volumes

Volume (ml·kg^{-1})	Fluid pH					
	1.0	1.4	1.8	2.5	3.5	5.8
0.2	20	0				
0.3	90	0	9			
0.4	90	40	9	0		
1.0	100	90	20	0	0	0
2.0	100	100	27	30	20	10
4.0	100	100	38	20	40	30

(Data from James CF, Modell JH, Gibbs CP, Kuck EJ, Ruiz BC. Pulmonary aspiration effects of volume and *p*H in the rat. Anesth Analg 1984; 63: 665–8; with permission.)

pneumonitis as long as the gastric fluid pH is elevated.

Particulate Antacids

Occasional failure of particulate antacids to elevate gastric fluid pH may reflect inadequate mixing with stomach contents or an unusually large volume of gastric fluid such that the standard dose of antacid is inadequate. Layering is common with particulate antacids (Holdsworth et al, 1980). Pneumonitis associated with functional and histologic changes in the lung may reflect a foreign body reaction to inhaled particulate antacid particles. Indeed, aspiration of a particulate antacid in a dog model produced changes comparable to those induced by acid (Gibbs et al, 1979). Clinical reports suggest that particulate antacids have caused or aggravated aspiration pneumonitis in humans (Bond et al, 1979; Heaney and Jones, 1979).

Nonparticulate Antacids

Nonparticulate (clear) antacids such as sodium citrate are less likely to cause a foreign body reaction if aspirated, and their mixing with gastric fluid is more complete than is that of particulate antacids (Gibbs et al, 1979; Holdsworth et al, 1980). Furthermore, the onset of effect is more rapid with sodium citrate than with particulate antacids that require longer times for adequate mixing with gastric fluid. Sodium citrate, 15 to 30 ml of 0.3 M solution administered 15 to 30 minutes before the induction of anesthesia, is effective in reliably elevating gastric fluid pH in pregnant and nonpregnant patients (Gibbs et al, 1982; Viegas et al, 1981). The pH of 0.3 M sodium citrate is approximately 8.4, accounting for its unpleasant taste and frequent addition of a flavoring agent to improve its palatability.

Bicitra is a nonparticulate antacid containing sodium citrate and citric acid that provides effective buffering of gastric fluid pH (Eyler et al, 1982). Polycitra is a nonparticulate antacid containing sodium citrate, potassium citrate, and citric acid that has greater buffering capacity than Bicitra (Conklin and Ziadlou-Rad, 1983). Bicitra and Polycitra are more palatable than sodium citrate, possibly due to their lower pHs of 4.5 and 5.2, respectively.

GASTROINTESTINAL PROKINETICS

Metoclopramide

Metoclopramide (methoxychloroprocainamide) is a dopamine antagonist that is structurally similar to procainamide but lacks local anesthetic activity (Fig. 26-1). Metoclopramide acts as a gastrointestinal prokinetic drug that stimulates motility of the upper gastrointestinal tract and increases lower esophageal sphincter tone by 10 to 20 cmH$_2$O in normal persons and parturients (Brock-Utne et al, 1978). Gastric acid secretion is not altered. The net effect is accelerated gastric clearance of liquids and solids (decreased gastric emptying time) and a shortened transit time through the small intestine.

Mechanism of Action

Metoclopramide produces selective cholinergic stimulation of the gastrointestinal tract (gastrokinetic effect) consisting of (1) increased smooth muscle tension in the lower esophageal sphincter and gastric fundus, (2) increased gastric and small intestinal motility, and (3) relaxation of the pylorus and duodenum during contraction of the stomach (Schulze-Delrieu, 1981). Cholinergic stimulating effects of metoclopramide are largely restricted to smooth muscle of the proximal gastrointestinal tract and require some background cholinergic activity. There is evidence that metoclopramide sensitizes gastrointestinal smooth muscle to the effects of acetylcholine, which explains why metoclopramide, unlike conventional cholinergic drugs, requires background cholinergic activity to be effective. Postsynaptic activity results from the ability of metoclopramide to cause the release of acetylcholine from cholinergic nerve endings. Indeed, atropine opposes metoclopramide-induced increases in lower esophageal sphincter tone and gastrointestinal hypermotility, indicating that metoclopramide acts on postganglionic cholinergic nerves intrinsic to the wall of the gastrointestinal tract. In the central nervous system, metoclopramide blocks dopamine receptors. As a result, metoclopramide induces secretion of prolactin, and extrapyramidal symptoms may occur.

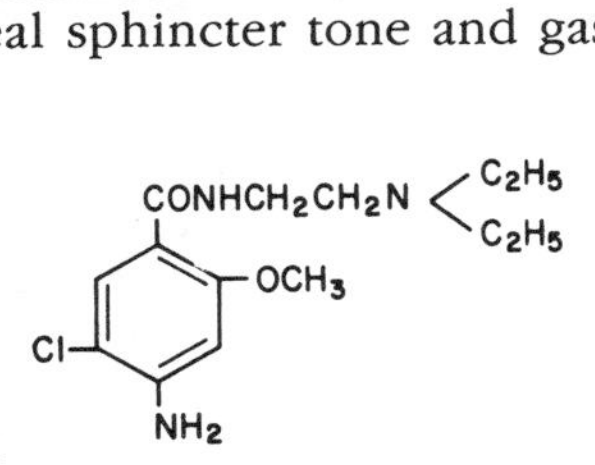

Pharmacokinetics

Metoclopramide is rapidly absorbed after oral administration, reaching peak plasma concentrations in 40 to 120 minutes (Schulze-Delrieu, 1981). Most patients achieve therapeutic plasma concentrations of 40 to 80 ng·ml^{-1} after 10 mg of metoclopramide administered orally. Intravenous doses of metoclopramide such as those used to speed gastric emptying are 10 to 20 mg. The elimination half-time is 2 to 4 hours. Approximately 85% of an oral dose of metoclopramide appears in the urine, equally divided among unchanged drug and sulfate and glucuronide conjugates. Impairment of renal function prolongs the elimination half-time and necessitates a reduction in metoclopramide dosage.

Clinical Uses

Clinical uses of metoclopramide include (1) preoperative reduction of gastric fluid volume, (2) treatment of gastroparesis, and (3) production of an antiemetic effect. Increased prolactin secretion evoked by metoclopramide has been proposed as a means to test the function of the anterior pituitary or to improve lactation in the postpartum period (Schulze-Delrieu, 1981). Metoclopramide has been used to improve the effectiveness of oral medication when other drugs or the patient's underlying condition slows gastric emptying. A possible benefit of metoclopramide in the management of patients with reflux esophagitis is suggested by the ability of this drug to increase lower esophageal sphincter tone. Indeed, metoclopramide reduces the incidence of heartburn. Nevertheless, lower esophageal sphincter tone has probably been overrated as a factor in reflux esophagitis.

PREOPERATIVE REDUCTION OF GASTRIC FLUID VOLUME. Metoclopramide, 10 to 20 mg IV, over 3 to 5 minutes at 15 to 30 minutes before induction of anesthesia, results in increased lower esopha-

FIGURE 26–1. Metoclopramide.

geal sphincter tone and decreased gastric fluid volume (Wyner and Cohen, 1982). More rapid intravenous administration may produce abdominal cramping. This gastric emptying effect of metoclopramide would be of particular benefit prior to the induction of anesthesia in (1) patients who have eaten, (2) trauma patients, (3) obese patients, (4) outpatients, and (5) parturients, especially those with a history of heartburn, suggesting lower esophageal sphincter dysfunction and gastric hypomotility. Nevertheless, beneficial effects of metoclopramide on gastric fluid volume may be difficult to document in otherwise normal patients with low gastric fluid volumes who are awaiting elective surgery (Table 26-4) (Cohen et al, 1984a). Regardless of the effect on gastric fluid volume, the administration of metoclopramide does not reliably alter gastric fluid pH. Furthermore, it is important to recognize that opioid-induced inhibition of gastric motility may not be reversible with metoclopramide. Likewise, the beneficial cholinergic stimulant effects of metoclopramide on the gastrointestinal tract may be offset by concomitant administration of atropine in the preoperative medication. Under no circumstances do metoclopramide or other protective drugs (antacids or H-2 receptor antagonists) replace the need for protection of the airway with a cuffed tracheal tube placed in the awake patient or following the appropriate induction of general anesthesia.

Table 26–4
Volume of Gastric Contents and pH in Study Groups (Mean ± SE)

	Metoclopramide (n = 30)	Placebo (n = 28)
Gastric Volume (range)	24 ± 2 ml (3–60)	30 ± 5 ml (4–155)
Volume >25 ml	16* (53%)	15* (54%)
Gastric pH (range)	2.86 ± 0.27 (1–6)	2.55 ± 0.24 (1–55)
pH <2.5	12* (40%)	16* (57%)

*Number of patients.
(Data from Cohen SE, Jasson J, Talafre M-L, Chauvelot-Moachon L, Barrier G. Does Metoclopramide decrease the volume of gastric contents in patients undergoing cesarean section? Anesthesiology 1984; 61: 604–7; with permission.)

TREATMENT OF GASTROPARESIS. Treatment of gastroparesis, as associated with diabetes mellitus, is with orally administered metoclopramide, 10 to 20 mg. Administration of metoclopramide, 10 to 20 mg IV, is indicated to facilitate small bowel intubation or to speed gastric emptying to improve radiographic examination of the small intestine. This dose should be administered over 3 to 5 minutes to reduce the likelihood of abdominal cramping.

PRODUCTION OF AN ANTIEMETIC EFFECT. The antiemetic property of metoclopramide probably results from antagonism of dopamine receptors in the chemoreceptor trigger zone. Additional antiemetic effects are provided by metoclopramide-induced increases in lower esophageal sphincter tone and facilitation of gastric emptying into the small intestine (these processes reverse gastric immobility and cephalad peristalsis that accompany the vomiting reflex). Gastric stasis induced by morphine is reversed by metoclopramide, and opioid-induced nausea and vomiting,which can accompany preoperative medication or postoperative pain management may be blunted by this drug. Administration of metoclopramide, 0.15 mg·kg^{-1} IV, following delivery of the infant greatly reduces the incidence of early postoperative nausea and vomiting in parturients undergoing elective cesarean section with epidural anesthesia (Fig. 26-2) (Chestnut et al, 1987). The usefulness of metoclopramide, 5 to 10 mg, administered orally before induction of anesthesia as prophylaxis against postoperative nausea and vomiting may be limited by its relatively brief duration of action. Indeed, reports of the antiemetic efficacy of metoclopramide administered preoperatively to prevent postoperative nausea and vomiting have been inconsistent (Cohen et al, 1984b; Pandit et al, 1989).

Side Effects

Side effects of metoclopramide are mild and infrequent but include sedation, dysphoria, agitation, dry mouth, glossal or periorbital edema, hirsutism, and urticarial or maculopapular rash. These side effects, including sedation, have not been observed following single doses of metoclopramide (Cohen et al, 1984a).

Extrapyramidal reactions are rare, occurring in approximately 1 in 500 patients. Although usu-

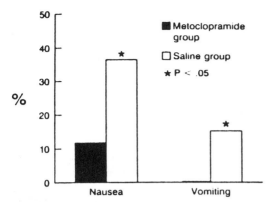

FIGURE 26–2. Incidence of intraoperative and post-delivery nausea and vomiting in parturients undergoing elective cesarean section with lumbar epidural anesthesia and receiving metoclopramide, 0.15 mg·kg^{-1} IV, or saline immediately after the umbilical cord was clamped. (From Chestnut DH, Vandewalker GE, Owen CL, Bates JN, Choi, WW. Administration of metoclopramide for prevention of nausea and vomiting during epidural anesthesia for elective cesarean section. Anesthesiology 1987;66:563–6; with permission.)

ally developing when large oral doses (40 to 80 mg daily) are administered chronically, there are reports of neurologic dysfunction related to the preoperative administration of metoclopramide (Barnes et al, 1982; Scheller and Sears, 1987). These extrapyramidal reactions are identical to the Parkinson's syndrome evoked by antipsychotic drugs that antagonize the central nervous system actions of dopamine (Grimes et al, 1982). Akathisia, a feeling of unease and restlessness in the lower limbs, seems to be related to plasma concentrations of metoclopramide of more than 100 ng·ml^{-1}. This response has been noted even with short-term use, particularly in young children or elderly patients with renal dysfunction.

Placental transfer of metoclopramide occurs rapidly, but adverse fetal effects with single doses have not been observed (Cohen et al, 1984a). The usual dopamine-induced inhibition of aldosterone secretion is prevented by metoclopramide. As a result, the possibility of sodium retention and hypokalemia should be considered, especially in patients who developed edema during chronic therapy. The major concern of chronic therapy with metoclopramide is stimulation of prolactin secretion and resulting galactorrhea. For this reason, patients with a history of carcinoma of

the breast probably should not be treated with metoclopramide.

Metoclopramide may increase the sedative actions of central nervous system depressants and the incidence of extrapyramidal reactions caused by certain drugs. For this reason, metoclopramide should not be given in combination with phenothiazine or butyrophenone drugs or to patients with extrapyramidal symptoms or epilepsy. Patients being treated with monoamine oxidase inhibitors or tricyclic antidepressants should not receive metoclopramide. This drug reduces the bioavailability of orally administered cimetidine by 25% to 50% (Gugler et al, 1981). Metoclopramide is contraindicated in the presence of gastrointestinal obstruction.

Metoclopramide has an inhibitory effect on plasma cholinesterase activity when tested *in vitro,* which may explain occasional observations of modestly prolonged responses to succinylcholine in patients receiving this drug (Kambam et al, 1988; Kao et al, 1990). Parturients may be at increased risk for this response considering the already reduced plasma cholinesterase activity associated with pregnancy. Likewise, the metabolism of ester local anesthetics could be slowed by metoclopramide-induced reductions in plasma cholinesterase activity.

Cisapride

Cisapride is a gastrointestinal prokinetic drug that stimulates gastric emptying and elevates lower esophageal sphincter tone (Rowbotham, 1989). This drug also enhances motility in the small and large intestine. In contrast to metoclopramide, this drug lacks dopamine antagonist effects. Instead, cisapride produces its gastrointestinal effects by enhancing the release of acetylcholine from nerve endings in the myenteric plexus in the wall of the gastrointestinal tract.

Opioid-induced gastric stasis, which may be an important cause of postoperative nausea and vomiting, is reversed by cisapride. The production rate and composition of gastric secretions are not affected by cisapride. Administration of cisapride before antagonism of neuromuscular blockade with atropine and neostigmine does not prevent the ability of atropine to decrease lower esophageal sphincter pressure (Jones et al, 1989).

ANTIEMETICS

(See also Chapters 19 and 21.)

Domperidone

Domperidone, like metoclopramide, is a dopamine receptor antagonist (Fig. 26-3). Unlike metoclopramide, domperidone does not easily cross the blood-brain barrier; thus its antidopaminergic activity is limited to peripheral sites. Indeed, extrapyramidal reactions do not accompany administration of domperidone. Restriction of antidopaminergic activity to peripheral sites allows domperidone to influence the chemoreceptor trigger zone, which is outside the blood-brain barrier, without affecting the basal ganglia. Domperidone increases lower esophageal sphincter tone and speeds gastric emptying (Brock-Utne, 1980).

Domperidone appears to be particularly effective in treating postprandial nausea and vomiting associated with gastroenteritis (Reyntjens, 1979). It may be useful for nausea and vomiting associated with dysmenorrhea, migraine headache, and radiation therapy. Domperidone is of no value for postoperative nausea and vomiting or that induced by opioids, and is of limited value against vomiting induced by chemotherapeutic drugs (Fragen and Caldwell, 1979).

Domperidone is rapidly absorbed after oral or intramuscular administration. Extensive metabolism occurs in the liver, and biliary excretion of inactive metabolites is the main route of elimination. The elimination half-time is approximately 7 hours.

Benzquinamide

Benzquinamide is a short-acting benzquinoline derivative that is used most often to prevent

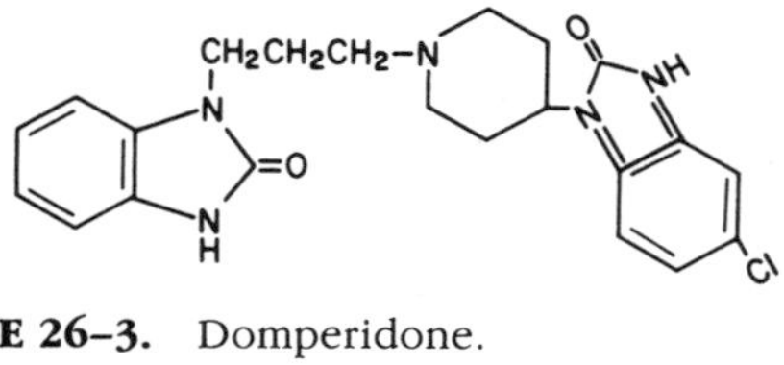

FIGURE 26–3.   Domperidone.

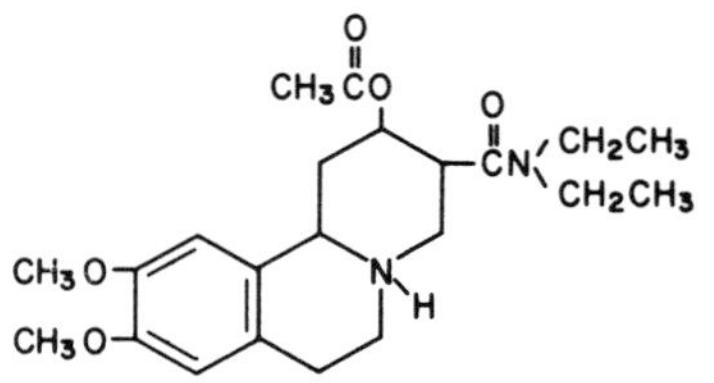

FIGURE 26–4.   Benzquinamide.

postoperative nausea and vomiting (Fig. 26-4). This drug apparently inhibits stimuli at the chemoreceptor trigger zone. The intramuscular dose is 0.5 to 1 $mg \cdot kg^{-1}$, injected at least 15 minutes prior to administration of antineoplastic drugs or emergence from anesthesia. The intravenous dose of benzquinamide is 0.2 to 0.4 $mg \cdot kg^{-1}$. The elimination half-time is approximately 40 minutes.

Side Effects

Drowsiness is noted frequently following administration of benzquinamide. Shivering, chills, and mild anticholinergic reactions have been observed. Benzquinamide directly relaxes vascular smooth muscle, producing reductions in systemic vascular resistance and hypotension that are compensated for by reflex activation of the sympathetic nervous system manifesting as increased circulating concentrations of norepinephrine (Fig. 26-5) (Smith et al, 1979). Reflex increases in heart rate and cardiac output are also possible. Indeed, sudden increases in blood pressure and cardiac dysrhythmias may accompany rapid intravenous administration of benzquinamide. Administration of benzquinamide to patients with moderate to severe hypertension or severe cardiovascular disease may be questionable, particularly if the drug is given intravenously during anesthesia. The modest ventilatory stimulant effect of benzquinamide may offset opioid-induced depression of ventilation (Mull and Smith, 1974). Conversely, phenothiazine antiemetics can potentiate opioid-induced depression of ventilation.

Benzquinamide has anticholinergic properties and can induce delirium (central anticholinergic syndrome) that is responsive to physostigmine (Chapin and Wingard, 1977). Conversely, in other patients, benzquinamide may produce dystonic extrapyramidal reactions. It is important

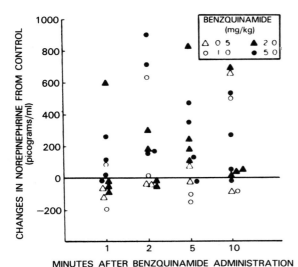

FIGURE 26–5. Intravenous administration of benzquinamide is accompanied by reflex activation of the sympathetic nervous system that often manifests as increased plasma concentrations of norepinephrine. (From Smith DJ, Rushin JM, Urquilla PR, et al. Cardiovascular effects of benzquinamide. Anesth Analg 1979; 58:189–94; with permission.)

to distinguish between those two responses because administration of physostigmine in the presence of extrapyramidal effects produced by benzquinamide could cause the symptoms to become worse. Likewise, treating a patient with drug-induced central anticholinergic syndrome with atropine would be deleterious. An important difference between these two reactions is the impairment of consciousness during anticholinergic excess but not during extrapyramidal responses.

Tetrahydrocannabinol (Dronabinol)

Tetrahydrocannabinol (THC) is the psychoactive component of marijuana that possesses antiemetic efficacy when given orally during cancer chemotherapy (Poster et al, 1981). This antiemetic effect is more effective in patients treated with methotrexate than in those treated with cyclophosphamide, doxorubicin, and cisplatin. Tetrahydrocannibol may also be effective as an antiemetic in patients who develop tolerance to metoclopramide, butyrophenones, or phenothiazines.

The antiemetic effect of THC lasts 2 to 3 hours, which parallels its psychoactive effects. The occasional dysphoric response or hallucinations limit the usefulness of THC as an antiemetic, particularly in patients with psychiatric disorders. Administration of THC to patients with epilepsy is questionable because it may enhance seizure activity. The drug may produce transient tachycardia, and large doses may cause orthostatic hypotension. These effects should be considered before THC is administered to patients with coronary artery disease or valvular heart disease. In animals, the acute intravenous administration of THC produces a transient dose-related reduction in anesthetic requirements (MAC) that parallels sedative effects (Stoelting et al, 1973; Vitez et al, 1973).

Tetrahydrocannibol is slowly and erratically absorbed from the gastrointestinal tract. The peak plasma concentration is reached in 60 to 90 minutes. Protein binding is extensive, accounting for 97% to 99% of the drug. Following systemic absorption, THC is converted to 11-hydroxyl-THC, which possesses equivalent pharmacologic activity. Subsequent metabolism results in inactive compounds that are excreted in the urine and feces. The elimination half-time of THC is approximately 19 hours, and that of its metabolites is approximately 48 hours.

Diphenidol

Diphenidol acts on the vestibular apparatus and is useful as an antiemetic for nausea and vomiting associated with radiation, chemotherapeutic drugs, and general anesthesia (Fig. 26-6). This drug is also effective in labyrinthine-induced vertigo following surgery on the middle and inner ear. Because of its central anticholinergic actions, diphenidol may induce visual or auditory hallucinations, disorientation, or confusion. Dryness of the mouth, sedation, and tachycardia may occur. More than 90% of diphenidol is eliminated by the kidney.

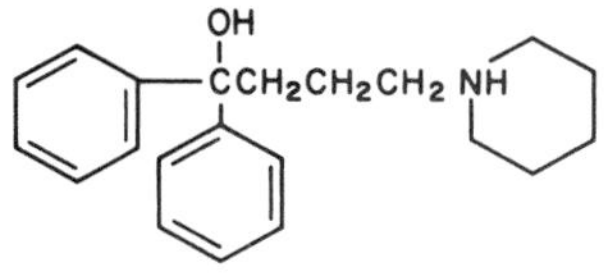

FIGURE 26-6. Diphenidol.

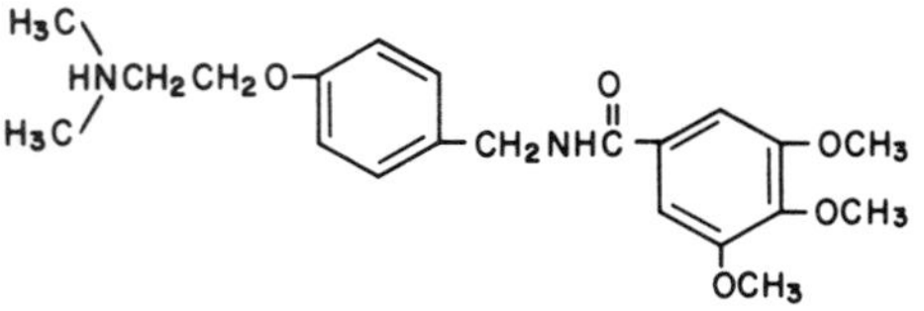

FIGURE 26-7. Trimethobenzamide.

Trimethobenzamide

Trimethobenzamide is useful as an antiemetic by inhibiting stimuli at the chemoreceptor trigger zone (Fig. 26-7). It is not as effective as phenothiazines in treating postoperative vomiting and has little or no value in the prevention or treatment of vertigo or motion sickness. Extrapyramidal reactions have been noted.

Fluphenazine

Fluphenazine is a piperazine phenothiazine that is effective in managing nausea and vomiting postoperatively and following radiation. Sedation is minimal, and awakening time after anesthesia is not altered when this drug is administered preoperatively. Fluphenazine does not prevent vertigo or motion sickness, and the incidence of extrapyramidal reactions is greater than with other phenothiazines.

Prochlorperazine

Prochlorperazine is a piperazine phenothiazine that is effective in managing postoperative nausea and vomiting and that which is due to radiation. Sedation and extrapyramidal reactions are undesirable side effects, especially with repeated doses. Prochlorperazine does not prevent vertigo or motion sickness.

REFERENCES

Alfrey AC, LeGendre GR, Kaehny WS. The dialysis encephalopathy syndrome. Possible aluminum intoxication. N Engl J Med 1976;294:184–8.

Barnes TRE, Brande WM, Hill DJ. Acute akathisia after oral droperidol and metoclopramide preoperative medication. Lancet 1982;2:48–9.

Berlyne GM, Ben-Ari J, Pest D, et al. Hyperaluminaemia from aluminum resins in renal failure. Lancet 1970;2:494–6.

Bond VK, Stoelting RK, Gupta CD. Pulmonary aspiration syndrome after inhalation of gastric fluid containing antacids. Anesthesiology 1979;51:452–3.

Brock-Utne JG, Dow TGB, Welman S, Dimopoulos GE, Moshal MG. The effect of metoclopramide on lower oesophageal sphincter tone in late pregnancy. Anaesth Intensive Care 1978;6:26–9.

Brock-Utne JG, Downing JW, Dimopoulos GE, Rubin J, Moshal MG. Effect of domperidone on lower esophageal sphincter tone in late pregnancy. Anesthesiology 1980;52:321–3.

Chapin JW, Wingard DW. Physostigmine reversal of benzquinamide-induced delirium. Anesthesiology 1977;46:364–5.

Chestnut DH, Vandewalker GE, Owen CL, Bates JN, Choi WW. Administration of metoclopramide for prevention of nausea and vomiting during epidural anesthesia for elective cesarean section. Anesthesiology 1987;66:563–6.

Clayman CB. The carbonate affair: Chalk one up (editorial). JAMA 1980;244:2554.

Cohen SE, Jasson J, Talafre M-L, Chauvelot-Moachon L, Barrier G. Does metoclopramide decrease the volume of gastric contents in patients undergoing cesearean section? Anesthesiology 1984a;61:604–7.

Cohen SE, Woods WA, Wyner J. Antiemetic efficacy of droperidol and metoclopramide. Anesthesiology 1984b;60:67–9.

Conklin KA, Ziadlou-Rad F. Buffering capacity of citrate antacids. Anesthesiology 1983;58:391–2.

Eyler SW, Cullen BF, Murphy ME, Welch WD. Antacid aspiration in rabbits: A comparison of Mylanta and Bicitra. Anesth Analg 1982;61:288–92.

Fragen RJ, Caldwell N. Antiemetic effectiveness of intramuscularly administered domperidone. Anesthesiology 1979;51:460–1.

Gibbs CP, Schwartz DJ, Wynne JW, Hood CI, Kuck EJ. Antacid pulmonary aspiration in the dog. Anesthesiology 1979;51:380–5.

Gibbs CP, Spohr L, Schmidt D. The effectiveness of sodium citrate as an antacid. Anesthesiology 1982;57:44–46.

Grimes JD, Hassan MN, Preston DN. Adverse neurologic effects of metoclopramide. Can Med Assoc J 1982;126:23–5.

Gugler R, Brand M, Somogyi A. Impaired cimetidine absorption due to antacids and metoclopramide. Eur J Clin Pharmacol 1981;20:225–8.

Heaney GAH, Jones HD. Aspiration syndrome in pregnancy (correspondence). Br J Anaesth 1979;51:266–7.

Holdsworth JD, Johnson K, Mascall G, Roulston RG, Tomlinson PA. Mixing of antacids with stomach contents. Anaesthesia 1980;35:641–50.

James CF, Modell JH, Gibbs CP, Kuck EJ, Ruiz BC. Pulmonary aspiration effects of volume and pH in the rat. Anesth Analg 1984;63:665–8.

Jones MJ, Mitchell WD, Hindocha N. Effects on the lower oesophageal sphincter of cisapride given before the combined administration of atropine and neostigmine. Br J Anaesth 1989;62:124–8.

Kambam JR, Parris WCV, Franks JJ, Sastry BVR, Naukam R, Smith BE. The inhibitory effect of metoclopramide on plasma cholinesterase activity. Can J Anaesth 1988;35:476–8.

Kao YJ, Teliez J, Turner DR. Dose-dependent effect of metoclopramide on cholinesterases and suxamethonium metabolism. Br J Anaesth 1990;65:220–4.

Mull TD, Smith TC. Comparison of the ventilatory effects of two antiemetics, benzquinamide and prochlorperazine. Anesthesiology 1974;40:581–7.

O'Sullivan GM, Bullingham RE. Noninvasive assessment by radiotelemetry of antacid effect during labor. Anesth Analg 1985;64:95–100.

Pandit SK, Kothary SP, Pandit UA, Randel G, Levy L. Dose-response study of droperidol and metoclopramide as antiemetics for outpatient anesthesia. Anesth Analg 1989;68:798–802.

Poster DS, Penta JS, Bruno S, MacDonald JS. Delta-nine-tetrahydrocannabinol in clinical oncology. JAMA 1981;245:2047–51.

Reyntjens A. Domperidone as antiemetic: Summary of research reports. Postgrad Med J 1979;55:50–4.

Rowbotham DJ. Cisapride and anaesthesia. Br J Anaesth 1989;62:121–3.

Scheller MS, Sears KL. Postoperative neurologic dysfunction associated with preoperative administration of metoclopramide. Anesth Analg 1987;66:274–6.

Schulze-Delrieuer. Drug therapy: Metoclopramide. N Engl J Med 1981;305:28–33.

Smith DJ, Rushin JM, Urquilla PR, et al. Cardiovascular effects of benzquinamide. Anesth Analg 1979;58:189–94.

Stoelting RK. Responses to atropine, glycopyrrolate, and Riopan of gastric fluid *p*H and volume in adult patients. Anesthesiology 1978;48:367–9.

Stoelting RK, Martz RC, Gartner J, Creasser C, Brown DJ, Forney RB. Effects of delta-9-tetrahydrocannabinol on halothane MAC in dogs. Anesthesiology 1973;38:521–4.

Taylor G. Acid pulmonary aspiration syndrome after antacids. Br J Anaesth 1975;47:615–6.

Tompkinson J, Turnbull A, Robson R, et al. Report on Confidential Enquiries into Maternal Deaths in England and Wales 1976–1978. London. Her Majesty's Stationery Office 1982;79–80.

Viegas OJ, Ravindran RS, Shumacker CA. Gastric fluid *p*H in patients receiving sodium citrate. Anesth Analg 1981;60:521–3.

Vitez TS, Way Wl, Miller RD, Eger EI. Effects of delta-9-tetrahydrocannabinol on cyclopropane MAC in the rat. Anesthesiology 1973;38:525–7.

Wyner J, Cohen SE. Gastric volume in early pregnancy: Effect of metoclopramide. Anesthesiology 1982;57:209–12.

Chapter

27

Anticoagulants

Anticoagulants are drugs that delay or prevent the clotting of blood by direct or indirect actions on the coagulation system (Stow and Burrows, 1987). These drugs, however, have no effect on the thrombus (clot) after it is formed. Antithrombotic drugs usually influence the formation of thrombus by acting on platelets. Thrombolytic drugs are those that possess inherent fibrinolytic effects or enhance the body's fibrinolytic system.

HEPARIN

Heparin is a negatively charged mucopolysaccharide organic acid that is present endogenously in high concentrations in the liver and granules of mast cells and basophils. It is one of the strongest acids occurring naturally in the body (Stow and Burrows, 1987). The designation "heparin" emphasizes the abundance of this substance in the liver.

Commercial Preparations

Heparin for clinical uses is most commonly prepared from bovine lung and bovine or porcine gastrointestinal mucosa. Standardization of heparin potency is based on *in vitro* comparison with a known standard. A *unit of heparin* is defined as the volume of heparin-containing solution that will prevent 1 ml of citrated sheep blood from clotting for 1 hour following the addition of 0.2 ml of 1:100 calcium chloride. Heparin must contain at least 120 United States Pharmacopeia units per ml. Because the potency of different commer-

cial preparations of heparin may vary greatly, the heparin dose should always be prescribed in units.

Clinical Uses

Commercially prepared solutions of heparin are used exclusively to produce an anticoagulant effect. Associated with this anticoagulant effect is a reduction in plasma triglyceride concentrations owing to heparin-induced release of lipid-hydrolyzing enzymes, such as lipoprotein lipase, into the circulation.

The onset of anticoagulant effect is almost instantaneous following intravenous injection of heparin and occurs 20 to 30 minutes after subcutaneous injection. In addition to providing anticoagulation during specific operative procedures, low-dose heparin is efficacious as a primary prophylaxis against postoperative deep vein thrombosis and pulmonary embolism. For example, the incidence of pulmonary embolism is reduced in patients older than 40 years of age who are undergoing abdominal or thoracic surgery and are treated with low-dose heparin (Cerrato et al, 1978). Treatment is initiated with 5000 units administered subcutaneously approximately 2 hours before surgery and repeated every 12 hours postoperatively. Low-dose heparin seems to be less protective against deep vein thrombosis following orthopedic surgery on the hip, femur, or leg, and that associated with immobility. In those instances an administration of heparin every 8 hours produces a slightly lower frequency of thrombosis but is associated with a higher incidence of hemorrhagic complications and therefore is not recommended (Stow and Burrows, 1987).

Continuous intravenous infusion of a solution containing a small amount of heparin is commonly used to maintain patency of intravascular catheters. Some catheters for intravascular use and tubing for cardiopulmonary bypass are impregnated with heparin to prevent deposition of thrombus on the surface of the material. Heparin has been recommended for use in the treatment of disseminated intravascular coagulation. The rationale is that heparin will arrest intravascular coagulation, which will allow normal amounts of coagulation factors to accumulate with subsequent cessation of bleeding. Conversely, heparin may aggravate symptoms of disseminated intravascular coagulation, making it difficult to select patients who would benefit from this unconventional therapeutic approach.

Mechanism of Action

The anticoagulant effect of heparin is due to its ability to stimulate the formation of antithrombin III, which is an alpha 2-globulin normally present in the plasma. Antithrombin III forms a complex with activated thrombin, resulting in neutralization of thrombin activity, thus preventing the conversion of fibrinogen to fibrin (see Fig. 57-1). Antithrombin III also neutralizes activated factor X, thus preventing conversion of prothrombin to thrombin (see Fig. 57-1). Thus, heparin functions as an anticoagulant by accelerating antithrombin III–induced neutralization of activated clotting factors. Low doses of heparin seem to exert predominant effects on factor X, whereas large doses of heparin have predominant effects on antithrombin III.

Route of Administration

Heparin is a poorly lipid-soluble, high–molecular weight substance that cannot cross lipid barriers in significant amounts. As a result, it is not effective when administered orally. Likewise, maternal administration of heparin does not result in passage across the placenta to the fetus. Deep subcutaneous (intrafat) injection of heparin is recommended when low-dose therapy is being administered for a prolonged effect in ambulatory patients. Intramuscular administration of

heparin is avoided owing to the risk of hematoma formation.

Administration of high doses of heparin is accomplished by intermittent or continuous intravenous infusion. Intermittent intravenous injection is often performed by means of an indwelling, rubber-capped needle (heparin lock). The size and frequency of the maintenance doses of heparin are based on the anticoagulant response to the previous dose as measured 1 hour previously. Continuous intravenous infusion of heparin is by means of constant infusion pump that delivers approximately 1000 units·h^{-1}.

Duration of Action

The duration of action of heparin depends on body temperature and the dose of drug administered. For example, intravenous doses of 100, 200, and 400 units·kg^{-1} have elimination half-times of 56, 96, and 152 minutes, respectively, and these durations are prolonged by reductions in body temperature below 37° C (Bull et al, 1975). The duration of action of heparin is also prolonged in the presence of hepatic and renal dysfunction. Conversely, patients with pulmonary embolism require larger doses because of more rapid clearance of the drug.

Clearance

Heparin is metabolized in the liver by the enzyme heparinase, and pharmacologically inactive metabolites are eliminated by the kidneys. A portion is also metabolized by depolymerization to an inactive product known as uroheparin. Unchanged heparin appears in the urine only after large doses are administered intravenously.

Laboratory Evaluation of Coagulation

Heparin effect is monitored by the partial thromboplastin time (PTT), activated coagulation (clotting) time (ACT), or both (Stow and Burrows, 1987). Bleeding time is not altered by heparin. Although it is generally believed that monitoring of low-dose heparin therapy is unnecessary, some clinicians recommend at least an initial laboratory evaluation in view of the wide variation in patient response to heparin.

Partial Thromboplastin Time

The PTT in the patient treated with heparin should be maintained approximately twice the patient's predrug value of 30 to 35 seconds. An excessively prolonged PTT (more than 120 seconds) is readily shortened by omitting a dose, since heparin has a short elimination half-time. When low-dose heparin therapy is used, laboratory tests may not be required to monitor treatment because the dosage and schedule are well known.

Activated Coagulation Time

Heparin effect and its antagonism by protamine are commonly monitored in patients undergoing surgical procedures by measuring the ACT. A baseline value for the ACT is determined (1) prior to the intravenous administration of heparin, (2) approximately 3 minutes after administration, and (3) at 30-minute intervals thereafter. A dose-response curve for heparin can be constructed with the dose of heparin in mg·kg⁻¹ on the vertical axis and the ACT in seconds on the horizontal axis (Fig. 27-1) (Bull et al, 1975). A line connecting the points before and 3 minutes after heparin is used to calculate the additional dose of heparin necessary to achieve an acceptable ACT.

The control ACT is usually 90 to 120 seconds. During cardiopulmonary bypass, the anticoagulant effect of heparin is often considered adequate when the ACT is more than 300 seconds, questionable with ACT times between 180 to 300 seconds, and inadequate at times less than 130 seconds. In animals, however, fibrin monomers may appear during cardiopulmonary bypass at ACT times less than 400 seconds (Young et al, 1978). The need to measure ACT is emphasized by the fourfold variation in heparin sensitivity between patients and the threefold variation in the rate at which heparin is metabolized.

Side Effects

Hemorrhage

Hemorrhage is the most serious complication associated with heparin therapy. This complication is minimized by dosage control based on laboratory measurement of heparin effect. Heparin should not be administered to patients with known bleeding tendencies or to persons undergoing intraocular or intracranial surgery. Placement of a needle or catheter in the lumbar subarachnoid or epidural space to inject a drug has been questioned for the patient who is receiving, or will subsequently receive, heparin. The concern is related to the possible occurrence of an epidural hematoma and compression of the spinal cord if a blood vessel were punctured during these injections. Likewise, hematomas and compression of peripheral nerves may be more likely to occur in association with performance of peripheral nerve blocks in patients being treated with heparin. Despite these concerns, a large retrospective study has not confirmed an increased

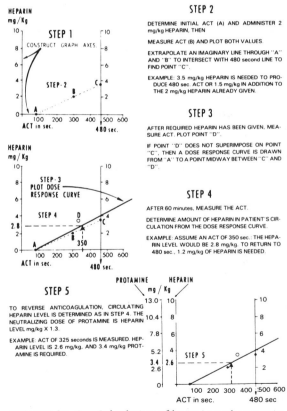

FIGURE 27–1. Calculation of heparin and protamine doses based on measurement of the activated coagulation time (ACT) (From Bull BS, Huse WM, Brauer FS, Korpman RA. Heparin therapy during extracorporeal circulation, II. The use of a dose–response curve to individualize heparin and protamine dosage. J Thorac Cardiovasc Surg 1975;69:685–9; with permission.)

incidence of epidural hematoma formation in patients receiving a spinal or epidural anesthetic followed by heparin anticoagulation (Rao and El-Etr, 1981).

Allergic Reactions

Heparin is obtained from animal tissues; thus, caution should be used in its administration to patients with a preexisting history of allergy. Indeed, fever, urticaria, and even cardiopulmonary changes occasionally occur after administration of heparin.

Thrombocytopenia

Thrombocytopenia owing to heparin administration can be divided into two syndromes (Stow and Burrows, 1987). The first and most common syndrome is mild, occurring in 30% to 40% of heparin-treated patients manifesting as platelet counts less than $100,000 \cdot mm^{-3}$. This mild thrombocytopenia is attributed to drug-induced platelet aggregation. It typically manifests on the second to fourth day of heparin therapy, is usually transient, and often remits even if heparin is continued.

A second, more severe and even life-threatening, syndrome develops in 0.5% to 6% of patients, manifesting as severe thrombocytopenia (less than $50,000 \cdot mm^{-3}$) often with associated resistance to the effects of heparin and the occurrence of thrombotic events (heparin-induced thrombocytopenia and thrombosis [HITT] syndrome). This severe response typically develops after 6 to 10 days of heparin therapy and is probably due to formation of heparin-dependent antiplatelet antibodies that trigger platelet aggregation and resulting thrombocytopenia. Indeed, platelet-associated immunoglobulin G (IgG) antibodies have been demonstrated in these patients. The diagnosis is confirmed by *in vitro* platelet aggregation studies. Heparin therapy must be immediately discontinued in these patients. All patients treated chronically with heparin (regardless of the route of administration) should be monitored with periodic platelet counts.

Patients with a history of life-threatening heparin-induced thrombocytopenia who subsequently require surgical procedures involving cardiopulmonary bypass present a therapeutic dilemma. One option is to administer warfarin for anticoagulation during cardiopulmonary bypass, but the difficulty posed in rapid reversal of this drug is a major disadvantage. Alternatively, vulnerable patients may be treated with prostacyclin analogues, which prevent platelet adhesion and aggregation, making reactions with antigens such as heparin impossible (Kraenzler and Starr, 1988). Vasodilation and severe hypotension may accompany administration of prostacyclin or its analogues.

Altered Protein Binding

Acute administration of heparin, as before cardiac catheterization or initiation of cardiopulmonary bypass, displaces alkaline drugs from protein binding sites. Evidence of this displacement is increased circulating concentrations of unbound fractions of propranolol and diazepam following the administration of heparin (Fig. 27-2) (Wood et al, 1980). It is conceivable that increased pharmacologic effects of propranolol and diazepam would accompany this heparin-induced reduction in protein binding. Certainly, measurement of plasma concentrations of drugs in heparinized blood must be interpreted differently than in the absence of heparin.

Cardiovascular Changes

Rapid intravenous infusion of large doses of heparin (300 units$\cdot kg^{-1}$) as administered prior to cardiopulmonary bypass may cause modest reductions in mean arterial pressure and pulmonary artery pressure (Konchigeri, 1984). These changes principally reflect decreases in systemic vascular resistance, perhaps owing to a direct heparin-induced relaxant effect on vascular smooth muscle. Ionized calcium (Ca^{2+}) concentrations are decreased in a dose-dependent manner by *in vitro,* but not *in vivo,* administration of heparin (Goto et al, 1985). These results indicate that blood pressure declines that are occasionally observed following administration of heparin are not related to changes in the plasma concentrations of ionized Ca^{2+}

Decreased Antithrombin III Concentrations

Paradoxically, patients who receive intermittent or continuous therapy with heparin manifest a progressive reduction of antithrombin III activity to values that approximate one third of normal

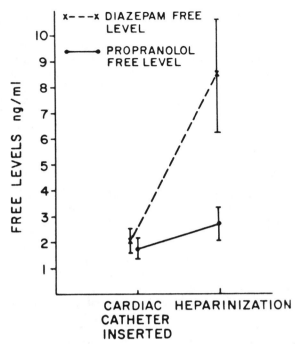

FIGURE 27–2. Administration of heparin displaces diazepam and propranolol from protein binding sites, leading to an increase in unbound (free) concentration of these drugs in the plasma. (From Wood AJJ, Robertson D, Robertson RM, Wilkinson GR, Wood M. Elevated plasma free drug concentration of propranolol and diazepam during cardiac catheterization. Circulation 1980;62:1119–22; with permission.)

(Marciniak and Gockerman, 1977). Thus, a heparin-induced reduction of the activity of antithrombin III may paradoxically increase the thrombotic tendency in humans. Estrogen-containing contraceptives also decrease concentrations of antithrombin III; this is consistent with the clinical impression that the incidence of thromboembolic episodes are increased in patients who take these drugs. Patients with genetically determined low levels of antithrombin III have a tendency to develop thromboembolism and may manifest increased dose requirements for heparin (Anderson, 1986). When heparin resistance is secondary to a deficiency in antithrombin III, administration of fresh frozen plasma restores the levels to normal and promotes the anticoagulant effects of heparin.

Altered Cell Morphology

Heparin added to whole blood distorts the morphology of leukocytes and erythrocytes. For this reason, heparinized blood is not acceptable for tests that involve complement, isoagglutinins, or erythrocyte fragility. Hematocrit, white blood cell count, and erythrocyte sedimentation rate are not altered by the presence of heparin.

Protamine

Protamine is the specific antagonist of heparin's anticoagulant effect. Protamines are strongly alkaline (nearly two thirds of the amino acid composition is arginine) polycationic low–molecular weight proteins found in sperm and testes of certain fish. The positively charged alkaline protamine combines with the negatively charged acidic heparin to form a stable complex that is devoid of anticoagulant activity. Despite the formation of this complex, the effect of heparin on platelet aggregation may persist and be responsible for continued bleeding, especially after cardiopulmonary bypass (Ellison et al, 1978). The dose of protamine required to antagonize heparin is 1 to 3 mg for every 100 units of heparin predicted to still be circulating. A more specific dose of protamine is calculated by *in vitro* titration of the patient's blood with protamine (Fig. 27-1) (Bull et al, 1975). A guideline is administration of 1.3 mg·kg^{-1} of protamine for each 100 units of heparin present as calculated from the ACT.

Protamine administered intravenously in the absence of heparin interacts with platelets and proteins, including fibrinogen. These interactions may manifest as an anticoagulant effect of protamine. Adverse cardiovascular responses to protamine include (1) hypotension, (2) pulmonary hypertension, and (3) allergic reactions (Horrow, 1985).

Hypotension

Rapid intravenous injection of protamine may be associated with histamine release, including facial flushing, tachycardia, and hypotension. Indeed, the alkaline characteristic of protamine makes it predictable that histamine release could occur, especially following rapid intravenous injection. Nevertheless, injection of protamine over at least 5 minutes is not associated with changes in circulating plasma concentrations of histamine, and blood pressure is not altered (Stoelting et al, 1984). Furthermore, there is no compelling evidence that protamine has direct negative inotropic effects (Conahan et al, 1981; Hines and Barash, 1986). Patients with poor left ventricular function, however, may be more susceptible to protamine-induced reductions in blood pressure because compensatory increases in cardiac output to offset peripheral vasodilation are limited (Michaels and Barash, 1983).

The site of intravenous administration may influence the subsequent circulatory changes evoked by protamine. For example, administration of protamine into the right atrium of anesthetized dogs is followed by (1) elevations in the plasma concentration of histamine, (2) increases in cardiac output, and (3) decreases in blood pressure and systemic vascular resistance (Casthely et al, 1986). These changes do not occur when protamine is injected into a peripheral vein or the left atrium. It is speculated that the heparin-protamine complex that evokes the release of histamine in the lungs is diluted before reaching the lungs when protamine is injected into a peripheral vein or the left atrium. Despite these animal data, intravenous or intra-atrial injection of protamine to patients has not been documented to produce different circulatory effects (Milne et al, 1983; Kronenfeld et al, 1987).

Pulmonary Hypertension

In rare cases, protamine neutralization of heparin can result in complement activation and thromboxane release manifesting as pulmonary vasoconstriction, pulmonary hypertension, and bronchoconstriction (Morel et al, 1987). These responses do not occur in patients manifesting blood pressure changes traditionally attributed to protamine-induced histamine release. Pretreatment with cyclooxygenase inhibitors such as indomethacin or aspirin blunts the increase in pulmonary vascular resistance (Conzen et al, 1989).

Allergic Reactions

Allergic reactions to protamine have been described most often in patients receiving protamine-containing insulin preparations (Doolan et al, 1981; Moorthy et al, 1980). For example, there

are approximately 2.8 mg of protamine per 100 units of protamine zinc insulin and 0.5 mg per 100 units of isophane (NPH) insulin. Presumably, chronic exposure to low doses of protamine in patients treated with protamine-containing insulin preparations evokes the production of antibodies against protamine. In this situation, the subsequent administration of large doses of protamine, as required to antagonize heparin-induced anticoagulation, may result in life-threatening allergic reactions. Patients allergic to fish may also be at increased risk for development of allergic reactions to protamine (Knape et al, 1981). The presence of circulating antisperm antibodies in vasectomized or infertile males has not been associated with allergic reactions to protamine (Horrow, 1985).

Patients known to be allergic to protamine and requiring heparin anticoagulation, as for cardiopulmonary bypass, present a unique problem (Campbell et al, 1984). Proposed options include (1) pretreatment with histamine receptor antagonists followed by a slow trial intravenous infusion of protamine; (2) complete avoidance of protamine, which allows the heparin effect to dissipate spontaneously; and (3) administration of an alternate heparin antagonist, hexadimethrine. Spontaneous dissipation of heparin effect may take several hours and is likely to be associated with substantial bleeding, requiring the administration of multiple blood transfusions. Hexadimethrine is the only drug alternative to protamine. In dogs, however, hexadimethrine produces hypotension, reductions in cardiac output, and increases in pulmonary vascular resistance that are more marked than hemodynamic derangements produced by protamine. In addition, hexadimethrine has an inherent anticoagulant effect resulting from inhibition of factor XII activation. For this reason, hexadimethrine must be administered by careful titration to avoid an exaggeration of the existing heparin-induced anticoagulant state. Most important, however, is the fact that hexadimethrine is not commercially available in the United States.

Ancrod

Ancrod is a defibrinogenating enzyme derived from snake venom that selectively depletes the plasma of fibrinogen. This anticoagulant has been used as an alternative to heparin during hemodialysis and cardiopulmonary bypass (Zulys et al, 1989). A specific antivenom is available.

ORAL ANTICOAGULANTS

Oral anticoagulants are derivatives of 4-hydroxy-coumarin (coumarin) (Fig. 27-3). The essential chemical characteristics of coumarin derivatives for anticoagulant activity are an intact d-hydroxy-coumarin residue with a carbon substitution at the number 3 position. Among the coumarin derivatives, warfarin is the most widely used drug (Table 27-1). Warfarin may be administered orally or parenterally.

Clinical Uses

Oral anticoagulants, in combination with dipyridamole, are commonly used to reduce the incidence of thromboembolism associated with prosthetic heart valves and atrial fibrillation in the presence of rheumatic heart disease. A frequent approach is an initial oral warfarin dose of 10 to 15 mg, followed by a daily maintenance dose of 1 to 15 mg as guided by the prothrombin time.

Mechanism of Action

The anticoagulant effect of coumarin derivatives reflects competitive inhibition of vitamin K, which is required for the formation of gamma carboxyglutamic acid in the liver. This amino acid is necessary for the normal synthesis of vitamin K–dependent clotting factors (factors II, VII, IX, and X) (see Fig. 57-1). Carboxyl groups of gamma carboxyglutamic acid are essential for the binding of Ca^{2+}, which normally forms the link between clotting factors and phospholipid. Because this link cannot be formed, there is impaired activation of the coagulation factors.

The anticoagulant effect of oral or intravenous warfarin is delayed for 8 to 12 hours, reflecting the onset of inhibition of clotting factor synthesis and the elimination half-time of previously formed clotting factors that are not altered by the oral anticoagulant. Peak effects of warfarin do not occur for 36 to 72 hours. Large initial doses of warfarin (approximately 0.75 $mg \cdot kg^{-1}$) hasten the onset of hypoprothrombinemia only to a limited extent.

Distribution and Clearance

Warfarin is rapidly and completely absorbed, with peak concentrations in plasma occurring within 1 hour after oral ingestion. It is 97% bound to albumin, and this contributes to its negligible urinary excretion and long elimination half-time of 24 to 36 hours after oral administration. The elimination half-time is prolonged by exposure to trace concentrations of anesthetic gases, presumably reflecting inhibition of warfarin metabolism (Ghoneim et al, 1975). Extensive protein bind-

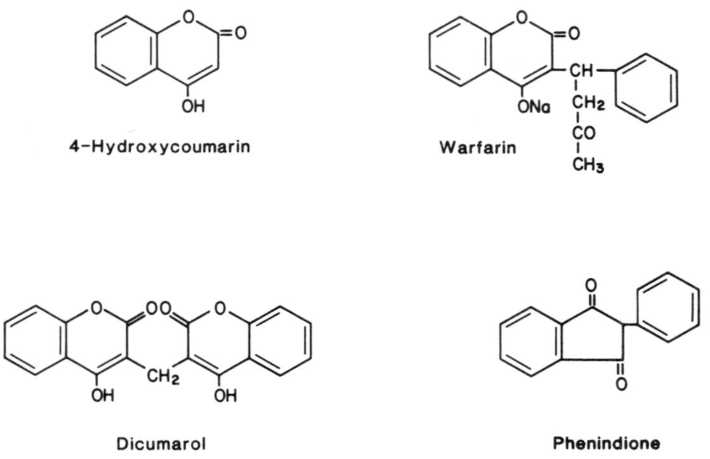

4-Hydroxycoumarin

Warfarin

Dicumarol

Phenindione

FIGURE 27-3. Oral anticoagulants are derivatives of 4-hydroxycoumarin.

Table 27–1
Comparative Pharmacology of Oral Anticoagulant

	Time to Peak Effect (h)	*Duration After Discontinuation (days)*	*Initial Adult Dose (mg)*	*Maintenance Adult Dose (mg)*
Warfarin	36–72	2–5	15, first day 10, second day 10, third day	2.5–10
Dicumarol	36–48	2–6	200–300, first day	25–200
Phenindione	18–24	1–2	300, first day 200, second day	25–200

ing prevents diffusion into erythrocytes, cerebrospinal fluid, and breast milk. Warfarin, however, does cross the placenta and produces exaggerated responses in the fetus who has a limited ability to synthesize clotting factors. Warfarin is metabolized to inactive metabolites that are conjugated with glucuronic acid and are ultimately excreted in the bile (enterohepatic circulation) and urine.

Laboratory Evaluation of Anticoagulation

Treatment with oral anticoagulants is best guided by the prothrombin time. The prothrombin time is particularly sensitive to three of the four vitamin K–dependent clotting factors (factors II, VII, and X). Conversion of the prothrombin time in seconds to percentage of normal prothrombin activity compensates for variations between different laboratories. Patients receiving oral anticoagulants should be maintained at a prothrombin time of approximately 25% of normal, which, in seconds, is approximately twice the normal baseline of 12 to 15 seconds. Prothrombin time is prolonged when plasma concentrations of fibrinogen are less than 100 mg·dl^{-1} or fibrin degradation products are present.

An excessively prolonged prothrombin time (more than 30 seconds) is not readily shortened by omitting a dose because of the long elimination half-time of oral anticoagulants. Likewise, an inadequate therapeutic effect is not readily corrected by increasing the dose because of the delayed onset of therapeutic effect. These slow responses of oral anticoagulants contrast with the rapid and predictable changes that are made possible by altering the dose of heparin.

Inadequate diet, disease of the small intestine, impaired delivery of bile into the gastrointestinal tract, preexisting liver disease, and advanced age are associated with enhanced effects of oral anticoagulants. Pregnancy is accompanied by increased activity of factors VII, VIII, IX, and X, and by a resulting decreased responsiveness to oral anticoagulants. Hereditary resistance to oral anticoagulants is an autosomal dominant trait.

Management Prior to Elective Surgery

Relatively minor surgical procedures can be safely performed in patients receiving oral anticoagulants. For major surgery, discontinuation of oral anticoagulants 1 to 3 days preoperatively is recommended to permit the prothrombin time to return to within 20% of the normal range (Tinker and Tarhan, 1978). This approach, followed by reinstitution of the oral anticoagulant regimen 1 to 7 days postoperatively, is not accompanied by an increased incidence of thromboembolic complications in vulnerable patients, such as those with prosthetic heart valves. In emergency situations, intravenous administration of vitamin K, fresh whole blood, or fresh frozen plasma may be necessary to abruptly counter the effects of oral anticoagulants.

Drug Interactions

Drug interactions occur between oral anticoagulants and salicylates, phenylbutazone, and barbiturates. For example, it is hazardous to administer any drug containing aspirin during anticoagulant therapy. Even a single 325-mg tablet of aspirin can impair platelet aggregation, and three aspirin tablets will prolong the bleeding time of most normal patients. Impairment of platelet aggregation owing to aspirin, plus inhibition of fibrin formation by oral anticoagulants, can result in catastrophic hemorrhage. Acetaminophen and sodium salicylate lack effects on platelets and therefore do not interact adversely when administered for antipyresis to patients being treated with oral anticoagulants.

Phenylbutazone impairs platelet aggregation, displaces warfarin from albumin, and inhibits the metabolism of warfarin, leading to an enhanced anticoagulant effect. Disulfiram inhibits drug metabolism and prolongs the anticoagulant effect. Cimetidine prolongs prothrombin time by an unknown mechanism (Flind, 1978). Clofibrate reduces adhesiveness of platelets and stimulates the metabolism of vitamin K–dependent clotting factors, enhancing responsiveness to oral anticoagulants.

Side Effects

Hemorrhage is the most serious side effect of oral anticoagulant therapy. The majority of deaths associated with coumarin therapy are due to massive gastrointestinal bleeding, usually in the presence of an unsuspected peptic ulcer or neoplasm. These drugs may increase the incidence of intracranial hemorrhage following a cerebrovascular accident. Bleeding may occur, even when the prothrombin time is in the desired therapeutic range. Compression neuropathy has been observed in treated patients following brachial artery puncture to obtain a sample for blood gas analysis. Treatment of mild hemorrhage is with administration of vitamin K (phytonadione), 10 to 20 mg orally, or 1 to 5 mg IV at a rate of 1 mg·min^{-1}, which will usually return the prothrombin time to a normal range within 4 to 24 hours. When immediate reversal of anticoagulation is required, the treatment is administration of fresh frozen plasma.

Warfarin crosses the placenta and is associated with serious teratogenic effects when administered during the first trimester of pregnancy. Indeed, approximately one third of infants exposed to coumarin derivatives are stillborn or are born with serious abnormalities such as nasal hypoplasia, stippled epiphyses, and blindness.

ANTITHROMBOTIC DRUGS

Antithrombotic drugs suppress platelet function and are used primarily for treatment of arterial thrombotic disease. In contrast, heparin and oral anticoagulants suppress function or synthesis of clotting factor and are used to control venous thromboembolic disorders. Platelet thrombi commonly occur in arterial walls, emphasizing the logic of using drugs that inhibit platelet aggregation in treating arterial thromboembolic diseases, especially those that lead to myocardial infarction or cerebrovascular accident. Oral anticoagulants have no effect on platelet function; thus, they are unlikely to be useful in the treatment of thrombotic disease in the arterial system. Examples of antithrombotic drugs are aspirin, dipyridamole, and dextran.

Aspirin

Aspirin inhibits thromboxane synthesis and the release of adenosine diphosphate by platelets and their subsequent aggregation. Despite rapid clearance from the body, the effects of aspirin on platelets are irreversible and last for the life of the platelet. Single doses of 325 mg of aspirin may prolong bleeding time for several days (Weiss, 1978). Aspirin may also inhibit synthesis of prostacyclin in vessel walls and thus tend to offset its effectiveness as an antithrombotic drug (Moncada and Vane, 1979).

Dipyridamole

Dipyridamole is a commonly prescribed antithrombotic drug that is commonly administered in combination with aspirin. Evidence that dipyridamole exerts an antithrombotic action by inhibiting platelet aggregation in humans is limited (Fitzgerald, 1987).

Dextran

Dextran-70 prolongs bleeding time, and polymerization of fibrin and platelet function may be impaired. For these reasons, dextran may have some value in prevention of postoperative thromboembolic disease.

THROMBOLYTIC DRUGS

Thrombolytic therapy begun soon after an acute myocardial infarction preserves left ventricular function and reduces mortality. Thrombolytic drugs, such as streptokinase, recombinant tissue plasminogen activator, urokinase, and anisoylated plasminogen activator, are proteins that promote the dissolution of thrombi by stimulating the conversion of endogenous plasminogen to plasmin (fibrinolysin). Plasmin is a proteolytic enzyme that hydrolyzes fibrin. The role of thrombolytic therapy is to restore circulation through a previously occluded vessel. The sooner therapy is initiated, the greater the likelihood of reperfusion, reflecting the fact that clots, as they age, become more resistant to lysis partly because of the alpha-chain cross-linking of the fibrin polymers. When administered intravenously within the first 3 hours following a myocardial infarction, a similar incidence of reperfusion is provided by all available thrombolytic drugs (Marder and Sherry, 1988; White et al, 1989). Reperfusion is reported to be 90% in pulmonary embolism and 65% in deep-vein thrombosis within the first 2 and 7 days, respectively, after the onset of symptoms (Marder and Sherry, 1988).

Spontaneous bleeding (especially intracranial hemorrhage) is the principal risk of thrombolytic drug therapy (Tiefenbrunn and Ludbrook, 1989). Bleeding is particularly likely in patients who have recently undergone surgery or invasive diagnostic procedures, emphasizing that these drugs do not distinguish between the fibrin of a thrombus and the fibrin of a hemostatic plug. Fever is common in treated patients and allergic reactions may occur.

Streptokinase is a catabolic product secreted by beta-hemolytic streptococci, making it potentially antigenic. Nevertheless, the commercial product is so highly purified that pyrogenic or allergic reactions are rarely serious. Most individuals, however, have some sensitivity as a result of previous streptococcal infections manifesting as fever in approximately one third of patients. Urokinase is produced by human fetal kidney cells in tissue culture and is not antigenic.

REFERENCES

Anderson EF, Heparin resistance prior to cardiopulmonary bypass. Anesthesiology 1986;64:504–7.

Bull BS, Huse WM, Brauer FS, Korpman RA. Heparin therapy during extracorporeal circulation, II. The use of a dose-response curve to individualize heparin and protamine dosage. J Thorac Cardiovasc Surg 1975;69:685–9.

Campbell FW, Goldstein MF, Atkins PC. Management of the patient with protamine hypersensitivity for cardiac surgery. Anesthesiology 1984;61:761–4.

Casthely PA, Goodman K, Fyman PN, Abrams LM, Aaron D. Hemodynamic changes after the administration of protamine. Anesth Analg 1986;65:78–80.

Cerrato D, Ariano C, Fiacchino F. Deep vein thrombosis and low-dose heparin prophylaxis in neurosurgical patients. J Neurosurg 1978;49:378–81.

Conahan TJ, Andrews RW, MacVaugh H. Cardiovascular effects of protamine sulfate in man. Anesth Analg 1981;60:33–6.

Conzen PF, Habazettl H, Gutmann R, Hobbhahn J, Goetz, AE, Peter K, Brendel W. Thromboxane mediation of pulmonary hemodynamic responses after neutralization of heparin by protamine in pigs. Anesth Analg 1989;68:25–31.

Doolan L, McKenzie L, Krafcheck J, Parsons B, Buxton B. Protamine sulfate hypersensitivity. Anaesth Intensive Care 1981;9:147–9.

Ellison N, Edmunds LH, Colman RW. Platelet aggregation following heparin and protamine administration. Anesthesiology 1978;48:65–8.

Fitzgerald GA. Dipyridamole. N Engl J Med 1987; 316:1247–57.

Flind AC. Cimetidine and oral anticoagulants. Br Med J 1978;2:1367.

Ghoneim MM, Delle M, Wilson WR, Ambre JJ. Alteration of warfarin kinetics in man associated with exposure to an operating-room environment. Anesthesiology 1975;43:333–6.

Goto H, Kushihashi T, Benson KT, Kato H, Fox DK, Arakawa K. Heparin, protamine, and ionized calcium *in vitro* and *in vivo*. Anesth Analg 1985;64:1081–4.

Hines RL, Barash PG. Protamine: Does it alter right ventricular function. Anesth Analg 1986;65:1271–4.

Horrow JC. Protamine: A review of its toxicity. Anesth Analg 1985;64:348–61.

Knape JA, Schuller JL, DeHaan P, DeJong AP, Bovill JG. An anaphylactic reaction to protamine in a patient allergic to fish. Anesthesiology 1981;55:324–5.

Konchigeri HN. Hemodynamic effects of heparin in patients undergoing cardiac surgery. Anesth Analg 1984;63:235.

Kraenzler EJ, Starr NJ. Heparin associated thrombocytopenia: Management of patients for open heart surgery. Case reports describing the use of Iloprost. Anesthesiology 1988;69:964–7.

Kronenfeld MA, Garguilo R, Weinberg P, Grant G, Thomas SJ, Turndorf H. Left atrial injection of protamine does not reliably prevent pulmonary hypertension. Anesthesiology 1987;67:578–80.

Marciniak E, Gockerman JP. Heparin-induced decrease in circulating antithrombin-III. Lancet 1977;2:581–4.

Marder VJ, Sherry S. Thrombolytic therapy: Current status. N Engl J Med 1988;318:1512–21; 1585–96.

Michaels IAL, Barash PG. Hemodynamic changes during protamine administration. Anesth Analg 1983; 62:831–5.

Milne B, Rogers K, Cervenko F, Salerno T. Haemodynamic effects of intra-aortic versus intravenous administration of protamine for reversal of heparin in man. Can Anaesth Soc J 1983;30:347–51.

Moncada S, Vane JR. Arachidonic acid metabolites and the interactions between platelets and blood vessel walls. N Engl J Med 1979;300:1142–7.

Moorthy SS, Pond W, Rowland RG. Severe circulatory shock following protamine (an anaphylactic reaction). Anesth Analg 1980;59:77–8.

Morel DR, Zapol WM, Thomas SJ, et al. C5a and thromboxane generation associated with pulmonary vaso- and broncho-constriction during protamine reversal of heparin. Anesthesiology 1987;66:597–604.

Rao TLK, El-Etr AA. Anticoagulation following placement of epidural and subarachnoid catheters: An evaluation of neurologic sequelae. Anesthesiology 1981;55:618–20.

Stoelting RK, Henry DP Verburg KM, McCammon RL, King RD, Brown JW. Haemodynamic changes and circulating histamine concentrations following protamine administration to patients and dogs. Can Anaesth Soc J 1984;31:534–40.

Stow PJ, Burrows FA. Anticoagulants in anaesthesia. Can J Anaesth 1987;34:632–49.

Tiefenbrunn AJ, Ludbrook PA. Coronary thrombolysis– It's worth the risk. JAMA 1989;261:2107–8.

Tinker JH, Tarhan S. Discontinuing anticoagulant therapy in surgical patients with cardiac valve prosthesis. Observations in 180 operations. JAMA 1978; 239:738–40.

Weiss HJ. Drug therapy. Antiplatelet therapy. N Engl J Med 1978;298:1344–7; 1403–6.

White HD, Rivers JT, Maslowski AH, et al. Effect of intravenous streptokinase as compared with that of tissue plasminogen activator on left ventricular function after first myocardial infarction. N Engl J Med 1989;320:817–21.

Wood AJJ, Robertson D, Robertson RM, Wilkinson GR, Wood M. Elevated plasma free drug concentrations of propranolol and diazepam during cardiac catheterization. Circulation 1980;62:1119–22.

Young JA, Kisker CT, Doty DB. Adequate anticoagulation during cardiopulmonary bypass determined by activated clotting time and the appearance of fibrin monomer. Ann Thorac Surg 1978;26:231–40.

Zulys VJ, Teasdale SJ, Michel ER, et al. Ancrod (Arvin) as an alternative to heparin anticoagulation for cardiopulmonary bypass. Anesthesiology 1989;71:870–77.

Chapter

28

Antibiotics

The therapeutic value and associated dangers of antibiotics are particularly relevant to the care of patients in the perioperative period and the intensive care unit who are at high risk for hospital-acquired infections. The choice of an antibiotic is determined by both the properties of the individual drug and the nature of the infecting organism as confirmed by bacteriologic investigation. In seriously ill patients or patients with decreased immune defense mechanisms, selection of bactericidal rather than bacteriostatic antibiotics is often recommended (Table 28-1). Narrow-spectrum antibiotics should be considered, before broad-spectrum antibiotics or combination antibiotic therapy is prescribed, to preserve normal bacterial flora of the patient (Table 28-2). These normal bacterial flora help prevent colonization by pathogens, because they will compete for nutrients and produce their own antibiotic substances. Normal bacterial flora assume special importance in hospitalized patients, because the hospital may serve as a reservoir of resistant bacteria from previously treated patients. It is inadvisable to use less than the recommended doses of antibiotics except in the presence of renal, and occasionally hepatic, dysfunction.

Antibiotics can be classified according to their mode of antibacterial action. For example, penicillins are drugs that exert antibacterial effects by inhibiting synthesis of bacterial cell walls. Amphotericin is a drug that affects permeability of bacterial cell membranes. Drugs that act by inhibiting bacterial synthesis of essential proteins include aminoglycosides, tetracyclines, erythromycin, clindamycin, and chloramphen-

icol. Alteration in nucleic acid production is the mechanism of action of rifampin. Sulfonamides and trimethoprim exert an antibacterial effect through an antimetabolite effect.

PROPHYLACTIC ANTIBIOTICS

Prophylactic antibiotics are indicated for most of the commonly performed surgical procedures (Table 28-3) (Kaiser, 1986). It is more cost effective to administer prophylactic antibiotics than it is to treat infections in untreated patients. Because of their antimicrobial spectrum and lack of toxicity, including a low incidence of allergic reactions, cephalosporins (most often cefazolin) are the antibiotics of choice for surgical procedures in which skin flora and the normal flora of the gastrointestinal and genitourinary tracts are the most likely pathogens. Timing of antibiotic administration must coincide with bacterial inoculation, emphasizing that the drug need not be given before the induction of anesthesia. Administration of the prophylactic antibiotic in the patient's room before transfer to surgery is illogical. Prolongation of prophylactic antibiotic therapy beyond the first postoperative day provides no additional protection. Emergence of resistant bacterial strains related to use of prophylactic antibiotics remains a concern, although there is lack of proof that short courses of perioperative antibiotics result in resistant strains (Kaiser, 1986). Pseudomembranous colitis is the most frequent complication of prophylactic antibiotics including the cephalosporins.

Table 28-1
Examples of Bactericidal and Bacteriostatic Antibiotics

Bactericidal	Bacteriostatic
Penicillins	Tetracyclines
Cephalosporins	Chloramphenicol
Aminoglycosides	Erythromycin
Colistin	Clindamycin
Vancomycin	Sulfonamides
Co-trimoxazole	

PENICILLINS

The basic structure of penicillins is a dicyclic nucleus (aminopenicillanic acid) that consists of a thiazolidine ring connected to a beta-lactam ring (Fig. 28-1) (Donowitz and Mandell, 1988). Benzylpenicillin (penicillin G) was the first penicillin derivative discovered (Fig. 28-2). This penicillin and its closely related cogener, phenoxymethylpenicillin (penicillin K), are highly active against gram-positive bacteria (streptococci). Both of these penicillins are readily hydrolyzed by bacteria-produced enzymes (penicillinases or beta-lactamases), thus rendering them ineffective against most strains of *Staphylococcus aureus.* Benzylpenicillin is five to ten times more active against gram-negative bacteria, especially *Neisseria,* than is phenoxymethyl penicillin.

The bacteriocidal action of penicillins reflects the ability of these antibiotics to interfere with the synthesis of *peptidoglycan,* which is an essential component of cell walls of susceptible bacteria. Penicillins also decrease the availability of an inhibitor of murein hydrolase such that the uninhibited enzyme can then destroy (lyse) the structural integrity of bacterial cell walls. Cell membranes of resistant gram-negative bacteria prevent penicillins from gaining access to sites where synthesis of peptidoglycan is taking place.

Benzylpenicillin

Benzylpenicillin is the drug of choice for treating pneumococcal, streptococcal, and meningococcal infections. The majority (60% to 80%) of staphylococcal infections are caused by bacteria that produce penicillinase and thus are resistant to treatment with most penicillins. Gonococci have gradually become more resistant to benzylpenicillin, requiring higher doses for adequate

Table 28-2
Examples of Narrow-Spectrum and Broad-Spectrum Antibiotics

Narrow-Spectrum	Broad-Spectrum
Benzylpenicillin	Ampicillin
Erythromycin	Cephalosporins
Clindamycin	Aminoglycosides
	Tetracyclines
	Chloramphenicol
	Sulfonamides
	Co-trimoxazole

Table 28-3
Examples of Surgical Procedures that May Benefit from Prophylactic Antibiotics

Gynecologic surgery
 Cesarean section
 Hysterectomy—abdominal or vaginal

Orthopedic surgery
 Arthroplasty of joints including replacement
 Open reduction of fractures

General surgery
 Cholecystectomy
 Colon surgery
 Appendectomy
 Gastric resection
 Penetrating abdominal trauma

Urologic surgery

Surgery on nose, mouth, and pharynx
 Tonsillectomy
 Incisions through oral or pharyngeal mucosa

Cardiothoracic and vascular surgery
 Coronary artery bypass graft
 Valve annuloplasty or replacement
 Pacemaker insertion
 Thoracotomy
 Peripheral vascular surgery (possible exception, carotid endarterectomy)

Neurosurgical procedures
 Shunt procedures
 Craniotomy

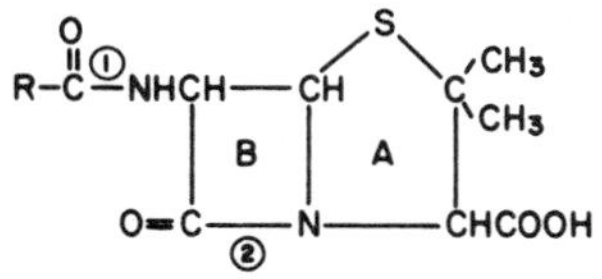

FIGURE 28–1. The basic structure of penicillins is a thiazolidine ring (A) connected to a beta-lactam ring (B). Breakdown of penicillin occurs at sites (1) and (2) by the actions of amidase and penicillinase, respectively.

treatment. Treatment of syphilis with benzylpenicillin is highly effective. Benzylpenicillin is the drug of choice for treating all forms of actinomycosis and clostridial infections causing gas gangrene.

Prophylactic administration of penicillin is highly effective against streptococcal infections, accounting for its value in patients with rheumatic fever. Transient bacteremia occurs in the majority of patients undergoing dental extractions, emphasizing the importance of prophylactic penicillin in patients with congenital or acquired heart disease undergoing dental procedures. Transient bacteremia may also accompany surgical procedures, such as tonsillectomy and operations on the genitourinary and gastrointestinal tracts, and vaginal delivery.

Route of Administration

Benzylpenicillin is more stable in an acidic medium than is phenoxymethylpenicillin following oral administration. Absorption after intramuscular injection is rapid but may result in sterile inflammatory responses at the site of injection. Benzylpenicillin can be administered intravenously or as a continuous infusion (6 to 20 million units daily). Thrombophlebitis may occur

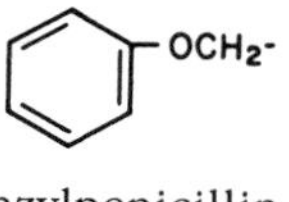

FIGURE 28–2. Benzylpenicillin (A) and phenoxymethylpenicillin (B). The structures shown are equivalent to R in Fig. 28–1.

along the vein used for intravenous administration. Potassium salts of penicillin are most commonly administered intravenously, with 1.7 mEq of potassium (K^+) being present in every 1 million units of penicillin. This amount of K^+ may result in hyperkalemia in patients who are in renal failure. Stability of benzylpenicillin is greatest at a pH of 6 to 7.2, which is important when considering a fluid diluent for continuous infusion. Other drugs should not be mixed with penicillin, because the combination may inactivate the antibiotic. Intrathecal administration of penicillins is not recommended, because these drugs are potent convulsants when administered by this route. Furthermore, arachnoiditis and encephalopathy may follow intrathecal penicillin administration.

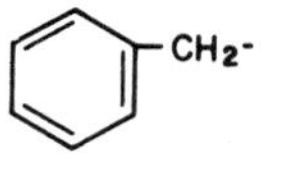

Excretion

Renal elimination of penicillin is rapid (60% to 90% of an intramuscular dose in the first hour), such that the concentration in plasma declines to half its peak value within 1 hour after injection. Approximately 10% is eliminated by glomerular filtration, and 90% is eliminated by renal tubular secretion. Anuria increases the elimination half-time of benzylpenicillin approximately tenfold.

Duration of Action

Methods to prolong the duration of action of penicillin include the simultaneous administration of *probenecid,* which blocks renal tubular secretion of penicillin. Alternatively, the intramuscular injection of poorly soluble salts of penicillin, such as procaine or benzathine, will delay absorption and thus prolong the duration of action. Procaine penicillin contains 120 mg of the local anesthetic for every 300,000 units of the antibiotic. Possible hypersensitivity to procaine must be considered when selecting this form of the antibiotic for administration.

PENICILLINASE-RESISTANT PENICILLINS

The most important mechanism of bacterial resistance to the penicillins is bacterial production of enzymes (penicillinases) that hydrolyze the cyclic amide bond of the beta-lactam ring and render it inactive (Fig. 28–1). Penicillinase-resistant penicillins are not susceptible to hydrolysis by staphylococcal penicillinases. Specific indications for these drugs are infections caused by staphylococci known or suspected to produce this enzyme. These antibiotics are less effective than benzyl-penicillin against infections caused by bacteria that do not produce penicillinase, including non-penicillinase-producing staphylococci.

Methicillin

Methicillin (dimethoxybenzylpenicillin) is bactericidal for nearly all strains of *S. aureus* that produce penicillinase. Oral administration is not effective because the drug is readily destroyed by acidic gastric fluid. Renal excretion, as with benzylpenicillin, is rapid.

Oxacillin and Cloxacillin

Oxacillin and cloxacillin, like methicillin, are markedly resistant to hydrolysis by penicillinase, but unlike methicillin, they are relatively stable in an acidic medium, resulting in adequate systemic absorption after oral administration. Nevertheless, variability of absorption from the gastrointestinal tract often dictates a parenteral route of administration for treatment of serious infections caused by penicillinase-producing staphylococci. Renal excretion is rapid, with up to 50% of the drug eliminated unchanged in the urine in the first 6 hours. Significant hepatic elimination into the bile also occurs. Hepatitis has been associated with high-dose oxacillin therapy.

Nafcillin

Nafcillin is highly resistant to penicillinase, being more active than oxacillin against benzylpenicillin-resistant *S. aureus*. Oral absorption of nafcillin is irregular because of variable inactivation of acidic gastric fluid. The usual parenteral dosage is 8 to 12 g daily, given in divided doses every 4 hours. There is selective sequestration of the drug in the liver, with peak concentrations in the bile exceeding those in the blood. Only approximately 10% of the drug appears unchanged in the urine. Penetration of nafcillin into the central nervous system is sufficient to treat staphylococcal meningitis.

BROAD-SPECTRUM PENICILLINS

Broad-spectrum penicillins, such as ampicillin, have a wider range of activity than other penicillins, being bactericidal against gram-positive and gram-negative bacteria. They are, nevertheless, all destroyed by penicillinase produced by certain gram-negative and gram-positive bacteria. Therefore, these drugs are not effective against most staphylococcal infections.

Ampicillin

Ampicillin (alpha-aminobenzylpenicillin) is considered the drug of choice for initial treatment of gonococcal urethritis. Upper respiratory tract infections caused by *Haemophilus influenzae* and streptococcal organisms and most urinary tract infections caused by enterococci respond to ampicillin. Acute bacterial meningitis in children is often treated with ampicillin, but since 5% to 30% of strains of *H. influenzae* may be resistant to ampicillin, it is recommended that chloramphenicol be administered concurrently until sensitivities of the infecting bacteria are determined.

Route of Administration

Ampicillin is stable in acid and thus is well absorbed after oral administration. Nevertheless, considerably higher blood levels can be obtained with intramuscular injections.

Among the penicillins, ampicillin is associated with the highest incidence (9%) of skin rash. This reaction is delayed, appearing 7 to 10 days after initiation of therapy. It is likely that a mechanism different from true penicillin hypersensitivity is responsible for this ampicillin-induced skin rash. Many ampicillin rashes are due to protein impurities that may be reduced by refinements in the manufacturing process.

Excretion

Approximately 50% of an oral dose of ampicillin is excreted unchanged by the kidney in the first 6 hours following administration, compared with approximately 70% of an intramuscular or intravenous dose in this same period. This emphasizes that renal function greatly influences the duration of action of ampicillin as well as the dose administered. Ampicillin also appears in the bile and undergoes enterohepatic circulation.

Carbenicillin

Carbenicillin (alpha-carboxybenzylpenicillin) is active against most infections caused by *Pseudomonas aeruginosa* and certain *Proteus* strains that are resistant to ampicillin. It is penicillinase susceptible and, therefore, ineffective against most strains of *S. aureus.*

Carbenicillin is not absorbed from the gastrointestinal tract; therefore, it must be given parenterally, often in large doses. The elimination half-time of carbenicillin in the presence of normal renal function is approximately 1 hour, and this time is prolonged to approximately 2 hours when there is hepatic dysfunction. Approximately 85% of the unchanged drug is recovered in the urine over 9 hours. Probenecid, by delaying renal excretion of the drug, increases the plasma concentration of carbenicillin by approximately 50%.

Cardiac failure may develop in patients treated with carbenicillin who are receiving excessive sodium. Hypokalemia may occur because of obligatory excretion with the large amount of nonreabsorbable carbenicillin. Carbenicillin interferes with normal platelet aggregation such that bleeding is prolonged but platelet count remains normal.

ALLERGY TO PENICILLINS

Allergic reactions are noted in 1% to 10% of patients treated with penicillins, making these antibiotics the most allergenic of all drugs (Pallasch, 1988). Patients allergic to penicillin are three to four times more likely to experience allergic reactions to other drugs unrelated to antibiotics.

The penicillin molecule itself is probably unable to form a complete antigen, but instead the ring structure of penicillin is opened to form a hapten metabolite, penicilloyl. Approximately 95% of patients allergic to penicillin form this penicilloyl-protein conjugate (the major antigenic determinant); the remaining allergic patients form 6-aminopenicillic acid and benzylpenamaldic acid (minor antigenic determi-

nants). Skin testing with a polyvalent skin test antigen, penicilloyl-polylysine, makes it possible to detect most patients who would develop a life-threatening allergic reaction if treated with a penicillin antibiotic. Nevertheless, minor antigenic determinants that would not be detected by skin testing may produce severe allergic reactions. Cephalosporins are often selected for treatment of patients who have a history of cutaneous reactions following treatment with penicillins (see the section entitled "Cross-Reactivity").

The most common manifestations of allergy to penicillins is a maculopapular or urticarial rash and fever. In a few patients, an immediate or accelerated life-threatening allergic reaction (hypotension; bronchospasm; or edema of the lips, tongue, and larynx) occurs. Fatal allergic reactions have occurred in patients receiving as little as 1 unit of penicillin for skin testing. Allergic reactions may occur in the absence of previous known exposure to any of the penicillins. This may reflect prior unrecognized exposure to penicillin presumably in ingested foods. Allergic reactions can occur with any dose or route of administration, although severe anaphylactic reactions are more often associated with parenteral than with oral administration. Some patients who experience cutaneous reactions may continue to receive the offending penicillin or receive the same penicillin in the future without experiencing a similar response.

Cross-Reactivity

The presence of a common nucleus (beta-lactam ring) in the structure of all penicillins means that allergy to one penicillin increases the likelihood of an allergic reaction to another penicillin (Fig. 28-1). Furthermore, there is potential cross-reactivity with cephalosporins that share a common beta-lactam ring (Fig. 28-3). Early estimates of cross-reactivity (patients allergic to penicillin who also are allergic to cephalosporins) between penicillin and cephalosporins were 5% to 15%. More recent estimates indicate a possible 1.1% to 1.7% cross-reactivity, which is similar to the incidence of allergy to the cephalosporins in the general population (Pallasch, 1988). Cephalosporins are often selected for administration to patients with a history of a cutaneous reaction following treatment with penicillins. It should be empha-

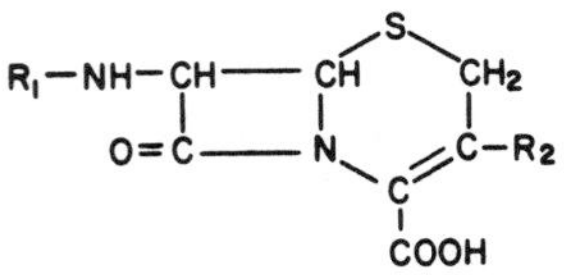

FIGURE 28–3. Basic structural formula of cephalosporins.

sized, however, that cephalosporins cannot be safely administered to patients with a history of an immediate or accelerated reaction (hypotension, bronchospasm, or angioedema) to any of the penicillins.

CEPHALOSPORINS

Cephalosporins are derived from 7-aminocephalosporanic acid (Fig. 28-3) (Donowitz and Mandell, 1988). These antibiotics inhibit bacterial cell wall synthesis in a manner similar to that of the penicillins. Resistance to cephalosporins, as to penicillins, may be due to an inability of the antibiotic to penetrate to its site of action. Bacteria can also produce cephalosporinases (beta-lactamases) that disrupt the beta-lactum structure of cephalosporins and thus inhibit their antibacterial activity.

Individual cephalosporins differ significantly with respect to extent of absorption following oral absorption, severity of pain produced by intramuscular injection, and protein binding. Intravenous administration of any of the cephalosporins can cause thrombophlebitis. Excretion of cephalosporins is principally by glomerular filtration and renal tubular secretion, emphasizing the need to reduce dosage of these drugs in the presence of renal dysfunction. Diacetyl metabolites of cephalosporins can occur, being associated with reduced antibiotic activity.

A positive Coombs' reaction frequently occurs in patients who receive large doses of cephalosporins. Hemolysis, however, is rarely associated with this response. Nephrotoxicity with cephalosporins, with the exception of cephaloridine, is less frequent than that following administration of aminoglycosides or polymyxins.

Allergy to cephalosporins, as with penicillins, is the most common adverse response associated with administration of these antibiotics. Nevertheless, the incidence of allergic reactions (fewer than 2% of patients) is much less than the incidence with penicillins (Donowitz and Mandell, 1988). When they do occur, however, they may be life-threatening with hypotension and bronchospasm (Beaupre et al, 1984).

The beta-lactam structure present in both penicillins and cephalosporins results in potential cross-reactivity between these two classes of antibiotics. Nevertheless, the incidence of cross-reactivity is low, and cephalosporins are a frequent alternative selection for patients with a history of cutaneous reactions following treatment with penicillins. Cephalosporins should not be administered to patients with a history of life-threatening allergic reactions to penicillins.

Classification

Cephalosporins have been categorized as first, second, and third generation on the basis of their activity spectrum against gram-negative rods (Table 28-4) (Donowitz and Mandell, 1988). First-generation cephalosporins are inexpensive, exhibit low toxicity, and are as active as second- and third-generation cephalosporins against staphylococci and nonenterococcal streptococci. For these reasons, first-generation cephalosporins have been extensively used for prophylaxis in cardiovascular, orthopedic, biliary, pelvic, and intraabdominal surgery (see the section entitled "Prophylactic Antibiotics"). Second-generation cephalosporins are more effective than first generation drugs against *Escherichia coli* and *Klebsiella*. Third-generation cephalosporins provide greater activity against aerobic gram-negative bacteria than is present with first- and

Table 28–4
Classification of Cephalosporins

First-Generation
   Cefazolin
   Cephalexin
   Cephalothin

Second-Generation
   Cefamandole
   Cefoxitin

Third-Generation
   Cefotaxime
   Cefoperazone

second-generation drugs and activity against gram-positive cocci is similar.

Cefazolin

Cefazolin, because it has a longer elimination half-time (2 hours) than other first-generation cephalosporins is viewed as the drug of choice for antibiotic prophylaxis in the perioperative period (Donowitz and Mandell, 1988). Elimination is principally by glomerular filtration. The drug is well tolerated after intramuscular or intravenous injection.

Cephalexin

Cephalexin is effective orally, being well absorbed from the gastrointestinal tract. The elimination half-time is approximately 50 minutes, with more than 90% of the drug excreted unchanged in the urine within 6 hours, primarily by renal tubular secretion. As such, probenecid is effective in slowing renal elimination of cephalexin and enhancing the duration of systemic antibiotic activity.

Cephalothin

Cephalothin is highly resistant to inactivation by cephalosporinases and is highly effective for treatment of severe staphylococcal infections (Fig. 28-4). Oral absorption is poor, and intramuscular injection is painful, accounting for its common administration by the intravenous route (1 gram over 20 to 30 minutes). Although cephalothin is present in many tissues and fluids, it does not enter the cerebrospinal fluid in significant amounts and should not be used for treatment of meningitis.

Approximately 50% of a dose of cephalothin is eliminated unchanged by the kidneys. Up to 30% is metabolized to a weakly antibacterial diacetyl metabolite, which is also excreted by the kidneys. Excretion of cephalothin is delayed

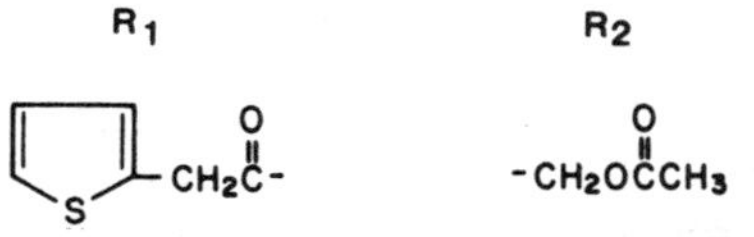

FIGURE 28–4. Cephalothin. R_1 and R_2 correspond to Fig. 28–3.

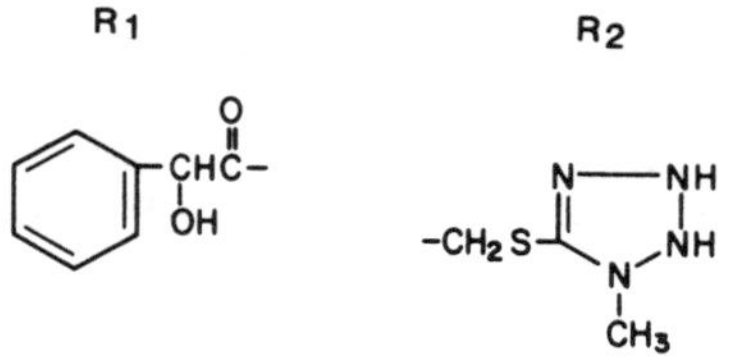

FIGURE 28–5. Cefamandole. R_1 and R_2 correspond to Fig. 28–3.

when there is renal dysfunction, requiring consideration of a decreased dosage or greater dosing intervals.

Cefamandole

Cefamandole is active against *H. influenzae* as well as most streptococci and staphylococci, making this antibiotic suitable for treating many cases of bacterial pneumonia (Fig. 28-5). The elimination half-time is approximately 50 minutes, and the drug is excreted unchanged by the kidneys.

Cefoxitin

Cefoxitin is highly resistant to cephalosporinases produced by gram-negative bacteria. It is effective in the treatment of urethritis due to penicillinase producing strains of *N. gonorrhoeae*. This drug is eliminated unchanged by the kidneys.

Cefotaxime

Cefotaxime, because of its resistance to hydrolysis by cephalosporinases, provides a potent and broad spectrum of activity against aerobic gram-negative bacteria. It inhibits more than 90% of strains of *Enterobacter,* including those resistant to aminoglycosides. Penetration through inflamed meninges is sufficient to produce therapeutic concentrations in the cerebrospinal fluid. Cefotaxime has only moderate activity against anaerobes. The elimination half-time is approximately 1 hour with clearance principally via the kidneys. An adjustment in dosage or dosing intervals is indicated when patients with renal dysfunction are being treated with this drug. Approximately 30% of cefotaxime is excreted as a desacetyl derivative that has antibacterial activity and is synergistic with the parent compound.

Cefoperazone

Cefoperazone is unique among cephalosporins in depending primarily on hepatic elimination for its clearance. Therefore, adjustments in dosage are unnecessary for treatment of patients with renal dysfunction. The elimination half-time is approximately 2 hours. Penetration across the meninges is not sufficient to produce therapeutic concentrations.

AZTREONAM

Aztreonam is a monolactam antibiotic whose chemical structure differs markedly from that of the penicillins and cephalosporins (Donowitz and Mandell, 1988). Because of this structural difference, aztreonam exhibits minimal cross-reactivity with other beta-lactam drugs and can be used in patients allergic to penicillins or cephalosporins. Aztreonam resembles aminoglycosides in that its spectrum of activity is limited to aerobic gram-negative bacilli. It is resistant to hydrolysis by penicillinases. Elimination is primarily renal with approximately two thirds of a dose excreted unchanged in the urine.

IMIPENEM

Imipenem is a carbapenem (beta-lactam) antibiotic with the broadest antibacterial spectrum of any antibiotic (Donowitz and Mandell, 1988). It is used in combination with cilastatin, a compound that inhibits the metabolism of imipenem by renal dipeptidases. In the presence of cilastatin, approximately 70% of the drug is excreted unchanged by the kidney. Toxic effects resemble those of other beta-lactam antibiotics, and allergic reactions occur in approximately 3% of patients.

AMINOGLYCOSIDES

Aminoglycosides are poorly lipid-soluble drugs that are rapidly bactericidal for aerobic gram-negative bacteria because of their ability to inhibit protein synthesis in bacterial ribosomes. To reach ribosomes, the antibiotic must be transported across bacterial cell membranes by an active process, because poor lipid solubility limits passive diffusion. This is an oxygen-dependent active transport system that is absent in anaerobic bacteria, explaining the resistance of these bacteria to the effects of aminoglycosides. Most of the acquired resistance to aminoglycosides results from inactivation of the antibiotic by enzymes located in bacterial cell membranes. Structurally, aminoglycosides contain three separate ring structures, two of which are substituted amino sugars with a glycosidic linkage.

Route of Administration

Less than 1% of an orally administered aminoglycoside is absorbed into the systemic circulation, reflecting the poor lipid solubility of these drugs. Orally administered drug is thus eliminated unchanged in the bile. Rapid systemic absorption occurs after intramuscular injection, with peak, plasma concentrations occurring in 30 to 90 minutes. Negligible binding to plasma proteins takes place, which is consistent with poor lipid solubility.

As would be predicted from poor lipid solubility, concentrations of aminoglycosides in secretions, the eyes, and the central nervous system are poor. The principal exception is the renal cortex, where high concentrations of aminoglycosides accumulate, thus likely contributing to adverse effects on the kidney. Inflammation improves penetration of aminoglycosides into peritoneal and pericardial cavities and the cerebrospinal fluid. For example, concentrations of aminoglycosides in the cerebrospinal fluid are less than 10% of those in plasma in the absence of inflammation. This value may approach 20% in the presence of meningitis. Nevertheless, these concentrations are usually inadequate, and intrathecal or intraventricular administration of the aminoglycoside is necessary.

Excretion

Aminoglycosides, because of their poor lipid solubility, have a volume of distribution similar to the extracellular fluid volume and undergo extensive renal excretion owing almost exclusively to glomerular filtration. Probenecid has no detectable effect on the rate of elimination, suggesting that renal tubular secretion mechanisms are not important. Approximately 60% of an aminoglycoside is eliminated unchanged by the kidneys during the first 24 hours and, eventually, all the drug is eliminated by the kidneys.

There is a linear relationship between the plasma creatinine concentration and the elimination half-time of aminoglycosides. In the presence of normal renal function, the elimination half-time of all aminoglycosides is 2 to 3 hours, and this is prolonged 20- to 40-fold in the presence of renal failure. Determination of the plasma concentration of aminoglycosides is an essential guide to the safe administration of these antibiotics.

Side Effects

Side effects of aminoglycosides that limit their clinical usefulness include ototoxicity, nephrotoxicity, skeletal muscle weakness, and potentiation of nondepolarizing neuromuscular blocking drugs. These side effects parallel the plasma concentration of aminoglycoside, emphasizing the need to reduce the dose of these drugs in patients with renal dysfunction.

Ototoxicity

Ototoxicity manifests as vestibular dysfunction, auditory dysfunction, or both, and parallels the accumulation of aminoglycosides in the perilymph of the inner ear. This accumulation of drug in the inner ear parallels the plasma concentration. The incidence of ototoxicity is 1% to 3% for patients treated with an aminoglycoside for less than 14 days. Prolonged administration, high doses, and advanced age, which is likely to be associated with preexisting auditory defects and renal disease increase the incidence of ototoxicity. Furosemide, mannitol, and probably other diuretics seem to accentuate the ototoxic effects of aminoglycosides.

Aminoglycoside-induced ototoxicity reflects progressive destruction of vestibular or cochlear sensory hair cells in a dose-dependent manner by the antibiotic. Streptomycin and gentamycin predominately produce vestibular toxicity manifesting as nystagmus, vertigo, nausea, and acute onset of Meniere's syndrome. Neomycin, kanamycin, and amikacin predominantly produce

auditory dysfunction manifesting as tinnitus or a sensation of pressure or fullness in the ears. Deafness may develop suddenly. Tobramycin adversely affects vestibular and cochlear function equally.

Nephrotoxicity

Aminoglycosides accumulate in the renal cortex; this correlates with the potential for these drugs to cause nephrotoxicity. As with ototoxicity, the incidence of nephrotoxicity depends on the specific drug, duration of treatment, total dose, and presence of predisposing factors such as advanced age and preexisting renal disease. Neomycin is the most nephrotoxic of the aminoglycosides and, for this reason, is not administered by the parenteral route. The incidence of nephrotoxicity with gentamicin is approximately 4%. Nephrotoxicity is estimated to occur in 3% to 8% of patients treated with kanamycin and amikacin and in 1% or fewer with tobramycin and streptomycin.

Nephrotoxicity induced by aminioglycosides is a form of acute renal tubular necrosis that initially manifests as an inability to concentrate urine and the appearance of proteinuria and red cell casts. This damage rarely manifests before 5 to 7 days of treatment. These changes are usually reversible if the drug is discontinued.

Skeletal Muscle Weakness

Skeletal muscle weakness can occur with intrapleural or intraperitoneal instillation of large doses of aminoglycosides. Patients with myasthenia gravis are particularly susceptible to this aminoglycoside effect with any route of administration. Patients with chronic obstructive airway disease may be susceptible to the skeletal muscle-weakening effects of aminoglycosides. Nevertheless, single doses of tobramycin or gentamicin lack clinically significant neuromuscular blocking effects when administered to otherwise healthy patients (Lippman et al, 1982).

The neuromuscular effects of aminoglycosides most likely reflect the ability of these drugs to inhibit the prejunctional release of acetylcholine while also reducing postsynaptic sensitivity to the neurotransmitter (Pittinger et al, 1970). Intravenous administration of calcium (Ca^{2+}) overcomes the effect of aminoglycosides at the neuromuscular junction.

Potentiation of Nondepolarizing Neuromuscular Blocking Drugs

Intravenous administration of aminoglycosides and associated high plasma concentrations are most likely to potentiate nondepolarizing neuromuscular blocking drugs (Sokoll and Gergis, 1981). Likewise, irrigation of the peritoneal or pleural cavities with large volumes of aminoglycoside-containing solutions can result in substantial systemic absorption and potentiation of previously administered neuromuscular blocking drugs. Reappearance of neuromuscular blockade is a possibility if aminoglycosides are administered systemically in the early postoperative period to a patient who has been judged to have adequately recovered from neuromuscular blocking drugs administered during anesthesia. Furthermore, the neuromuscular blocking effects of lidocaine are enhanced in the presence of neuromuscular blocking drugs and aminoglycosides. Conceivably, administration of lidocaine in the early postoperative period could produce skeletal muscle weakness in a patient who had previously received a neuromuscular blocking drug and an aminoglycoside (Bruckner et al, 1980).

Neostigmine or Ca^{2+}-induced antagonism of aminoglycoside-potentiated neuromuscular blockade may be incomplete or transient. (Sokoll and Gergis, 1981). Speculation that reversal of antibiotic-induced neuromuscular blockade would also antagonize antibiotic effects, however, has not been demonstrated (Booij et al, 1980). Clinical evaluation, as well as electrophysiologic criteria, are necessary to evaluate aminoglycoside-potentiated neuromuscular blockade. The importance of clinical observation is the fact that neuromuscular blockade in the presence of neomycin can be characterized by a sustained response to continuous electrical stimulation and a train-of-four ratio near 1, despite a greatly decreased single twitch response (Lee et al, 1976).

Effects of antibiotics at the neuromuscular junction probably involve multiple sites of action (Fig. 28-6) (Sokoll and Gergis, 1981). In terms of producing clinically significant skeletal muscle effects with therapeutic doses, the penicillins, cephalosporins, tetracyclines, and erythromycin are devoid of effects at the neuromuscular junction. The mechanism of the neuromuscular blocking effects of polymyxins is complex but is most likely postsynaptic. Neomycin and genta-

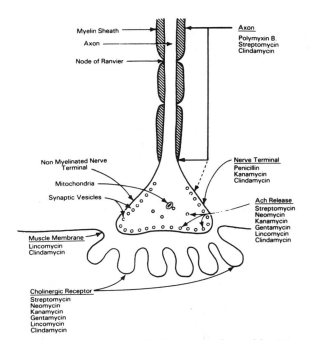

FIGURE 28–6. Schematic depiction of possible sites of action of antibiotics at the neuromuscular junction. (From Sokoll MD, Gergis SD. Antibiotics and neuromuscular function. Anesthesiology 1981; 55:148–59; with permission.)

micin reduce the amount of acetylcholine released by presynaptic motor nerves and decrease the sensitivity of the postsynaptic motor endplate to the depolarizing action of acetylcholine. Oral neomycin, which is used to reduce the bacterial population of the gastrointestinal tract prior to abdominal surgery, is unlikely to produce effects at the neuromuscular junction, because this antibiotic is not absorbed into the systemic circulation. Nevertheless, prolonged oral administration of neomycin has been associated with antibiotic-induced neuromuscular blockade (Pittinger et al, 1970).

Streptomycin

Streptomycin is most often used in combination with other antibiotics to treat specific but unusual infections. For example, streptomycin and penicillin produce a synergistic bactericidal effect in the treatment of bacterial endocarditis. Brucellosis is treated with the combination of streptomycin and tetracycline. Tularemia and all forms of plague are treated with streptomycin. Streptomycin is occasionally administered for treatment of tuberculosis. Diffusion of streptomycin occurs readily into most tissues, but the drug does not enter the cerebrospinal fluid.

Deep intramuscular injection of streptomycin, 15 to 25 mg·kg^{-1} daily in two divided doses, is the most common method of parenteral administration. Intramuscular injection is painful and may be associated with tender masses in the injected area. Skin eruptions occur in approximately 5% of patients. Neutropenia occurs in fewer than 1% of patients. Streptomycin is the least likely of all the aminoglycosides to produce nephrotoxicity, although excretion occurs primarily by glomerular filtration. Up to 15% of patients receiving the drug for more than 1 week, however, manifest a measurable decrease in hearing.

Gentamicin

Gentamicin, because of its potential to cause ototoxicity, is used for the treatment of only life-threatening gram-negative infections. For example, this antibiotic administered alone or in combination with ampicillin provides effective initial treatment of the critically ill patient with a gram-negative urinary tract infection. Patients with impaired immune defense mechanisms and requiring mechanical ventilation of the lungs have an increased incidence of gram-negative pneumonia. In these patients, gentamicin in combination with a penicillin or cephalosporin antibiotic is effective, especially if the invading bacteria is *Klebsiella* or *Pseudomonas aeruginosa*. Intrathecal administration of gentamicin is necessary for the treatment of meningitis caused by bacteria sensitive to this antibiotic. Resistance to the antibiotic effects of gentamicin is likely to develop in critically ill patients in burn units and in intensive care units.

Intramuscular administration of gentamicin in three divided doses is the recommended route of administration. Periodic determination of the plasma concentration of gentamicin is necessary to guide therapy, especially in the presence of preexisting renal disease.

Tobramycin

Tobramycin closely resembles the antibiotic effects of gentamicin. Ototoxicity and nephrotoxicity, however, are less likely following the administration of tobramycin as compared with gentamicin. Tobramycin can be administered intramuscularly or intravenously. Indications for the use of tobramycin are similar to those for gentamicin. In contrast to other aminoglycosides, tobramycin is ineffective against mycobacteria.

Amikacin

Amikacin in uniquely resistant to hydrolysis by aminoglycoside-inactivating enzymes, making it a useful drug in hospitalized patients where gentamycin-resistant bacteria are prevalent. This antibiotic may be administered intramuscularly or intravenously.

Kanamycin

Kanamycin has a limited spectrum of activity compared with other aminoglycosides and, as a result, is not frequently used. Oral administration of kanamycin, 6 to 8 g daily, is used as an adjunct to the treatment of hepatic coma and to suppress intestinal flora prior to surgery on the gastrointestinal tract.

Neomycin

Neomycin is commonly used for topical application to treat infections of the skin (as after burn injury), the cornea, and the mucous membranes. Continuous irrigation of the bladder with neomycin solution is used to prevent bacteriuria and bacteremia associated with the use of indwelling bladder catheters. Oral neomycin, 4 to 8 g daily, does not undergo systemic absorption and is thus administered to decrease bacterial flora in the intestine prior to gastrointestinal surgery and as an adjunct to the therapy of hepatic coma. Indeed, blood ammonia concentrations in the presence of hepatic failure are reduced by oral therapy with neomycin. Nephrotoxicity and ototoxicity associated with plasma concentrations of neomycin that occur after parenteral administration have caused administration of the drug by this route to be abandoned.

Allergic reactions occur in 6% to 8% of patients treated with topical neomycin. Oral administration of neomycin may result in suprainfection and intestinal malabsorption. Oral, but not parenteral, administration of neomycin produces a marked decrease in the plasma concentration of cholesterol. Neuromuscular blockade produced by neomycin is similar to that produced by hypermagnesemia. Delayed awakening from anesthesia has been reported in a single patient in association with irrigation of the bladder with neomycin (Yao et al, 1980). It was speculated that neomycin decreased the release of acetylcholine in the central nervous system by competing with Ca^{2+} necessary for release of neurotransmitter. Indeed, neomycin has been shown to bind Ca^{2+}, but the serum-ionized Ca^{2+} concentration is unaltered by this antibiotic.

VANCOMYCIN

Vancomycin is a glycopeptide antibiotic that is bactericidal for gram-positive cocci, including strains of *S. aureus* that produce penicillinase or are resistant to methicillin. Indeed, vancomycin is the only clinically effective treatment of methicillin-resistant staphylcoccal infection. Patients who are allergic to penicillin or cephalosporin antibiotics are likely to receive vancomycin when a staphylococcal infection is present. Furthermore, vancomycin is a useful prophylactic antibiotic, especially in cardiac, orthopedic, and neurosurgical procedures where a foreign body is implanted (Kaiser, 1986; Dempsey et al, 1988). Nevertheless, the cost of this antibiotic and its increased incidence of cardiovascular side effects cause most physicians to reserve prophylactic use of vancomycin to operations where the risk of methicillin-resistant staphylococcal infection is high or the patient is allergic to cephalosporins. When vancomycin is administered intravenously, the recommendation is to infuse the calculated dose (10 to 15 $mg \cdot kg^{-1}$) over 60 minutes so as to minimize the occurrence of cardiovascular side effects. Vancomycin is administered orally to treat colitis associated with the overgrowth of exotoxin-producing bacteria in patients being treated with other antibiotics. Penetration into the cerebrospinal fluid is substantial.

Vancomycin acts by inhibiting synthesis of cell walls of sensitive bacteria. Oral absorption of the drug is poor, with large amounts being excreted in the feces. Intravenous infusion over 60 minutes produces sustained plasma concentrations for up to 12 hours. Vancomycin is principally excreted by the kidneys, with 90% of a dose being recovered unchanged in the urine. The elimination half-time is approximately 6 hours and this may be greatly prolonged in the presence of renal failure.

Side Effects

Rapid intravenous infusion (less than 15 to 30 minutes) of vancomycin has been associated with profound hypotension and even, rarely, cardiac arrest (Lyon and Bruce, 1988; Mayhew and Deutsch, 1985; Miller and Tausk, 1977; Southorn et al, 1986; Symons et al, 1985). Hypotension is typically accompanied by signs of histamine release often characterized by intense facial and truncal erythema ("red-neck syndrome"). The red-neck syndrome may occur even with slow infusion of vancomycin and is not always associated with hypotension (Davis et al, 1985). Cardiovascular side effects most likely reflect nonimmunologic histamine release induced by vancomycin (Fig. 28-7) (Levy et al, 1987). Although drug-induced histamine release initially causes increases in myocardial contractility, this effect is rapidly followed by venodilation, a sudden decrease in left ventricular filling, and decreased contractility. Histamine produces hypotension in humans by directly dilating peripheral blood vessels. Direct myocardial depression produced by vancomycin does not seem to be important in causing hypotension in humans (Levy et al, 1987). Conclusions that anesthesia increases the incidence and severity of vancomycin-induced hypotension are not supported by scientific data. The importance of slow intravenous infusion of vancomycin (recommendation is 60 minutes) to awake or anesthetized patients to minimize the likelihood of histamine release must be emphasized. Indeed, administration of vancomycin over 10 minutes is associated with a 25% to 50% reduction in systolic blood pressure in 20% of patients, whereas hypotension does not occur in patients receiving the drug for more than 30 minutes (Newfield and Roizen, 1979). Nevertheless, in another report, vancomycin, 1 g, administered intravenously over 30 minutes to 16 patients follow-

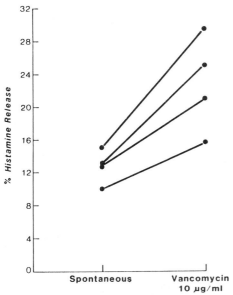

FIGURE 28–7. Histamine release (%) from dispersed human cutaneous mast cells following the administration of vancomycin. Spontaneous release averaged 12.9 ± 1% (mean ± SEM) and increased to 22.9 ± 2.3% (P < .025) following the administration of 10 µg·ml⁻¹ vancomycin (3 × 10⁻³ M). (From Levy JH, Kettlekamp N, Goertz P, Hermens J, Hirshman CA. Histamine release by vancomyein. A mechanism for hypotension in man. Anesthesiology 1987;67:122-5; with permission.)

ing coronary artery bypass graft surgery was unassociated with hemodynamic changes, and there was no correlation between plasma antibiotic levels and the release of histamine (Stier et al, 1990).

Vancomycin may produce allergic reactions characterized as anaphylactoid with associated hypotension, erythema, and occasionally bronchospasm (Symons et al, 1985). Potentiation of nondepolarizing neuromuscular blocking drugs is a consideration. Ototoxicity is likely when excessively high plasma concentrations (more than 30 µg·ml⁻¹) are present. The incidence of nephrotoxicity is low.

TETRACYCLINES

Tetracyclines consist of four interconnected carbon rings with side chains on which various substitutions are made (Fig. 28-8). These drugs possess a wide range of antibiotic activity against gram-positive and gram-negative bacteria. For example, tetracycline antibiotics are frequently administered in the treatment of chronic bronchitis. Prophylactic administration of tetracyclines may reduce the number of acute pulmonary infections in patients with chronic obstructive airway disease. These drugs are effective against mycoplasma, which causes pneumonia; chlamydia, which causes nonspecific urethritis; *Rickettsia,* which causes Rocky Mountain spotted fever; and lymphogranuloma venereum. Tetracyclines have been administered in small oral doses to treat acne, presumably producing a beneficial effect by reducing the fatty acid content of sebum.

Mechanism of Action

Therapeutic concentrations of tetracyclines are bacteriostatic, affecting only multiplying bacteria. Nevertheless, high plasma concentrations may be bactericidal. The site of action of tetracyclines is the bacterial ribosome where the antibiotic acts by inhibiting protein synthesis. Both passive diffusion and an energy-dependent active transport system are necessary for tetracyclines to cross bacterial cell membranes and reach ribosomes. Resistance to tetracyclines can develop by way of genetic changes in bacteria that affect active transport of the drug into bacterial cells.

Route of Administration

Tetracyclines are adequately but incompletely absorbed from the gastrointestinal tract. The percentage of an oral dose that is absorbed when the stomach is empty is 30% for chlorotetracycline; 60% to 80% for oxytetracycline, demeclocycline, and tetracycline; and almost 100% for doxycycline and minocycline. Most absorption occurs from the stomach and upper small intestine. Absorption is impaired by the presence of milk and particulate antacids, presumably reflecting chelation and an increase in gastric pH.

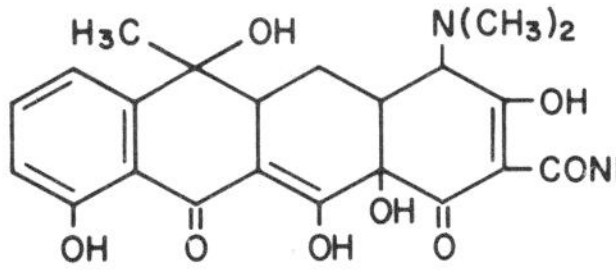

FIGURE 28–8. Tetracyclines consist of four interconnected carbon rings with side chains.

Indications for intravenous administration for tetracyclines are few because more acceptable alternatives exist. Thrombophlebitis is likely to occur following intravenous injection of these drugs. The advantage of intravenous injection is rapid penetration of these lipid-soluble antibiotics into tissues and fluids. The greater lipid solubility of minocycline compared with other tetracyclines results in unique penetration into the central nervous system to eradicate the meningococcal carrier state. Local irritation and poor absorption generally make intramuscular administration of tetracyclines unacceptable. Topical administration, except for use in the eye, is not recommended because of a high incidence of sensitization.

Excretion

All tetracyclines are concentrated in the liver and excreted by way of bile into the small intestine, from which they are partially reabsorbed. Chloro tetracycline depends more on biliary excretion for its elimination from the body than do any of the other tetracyclines. Decreased hepatic function or obstruction of the common bile duct results in reduced biliary excretion and persistence in the blood. Enterohepatic circulation of the tetracyclines ensures the presence of antibiotic in the blood for prolonged periods following the cessation of therapy. The elimination half-time is prolonged, averaging 6 to 9 hours for chlorotetracycline, oxytetracycline, and tetracycline; 16 hours for demeclocycline; and 17 to 20 hours for doxycycline and minocycline.

Glomerular filtration and renal tubular secretion are also important for the excretion of tetracyclines. Minocycline is an exception in that renal clearance is low and hepatic metabolism seems to be extensive. Doxycycline is unique in that it does not accumulate significantly in the plasma of patients in renal failure, making it an attractive drug for treatment of extrarenal infections in patients with renal dysfunction. This drug is excreted in the bile largely as an inactive conjugate or possibly as a chelate, accounting for its modest impact on intestinal bacterial flora.

Side Effects

Gastrointestinal distress and the possibility of tetracycline-resistant bacterial enteritis limit the oral dose of these antibiotics. Tetracyclines evoke a catabolic effect, presumably owing to a generalized inhibition of amino acid use for protein synthesis. This catabolic effect may contribute to additional weight loss in critically ill patients, and the associated increase in urea excretion is undesirable in the presence of renal dysfunction. *Phototoxicity,* characterized by increased sensitivity of the skin to sunlight, occurs in patients treated with tetracycline. Fatty liver infiltration has been observed, and parturients seem to be uniquely susceptible (Schultz et al, 1963). Cross-sensitization occurs between tetracyclines, requiring the use of a different class of antibiotics if an allergic reaction occurs following administration of a tetracycline. Tetracyclines may cause increased intracranial pressure (pseudotumor cerebri), especially when administered to infants (Stuart and Litt, 1978). Outdated tetracyclines have been associated with a form of Fanconi's syndrome (nausea, polyuria, polydipsia, or proteinuria), emphasizing the importance of discarding unused supplies of the drug.

Tetracycline is deposited in the enamel of teeth, including unerupted teeth, when given to children between the ages of 2 months and 5 years, resulting in hypoplasia and brown discoloration of the tooth. Even treatment of parturients with tetracyclines can produce discoloration in the offspring's teeth. Deposition of tetracycline in teeth and bones is probably due to its chelating property and the formation of a tetracycline-orthophosphate-Ca^{2+} complex.

CHLORAMPHENICOL

Chloramphenicol is unique among antibiotics in that it contains a nitrobenzene moiety and is a derivative of dichloroacetic acid (Fig. 28-9). The drug is actively transported into bacterial cells, where it inhibits protein synthesis. Chloramphenicol possesses a wide range of antibacterial activity, including all anaerobic bacteria and gram-negative rods. It is primarily bacteriostatic, although it is bactericidal to certain bacterial strains such as *H. influenzae.* The risk of aplastic anemia dictates that use of chloramphenicol be reserved for treatment of diseases unresponsive to other antibiotics. For example, ampicillin-resistant strains of *H. influenzae* causing meningitis may be an indication for treatment with chloramphenicol. Chloramphenicol is the drug of choice for treatment of typhoid fever. Resis-

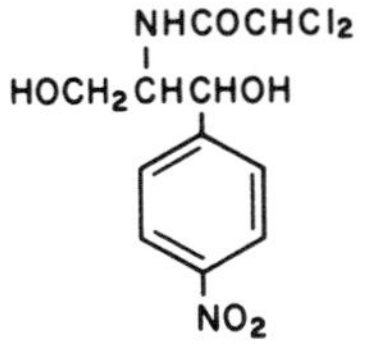

$$NHCOCHCl_2$$
$$HOCH_2CHCHOH$$

FIGURE 28–9. Chloramphenicol.

tance to chloramphenicol develops when a specific bacterial acetyltransferase acetylates the drug to a form that cannot bind to bacterial ribosomes.

Route of Administration

Chloramphenicol is rapidly absorbed from the gastrointestinal tract. The preparation of chloramphenicol for intravenous administration is the inactive succinate ester, which is rapidly hydrolyzed *in vivo* to the biologically active drug. Absorption after intramuscular administration is unpredictable. Chloramphenicol is distributed in body fluids and achieves therapeutic concentrations in the cerebrospinal fluid. This drug readily crosses the placenta.

Excretion

Chloramphenicol is inactivated primarily in the liver by glucuronyl transferase. The elimination half-time is 1.5 to 3.5 hours, and this is prolonged in the presence of liver disease. Over a 24-hour period, 75% to 90% of an orally administered dose of chloramphenicol, of which 5% to 10% is the unchanged drug, is excreted in the urine. The unchanged drug is eliminated mainly by glomerular filtration, whereas inactive metabolites undergo renal tubular secretion. The elimination half-time of the active drug is only slightly prolonged by renal failure, necessitating the administration of usual doses to maintain a therapeutic concentration. Conversely, inactive metabolites accumulate in anuric patients.

Side Effects

The most important side effect of chloramphenicol is bone marrow depression, which occurs in approximately 1 of every 30,000 treated

patients and manifests as leukopenia, thrombocytopenia, and ultimately, fatal aplastic anemia. The incidence of this adverse response is not related to the dose of chloramphenicol but does seem to occur more commonly in patients who undergo prolonged therapy or who are exposed more than once to chloramphenicol. An allergic reaction or genetically determined idiosyncratic response to the drug may be responsible for bone marrow depression.

Chloramphenicol can inhibit hepatic microsomal enzymes and prolong the duration of action of drugs such as dicumarol, phenytoin, and tolbutamide. This hepatic microsomal enzyme inhibitory effect may protect the liver from toxic effects of known hepatotoxins, such as carbon tetrachloride, by inhibiting metabolism.

ERYTHROMYCIN

Erythromycin is an orally effective antibiotic that may be bacteriostatic or bactericidal for gram-positive bacteria depending on the microorganism and concentration. It has moderate activity against *H. influenzae* and excellent activity against most strains of *N. gonorrhoeae*. Erythromycin, administered orally, reduces the duration of fever caused by mycoplasma pneumoniae. Legionnaires' disease is effectively treated with erythromycin. This drug also predictably eradicates the diphtheria carrier state. Streptococcal infections, including pharyngitis and scarlet fever, and pneumococcal pneumonia respond promptly to erythromycin.

Erythromycin diffuses readily into intracellular fluids; and antibiotic activity can be achieved at essentially all sites except the brain and cerebrospinal fluid. This is one of the few antibiotics that penetrate into prostatic fluid, achieving concentrations that are approximately 50 % of those present in the circulation. An important use of oral erythromycin, 250 mg every 6 hours, is as an alternative to benzylpenicillin in patients who are allergic to penicillin antibiotics. Intramuscular injections of erythromycin are painful, and intravenous administration often results in thrombophlebitis.

Mechanism of Action

Erythromycin is a structurally complex macrolide antibiotic containing a many-membered lactone ring to which are attached one or more deoxy-sugars (Fig. 28-10). Erythromycin inhibits protein synthesis by bacterial ribosomes.

Route of Administration and Excretion

Erythromycin is absorbed from the upper part of the small intestine but is inactivated by gastric fluid, requiring its administration as an enteric-coated tablet that dissolves in the duodenum. Only 2% to 5% of orally administered drug is excreted unchanged by the kidneys. The antibiotic is concentrated in the liver and bile. Some drug may be inactivated by demethylation in the liver. The elimination half-time is approximately 1.4 hours.

Side Effects

Erythromycin is one of the safest antibiotics available, having minimal side effects. Cholestatic hepatitis with jaundice is the most serious side effect and is caused primarily by erythromycin estolate and only rarely by other preparations. Indeed, the syndrome may represent an allergic reaction to the estolate ester. Pain associated with onset of hepatic dysfunction may mimic acute cholecystitis. Hepatic dysfunction is reversible when erythromycin is discontinued.

CLINDAMYCIN

Clindamycin resembles erythromycin in antibacterial activity except that it is more active against many anaerobic bacteria (Fig. 28-11). A number of gram-positive cocci are sensitive to clindamy-

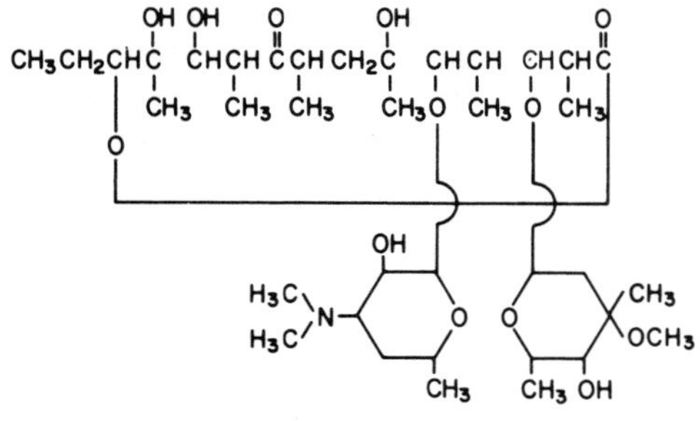

FIGURE 28–10.   Erythromycin.

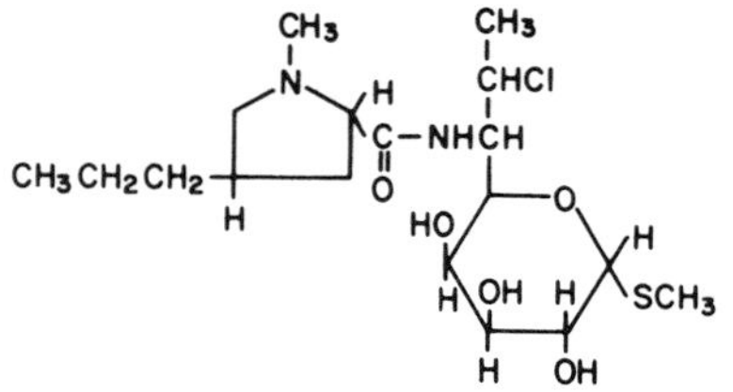

FIGURE 28–11.   Clindamycin.

cin, but a high incidence of gastrointestinal side effects limits its use to infections in which it is clearly superior to other antibiotics. Intravenous administration is useful in the treatment of staphylococcal osteomyelitis.

Antibiotic activity of clindamycin is due to suppression of protein synthesis by bacterial ribosomes. Oral absorption of the drug is nearly complete, and the elimination half-time is approximately 24 hours. Significant concentrations of clindamycin are not achieved in the cerebrospinal fluid.

Clindamycin is occasionally associated with pseudomembranous colitis, which is presumably caused by elaboration of an exotoxin by clindamycin-resistant bacteria. If diarrhea occurs, clindamycin should be discontinued and vancomycin should be administered orally. Skin rashes occur in approximately 10% of patients treated with clindamycin.

POLYMYXIN AND COLISTIN

Polymyxin B and colistin are basic peptides with molecular weights near 1000 that are effective against gram-negative bacteria, including *E. coli*, *Klebsiella*, and *P. aeruginosa*. *Proteus* and most strains of *Neisseria* are resistant to these drugs. Polymyxin B and colistin are used primarily to treat severe urinary tract infectious caused by *P. aeruginosa* and other gram-negative bacteria that are not susceptible to other antibiotics. Meningeal infections caused by similar organisms are treated with intrathecal administration of polymyxin B, because systemically administered drug does not enter the cerebrospinal fluid. Infections of the skin, mucous membranes, eyes, and ears can be effectively treated with topical application. Indeed, *P. aeruginosa* is a common cause of corneal ulcers.

Polymyxin B and colistin are surface-active antibiotics that interact with phospholipids and penetrate into and disrupt the structure of bacterial cell membranes. Oral or mucous membrane absorption is inadequate such that these drugs are administered intramuscularly. Pain after intramuscular injection is common and may follow the distribution of a nearby peripheral nerve. Elimination is predominantly by the kidneys, and these drugs accumulate in patients with renal failure.

Side Effects

Polymyxin applied to intact or denuded skin is not absorbed systemically and, therefore, allergic reactions are unlikely to occur. Like aminoglycosides, polymyxin B can produce skeletal muscle weakness resembling nondepolarizing neuromuscular blockade, particularly in the presence of high plasma concentrations of drugs such as are likely to occur in patients with renal dysfunction. Neostigmine or Ca^{2+} does not antagonize this drug-induced effect at the neuromuscular junction, which contrasts with the ability of these drugs to reverse aminoglycoside-induced skeletal muscle weakness (Sokoll and Gergis, 1981). This antibiotic-induced neuromuscular effect may also manifest as marked potentiation of nondepolarizing neuromuscular blocking drugs.

The most significant side effect of these antibiotics is nephrotoxicity, with polymyxin B being more toxic than colistin. For this reason, these antibiotics should not be used in patients with renal disease if alternative drugs are available.

BACITRACIN

Bacitracins are a group of polypeptide antibiotics effective against a variety of gram-positive bacteria. Bacitracin inhibits bacterial cell wall synthesis. Its use is limited to topical application in ophthalmologic and dermatologic ointments. An advantage of bacitracin compared with other antibiotics is that its topical application rarely results in allergic reactions. Established topical uses of bacitracin include treatment of furunculosis, carbuncle, impetigo, suppurative conjunctivitis, and infected corneal ulcer.

SULFONAMIDES

Sulfonamides are drugs that are derivatives of sulfanilamide. These drugs were the first antibiotics that exhibited a wide range of bacteriostatic activity against gram-positive and gram-negative bacteria. The important structural features for antibacterial activity are the benzene ring and the para-amino group (Fig. 28-12). The para-amino group can be replaced only by radicals capable of conversion in the tissues to a free amino group.

Mechanism of Action

Antibiotic activity of sulfonamides is due to the ability of these drugs to prevent normal use of para-aminobenzoic acid by bacteria to synthesize folic acid (pteroylglutamic acid). Specifically, sulfonamides act as competitive inhibitors of the bacterial enzyme responsible for the incorporation of para-aminobenzoic acid into the immediate precursor of folic acid. Bacteria that do not require folic acid or normal mammalian cells that can use preformed folic acid that is absorbed from the gastrointestinal tract are unaffected by sulfonamides. Bacteriostatic effects of sulfonamides are counteracted by para-aminobenzoic acid. For example, ester local anesthetics that are hydrolyzed to para-aminobenzoic acid antagonize the *in vivo* antibacterial effects of sulfonamides. Indeed, resistance that develops to the antibacterial effects of sulfonamides may reflect the development of the ability of bacteria to synthesize para-aminobenzoic acid.

Route of Administration

Except for sulfonamides that are especially designed for their local effects in the bowel, these antibiotics are rapidly and highly absorbed (70% to 100%) from the gastrointestinal tract, primarily from the small intestine. Sulfonamides readily enter pleural, peritoneal, synovial, ocular, and cerebrospinal fluid, reaching concentrations similar to those in the blood. Passage across the placenta is prompt.

Excretion

Metabolism of sulfonamides is predominantly by acetylation in the liver to pharmacologically inac-

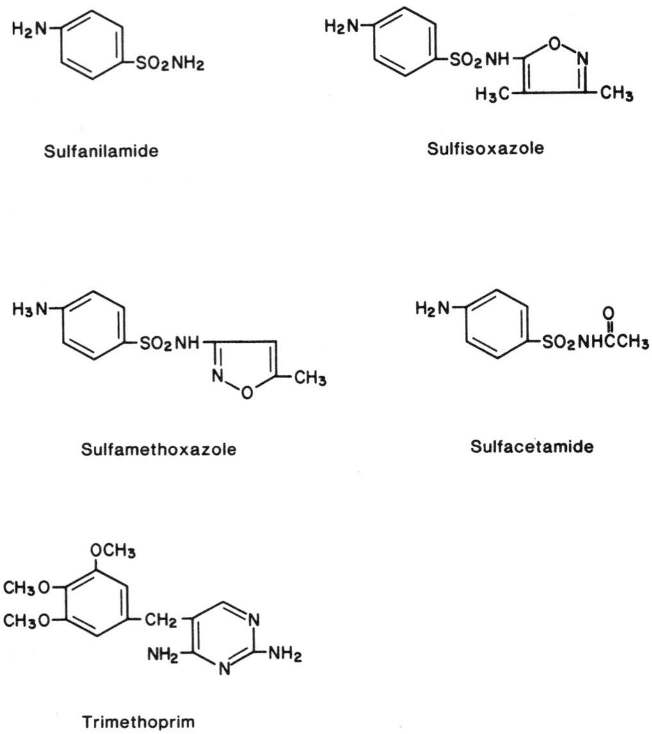

FIGURE 28–12. Sulfonamides are derivatives of sulfanilamide.

tive compounds. Acetyl metabolites, however, are often less soluble, which increases the likelihood of crystalluria. The magnitude of acetylation varies greatly among the various sulfonamides. Elimination of unchanged and acetylated drug is primarily by glomerular filtration, with renal tubular secretion being of variable importance. The elimination half-time of sulfonamides depends on renal function.

Side Effects

Side effects that may follow administration of sulfonamides are numerous and varied. Allergic reactions ranging from skin rash to anaphylaxis are possible with any of the sulfonamides, and cross-sensitivity may or may not occur. Drug fever is a common side effect of sulfonamide treatment. Hepatotoxicity resulting from direct toxicity or sensitization occurs in less than 0.1% of patients. Acute hemolytic anemia and agranulocytosis are rare, but possible, adverse effects of treatment

with sulfonamides. Formation and deposition of crystalline aggregates in the kidneys and ureter are infrequent with the use of highly soluble sulfonamides. Administration of sulfonamides may increase the effect of oral anticoagulants, methotrexate, sulfonylurea hypoglycemic drugs, and thiazide diuretics, probably by displacement of these drugs from binding sites on plasma albumin. Likewise, sulfonamides can compete for the same protein binding sites as bilirubin, enhancing the risk of jaundice in premature infants. Conversely, indomethacin, probenecid, and salicylates may displace sulfonamides from plasma albumin and increase the concentrations of free drug in the plasma. Hemolytic anemia may occur in patients with glucose-6-phosphatase deficiency who receive sulfonamides.

Sulfisoxazole

Sulfisoxazole administered orally is rapidly absorbed from the gastrointestinal tract (Fig. 28-

12). The usual adult oral dose is 2 to 4 g initially, followed by 1 g every 4 to 6 hours. Sulfisoxazole is primarily used as a treatment for urinary tract infections. In susceptible patients who are allergic to penicillin antibiotics, sulfisoxazole can be used as prophylaxis against streptococcal infections and recurrences of rheumatic fever. Its high water solubility minimizes the hazards of renal toxicity such as crystalluria. Approximately 95% of a single oral dose is excreted by the kidneys in 24 hours. Concentrations of sulfisoxazole in the urine greatly exceed those in the blood and may be bactericidal. The cerebrospinal fluid concentration averages approximately one third of that in the plasma.

Sulfamethoxazole

Sulfamethoxazole is a congener of sulfisoxazole, but its rate of absorption and urinary excretion are slower (Fig. 28-12). Crystalluria is a risk with sulfamethoxazole, and anuria may occur through precipitation of crystals of the acetylated drug in the renal tubules and ureter. Alkalinization of the urine or increased fluid intake is effective in preventing such precipitation.

Sulfasalazine

Sulfasalazine is poorly absorbed from the gastrointestinal tract. For this reason, it is used in the treatment of ulcerative colitis and regional enteritis.

Sulfacetamide

Sulfacetamide is frequently used for topical application as an ointment or solution for treatment of ophthalmic infections (Fig. 28-12). The preparation has a pH of 7.4, is nonirritating, and penetrates into ocular fluid in high concentrations.

Co-trimoxazole

Co-trimoxazole is a combination of trimethoprim with sulfamethoxazole that results in a synergistic antibacterial action (Fig. 28-12). The usual combination is 800 mg sulfamethoxazole plus 160 mg of trimethoprim (5:1 ratio). Chronic and recurrent urinary tract infections are particularly responsive to treatment with this combination. In females, this may be related to the presence of therapeutic concentrations of trimethoprim in vaginal secretions. Trimethoprim is also found in prostatic secretions and is often effective for treating bacterial prostatitis. Acute exacerbations of chronic bronchitis are effectively treated with this combination. Infection by *Pneumocystis carinii* is eradicated by high doses, whereas low doses provide protection against this infection in immunosuppressed hosts. Acute gonococcal urethritis, but not syphilis, is effectively treated. In fact, this combination appears to be as effective as 4.8 million units of benzylpenicillin plus 1 g of probenecid for the treatment of gonorrhea.

Mechanism of Action

The antimicrobial activity of this drug combination results from its actions on two sequential steps of the enzymatic pathway for the synthesis of tetrahydrofolic acid. Sulfamethoxazole inhibits the incorporation of para-aminobenzoic acid into folic acid, and trimethoprim prevents the reduction of dihydrofolate to tetrahydrofolate by selectively inhibiting dihydrofolate reductase. The dihydrofolate reductase of the host is many thousands of times less sensitive to trimethoprim than are the bacterial enzymes, accounting for the selectivity of this drug. Development of resistance to the combination is lower than if either of the drugs were used alone. This is predictable, because bacteria that have acquired resistance to one of the components may still be destroyed by the other.

Excretion

After a single oral dose of the combined preparation, trimethoprim is absorbed more rapidly than sulfamethoxazole. The elimination half-time of both trimethoprim and sulfamethoxazole is approximately 9.5 hours. Trimethoprim is rapidly distributed and concentrated in tissues, achieving a volume of distribution that is approximately six times that of sulfamethoxazole. It enters cerebrospinal fluid and sputum readily. Up to 60% of administered trimethoprim and from 25% to 50% of sulfamethoxazole are excreted in the urine as metabolites and unchanged drug.

Side Effects

The most common side effects of this combined preparation are skin rashes, glossitis, and stomatitis. Mild and transient jaundice with histologic features resembling allergic cholestatic hepatitis have been observed. Impairment of renal function may follow administration of this drug combination to patients with renal disease, and a reversible decrease in creatinine clearance has been noted in patients with normal renal function.

There is no evidence that co-trimoxazole induces folate deficiency in normal persons, but the margin between toxicity for bacteria and patients may be narrow when the cells of the patient are already deficient in folate. In this situation, the drug combination may cause or precipitate megaloblastic anemia, leukopenia, or thrombocytopenia. Accordingly, complete blood counts should be followed in patients being treated longer than 2 weeks. Previous or simultaneous administration of diuretics may increase the likelihood of thrombocytopenia, particularly in elderly patients.

URINARY TRACT ANTISEPTICS

Urinary tract antiseptics are drugs that are concentrated in the renal tubules, making them effective for the treatment of infections in the kidney and bladder. Because these drugs are selectively concentrated in the renal tubules, their plasma concentrations do not reach adequate levels to be effective against systemic infections.

Methenamine

Methenamine is a urinary tract antiseptic that decomposes in water, at a pH below 7.4, to formaldehyde (Fig. 28-13). Formaldehyde is responsible for the antibacterial action. *Proteus* orga-

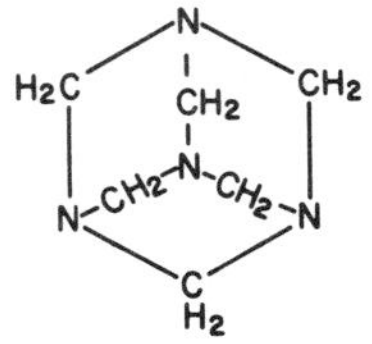

FIGURE 28–13. Methenamine.

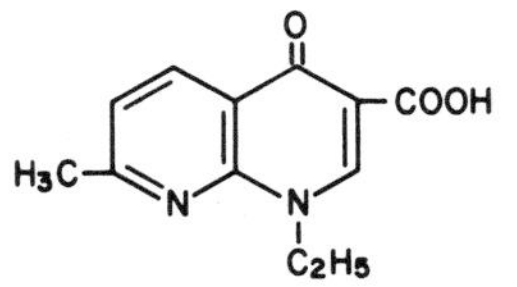

FIGURE 28–14. Nalidixic acid.

nisms, as urea-splitting bacteria, often raise the pH of urine above 5.5 and thus inhibit the release of formaldehyde. Bacteria do not develop resistance to formaldehyde. Methenamine is not used as a treatment of acute urinary tract infections but is of value for chronic suppressive treatment.

Nalidixic Acid

Nalidixic acid is bactericidal to most of the common gram-negative bacteria that cause urinary tract infections (Fig. 28-14). It appears to act by inhibiting deoxyribonucleic acid (DNA) synthesis. Therapeutic concentrations do not occur in prostatic fluid, which may account for reinfection of the urinary tract. Resistance may develop rapidly.

Nitrofurantoin

Nitrofurantoin is active against many strains of *E. coli* in the urine, and its antibacterial activity is higher in acidic urine (Fig. 28-15). In addition to use for treatment of urinary tract infections, this drug is used for the prevention of bacteriuria after prostatectomy.

Chronic active hepatitis is a rare complication (Tolman, 1980). Acute pneumonitis with fever, chills, dyspnea, and chest pain may accompany administration of this drug. Elderly patients are especially susceptible to the pulmonary toxicity of nitrofurantoin. Neuropathies are most likely to occur in patients with impaired renal function.

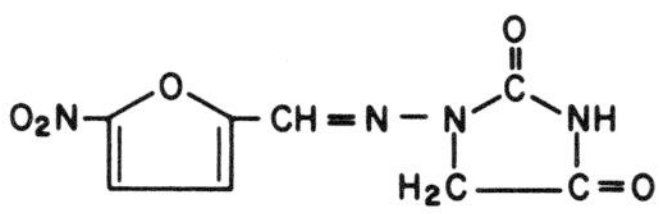

FIGURE 28–15. Nitrofurantoin.

Phenazopyridine

Phenazopyridine is not a urinary antiseptic but provides an analgesic action on the urinary tract that alleviates symptoms of dysuria, frequency, and urgency. The compound is an azo dye, and the urine is colored orange or red. Overdose may result in methemoglobinemia. This drug may be marketed in combination with sulfisoxazole or sulfamethoxazole.

DRUGS FOR TREATMENT OF TUBERCULOSIS

The majority of patients with tuberculosis can be successfully treated with drugs such as isoniazid, rifampin, ethambutol, and streptomycin. Administration of isoniazid in combination with rifampin or ethambutol represents optimal therapy for all forms of disease caused by sensitive strains of *Mycobacterium* tuberculosis. Treatment must include at least two drugs to which the mycobacteria are sensitive to offset the impact of resistance that commonly develops during therapy. Isoniazid alone is used for prophylaxis. For example, patients without apparent disease, but whose skin test has changed from negative to positive, should be treated with isoniazid for 12 months.

Isoniazid

Isoniazid is the hydrazide derivative of isonicotinic acid and is considered the primary drug for the chemotherapy of tuberculosis (Fig. 28-16). A congener of isoniazid is the isopropyl derivative iproniazid, which markedly inhibits the multiplication of the tubercle bacillus and is also a potent inhibitor of monoamine oxidase. Isoniazid is both tuberculostatic and tuberculocidal. Resistance during therapy can occur, presumably as a result of emergence of strains that do not take up the drug. Cross-resistance, however, between isoniazid and other tuberculostatic drugs does not occur. The mechanism of action of isoniazid is unknown but may reflect drug-induced inhibition of synthesis of mycolic acids, which are important constituents of the mycobacterial cell wall.

Excretion

Isoniazid is readily absorbed when administered orally or parenterally. The drug diffuses into all body fluids and cells. Up to 95% of a dose of isoniazid is excreted in the urine over 24 hours entirely as metabolites. The primary route of metabolism is hepatic acetylation of acetylisoniazid. There is a genetic determination of the rate of isoniazid acetylation, with patients being categorized as slow or rapid acetylators. Rapid acetylation is inherited as an autosomal dominant trait. Rapid acetylators are homozygous. The average concentration of active isoniazid in the plasma of rapid acetylators is 30 to 50 times less than that present in the plasma of slow acetylators. The elimination half-time of isoniazid averages approximately 1.5 hours in rapid acetylators and 3 hours in patients who are slow acetylators.

The clearance of isoniazid is dependent to only a small degree on the status of renal function, but patients who are slow acetylators may be susceptible to accumulation of toxic concentrations if renal function is impaired.

Side Effects

Side effects can be minimized by prophylactic therapy with pyridoxine and careful surveillance of the patient. For example, pyridoxine, 10 mg daily, is administered with isoniazid to minimize the occurrence of peripheral neuritis and anemia. The protective effect of pyridoxine is based on the fact that isoniazid increases the excretion of pyridoxine, resulting in a deficiency of this vitamin. Isoniazid may precipitate seizures in patients with epilepsy and rarely in patients with no prior history of seizures. Optic neuritis has occurred during therapy with this drug. Mental changes during treatment with isoniazid include euphoria, impairment of memory, and occasionally psychoses. Excessive sedation may occur in slow acetylators given isoniazid who are also receiving phenytoin, reflecting isoniazid-induced inhibition of anticonvulsant metabolism.

Severe hepatic injury characterized pathologically by bridging and multilobular necrosis

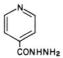

FIGURE 28–16. Isoniazid.

(similar to the changes associated with halothane) can occur (Garibaldi et al, 1972). The mechanism for hepatotoxicity is not known, although a metabolite of isoniazid, acetylisoniazid, is a known hepatotoxin (Mitchell et al, 1976). Rapid acetylators who produce more acetylisoniazid may be more vulnerable to isoniazid-induced hepatotoxicity than those who do not. Age seems to be an important determinant in the incidence of isoniazid-induced hepatic dysfunction, with an incidence of 0.3% in patients 20 to 34 years old, 1.2% in patients 35 to 49 years old, and 2.3% in patients 50 years old or older. Up to 12% of patients treated with isoniazid manifest elevated plasma transaminase enzyme levels. A greater than threefold elevation in the serum glutamic-oxaloacetic transaminase activity is cause for discontinuation of isoniazid.

Isoniazid treatment significantly enhances defluorination of volatile anesthetics, presumably by inducing the necessary hepatic microsomal enzymes (Mazze et al, 1982). Following enflurane anesthesia, the magnitude of increase in serum fluoride concentrations in isoniazid-treated patients is variable, presumably reflecting different levels of enzyme induction among rapid and slow acetylators (Fig. 28-17) (Mazze et al, 1982). Serum fluoride concentrations may be in a nephrotoxic range in those patients presumed to be rapid acetylators.

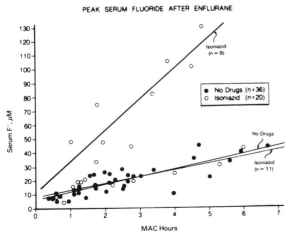

FIGURE 28–17. Isoniazid enhances defluorination of enflurane in patients who are rapid acetylators. (From Mazze RI, Woodruff RE, Heerdt ME. Isoniazid-induced enflurane defluorination in humans. Anesthesiology 1982;57:5–8; with permission.)

Rifampin

Rifampin is a complex macrocyclic antibiotic that inhibits the growth of most gram-positive bacteria as well as many gram-negative bacteria. This antibiotic is the drug of choice for prophylaxis against meningococcal disease in household contacts of patients with such infections. Resistance to the antibacterial effects of rifampin develops rapidly (within 48 hours), emphasizing that this drug must not be used alone in the chemotherapy of tuberculosis. Rifampin is effective because of its ability to inhibit ribonucleic acid synthesis in bacteria at concentrations far below those that produce this effect in normal cells.

Route of Administration

Oral absorption of rifampin is adequate but often highly variable. Salicylates may delay absorption and prevent achievement of therapeutic plasma concentrations. Rifampin penetrates tissues and body fluids, including cerebrospinal fluid, imparting a red color to the urine and saliva of patients treated with this drug.

Excretion

Rifampin undergoes hepatic deacetylation, and the resulting metabolite, which has antibacterial activity similar to the parent compound, enters bile where enterohepatic circulation occurs. The elimination half-time of rifampin varies from 1.5 to 5 hours and is prolonged in patients with hepatic dysfunction.

Side Effects

Side effects of rifampin are infrequent but with high doses may include thrombocytopenia, anemia, hepatic dysfunction with jaundice, and occasionally hepatorenal syndrome. Elevations of the serum glutamic-oxaloacetic transaminase activity and alkaline phosphatase concentrations may occur. Hepatic dysfunction rarely occurs in patients with normal hepatic function; it is more likely to occur in elderly patients with preexisting liver disease, especially that related to alcohol abuse.

Biliary excretion of rifampin competes with that of contrast media used for the study of the gallbladder. Rifampin, by an unknown mechanism, interferes with the anticoagulant effect of coumarin drugs. Methadone metabolism is accelerated by rifampin, and the likelihood of an opioid withdrawal syndrome may be increased. Rifampin appears to speed the breakdown of glucocorticoids and estrogens, which may decrease the reliability of oral contraceptives. Central and peripheral nervous system effects associated with rifampin administration include fatigue, generalized numbness, skeletal muscle weakness, and pain in the extremities.

Ethambutol

Ethambutol is tuberculostatic to mycobacteria but not to other bacteria (Fig. 28-18). It is used in combination with isoniazid for the treatment of active tuberculosis. Absorption after oral administration approaches 85% of the drug. Ethambutol is concentrated in erythrocytes, which may serve as a depot of drug to maintain a therapeutic concentration as the plasma level declines.

Excretion

Approximately 50% of an ingested dose of ethambutol is excreted unchanged by the kidneys in 24 hours. The high renal clearance of ethambutol confirms that the drug is excreted by renal tubular secretion as well as by glomerular filtration. The elimination half-time is 3 to 4 hours. Accumulation of ethambutol is likely in patients with renal dysfunction.

Side Effects

The most important side effect of therapy with ethambutol is optic neuritis, resulting in a decrease in visual acuity and loss of ability to perceive the color green. The incidence of this complication is dose related, occurring in approximately 5% of patients treated with 25 mg·kg^{-1} daily and in fewer than 1% of patients receiving daily doses less than 15 mg·kg^{-1}. There is decreased renal excretion of uric acid, resulting in increased blood concentration of urate in approximately 50% of patients.

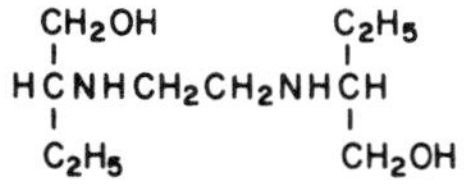

$$CH_2OH \qquad C_2H_5$$
$$HCNHCH_2CH_2NHCH$$
$$C_2H_5 \qquad CH_2OH$$

FIGURE 28–18. Ethambutol.

ANTIFUNGAL DRUGS

Nystatin

Nystatin is a polyene antibiotic that is both fungistatic and fungicidal but lacks effects on bacteria. This drug increases the permeability of the membrane of sensitive fungi such that small molecules escape. Absorption of nystatin via the skin, mucous membranes, or gastrointestinal tract is negligible. Nystatin is used primarily to treat *Candida* infections and is available as oral tablets, vaginal tablets, and ointments. Paronychia, vaginitis, and stomatitis (thrush) caused by *Candida* organisms usually respond to topical therapy. Oral, esophageal, and gastric *Candida* infections are common in patients receiving immunosuppressive therapy and certain antibiotics such as the tetracyclines. These infections usually respond to oral nystatin. Side effects are rare. For example, allergic reactions have not been reported. Because nystatin has no effect on bacteria, superinfections do not occur.

Amphotericin B

Amphotericin B, like nystatin, is a polyene antibiotic that exerts maximal antifungal effects between pH 6 and 7.5. This is the most effective antifungal drug for managing infections due to yeasts and fungi. Cryptococcal infection of the lungs or meninges, histoplasmosis, coccidioidomycosis, blastomycosis, sporotrichosis, and disseminated candidiasis are treated with amphotericin B.

Oral absorption is poor, accounting for the need to administer amphotericin B intravenously if therapeutic concentrations in infected tissues are to be achieved. The drug does not penetrate into the cerebrospinal fluid or vitreous humor. Intrathecal injection may be necessary for treatment of *Coccidioides* meningitis. Renal excretion is slow, with detectable drug being present for up to 8 weeks after discontinuation of therapy.

Side Effects

Side effects are common with the use of amphotericin B. For example, renal function is impaired in more than 80% of treated patients, and some permanent reduction in glomerular filtration rate is likely. During therapy, plasma creatinine concentrations should be monitored, and the dose of amphotericin B should be reduced when creatinine levels are more than 3.5 mg·dl^{-1}. Hypokalemia and hypomagnesemia may occur. Fever, chills, dyspnea, and hypotension are common during intravenous infusion of amphotericin B. Allergic reactions, seizures, anemia, and thrombocytopenia may occur. Hepatotoxicity is not documented as a side effect of treatment with amphotericin B.

Flucytosine

Flucytosine is converted to fluorouracil exclusively in fungal cells by the enzyme cytosine deaminase (Fig. 28-19). This selective effect avoids cytotoxicity of fluorouracil on normal cells. The drug is well absorbed from the gastrointestinal tract. Penetration into the cerebrospinal fluid and aqueous humor is excellent. Approximately 80% of flucytosine is excreted unchanged in the urine by glomerular filtration. The elimination half-time is 3 to 6 hours, but this is greatly prolonged in the presence of renal failure. In approximately 5% of patients, liver transaminase enzymes are increased and hepatomegaly occurs.

Flucytosine is available only for oral administration. It is used predominantly in combination with amphotericin B, because rapid emergence of resistant strains limits the use of flucytosine as a single drug.

Griseofulvin

Griseofulvin inhibits mitosis in certain fungi, accounting for its fungistatic effects, especially in dermatophytes (Fig. 28-20). Mycotic diseases of the skin, hair, and nails respond to griseofulvin. Symptomatic relief of skin infections usually occurs in 48 to 96 hours. There is no effect on bacteria.

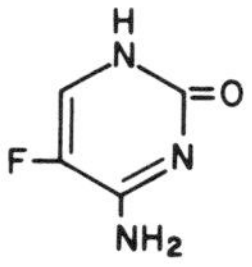

FIGURE 28-19.   Flucytosine.

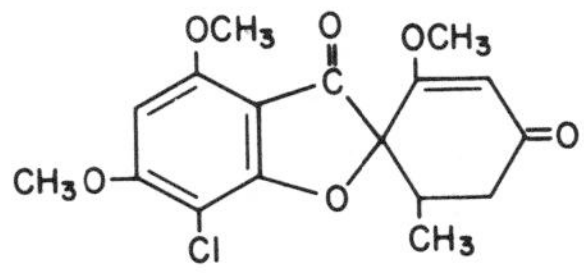

FIGURE 28-20.   Griseofulvin.

Oral absorption of griseofulvin is adequate but highly variable. Approximately 50% of an oral dose appears in the urine, mostly in the form of metabolites. The drug has greater affinity for cells of diseased skin than of normal skin, accounting for the prompt appearance of new growth of hair or nails.

Side Effects

Headache, which may be severe, occurs in as many as 15% of patients. Other nervous system manifestations include peripheral neuritis, fatigue, blurred vision, and syncope. Hepatotoxicity has been observed. Renal effects include proteinuria without evidence of renal insufficiency. Griseofulvin appears to reduce the activity of warfarin-like anticoagulants.

ANTIVIRAL DRUGS

Development of antiviral drugs has been hampered by the fact that viruses, in contrast to bacteria, are obligate intracellular parasites that use many of the biochemical mechanisms of the host cells. Therefore, it is difficult to achieve antiviral activity without also affecting some aspect of normal host cell metabolism and thus causing toxic effects in uninfected host cells. Nevertheless, there are host cell surface receptors and enzymes that are unique for viruses, providing a mechanism for the development of antiviral drugs with selective activity.

Viruses are composed of a nucleic acid core surrounded by a protein-containing outer coat. The viral genome contains either RNA or DNA but never both, and viruses are classified on this basis (Table 28-5) (Melnick, 1980).

Idoxuridine

Idoxuridine is a halogenated pyrimidine that resembles thymidine. Following phosphorylation

Table 28-5
Classification of Viruses and Associated Diseases

RNA viruses
Picornaviruses—polio, encephalitis, common cold
Reoviruses—diarrhea
Togaviruses—encephalitis, rubella
Orthomyxoviruses—influenza
Paramyxoviruses—croup, bronchitis, mumps, measles
Retroviruses—acquired immunodeficiency syndrome,
   leukemia

DNA viruses
Papovaviruses—warts
Adenoviruses—acute respiratory diseases, keratitis
Herpesviruses—cold sores, keratitis, genital lesions,
   varicella, shingles, cytomegalic inclusion disease,
   infectious mononucleosis

in the cells, the triphosphate derivative is incorporated into both viral and mammalian DNA. As such, the antiviral activity of idoxuridine is mainly limited to DNA viruses, usually of the herpes simplex group. The primary clinical use of this drug is topical treatment of herpes simplex keratitis lesions of the skin, conjunctiva, and mucous membranes. Rapid inactivation by nucleotidases precludes its use by routes other than intravenous or topical administration. After intravenous injection, most of the drug disappears from the blood in approximately 30 minutes.

Amantadine

Amantadine is a synthetic tricyclic amine antiviral drug that inhibits replication of strains of influenza A virus. It has no clinical activity against influenza B viruses. Amantadine is almost completely absorbed after oral administration, with 90% of the dose appearing unchanged in the urine. Amantadine has prophylactic value when administered to persons who have had contact with an active case of influenza A virus. Approximately 70% of treated patients exposed to influenza A are protected. This drug also has therapeutic value in the treatment of patients with Parkinson's disease (see Chapter 31).

Amantadine accumulates in patients with impaired renal function. Excessive plasma concentrations are associated with central nervous system toxicity, including seizures and coma.

Vidarabine

Vidarabine is an analogue of adenosine that is effective in the treatment of herpes simplex encephalitis and keratoconjunctivitis (Fig. 28-21) (Whitley et al, 1986). Severe infections with herpes simplex virus in neonates may also respond to vidarabine. It is ineffective in varicella, cytomegalic inclusion disease, and recurrent or primary genital herpes. The drug acts by inhibiting viral DNA polymerase, whereas DNA synthesis in noninfected cells is inhibited less. Because vidarabine is poorly soluble in water, large volumes (2.5 L) are needed to dissolve the drug for intravenous infusion and treatment of encephalitis. Topical ointment is used for treatment of conjunctivitis. Vidarabine may be both mutagenic and carcinogenic.

Interferon

Interferon is a general term used to designate glycoproteins produced by cells in response to viral infection. Binding of interferons by specific receptors on cell membranes is the first step in establishing their antiviral effect, which may include degradation of viral RNA. In addition to antiviral effects, interferons inhibit cell proliferation and enhance tumoricidal activities of macrophages. Interferons produced by recombinant DNA techniques in bacteria are effective when administered as a nasal spray against rhinovirus infections (Hayden et al, 1986). Treatment with interferons may be associated with fever, headache, malaise, myalgia, and transient leukopenia, especially following intravenous or intramuscular administration. Nasal irritation may accompany intranasal administration.

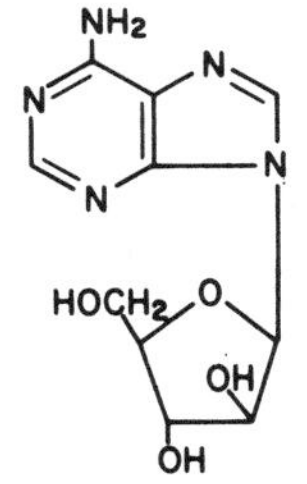

FIGURE 28-21. Vidarabine.

Acyclovir

The antiviral spectrum of acyclovir is limited to herpes viruses (Fig. 28-22). Acyclovir administered topically or orally is effective in the initial and recurrent treatment of genital herpes. Intravenous or oral administration of acyclovir will reduce the duration of viral shedding, decrease pain, and accelerate healing of herpes zoster in immunosuppressed patients. There is no apparent effect, however, on postherpetic neuralgia. Patients with chronic fatigue syndrome and persisting antibodies to Epstein-Barr virus failed to experience a beneficial response when treated with acyclovir (Straus et al, 1988).

Following intravenous administration, acyclovir is widely distributed it tissues and body fluids, attaining concentrations in the cerebrospinal fluid that are approximately 50% of those in plasma. Excretion is by glomerular filtration and renal tubular secretion, principally of unchanged drug. The elimination half-time is approximately 2.5 hours in the presence of normal renal function.

Side Effects

Elevations in blood urea nitrogen and serum creatinine have occurred following rapid intravenous administration of acyclovir. This may reflect crystallization of acyclovir in renal tubules. Thrombophlebitis may occur at the site of intravenous administration. A frequent nonspecific complaint in patients treated with oral acyclovir is headache.

Zidovudine

Zidovudine inhibits replication of some retroviruses including human immunodeficiency virus (Yarchoan et al, 1989). Treatment with this drug reduces the risk of developing opportunistic infections associated with acquired immunodeficiency syndrome. Granulocytopenia and anemia occur in nearly one third of patients, necessitating either a dose reduction or discontinuation of the drug. Blood counts are recommended every 3 to 4 days in patients being treated with this drug. Other toxic effects of the drug include nausea and vomiting, myalgia, hepatic dysfunction, and bluish nail pigmentation. Following glucuronidation in the liver, the drug is primarily eliminated by the kidneys. As estimated, 15% to 20% of the drug is excreted unchanged by the kidneys. Probenecid inhibits both hepatic glucuronidation and renal excretion, thus reducing total-body clearance of zidovudine by 65%. Other drugs that undergo hepatic glucuronidation and may therefore inhibit the metabolism of zidovudine include nonsteroidal anti-inflammatory drugs and opioids (Yarchoan et al, 1989). Nephrotoxicity is possible especially when zidovudine is co-administered with other toxic drugs.

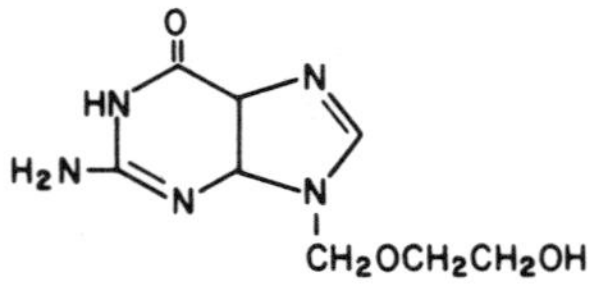

REFERENCES

Beaupre PN, Roizen MF, Cahalan MK, Alpert RA, Cassorla L, Schiller NB. Hemodynamic and two-dimensional transesophageal echocardiographic analysis of an anaphylactic reaction in a human. Anesthesiology 1984;60:482–4.

Booij LHDJ, VanderPloeg GCJ, Crul JF, Muytijens HL. Do neostigmine and 4-aminopyridine inhibit the antibacterial activity of antibiotics? Br J Anaesth 1980;52:1097–9.

Bruckner J, Thomas KC, Bikhazi GB, Foldes FF. Neuromuscular drug interactions of clinical importance. Anesth Analg 1980;59:678–82.

Davis RL, Smith AL, Koup JR. The "red-man's syndrome" and slow infusion of vancomycin. N Engl J Med 1985;313:756–7.

Dempsey R, Rapp RP, Young B, Johnston S, Tibbs P. Prophylactic parenteral antibiotics in clean neurosurgical procedures: A review. J Neurosurg 1988;69:52–7.

Donowitz GR, Mandell GL. Beta-lactam antibiotics. N Engl J Med 1988;318:419–6;490–99.

Garibaldi RA, Drusin RE, Ferebee SH, Gregg MB. Isoniazid-associated hepatitis. Report of an outbreak. Am Rev Respir Dis 1972;106:357–65.

Hayden FG, Albrecht JK, Kaiser DL, Gwaltney JM. Prevention of natural colds of contact prophylaxis with intranasal alpha$_2$ interferon. N Engl J Med 1986;314:71–5.

Kaiser AB. Antimicrobial prophylaxis in surgery. N Engl J Med 1986;315:1129–38.

Lee C, Chen D, Barnes A, Katz RL. Neuromuscular block by neomycin in the cat. Can Anaesth Soc J 1976;23:527–33.

FIGURE 28–22. Acyclovir.

Levy JH, Kettlekamp N, Goertz P, Hermens J, Hirshman CA. Histamine release by vancomycin: A mechanism for hypotension in man. Anesthesiology 1987; 67:122–5.

Lippmann M, Yang E, Au E, Lee C. Neuromuscular blocking effects of tobramycin, gentamicin, and cefazolin. Anesth Analg 1982;61:767–70.

Lyon GD, Bruce DL. Diphenhydramine reversal of vancomycin-induced hypotension. Anesth Analg 1988;67:1109–10.

Mazze RI, Woodruff RE, Heerdt ME. Isoniazid-induced enflurane defluorination in humans. Anesthesiology 1982;57:5–8.

Mayhew JF, Deutsch S. Cardiac arrest following administration of vancomycin. Can Anaesth Soc J 1985; 32:65–6.

Melnick JL. Taxonomy of viruses, 1980. Prog Med Virol 1980;26:214–32.

Miller R, Tausk HC. Anaphylactoid reaction to vancomycin during anesthesia. Anesth Analg 1977; 56:870–2.

Mitchell JR, Zimmerman HJ, Ishak KG, et al. Isoniazid liver injury: Clinical spectrum, pathology, and probable pathogenesis. Ann Intern Med 1976;84:181–92.

Newfield P, Roizen MF. Hazards of rapid administration of vancomycin. Ann Intern Med 1979;91:581.

Pallasch TJ. Principles of pharmacotherapy: III. Drug allergy. Anesth Prog 1988;35:178–89.

Pittinger CP, Eryasa T, Adamson R. Antibiotic-induced paralysis. Anesth Analg 1970;49:487–501.

Schultz JC, Adamson JS, Workman WW, Norman TD. Fatal liver disease after intravenous administration of tetracycline in high dosage. N Engl J Med 1963; 269:999–1004.

Sokoll MD, Gergis SD. Antibiotics and neuromuscular function. Anesthesiology 1981;55:148–59.

Southorn PA, Plevak DJ, Wilson WR. Adverse effects of vancomycin administered in the perioperative period. Mayo Clinic Proc 1986;61:721–4.

Stier GR, McGory RW, Spotnitz WD, Schwenzer KJ. Hemodynamic effects of rapid vancomycin infusion in critically ill patients. Anesth Analg 1990;71:394–9.

Straus SE, Dale JK, Tobi M, et al. Acyclovir treatment of the chronic fatigue syndrome of efficacy in a placebo-controlled trial. N Engl J Med 1988;319:1692–8.

Stuart BH, Litt TF. Tetracycline-associated intracranial hypertension in an adolescent: A complication of systemic acne therapy. J Pediatr 1978;92:679–80.

Symons NLP, Hobbes AFT, Leaver HK. Anaphylactoid reactions to vancomycin. Can Anaesth Soc J 1985; 32:65–6.

Tolman KG. Nitrofurantoin and chronic active hepatitis. Ann Intern Med 1980;92:2119–20.

Whitley RJ, Alford C, Hirsch MS, et al. Vidarabine versus acyclovir therapy in herpes simplex encephalitis. N Engl J Med 1986;314:144–9.

Yao F-S, Saidman SF, Artusio JF. Disturbance of consciousness and hypocalcemia after neomycin irrigation, and reversal by calcium and physostigmine. Anesthesiology 1980;53:69–71.

Yarchoan R, Mitsuya H. Myers CE, Broder S. Clinical pharmacology of 3'-azido-2',3'-dideoxythymidine (Zidovudine), and related dideoxynucleosides. N Engl J Med 1989;321:726–37.

29

Chemotherapeutic Drugs

Chemotherapy is the best available therapeutic approach for the eradication of malignant cells that can occur anywhere in the body. Effectiveness of chemotherapy requires that there be complete destruction (total cell-kill) of all cancer cells, because a single surviving clonogenic cell can give rise to sufficient progeny to ultimately kill the host. The logical outgrowth of the recognition for the need of total cell-kill is use of several chemotherapeutic (antineoplastic) drugs concurrently or in a planned sequence. The goal of combination chemotherapy is to administer the largest possible doses of chemotherapeutic drugs, each working by different mechanisms and not sharing similar toxic effects. Using a combination of chemotherapeutic drugs with different mechanisms of action also reduces the chances that drug-resistant tumor cell populations will emerge. Chemotherapeutic drugs used in combination are usually administered over short periods at specific treatment intervals rather than as continuous therapy. This approach is based on the empiric observation that normal cells usually recover more rapidly from a pulse of maximal chemotherapy than do malignant cells. Furthermore, immunosuppression is less with intermittent chemotherapy.

Malignant cells are often characterized by rapid division and synthesis of deoxyribonucleic acid (DNA). Most chemotherapeutic drugs exert their antineoplastic effects on those cells that are actively undergoing division (mitosis) or DNA synthesis. Slow-growing malignant cells with a slow rate of division, such as carcinoma of the lung and colon, are often unresponsive to chemotherapeutic drugs. Conversely, rapidly dividing normal cells, as in the bone marrow, gas-trointestinal mucosa, skin, and hair follicles, are vulnerable to the toxic effects of chemotherapeutic drugs. It is predictable, therefore, that clinical manifestations of toxicity as a result of chemotherapeutic drugs may include myelosuppression (leukopenia, thrombocytopenia, or anemia), nausea, vomiting, diarrhea, mucosal ulceration, dermatitis, and alopecia. Often, myelosuppression is the dose-limiting factor for chemotherapeutic drugs and is the indication for temporary or permanent withdrawal of therapy. Fortunately, this drug-induced myelosuppression is usually reversible with discontinuation of chemotherapeutic drug therapy.

CLASSIFICATION

Chemotherapeutic drugs are classified as (1) alkylating drugs, (2) antimetabolites, (3) *Vinca* alkaloids, (4) antibiotics, (5) enzymes, (6) synthetics, and (7) hormones (Table 29-1) (Selvin; 1981).

Knowledge of drug-induced adverse effects and evaluation of appropriate laboratory tests (hemoglobin and platelet count, white blood cell count, coagulation profile, arterial blood gases, blood glucose, plasma electrolytes, liver and renal function tests, electrocardiogram [ECG], and radiograph of the chest) are useful in the preoperative evaluation of patients being treated with chemotherapeutic drugs (Table 29-1) (Selvin, 1981). Attention to asepsis is essential, because immunosuppression makes these patients susceptible to iatrogenic infection. A history of severe diarrhea may be associated with electrolyte disturbances and decreased intravascular fluid volume. The existence of stomatitis makes placement of pharyngeal airways and esophageal catheters questionable. The response to inhaled and injected drugs may be altered by drug-induced cardiac, hepatic, or renal dysfunction. The response to nondepolarizing neuromuscular blocking drugs may be altered by impaired renal function. Furthermore, effects of succinylcholine may be prolonged if plasma cholinesterase activity is decreased by chemotherapeutic drugs. An increased incidence of spontaneous abortions has been reported in female personnel who handle certain chemotherapeutic drugs during the first trimester of pregnancy (Selevan et al, 1985).

ALKYLATING DRUGS

Alkylating drugs include nitrogen mustards, alkyl sulfonates, and nitrosoureas. These chemotherapeutic drugs have the common property of undergoing electrophilic chemical reactions that result in the formation of covalent linkages (alkylation) with various nucleophilic substances, principally DNA. The 7-nitrogen atom of guanine residues in DNA is particularly susceptible to formation of a covalent bond. The result is a miscoding of DNA information or opening of the purine ring with damage to the DNA molecule. Although alkylating drugs depend on cell division, they are not cycle-specific, acting on the DNA molecule at any stage of the division. Acquired resistance to alkylating drugs is a common occurrence and may reflect decreased cell membrane permeability to the drugs and increased production of nucleophilic substances that can compete with target DNA for alkylation.

Side Effects

Bone marrow suppression is the most important dose-limiting factor in the clinical use of alkylating drugs. Cessation of mitosis is evident within 6 to 8 hours. Lymphocytopenia is usually present within 24 hours. Variable degrees of depression of platelet and erythrocyte counts may occur. Hemolytic anemia is predictably present. Gastrointestinal mucosa is sensitive to the effects of alkylating drugs, manifesting as mitotic arrest, cellular hypertrophy, and desquamation of the epithelium. Nevertheless, mucosal irritation

is less common than with antimetabolites. Damage to hair follicles, often leading to alopecia, is a common side effect. Increased skin pigmentation is frequent. All alkylating drugs are powerful central nervous system stimulants, manifesting most often as nausea and vomiting. Skeletal muscle weakness and seizures may be present. Pneumonitis and pulmonary fibrosis are potential adverse effects of alkylating drugs. Inhibition of plasma cholinesterase activity may be responsible for prolonged skeletal muscle paralysis following administration of succinylcholine (Zsigmond and Robins, 1972).

Rapid drug-induced destruction of malignant cells can produce increased purine and pyrimidine breakdown leading to uric acid nephropathy. To minimize the likelihood of this complication, it is recommended that adequate fluid intake, alkalinization of the urine, and administration of allopurinol be established prior to drug treatment.

Nitrogen Mustards

The most commonly used nitrogen mustards are mechlorethamine, cyclophosphamide, melphalan, and chlorambucil (Fig. 29-1).

Mechlorethamine

Mechlorethamine is a rapidly acting nitrogen mustard administered intravenously to minimize local tissue irritation. This drug must be freshly prepared before each administration. Mechlorethamine and other nitrogen mustards are intensely powerful vesicants, requiring that gloves be worn by personnel handling the drug. A course of therapy with mechlorethamine consists of the injection of a total dose of 0.4 mg·kg^{-1}. The drug undergoes rapid chemical transformation in tissues such that active drug is no longer present after a few minutes. For this reason, it is possible to prevent tissue toxicity from the drug by isolating the blood supply to that tissue. Alternatively, it is theoretically possible to localize the action of mechlorethamine in a specific tissue by injecting the drug into the arterial blood supply to the tissue.

CLINICAL USES. Mechlorethamine produces beneficial effects in the treatment of Hodgkin's disease and, less predictably, in other lymphomas. The

(text continues on page 508)

Table 29-1
Classification of Chemotherapeutic Drugs and Associated Side Effects

	Immuno-suppression	Thrombo-cytopenia	Leuko-penia	Anemia	Cardiac Toxicity	Pulmon-ary Toxicity	Renal Toxicity	Hepatic Toxicity	Nervous System Toxicity	Stomatitis	Plasma Cholinesterase Inhibition
Alkylating Drugs											
Nitrogen Mustards											
Mechlorethamine	+	+++	+++			+			++		++
Cyclophosphamide	++++	+	++	+			+	+		+	++
Melphalan	+	++	++	++		+					+
Chlorambucil	+	++	++	++		+		+	+		+
Alkyl Sulfonates											
Busulfan	+	+++	+++	+++		++	++			+	+
Nitrosoureas											
Carmustine		++	++	++		+	+			+	
Lomustine		+++	+++	++				+		+	
Semustine		++	++	++				+		+	
Streptozocin		+	+	+			+++	+++			
Antimetabolites											
Folic Acid Analogues											
Methotrexate	+++	+++	+++	+++		+	++	+		+++	
Pyrimidine Analogues											
Fluorouracil	++++	+++	+++	+++					+	+++	
Cytarabine	+++	+++	+++			+		+		+	

Purine Analogues

Drug						
Mercaptopurine	+++	++	++		++	+
Azathioprine	++++	+++	+++		++	++
Thioguanine	+++	+	++		++	+

Vinca Alkaloids

Drug						
Vinblastine	++	+	+		+	+
Vincristine	++	+	+		++	++

Antibiotics

Drug							
Dactinomycin	+++	+++	+++		+++	+++	+++
Daunorubicin	++	+++	++	++	++	++	++
Doxorubicin	+	+++	++	++		++	++
Bleomycin	+	+	+		+	+	
Plicamycin	++++	++++	+++		++	++	+++
Mitomycin	+++	++++	++++	+	+++	++	+++

Enzymes

Drug						
Asparaginase	++	+	+	+	+	+

Synthetics

Drug						
Cisplatin	+	++	++	+	++++	++
Hydroxyurea	+	+++	++		+++	++	++
Procarbazine	+	+++	++		+	+	++
Mitotane			++				+

Hormones

Drug		
Corticosteroids	+++	+++
Progestins		
Estrogens/Androgens		

+, minimal; ++, mild; +++, moderate; ++++, marked.

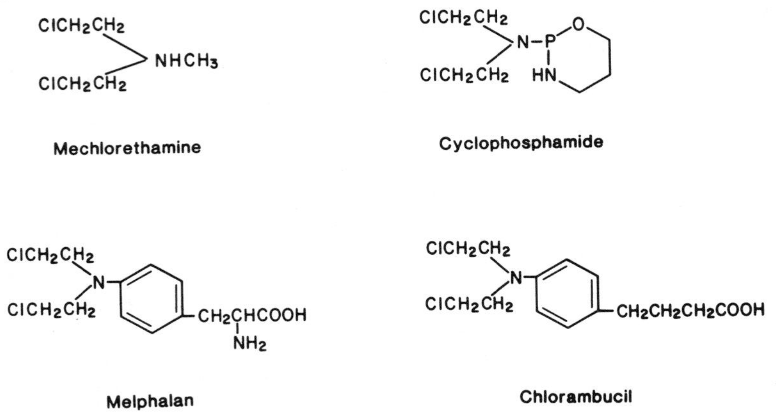

Mechlorethamine

Cyclophosphamide

Melphalan

Chlorambucil

FIGURE 29–1. Nitrogen mustards.

drug is most often used in combination with vincristine, procarbazine, and prednisone (MOPP regimen) for treatment of Hodgkin's disease.

SIDE EFFECTS. The major side effects of mechlorethamine include nausea, vomiting, and myelosuppression. Leukopenia and thrombocytopenia constitute the principal limitation on the amount of drug that can be given. Herpes zoster is a type of skin lesion frequently associated with nitrogen mustard therapy. Latent viral infections may be unmasked by treatment with mechlorethamine. Thrombophlebitis is a potential complication, and extravasation of the drug results in severe local tissue reaction with brawny and tender induration that may persist for prolonged periods.

Cyclophosphamide

Cyclophosphamide is well absorbed after oral administration and is subsequently activated in the liver to aldophosphamide for transport to target tissues. Parenteral administration is also effective. Target cells are able to convert aldophosphamide to highly cytotoxic metabolites, phosphoramide, and acrolein that then alkylate DNA. Maximal concentrations of cyclophosphamide in plasma are achieved 1 hour after oral administration, and the elimination half-time is 6 to 7 hours. Urinary elimination accounts for approximately 14% of this drug in an unchanged form.

CLINICAL USES. The clinical spectrum of cyclophosphamide activity is broad, making it one of the most frequently used chemotherapeutic drugs. Its versatility is improved because of its effectiveness after oral as well as parenteral administration. Given in combination with other drugs, favorable responses have been shown in patients with Hodgkin's disease, lymphosarcoma, Burkitt's lymphoma, and acute lymphoblastic leukemia of childhood. Cyclophosphamide is frequently used in combination with methotrexate and fluorouracil as adjuvant therapy after surgery for carcinoma of the breast when there is involvement of axillary nodes. Cyclophosphamide has potent immunosuppressive properties, leading to its use in nonneoplastic disorders associated with altered immune reactivity, including Wegener's granulomatosis and rheumatoid arthritis.

SIDE EFFECTS. Cyclophosphamide differs from other nitrogen mustards in that significant degrees of thrombocytopenia are less common but alopecia is more frequent. Nausea and vomiting occur with equal frequency regardless of the route of administration. Mucosal ulcerations, increased skin pigmentation, interstitial pulmonary fibrosis, and hepatotoxicity are possible side effects. Sterile hemorrhagic cystitis occurs in 5% to 10% of patients, presumably reflecting chemical irritation produced by reactive metabolites of cyclophosphamide. Dysuria or hematuria are indications to discontinue the drug. Inappropriate secretion of antidiuretic hormone has been observed in patients receiving cyclophosphamide, usually with doses more than 50 mg·kg^{-1}. It is important to consider the possibility of water intoxication because these patients are usually being hydrated to minimize the likelihood that hemorrhagic cystitis will develop. Extravasation of the drug does not produce local reactions, and thrombophlebitis does not complicate intravenous administration.

Melphalan

Melphalan is a phenylalanine derivative of nitrogen mustard with a range of activity similar to other alkylating drugs. It is not a vesicant. Oral absorption is excellent, resulting in drug concentrations similar to those achieved by the intravenous route of administration. The elimination half-time is approximately 1.5 hours, and up to 15% of the drug is eliminated unchanged in the urine.

It is usually necessary to maintain a significant degree of bone marrow depression (leukocyte count 3000 to 3500 cells·mm^{-3}) in order to achieve optimal therapeutic effects. Beneficial effects of melphalan therapy have been observed in the treatment of multiple myeloma, malignant melanoma, and carcinoma of the breast and ovary.

Side effects of melphalan are primarily hematologic and are similar to other alkylating drugs. Nausea and vomiting are infrequent. Alopecia does not occur, and changes in renal or hepatic function have not been reported.

Chlorambucil

Chlorambucil is the aromatic derivative of mechlorethamine. Oral absorption is adequate. The drug has an elimination half-time of approximately 1.5 hours and is almost completely metabolized. Chlorambucil is the slowest-acting nitrogen mustard in clinical use. It is the treatment of choice in chronic lymphocytic leukemia and in primary (Waldenström's) macroglobulinemia. A marked increase in the incidence of leukemia and other tumors has been noted with the use of this drug for the treatment of polycythemia vera.

Cytotoxic effects of chlorambucil on the bone marrow, lymphoid organs, and epithelial tissues are similar to those observed with the other alkylating drugs. Its myelosuppressive action is usually moderate, gradual, and rapidly reversible. Nausea and vomiting are frequent. Central nervous system stimulation can occur but has been observed only with large doses. Hepatotoxicity may rarely occur.

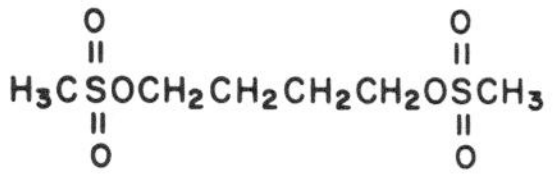

FIGURE 29–2. Busulfan.

Alkyl Sulfonates

Busulfan

Busulfan is well absorbed after oral administration (Fig. 29-2). Intravenous administration is also effective. Almost all of the drug is eliminated by the kidneys as methanesulfonic acid. Busulfan produces remissions in up to 90% of patients with chronic granulocytic leukemia. The drug is of no value in the treatment of acute leukemia.

Myelosuppression and thrombocytopenia are the major side effects of busulfan. Nausea, vomiting, and diarrhea occur. Hyperuricemia resulting from extensive purine catabolism accompanying the rapid cellular destruction and renal damage from precipitation of urates have been noted. Allopurinol is recommended to minimize renal complications.

Nitrosoureas

Nitrosoureas, represented by carmustine, lomustine, semustine, and streptozocin, possess a wide spectrum of activity for human malignancies (Fig. 29-3). These drugs appear to act by alkylation of nucleic acids and carboxylation. Their high lipid solubility results in passage across the blood-brain barrier and efficacy in the treatment of meningeal leukemias and brain tumors. With

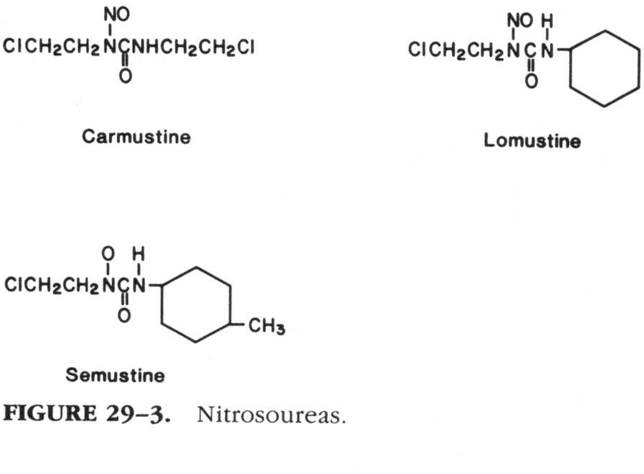

FIGURE 29–3. Nitrosoureas.

the exception of streptozocin, the clinical use of nitrosoureas is limited by profound drug-induced myelosuppression.

Carmustine

Carmustine is capable of inhibiting synthesis of both ribonucleic acid (RNA) and DNA. Although oral absorption is rapid, the drug is injected intravenously because tissue uptake and metabolism occur quickly. Local burning may accompany intravenous infusion. Carmustine disappears from plasma in 5 to 15 minutes. Because of its ability to rapidly cross the blood-brain barrier, carmustine is used to treat meningeal leukemia and primary as well as metastatic brain tumors.

A unique side effect of carmustine is a delayed onset (after approximately 6 weeks of treatment) of leukopenia and thrombocytopenia. Active metabolites may be responsible for this toxicity. Central nervous system toxicity, nausea and vomiting, flushing of the skin and conjunctiva, interstitial pulmonary fibrosis, nephrotoxicity, and hepatotoxicity have been reported.

Lomustine and Semustine

Lomustine and its methylated analogue semustine possess similar clinical toxicity to carmustine, including delayed bone marrow depression manifesting as leukopenia and thrombocytopenia. Lomustine appears to be more effective than carmustine in the treatment of Hodgkin's disease.

Streptozocin

Streptozocin has a methylnitrosourea moiety attached to the number 2 carbon atom of glucose. It has a unique affinity for beta cells of the islets of Langerhans and has proved useful in the treatment of human pancreatic islet cell carcinoma and malignant carcinoid. In animals, the drug is used to produce experimental diabetes mellitus.

Approximately 70% of patients receiving this drug develop hepatic or renal toxicity. Renal toxicity may manifest as tubular damage and progress to renal failure and death. Hyperglycemia can occur as a result of selective destruction of pancreatic beta cells and resultant hypoinsulinism (Selvin, 1981). Myelosuppression is not produced by this drug.

ANTIMETABOLITES

Antimetabolites include folic acid analogues, pyrimidine analogues, and purine analogues. Typically, these chemotherapeutic drugs are structural analogues of normal metabolites required for cell function and replication. These drugs interact directly with specific enzymes, leading to inhibition of that enzyme and subsequent synthesis of an aberrant molecule that cannot function normally. The principal targets for the antimetabolite chemotherapeutic drugs are the proliferating bone marrow cells and gastrointestinal epithelial cells. The majority of these drugs are also potent immunosuppressants.

Folic Acid Analogues

Methotrexate

Methotrexate is a poorly lipid soluble folic acid analogue and is classified as an antimetabolite (folic acid antagonist) (Fig. 29-4). Folic acid is an essential dietary factor that is the source of *tetrahydrofolic acid,* which is an essential co-enzyme necessary for the transfer of 1-carbon units. The enzyme dihydrofolate reductase seems to be the primary site of action of most folic acid analogues. Inhibition of dihydrofolate reductase by methotrexate prevents the formation of tetrahydrofolic acid and causes disruption of cellular metabolism by producing an acute intracellular deficiency of folate enzymes. As a result, 1-carbon transfer reactions necessary for the eventual synthesis of DNA and RNA cease.

Methotrexate is readily absorbed after oral administration. Significant metabolism of methotrexate does not seem to occur, with more than 50% of the drug appearing unchanged in the urine. Renal excretion reflects glomerular filtration and tubular secretion. Toxic concentrations of methotrexate may occur in patients with renal insufficiency. Methotrexate remains in tissues for

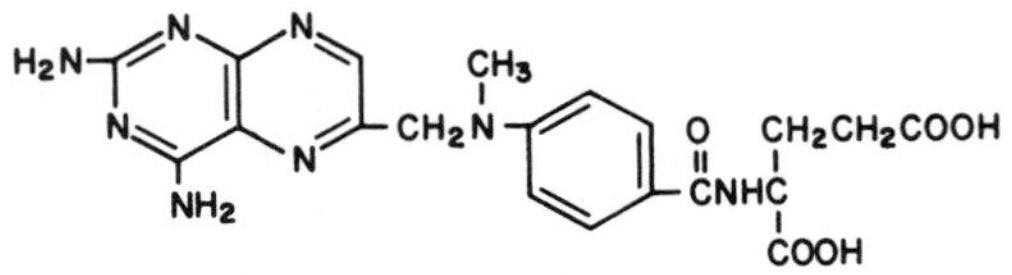

FIGURE 29-4.   Methotrexate.

weeks, suggesting binding of the drug to dihydrofolate reductase.

CLINICAL USES. Methotrexate is a useful drug in the management of acute lymphoblastic leukemia in children but not in adults. It is of established value in choriocarcinoma. Improvement in the treatment of psoriasis reflects the effect of methotrexate on rapidly dividing epidermal cells characteristic of this disease. This drug may also be useful in the treatment of rheumatoid arthritis.

Methotrexate is poorly transported across the blood-brain barrier, and neoplastic cells that have entered the central nervous system probably are not affected by usual concentrations of drug in the plasma. Intrathecal injection is used to treat cerebral involvement with either leukemia or choriocarcinoma.

Acquired resistance to methotrexate develops as a result of (1) impaired transport of methotrexate into cells, (2) production of altered forms of dihydrofolate reductase that have decreased affinity for the drug, and (3) increased concentrations of intracellular dihydrofolate reductase.

SIDE EFFECTS. The most important side effects of methotrexate occur in the gastrointestinal tract and bone marrow. Leukopenia and thrombocytopenia reflect bone marrow depression. Ulcerative stomatitis and diarrhea are frequent side effects and require interruption of treatment. Hemorrhagic enteritis and death from intestinal perforation may occur. Other toxic manifestations include alopecia, dermatitis, pneumonitis, nephrotoxicity, and hepatic dysfunction. Hepatic dysfunction is usually reversible but may sometimes lead to cirrhosis.

Normal cells can be protected from lethal damage by folate antagonists with concomitant administration of leucovorin, thymidine, or both. This approach has been termed the "rescue technique." Folic acid antagonists also interfere with embryogenesis, emphasizing the risk in administering these drugs to pregnant patients.

Pyrimidine Analogues

Pyrimidine analogues have in common the ability to prevent the biosynthesis of pyrimidine nucleotides or to mimic these natural metabolites to such an extent that they interfere with vital cellular activities such as the synthesis and functioning of nucleic acids. Examples of antimetabolite chemotherapeutic drugs that function as pyrimidine analogues are fluorouracil and cytarabine (Fig. 29-5).

Fluorouracil

Fluorouracil lacks significant inhibitory activity on cells and must be converted enzymatically to a 5'-monophosphate nucleotide. Administration of fluorouracil is usually by intravenous injection, because absorption after oral ingestion is unpredictable and incomplete. Metabolic degradation occurs primarily in the liver, with an important metabolite being adenine. Only approximately 10% of fluorouracil appears unchanged in the urine. Fluorouracil readily enters the cerebrospinal fluid, with therapeutic concentrations being present within 30 minutes after intravenous administration.

CLINICAL USES. Fluorouracil may be of palliative value in certain types of carcinoma, particularly of the breast and gastrointestinal tract. The drug is often used for the topical treatment of premalignant keratoses of the skin and superficial basal cell carcinomas.

SIDE EFFECTS. Side effects caused by fluorouracil are difficult to anticipate because of their delayed appearance. Stomatitis manifesting as a white patchy membrane that ulcerates and becomes necrotic is an early sign of toxicity, and warns of the possibility that similar lesions may be developing in the esophagus and gastrointestinal tract. Myelosuppression, most frequently

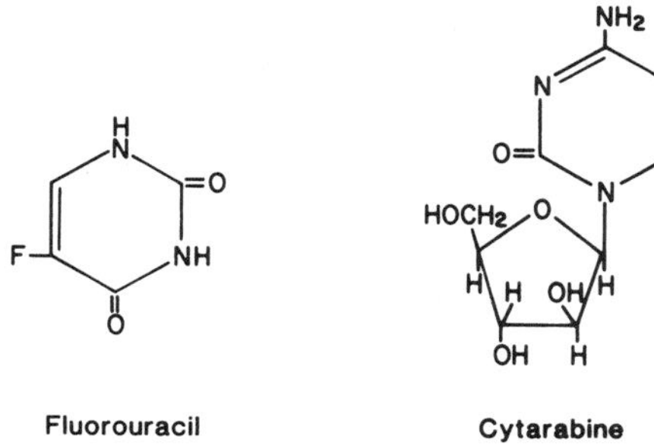

Fluorouracil   Cytarabine

FIGURE 29-5. Pyrimidine analogues.

manifesting as leukopenia between 9 and 14 days of therapy, is a serious side effect. Thrombocytopenia and anemia may complicate treatment with fluorouracil. Loss of hair progressing to total alopecia, nail changes, dermatitis, and increased pigmentation and atrophy of the skin may occur. Neurologic manifestations, including an acute cerebellar syndrome, have been reported.

Cytarabine

Cytarabine, like other pyrimidine antimetabolites, must be activated by conversion to the 5′-monophosphate nucleotide before inhibition of DNA synthesis can occur. Both natural and acquired resistance to cytarabine develop, reflecting the activity of cytidine deaminase, an enzyme capable of converting cytarabine to the inactive metabolite arabinosyl uracil.

In addition to its chemotherapeutic activity, particularly in acute leukemia in children or adults, cytarabine has potent immunosuppressive properties. The drug is particularly useful in chemotherapy of acute granulocytic leukemia in adults. Intravenous administration of cytarabine is recommended, since oral absorption is poor and unpredictable. Thrombophlebitis at the site of intravenous infusion is common.

Cytarabine is a potent myelosuppressive drug capable of producing severe leukopenia, thrombocytopenia, and anemia. Other side effects include gastrointestinal disturbances, stomatitis, and hepatic dysfunction.

Purine Analogues

Antimetabolite chemotherapeutic drugs that function as purine analogues include mercaptopurine, azathioprine, and thioguanine (Fig. 29-6). Mercaptopurine and thioguanine are analogues of the natural purines hypoxanthine and guanine, respectively.

It seems likely that this class of drugs acts by multiple mechanisms, including effects on purine nucleotide synthesis and metabolism as well as alterations in the synthesis and function of RNA and DNA. As with other antimetabolites, the occurrence of acquired resistance represents a major obstacle in the successful use of purine analogues.

Mercaptopurine

Mercaptopurine is most useful in the treatment of acute leukemia in children. This drug has not been of value in the treatment of chronic lymphocytic leukemia and Hodgkin's disease. Although it is active as an immunosuppressant, its use has been largely superseded by azathioprine.

Mercaptopurine is readily absorbed after oral ingestion, and the gastrointestinal epithelium is not damaged. The elimination half-time is brief (approximately 90 minutes) owing to rapid tissue uptake, renal excretion, and hepatic metabolism. One pathway of metabolism is methylation and subsequent oxidation of the methylated derivatives. A second pathway involves the enzyme xanthine oxidase, which oxidizes mercaptopurine to 6-thiouric acid. Allopurinol, as an inhibitor of xanthine oxidase, prevents conversion of mercaptopurine to 6-thiouric acid and thus increases the exposure of cells to mercaptopurine.

The principal side effect of mercaptopurine is a gradual development of bone marrow depression manifesting as thrombocytopenia, granulocytopenia, or anemia several weeks after initiation of therapy. Anorexia, nausea, and vomiting are common side effects; stomatitis and diarrhea rarely occur. Jaundice occurs in approximately one third of patients and is associated with bile stasis and occasional hepatic necrosis. Hyperuricemia and hyperuricosuria may occur during treatment with mercaptopurine, presumably reflecting destruction of cells. This effect may require the use of allopurinol.

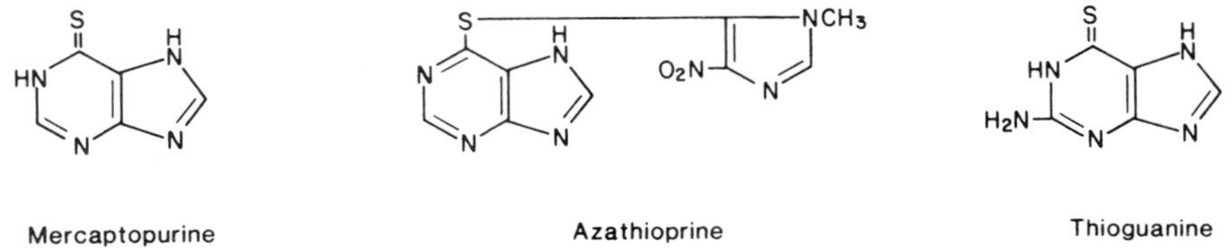

Mercaptopurine   Azathioprine   Thioguanine

FIGURE 29-6. Purine analogues.

Azathioprine

Azathioprine is a derivative of mercaptopurine. It is a potent immunosuppressant and is used as an adjunct (often with corticosteroids) to prevent rejection following organ transplantation. The oral dose may need to be reduced in patients with impaired renal function to prevent dangerous accumulation of the drug. If allopurinol is administered concurrently, the dose of azathioprine should be reduced, because inhibition of xanthine oxidase impairs the conversion of azathioprine to 6-thiouric acid and may greatly increase tissue exposure to the drug.

Leukopenia as a manifestation of bone marrow depression is the most common side effect of azathioprine therapy. Infection is a predictable complication of any form of immunosuppressive therapy. Biliary stasis and hepatic necrosis have been described. Infrequent complications include stomatitis, dermatitis, fever, alopecia, and diarrhea. An increase in lymphoma, reticulum cell sarcoma, and other neoplasms has been noted in renal transplant patients treated with this drug.

Thioguanine

Thioguanine is of particular value in the treatment of acute granulocytic leukemia, especially when given with cytarabine. Following oral administration, thioguanine appears in the urine as a methylated metabolite and inorganic sulfate. Minimal amounts of 6-thiouric acid are formed, suggesting that deamination is not important in the metabolic inactivation of thioguanine. For this reason, thioguanine may be administered concurrently with allopurinol without a reduction in dosage, unlike mercaptopurine and azathioprine. Toxic manifestations of thioguanine treatment include bone marrow depression and, occasionally, gastrointestinal effects.

VINCA ALKALOIDS

Useful *Vinca* alkaloids derived from the periwinkle plant are vinblastine and vincristine. These drugs block mitosis in rapidly dividing cells. Nevertheless, most of the biologic activity of *Vinca* alkaloids is due to their ability to bind with an essential protein component of microtubules. Disruption of microtubules of the mitotic apparatus arrests cell division in metaphase. Despite their structural similarity, there is a remarkable lack of cross-tolerance between individual *Vinca* alkaloids.

Oral absorption of vinblastine is unpredictable; thus, intravenous infusion is recommended. Subcutaneous extravasation can cause painful inflammatory changes. Vincristine and vinblastine can be infused into the arterial blood supply of tumors in doses far greater than are permissible via the intravenous route, suggesting that local tissue uptake or metabolism is rapid. Excretion of the *Vinca* alkaloids appears to be primarily into the bile, with minimal amounts of drug appearing in the urine. Indeed, toxicity is increased when vincristine is administered to patients with obstructive jaundice.

Clinical Uses

The most important clinical use of vinblastine is with bleomycin and cisplatin in the treatment of metastatic testicular tumors (Einhorn and Donahue, 1977). Lymphomas, including Hodgkin's disease, are responsive, even when the disease is refractory to alkylating drugs. Vincristine combined with corticosteroids is an effective treatment to induce remissions in childhood leukemia. An important feature of *Vinca* alkaloids is the lack of cross-resistance between these drugs. The rapid action of vincristine and its reduced tendency for myelosuppression render it a more desirable drug for therapy in the presence of pancytopenia or in conjunction with other myelotoxic drugs. Vincristine apparently does not cross the blood-brain barrier as evidenced by persistence of central nervous system leukemia despite hematopoietic remission. Intrathecal administration of vincristine is not used. The rapid onset of action of *Vinca* alkaloids often necessitates the concomitant administration of allopurinol to prevent the complications of hyperuricemia.

Side Effects

Myelosuppression manifesting as leukopenia, thrombocytopenia, and anemia are the most prominent side effects of *Vinca* alkaloids, appearing 7 to 10 days after initiation of treatment. Vincristine is less likely than vinblastine to cause bone marrow depression. Alopecia appears to occur more frequently with vincristine than with vinblastine.

Neuromuscular abnormalities, including skeletal muscle weakness, ataxia, and tremors, are frequently observed during treatment with vincristine. Peripheral neuropathy manifesting as tingling and weakness of the extremities, foot drop, and neuritic pains occur frequently. Weakness of the extraocular muscles and larynx manifesting as hoarseness have been observed. The syndrome of hyponatremia associated with high urinary sodium and inappropriate secretion of antidiuretic hormone has occasionally been observed during vincristine therapy. An effect on the autonomic nervous system may be responsible for paralytic ileus and abdominal pain that frequently develops during vincristine, but only rarely during vinblastine, therapy. Urinary retention, tenderness of the parotid glands, dryness of the mouth, and sinus tachycardia are other occasionally experienced manifestations of altered autonomic nervous system activity. Transient mental depression is most likely to occur on the second or third day of treatment with vinblastine.

ANTIBIOTICS

Clinically useful chemotherapeutic antibiotics are natural products of certain soil fungi. Chemotherapeutic effects are produced by formation of relatively stable complexes with DNA, thereby inhibiting DNA synthesis, RNA synthesis, or both.

Dactinomycin

Dactinomycin (actinomycin D) is an antibiotic with chemotherapeutic activity resulting from its ability to bind to DNA, especially in rapidly proliferating cells. As a result of this binding, the function of RNA polymerase, and thus the transcription of the DNA molecule, are blocked. Following intravenous injection, dactinomycin rapidly leaves the circulation. In animals, approximately 50% of an injected dose is excreted unchanged in the bile, and 10% in the urine. There is no evidence that the drug undergoes metabolism. Dactinomycin does not cross the blood-brain barrier in amounts sufficient to produce a pharmacologic effect.

Clinical Uses

The most important clinical use of dactinomycin is the treatment of Wilms' tumor in children and of rhabdomyosarcoma. It may be effective in some women with methotrexate-resistant choriocarcinoma. Occasionally, this drug is used to inhibit immunologic responses associated with organ transplantation.

Side Effects

Toxic effects of dactinomycin include the early onset of nausea and vomiting, often followed by myelosuppression manifesting as pancytopenia 1 to 7 days after completion of therapy. Pancytopenia may be preceded by thrombocytopenia as the first manifestation of bone marrow suppression. Glossitis, ulcerations of the oral mucosa, diarrhea, alopecia, and cutaneous erythema are commonly associated with dactinomycin therapy.

Daunorubicin and Doxorubicin

Daunorubicin and doxorubicin are anthracycline antibiotics. Structurally, these anthracycline antibiotics contain a tetracycline ring attached to the sugar daunosamine by a glycosidic linkage (Fig. 29-7). These drugs most likely act by binding to DNA, which results in changes in the DNA helix that inhibit the template activity of the nucleic acid. These drugs also likely cause disruptive effects on cellular membranes. Free radicals that attack unsaturated free fatty acids in the heart may play a role in cardiotoxicity. Evidence that free

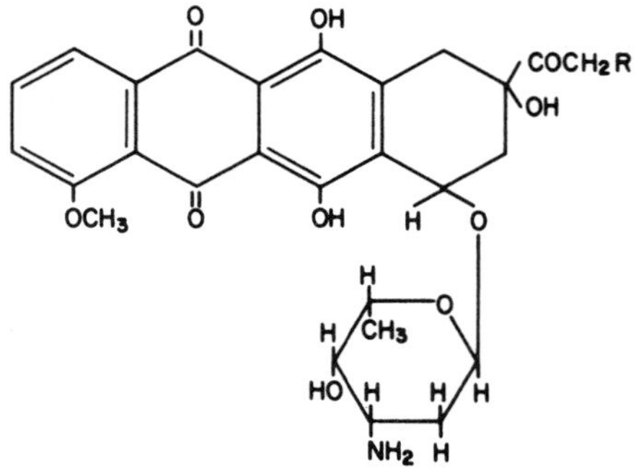

FIGURE 29–7. Anthracycline antibiotics contain a tetracycline ring attached to a sugar by a glycosidic linkage.

radicals have a role is the protective effect of free radical scavengers such as vitamin E.

Daunorubicin and doxorubicin are administered intravenously, with care taken to prevent extravasation, because local vesicant action may result. There is rapid clearance from the plasma into the heart, kidneys, lungs, and liver. These drugs do not cross the blood-brain barrier to any significant extent. The urine may become red for 1 to 2 days after administration of these drugs.

Daunorubicin is metabolized primarily to daunorubiconol, whereas doxorubicin is excreted unchanged and as metabolites, including adriamycinol in the urine. Ultimately, approximately 40% of the drugs are metabolized. Indeed, clinical toxicity may result in patients with hepatic dysfunction.

Clinical Uses

Daunorubicin is used primarily in the treatment of acute lymphocytic and granulocytic leukemia. Doxorubicin, which differs from daunorubicin only by a single hydroxyl group on the number 14 carbon atom, is also effective against a wide range of solid tumors (Fig. 29-7). For example, doxorubicin is one of the most active single drugs for treating metastatic adenocarcinoma of the breast, carcinoma of the bladder, bronchogenic carcinoma, metastatic thyroid carcinoma, oat cell carcinoma, and osteogenic carcinoma.

Resistance is observed to the anthracycline antibiotics, as with other chemotherapeutic drugs. Furthermore, cross-tolerance occurs between daunorubicin and doxorubicin. Cross-resistance also occurs between these antibiotics and the *Vinca* alkaloids, suggesting that an alteration of cellular permeability may be involved.

Side Effects

Cardiomyopathy is a unique dose-related and often irreversible side effect of the anthracycline antibiotics. Two types of cardiomyopathies may occur (Selvin, 1981). An acute form occurs in approximately 10% of patients and is characterized by relatively benign changes on the ECG that include nonspecific ST-T changes and decreased QRS voltage. Other cardiac changes include premature ventricular contractions, supraventricular tachydysrhythmias, cardiac conduction abnormalities, and left axis deviation. These abnormal-

ities occur during therapy at all dose levels and, except for decreased QRS voltage on the ECG, resolve 1 to 2 months after discontinuation of therapy. There is an associated acute reversible reduction in the ejection fraction within 24 hours after a single dose.

The second form of cardiomyopathy is characterized by the insidious onset of symptoms such as dry nonproductive cough, suggesting bronchitis, followed by rapidly progressive heart failure that is unresponsive to inotropic drugs and mechanical ventricular assistance (Selvin, 1981). This severe form of cardiomyopathy occurs in almost 2% of treated patients and is fatal approximately 3 weeks after the onset of symptoms in nearly 60% of affected patients. Predictive tests to permit early recognition of impending cardiomyopathy are not available, although diminution in QRS voltage on the ECG is consistent with the diffuse character of the myocardial damage. Serum enzyme elevations occur late in the course of cardiac failure and are of limited value in achieving an early diagnosis. Systolic time intervals and echocardiograms have been used to detect cardiotoxicity before the occurrence of clinically significant damage.

The incidence of cardiomyopathy is negligible when the total dose of these drugs is less than 200 mg·m^{-2} of body surface area. Prior mediastinal irradiation or previous treatment with cyclophosphamide increases the subsequent risk of cardiomyopathy in response to administration of an anthracycline antibiotic. Marked impairment of a left ventricular function for as long as 3 years after discontinuing doxorubicin has been observed. Acute left ventricular failure 2 months after the cessation of treatment with doxorubicin has been described during general anesthesia (Borgeat et al, 1988).

Myelosuppression is another serious side effect of chemotherapeutic antibiotics, with leukopenia typically manifesting during the second week of therapy. Thrombocytopenia and anemia occur but are usually less pronounced. Stomatitis, gastrointestinal disturbances, and alopecia are common side effects.

Bleomycin

Bleomycins are water-soluble glycopeptides that differ from one another (there are more than 200 congeners) in their terminal amine moiety. The terminal amine is coupled through an amide linkage to a carboxylic acid. The mechanism of action is most likely related to the ability of these drugs to cause fragmentation of DNA.

Bleomycin is administered intravenously, and high concentrations occur in the skin and lungs. The drug accumulates in tumors, suggesting the presence of a lower level of inactivating enzyme. Approximately two thirds of the unchanged drug is excreted by the kidneys, probably by glomerular filtration. Indeed, excessive concentrations of drug occur if usual doses are given to patients with impaired renal function.

Clinical Uses

Bleomycin is effective in the treatment of testicular carcinoma, particularly when administered in combination with vinblastine (Einhorn and Donahue, 1977). It is also useful in the palliative treatment of squamous cell carcinomas of the head, neck, esophagus, skin, and genitourinary tract.

Side Effects

The most commonly encountered side effects of bleomycin are mucocutaneous reactions, including stomatitis, alopecia, pruritic erythema, and hyperpigmentation, which occur in approximately 45% of patients. In contrast to other chemotherapeutic drugs, bleomycin causes minimal myelosuppression. Unexplained exacerbations of rheumatoid arthritis have occurred.

Patients with lymphomas who are receiving bleomycin may develop an acute reaction characterized by hyperthermia, hypotension, and hypoventilation. The likely mechanism is release of an endogenous pyrogen, presumably from destroyed tumor cells. An initial small test dose of bleomycin is recommended to minimize the occurrence of this syndrome.

PULMONARY TOXICITY. The most serious side effect of bleomycin is pulmonary toxicity. It is estimated that 5% to 10% of patients treated with bleomycin develop pulmonary toxicity, and 1% to 2% of all patients receiving bleomycin die from this complication.

The first signs of pulmonary toxicity are cough, dyspnea, and basilar rales, which progress in one of two directions. A mild form of pulmonary toxicity is characterized by exertional dyspnea and a normal resting PaO_2. A more severe form of arterial hypoxemia at rest is associated with radiographic findings of intestitial pneumonitis and fibrosis. Lesions are found more frequently in lower lobes and subpleural areas, and radiographs of the chest often reveal bilateral basilar and perihilar infiltrates. The alveolar-to-arterial difference for oxygen is increased, and pulmonary diffusion capacity may be reduced.

Pulmonary function studies have been of no greater value than clinical signs in detecting the onset of pulmonary toxicity. The likelihood of developing pulmonary toxicity is greater when the total dose of bleomycin is more than 400 units administered to patients older than 70 years of age with underlying pulmonary disease. Prior radiotherapy may also predispose the patient to pulmonary toxicity. Skin toxicity may parallel the more serious pulmonary toxicity. Patients who develop pulmonary toxicity despite low-dose therapy may be manifesting an idiosyncratic or immune response in contrast to the more predictable reaction noted with higher doses (Iacovino et al, 1976).

Patients treated with bleomycin who have undergone anesthesia and surgery appear to be at increased risk for developing adult respiratory distress syndrome in the postoperative period (Goldiner et al, 1978). One speculation is that acutely increased inhaled concentrations of oxygen facilitate production of superoxide and other free radicals in the presence of bleomycin. For this reason, it has been recommended that inhaled concentrations of oxygen during surgery be maintained below 30% in bleomycin-treated patients. Nevertheless, data from animals and patients do not demonstrate enhanced pulmonary toxicity in the presence of bleomycin therapy and high concentrations of oxygen (Douglas and Coppin, 1980; LaMantia et al, 1984; Matalon et al, 1986). Another recommendation is replacement of fluids with colloids rather than crystalloids to decrease or prevent pulmonary interstitial edema in bleomycin-treated patients undergoing surgery (Goldiner et al, 1978). Accumulation of interstitial fluid may reflect impaired lymphatic function caused by bleomycin-induced fibrotic changes in the lung.

Plicamycin

Plicamycin (formerly named mithramycin) is a highly toxic antibiotic that acts by inhibiting the synthesis of RNA without altering the synthesis of DNA. The drug has a specific effect on osteoclasts and lowers the plasma concentration of calcium in patients who are hypercalcemic as a result of metastatic bone tumors or tumors that produce parathyroid hormone–like substances. In patients with Paget's disease treated with plicamycin, the plasma alkaline phosphatase activity is decreased and pain is reduced. Plicamycin is adminstered by slow intravenous infusion over 4 to 6 hours. Extravasation can cause local irritation and cellulitis.

Side Effects

Plicamycin is extremely toxic to the gastrointestinal tract and bone marrow. A fatal hemorrhagic diathesis occurs in 1% to 5% of treated patients. This hemorrhagic diathesis may reflect impaired synthesis of clotting factors in addition to thrombocytopenia. Prolongation of the prothrombin time and an increase in fibrinolytic activity are likely. Epistaxis may be the first manifestation of the presence of a drug-induced coagulopathy. Adverse neurologic and cutaneous side effects are frequently observed. Irreversible hepatic or renal toxicity may occur, especially in patients with preexisting disease.

Mitomycin

Mitomycin inhibits synthesis of DNA and is of value in the palliative treatment of gastric adenocarcinoma in combination with fluorouracil and doxorubicin. The drug is administered intravenously and is widely distributed in tissue but does not readily enter the central nervous system. Metabolism is in the liver, with less than 10% of mitomycin excreted unchanged in the bile or urine.

Side Effects

Myelosuppression is a prominent side effect of mitomycin and is characterized by severe leukopenia and thrombocytopenia, which may be delayed in appearance. Interstitial pneumonia and glomerular damage resulting in renal failure are rare but well-recognized complications.

ENZYMES

Asparaginase

Asparaginase is an enzyme with chemotherapeutic activity that is effective in the treatment of acute lymphoblastic leukemia. This drug acts by catalyzing the conversion of asparagine to aspartic acid and ammonia, thus depriving malignant cells of necessary extracellular supplies of asparagine. Malignant cells that lack the enzyme necessary to form this amino acid cannot survive in the absence of exogenous sources.

Side Effects

In contrast to other chemotherapeutic drugs, asparaginase has minimal effects on the bone marrow, and it does not damage oral or gastrointestinal mucosa or hair follicles. Conversely, severe toxicity manifests at the liver, kidneys, pancreas, and the central nervous system, and this drug inhibits clotting mechanisms. For example, hepatic dysfunction associated with elevated blood concentrations of ammonia occurs, and approximately 5% of treated patients develop overt hemorrhagic pancreatitis. Impaired sensorium and coma may develop. Presumably, all these side effects result from widespread inhibition of protein synthesis in various tissues of the body. Because asparaginase is a relatively large foreign protein, it is antigenic, and hypersensitivity phenomena ranging from mild allergic reactions to anaphylactic shock occur in as many as 20% of treated patients.

SYNTHETICS

Examples of synthetic chemotherapeutic drugs include cisplatin, hydroxyurea, procarbazine, and mitotane (Fig. 29-8).

Cisplatin

Cisplatin is an inorganic platinum-containing complex that enters cells by diffusion and dis-

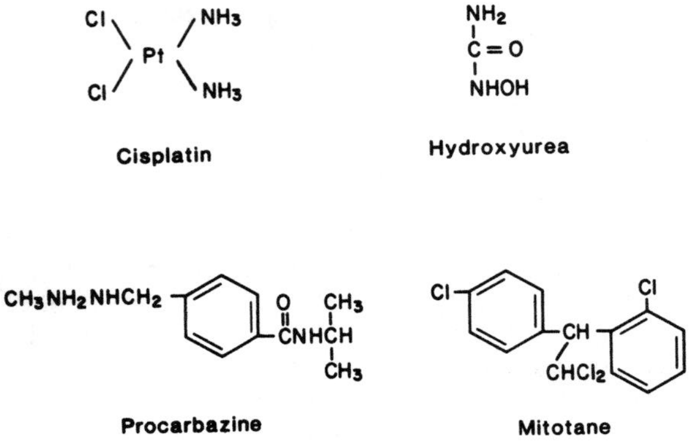

FIGURE 29–8. Synthetic chemotherapeutic drugs.

rupts the DNA helix. The drug must be administered intravenously, because oral ingestion is ineffective. High concentrations of cisplatin are found in the kidneys, liver, intestines, and testes, but there is poor penetration into the central nervous system. Cisplatin is frequently used with other drugs, especially in chemotherapy of metastatic testicular and ovarian carcinoma (Einhorn and Donahue, 1977).

Side Effects

Renal toxicity is prominent, and hydration prior to and following administration of cisplatin is indicated. Decreased renal tubular function produced by cisplatin is dose related and typically occurs during the second week of treatment. Ototoxicity caused by cisplatin is manifested by tinnitus and hearing loss in the high-frequency range. Marked nausea and vomiting occurs in almost all patients. Mild to moderate myelosuppression may develop with transient leukopenia and thrombocytopenia. Hyperuricemia, peripheral neuropathies, seizures, and cardiac dysrhythmias have been observed. Allergic reactions characterized by facial edema, bronchoconstriction, tachycardia, and hypotension may occur minutes after injection of the drug.

Hydroxyurea

Hydroxyurea acts on the enzyme ribonucleoside diphosphate reductase to interfere with the synthesis of DNA. Oral absorption is excellent, and approximately 80% of the drug appears in the urine within 12 hours after oral or intravenous administration. The primary use of hydroxyurea is in the treatment of chronic granulocytic leukemia. Temporary remissions in patients with metastatic malignant melanoma have been reported. Myelosuppression manifesting as leukopenia, megaloblastic anemia, and occasionally thrombocytopenia is the major side effect produced by hydroxyurea. Stomatitis and alopecia occur infrequently.

Procarbazine

Procarbazine inhibits DNA synthesis and is of greatest efficacy in the treatment of Hodgkin's disease, particularly when given in combination with other drugs. Oral absorption is excellent, and the drug is widely distributed, entering the cerebrospinal fluid. Oxidative metabolism is extensive, with less than 5% of procarbazine excreted unchanged in the urine.

Side Effects

The most common side effects of procarbazine include nausea, vomiting, leukopenia, and thrombocytopenia, which occur in more than 50% of treated patients. Sedative effects are prominent. Synergism occurs with phenothiazine derivatives, barbiturates, opioids, and sedative-producing antihypertensive drugs. Ingestion of alcohol may cause intense warmth and reddening of the face, resembling the acetaldehyde syndrome as produced by disulfiram. Procarbazine is a weak monoamine oxidase inhibitor. For this reason, administration of sympathomimetic drugs and tricyclic antidepressants or ingestion of foods containing tyramine may evoke hypertensive reactions. Hypersensitivity reactions, including pleural and pulmonary changes, can occur.

Mitotane

Mitotane is chemically similar to insecticides such as DDT. This drug produces selective destruction of normal or malignant adrenocortical cells, leading to a prompt reduction in the circulating concentration of corticosteroids. The specific effect on the adrenal cortex is the basis for the use of this drug in the palliative treatment of inoperable adrenocortical carcinoma. After discontinuation of treatment, plasma concentrations of mitotane are present for up to 9 weeks, reflecting storage in fat.

Damage to the bone marrow, kidneys, or liver has not been observed. Anorexia and nausea occur in the majority of treated patients. Somnolence and lethargy are present in approximately one third of patients. The need for supplemental administration of corticosteroids should be considered when patients treated with mitotane undergo anesthesia and surgery.

HORMONES

Hormones, including corticosteroids, progestins, estrogens, and androgens, may have use in the treatment of neoplastic disease.

Corticosteroids

Corticosteroids, because of their lympholytic effects and their ability to suppress mitosis in lymphocytes, have value in the treatment of acute leukemia in children (not adults) and malignant lymphoma. These hormones are particularly effective in the management of hemolytic anemia and thrombocytopenia that frequently accompany leukemia and lymphoma. Prednisone is commonly administered orally in high doses (0.5 to 1.5 mg·kg^{-1}), which are then gradually reduced to maintenance levels.

Progestins

Progestational agents are useful in the management of patients with endometrial carcinoma.

Presumably, unopposed overstimulation of the endometrium is responsible for neoplastic changes.

Estrogens and Androgens

Malignant changes in the prostate and breast are often dependent on hormones for their continued growth. For example, prostatic cancer is stimulated by androgens, whereas orchiectomy or estrogens (diethylstilbestrol) slow the growth of the tumor. Eventually, prostatic tumors become insensitive to lack of androgen or the presence of estrogen, presumably because of the survival of progressively undifferentiated cells that favor the emergence of cell types that no longer depend on androgens.

Estrogens and androgens have value in the treatment of advanced breast carcinoma. Malignant tissues that are responsive to estrogens contain receptors for the hormone, whereas malignant tissues lacking these receptors are unlikely to respond to hormonal manipulation. The onset of action of hormone therapy is slow, requiring 8 to 12 weeks.

Hypercalcemia may be associated with androgen or estrogen therapy, requiring adequate hydration in an attempt to facilitate renal excretion of calcium. Plasma calcium concentrations should be determined routinely in patients receiving treatment with these hormones.

Antiestrogens

Tamoxifen binds to estrogen receptors and inhibits continued growth of estrogen-dependent tumors. As such, this drug is useful in the palliative treatment of advanced carcinoma of the breast in postmenopausal women. Toxicity is minimal, and side effects include hot flashes, nausea, and vomiting. Hypercalcemia is an infrequent complication.

REFERENCES

Borgeat A, Chiolero R, Baylon P, Freeman J, Neff R. Perioperative cardiovascular collapse in a patient previously treated with doxorubicin. Anesth Analg 1988;67:1189–91.

Douglas MJ, Coppin CML. Bleomycin and subsequent anaesthesia: A retrospective study at Vancouver General Hospital. Can Anaesth Soc J 1980; 27:449–52.

Einhorn LH, Donahue J. Cis-diaminedichloroplatinum, vinblastine, and bleomycin: Combination chemotherapy in disseminated testicular cancer. Ann Intern Med 1977;87:293–8.

Goldiner PL, Carlon G, Cvitkovic E, Schweizer O, Howland WS. Factors influencing postoperative morbidity and mortality in patients with bleomycin. Br Med J 1978;1:1664–7.

Iacovino JR, Leitner J, Abbas AK, et al. Fatal pulmonary reaction from low doses of bleomycin: An idiosyncratic tissue response. JAMA 1976;235:1253–5.

LaMantia KR, Glick JH, Marshall BE. Supplemental oxygen does not cause respiratory failure in bleomycin-treated surgical patients. Anesthesiology 1984;60:65–7.

Matalon S, Harper WV, Nickerson PA, Olszowka J. Intravenous bleomycin does not alter the toxic effects of hyperoxia in rabbits. Anesthesiology 1986;64:614–9.

Rudders RA, Mensley GT. Bleomycin pulmonary toxicity. Chest 1973;63:626–8.

Selevan SG, Lindbohm M-L, Hornung RW, Hemminki K. A study of occupahonal exposure to antineoplastic drugs and fetal loss in nurses. N Engl J Med 1985;313:1173–78.

Selvin BF. Cancer chemotherapy: Implications for the anesthesiologist. Anesth Analg 1981;60:425–34.

Zsigmond EK, Robins G. The effect of a series of anticancer drugs on plasma cholinesterase activity. Can Anaesth Soc J 1972;19:75–82.

30

Antiepileptic Drugs

Epilepsy is a collective term used to designate a group of chronic central nervous system disorders characterized by the onset of sudden disturbances of sensory, motor, autonomic, or psychic origin. These disturbances are usually transient and are almost always associated with abnormal discharges of the electroencephalogram. The incidence of epilepsy is between 0.3% and 0.6% of the population (Hauser, 1978). The antiepileptic drug selected to treat epilepsy is determined by the characteristics of the seizure experienced by the patient. Epilepsy is classified as (1) grand mal epilepsy, (2) petit mal epilepsy, (3) focal epilepsy, and (4) psychomotor epilepsy (see Chapter 41). Febrile seizures typically occur between 3 months and 5 years of age in the absence of any known cause other than an association with fever. Daily administration of antiepileptic drugs prevents recurrence of febrile seizures. Seizures are sometimes a result of withdrawal from drugs such as barbiturates and alcohol.

MECHANISM OF SEIZURE ACTIVITY

Seizure activity in most patients with epilepsy has a localized or focal origin. The reason for the high frequency and synchronous firing in a seizure focus is unknown. Possible explanations include (1) local biochemical changes, (2) ischemia, (3) loss of cellular inhibitory systems, (4) infections, and (5) head trauma.

Neurons in a chronic seizure focus exhibit a type of denervation hypersensitivity with regard to excitatory stimuli. The spread of seizure activity to neighboring normal cells is presumably re-strained by normal inhibitory mechanisms. Factors such as changes in blood glucose concentration, PaO_2, $PaCO_2$, pH, electrolyte balance, endocrine function, stress, and fatigue may result in spread of a seizure focus into areas of normal brain. If the spread is sufficiently extensive, the entire brain is activated and a tonic-clonic seizure with unconsciousness ensues. Conversely, if the spread is localized, the seizure produces signs and symptoms characteristic of the anatomic focus. Once initiated, a seizure is most likely maintained by reentry of excitatory impulses in a closed feedback pathway that may not even include the original seizure focus.

MECHANISM OF DRUG ACTION

Most antiepileptic drugs act by reducing the spread of excitation from a seizure focus to normal neurons. The mechanism by which these drugs prevent spread of abnormal activity is unknown but may involve (1) posttetanic potentiation, (2) reductions in movement of sodium (Na^+) or calcium ions (Ca^{2+}), (3) potentiation of presynaptic or postsynaptic inhibition, or (4) reduction of responsiveness of various monosynaptic or polysynaptic pathways. Inhibition of postsynaptic neurons by some drugs may reflect binding to gamma-aminobutyric acid (GABA) receptors and may lead to greater chloride ion influx through chloride channels.

Initial drug therapy is based principally on seizure pattern (Table 30-1). Complete drug-induced control of seizures can be achieved in up to 50% of patients, in addition to significant im-

Table 30–1
Selection of Drug Based on Seizure Type

Seizure Type	Drug Therapy
Focal seizures	Phenytoin
	Phenobarbital
	Primidone
	Carbamazepine
Petit mal (absence) seizures	Ethosuximide
	Valproic acid
	Clonazepam
Grand mal (tonic-clonic) seizures	Phenytoin
	Phenobarbital
	Carbamazepine
	Valproic acid
Myoclonic seizures	Valproic acid
	Clonazepam
	Corticosteroids

provement in 25% of patients. Multiple drug therapy is often required because two or more seizure types may occur in the same patient.

PLASMA CONCENTRATIONS

Measurement of plasma concentrations of antiepileptic drugs greatly facilitates treatment of seizure disorders, especially when multiple drug therapy is used (Table 30-2). Nevertheless, interpretation of plasma concentrations must be cautious because clinical effects do not always parallel these levels. Furthermore, the method of measurement may not distinguish protein-bound drug from the free and pharmacologically active fraction.

HYDANTOINS

Hydantoin derivatives used as antiepileptic drugs include phenytoin, mephenytoin, and phenacemide.

Phenytoin

Phenytoin is the prototype of hydantoins and is the drug administered for treatment of focal seizures and grand mal seizures (Fig. 30-1). Phenytoin can induce complete suppression of these forms of epilepsy but does not completely eliminate the sensory aura or other prodromal signs. The antiepileptic activity of phenytoin is not accompanied by sedation.

Mechanism of Action

Phenytoin limits the development and spread of activity from a seizure focus. Elevation of seizure

Table 30–2
Pharmacokinetics of Antiepileptic Drugs

	Plasma Therapeutic Concentration ($\mu g \cdot ml^{-1}$)	Protein Binding (%)	Volume of Distribution ($L \cdot kg^{-1}$)	Elimination Half-Time (h)	Clearance ($ml \cdot kg^{-1} \cdot min^{-1}$)	Site of Clearance and Percent
Phenytoin	10–20	90	0.64	24	Dose dependent	Hepatic, 98%
Phenobarbital	10–20	40–60	0.8	90	0.09	Hepatic, 75% Renal, 25%
Primidone	5–10	20	0.8	8	0.78	Hepatic, 60% Renal, 40%
Carbamazepine	4–12	80	1.4	13–17	0.58	Hepatic, 98%
Ethosuximide	40–100	Insignificant	0.72	60	0.26	Hepatic, 80% Renal, 20%
Valproic Acid	50–100	80–90	0.13	12	0.12	Hepatic, >70%
Clonazepam	0.02–0.08	50	3.2	24–36	0.92	Hepatic, 98%

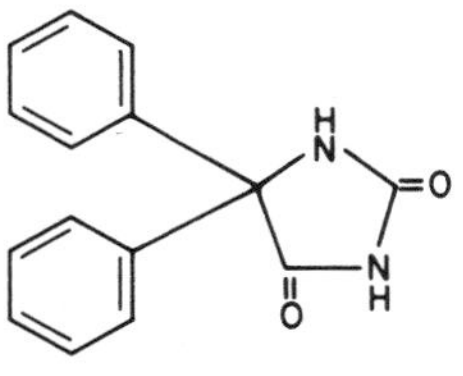

FIGURE 30–1. Phenytoin.

threshold is relatively selective for the cerebral cortex. A stabilizing effect of phenytoin is apparent on all neuron cell membranes, including peripheral nerves. This stabilizing effect is most likely a result of drug-induced alterations in the movement of ions across cell membranes. For example, phenytoin decreases fluxes of Na^+ that occur during action potentials. In addition, influx of Ca^{2+} during depolarization is decreased—possibly due to reduced intracellular concentrations of Na^+. Phenytoin can also delay the activation of outward potassium ion current during an action potential, leading to an increased refractory period and a decrease in repetitive firing.

Pharmacokinetics

Phenytoin is a weak acid with a pK of approximately 8.3 (Table 30-2). Its poor water solubility may result in slow and sometimes variable absorption from the gastrointestinal tract (30% to 97%). Initial daily adult dosage is 3 to 4 mg·kg^{-1}. Doses more than 500 mg daily are rarely tolerated. The long duration of action of phenytoin allows a single daily dosage, but gastric intolerance may necessitate divided dosage. Following intramuscular injection, the drug precipitates at the injection site and is only slowly absorbed. For this reason, intramuscular administration is not recommended. Intravenous infusion of phenytoin should probably not exceed 5 mg·min^{-1}.

PLASMA CONCENTRATIONS. Control of seizures is usually obtained with plasma concentrations of phenytoin 10 to 20 μg·ml^{-1}. In the control of digitalis-induced cardiac dysrhythmias, phenytoin, 0.5 to 1 mg·kg^{-1} IV, is administered every 15 to 30 minutes until a satisfactory response is achieved or a maximum dose of 15 mg·kg^{-1} is administered. A plasma phenytoin concentration of 8 to 16 μg·ml^{-1} is usually sufficient to suppress cardiac dysrhythmias. Adverse side effects of phenytoin such as nystagmus and ataxia are likely when the plasma concentration of drug is more than 20 μg·ml^{-1}.

PROTEIN BINDING. Phenytoin is bound approximately 90% to plasma albumin. A greater fraction of phenytoin remains unbound in neonates, in patients with hypoalbuminemia, and in uremic patients (Reindenberg et al, 1971).

METABOLISM. Metabolism of phenytoin is by hepatic microsomal enzymes that are susceptible to stimulation or inhibition by other drugs. When the plasma concentration is less than 10 μg·ml^{-1}, metabolism of phenytoin follows first-order kinetics, and the elimination half-time averages 24 hours. At a plasma concentration of more than 10 μg·ml^{-1}, the enzymes necessary for metabolism of phenytoin become saturated, and the elimination half-time becomes dose dependent (zero-order kinetics). Zero-order kinetics resembles the metabolism of alcohol.

An estimated 98% of phenytoin is metabolized principally to the inactive derivative parahydroxyphenyl. This metabolite appears in the urine as a glucuronide. Approximately 2% of phenytoin is recovered unchanged in the urine. A genetically determined inability to metabolize phenytoin may be present.

Side Effects

Side effects associated with chronic phenytoin therapy include (1) cerebellar-vestibular dysfunction, (2) peripheral neuropathy, (3) gingival hyperplasia, (4) allergic reactions, (5) megaloblastic anemia, and (6) gastrointestinal irritation. Central nervous system toxicity is the most consistent effect of phenytoin overdosage. Administration of phenytoin during pregnancy may result in the fetal hydantoin syndrome, which manifests as wide-set eyes, broad mandible, and finger deformities. Phenytoin-induced hepatotoxicity, although rare, may occur in genetically susceptible persons who lack the enzyme phenytoin epoxide (Spielberg et al, 1981). This enzyme is necessary to convert an electrophilic intermediate formed after the oxidative metabolism of phenytoin to an inert and nontoxic product.

Nystagmus, ataxia, diplopia, and vertigo are likely when the plasma concentration of phenytoin is more than 20 μg·ml^{-1}. These are symptoms of cerebellar-vestibular dysfunction. Peripheral neuropathy has been reported in up to 30% of patients. Gingival hyperplasia occurs in approximately 20% of patients and is probably the most common manifestation of phenytoin toxicity in children and young adolescents. This complication is minimized by improved oral hygiene and does not necessarily require discontinuation of phenytoin therapy. Hyperglycemia and glycosuria appear to be due to phenytoin-induced inhibition of insulin secretion (Kiser et al, 1970). Allergic reactions include morbilliform rash in 2% to 5% of patients. Megaloblastic anemia is rare and has been attributed to altered folic acid absorption but probably also involves altered folic acid metabolism. Gastrointestinal irritation is due to alkalinity of the drug; this may be minimized by taking phenytoin after meals.

Mephenytoin

Mephenytoin is a hydantoin derivative which, unlike phenytoin, is rapidly absorbed after oral administration. Its antiepileptic spectrum is the same as that of phenytoin, and it may exacerbate petit mal epilepsy. Ataxia, gingival hyperplasia, and gastric distress are less likely than with phenytoin therapy. Conversely, serious toxicity, including morbilliform rash, fever, pancytopenia, aplastic anemia, and hepatotoxicity, are more likely and greatly limit the use of this drug.

Phenacemide

Phenacemide is the straight-chain analogue of 5-phenylhydantoin, which is used in the treatment of psychomotor epilepsy only when other less toxic drugs are ineffective. Toxicity may manifest as hepatic, renal, and bone marrow dysfunction.

BARBITURATES

Phenobarbital, mephobarbital, and metharbital are the barbiturates used as antiepileptic drugs.

Phenobarbital

Phenobarbital is an effective antiepileptic drug for suppression of grand mal epilepsy and focal epilepsy and is the drug used most frequently for prophylaxis against the recurrence of febrile seizures (see Fig. 4-2). Although most barbiturates have antiepileptic activity, phenobarbital is unique in producing this effect at doses less than those that usually produce sedation. Phenobarbital limits the spread of seizure activity and also elevates seizure threshold. The ability to reduce the spread of seizures may depend on the potentiation of inhibitory pathways. Sedation, when it occurs, may be due to stimulation of GABA activity.

Pharmacokinetics

Oral absorption of phenobarbital is slow but nearly complete, with peak concentrations occurring 12 to 18 hours after a single dose (Table 30-2). Plasma protein binding is 40% to 60%. Approximately 25% of phenobarbital is eliminated by pH-dependent renal excretion, with the remainder inactivated by hepatic microsomal enzymes. The major metabolite is an inactive parahydroxyphenyl derivative that is excreted in the urine as a sulfate conjugate. The elimination half-time is approximately 90 hours.

The usual daily dosage of phenobarbital is 1 to 5 $mg \cdot kg^{-1}$. Plasma phenobarbital concentrations of 10 to 20 $\mu g \cdot ml^{-1}$ are usually necessary for control of seizures.

Side Effects

Sedation is the most common undesired side effect resulting from phenobarbital therapy. Tolerance to sedation develops, however, with chronic therapy. Phenobarbital sometimes produces irritability and hyperactivity in children and confusion in the elderly. Scarlatiniform or morbilliform rash occurs in up to 2% of patients. Megaloblastic anemia that responds to folic acid administration and osteomalacia that responds to vitamin D therapy may occur during chronic phenobarbital therapy as well as during treatment with pheny-

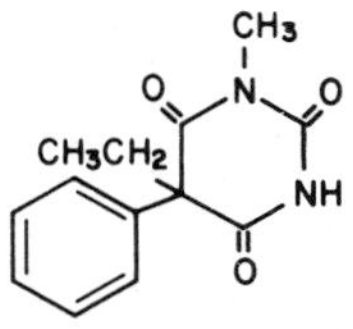

FIGURE 30–2.   Mephobarbital.

toin. Nystagmus and ataxia are likely when the plasma phenobarbital concentration is more than 30 $\mu g \cdot ml^{-1}$.

Congenital malformations may occur when phenobarbital is administered chronically during pregnancy. A coagulation defect and hemorrhage in the neonate must be considered. Interactions between phenobarbital and other drugs usually involve induction of the hepatic microsomal enzymes by phenobarbital.

Mephobarbital

Mephobarbital undergoes N-demethylation to phenobarbital (Fig. 30-2). Consequently, the pharmacologic properties, clinical uses, and side effects of mephobarbital are identical to those of phenobarbital. Oral absorption of mephobarbital, however, is often incomplete, and the dose is approximately twice that of phenobarbital.

Metharbital

Metharbital undergoes N-demethylation to barbital, which is responsible for its pharmacologic activity. This drug has greater sedative and less antiepileptic activity than does phenobarbital.

PRIMIDONE

Primidone is a deoxybarbiturate that is principally used in the treatment of focal epilepsy. It is ineffective against petit mal epilepsy but is sometimes effective in the management of myoclonic seizures in children. Primidone may be administered alone but seems to be more effective when combined with phenytoin. Structurally, primidone is a congener of phenobarbital in which the carbonyl oxygen of the urea moiety is replaced by two hydrogen atoms (Fig. 30-3).

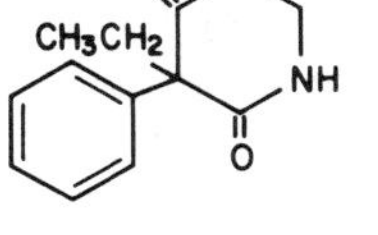

Pharmacokinetics

Primidone is rapidly and almost completely absorbed after oral administration, with peak plasma concentrations occurring in approximately 3 hours. The elimination half-time is approximately 8 hours. Active metabolites of primidone are phenobarbital (elimination half-time 48 to 120 hours) and phenylethylmalonamide (elimination half-time 24 to 48 hours). Both these metabolites accumulate with chronic therapy. Approximately 40% of the drug is excreted unchanged in the urine.

Side Effects

Sedation, nystagmus, vertigo, nausea, and vomiting are common side effects of primidone. Maculopapular rash, leukopenia, thrombocytopenia, megaloblastic anemia, and osteomalacia have been described, although these responses are rare. Ataxia and sedation usually occur when the plasma primidone concentration is more than 12 $\mu g \cdot ml^{-1}$.

The dose of primidone is adjusted on the basis of the plasma concentrations of primidone and phenobarbital. Therapeutic plasma concentrations of primidone are 5 to 10 $\mu g \cdot ml^{-1}$ and a phenobarbital concentration of 2 $\mu g \cdot ml^{-1}$ for every $mg \cdot kg^{-1}$ of the daily dose of primidone.

CARBAMAZEPINE

Carbamazepine is useful in the treatment of psychomotor epilepsy. In addition, this drug is highly effective in the management of patients with trigeminal and glossopharyngeal neuralgias (Crill, 1973). Structurally, carbamazepine is related to the tricyclic antidepressant imipramine (Fig. 30-4).

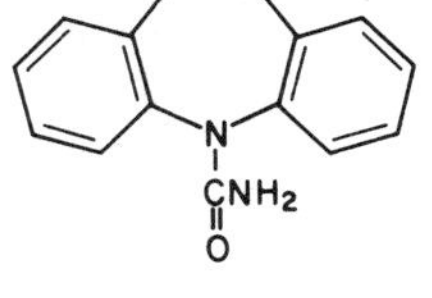

FIGURE 30–3. Primidone.

FIGURE 30–4. Carbamazepine.

Pharmacokinetics

Oral absorption is rapid, with peak concentrations in plasma occurring 2 to 6 hours after ingestion (Table 30-2). Plasma protein binding approximates 80%. The plasma elimination half-time is 13 to 17 hours. An active metabolite has a shorter elimination half-time. The relatively short elimination half-time necessitates dosing intervals every 6 to 8 hours to minimize fluctuations in plasma concentrations. The usual therapeutic plasma concentration of carbamazepine is 4 to 12 $\mu g \cdot ml^{-1}$.

Side Effects

Sedation, vertigo, diplopia, nausea, vomiting, and ataxia are the most frequent side effects of carbamazepine therapy. Aplastic anemia, thrombocytopenia, hepatocellular and cholestatic jaundice, oliguria, hypertension, and acute left ventricular failure are potential life-threatening complications. For these reasons, bone marrow, hepatic, renal, and cardiac function must be monitored in patients treated with this drug. Skin rash, often with other manifestations of drug allergy, occurs in approximately 3% of patients. Carbamazepine may enhance the metabolism of phenytoin, whereas phenobarbital may enhance the metabolism of carbamazepine.

SUCCINIMIDES

Ethosuximide, methsuximide, and phensuximide are examples of succinimides that are uniquely effective in the treatment of petit mal epilepsy.

Ethosuximide

Ethosuximide with alkyl substituents resembles other antiepileptic drugs (Fig. 30-5). This drug

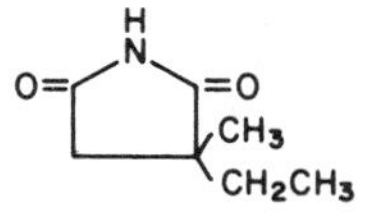

FIGURE 30–5.   Ethosuximide.

has a characteristic effect on thalamocortical excitation when compared with phenytoin. This is consistent with the speculated importance of the thalamocortical system in the etiology of petit mal epilepsy.

Pharmacokinetics

Oral absorption of ethosuximide is adequate, with peak concentrations occurring in 1 to 7 hours (Table 30-2). Ethosuximide is not significantly bound to albumin. Approximately 20% of the drug is excreted unchanged in the urine, and the remainder is metabolized to inactive metabolites by the hepatic microsomal enzymes. The elimination half-time is approximately 60 hours. The usual maintenance dose of ethosuximide is 20 to 40 $mg \cdot kg^{-1}$. A plasma concentration of 40 to 100 $\mu g \cdot ml^{-1}$ is required for satisfactory suppression of petit mal epilepsy.

Side Effects

The most common side effects of ethosuximide are nausea, vomiting, sedation, headache, and hiccough. Parkinson-like symptoms and photophobia have been reported. Urticaria, thrombocytopenia, and aplastic anemia have been described. Renal or hepatic toxicity has not been a problem with this drug.

Methsuximide

Methsuximide is effective in the treatment of petit mal epilepsy but less so than ethosuximide. Combined with other drugs, methsuximide may also be useful in the treatment of psychomotor epilepsy. An N-dimethyl metabolite has been implicated in the production of coma following an overdose (Karch, 1973). The usual daily dosage is 600 to 1200 mg. Side effects are similar to those described for ethosuximide.

Phensuximide

Phensuximide has a low efficacy and is seldom used. A dreamlike state, skin rash, fever, leukopenia, and reversible nephropathy have been reported.

VALPROIC ACID

Valproic acid is a branched chain carboxylic acid that is effective in the treatment of petit mal epilepsy (Fig. 30-6). Its mechanism of action is unknown but may involve an interaction with the metabolism of GABA (Browne, 1980).

Pharmacokinetics

Valproic acid is rapidly absorbed, with peak concentrations in plasma observed after 1 to 4 hours. Binding to plasma proteins is more than 80%. More than 70% of the drug can be recovered as inactive glucuronide conjugates. The elimination half-time is approximately 12 hours. The usual daily dosage of valproic acid is 1 to 3 g to achieve a therapeutic plasma concentration of 50 to 100 $\mu g \cdot ml^{-1}$.

Side Effects

Side effects produced by valproic acid are infrequent, but nausea and vomiting do occur (Browne, 1980). Sedation and ataxia are less frequent than after administration of other antiepileptic drugs. Valproic acid may affect platelet aggregation, and bleeding time should be determined prior to initiating therapy as well as preoperatively. Because valproic acid is partly eliminated as a ketone-containing metabolite, the urine ketone test may show false-positive results. The most serious side effect is hepatotoxicity, emphasizing the need to monitor liver function during chronic therapy with this drug.

Valproic acid can displace phenytoin and diazepam from protein binding sites, resulting in increased pharmacologic effects produced by these drugs. The metabolism of phenytoin is also inhibited by valproic acid. Finally, this drug causes the plasma concentration of phenobarbital to increase almost 50%, presumably owing to inhibition of hepatic microsomal enzymes.

OXAZOLIDINEDIONES

Trimethadione and paramethadione are examples of oxazolidinediones that are effective in the treatment of petit mal epilepsy. Thalamic nuclei are particularly sensitive to these drugs, which is consistent with the speculated importance of the thalamocortical system in the etiology of petit mal epilepsy.

Trimethadione

Trimethadione contains structural characteristics common to other classes of antiepileptic drugs, including alkyl substitutes on the number 5 carbon atom (Fig. 30-7).

Pharmacokinetics

Trimethadione is rapidly absorbed from the gastrointestinal tract, producing peak plasma concentrations in 1 to 2 hours. Plasma protein binding is insignificant. Hepatic microsomal enzymes are responsible for demethylation of trimethadione to its active metabolite dimethadione. Dimethadione is not further metabolized but is excreted unchanged in the urine, with an elimination half-time of 6 to 13 days. During chronic therapy, dimethadione accumulates and is responsible for the pharmacologic activity of the parent drug.

The usual daily dosage of trimethadione is 0.9 to 2.1 g. Plasma concentrations of the active metabolite dimethadione are used to guide therapy and adjust the maintenance dose of trimethadione. The plasma concentration of dimethadione must usually be maintained above 700 $\mu g \cdot ml^{-1}$ to control petit mal epilepsy.

Side Effects

The most common side effects of trimethadione therapy are sedation and blurring of vision in bright light (hemeralopia). Sedation tends to diminish with chronic therapy. Less common, but

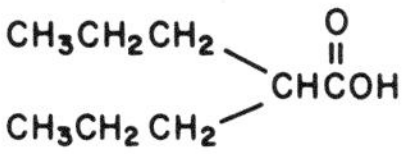

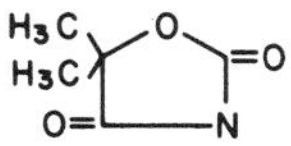

FIGURE 30–6. Valproic acid.

FIGURE 30–7. Trimethadione.

more serious, side effects include exfoliative dermatitis, neutropenia, aplastic anemia, hepatitis, and nephrosis. A myasthenic syndrome has also been reported (Booker et al, 1968).

Paramethadione

Paramethadione differs from trimethadione only in replacement of one of the methyl groups on the number 5 carbon atom with an ethyl substituent. An active metabolite results from N-demethylation and is likely to be responsible for the antiepileptic activity of the drug. The pharmacologic properties, therapeutic uses, dosage, and toxicity are similar to those of trimethadione. Nevertheless, patients who do not tolerate trimethadione may tolerate paramethadione and vice versa.

BENZODIAZEPINES

A large number of benzodiazepines have broad antiepileptic properties, but only clonazepam and diazepam are commonly used (see Fig. 5-1). The antiepileptic actions of benzodiazepines as well as barbiturates and valproic acid may involve drug-induced increases in the activity of inhibitory neurotransmitters such as GABA. In low doses, benzodiazepines suppress polysynaptic activity in the spinal cord and decrease neuronal activity in the mesencephalic reticular system.

Clonazepam

Clonazepam is useful in the therapy of petit mal epilepsy as well as myoclonic seizures in children (Browne, 1978).

Pharmacokinetics

Absorption of clonazepam after oral administration is rapid, with peak plasma concentrations occurring within 2 to 4 hours (Table 30-2). Intravenous administration of clonazepam results in rapid central nervous system effects. Approximately 50% of the drug is bound to plasma proteins. Clonazepam is extensively metabolized to inactive products, with less than 2% of an injected dose appearing unchanged in the urine. The elimination half-time is 24 to 36 hours. The oral maintenance dose of clonazepam should not exceed approximately 0.25 $mg \cdot kg^{-1}$ Therapeutic plasma concentrations of clonazepam are 0.02 to 0.08 $\mu g \cdot ml^{-1}$.

Side Effects

Side effects are infrequent after oral administration. Sedation is present in approximately 50% of patients but tends to subside with chronic administration. Skeletal muscle incoordination and ataxia occur in approximately 30% of patients. Hypotonia, dysarthria, and dizziness have been described. Personality changes occur in approximately 25% of patients, manifesting as behavioral disturbances, including hyperactivity, irritability, and difficulty in concentration. Increased salivary and bronchial secretions may be particularly prominent in children. Seizures are exacerbated in some patients, and status epilepticus may be precipitated if the drug is discontinued abruptly. Cardiovascular and respiratory depression have occurred after intravenous administration.

Diazepam

Diazepam is effective in the treatment of status epilepticus and local anesthetic-induced seizures. The usual approach is the administration of 0.1 $mg \cdot kg^{-1}$ IV every 10 to 15 minutes until seizure activity has been suppressed or a maximum dose of 30 mg has been administered (see Chapter 5).

ACETAZOLAMIDE

Acetazolamide is a carbonic anhydrase inhibitor that may be effective in the treatment of petit mal epilepsy. Its effectiveness, however, is limited by the rapid development of tolerance.

REFERENCES

Booker HE, Chun RWM, Sanguino M. Myasthenia syndrome associated with trimethadione. Neurology 1968;18:274.

Browne TR. Clonazepam. N Engl J Med 1978; 299:812–6.

Browne TR. Valproic acid. N Engl J Med 1980; 302:661–6.

Crill WE. Carbamazepine. Ann Intern Med 1973; 79:844–7.

Hauser WA. Epidemiology of epilepsy. Adv Neurol 1978;19:313–39.

Karch SB. Methsuximide overdose: Delayed onset of profound coma. JAMA 1973;223:1463–5.

Kiser JS, Vargas-Cordon M, Brendel K, Bressler R. The *in vitro* inhibition of insulin secretion by diphenylhydantoin. J Clin Invest 1970;49:1942–8.

Reidenberg MM, Odar-Cedarlof, VonBahr C, Borga O, Sjoqvist F. Protein binding of diphenylhydantoin and desmethylimipramine in plasma from patients with poor renal function. N Engl J Med 1971; 285:264–7.

Spielberg SP, Gordon GB, Blake DA, Goldstein DA. Herlong HF. Predisposition to phenytoin hepatotoxicity assessed *in vitro*. N Engl J Med 1981; 305:722–7.

Chapter

31

Drugs Used for Treatment of Parkinson's Disease

Parkinson's disease is a manifestation of an imbalance between dopaminergic and cholinergic activity transmitted by the extrapyramidal nervous system. Conceptually, dopamine is believed to act principally as an inhibitory neurotransmitter and acetylcholine as an excitatory neurotransmitter in the extrapyramidal system. Although dopamine is more important, a proper balance with the cholinergic neurotransmitter is also necessary for normal function. The goal of treating Parkinson's disease is to enhance the inhibitory effect of dopamine or reduce the stimulatory effect of acetylcholine by the administration of centrally acting drugs. Often combinations of drugs with effects on the dopaminergic and cholinergic components of the extrapyramidal nervous system are also used. Regardless of the drug or drugs selected, treatment of Parkinson's disease is always palliative and never curative, emphasizing that therapy does not halt progression of neuronal degeneration. Indeed, the gradual loss of responsiveness to drug therapy that occurs over 1 to 5 years may be caused in part by the decreasing capacity of nigrostriatal neurons to synthesize and store dopamine.

The most common causes of Parkinson's disease are cerebral atherosclerosis, viral encephalitis, and drugs that prevent the action of dopamine in the basal ganglia (butyrophenones or phenothiazines) (Severn, 1988). A neurotoxin (MPTP) causes Parkinson's disease in primates, leading to the search for environmental toxins similar to MPTP. It is interesting that the lower incidence of Parkinson's disease in cigarette smokers has been attributed to inhibition of monoamine oxidase Type B enzyme by products of tobacco combustion (Severn, 1988).

Approximately 80% of the dopamine in the brain is concentrated in the basal ganglia, mostly in the caudate nucleus and putamen. In patients with Parkinson's disease, the basal ganglia content of dopamine is only approximately 10% of normal. As a result, there is an excess of excitatory cholinergic activity manifesting as tremor, skeletal muscle rigidity, bradykinesia, and disturbances of posture. In addition to these classic peripheral manifestations of Parkinson's disease, approximately one fifth of afflicted patients become mentally depressed and one third develop cognitive and memory deficits that may progress to delirium. Alzheimer's disease is six times more frequent in patients with Parkinson's disease (Boller et al, 1980).

LEVODOPA

Levodopa, as the immediate metabolic precursor of dopamine, acts by replenishing the depleted stores of dopamine in the basal ganglia (Fig. 31-

1). Indeed, approximately 75% of patients with Parkinson's disease respond favorably to treatment with levodopa. An optimal therapeutic response, however, may not occur in some patients until the completion of 1 to 6 months of therapy. The beneficial therapeutic response to levodopa typically diminishes after 2 to 5 years of treatment, presumably reflecting progression of the disease process and continuing loss of nigrostriatal neurons with a capacity to store dopamine.

The usual daily maintenance dosage of levodopa is 3 to 8 g administered orally in at least four divided doses. Absorption from the gastrointestinal tract is efficient using an active transport system. Maximal plasma concentrations of levodopa occur 0.5 to 2 hours after administration, but the brief elimination half-time of 1 to 3 hours requires frequent dosing intervals to maintain a therapeutic tissue concentration. Slowed gastric emptying, as caused by opioids or anticholinergics and increased gastric acidity, reduces absorption of levodopa from the gastrointestinal tract. An intravenous formulation of levodopa is not available.

Abrupt discontinuation of levodopa therapy may result in a precipitous return of symptoms of Parkinson's disease. For this reason, levodopa should be continued throughout the perioperative period, being included in the preoperative medication.

Metabolism

Approximately 95% of orally administered levodopa is rapidly decarboxylated to dopamine by a hepatic first-pass effect, reflecting the activity of the enzyme dopa decarboxylase. The resulting dopamine cannot easily cross the blood-brain barrier to exert a beneficial therapeutic effect, whereas increased plasma concentrations of dopamine often lead to undesirable side effects. Inhibition of the peripheral activity of dopa decarboxylase enzyme greatly increases the fraction of administered levodopa that remains unmetabolized and available to cross the blood-brain barrier.

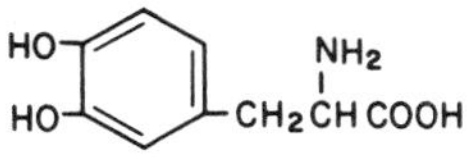

FIGURE 31–1. Levodopa.

At least 30 metabolites of levodopa have been identified. Most are converted to dopamine, small amounts of which are subsequently metabolized to norepinephrine and epinephrine. Metabolism of dopamine yields 3,4-dihydroxyphenylacetic acid and 3-methoxy-4-hydroxyphenylacetic acid (homovanillic acid). Dietary methionine is necessary as a source of methyl donors to permit continued activity of catechol-o-methyl transferase, which is necessary for the metabolism of the excess amounts of dopamine that result from high doses of levodopa. Most metabolites of dopamine are excreted by the kidneys.

Side Effects

Most patients with Parkinson's disease who are treated with levodopa experience side effects. These side effects are typically dose dependent and reversible. Presumably, increased formation of catecholamines, particularly dopamine, in both the central nervous system and the periphery is responsible for these side effects.

Gastrointestinal Dysfunction

A most common side effect early in therapy with levodopa is anorexia, nausea, and vomiting occurring in approximately 80% of patients. Nausea and vomiting presumably reflect dopamine-induced stimulation of the chemoreceptor trigger zone, which is not protected by the blood-brain barrier. Antiemetic drugs are not indicated, because they may interfere with the action of dopamine at basal ganglia. Gastrointestinal side effects tend to disappear with continuing therapy as tolerance develops.

Abnormal Involuntary Movements

Abnormal involuntary movements are the most common side effect of levodopa therapy, appearing in approximately 50% of patients within 1 to 4 months after initiation of treatment. This incidence increases to approximately 80% of patients on therapeutic doses of levodopa for more than 1 year. These involuntary movements may include faciolingual tics, grimacing, and rocking movements of the arms, legs, or trunk. Rarely, exaggerated respiratory movements can produce an irregular gasping pattern of breathing, presumably reflecting dyskinesias of the diaphragm and intercostal muscles. Tolerance does not develop to this side effect. Abnormal voluntary movements are reduced or abolished by a decrease in the dose of levodopa or administration of pyridoxine, both of which also reduce the efficacy of levodopa. The goal is to titrate the dose of levodopa to maximize the therapeutic benefit while minimizing this side effect.

Behavioral Disturbances

Serious behavioral disturbances characterized by confusion and even delirium occur in approximately 15% of patients treated with levodopa. Excessive sexual behavior may reflect actions of levodopa on the hypothalamus. Elderly patients receiving combinations of levodopa and anticholinergic drugs are particularly vulnerable to the development of psychiatric disturbances.

Cardiovascular Changes

Cardiovascular changes associated with levodopa most likely reflect alpha- and beta-adrenergic responses evoked by increased plasma concentrations of dopamine. Furthermore, large doses of levodopa cause hypokalemia associated with increased plasma concentrations of aldosterone.

CARDIAC DYSRHYTHMIAS. Cardiac dysrhythmias, including sinus tachycardia, atrial and ventricular premature contractions, atrial fibrillation, and ventricular tachycardia, although rare, have been associated with levodopa therapy. Presumably, the potential beta-adrenergic effects of dopamine on the heart contribute to cardiac dysrhythmias, although a cause-and-effect relationship has not been documented. Patients with preexisting disturbances of cardiac conduction or coronary artery disease are most likely to develop cardiac dysrhythmias in association with levodopa therapy. Propranolol is an effective treatment when cardiac dysrhythmias occur in these patients.

ORTHOSTATIC HYPOTENSION. For unknown reasons, approximately 30% of patients develop orthostatic hypotension early in therapy. As a result, some patients experience vertigo and, rarely, syncope. Orthostatic hypotension becomes less prominent with continued therapy. It is of interest that dopamine resulting from levodopa may displace norepinephrine from peripheral sympathetic nerve endings and interfere with adrenergic transmission. Transient flushing of the skin is common during levodopa therapy.

Endocrine Effects

Dopamine inhibits the secretion of prolactin, presumably by stimulating the release of a prolactin inhibitory factor. The release of growth hormone that occurs in response to the administration of levodopa to normal patients is minimal or absent when levodopa is administered to patients with Parkinson's disease. Indeed, signs of acromegaly or diabetes mellitus do not occur in patients treated chronically with levodopa. Large doses of levodopa may cause hypokalemia associated with increased plasma levels of aldosterone.

Laboratory Measurements

Urinary metabolites of levodopa cause false-positive tests for ketoacidosis. These metabolites also color the urine red and then black on exposure to air. Mild, transient elevations of blood urea nitrogen occur and usually can be controlled by increasing oral fluid intake. Elevated liver transaminase enzymes occasionally occur. Positive Coombs' tests have been attributed to levodopa therapy in a few patients.

Reduced Anesthetic Requirements

Intravenous administration of levodopa to animals reduces halothane anesthetic requirements (MAC) (Johnston et al, 1975). It is speculated that dopamine derived from levodopa in the central nervous system acts as an inhibitory neurotransmitter. Conversely, chronic treatment of animals with levodopa does not consistently alter anesthetic requirements.

Drug Interactions

Drug interactions may occur in patients being treated with levodopa, resulting in enhanced or reduced therapeutic effects.

Antipsychotic Drugs

Antipsychotic drugs such as butyrophenones and phenothiazines can antagonize the effects of dopamine. For this reason, these drugs should not be administered to patients with known or suspected Parkinson's disease. Indeed, administration of droperidol to patients being treated with levodopa has produced severe skeletal muscle rigidity and even pulmonary edema, presumably reflecting sudden antagonism of dopamine (Ngai, 1972). Droperidol has even produced a Parkinson's disease–like syndrome in otherwise healthy patients (Rivera et al, 1975). Metoclopramide may also interfere with dopamine activity.

Monoamine Oxidase Inhibitors

Nonspecific monoamine oxidase inhibitors interfere with the inactivation of catecholamines, including dopamine. As a result, these drugs can exaggerate the peripheral and central nervous system effects of levodopa. Hypertension and hyperthermia are side effects associated with the concurrent administration of these drugs.

Anticholinergic Drugs

Anticholinergic drugs act synergistically with levodopa to improve certain symptoms of Parkinson's disease, especially tremor. Large doses of anticholinergics, however, can slow gastric emptying time such that absorption of levodopa from the gastrointestinal tract is reduced.

Methyldopa

Methyldopa is a weak dopa decarboxylase inhibitor manifesting as potentiation of the central nervous system actions of levodopa including antiparkinson, emetic, and hypotensive effects.

Pyridoxine

Pyridoxine, in doses as low as 5 mg as present in multivitamin preparations, can abolish the therapeutic efficacy of levodopa by enhancing the activity of pyridoxine-dependent dopa decarboxylase and thus increasing the peripheral metabolism of levodopa. As a result, even less dopamine is available to enter the central nervous system.

CARBIDOPA

Carbidopa is an effective inhibitor of the peripheral enzyme activity of dopa decarboxylase (Fig. 31-2). Enzyme activity is not altered in the brain because carbidopa does not cross the blood-brain barrier. Concurrent administration of carbidopa with levodopa results in increased peripheral availability of levodopa to enter the central nervous system, where it is converted to dopamine. This increased availability of levodopa reflects reduced extracerebral metabolism owing to carbidopa-induced inhibition of dopa decarboxylase activity. Indeed, plasma concentrations of levodopa are higher and the elimination half-time is prolonged following concurrent administration of carbidopa and levodopa compared with levodopa alone. As a result of this combination therapy, the dose of levodopa can be decreased by up to 75% while maintaining beneficial central nervous system effects and, at the same time, reducing the likelihood of dose-dependent side effects resulting from excessive plasma concentrations of dopamine. For example, nausea, vomiting, and cardiac dysrhythmias are diminished or absent in the presence of carbidopa compared with the incidence of these side effects in patients treated only with levodopa. Antagonism of the therapeutic effect of levodopa by pyridoxine therapy does not occur during combination therapy. The incidence of abnormal involuntary movements and behavioral disturbances, however, is not influenced by carbidopa. Administered alone, carbidopa lacks pharmacologic activity.

AMANTADINE

Amantadine is an antiviral drug used for prophylaxis against infection with influenza A. This drug also produces symptomatic improvement in patients with Parkinson's disease, presumably by facilitating the release of dopamine from intact dopaminergic terminals that remain in the nigrostriatum of patients with this disease

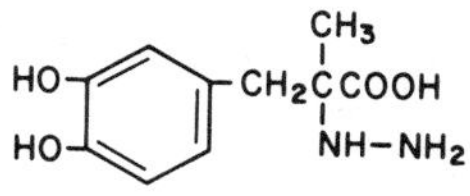

FIGURE 31–2. Carbidopa.

(Schwab et al, 1971). In addition, amantadine delays uptake of dopamine back into nerve endings and exerts anticholinergic effects.

Amantadine is well absorbed after oral administration, and the elimination half-time is approximately 12 hours. More than 90% of the drug is excreted unchanged by the kidneys, necessitating dosage adjustments in patients with renal dysfunction.

Side Effects

Side effects of amantadine therapy, such as nausea and vomiting, are mild and infrequent. Approximately 25% of patients develop difficulty in concentration as well as confusion and anxiety. The peripheral and central adverse effects of anticholinergic drugs are increased by amantadine. Combined therapy has induced psychotic reactions identical to those caused by atropine poisoning. Livedo reticularis (mottling of the skin) is relatively common in patients (especially females) receiving amantadine for more than 1 month. Long-term use of amantadine may be associated with erythromelalgia (red, tender, and edematous lower extremities) with or without cardiac failure (Pearce et al, 1974).

BROMOCRIPTINE

Bromocriptine is a direct-acting dopamine receptor agonist effective in the treatment of galactorrhea, hyperprolactinemia, and acromegaly (Fig. 31-3). The effectiveness of bromocriptine in the treatment of acromegaly reflects the paradoxical inhibitory effect of dopamine agonists on secretion of growth hormone. Bromocriptine also suppresses excess prolactin secretion that is often

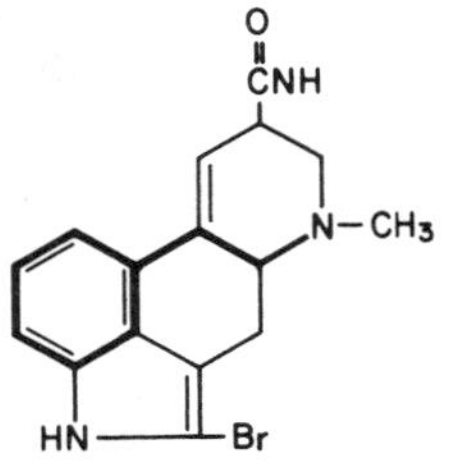

associated with growth hormone secretion. Large doses of bromocriptine are necessary to control the symptoms of Parkinson's disease. As a result, bromocriptine in small doses may be used to supplement treatment regimens that depend primarily on levodopa (Lang and Blair, 1984).

Absorption of bromocriptine from the gastrointestinal tract is rapid but incomplete. Extensive hepatic first-pass metabolism occurs and more than 90% of the metabolites are excreted in the bile, whereas less than 10% of the drug is excreted unchanged or as inactive metabolites in the urine.

Side Effects

Visual and auditory hallucinations, hypotension, dyskinesia, and erythromelalgia occur more frequently with bromocriptine than with levodopa therapy. Asymptomatic elevations of serum transaminase and alkaline phosphatase concentrations have been reported. Vertigo and nausea are occasionally associated with bromocriptine therapy.

SELEGILINE

Selegiline is a highly selective inhibitor of monoamine oxidase Type B enzyme (Fig. 31-4) (see Chapter 19). This drug is effective in the treatment of Parkinson's disease because it inhibits the intracerebral metabolism of dopamine, thus maximizing the therapeutic efficacy of concomitantly administered levodopa. In contrast to nonspecific monoamine oxidase inhibitors, selegiline does not result in life-threatening potentiation of the effects of catecholamines when administered concurrently with a centrally active amine (Severn, 1988). This reflects the fact that metabolism of norepinephrine in peripheral nerve endings is not altered by selegiline, which minimizes the likelihood of adverse responses during anesthesia in response to sympathomimetics. The most common side effect of com-

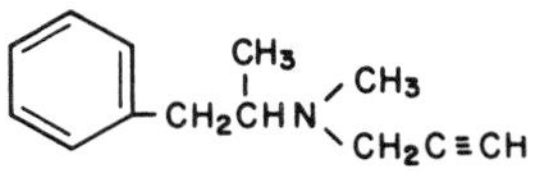

FIGURE 31-3. Bromocriptine. The darkened portion corresponds to the structure of dopamine.

FIGURE 31-4. Selegiline.

bined therapy, including selegiline, is an increased incidence of dyskinesia. Mental depression and paranoid ideation are also common side effects.

ANTICHOLINERGIC DRUGS

Centrally active anticholinergic drugs, such as benztropine, cycrimine, and trihexyphenidyl, are useful in patients with minimal symptoms caused by Parkinson's disease and in those who do not tolerate or respond to levodopa. More than 50% of patients who respond to levodopa manifest additional beneficial effects when therapy is supplemented with anticholinergic drugs. Anticholinergic drugs are also useful in the treatment of Parkinson's disease–like symptoms induced by antipsychotic drugs that presumably act by blocking dopaminergic receptors. In this regard, levodopa would not be effective in reversing drug-induced parkinsonism symptoms, because the increase in brain dopamine concentrations produced by levodopa is insufficient to overcome receptor blockade. The presumed mechanism of action of anticholinergic drugs is the ability of these drugs to blunt the effects of the excitatory neurotransmitter acetylcholine.

Certain antihistamines that are structurally related to diphenhydramine possess modest central anticholinergic properties. These drugs are less effective than anticholinergic drugs in the treatment of Parkinson's disease but are well tolerated, especially by elderly patients. Sedative effects of these drugs may be useful in countering the insomnia produced by levodopa and potent anticholinergic drugs.

Trihexyphenidyl

Trihexyphenidyl is the prototype of anticholinergic drugs that are particularly useful in reducing the tremor and excess salivation associated with Parkinson's disease (Fig. 31-5). Rigidity and bradykinesia are less effectively blunted. Although the peripheral and central nervous system actions of this synthetic drug are less prominent than those of atropine, side effects such as mydriasis, cycloplegia, dry mouth, tachycardia, adynamic ileus, urinary retention, sedation, hallucinations, confusion, and delirium may still occur. Because of the mydriatic effect, trihexyphenidyl could precipitate acute glaucoma in a susceptible patient.

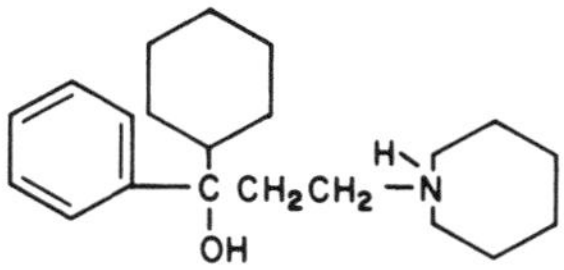

FIGURE 31–5.   Trihexyphenidyl.

REFERENCES

Boller F, Mizatani T, Roessmann U, Gambetti P. Parkinson disease, dementia and Alzheimer's disease: Clinicopathological correlations. Ann Neurol 1980;7:329–35.

Johnston RR, White PF, Way WL, Miller RD. The effect of levodopa on halothane anesthetic requirement. Anesth Analg 1975;54:178–81.

Lang AE, Blair RDG. Parkinson's disease in 1984: Update. Can Med Assoc J 1984;131:1031–7.

Ngai SH. Parkinsonism, levodopa, and anesthesia. Anesthesiology 1972;37:344–51.

Pearce LA, Waterbury LD, Green HD. Amantadine hydrochloride: Alteration in peripheral circulation. Neurology 1974;24:46–8.

Rivera VM, Keichian AH, Oliver RE. Persistent parkinsonism following neuroleptanalgesia. Anesthesiology 1975;43:635–7.

Schwab RS, Poskanzer DC, England AC, Young RR. Amantadine in Parkinson's disease. Review of more than two years' experience. JAMA 1971;222:792–5.

Severn AM. Parkinsonism and the anaesthetist. Br J Anaesth 1988;61:761–70.

Chapter

32

Drugs Used to Treat Hyperlipoproteinemia

Lipoproteins are categorized as (1) chylomicrons, (2) very low-density lipoproteins (VLDL), (3) intermediate-density lipoproteins (IDL), (4) low-density lipoproteins (LDL), and (5) high-density lipoproteins (HDL). Hyperlipoproteinemia is classified according to the type of lipoprotein that is increased (Table 32-1). Hypercholesterolemia can occur from elevations in the plasma concentrations of any of these lipoproteins. Cholesterol is an essential structural component of biologic membranes and a precursor of the steroid hormones and other important molecules. Humans derive cholesterol both exogenously, from the consumption of animal products, and endogenously, from synthesis in the liver and other tissues.

Elevation of blood cholesterol is a major risk factor for the development of atherosclerosis and, in particular, for death from coronary artery disease and nonhemorrhagic stroke (Grundy, 1986; Iso et al, 1989; Steinberg et al, 1989). Because LDL are the principal cholesterol-carrying lipoproteins in plasma, there is a predictable association between elevations in the plasma concentrations of LDL-cholesterol (type IIa hyperlipoproteinemia) and accelerated atherogenesis (coronary artery disease). Conversely, there is an inverse relationship between plasma cholesterol levels and the risk of intracranial hemorrhage (Iso et al, 1989).

Removal of LDL-cholesterol from the plasma, and, thus, control of the plasma cholesterol concentration, occurs principally by attachment to LDL receptors on the surfaces of liver cells. These receptors invaginate and internalize LDL-cholesterol by endocytosis where lysosomal hydrolytic enzymes subsequently exert their effects. Synthesis of these receptors is genetically determined, with one gene inherited from each parent. Inheritance of one nonfunctional and one normal gene (heterozygous) for LDL receptors results in plasma cholesterol levels that are approximately twice the normal level. The incidence of heterozygous familial hypercholesterolemia is approximately 1 in 500 persons and affected persons are prone to premature coronary artery disease. Less common is homozygous familial hypercholesterolemia in which abnormal genes are inherited from both parents, plasma cholesterol concentrations are approximately four times normal, and early atherosclerosis is likely.

The ideal plasma cholesterol level for Americans older than 30 years of age is 200 mg·dl^{-1} or less (Consensus Conference, 1985). Attempts should be made to lower plasma cholesterol concentrations in middle-aged men when those concentrations exceed 240 mg·dl^{-1}. Addition of the risk factor from smoking is equivalent to increasing the plasma cholesterol concentration 50 to 100 mg·dl^{-1}. Other risk factors that increase the

Table 32–1
Classification of Hyperlipoproteinemia

Plasma Concentration of Lipoprotein that Is Increased	Type
Chylomicrons	I
Low-density lipoprotein	IIa
Low-density lipoproteins and very low-density lipoproteins	IIb
Intermediate-density lipoproteins	III
Very low-density lipoproteins	IV
Chylomicrons and very low-density lipoproteins	V

relative equivalent of the plasma LDL-cholesterol concentrations include hypertension, obesity, family history of premature coronary artery disease (before age 55 to 60 years), diabetes mellitus, male sex, and advancing age. Reducing risk factors, especially cessation of smoking and control of hypertension in combination with efforts to lower the plasma concentrations of cholesterol, is effective in retarding the progression of atherosclerosis even in patients with established coronary artery disease. It is estimated that 15% to 20% of the population has hypercholesterolemia. There is compelling evidence that successful attempts to reduce plasma cholesterol concentrations will decrease the risk of coronary artery disease.

Diet and weight reduction are the mainstays of lipid-lowering treatment and should always be tried first, although diets sufficiently palatable to be accepted by most patients typically only lower plasma cholesterol levels by 10% or less. Emphasis is on avoidance of foods high in cholesterol or saturated animal fat content.

DRUGS THAT LOWER PLASMA CONCENTRATIONS OF CHOLESTEROL

Drugs available to reduce plasma concentrations of cholesterol act by a variety of mechanisms including bile acid sequestration and inhibition of the rate-limiting enzyme in cholesterol synthesis. Often there is insufficient efficacy at tolerated doses and, in some cases, a high incidence of unacceptable side effects. Dietary regulation and weight reduction must continue during drug therapy, because the effects of diet and drugs are additive.

NICOTINIC ACID

Nicotinic acid is a water-soluble vitamin that reduces the production of VLDL, which results in a subsequent 10% to 15% decrease in the concentration of LDL-cholesterol. The mechanism by which nicotinic acid lowers VLDL production is uncertain, but it is probably related to several diverse actions of the drug, including inhibition of lipolysis in adipose tissue, decreased esterification of triglycerides in the liver, and increased activity of lipoprotein lipase. Nicotinic acid does not produce any detectable changes in synthesis of cholesterol nor does it alter excretion of bile acids (Grundy et al, 1981).

Side Effects

Hepatic dysfunction manifesting as increased plasma transaminase activity and cholestatic jaundice may be associated with large doses of nicotinic acid. Although the mechanism by which nicotinic acid or one of its metabolites induces hepatic injury is unknown, evidence exists to suggest a dose-related, direct toxic effect rather than an idiosyncratic drug reaction. Furthermore, crystalline preparations of nicotinic acid are less likely than sustained release preparations to cause hepatotoxicity. Hyperglycemia and abnormal glucose tolerance occur in nondiabetic patients receiving nicotinic acid. Plasma concentrations of uric acid are elevated, and the incidence of gouty arthritis is increased. For these reasons, nicotinic acid should be used with caution, if at all, in patients with liver disease, diabetes mellitus, or gout. Finally, nicotinic acid may also exaggerate vasodilation and orthostatic hypotension caused by ganglionic blocking and antihypertensive drugs. Intense cutaneous flushing and pruritus occur initially in almost all treated patients and persist in 10% to 15% of patients. This flushing is due to prostaglandin release and can be ameliorated by concomitant administration of aspirin. Peptic ulcer disease may be reactivated by nicotinic acid therapy of hyperlipoproteinemia.

CLOFIBRATE

Clofibrate characteristically reduces plasma concentrations of triglycerides by enhancing the

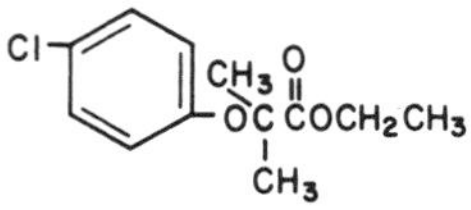

FIGURE 32–1.   Clofibrate.

intravascular breakdown of VLDL and IDL, as well as by accelerating the rate of removal of these lipoproteins from the circulation (Fig. 32-1). In addition, the plasma concentration of cholesterol and LDL often decline, although the decrease in cholesterol concentration may be minimal. Clofibrate has no effect on chylomicronemia nor does it alter plasma concentrations of HDL. This drug is used almost exclusively to treat type III hyperlipoproteinemia. Clofibrate is occasionally useful in treatment of patients with severe hypertriglyceridemia who do not respond to nicotinic acid or gemfibrozil.

Pharmacokinetics

Clofibrate is completely absorbed from the gastrointestinal tract following oral administration. Following absorption, clofibrate rapidly undergoes hydrolysis, with peak plasma concentrations appearing as the active metabolite chlorophenoxyisobutyric acid within 4 hours. Urinary excretion accounts for clearance of approximately 60% of the drug as a glucuronide conjugate. The elimination half-time of clofibrate is approximately 15 hours.

Side Effects

Clofibrate therapy may be associated with a flu-like syndrome, including skeletal muscle myalgia and weakness. Often, this syndrome is accompanied by elevations in the plasma concentrations of creatine phosphokinase and liver transaminases (Langer and Levy, 1968). The lithogenicity of bile is enhanced, and there is an increased incidence of cholelithiasis and cholecystitis. Patients with coronary artery disease may be at increased risk for drug-induced cardiac dysrhythmias and exaggerated angina pectoris. Clofibrate enhances the pharmacologic effect of other acidic drugs such as phenytoin, tolbutamide, and oral anticoagulants, presumably by displacing these drugs from binding sites on al-

bumin. Other less serious side effects of clofibrate include nausea, diarrhea, skin rashes, alopecia, and decreased libido.

GEMFIBROZIL

Gemfibrozil is a homologue of clofibrate that decreases synthesis of VLDL by reducing incorporation of long-chain fatty acids into newly formed triglycerides (Fig. 32-2) (Hall et al, 1981). Effects on the plasma concentrations of triglycerides are similar to those produced by clofibrate. This drug is accompanied by an increase in the plasma concentrations of HDL-cholesterol while plasma levels of LDL cholesterol are typically reduced by less than 10%.

The elimination half-time of gemfibrozil is approximately 1.5 hours, with approximately 70% of a single dose appearing unchanged in the urine. Considering the dependence on renal excretion for elimination and occasional transient elevations in plasma transaminases, it is probably prudent to avoid administration of this drug to patients with preexisting renal or hepatic disease. Other side effects associated with gemfibrozil are similar to those observed during treatment with clofibrate.

CHOLESTYRAMINE

Cholestyramine is the chloride salt of an ion exchange resin originally used to control pruritus in patients with elevated plasma concentrations of bile acids resulting from cholestasis (Fig. 32-3). In addition, cholestyramine, by binding bile acids in the small intestine, reduces the circulating level of bile acids, which, in turn, increases the rate of conversion of cholesterol to bile acids in the liver. The result is a decrease in the circulating plasma concentrations of cholesterol. Cholestyramine also increases the rate of LDL clearance by increasing LDL receptor activity.

Cholestyramine is considered by many to be the drug of choice for treatment of patients with

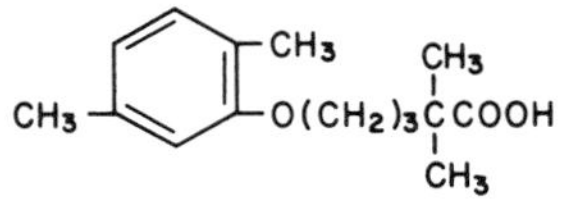

FIGURE 32–2.   Gemfibrozil.

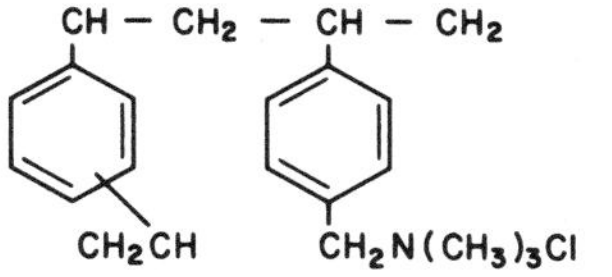

FIGURE 32-3. Cholestyramine.

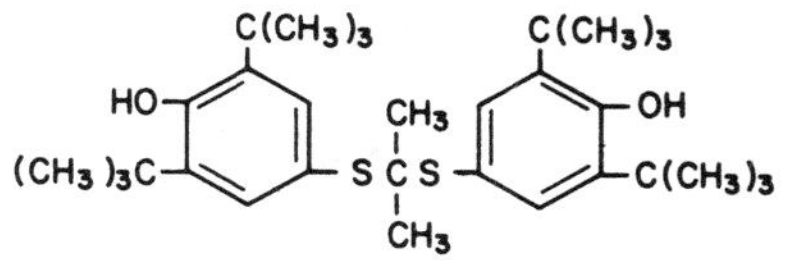

FIGURE 32-4. Probucol.

elevated plasma concentrations of LDL-cholesterol (type IIa hyperlipoproteinemia). When administered with a diet low in cholesterol and saturated fats, this drug lowers plasma LDL levels 15% to 20% and decreases morbidity and mortality associated with coronary artery disease. When combined with nicotinic acid or lovastatin, a decrease in plasma LDL concentrations in the range of 50% can be achieved (Bilheimer et al, 1983).

Side Effects

Nausea, abdominal pain, and constipation are frequent side effects of cholestyramine therapy. A high fluid intake is useful in minimizing constipation. There may be transient increases in the plasma concentrations of alkaline phosphatase and transaminases. Because cholestyramine is a chloride form of an ion exchange resin, hyperchloremic acidosis can occur, especially in younger and smaller patients in whom the relative dose is larger. Absorption of fat-soluble vitamins may be impaired, and hypoprothrombinemia has been observed. Cholestyramine may bind other drugs in the gastrointestinal tract and impair their absorption. For this reason, other drugs should be given at least 1 hour before or 4 hours after administration of cholestyramine. Cholestyramine has a gritty quality that may reduce patient compliance. Despite these side effects, cholestyramine is considered one of the safest drugs available for treatment of hypercholesterolemia.

COLESTIPOL

Colestipol is a bile-sequestering drug with pharmacologic effects similar to those of cholestyramine.

PROBUCOL

Probucol lowers plasma concentrations of cholesterol by decreasing LDL levels (Fig. 32-4).

Therefore, like cholestyramine, this drug is useful in the management of patients with elevated LDL levels. Probucol is also a powerful antioxidant, resulting in inhibition of LDL oxidation and production of a protective effect against atherogenesis even in the absence of drug-induced changes in plasma cholesterol levels (Steinberg et al, 1989).

Despite its lipid solubility, less than 10% of an oral dose of probucol is absorbed from the gastrointestinal tract. Elimination is by way of the bile, with renal excretion being minimal. Nausea and diarrhea are occasional side effects. Transient elevations of plasma transaminases, alkaline phosphatase, uric acid, blood urea nitrogen, and blood glucose have been observed.

LOVASTATIN

Lovastatin is a fungal metabolite that acts as a specific and reversible inhibitor of the rate-limiting enzyme 3-hydroxy-3 methylglutaral coenzyme A (HMG-CoA) for the synthesis of cholesterol (Fig. 32-5). Inhibition of cholesterol synthesis in the liver triggers an increase in synthesis of hepatic LDL surface receptors, leading to an increase in hepatic uptake of cholesterol and a subsequent lowering of the plasma concentrations of LDL-cholesterol. In patients with nonfamilial hypercholesterolemia, administration of lovastatin decreases LDL-cholesterol concentrations approximately 35% (The Lova-

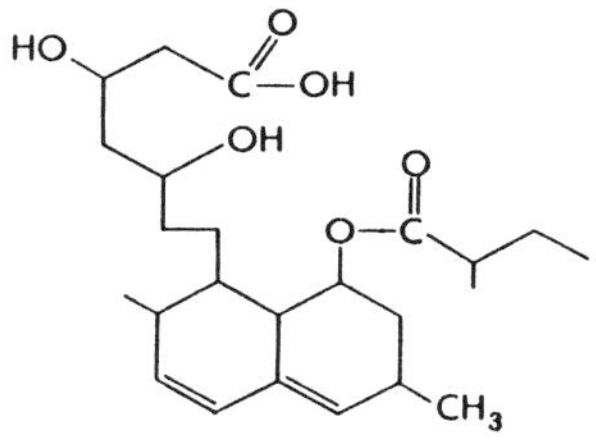

FIGURE 32-5. Lovastatin.

statin Study Group, 1986). Plasma triglyceride concentrations decrease moderately and HDL-cholesterol increases slightly. Combination of lovastatin with a bile acid-binding resin produces a greater decrease of plasma LDL-cholesterol concentrations than can be obtained with either drug along (Bilheimer et al, 1983).

Pharmacokinetics

Lovastatin is rapidly absorbed after oral administration and undergoes extensive hepatic metabolism. Metabolites are excreted through the biliary tract with virtually none of the drug or its metabolites appearing in the urine.

Side Effects

Lovastatin seems to be well tolerated with no adverse effects that require discontinuation of therapy (The Lovastatin Study Group, 1986).

COMPACTIN

Compactin is an HMG-CoA inhibitor that differs structurally from lovastatin only by the absence of a methyl group.

DEXTROTHYROXINE

Dextrothyroxine reduces plasma concentrations of LDL by up to 30% by increasing LDL receptor activity in euthyroid and hypothyroid patients. Mortality, however, is increased in patients with coronary atherosclerosis who are treated with this drug. Adverse side effects reflect metabolic stimulation.

REFERENCES

Bilheimer DW, Grundy SM, Brown MS, Goldstein JL. Mevinolin and colestipol stimulate receptor mediated clearance of low density lipoprotein from plasma in familial hypercholesterolemia heterozygotes. Proc Natl Acad Sci USA 1983;80:4124–8.

Concensus Conference. Lowering blood cholesterol to prevent heart disease. JAMA 1985;253:2080–90.

Grundy SM. Cholesterol and coronary heart disease: A new era. JAMA 1986;256:2849–58.

Grundy SM, Mok HYI, Zech L, Berman M. Influence of nicotinic acid on metabolism of cholesterol and triglycerides in man. J Lipid Res 1981;22:24–36.

Hall MJ, Nelson LM, Russell RI, Howard AN. Gemfibrozil: Effect on biliary cholesterol saturation of new lipid-lowering agent and comparison with clofibrate. Atherosclerosis 1981;39:511–6.

Iso H, Jacobs DR, Wentworth D, et al. Serum cholesterol levels and six-year mortality from stroke in 350,977 men screened for multiple risk factor intervention trial. N Engl J Med 1989;320:904–10.

Langer T, Levy RI. Acute muscular syndrome associated with administration of clofibrate. N Engl J Med 1968;279:856–8.

The Lovastatin Study Group. Therapeutic response to lovastatin (Mevinolin) in nonfamilial hypercholesterolemia. A multicenter study. JAMA 1986;256:2829–34.

Steinberg D, Parthasarathy S, Carew TE, Khoo JC, Witztum JL. Beyond cholesterol: Modifications of low-density lipoprotein that increases its atherogenicity. N Engl J Med 1989;320:915–24.

Chapter

33

Central Nervous System Stimulants and Muscle Relaxants

CENTRAL NERVOUS SYSTEM STIMULANTS

Drugs that stimulate the central nervous system as their primary action are classified as analeptics or convulsants. Analeptics were previously used in the treatment of generalized central nervous system depression accompanying deliberate drug overdoses. This practice, however, has been abandoned because these drugs lack specific antagonist properties and their margin of safety is narrow.

The excitability of the central nervous system reflects a balance between excitatory and inhibitory influences that is normally maintained within relatively narrow limits. Analeptics can increase excitability either by blocking inhibition or by enhancing excitation. Strychnine and picrotoxin selectively block inhibition in the central nervous system. As such, these drugs lack clinical value but, rather, are useful as research tools to study inhibitory neurotransmitters such as gamma-aminobutyric acid (GABA) and corresponding receptors.

Doxapram

Doxapram is a centrally acting analeptic that selectively increases minute ventilation by activating the carotid bodies (Fig. 33-1) (Mitchell and Herbert, 1975). Lack of a direct stimulant effect on the medullary respiratory center is emphasized by the lack of doxapram effect on ventilation when carotid body activity is absent. The stimulus to ventilation produced by administration of doxapram, 1 mg·kg^{-1} IV is similar to that produced by a PaO$_2$ of 38 mmHg acting on the carotid bodies (Hirsh and Wang, 1974). An increase in tidal volume, more than an increase in breathing frequency, is responsible for the doxapram-induced increase in minute ventilation. Oxygen consumption is increased concomitantly with the increase in minute ventilation.

Doxapram has a large margin of safety as reflected by a 20- to 40-fold difference in the dose that stimulates ventilation and the dose that produces seizures (Sebel et al, 1980). Nevertheless, continuous intravenous infusion of doxapram, as required to produce a sustained effect on ventilation, often results in evidence of subconclusive central nervous system stimulation (hypertension, tachycardia, cardiac dysrhythmias, vomiting, and increased body temperature). These changes are consistent with increased sympathetic nervous system outflow from the brain.

Doxapram is extensively metabolized, with less than 5% of an intravenous dose being excreted unchanged in the urine. A single intravenous dose produces an effect on ventilation that lasts only 5 to 10 minutes.

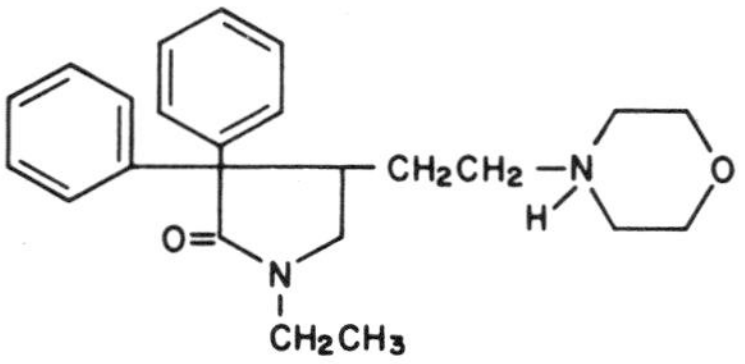

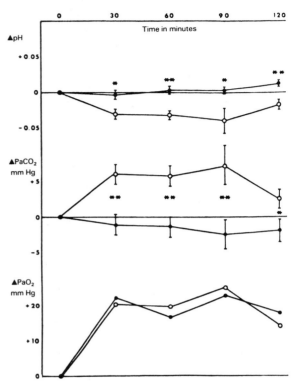

FIGURE 33–1.   Doxapram.

Clinical Uses

Doxapram administered as a continuous intravenous infusion (2 to 3 mg·min⁻¹) has been used as a temporary measure to maintain ventilation during administration of supplemental oxygen to patients with chronic obstructive airway disease who otherwise depend on a hypoxic drive to maintain an adequate minute ventilation (Fig. 33-2) (Moser et al, 1973). Administered concomitantly with intramuscular meperidine, doxapram prevents the ventilatory depression produced by the opioid without altering analgesia, suggesting a possible benefit in the early postoperative period (Ramamurthy et al, 1975). Because controlled ventilation of the lungs and standard supportive therapy are effective in managing ventilatory failure, doxapram should not be used in patients with drug-induced coma or exacerbation of chronic lung disease. More specific tests (peripheral nerve stimulator, airway pressures, or head-lift) render the diagnostic use of doxapram in postanesthetic apnea or hypoventilation of minimal clinical value. Arousal from residual effects of inhaled anesthetics follows administration of doxapram, but the effect is transient, nonselective, and not recommended.

Methylphenidate

Methylphenidate is structurally related to amphetamine (Fig. 33-3). This drug is a mild central nervous system stimulant, with more prominent effects on mental than on motor activities. Large doses, however, produce generalized central nervous system stimulation and seizures. Absorption after oral administration is rapid, and concentrations of methylphenidate in the brain exceed those in the plasma. The abuse potential

FIGURE 33–2.   Doxapram, as a continuous intravenous infusion (●), may be used to maintain alveolar ventilation during administration of supplemental oxygen to patients with chronic obstructive airway disease. (From Moser KM, Luchsinger PC, Adamson JS, et al. Respiratory stimulation with intravenous doxapram in respiratory failure. N Engl J Med 1973; 288: 428–31; with permission.)

of methylphenidate is the same as that of amphetamine.

Clinical Uses

Methylphenidate is useful in the treatment of hyperkinetic syndromes in children characterized as having minimal brain dysfunction. There have, however, been reports of bradycardia, hallucinations, and growth suppression in patients treated with methylphenidate. Methylphenidate may also be effective in the treatment of narcolepsy, either alone or in combination with tricyclic antidepressants.

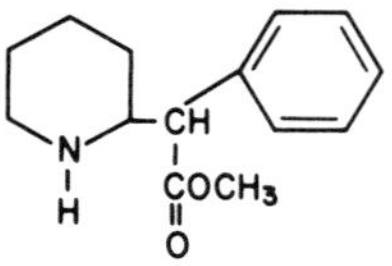

FIGURE 33–3. Methylphenidate.

Methylxanthines

Methylxanthines are represented by caffeine, theophylline, and theobromine (Fig. 33-4). Solubility of methylxanthines is low and is enhanced by formation of complexes as represented by the combination of theophylline with ethylenediamine to form aminophylline. Methylxanthines have in common the ability to (1) stimulate the central nervous system, (2) produce diuresis, (3) increase myocardial contractility, and (4) relax smooth muscle, especially that in the airways (see Chapter 12).

The best-characterized cellular action of methylxanthines is antagonism of receptor-mediated actions of adenosine. Theophylline is more active than caffeine or theobromine as an antagonist at these receptors. Methylxanthines are eliminated primarily by metabolism in the liver. Unlike adults, premature infants metabolize theophylline in part to caffeine. Furthermore, the clearance of methylxanthines is greatly prolonged in the neonate compared with that in the adult. This slowed metabolism is important to consider when methylxanthines are used as analeptics to treat primary apnea of prematurity. Theophylline preparations are most commonly used to relax bronchial smooth muscle in the treatment of asthma (see Chapter 12).

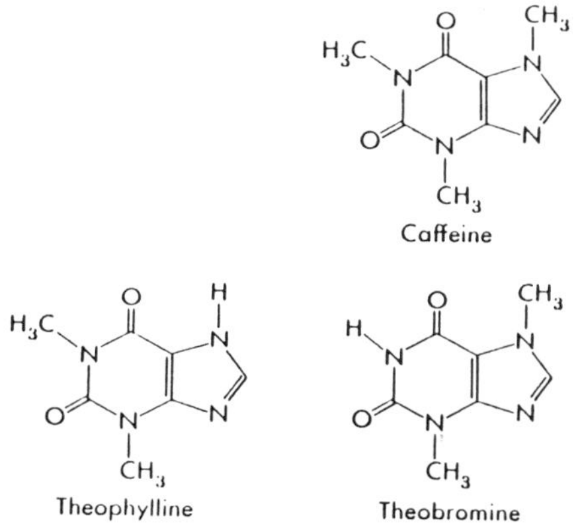

Caffeine

Caffeine is present in a variety of beverages and nonprescription medications (Table 33-1) (Bunker and McWilliams, 1979). A prominent effect of caffeine is central nervous system stimulation. In addition, this substance acts as a cerebral vasoconstrictor and may cause secretion of acidic gastric fluid. Caffeine may increase plasma glucose concentrations.

Pharmacologic uses of caffeine include administration to neonates experiencing apnea of prematurity. Postdural puncture headache may respond to administration of caffeine, 300 mg orally (Camman et al, 1990). Presumably, a cerebral vasoconstriction effect accounts for the occasional efficacy of caffeine in alleviating symptoms of postdural puncture headache as well as migraine headache. Caffeine may be included in common cold remedies in an attempt to offset the sedating effects of antihistamines.

FIGURE 33–4. Methylxanthines.

Table 33–1
Caffeine Content of Common Substances

Substance	Caffeine (mg)
Coffee (150 ml)	
Freeze dried	66
Percolator	107
Drip grind	142
Tea (150 ml)	15–47
Cocoa (150 ml)	13
Coca-Cola® (360 ml)	65
Pepsi-Cola® (360 ml)	43
Dr. Pepper® (360 ml)	61
Mountain Dew® (360 ml)	55
Jolt® Cola	71
Candy bar (1.2 oz)	5
No-Doz®	100

(Data from Bunker ML, McWilliams M. Caffeine content of common beverages. J Am Diet Assoc 1979;74: 28–72; with permission.)

Nicotine

Nicotine has no therapeutic action, but its toxicity and presence in tobacco have lent it medical importance. An estimated 56 million Americans smoke cigarettes. Smoking is the single most important preventable cause of death, being responsible for more than one in every six fatalities (Rigotti, 1989). The highly addictive nature of nicotine results in a withdrawal syndrome that presents a major barrier to successful cessation. Nicotine is readily absorbed from the respiratory tract and buccal mucous membranes and through the skin. As an alkaloid, nicotine is absorbed minimally from the acidic environment of the stomach. Nicotine is metabolized in the lungs and liver after inhalation and oral administration, respectively. A principal metabolite is cotinine, which has approximately one fifth the pharmacologic activity of nicotine. Nicotine and cotinine are rapidly eliminated by the kidneys and, in parturients, in breast milk. The elimination half-time of nicotine is 30 to 60 minutes.

Cigarette smoking alters the activity of many drugs, presumably reflecting induction of liver microsomal enzymes by polycyclic hydrocarbons in cigarette smoke. This enzyme activity differs from that produced by phenobarbital. Enzyme activity remains elevated for up to 6 months after cessation of cigarette smoking.

Effects on Organ Systems

The complex and often unpredictable pharmacologic effects of nicotine may reflect its stimulant and depressant actions. The primary action of nicotine is an initial stimulation quickly followed by persistent depression of autonomic ganglia. Nicotine markedly stimulates the central nervous system, manifesting initially as tremor. Stimulation of ventilation by small doses reflects nicotine-induced excitation of aortic and carotid body chemoreceptors. Nicotine characteristically increases heart rate and blood pressure and evokes peripheral vasoconstriction. These responses most likely reflect stimulation of sympathetic nervous system ganglia and the adrenal medulla.

In contrast to the effects on the cardiovascular system, the effects of nicotine on the gastrointestinal tract are largely due to parasympathetic nervous system stimulation leading to vomiting and diarrhea. Nicotine causes an initial stimulation of salivary and bronchial secretions that is followed by inhibition. Salivation caused by smoking is reflexively produced by irritant smoke rather than by a systemic effect of nicotine.

Overdose

Overdose from nicotine may occur from ingestion of insecticide sprays containing nicotine or from ingestion of tobacco products. The fatal dose of nicotine in adults is approximately 60 mg. Individual cigarettes deliver up to 2.5 mg of nicotine. Gastric absorption of nicotine is minimized by vomiting due to the central emetic effect of the initially absorbed material.

The onset of symptoms of nicotine overdose is rapid and characterized by nausea, salivation, abdominal cramps, vertigo, mental confusion, and skeletal muscle weakness. Hypotension and difficulty in breathing ensue, the heart rate is rapid, and terminal seizures may occur. Paralysis of the intercostal muscles may cause apnea. Treatment is supportive, including attempts to remove any residual nicotine from the stomach.

Almitrine

Almitrine is a peripheral chemoreceptor agonist that improves PaO_2 and decreases $PaCO_2$ in patients with chronic respiratory failure associated with obstructive pulmonary disease. It is presumed that this improvement in gas exchange is due to enhancement of hypoxic pulmonary vasoconstriction. Indeed, in animals, intravenous administration produces dose-dependent enhancement of hypoxic pulmonary vasoconstriction (Chen et al, 1990).

CENTRALLY ACTING MUSCLE RELAXANTS

Centrally acting muscle relaxants act in the central nervous system or directly on skeletal muscle to relieve spasticity. Spasticity of skeletal muscle occurs when there is an abnormal increase in resistance to passive movement of a muscle group as a result of hyperactive proprioceptive or stretch reflexes. Spasticity occurs in a wide variety of neurologic conditions and is highly variable in its etiology and presentation.

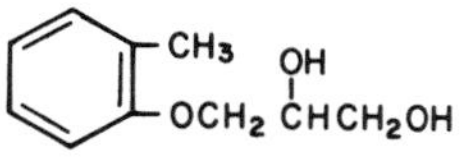

FIGURE 33-5. Mephenesin.

Mephenesin

The relative efficacy of centrally acting muscle relaxants that are related to mephenesin has not been determined (Fig. 33-5). As a result, selection of one of these drugs over another remains highly empirical and subjective. These drugs produce skeletal muscle relaxation by an unknown mechanism in the central nervous system. A prominent effect of centrally acting muscle relaxants is depression of spinal polysynaptic reflexes. Nevertheless, the importance of this effect in the mechanism of skeletal muscle relaxation is not documented. Sedation is not a prominent side effect of these drugs.

Benzodiazepines

Benzodiazepines are widely used as centrally acting skeletal muscle relaxants. These drugs appear to have a more selective action on reticular neuronal mechanisms that control skeletal muscle tone than on spinal interneuronal activity (Tseng and Wang, 1971). Sedation may limit the efficacy of diazepam as a muscle relaxant.

Baclofen

Baclofen is a GABA analogue that is often administered for treatment of spasticity resulting from disease or injury of the spinal cord (Fig. 33-6). It has no direct effect on the neuromuscular junction but diminishes transmission of monosynaptic extensor and polysynaptic flexor reflexes in the spinal cord. This effect may reflect a drug-induced inhibition of excitatory neurotransmitters such as glutamic acid and aspartic acid. Baclofen is particularly effective in the treatment of flexor spasms and skeletal muscle rigidity associated with spinal cord injury or multiple sclerosis. Intrathecal administration of baclofen may be an effective treatment of spinal spasticity that has not responded to oral administration of the drug (Penn et al, 1989). An analgesic effect is demonstrable in animals, but the dose required is large.

Baclofen is rapidly and almost completely absorbed from the gastrointestinal tract. The elimination half-time is 3 to 6 hours, with approximately 80% of the drug excreted unchanged in the urine, emphasizing the need to modify the dose in patients with renal dysfunction. Therapeutic plasma concentrations are 80 to 400 ng·ml^{-1} (Young and Delwaide, 1981).

Use of baclofen is limited by its side effects, which include sedation, skeletal muscle weakness, and confusion. Sudden discontinuation of chronic baclofen therapy may result in tachycardia and both auditory and visual hallucinations. Coma, depression of ventilation, and seizures may accompany an overdose of baclofen. The threshold for initiation of seizures may be lowered in patients with epilepsy. Mild hypotension may occur in awake patients being treated with baclofen, whereas bradycardia and hypotension have been observed when general anesthesia is induced in these patients (Sill et al, 1986). A decrease in sympathetic nervous system outflow from the central nervous system mediated by a GABA-baclofen sensitive system might contribute to this hemodynamic response. Rarely, elevations of liver transaminases and blood glucose levels have occurred.

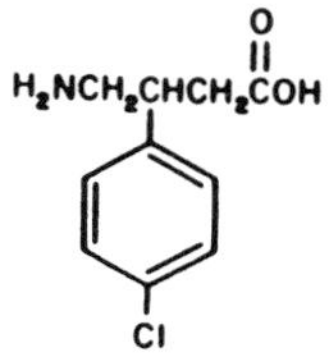

Cyclobenzaprine

Cyclobenzaprine is related structurally and pharmacologically to tricyclic antidepressants (Fig. 33-7). Anticholinergic effects are similar to those

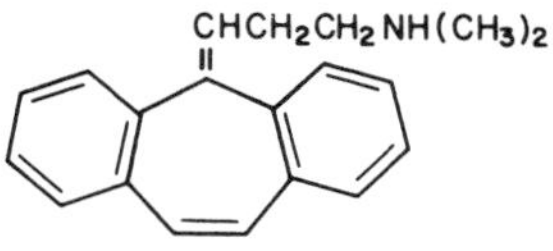

FIGURE 33-6. Baclofen.

FIGURE 33-7. Cyclobenzaprine.

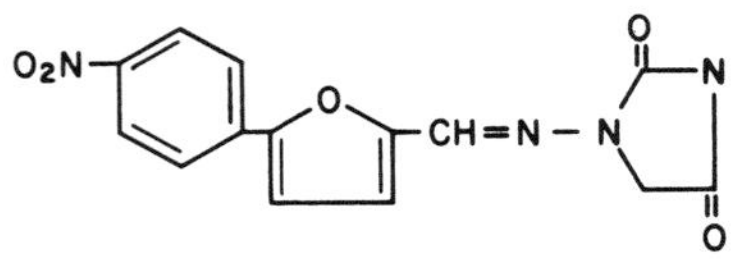

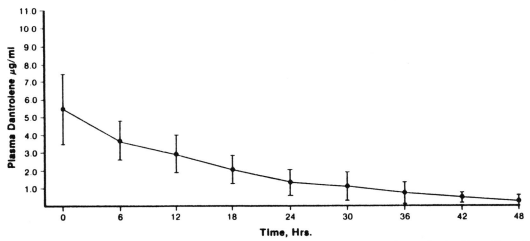

FIGURE 33–8.   Dantrolene.

of tricyclic antidepressants and can include dry mouth, tachycardia, blurred vision, and sedation. The mechanism of skeletal muscle relaxant effects produced by cyclobenzaprine is unknown.

Cyclobenzaprine must not be administered in the presence of monoamine oxidase inhibitors. In view of the potential adverse side effects of some tricyclic antidepressant drugs on the heart, the use of cyclobenzaprine may be questionable in patients with cardiac dysrhythmias or altered conduction of cardiac impulses.

Dantrolene

Dantrolene produces skeletal muscle relaxation by a direct action on excitation–contraction coupling, presumably by decreasing the amount of calcium released from the sarcoplasmic reticulum (Fig. 33-8). Neuromuscular transmission and electrical properties of the skeletal muscle membranes are not altered. Unlike nondepolarizing muscle relaxants, dantrolene cannot decrease contractile activity by more than 80%. Therapeutic doses have little or no effect on cardiac and smooth muscles. In contrast to centrally acting skeletal muscle relaxants, dantrolene does not impair polysynaptic reflexes.

Pharmacokinetics

Absorption of dantrolene from the gastrointestinal tract as well as intravenous injection provides sustained dose-released concentrations of drug in the plasma (Figs. 33-9 and 33-10) (Allen et al, 1988; Lerman et al, 1989). The intravenous preparation of dantrolene is alkaline (pH 9.5) and phlebitis may follow its injection. Extravasation of dantrolene may result in tissue necrosis. Diuresis may accompany intravenous administration, reflecting addition of mannitol to the dantrolene powder to make the solution isotonic. For this reason, it is recommended that patients receiving intravenous dantrolene also have a uri-

FIGURE 33–9.   Plasma dantrolene concentrations following induction of anesthesia (time 0) and until 48 hours postoperatively in 10 malignant hyperthermia-susceptible patients. The total dose of dantrolene was 5 mg·kg⁻¹ orally in three or four divided doses with the last dose 4 hours before induction of anesthesia. All patients had plasma concentrations of dantrolene more than 2.8 μg·ml⁻¹ for at least 6 hours following induction of anesthesia. (From Allen GC, Cattrain CB, Peterson RG, Lakende M. Plasma levels of dantrolene following oral administration in malignant hyperthermia-susceptible patients. Anesthesiology 1988;67:900–4; with permission.)

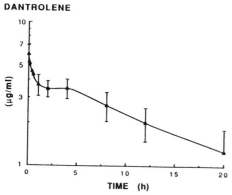

DANTROLENE

FIGURE 33–10. Plasma concentrations of dantrolene in venous blood following induction of anesthesia and administration of dantrolene 2.4 mg·kg⁻¹ IV to 10 children. Mean ± SD. (From Lerman J, McLeod ME, Strong HA. Pharmacokinetics of intravenous dantrolene in children. Anesthesiology 1989; 70:625–9; with permission.)

nary catheter in place (Flewellen et al, 1983).

Dantrolene is metabolized in the liver principally to 5-hydroxydantrolene, which is 30% to 50% as effective in depressing the twitch response. Less than 1% of dantrolene appears unchanged in the urine. The elimination half-time of dantrolene is 5 to 8 hours. The minimal effective blood level of dantrolene is not known, although plasma concentrations of 2.8 μg·ml⁻¹ or greater in animals are associated with near-maximal depression of skeletal muscle contractile activity (Allen et al, 1988). For this reason, it seems prudent to maintain blood levels of dantrolene of at least 2.8 μg·ml⁻¹ when the drug is being administered for prophylaxis against or treatment of malignant hyperthermia (Duncan, 1985).

Clinical Uses

Dantrolene is useful in the management of patients with skeletal muscle spasticity owing to upper motor neuron lesions. The maximum oral dose is 400 mg administered in four divided doses. Associated dantrolene-induced skeletal muscle weakness, however, often negates any significant improvement, despite reductions in skeletal muscle spasticity.

Dantrolene is effective in the prevention and treatment of malignant hyperthermia (Duncan,

1985). Prophylaxis in malignant hyperthermia-susceptible patients may be with oral administration of dantrolene 5 mg·kg⁻¹ in three or four divided doses every 6 hours with the last dose 4 hours preoperatively. This regimen results in plasma levels of dantrolene more than 2.8 μg·ml⁻¹ at the time of induction of anesthesia and for at least 6 hours (Fig. 33-9) (Allen et al, 1988). Alternatively, dantrolene, 2.4 mg·kg⁻¹ IV, may be administered over 10 to 30 minutes as prophylaxis just prior to induction of anesthesia, and for continued protection, one half the dose is repeated in 6 hours (Fig. 33-10) (Lerman et al, 1989). For treatment of malignant hyperthermia, the dose of dantrolene is 2 mg·kg⁻¹ IV, with repeated doses until symptoms subside or a cumulative dose of 10 mg·kg⁻¹ is reached. Despite the efficacy of dantrolene, it must be recognized the drug is not 100% effective and known triggering drugs must be avoided even when dantrolene prophylaxis is used (Fitzgibbon, 1981; Ruhland and Hinkle, 1984).

Side Effects

The most common side effect of dantrolene administration is skeletal muscle weakness. Skeletal muscle weakness may be sufficient to interfere with adequate ventilation or protection of the lungs from aspiration of gastric fluid (Watson et al, 1986). Large doses of dantrolene administered acutely as for prophylaxis against malignant hyperthermia may cause nausea, diarrhea, and blurred vision as well as skeletal muscle weakness. Uterine atony has been observed in a malignant hyperthermia-susceptible patient treated with dantrolene following cesarean section (Weingarten et al, 1987). Dantrolene administered to animals with or without verapamil has been associated with hyperkalemia (San Juan et al, 1988) (see Chapter 18).

Dantrolene produces hepatitis in approximately 0.5% of patients treated for more than 60 days. Fatal hepatitis occurs in 0.1% to 0.2% of patients treated chronically. For this reason, hepatic function should be monitored when dantrolene therapy is continued for more than 45 days. Pleural effusion may also occur with chronic therapy. Short-term use of dantrolene in preparation or treatment of malignant hyperthermia-susceptible patients is not associated with hepatotoxicity or pleural effusion.

REFERENCES

Allen GC, Cattran CB, Peterson RG, Lalande M. Plasma levels of dantrolene following oral administration in malignant hyperthermia-susceptible patients. Anesthesiology 1988;69:900–4.

Bunker ML, McWilliams M. Caffeine content of common beverages. J Am Diet Assoc 1979;74:28–32.

Camman WR, Murray RS, Mushlin PS, Lambert DH. Effects of oral caffeine on postdural puncture headache. A double-blind, placebo-controlled trial. Anesth Analg 1990;70:181–4.

Chen L, Miller FL, Malmkvist G, Clarke WR, Clergue FX, Marshall C, Marshall BE. Low-dose almitrine bismesylate enhances hypoxic pulmonary vasoconstriction in closed-chest dogs. Anesth Analg 1990;71:475–83.

Duncan PG. Availability of dantrolene in Canadian hospitals. Can Anaesth Soc J 1985;32:205–9.

Fitzgibbon DC. Malignant hyperthermia following preoperative oral administration of dantrolene. Anesthesiology 1981;54:73–5.

Flewellen EH, Nelson TE, Jones WP, Arens JF, Wagner DL. Dantrolene dose response in awake man. Implications for management of malignant hyperthermia. Anesthesiology 1983;59:275–80.

Hirsh WH, Wang SC. Selective respiratory stimulating action of doxapram compared to pentylenctetrazol. J Pharmacol Exp Ther 1974;189:1–11.

Lerman J, McLeod ME, Strong HA. Pharmacokinetics of intravenous dantrolene in children. Anesthesiology 1989;70:625–9.

Mitchell RM, Herbert DA. Potencies of doxapram and hypoxia in stimulating carotid-body chemoreceptors and ventilation in anesthetized cats. Anesthesiology 1975;42:559–66.

Moser KM, Luchsinger PC, Adamson JS, et al. Respiratory stimulation with intravenous doxapram in respiratory failure. N Engl J Med 1973;288:428–31.

Penn RD, Savoy SM, Corcos D, Latash M, Gottlieb G, Parke B, Kroin JS. Intrathecal baclofen for severe spinal spasticity. N Engl J Med 1989;320:1517–21.

Ramamurthy S, Steen SN, Winnie AP. Doxapram antagonism of meperidine-induced respiratory depression. Anesth Analg 1975;54:352–6.

Rigotti NA. Cigarette smoking and body weight. N Engl J Med 1989;320:931–3.

Ruhland G, Hinkle AJ. Malignant hyperthermia after oral and intravenous pretreatment with dantrolene in a patient susceptible to malignant hyperthermia. Anesthesiology 1984;60:159–60.

San Juan AC, Wong KC, Port JD. Hyperkalemia after dantrolene and verapamil-dantrolene administration in dogs. Anesth Analg 1988;67:759–62.

Sebel PS, Kershaw EJ, Rao WS. Effects of doxapram on postoperative pulmonary complications following thoracotomy. Br J Anaesth 1980;52:81–4.

Sill JC, Schumacher K, Southorn PA, Reuter J, Yaksh TL. Bradycardia and hypotension associated with baclofen used during general anesthesia. Anesthesiology 1986;64:255–8.

Tseng TC, Wang SC. Locus of action of centrally acting muscle relaxants, diazepam and tybamate. J Pharmacol Exp Ther 1971;178:350–60.

Watson CB, Reierson N, Norfleet EA. Clinically significant muscle weakness induced by oral dantrolene sodium prophylaxis for malignant hyperthermia. Anesthesiology 1986;65:312–4.

Weingarten AE, Korsh JI, Neuman GG, Stern SB. Postpartum uterine atony after intravenous dantrolene. Anesth Analg 1987;66:269–70.

Young RR, Delwaide PJ. Drug therapy-spasticity. N Engl J Med 1981;304:96–9.

Chapter

34

Vitamins

Vitamins are a group of structurally diverse organic substances that must be provided in small amounts in the diet for the subsequent synthesis of cofactors that are essential for various metabolic reactions. Food is the best source of vitamins, and healthy persons consuming an adequate balanced diet will not benefit from additional vitamins. Nevertheless, many otherwise healthy persons take supplemental vitamins, despite the absence of scientific evidence that these substances are necessary or useful (Herbert, 1980). Often, the patient's intake of vitamins remains undiscovered when a preoperative drug history is elicited. Excessive intake of fat-soluble vitamins, particularly vitamins A and D, is more likely to cause toxicity than is intake of water-soluble vitamins (Lewis, 1980). For example, unrecognized vitamin A–induced hydrocephalus may result in unnecessary neurosurgery. Excessive intake of vitamin D may lead to hypercalcinosis. High intake of water-soluble vitamins can elevate circulating plasma concentrations of administered salicylates and interfere with the anticoagulant action of warfarin.

The use of dietary vitamin supplements is medically indicated in situations associated with inadequate intake, malabsorption, increased tissue needs, or inborn errors of metabolism. Inadequate vitamin intake may reflect socioeconomic conditions, self-imposed dieting, or food faddism. Disturbances of vitamin absorption may occur in diseases of the liver and biliary tract, diarrhea, hyperthyroidism, small-bowel bypass surgery for treatment of obesity, and alcoholism. Antibiotic therapy may alter the usual bacterial flora of the gastrointestinal tract necessary for the synthesis of vitamin K. Loss of vitamins may occur

during hemodialysis or hyperalimentation. Indeed, multivitamin preparations for parenteral administration are essential during long-term hyperalimentation (Nichoalds et al, 1977). Infants require vitamins to support normal growth. Vitamin supplementation is also indicated for people who are on low-calorie diets. Healthy adults, however, require no vitamin supplementation except during pregnancy and lactation.

WATER-SOLUBLE VITAMINS

Water-soluble vitamins include members of the vitamin B complex (thiamine, riboflavin, nicotinic acid, pyridoxine, pantothenic acid, biotin, cyanocobalamin, and folic acid) and ascorbic acid (Fig. 34-1).

Thiamine (Vitamin B_1)

Thiamine is converted to a physiologically active coenzyme known as thiamine pyrophosphate. This coenzyme is essential for the decarboxylation of alpha-keto acids such as pyruvate and in the use of pentose in the hexose-monophosphate shunt pathway. Indeed, increased plasma concentrations of pyruvate are a diagnostic sign of thiamine deficiency.

Causes of Deficiency

The requirement for thiamine is related to the metabolic rate and is greatest when carbohydrate is the source of energy. This is important in patients maintained by hyperalimentation in which

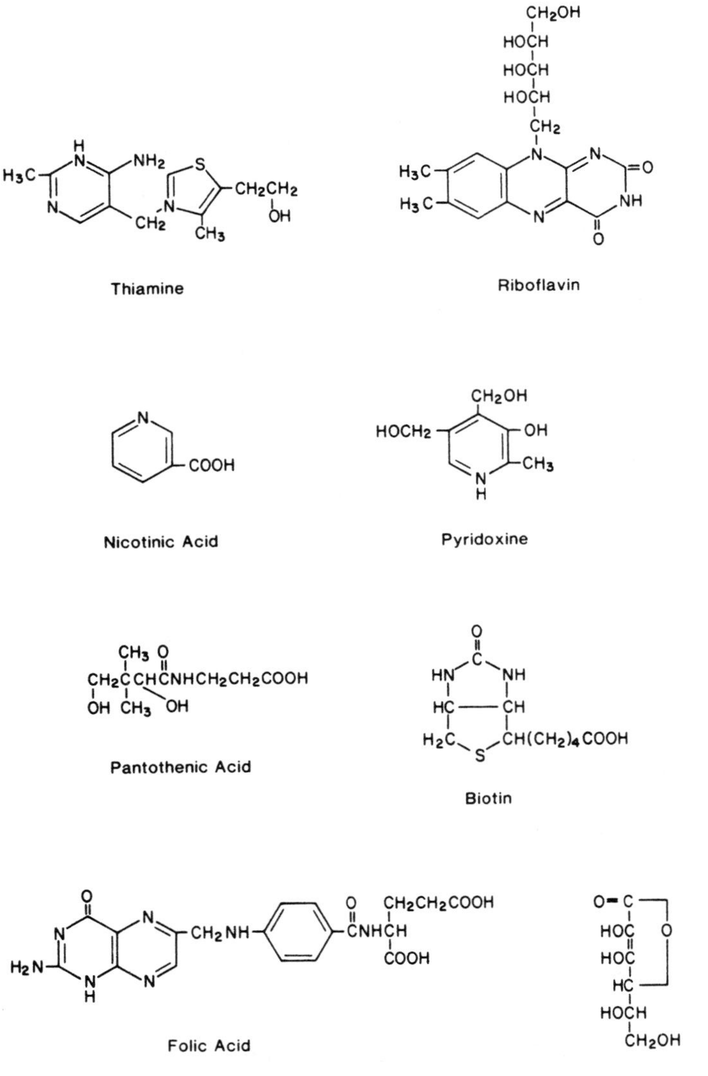

Thiamine

Riboflavin

Nicotinic Acid

Pyridoxine

Pantothenic Acid

Biotin

Folic Acid

Ascorbic Acid **FIGURE 34–1.** Water-soluble vitamins.

the majority of calories are provided in the form of glucose. Such patients should receive supplemental amounts of thiamine. Thiamine requirements are also increased during pregnancy and lactation.

Symptoms of Deficiency

Symptoms of mild thiamine deficiency (beriberi) include loss of appetite, skeletal muscle weak-ness, a tendency to develop peripheral edema, decreased blood pressure, and low body temper-ature. Severe thiamine deficiency (Korsakoff's syndrome), which often occurs in alcoholics, may be associated with peripheral polyneuritis, including areas of hyperesthesia and anesthesia of the legs, impairment of memory, and enceph-alopathy. High-output cardiac failure with exten-sive peripheral edema reflecting hypoprotein-emia is often prominent. There is flattening or inversion of the T wave and prolongation of the Q-T interval on the electrocardiogram.

Treatment of Deficiency

Severe thiamine deficiency is treated with intravenous administration of the vitamin. Once severe thiamine deficiency has been corrected, oral supplementation is acceptable.

Riboflavin (Vitamin B₂)

Riboflavin is converted in the body to one of two physiologically active coenzymes: flavin mononucleotide or flavin adenine dinucleotide. These coenzymes primarily influence hydrogen ion (H^+) transport in oxidative enzymes systems, including cytochrome C reductase, succinic dehydrogenase, and xanthine oxidase. Chlorpromazine and tricyclic antidepressants interfere with the flavokinase reaction necessary to convert riboflavin to its active coenzymes, thus increasing requirements. Tissue storage of this water-soluble vitamin is not extensive.

Symptoms of Deficiency

Pharyngitis and angular stomatitis are typically the first signs of riboflavin deficiency. Later, glossitis, red denuded lips, seborrheic dermatitis of the face, and dermatitis over the trunk and extremities occur. Anemia and peripheral neuropathy may be prominent. Corneal vascularization and cataract formation occur in some subjects. Treatment is with oral vitamin supplements that contain riboflavin.

Nicotinic Acid (Niacin)

Nicotinic acid is converted to the physiologically active coenzyme nicotinamide adenine dinucleotide (NAD) and nicotinamide adenine dinucleotide phosphate (NADP). These coenzymes are necessary to catalyze oxidation-reduction reactions essential for tissue respiration.

Symptoms of Deficiency

Nicotinic acid is an essential dietary constituent, the lack of which leads to dermatitis, diarrhea, and dementia. Pellagra is the all-inclusive term for the symptoms of nicotinic acid deficiency. The skin characteristically becomes erythematous and rough in texture, especially in areas exposed to sun, friction, or pressure. The chief symptoms referable to the digestive tract are stomatitis, enteritis, and diarrhea. The tongue becomes very red and swollen. Salivary secretions are excessive, and nausea and vomiting are common. In addition to dementia, motor and sensory disturbances of the peripheral nerves also occur, mimicking changes that accompany a deficiency of thiamine.

The dietary requirement for niacin can be satisfied not only by nicotinic acid but also by nicotinamide and the amino acid tryptophan. The relationship between nicotinic acid requirement and the intake of tryptophan explains the association of pellagra with tryptophan-deficient corn diets. Carcinoid syndrome is associated with diversion of tryptophan from the synthesis of nicotinic acid to the production of serotonin (5-hydroxytryptamine), leading to symptoms of pellagra. Isoniazid inhibits incorporation of nicotinic acid into NAD and may produce pellagra.

Pellagra is uncommon in the United States, reflecting the supplementation of flour with nicotinic acid. Common causes of pellagra include chronic gastrointestinal disease and alcoholism, which are characteristically associated with multiple nutritional deficiencies. When pellagra is severe, intravenous administration of nicotinic acid is indicated. In less severe cases, oral administration of nicotinic acid is adequate. The response to nicotinic acid is dramatic, with symptoms waning within 24 hours after initiation of therapy.

Toxic effects of nicotinic acid include flushing, pruritus, hepatotoxicity, hyperuricemia, and activation of peptic ulcer disease. Nicotinic acid has also been used to lower the plasma concentration of cholesterol (see Chapter 32).

Pyridoxine (Vitamin B₆)

Pyridoxine is converted to its physiologically active form, pyridoxal phosphate, by the enzyme pyridoxal kinase. Pyridoxal phosphate serves an important role in metabolism as a coenzyme for conversion of tryptophan to serotonin and methionine to cysteine.

Symptoms of Deficiency

Pyridoxine deficiency is frequent in alcoholics (estimated incidence 30%), manifesting as alterations in the skin, central nervous system dysfunction, and anemia. Seborrhea-like skin lesions about the eyes, nose, and mouth accompanied by glossitis and stomatitis occur. Seizures accompany deficiency of pyridoxine, and peripheral neuritis such as carpal tunnel syndrome is common. The lowered seizure threshold may reflect decreased concentrations of the inhibitory neurotransmitter gamma-aminobutyric acid, the synthesis of which requires a pyridoxal phosphate-requiring enzyme.

It is presumed that a person with a deficiency of other B vitamins may also have a relative deficiency of pyridoxine. For this reason, pyridoxine is incorporated into many multivitamin preparations for prophylactic use. Pyridoxine is unpredictably effective in the treatment of sideroblastic anemias (deficiency of hemoglobin synthesis and accumulation of iron in the mitochondria).

Drug Interactions

Isoniazid and hydralazine act as potent inhibitors of pyridoxal kinase, thus preventing synthesis of the active coenzyme form of the vitamin. Indeed, administration of pyridoxine reduces the incidence of the neurologic side effects associated with the administration of these drugs. Pyridoxine enhances the peripheral decarboxylation of levodopa and reduces its effectiveness for the treatment of Parkinson's disease. There is a decrease in the plasma concentration of pyridoxal phosphate in patients taking oral contraceptives.

Pantothenic Acid

Pantothenic acid is converted to its physiologically active form, coenzyme A, which serves as a cofactor for enzyme-catalyzed reactions involving transfer of two-carbon (acetyl) groups. Such reactions are important in the oxidative metabolism of carbohydrates, gluconeogenesis, and the synthesis and degradation of fatty acids.

Pantothenic acid deficiency in humans is rare, reflecting the ubiquitous presence of the vitamin in ordinary foods as well as its production by intestinal bacteria. No clearly defined uses of pantothenic acid exist, although it is commonly included in multivitamin preparations and in products for hyperalimentation.

Biotin

Biotin is an organic acid that functions as a coenzyme for enzyme-catalyzed carboxylation reactions and fatty acid synthesis. In adults, a deficiency of biotin manifests as glossitis, anorexia, dermatitis, and mental depression. Seborrheic dermatitis of infancy is most likely a form of biotin deficiency. For this reason, it is recommended that formulas contain supplemental biotin. Prolonged hyperalimentation may result in a deficiency of biotin.

Cyanocobalamin (Vitamin B_{12})

Cyanocobalamin and vitamin B_{12} are generic terms that are used interchangeably to designate several cobalt-containing compounds (cobalamins). Dietary vitamin B_{12} in the presence of H^+ in the stomach is released from proteins and subsequently binds to a glycoprotein intrinsic factor. This vitamin-intrinsic factor complex travels to the ileum, where it interacts with a specific receptor and is transported into the circulation. Following absorption, vitamin B_{12} binds to a beta globulin, transcobalamin II, for transport to tissues, especially the liver, which serves as a storage depot.

Causes of Deficiency

Although humans depend on exogenous sources of vitamin B_{12}, a deficient diet is rarely the cause of a deficiency state. Instead, gastric achlorhydria and decreased gastric secretion of intrinsic factor are more likely to be causes of vitamin B_{12} deficiency in adults. Antibodies to intrinsic factor may interfere with attachment of the complex to gastrin receptors in the ileum (DeAizpurua et al, 1985). Bacterial overgrowth may prevent an adequate amount of vitamin B_{12} from reaching the ileum. Surgical resection or disease of the ileum predictably interferes with the absorption of vitamin B_{12}. Finally, nitrous oxide irreversibly oxidizes the cobalt atom of vitamin B_{12} such that the activity of two vitamin B_{12}-dependent enzymes, methionine synthetase and thymidylate synthetase, are reduced (see Chapter 2).

Diagnosis of Deficiency

The plasma concentration of vitamin B_{12} is less than 200 pg·ml^{-1} when there is a deficiency state. Measurements of gastric acidity may provide indirect evidence of a defect in gastric parietal cell function, whereas the Schilling test (radioactivity in urine measured after oral administration of labeled vitamin B_{12}) can be used to quantitate ileal absorption of vitamin B_{12}. Finally, observation of reticulocytosis following a therapeutic trial of vitamin B_{12} confirms the diagnosis.

Symptoms of Deficiency

Deficiency of vitamin B_{12} results in defective synthesis of deoxyribonucleic acid (DNA), especially in tissues with the greatest rate of cell turnover. In this regard, symptoms of vitamin B_{12} deficiency manifest most often on the hematopoietic and nervous systems. Changes in the hematopoietic system are most apparent in erythrocytes, but when deficiency of vitamin B_{12} is severe, a pronounced cytopenia may occur. Clinically, the earliest sign of vitamin B_{12} deficiency is megaloblastic (pernicious) anemia. Anemia may be so severe that cardiac failure occurs, especially in elderly patients with limited cardiac reserves. Damage to the myelin sheath is the most obvious symptom of nervous system dysfunction associated with vitamin B_{12} deficiency. Demyelination and cell death occur in the spinal cord and cerebral cortex, manifesting as paresthesias of the hands and feet and diminution of sensation of vibration and proprioception with resultant unsteadiness of gait. Deep tendon reflexes are decreased, and, in advanced stages, loss of memory and mental confusion occur. Indeed, vitamin B_{12} deficiency should be considered as a possibility in elderly patients with psychosis. Folic acid therapy will correct the hematopoietic, but not the nervous system, effects produced by vitamin B_{12} deficiency.

Treatment of Deficiency

Vitamin B_{12} is available in a pure form for oral or parenteral use or in combination with other vitamins for oral administration. These preparations are of little value in the treatment of patients with deficiency of intrinsic factor or ileal disease. In the presence of clinically apparent vitamin B_{12} deficiency, oral absorption cannot be relied on; the preparation of choice is cyanocobalamin administered intramuscularly. For example, in the patient with neurologic changes, leukopenia, or thrombocytopenia, treatment must be aggressive. Initial treatment is with intramuscular administration of vitamin B_{12} and oral administration of folic acid. An increase in hematocrit does not occur for 10 to 20 days. The plasma concentration of iron, however, usually declines within 48 hours, because iron is now used in the formation of hemoglobin. Platelet counts can be expected to reach normal levels within 10 days of treatment; the granulocyte count requires a longer period to normalize. Memory and sense of well-being may improve within 24 hours after initiation of therapy. Neurologic signs and symptoms that have been present for prolonged periods, however, often regress slowly and may never return to completely normal function. Indeed, neurologic damage from pernicious anemia that is not reversed after 12 to 18 months of treatment is likely to be permanent.

Once initiated, vitamin B_{12} therapy must be continued indefinitely at monthly intervals. It is important to monitor plasma concentrations of vitamin B_{12} and examine the peripheral blood cells every 3 to 6 months to confirm the adequacy of therapy.

Hydroxocobalamin has hematopoietic activity similar to that of vitamin B_{12} but appears to offer no advantage despite its somewhat longer duration of action. Furthermore, some patients develop antibodies to the complex of hydroxocobalamin and transcobalamin II. Large doses of hydroxocobalamin have been proposed for treatment of cyanide poisoning owing to nitroprusside (see Chapter 16). Conceptually, cyanide reacts with hydroxocobalamin to form cyanocobalamin.

Folic Acid

Folic acid is transported and stored as 5-methylhydrofolate following absorption from the small intestine, principally the jejunum. Conversion to the metabolically active form, tetrahydrofolate, is dependent on the activity of vitamin B_{12}. Tetrahydrofolate acts as an acceptor of one-carbon units necessary for (1) conversion of homocysteine to methionine, (2) conversion of serine to glycine, (3) synthesis of DNA, and (4) synthesis of purines. Supplies of folic acid are maintained by ingestion of food and by enterohepatic circulation of the vitamin. Virtually all foods contain folic acid, but protracted cooking can destroy up to 90% of the vitamin.

Causes of Deficiency

Folic acid deficiency is a common complication of diseases of the small intestine, such as sprue, that interfere with absorption of the vitamin and its enterohepatic recirculation. Alcoholism reduces intake of folic acid in food, and enterohepatic recirculation may be damaged by the toxic effect of alcohol on hepatocytes. Indeed, alcoholism is the most common cause of folic acid deficiency, with reductions in the plasma concentration of folic acid manifesting within 24 to 48 hours of steady alcohol ingestion. Drugs that inhibit dehydrofolate reductase (methotrexate or trimethoprim) or interfere with absorption and storage of folic acid in tissue (phenytoin) may cause folic acid deficiency.

Symptoms of Deficiency

Megaloblastic anemia is the most common manifestation of folic acid deficiency. This anemia cannot be distinguished from that caused by a deficiency of vitamin B_{12}. Folic acid deficiency, however, is confirmed by the presence of a folic acid concentration in the plasma of less than 4 ng·ml^{-1}. Furthermore, the rapid onset of megaloblastic anemia produced by folic acid deficiency (1 to 4 weeks) reflects the limited *in vivo* stores of this vitamin and contrasts with the slower onset (2 to 3 years) of symptoms of vitamin B_{12} deficiency.

Treatment of Deficiency

Folic acid is available as an oral preparation alone or in combination with other vitamins and as a parenteral injection. The therapeutic uses of folic acid are limited to the prevention and treatment of deficiencies. For example, pregnancy is associated with increased folic acid requirements, and oral supplementation, usually in a multivitamin preparation, is indicated. In the presence of megaloblastic anemia as a result of folic acid deficiency, the administration of the vitamin is associated with a decrease in the plasma concentration of iron within 48 hours, reflecting new erythropoiesis. Likewise, the reticulocyte count begins to rise within 48 to 72 hours, and the

hematocrit begins to increase during the second week of therapy.

LEUCOVORIN. Leucovorin (citrovorum factor) is a metabolically active, reduced form of folic acid. Following treatment with folic acid antagonists, such as methotrexate, patients may receive leucovorin (rescue therapy), which serves as a source for tetrahydrofolate that cannot be formed owing to drug-induced inhibition of dihydrofolate reductase (see Chapter 29). It is possible that nitrous oxide, by inhibiting vitamin B_{12}-dependent enzymes, would impair the efficacy of leucovorin as a source for tetrahydrofolate (see Chapter 2) (Ueland et al, 1986).

Ascorbic Acid (Vitamin C)

Ascorbic acid is a six-carbon compound structurally related to glucose. This vitamin acts as a coenzyme and is important in a number of biochemical reactions, mostly involving oxidation. For example, ascorbic acid is necessary for the synthesis of collagen, cornitine, and corticosteroids. Ascorbic acid is readily absorbed from the gastrointestinal tract and many foods, such as orange juice and lemon juice, have a high content of ascorbic acid. When gastrointestinal absorption is impaired, ascorbic acid can be administered intramuscularly or intravenously. Apart from its role in nutrition, ascorbic acid is commonly used as an antioxidant to protect the natural flavor and color of many foods.

Despite contrary claims, controlled studies do not support the efficacy of even large doses of ascorbic acid in treating cancer of the colon or viral respiratory tract infections (Moertel et al, 1985; Pitt and Costrini, 1979). A risk of large doses of ascorbic acid is the formation of kidney stones resulting from the excessive excretion of oxalate. Excessive ascorbic acid doses can also enhance the absorption of iron and interfere with anticoagulant therapy.

Symptoms of Deficiency

A deficiency of ascorbic acid is known as scurvy. Humans, in contrast to many other mammals, are unable to synthesize ascorbic acid, emphasizing the need for dietary sources of the vitamin to prevent scurvy. Specifically, humans lack the hepatic enzyme necessary to produce ascorbic acid from gluconate (Crandon et al, 1940). Manifestations of scurvy include gingivitis, rupture of capillaries with formation of numerous petechiae, and failure of wounds to heal. An associated anemia may reflect a specific function of ascorbic acid on hemoglobin synthesis. Scurvy is evident when the plasma concentration of ascorbic acid is less than 0.15 mg·dl^{-1}.

Scurvy is encountered among the elderly, alcoholics, and drug addicts. Ascorbic acid requirements are increased during pregnancy, lactation, and stresses such as infection or following surgery. Infants receiving formula diets with inadequate concentrations of ascorbic acid can develop scurvy. Patients receiving hyperalimentation should receive supplemental ascorbic acid. Urinary loss of infused ascorbic acid is large, necessitating daily doses of 200 mg to maintain normal concentrations in plasma of 1 mg·dl^{-1} (Nicholalds et al, 1977). Increased urinary excretion of ascorbic acid is caused by salicylates, tetracyclines, and barbiturates.

FAT-SOLUBLE VITAMINS

Fat-soluble vitamins are vitamins A, D, E, and K (Fig. 34-2). They are absorbed from the gastrointestinal tract by complex processes that parallel absorption of fat. Thus, any condition that causes malabsorption of fat, such as obstructive jaundice, may result in deficiency of one or all these vitamins. Fat-soluble vitamins are stored principally in the liver and excreted in the feces. Because these vitamins are metabolized very slowly, overdose may produce toxic effects. Vitamin D, despite its name, functions as a hormone.

Vitamin A

Vitamin A exists in a variety of forms, including retinol and 3-dehydroretinol. This vitamin is important in the function of the retina, integrity of mucosal and epithelial surfaces, bone development and growth, reproduction, and embryonic development. It also has a stabilizing effect on various membranes and regulates membrane permeability. Vitamin A may exert transcriptional control of the production of specific proteins, a process that has important implications with respect to regulation of cellular differentiation and development of malignancies. Limitations in the therapeutic use of vitamin A for antineoplastic uses are the associated hepatotoxicity and its failure to distribute to specific organs (Smith and Goodman, 1976).

Major dietary sources of vitamin A are liver, butter, cheese, milk, certain fish, and various

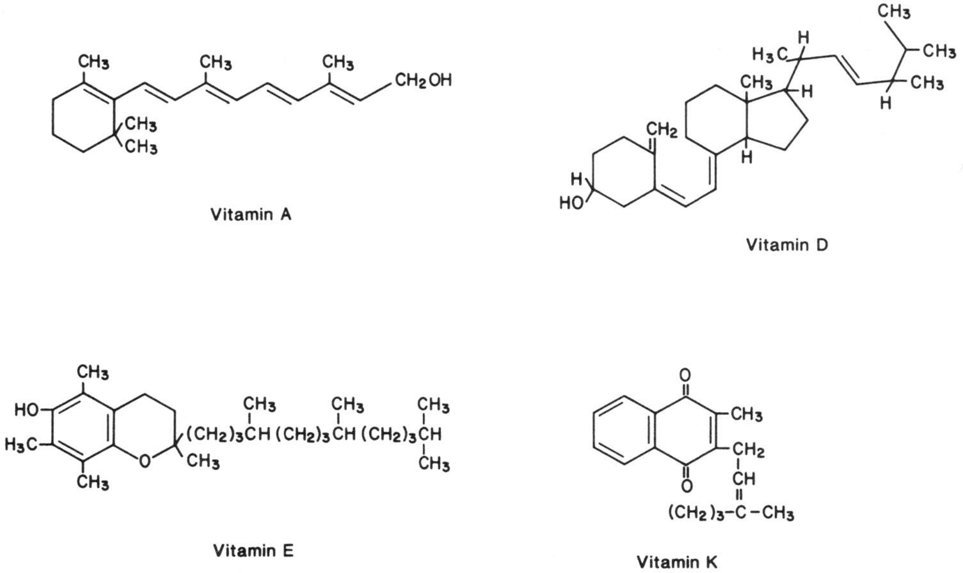

FIGURE 34-2. Fat-soluble vitamins.

yellow or green fruits and vegetables. Fish liver oils contain large amounts of vitamin A. Sufficient vitamin A is stored in the liver of well-nourished persons to satisfy requirements for several months. Plasma concentrations of vitamin A are maintained at the expense of hepatic reserves and thus do not always reflect a person's vitamin A status. Vitamin A may interact with cellular proteins, which function analogously to receptors for estrogens and other steroids.

Symptoms of Deficiency

In the United States, it is estimated that approximately 15% of the population has plasma concentrations of vitamin A less than 20 $\mu g \cdot dl^{-1}$, indicating a risk of deficiency (Roels, 1970). Most of these people are infants or children. Signs and symptoms of mild vitamin A deficiency are easily overlooked. Skin lesions such as follicular hyperkeratosis and infections are often the earliest signs of deficiency. Nevertheless, the most recognizable manifestation of vitamin A deficiency is night blindness (nyctalopia), which occurs only when depletion is severe. Respiratory infections are increased as bronchial epithelium for mucous secretion undergoes keratinization. Keratinization and drying of the epidermis occur. Urinary calculi are frequently associated with vitamin A deficiency, which may reflect epithelial changes that provide a nidus around which a calculus is formed. Abnormalities of reproduction include impairment of spermatogenesis and spontaneous abortion. Impairment of taste and smell is common in patients with vitamin A deficiency, presumably reflecting a keratinizing effect. Decreased erythropoiesis may be masked by abnormal losses of fluids.

Hypervitaminosis A

Hypervitaminosis A is the toxic syndrome that results from excessive ingestion of vitamin A, particularly in children (James et al, 1982). Typically, high vitamin A intakes have resulted from overzealous prophylactic vitamin therapy. Plasma concentrations of vitamin A more than 300 $\mu g \cdot dl^{-1}$ are diagnostic of hypervitaminosis A. Treatment consists of withdrawal of the vitamin source, which is usually followed within 7 days by disappearance of the manifestations of excess vitamin activity.

Early signs and symptoms of vitamin A toxicity include irritability, vomiting, and dermatitis. Fatigue, myalgia, loss of body hair, diplopia, nystagmus, gingivitis, stomatitis, and lymphadenopathy have been observed. Hepatosplenomegaly is accompanied by cirrhosis, portal vein hypertension, and ascites. Intracranial pressure may be increased, and neurologic symptoms, including papilledema, may mimic those of a brain tumor (pseudotumor cerebri). The diagnosis is confirmed by radiologic demonstration of hyperostoses underlying tender hard swellings on the extremities and the occipital region of the head. The activity of plasma alkaline phosphatase is increased, reflecting osteoblastic activity. Hypercalcemia may occur as a result of bone destruction. Bones continue to grow in length but not in thickness, with increased susceptibility to fractures. Congenital abnormalities may occur in infants whose mothers have consumed excessive amounts of vitamin A during pregnancy. Psychiatric disturbances may mimic depression or schizophrenia.

Vitamin D

Vitamin D is the generic designation for several sterols and their metabolites that act as hormones to maintain plasma concentrations of calcium (Ca^{2+}) and phosphate ions in an optimal range for normal neuromuscular function, mineralization of bone, and other Ca^{2+}-dependent functions. This regulation of plasma concentrations of Ca^{2+} and phosphate ions reflects the ability of vitamin D to facilitate absorption of these ions from the gastrointestinal tract and enhance the mobilization of Ca^{2+} from bone. In addition, there may be a direct effect of vitamin D on proximal renal tubules that results in increased retention of Ca^{2+} and phosphate ions.

The principal provitamin of vitamin D in tissues, 7-dehydrocholesterol, is synthesized in the skin and converted to vitamin D on exposure of the skin to sunlight. Vitamin D is also absorbed from the gastrointestinal tract following oral administration. Bile salts are necessary for this absorption, emphasizing that hepatic or biliary dysfunction may impair passage of vitamin D into the circulation. Absorbed vitamin D is hydroxylated in the liver to calcifediol, which is further hydroxylated in the kidneys to calcitriol, the active form of vitamin D. This conversion to calcitriol is regulated in a negative feedback manner by the plasma Ca^{2+} concentration. The elimination half-time of calcitriol is 3 to 5 days.

Symptoms of Deficiency

A deficiency of vitamin D results in reduced concentrations of Ca^{2+} and phosphate ions, with the subsequent stimulation of parathyroid hormone secretion. Parathyroid hormone acts to restore plasma Ca^{2+} concentrations at the expense of bone Ca^{2+}. In infants and children, this results in failure to mineralize newly formed osteoid tissue and cartilage, causing the formation of soft bone, which, with weight bearing, results in deformities known as rickets. In adults, vitamin D deficiency results in osteomalacia. Anticonvulsant therapy with phenytoin increases target organ resistance to vitamin D, resulting in an increased incidence of rickets and osteomalacia.

Hypervitaminosis D

Administration of excessive amounts of vitamin D results in hypervitaminosis manifesting as hypercalcemia, skeletal muscle weakness, fatigue, headache, and vomiting. Early impairment of renal function from hypercalcemia manifests as polyuria, polydipsia, proteinuria, and decreased urine concentrating ability. In addition to withdrawal of the vitamin, treatment includes increased fluid intake and administration of corticosteriods.

Vitamin E (Tocopherol)

Vitamin E is a group of fat-soluble substances occurring in plants. There is little persuasive evidence that vitamin E is nutrtionally significant in humans or of any value in therapy (Roberts, 1981). Alpha-tocopherol is the most abundant and important of the eight naturally occurring tocopherols that constitute vitamin E. An important chemical feature of the tocopherols is that they are antioxidants. In acting as an antioxidant, vitamin E presumably prevents oxidation of essential cellular constituents or prevents the formation of toxic oxidation products. There seems to be a relationship between vitamins A and E in which vitamin E facilitates the absorption, hepatic storage, and use of vitamin A. In addition, vitamin E seems to protect against the development of hypervitaminosis A by enhancing use of the vitamin. Vitamin E is stored in adipose tissue and is thought to stabilize the lipid portions of cell membranes. Other functions attributed to vitamin E are inhibition of prostaglandin production and stimulation of an essential cofactor in corticosteroid metabolism.

Vitamin E requirements may be increased in people exposed to high oxygen environments or in those taking therapeutic doses of iron or large doses of thyroid replacement. The severity of retrolental fibroplasia is alleged to be less in premature infants given large daily doses of vitamin E (Hittner et al, 1981). Vitamin E may be important in hematopoiesis, with occasional forms of anemia responding favorably to the administration of alpha-tocopherol.

Despite absence of conclusive supportive evidence, vitamin E has been used in females for treatment of recurrent abortion and for sterility in both sexes. In animals, vitamin E deficiency leads to the development of muscular dystrophy, but there is no evidence that similar events occur in humans. Changes similar to those observed in skeletal muscle have occurred in cardiac muscle of animals. Nevertheless, carefully controlled studies have failed to show any value in the treatment of cardiac failure in patients. There are data that support an association between low plasma levels of vitamin E and the risk of developing lung cancer (Menkes et al, 1986).

Vitamin K

Vitamin K is a lipid-soluble dietary principal essential for the biosynthesis of several factors required for normal blood clotting (see Chapter 57). Phytonadione (vitamin K_1) is present in a variety of foods and is the only natural form of vitamin K available for therapeutic use. Vitamin K_2 represents a series of compounds that are synthesized by gram-positive bacteria in the gastrointestinal tract. Synthesis of vitamin K provides approximately 50% of the estimated daily requirement of vitamin K; the rest is supplied by the diet. Vitamin K is absorbed from the gastrointestinal tract only in the presence of adequate quantities of bile salts. Vitamin K accumulates in the liver, spleen, and lungs, but, despite its lipid solubility, significant amounts are not stored in the body for prolonged periods.

Mechanism of Action

Vitamin K functions as an essential cofactor for the hepatic microsomal enzyme system that converts glutamic acid residues to gamma-carboxyglutamic acid residues in factors II (prothrombin), VII, IX, and X. The gamma-carboxyglutamic acid residues make it possible for these coagulation factors to bind Ca^{2+} and attach to phospholipid surfaces, leading to clot formation. If vitamin K deficiency occurs, the plasma concentrations of these coagulation factors decrease and a hemorrhagic disorder develops. This disorder is characterized by ecchymoses, epistaxis, hematuria, and gastrointestinal bleeding; postoperative hemorrhage is also a possibility. Prothrombin time is used to monitor vitamin K activity.

Clinical Uses

Vitamin K is administered to treat its deficiency and attendant reduction in plasma concentrations of prothrombin and related clotting factors. Deficiency of vitamin K may be due to (1) inadequate dietary intake, (2) decreased bacterial synthesis owing to antibiotic therapy, (3) impaired gastrointestinal absorption resulting from obstructive biliary tract disease and absence of bile salts, or (4) hepatocellular disease. Neonates have hypoprothrombinemia owing to vitamin K deficiency until adequate dietary intake of the vitamin occurs and normal intestinal bacterial flora are established. Indeed, at birth, the normal infant has only 20% to 40% of the adult plasma concentrations of clotting factors II, VII, IX, and X. These plasma concentrations decline even further during the first 2 to 3 days after birth, then begin to increase toward adult values after approximately 6 days. In premature infants, plasma concentrations of clotting factors are even lower. Human breast milk has low concentrations of vitamin K. Administration of vitamin K, 0.5 to 1 mg IM at birth, to the normal neonate prevents the decline in concentration of vitamin K–dependent clotting factors in the first days following birth but does not increase these concentrations to adult levels.

Vitamin K replacement therapy is not effective when severe hepatocellular disease is responsible for decreased production of clotting factors. In the absence of severe hepatocellular disease and the presence of adequate bile salts, the administration of oral vitamin K preparations is effective in reversing hypoprothrombinemia. Phytonadione and menadione are the vitamin K preparations most often used to treat hypoprothrombinemia.

PHYTONADIONE. Phytonadione (vitamin K_1) is the preferred drug to treat hypoprothrombinemia, particularly when large doses or prolonged therapy is necessary. Hypoprothrombinemia of the neonate is treated with phytonadione, 0.5 to 1 mg IM, within 24 hours of birth. A frequent indication for phytonadione is to reverse the effects of oral anticoagulants. For example, phytonadione, 10 to 20 mg orally or administered intravenously at a rate of 1 mg·min^{-1}, is usually adequate to reverse the effects of oral anticoagulants (see Chapter 27). The oral and intramuscular routes of administration are less likely than intravenous injections of phytonadione to cause side effects and are thus preferred for nonemergency reversal of oral anticoagulants. Even large doses of phytonadione are ineffective against heparin-induced anticoagulation. Vitamin K supplementation is also indicated for patients receiving prolonged parenteral hyperalimentation, especially if antibiotics are concomitantly administered.

Intravenous injection of phytonadione may cause life-threatening allergic reactions characterized by hypotension and bronchospasm. Intramuscular administration may produce local hemorrhage at the injection site in hypoprothrombinemic patients. In neonates, doses of phytonadione more than 1 mg may cause hemolytic anemia and increase plasma concentrations of unbound bilirubin, thus increasing the risk of kernicterus. The occurrence of hemolytic anemia reflects a deficiency of glycolytic enzymes in some neonates.

MENADIONE. Menadione has the same actions and uses as phytonadione (Fig. 34-3). Water-soluble salts of menadione do not require the presence of bile salts for their systemic absorption following oral administration. This characteristic becomes important when malabsorption of vitamin K is due to biliary obstruction.

Menadione hemolyzes erythrocytes in patients genetically deficient in glucose-6-phosphate dehydrogenase as well as in neonates, particularly the premature infant. This hemolysis and occasionally hepatic toxicity reflects combination of menadione with sulfhydryl groups in

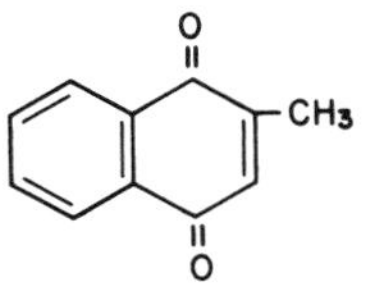

FIGURE 34–3. Menadione.

tissues. Kernicterus has occurred following menadione administration of neonates. For this reason, menadione is not recommended for treatment of hemorrhagic disease of the neonate. Administration of large doses of menadione or phytonadione may depress liver function, particularly in the presence of preexisting liver disease.

REFERENCES

Crandon JH, Lund CC, Dill DB. Experimental human scurvy. N Engl J Med 1940;223:353–69.

DeAizpurua HJ, Ungar B, Toh B-H. Autoantibody to the gastrin receptor in pernicious anemia. N Engl J Med 1985;313:479–83.

Herbert V., The vitamin craze. Arch Intern Med 1980;140:173–80.

Hittner HM, Godio LB. Rudolph AJ, et al. Retrolental fibroplasia: Efficacy of vitamin E in double-blind clinical study of preterm infants. N Engl J Med 1981;305:1365–71.

James MB, Leonard JC, Fraser JJ, Stuemby JH. Hypervitaminosis A: Case report. Pediatrics 1982;69:112–5.

Lewis JG. Adverse reactions to vitamins. Adverse Drug React Acute Poisoning Rev 1980;82:296–9.

Menkes MS, Comstock GW, Vuilleumier JP, Helsing KJ, Rider AA, Brookmeyer R. Serum beta-carotene, vitamins A and E, selenium, and the risk of lung cancer. N Engl J Med 1986;315;1250–4.

Moertel CG, Fleming TR, Creagan ET, Rubin J, O'Connell MJ, Ames MM. High-dose vitamin C versus placebo in the treatment of patients with advanced cancer who have had no prior chemotherapy. N Engl J Med 1985;312:137–41.

Nichoalds GE, Meng HC, Caldwell MD. Vitamin requirements in patients receiving total parenteral nutrition. Arch Surg 1977;112:1061–4.

Pitt HA, Costrini AM. Vitamin C prophylaxis in marine recruits. JAMA 1979;241:908–11.

Roberts HJ. Perspective on vitamin E as therapy. JAMA 1981;246:129–31.

Roels OA. Vitamin A physiology. JAMA 1970;214:1097–1102.

Smith FR, Goodman DS. Vitamin A transport in human vitamin A toxicity. N Engl J Med 1976;294:805–8.

Ueland PM, Refsum H, Wesenberg F, Kvinnsland S. Methotrexate therapy and nitrous oxide anesthesia. N Engl J Med 1986;314:1514.

Minerals

Many minerals function as essential constituents of enzymes and regulate a variety of physiologic functions including (1) maintenance of osmotic pressure, (2) transport of oxygen, (3) skeletal muscle contraction, (4) integrity of the central nervous system, (5) growth and maintenance of tissues and bones, and (6) hematopoiesis. Elements present in the body in large amounts include calcium, phosphorus, sodium, potassium, magnesium, sulfur, and chloride. Iron, cobalt in vitamin B_{12}, copper, zinc, chromium, selenium, manganese, and molybdenum are present in trace amounts (Ulmer, 1977). Nickel, tin, silicon, and arsenic also are considered essential elements.

In the absence of absorption abnormalities, severe mineral deficiency is unlikely because most minerals, with the exception of zinc, are present in foods. Nevertheless, iron deficiency is common especially in infants and females consuming inadequate diets. Modest zinc and copper deficiencies also occur frequently.

A balanced, varied diet supplies adequate amounts of trace elements, and dietary supplements containing minerals should be used only when evidence of deficiency exists or when demands are known to be increased, as during pregnancy and lactation. Mineral deficiencies may develop during prolonged hyperalimentation, emphasizing the importance of monitoring plasma concentrations of trace metals in these patients.

CALCIUM

Calcium is present in the body in greater amounts than any other mineral. The plasma concentration of calcium is maintained between 4.5 and 5.5 $mEq \cdot L^{-1}$ (8.5 to 10.5 $mg \cdot dl^{-1}$) by an endocrine control system that includes vitamin D, parathyroid hormone, and calcitonin (see Chapter 52). Total plasma calcium consists of (1) calcium bound to albumin, (2) calcium complexed with citrate and phosphate ions, and (3) freely diffusible ionized calcium. It is the ionized fraction of calcium that produces physiologic effects.

The ionized fraction of calcium represents approximately 45% of the total plasma concentration. Therefore, a normal plasma ionized calcium concentration is 2 to 2.5 $mEq \cdot L^{-1}$. Symptoms due to altered concentrations of calcium reflect changes in the plasma level of ionized calcium. This emphasizes the need to evaluate disturbances in calcium homeostasis by measuring ionized calcium. It must be remembered that the concentration of ionized calcium is dependent on arterial pH, with acidosis increasing and alkalosis decreasing the concentration. Likewise, the plasma albumin concentration must be considered when interpreting plasma calcium measurements. For example, albumin in plasma binds nonionized calcium. When the serum albumin concentration is decreased, there will be less calcium bound to protein. As a result, nonionized calcium is free to return to storage sites such as bone. Therefore, the total plasma calcium concentration can be reduced in the presence of hypoalbuminemia, but symptoms of hypocalcemia do not occur unless the ionized calcium concentration is also reduced. For example, hypocalcemia due to hypoproteinemia is not accompanied by signs of hypocalcemia unless the ionized fraction of calcium in the plasma is also decreased. For this reason, accurate interpretation of the plasma concentration of calcium is not possible without knowledge of the plasma albumin concentration.

Role of Calcium

Calcium is important for (1) neuromuscular transmission, (2) skeletal muscle contraction, (3) cardiac muscle contractility, (4) blood coagulation, and (5) exocytosis necessary for release of neurotransmitters and autocoids. In addition, calcium is a principal component of bone (see the section entitled "Bone Composition"). The cytoplasmic concentration of ionized calcium is maintained at low levels by extrusion from the cell and sequestration of this ion within cellular organelles, particularly mitochondria, and in skeletal muscle, the sarcoplasmic reticulum. The large gradient for calcium across cell membranes contributes to the use of this ion for transmembrane signaling in response to various electrical or chemical stimuli.

Cardiovascular Effects

Calcium chloride, 7 mg·kg^{-1} IV, transiently increases myocardial contractility and cardiac output in halothane-anesthetized volunteers (Denlinger et al, 1975). At the same time, heart rate decreases while mean arterial pressure and central venous pressure are unchanged. The net effect of these changes is a decrease in calculated systemic vascular resistance. Calcium administered in the presence of an artificial mechanical heart (myocardial contractility constant) also produces transient dose-related reductions in systemic vascular resistance (Stanley et al, 1976). Heart rate slowing may reflect a calcium-mediated increase in vagal activity or a delay in transmission of the cardiac impulse through the atrioventricular node. Absence of an effect of calcium on pulmonary blood flow is suggested by the lack of change in shunt fraction following the intravenous injection of calcium (Gallagher et al, 1984).

It is possible that anesthetics could alter the effect of calcium on the heart. For example, anesthetics that produce peripheral vasoconstriction or vasodilation could augment or diminish the peripheral vascular effects of calcium. Volatile anesthetics may induce myocardial depression by

inhibiting calcium uptake by the sarcoplasmic reticulum (Su and Kerrick, 1980). The direct dilating effect of ketamine on cerebral arteries may be in part due to interference with the transmembrane influx of calcium (Fukada et al, 1983).

Hypocalcemia

The most common cause of hypocalcemia (plasma concentration of calcium less than 4.5 mEq·L^{-1}) is a reduced plasma concentration of albumin. Other causes of hypocalcemia include hypoparathyroidism, acute pancreatitis, vitamin D deficiency, and chronic renal failure associated with hyperphosphatemia. Malabsorption states resulting in deprivation of calcium and vitamin D readily lead to hypocalcemia.

Citrate binding of calcium can result in hypocalcemia, but this is unlikely in adults because the rate of whole blood infusion must be more than 50 ml·70 kg^{-1}·min^{-1} before a reduction in the plasma concentration of ionized calcium occurs (Fig. 35-1) (Denlinger et al, 1976). This reflects mobilization of calcium from bone and the ability of the liver to metabolize rapidly citrate to bicarbonate ions. Therefore, the arbitrary intravenous administration of supplemental calcium to adults receiving stored blood is not indi-

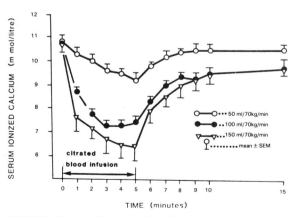

FIGURE 35–1. Citrate-induced reductions in serum-ionized calcium concentrations do not occur unless the rate of whole blood infusion is more than 50 ml·70 kg^{-1}·min^{-1}. (From Denlinger JK, Kaplan JA, Lecky JH, Wollman H. Cardiovascular responses to calcium administered intravenously to man during halothane anesthesia. Anesthesiology 1975;42:390–7; with permission).

cated in the absence of objective evidence for hypocalcemia. Supplemental intravenous administration of calcium, however, is indicated to prevent citrate-induced hypocalcemia in the neonate receiving stored blood. Furthermore, in the presence of hypothermia or severe liver dysfunction, the ability to metabolize citrate to bicarbonate may be reduced and the administration of supplemental calcium may be indicated.

Symptoms

Symptoms of hypocalcemia include (1) tetany, (2) circumoral paresthesias, (3) increased neuromuscular excitability, (4) laryngospasm, and (5) seizures. Abrupt reductions in the ionized portions of the total plasma concentration of calcium are associated with hypotension and increased left ventricular end-diastolic pressure (Fig. 35-2) (Denlinger and Nahrwold, 1976; Scheidegger and Drop, 1979). The Q-T interval on the electrocardiogram (ECG) may be prolonged, but this is not a consistent observation. For this reason, monitoring the Q-T interval on the ECG may not be a clinically reliable guide to the presence or absence of hypocalcemia.

Treatment

Treatment of hypocalcemia is with a commercially available preparation of calcium (calcium chloride, calcium gluconate, or calcium glucept-ate) administered intravenously. In this regard, equal elemental doses of calcium chloride and calcium gluconate are approximately 1:3 (Cote et al, 1987). For example, calcium chloride contains 27 mg·ml^{-1} of calcium and calcium gluconate contains 9 mg·ml^{-1} of calcium. Administered intravenously over 5 to 15 minutes, equivalent doses of calcium chloride (3 to 6 mg·kg^{-1}) and calcium gluconate (7 to 14 mg·kg^{-1}) produce similar effects on the plasma concentrations of calcium. Calcium chloride is irritating to veins and may cause discomfort in an awake patient. Calcium gluceptate contains 23 mg·ml^{-1} of calcium and may be injected intramuscularly as well as intravenously.

HYPERKALEMIA.   Life-threatening hyperkalemia is initially treated by intravenous administration of calcium. Calcium counteracts the effects of hyperkalemia by activation of calcium channels so that ion flux through these channels generates an action potential and restores myocardial contractil-

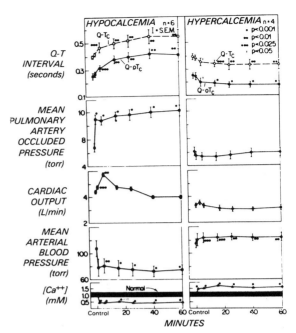

FIGURE 35–2. Abrupt reductions in the plasma concentration of calcium result in an increased Q–T interval on the electrocardiogram, increased mean pulmonary artery occlusion pressure, and decreased mean arterial pressure. Hypercalcemia results in a decreased Q–T interval on the electrocardiograms. (From Scheidegger D, Drop LJ. The relationship between duration of Q–T interval and plasma ionized calcium concentration: Experiments with acute, steady-state Ca^{++} changes in the dog. Anesthesiology 1979; 51:143–8; with permission.)

ity. For example, intravenous administration of 10 to 20 ml of a 10% calcium chloride solution restores myocardial contractility in 1 to 2 minutes. This effect lasts 15 to 20 minutes. Serum potassium concentrations are not significantly changed by intravenous administration of calcium.

Other measures to treat hyperkalemia include intravenous infusion of sodium bicarbonate and glucose-insulin mixtures. Sodium bicarbonate (0.5 to 1 mEq·kg^{-1}) causes a shift of potassium into cells in approximately 5 minutes. Serum potassium will be decreased as long as pH is increased. Glucose-insulin infusion (50 ml of 50% glucose plus 10 units of regular insulin) produces a sustained transfer of potassium into cells resulting in a 1.5 to 2.5 mEq·L^{-1} decrease in serum potassium concentration after approximately 30 minutes.

Hypercalcemia

Neoplasms are the most common cause of life-threatening hypercalcemia (plasma calcium concentration more than 5.5 mEq·L^{-1}), presumably reflecting secretion by tumors of a substance that stimulates resorption of bone. The most common cause of mild hypercalcemia is hyperparathyroidism. Hyperparathyroidism due to chronic renal failure may manifest as hypercalcemia following successful renal transplantation. Sarcoidosis is associated with hypercalcemia in approximately 20% of patients.

Symptoms

Early symptoms of hypercalcemia include sedation and vomiting. When the plasma concentration of calcium exceeds approximately 10 mEq·L^{-1}, cardiac conduction disturbances, characterized on the ECG as a prolonged P-R interval, a wide QRS complex, and a shortened Q-T interval, occur. The most serious adverse effect of persistent hypercalcemia is renal damage.

Treatment

Asymptomatic patients with mild hypercalcemia are managed with intravenous administration of saline and furosemide to speed the renal excretion of calcium. When the plasma concentration of calcium is more than 10 mEq·L^{-1}, aggressive therapy is necessary. In this situation, administration of plicamycin (formerly named mithramycin), a cytotoxic antibiotic, lowers plasma concentrations of calcium in 24 to 48 hours at doses one tenth those used for chemotherapy. This calcium-lowering property reflects the ability of plicamycin to reduce the responsiveness of osteoclasts to parathyroid hormone. Calcitonin is also potentially useful for lowering the plasma concentration of calcium. Corticosteroids, such as prednisone, reduce the absorption of calcium from the gastrointestinal tract by antagonizing the actions of vitamin D. The onset of calcium-lowering effects by this mechanism, however, is often slow (7 to 14 days) and unpredictable. Edetate disodium (EDTA) is a chelating agent that forms soluble complexes with calcium in the blood and results in a rapid decrease in the plasma concentration of ionized calcium. Hypocalcemia may be so abrupt, however, that seizures occur. For this reason, EDTA is rarely used except as a slow intravenous infusion.

Bone Composition

Bone is composed of an organic matrix that is strengthened by deposits of calcium salts. The organic matrix is more than 90% collagen fibers, and the remainder is a homogenous material called ground substance. *Ground substance* is composed of proteoglycans that include chondroitin sulfate and hyaluronic acid.

Salts deposited in the organic matrix of bone are composed principally of calcium and phosphate ions in a combination known as *hydroxyapatites*. Many different ions can conjugate to these bone crystals, explaining deposition of radioactive substances in bone that may lead to an osteogenic sarcoma from prolonged irradiation.

The initial stage of bone production is the secretion of collagen and ground substance of osteoblasts. Calcium salts precipitate on the surfaces of collagen fibers, forming nidi that develop into hydroxyapatite crystals. Bone is continually being deposited by osteoblasts and is constantly being absorbed where osteoclasts are active. Parathyroid hormone controls the bone absorptive activity of osteoclasts. Except in growing bones, the rates of bone deposition and absorption are equal so the total mass of bone remains constant.

Bone is deposited in proportion to the compressional load that the bone must carry. For example, continual physical stress stimulates new bone formation. The deposition of bone at points of compression may be caused by a piezoelectric effect. Indeed, small amounts of electrical current flowing in bone cause osteoblastic activity at the negative end of the current flow. Fracture of a bone maximally activates osteoblasts involved in the break. The resulting bulge of osteoblastic tissue and new bone matrix is known as the callus.

Osteoblasts secrete large amounts of alkaline phosphatase when they are actively depositing bone matrix. As a result, the rate of new bone formation is mirrored by measurement of the plasma concentration of alkaline phosphatase. Alkaline phosphatase is also elevated by any disease process that causes destruction of bone (osteomalacia or rickets).

Calcium salts almost never precipitate in normal tissues other than bone. A notable exception, however, is atherosclerosis, in which calcium precipitates in the walls of large arteries. Calcium salts are also frequently deposited in degenerating tissues or in old blood clots.

Exchangeable Calcium

Exchangeable calcium is that calcium in the body which is in equilibrium with calcium in the extracellular fluid. Most of this exchangeable calcium is in bone, providing a rapid buffering mechanism to keep the calcium concentration in the extracellular fluid from changing excessively in either direction. The movement of exchangeable calcium in either direction is so rapid that a single passage of blood containing excess calcium through bone will remove almost all the excess calcium. It is estimated that approximately 5% of the cardiac output flows through bone.

Teeth

The major functional parts of teeth are the enamel, dentine, cementum, and pulp (Fig. 35-3) (Guyton, 1986). The tooth can also be divided into (1) the crown, which is the portion that protrudes above the gum; (2) the root, which protrudes into the bony sockets of the jaw; and (3) the neck, which separates the crown from the root.

STRUCTURE. Dentine is the main body of the tooth and is composed principally of hydroxyapatite crystals similar to those in bone. In contrast to bone, dentine lacks osteoblasts, osteoclasts, or spaces for nerves or blood vessels.

The outer surface of the tooth is covered by a layer of enamel that is formed prior to eruption of the tooth by special epithelial cells. Once the tooth has erupted, no more enamel is formed. Enamel is a protein that is extremely hard and resistant to corrosive agents such as acids or enzymes.

Cementum is a body substance secreted by cells that line the socket of the tooth. This substance is important in holding the tooth in place in the body socket. Cementum has characteristics similar to normal bone including the presence of osteoblasts and osteoclasts.

The inside of each tooth is filled with pulp containing nerves, blood vessels, and lymphatics.

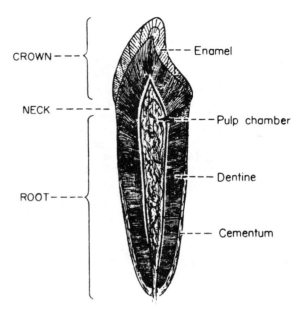

FIGURE 35–3.   Schematic depiction of the functional parts of a tooth. (From Guyton AC. Textbook of Medical Physiology, 6th ed. Philadelphia: WB Saunders, 1986; with permission.)

DENTITION.   Each human forms two sets of teeth. The first set of 20 teeth are known as deciduous teeth. These deciduous teeth erupt between the ages of 7 and 24 months and remain in place until 6 to 13 years of age. After each deciduous tooth is lost, a permanent tooth replaces it. An additional 8 to 12 molars appear posteriorly in the mandible and maxilla, making a total of 28 to 32 permanent teeth.

DENTAL CARIES.   Dental caries result from the action of bacteria, the most common of which are streptococci. The first event in the development of caries is deposit of *plaque,* which is a film of precipitated products of saliva and food. Bacteria inhabit this plaque, setting the stage for the development of caries. Formation of acids by bacteria is the most important event leading to the development of caries. Enamel is very resistant to demineralization by acids and thus serves as a primary barrier to the development of caries. Once the carious process has penetrated through enamel of dentine, it proceeds rapidly, reflecting the high solubility of the dentine salts.

Bacteria depend on carbohydrates for survival, explaining the association between caries and the frequent ingestion of food containing glucose. If carbohydrates are eaten in small amounts through the day, such as in the form of candy, bacteria are supplied with their preferential metabolic substrate for many hours of the day. Conversely, ingestion of carbohydrates only at meals followed by brushing of the teeth limits the availability of metabolic substrate to the bacteria and thus reduces the likelihood of caries formation.

Teeth formed in children who drink fluorinated water develop enamel that is approximately three times more resistant than normal to the formation of caries. Fluorine does not make the enamel harder than usual, but instead displaces hydroxyl ions in the hydroxyapatite crystals; this in turn makes the enamel less soluble.

PHOSPHATE

Inorganic phosphate exists in two forms in the plasma. Because it is difficult to measure the exact amounts of each ion, it is common to express the total quantity of phosphate as $mg \cdot dl^{-1}$ of phosphorus. The total quantity of inorganic phosphorus represented by both phosphate ions is 3.0 to 4.5 $mg \cdot dl^{-1}$.

Phosphate is important in energy metabolism and maintenance of acid-base balance. For example, phosphate ions are the most abundant buffer in the distal renal tubule, allowing excretion of large quantities of hydrogen ions. These ions are also important intracellular buffers.

Vitamin D stimulates the systemic absorption of phosphate from the gastrointestinal tract. This absorbed phosphate is almost entirely excreted by the kidneys since parathyroid hormone blocks reabsorption from the renal tubules. Conversely, vitamin D facilitates reabsorption of phosphate from the proximal renal tubules.

A decrease in the plasma concentration of phosphate permits the presence of a greater plasma concentration of calcium and inhibits deposition of new bone salts. Hypophosphatemia (phosphorus concentration less than 1.5 $mg \cdot dl^{-1}$) causes a decrease in the concentration of adenosine triphosphate and 2,3-diphosphoglycerate in erythrocytes. Profound skeletal muscle weakness sufficient to contribute to ventilatory failure may be a manifestation of hypophosphatemia (Aubier et al, 1985). Central nervous system dysfunction and peripheral neuropathy may accompany hy-

pophosphatemia. Alcohol abuse and prolonged parenteral nutrition are causes of phosphorus deficiency.

MAGNESIUM

Magnesium is the fourth most plentiful cation in the body and the second most plentiful intracellular cation after potassium. Only 1% of magnesium is present in the extracellular fluid compartment and 30% of this is bound to protein. Approximately one half of total body magnesium is present in bone and 20% in skeletal muscle. Normal plasma concentrations of magnesium are achieved and maintained by absorption from the small intestine and renal excretion.

Magnesium is an obligatory cofactor in all cells that contain adenosine triphosphate (ATP). Membrane sodium–potassium-dependent ATPase, which is necessary for maintaining normal intracellular concentrations of potassium, requires magnesium. Adenylate cyclase mediated production of adenosine monophosphate is magnesium dependent. An inhibitory action on smooth muscle contraction is suggested by bronchodilation in asthmatic patients (Okayama et al, 1987). Magnesium is necessary for the presynaptic release of acetylcholine from nerve endings and may produce effects similar to calcium-entry–blocking drugs.

Abnormalities of plasma and cellular magnesium concentrations frequently accompany other electrolyte abnormalities. For example, there is a strong correlation between hypomagnesemia and hypokalemia. Including measurement of plasma magnesium concentrations with that of other electrolytes has been recommended because more than 8% of patients with hypomagnesemia or hypermagnesemia are currently clinically unrecognized (Whang and Ryder, 1990).

Hypomagnesemia

Hypomagnesemia (serum magnesium concentration less than 1.6 $mEq \cdot L^{-1}$) may be the most common unrecognized electrolyte deficiency (Gambling et al, 1988). Patients at increased risk for hypomagnesemia include chronic alcoholics (because of magnesium-poor diets and increased renal losses of magnesium from alcohol) and those in critical care units maintained on hyperalimentation solutions containing inadequate amounts of magnesium. Malabsorption syndromes and protracted vomiting or diarrhea may also lead to hypomagnesemia. Patients undergoing cardiac surgery requiring cardiopulmonary bypass may be vulnerable to hypomagnesemia owing to dilutional effects from pump-priming solutions or preexisting effects of diuretic therapy. Also, secondary aldosteronism associated with chronic congestive heart failure increases renal excretion of magnesium. Increased fluxes of magnesium may occur in organ donors owing to large-volume infusion of non-electrolyte solutions to prevent hypernatremia that can occur secondary to diabetes insipidus. In this regard, organ transplant recipients may experience cyclosporin-induced loss of magnesium via the kidneys, resulting in hypomagnesemia. There is a strong correlation between hypokalemia and hypomagnesemia. Repletion of cellular potassium concentrations is impaired in the presence of unrecognized and untreated hypomagnesemia, perhaps reflecting impaired ion pump activity. A low serum magnesium concentration is almost always due to a total body depletion of this cation.

Manifestations of hypomagnesemia on the ECG are nonspecific and mimic those associated with hypokalemia. Ventricular cardiac dysrhythmias are a frequent symptom of hypomagnesemia that may manifest for the first time during anesthesia. Neuromuscular manifestations (Chvostek's and Trousseau's signs, carpopedal spasm, stridor, and skeletal muscle weakness) resemble hypocalcemia. Severe deficiency may lead to seizures, coma, or both. Chronic hypomagnesemia is more likely to be symptomatic than an acute deficiency, suggesting a normalization of the intracellular to extracellular magnesium ratio with time similar to chronic hypokalemia. Emergency treatment of life-threatening hypomagnesemia is infusion of magnesium, 10 to 20 mg·kg^{-1} IV, administered over 10 to 20 minutes.

Hypermagnesemia

Hypermagnesemia is present when the plasma concentration of magnesium is more than 2.6 mEq·L^{-1}. The most common cause is administration of magnesium to treat toxemia of pregnancy (pregnancy-induced hypertension). Therapeutic plasma concentrations of magnesium for treating toxemia of pregnancy are 4 to 6 mEq·L^{-1}. Patients with chronic renal dysfunction are at an increased risk for developing hypermagnesemia because excretion of magnesium is dependent on glomerular filtration rate.

Hypermagnesemia is associated with sedation, cardiac depression, and suppression of peripheral neuromuscular function due to reductions in acetylcholine release from motor nerve endings as well as decreased responsiveness of the postjunctional membrane to acetylcholine. Furthermore, magnesium exerts a direct relaxant effect on skeletal muscles. Deep tendon reflexes diminish when the plasma concentration of magnesium is more than 10 mEq·L^{-1}. Paralysis of respiratory muscles and heart block may appear at concentrations that are more than 12 mEq·L^{-1}. Treatment of life-threatening hypermagnesemia is with calcium gluconate, 10 to 15 mg·kg^{-1} IV, followed by fluid loading and drug-induced diuresis.

Magnesium enhances the effects of nondepolarizing muscle relaxants, emphasizing the need to reduce the usual dose of these muscle relaxants by one half to one third in patients being treated with magnesium sulfate (Ghoneim and Long, 1970) (see Chapter 8). Potentiation of succinylcholine by magnesium sulfate therapy is not a consistent observation (Gambling et al, 1988). Calcium administered intravenously is not predictably effective in antagonizing magnesium-enhanced neuromuscular blockade.

IRON

Iron present in food is absorbed from the proximal small intestine, especially the duodenum, into the circulation where it is bound to transferrin. *Transferrin* is a glycoprotein that delivers iron to specific receptors on cell membranes. Approximately 80% of the iron in plasma enters the bone marrow to be incorporated into new erythrocytes. In addition to bone marrow, iron is incorporated into reticuloendothelial cells of the liver and spleen. Iron is also an essential component of many enzymes necessary for energy transfer. A normal range for the plasma iron concentration is 50 to 150 µg·dl^{-1}.

Iron that is stored in tissues is bound to protein as ferritin or in an aggregated form known as hemosiderin. Hemoglobin synthesis is the principal determinant of the plasma iron turnover rate. When blood loss occurs, hemoglobin concentration is maintained by mobilizaton of tissue iron stores. Indeed, hemoglobin concentrations become chronically decreased only after these iron reserves are depleted. For this reason, the presence of a normal hemoglobin concentration is not a sensitive indicator of tissue iron stores. The infant, parturient, and menstruating female may have iron requirements that exceed amounts available in the diet. Absorption of iron from the gastrointestinal tract is increased by ascorbic acid or the presence of iron deficiency. Antacids bind iron and impair its absorption.

Iron Deficiency

Iron deficiency is estimated to be present in 20% to 40% of menstruating females and in fewer than 5% of adult males and postmenopausal females. Attempts to achieve better iron balance in large parts of the population are evidenced by addition of iron to flour, use of iron-fortified formulas for infants, and the prescription of iron-containing vitamin supplements during pregnancy.

Causes

Causes of iron deficiency anemia include inadequate dietary intake of iron (nutritional) or increased iron requirements due to pregnancy, blood loss, or interference with absorption from the gastrointestinal tract. Most nutritional iron deficiency in the United States is mild. Severe iron deficiency is usually the result of blood loss, either from the gastrointestinal tract or, in females from the uterus. Partial gastrectomy and sprue are causes of inadequate iron absorption.

Diagnosis

Iron deficiency initially results in a reduction of iron stores and a parallel decrease in erythrocyte content of iron. Depleted iron stores are indicated by decreased plasma concentrations of ferritin and the absence of reticuloendothelial hemosiderin in the bone marrow aspirate. Plasma ferritin concentrations less than $12 \ \mu g \cdot dl^{-1}$ are diagnostic of iron deficiency. Iron deficiency anemia is present when depletion of total body iron is associated with a recognizable decrease in the blood concentration of hemoglobin. The large physiologic variation in hemoglobin concentra-

tion, however, makes it difficult to reliably identify all individuals with iron deficiency anemia.

The frequency of iron deficiency anemia in infancy and in the menstruating or parturient female makes an exhaustive search for the cause of mild anemia less important. Conversely, in males and postmenopausal females, in whom iron balance should be favorable, it becomes more important to pursue the search for a site of bleeding whenever anemia is present.

Treatment

Prophylactic use of iron preparations should be reserved for individuals at high risk for developing iron deficiency, such as pregnant and lactating females, low-birth-weight infants, and females with heavy menses. The inappropriate prophylactic use of iron should be avoided in adults because of excessive accumulation of iron, which may damage tissues.

Administration of medicinal iron is followed by an increased rate of erythrocyte production that manifests as an improved hemoglobin concentration within 72 hours. If the concentration of hemoglobin before treatment is reduced by more than $3 \ g \cdot dl^{-1}$, an average daily incremental increase of $0.2 \ g \cdot dl^{-1}$ of hemoglobin is achieved with the usual therapeutic doses of oral or parenteral iron. An increase of $2 \ g \cdot dl^{-1}$ or more in the plasma concentration of hemoglobin within 3 weeks is evidence of a positive response to iron. If a positive response does not occur within this time, the presence of (1) continuous bleeding, (2) an infectious process, or (3) impaired gastrointestinal absorption of iron should be considered.

There is no justification for continuing iron therapy beyond 3 weeks if a favorable response in the hemoglobin concentration has not occurred. Once a response to iron therapy is demonstrated, the medication should be continued until the hemoglobin concentration is normal. Iron therapy may be continued beyond this point for 4 to 6 weeks if it is desired to reestablish tissue iron stores. The replenishment of tissue iron stores requires several months of therapy.

ORAL IRON. Ferrous sulfate administered orally is the most frequently used approach for the treatment of iron deficiency anemia. Ferric salts are less efficiently absorbed than ferrous salts from the gastrointestinal tract. Ferrous sulfate is available as syrup, pills, or tablets. Although other salts of the ferrous form of iron are available, they offer little, or no advantage, over sulfate preparations. The usual therapeutic dose of iron for adults to treat iron deficiency anemia is 2 to 3 mg·kg^{-1} (200 mg daily) in three divided doses. Prophylaxis and treatment of mild nutritional iron deficiency can be achieved with modest dosages of iron such as 15 to 30 mg daily if the object is the prevention of iron deficiency in pregnant patients.

Nausea and upper abdominal pain are the most frequent side effects of oral iron therapy particularly if the dosage is more than 200 mg daily. Hemochromatosis is unlikely to result from oral iron therapy that is administered to treat nutritional anemia. Fatal poisoning from overdose of iron is rare, but children 1 to 2 years of age are most vulnerable. Symptoms of severe iron poisoning may manifest within 30 minutes as vomiting, abdominal pain, and diarrhea. In addition, there may be sedation, hyperventilation due to acidosis, and cardiovascular collapse. Hemorrhagic gastroenteritis and hepatic damage are often prominent at autopsy. When iron overdose is suspected, a plasma concentration more than 0.5 mg·dl^{-1} confirms the presence of a life-threatening situation that should be treated with deferoxamine.

PARENTERAL IRON. Parenteral iron acts similarly to oral iron but should be used only when patients cannot tolerate or do not respond to oral therapy (continuing loss is greater than can be replaced because of limitations to oral absorption). For example, parenteral iron therapy is necessary when disease processes, such as sprue, impair gastrointestinal absorption of iron. In addition, tissue iron stores may be rapidly restored by administration of parenteral iron in contrast to the slow response with oral therapy. There is no evidence, however, that the therapeutic response to parenteral iron is more prompt than that achieved with oral iron.

Iron dextran injection contains 50 mg·ml^{-1} of iron and is available for intramuscular or intravenous use. After absorption, the iron must be split from the glucose molecule of the dextran before it becomes available to tissue. Intramuscular injection is painful, and there is concern about malignant changes at the injection site. For these reasons, intravenous administration of iron is preferred over intramuscular injection. A dose of 500

mg of iron can be infused intravenously over 5 to 10 minutes.

The principal side effect of parenteral iron therapy is the rare occurrence of a severe allergic reaction, presumably owing to the presence of dextran. Less severe reactions include headache, fever, generalized lymphadenopathy, and arthralgias. Hemosiderosis is more likely to occur with parenteral iron therapy that bypasses gastrointestinal regulatory mechanisms.

COPPER

Copper is present in ceruloplasmin and is a constituent of other enzymes, including dopamine beta-hydroxylase and cytochrome C oxidase. It is bound to albumin and is an essential component of several proteins. Copper is thought to act as a catalyst in the storage and release of iron to form hemoglobin. It is believed to be essential for the formation of connective tissues, hematopoiesis, and function of the central nervous system. Copper deficiency is rare in the presence of an adequate diet. Supplements of copper should be given during prolonged hyperalimentation.

ZINC

Zinc is a cofactor of enzymes and is essential for cell growth and synthesis of nucleic acid, carbohydrates, and proteins. Adequate zinc is provided by a diet containing sufficient animal protein. Diets in which protein is obtained primarily from vegetable sources may not supply adequate zinc.

Zinc deficiency may occur in elderly or debilitated patients or during periods of increased requirements as in growing children, pregnancy, lactation, or infection. Severe zinc deficiency is most likely in the presence of malabsorption syndromes. Based on animal evidence, it has been suggested that maternal zinc deficiency during pregnancy may have teratogenic effects. Cutaneous manifestations of zinc deficiency may occur during prolonged hyperalimentation, emphasizing the need for zinc supplements in these patients. During hemodialysis, zinc chloride may be added to the dialysis bath. Symptoms of zinc deficiency include disturbances in taste and smell, suboptimal growth in children, hepatosplenomegaly, alopecia, cutaneous rashes, glossitis, and stomatitis.

CHROMIUM

Chromium is important in a cofactor complex with insulin and thus is involved in normal glucose use. Deficiency has been accompanied by a diabetes-like syndrome, peripheral neuropathy, and encephalopathy.

SELENIUM

Selenium is a constituent of several metabolically important enzymes. A selenium-dependent glutathione peroxidase is present in human erythrocytes. There seems to be a close relationship between vitamin E and selenium. Deficiency of selenium has been associated with cardiomyopathy, suggesting the need to add this trace element to supplements administered during prolonged hyperalimentation.

MANGANESE

Manganese is concentrated in mitochondria, especially in the liver, pancreas, kidneys, and pituitary. It influences the synthesis of mucopolysaccharides, stimulates hepatic synthesis of cholesterol and fatty acids, and is a cofactor in many enzymes. Deficiency is unknown clinically, but supplementation is recommended during prolonged hyperalimentation.

MOLYBDENUM

Molybdenum is an essential constituent of many enzymes. It is well absorbed from the gastrointestinal tract and is present in bones, liver, and kidneys. Deficiency is rare, whereas excessive ingestion has been associated with a gout-like syndrome.

REFERENCES

Aubier M, Murciano D, Lecocguic Y, et al. Effect of hypophosphatemia on diaphragmatic contractility in patients with acute respiratory failure. N Engl J Med 1985;313:420–4.

Cote CJ, Drop LJ, Daniels AL, Hoaglin DC. Calcium chloride versus calcium gluconate: Comparison of ionization and cardiovascular effects in children and dogs. Anesthesiology 1987;66:465–70.

Denlinger JK, Kaplan JA, Lecky JH, Wollman H. Cardiovascular responses to calcium administered intravenously to man during halothane anesthesia. Anesthesiology 1975;42:390–7.

Denlinger JK, Nahrwold ML. Cardiac failure associated with hypocalcemia. Anesth Analg 1976; 55:34–6.

Denlinger JK, Nahrwold ML, Gibbs PS, Lecky JH. Hypocalcemia during rapid blood transfusion in anesthetized man. Br J Anaesth 1976;48: 995–1000.

Fukada S. Murakawa T, Takeshita H, Toda N. Direct effects of ketamine on isolated canine cerebral and mesenteric arteries. Anesth Analg 1983; 62:553–8.

Gallagher JD, Geller EA, Moore RA, Botros SB, Jose AB, Clark DL. Hemodynamic effects of calcium chloride in adults with regurgitant valve lesions. Anesth Analg 1984;63:723–8.

Gambling DR, Birmingham CL, Jenkins LC. Magnesium and the anaesthetist. Can J Anaesth 1988; 35:644–54.

Ghoneim MM, Long JP. The interaction between magnesium and other neuromuscular blocking agents. Anesthesiology 1970;32:23–7.

Guyton AC. Textbook of Medical Physiology. 6th ed. Philadelphia. WB Saunders, 1986.

Okayama H, Aikawa T, Okayama M, Sasaka H, Mue S, Takishima T. Bronchodilating effect of intravenous magnesium sulfate in bronchial asthma. JAMA 1987;257:1076–8.

Scheidegger D, Drop LJ. The relationship between duration of Q-T interval and plasma ionized calcium concentration: Experiments with acute, steady-state (Ca++) changes in the dog. Anesthesiology 1979; 51:143–8.

Stanley TH, Isern-Amaral J, Liu W-S, Lunn JK, Gentry S. Peripheral vascular versus direct cardiac effects of calcium. Anesthesiology 1976;45:46–58.

Su JY, Kerrick WGL. Effects of enflurane and functionally skinned myocardial fibers from rabbits. Anesthesiology 1980;52:385–9.

Ulmer DD. Trace elements. N Engl J Med 1977; 297:318–21.

Whang R, Ryder KW. Frequency of hypomagnesemia and hypermagnesemia. JAMA 1990;263:3063–4.

36

Blood Components and Substitutes

INTRODUCTION

Blood components and certain drugs are most often administered systemically to overcome specific coagulation defects. Topical application of hemostatics is used to control surface bleeding and capillary oozing. Blood substitutes lack coagulation activity but are administered systemically to replace and maintain intravascular fluid volume.

BLOOD COMPONENTS

The advantages of blood components include (1) replacement of only the deficient blood procoagulant, cell, or protein; (2) minimization of the likelihood of circulatory overload; and (3) avoidance of transfusion of unnecessary donor plasma, which may contain undesirable antigens or antibodies. Administration of specific components is recommended in all circumstances other than acute hemorrhage. In the presence of acute hemorrhage, whole blood is indicated to replace both oxygen-carrying capacity and intravascular fluid volume. A unit of whole blood can be divided into several components (Table 36-1).

Packed Erythrocytes

Packed erythrocytes are prepared by removing most of the plasma from whole blood at any time during the dating period. The resulting volume is about 300 ml, and the hematocrit is 70% to 80%. Preparation of packed erythrocytes from whole blood just prior to transfusion results in the infusion of less sodium (Na^+) and potassium (K^+) ions, ammonia, citrate, and lactic acid. As a result, packed erythrocytes so prepared are useful for administration to patients with renal or hepatic dysfunction. The decreased amount of plasma infused with packed erythrocytes reduces the likelihood of allergic transfusion reactions as compared with whole blood. Packed erythrocytes are stored at 1 to 6 C. The expiration date for these cells is not different from that of the whole blood from which they are derived. The addition of adenine to the citrate-phosphate-dextrose preservative (CPD-A) can prolong the expiration date from 21 days to at least 35 days, as reflected by the fact at least 70% of the erythrocytes remain viable at the time of transfusion. Adenine increases erythrocyte survival by allowing cells to resynthesize adenosine triphosphate (ATP) needed to drive metabolic reactions. Glucose is also added to maintain glycolysis during prolonged storage with adenine. Nephrotoxicity from precipitation of a metabolite of adenine in the renal tubules is unlikely considering the estimated amount of CPD-A blood (60 units) that would be required before toxic levels occurred. Adenine-glucose-mannitol-sodium chloride (ADSOL) preservative extends the shelf life of blood to 49 days.

The expiration date for frozen erythrocytes stored at 65 C is 3 years. Once the unit has been thawed and deglycerolized or saline washed, however, it is outdated in 24 hours. The normal function of frozen packed erythrocytes after prolonged storage reflects the maintenance of concentrations of 2,3-diphosphoglycerate and ATP in the erythrocyte at levels near those present at the time the cells were frozen. At present, the major indication for frozen erythrocytes is as a source of rare blood types (Chaplin, 1984). Otherwise, the cost of frozen erythrocytes is too great to justify their more frequent use. Furthermore, transmission of viral hepatitis still can occur following administration of frozen erythrocytes (Alter et al, 1978).

Packed erythrocytes are the product of choice when the goal is to increase oxygen-carrying capacity in the absence of preexisting hypovolemia. Many clinicians believe that packed erythrocytes may be used to replace blood loss that is less than 1500 ml in an adult. One unit of packed erythrocytes typically elevates the hemoglobin concentration 1 $g \cdot dl^{-1}$. Administration of packed erythrocytes is facilitated by reconstituting them with crystalloid solutions (5% dextrose in 0.9% saline, 0.9% saline, Normosol) so as to reduce viscosity. Lactated Ringer's solution should probably not be used for this purpose because the calcium ions that are present could induce clotting. A diluent that is hypotonic with respect to plasma (glucose solutions) may cause osmotic lysis of infused erythrocytes.

Table 36–1
Components Available from Whole Blood

Component	Content	Approximate Volume (ml)	Shelf Life
Packed erythrocytes	Erythrocytes Leukocytes Plasma Clotting factors	300	35 days in CPD-A 49 days in ADSOL
Fresh frozen plasma	Clotting factors	225	Frozen—1 year Thawed—6 hours
Cryoprecipitated antihemophiliac factor	Factor VIII	Lyphilized powder	Determined by manufacturer
Factor IX concentrate	Factor IX Some of factors II, VII, and X	Lyphilized powder	Determined by manufacturer
Fibrinogen	Fibrinogen		
Platelet concentrates	Platelets Few leukocytes Some plasma Few erythrocytes	50	1–5 days
Granulocyte concentrates	Leukocytes Platelets Few erythrocytes	50–300	24 hours
Albumin	5% Albumin 25% Albumin	250 or 500 50 or 100	3 years
Plasma protein	Albumin Alpha- and beta-globulins	500	3 years
Immune globulin	Gamma-globulin	1–2	3 years

CPD-A, citrate-phosphate-dextrose–adenine; ADSOL, adenine-glucose-mannitol-sodium chloride.

Fresh Frozen Plasma

Fresh frozen plasma is the liquid portion of a single unit of whole blood that has been separated from the erythrocytes within 6 hours and frozen promptly. It may be stored at −18 C for up to 1 year. After thawing in a water bath at 37 C, the unit must be administered within a few hours.

Fresh frozen plasma contains all procoagulants except platelets in a concentration of 1 unit·ml^{-1} and is specifically indicated for patients with documented deficiencies of labile plasma coagulation factors. Fresh frozen plasma is also effective for the rapid reversal of oral anticoagulants. An infrequent use of fresh frozen plasma is for management of patients with antithrombin III deficiency who require heparin for surgery or treatment of thrombosis. Consistent with the ability of fresh frozen plasma to provide supplemental antithrombin III is the observation that infusion of this material potentiates the effects of systemic heparinization (Fig. 36-1) (Barnette et al, 1988). There is no documentation that fresh frozen plasma has a beneficial effect when used as part of the transfusion management of patients with massive hemorrhage but in the absence of a documented clotting factor deficiency (Bove, 1985). Even when packed erythrocytes are used to replace blood loss equivalent to one blood volume, clotting factors in the form of fresh frozen plasma may not be necessary to maintain the prothrombin time or plasma thromboplastin time at normal levels (Murray et al, 1988).

A substantial Na$^+$ load is associated with the administration of fresh frozen plasma. Dosage of fresh frozen plasma is determined by clinical response and, when possible, by laboratory measurements of plasma concentrations of appropriate coagulation factors. Compatibility for ABO antigens is desirable, but cross-matching is not necessary. Life-threatening allergic reactions may occur, and transmission of diseases, including hepatitis and acquired immunodeficiency syndrome, is possible (Bove, 1985).

Plasma

Plasma is the liquid portion of a single unit of citrated whole blood separated during the dating period. Storage is at 1 to 6 C for no more than 5 days beyond the expiration date of the whole blood from which it was derived. Plasma is used as a volume expander in treatment of burns and,

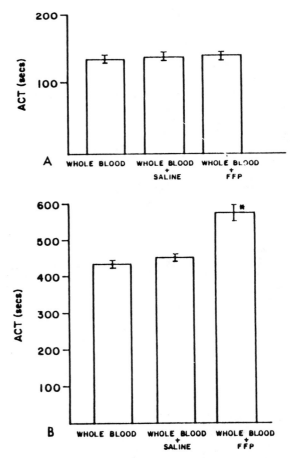

FIGURE 36–1. The *in vitro* addition of fresh frozen plasma (*FFP*) to blood containing heparin significantly (*P < 0.05) prolongs the activated coagulation time (*ACT*). (From Barnette RB, Shupak RC, Pontius J, Rao AK. *In vitro* effect of fresh frozen plasma on the activated coagulation time in patients undergoing cardiopulmonary bypass. Anesth Analg 1988; 67:57–60; with permission.)

occasionally, as a source of stable clotting factors II, VII, IX, and X. Cross-matching is desirable but not mandatory. Dosage of plasma is determined by clinical response and, when possible, by measurements of the plasma concentration of appropriate coagulation factors.

Cryoprecipitated Antibemophiliac Factor

Cryoprecipitated antihemophiliac factor (factor VIII) is that fraction of plasma that precipitates when fresh frozen plasma is thawed (Hoyer, 1981). This fraction can then be stored for future use. Cryoprecipitate is useful for treating hemophilia A because it contains high concentrations of factor VIII (80 to 120 units) in a volume of only about 10 ml. This preparation does not contain factor IX, and the content of factor VIII varies from donor to donor. Cryoprecipitate should be kept at room temperature after thawing and used within 3 hours.

Commercial factor VIII concentrates, in contrast to single-donor cryoprecipitate, contain a standardized amount of antihemophiliac factor (Hoyer, 1981). These preparations, however, are more expensive than cryoprecipitated antihemophiliac factor and have a potentially greater risk for transmitting viral diseases because they are prepared from pooled plasma derived from a large number of donors. Indeed, hepatitis is the most common adverse side effect of pooled plasma products, reflecting the multiple donor sources of the fibrinogen that are present.

Hemolytic anemia may occur when cryoprecipitated antihemophiliac factor is given to individuals with group A, B, or AB erythrocyte antigens. These patients should be treated with cryoprecipitate from type-specific or type O donors who have low titers of antibodies. About 10% to 15% of patients with hemophilia A develop an immunoglobulin inhibitor that inactivates infused antihemophiliac factor. Assay for this inhibitor should be performed in all hemophiliacs prior to cryoprecipitate infusion, especially preoperatively. Multiple transfusions of cryoprecipitate may result in hyperfibrinogenemia, emphasizing the substantial fibrinogen content of these preparations.

The major portion of transfused cryoprecipitate remains in the intravascular space with an elimination half-time of about 12 hours. Hemophilia A patients with factor VIII levels that are greater than 5% of normal usually do not experience spontaneous bleeding. Effective hemostasis during and after major surgery, however, requires maintenance of a factor VIII level of at least 40% of normal for 7 to 10 days (Ellison, 1977).

Desmopressin

Desmopressin, a synthetic analogue of antidiuretic hormone, greatly increases factor VIII activity in patients with mild to moderate hemophilia and von Willebrand's disease (see Chapter 23). Doses of 0.3 to 0.5 μg·kg^{-1} IV given before

and soon after dental surgery have prevented abnormal bleeding. Even cholecystectomy, thoracotomy, and tonsillectomy have been performed successfully in hemophiliac patients treated with desmopressin. This drug has been administered to improve hemostasis following complex cardiopulmonary bypass procedures, perhaps reflecting desmopressin-induced release of von Willebrand factor necessary for adequate activity of factor VIII and optimal adhesion of platelets (Czer et al, 1987; Salzman et al, 1986). Nevertheless, routine administration of desmopressin to patients undergoing elective cardiac surgery does not alter blood loss following cardiopulmonary bypass (Hackman et al, 1989). Decreases in blood pressure associated with evidence of peripheral vasodilation may occur in association with infusion of desmopressin (D'Alauro and Johns, 1988). In contrast to blood components, desmopressin administration does not introduce the risk of transmission of viral diseases.

Factor IX Concentrate

Factor IX concentrate (prothrombin complex, plasma thromboplastin component) is prepared from pooled plasma. Cryoprecipitated antihemophiliac factor preparations do not contain factor IX. Factor IX concentrates can be infused without typing or cross-matching. Hypervolemic reactions do not occur because of the concentrated nature of these products and the small amount of fluid needed for administration. Factor IX concentrates are stable for at least 12 hours at room temperature following reconstitution.

Factor IX concentrates have a significant potential to cause hepatitis because of the pooled origin of these products. In addition, there is a high risk of thrombotic complications associated with infusion, presumably reflecting the high concentrations of prothrombin and factor X that result from factor IX (Fuerth and Mahrer, 1981). This complication seems particularly likely and severe in patients with preexisting liver disease.

Fibrinogen

Fibrinogen preparations carry a high risk of hepatitis and, for this reason, are no longer commercially available. If fibrinogen is required, cryoprecipitated antihemophiliac factor may be administered. More important than administration of cryoprecipitate is control of the underlying defect leading to hypofibrinogenemia. Hypofibrinogenemia is most often due to decreased synthesis by a diseased liver or increased utilization associated with disseminated intravascular coagulation.

Fibrin Glue

Fibrin glue, or cryoprecipitated fibrinogen, is prepared from bovine thrombin and human fibrinogen, which, when combined, form a clot. This glue has been used for sealing suture holes as associated with vascular anastomoses. An allergic reaction to fibrin glue has been reported (Milde, 1989).

Aminocaproic Acid

Aminocaproic acid may be of benefit in the control of hemorrhage associated with excessive fibrinolysis caused by increased plasminogen activation. This drug is a monoaminocarboxylic acid that acts as a competitive inhibitor of plasminogen activators and, to a lesser degree, inhibits plasmin (Fig. 36-2). As a result, aminocaproic acid prevents formation of excessive plasmin, which could destroy fibrinogen.

PHARMACOKINETICS. Aminocaproic acid is efficiently absorbed following oral administration and may also be administered intravenously. The usual adult dose is 5 to 6 g IV slowly every 6 hours. This dosage produces therapeutic plasma concentrations of about 13 mg·dl^{-1}. After prostatic surgery, a dose of 6 g administered over 24 hours is effective because the drug is concentrated in the urine. Indeed, unchanged aminocaproic acid is rapidly excreted by the kidneys.

CLINICAL USES. Aminocaproic acid is useful for the treatment of hypofibrinogenemia that is due to primary fibrinolysis and not secondary fibrinolysis owing to disseminated intravascular coagulation. A normal platelet count in the presence of hypofibrinogenemia supports the diagnosis of primary fibrinolysis. Nevertheless, isolated primary fibrinolysis is rare, and administration of aminocaproic acid in the presence of disseminated intravascular coagulation may cause fatal side effects.

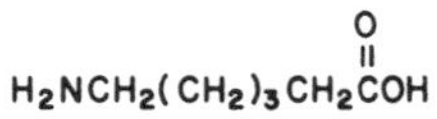

Aminocaproic acid is useful in surgical and nonsurgical hematuria arising from the bladder, prostate, or urethra. For example, postoperative hematuria following transurethral and suprapubic prostatectomy is reduced by aminocaproic acid. This drug, however, is recommended only when hemorrhage is severe and correctable causes have been eliminated.

Aminocaproic acid has been used to treat hemorrhage in patients with hereditary angioedema or subarachnoid hemorrhage. This drug has also been administered before and during surgery for ruptured intracranial aneurysms, although the value in this situation and in patients following a subarachnoid hemorrhage is not convincingly documented. Aminocaproic acid does not control hemorrhage caused by thrombocytopenia or most other coagulation defects. Nevertheless, aminocaproic acid has been useful in hemophiliacs prior to and following dental extractions.

SIDE EFFECTS. Aminocaproic acid administered to a patient with disseminated intravascular coagulation may cause serious or even fatal thrombus formation. Nausea, vomiting, and diarrhea are frequent side effects of aminocaproic acid therapy. When aminocaproic acid is given during surgery, it is important to eliminate blood clots from the bladder because the drug accumulates in these clots and inhibits their dissolution. Administration of aminocaproic acid in the presence of renal or ureteral bleeding is not recommended because ureteral clot formation, and possibly obstruction, may result.

Platelet Concentrates

Platelet concentrates are prepared by centrifugation of citrated whole blood within 4 hours after collection. An average single unit of platelets contains more than 5.5 million platelets. One unit of platelet concentrate will increase the platelet count 5000 to 10,000 mm^3. Platelets stored at room temperature (20 to 24 C) are viable for up to 7 days, and bacterial contamination does not seem to occur. When preserved at 4 C, platelets appear to be effective only when transfused within 24 hours. Multiple units of platelets

$$H_2NCH_2(CH_2)_3CH_2\overset{\overset{\displaystyle O}{\|}}{C}OH$$

FIGURE 36–2. Aminocaproic acid.

may be obtained from a single donor by platelet-pheresis. Single-donor platelets obtained by plateletpheresis must be used within 24 hours after collection.

Although platelet concentrates contain only a few erythrocytes, they do contain large amounts of plasma and administration on the basis of ABO plasma compatibility is desirable. Likewise, the small quantity of erythrocytes present can cause Rh immunization if platelets from an Rh-positive donor are administered to an Rh-negative recipient. For this reason, Rh-compatible platelets should be used in females of childbearing age. Platelets possess HLA antigens on their cell membranes, and patients sensitized to these antigens will destroy infused platelets, thus manifesting as the absence of a therapeutic response. In these patients, the administration of type-specific HLA platelets is the only effective treatment.

Granulocyte Concentrates

Leukapheresis is continuous or intermittent flow centrifugation to obtain granulocytes for infusion to treat infection (Higby and Burnett, 1980). Granulocytes have been beneficial in patients recovering from bone marrow transplants. Phagocytic and microbicidal functions of collected granulocytes persist for about 48 hours.

Fever often accompanies granulocyte transfusion and can be ameliorated by administration of an antihistamine and an antipyretic. Granulocytes should be administered slowly to avoid pulmonary insufficiency that may be caused by sequestration of granulocytes in the pulmonary capillaries. Acute dyspnea, arterial hypoxemia, and interstitial infiltrates may be more likely when patients treated with amphotericin B receive granulocyte transfusions (Wright et al, 1981). Cytomegalovirus infections frequently are observed following granulocyte transfusions because the virus is concentrated in granulocytes.

Albumin

Albumin is obtained by fractionating human plasma that is nonreactive for hepatitis B surface antigen. Coagulation factors and blood group antibodies are not present. In fact, an albumin-induced increase in the intravascular fluid volume may actually dilute the plasma concentra-

tions of coagulant factors. Albumin is heated for 10 hours at 60 C, which appears to remove the hazard of viral hepatitis. Albumin preparations contain sodium capylate, acetyltryptophanate, or both as stabilizers, allowing storage for about 3 years.

Albumin, 25 g, is equivalent osmotically to about 500 ml of plasma but contains only about one seventh the amount of Na^+ present in the same volume of plasma. Hypoalbuminemia is the most frequent indication for the administration of albumin. Albumin also binds bilirubin and has been used during exchange transfusions to treat hyperbilirubinemia. Administration of hypertonic 25% albumin will draw 3 to 4 ml of fluid from the interstitial space into the intravascular fluid space for every 1 ml of albumin administered. This is the reason 25% albumin is not recommended for administration to patients in cardiac failure or in the presence of anemia. The 5% solution of albumin is isotonic with plasma and is most often administered undiluted at a rate of 2 to 4 ml·min^{-1}.

Plasma Protein Fraction

Plasma protein fraction is a 5% pooled solution of stabilized human plasma proteins in saline containing at least 83% albumin and no more than 17% globulins, of which less than 1% are gamma globulins. Each 100 ml of solution provides 5 g of proteins. The preparation is equivalent osmotically to an equal volume of plasma. Although plasma protein fraction is prepared from large pools of normal human plasma, viral hepatitis is not a hazard because of heating to 60 C for 10 hours. It must be recognized that plasma protein fraction does not contain any coagulation factors and may even dilute the plasma concentration of existing coagulants.

Plasma protein fraction is used to treat hypovolemic shock and provide protein to patients with hypoproteinemia. It is also effective for the initial treatment of shock in infants and small children with dehydration, hemoconcentration, and electrolyte deficiency caused by diarrhea. Although dosage is guided by individual response, the usual treatment of hypovolemia or hypoproteinemia is with 20 to 30 ml·kg^{-1} of plasma protein fraction (75 to 100 g of protein).

Hypotension that may accompany rapid infusion of plasma protein fraction has been attributed to the presence of a prekallikrein activator that leads to production of bradykinin with resultant peripheral vasodilatation (Bland et al, 1973; Isbister and Fisher, 1980). The level of prekallikrein activator in plasma protein fraction has been decreased since these reports, and hypotension no longer seems to occur.

Signs of hypervolemia may occur when plasma protein fraction is administered to patients with increased intravascular fluid volumes. Administration of large quantities of plasma protein fraction to patients with impaired renal function has been reported to cause electrolyte imbalances resulting in metabolic alkalosis (Rahilly and Berl, 1979).

Immune Globulin

Immune globulin is a concentrated solution of globulins, primarily immunoglobulins, prepared from large pools of human plasma. This preparation protects against clinical manifestations of hepatitis A when administered before or within 2 weeks after exposure. Replacement therapy for patients with hypogammaglobulinemia is another use of immune globulin. Immune globulin prevents or modifies rubeola, rubella, and varicella. Low concentrations of immunoglobulin A are present in immune globulin, emphasizing the need to avoid administration of this preparation to patients with anti-immunoglobulin A. Hepatitis B immune globulin is a special preparation with a high antibody titer that delays the onset of hepatitis B and ameliorates the severity of the disease (Prince, 1978).

TOPICAL HEMOSTATICS

Topical hemostatics include absorbable gelatin sponge or film, oxidized cellulose, microfibrillar collagen and hemostat, and thrombin. These substances may help to control surface bleeding and capillary oozing as associated with biliary tract surgery; partial hepatectomy; resection or injuries of the pancreas, spleen or kidneys; and oral, neurologic, and otolaryngologic surgery. Although usually innocuous, the presence of bacterial contamination at the site of application of topical hemostatics may exacerbate infections.

Absorbable Gelatin Sponge (Gelfoam)

This sterile gelatin-base surgical sponge controls bleeding in highly vascular areas that are difficult to suture. The preparation may be left in place following closure of a surgical wound. Absorption is complete in 4 to 6 weeks, and scar formation or cellular reaction is minimal. When this material is placed into closed tissue spaces, it must be remembered that the material absorbs fluid and expands, which could cause pressure on neighboring structures.

Absorbable Gelatin Film (Gelfilm)

This sterile thin film is used primarily in neurologic and thoracic surgery for nonhemostatic purposes to repair defects in the dura and pleural membranes. It is also used in ocular surgery. Absorption is complete within 6 months of implantation.

Oxidized Cellulose (Oxycel) and Oxidized Regenerated Cellulose (Surgical)

These celluloses do not enter into the normal clotting cascade, but when exposed to blood, they expand and are converted to a reddish-brown or black gelatinous mass that forms an artificial clot. Oxidized cellulose has a low pH, which contributes to a local cauterizing action. The hemostatic action of these celluloses is not enhanced by other hemostatic agents, and thrombin is destroyed by the low pH. Absorption of these products may require 6 weeks or longer. Some stenosis of arterial anastomoses may occur, apparently from cicatricial contraction. These products should not be used for permanent packing or implantation in fractures because they may interfere with bone regeneration and cause cyst formation.

Microfibrillar Collagen Hemostat (Avitene)

When applied directly onto a bleeding surface, this water-insoluble, fibrous material attracts and entraps platelets to initiate formation of a platelet plug and development of a natural clot. Absorption without cellular reaction occurs in about 7 weeks. This topical hemostatic appears to retain its effectiveness in heparinized patients, in those receiving oral anticoagulants, and in the presence of moderate thrombocytopenia. Microfibrillar collagen hemostat is a useful adjunct to therapy in the oral cavity of patients with hemophilia. This material can be used on skin graft donor sites, around a vascular anastomosis where only minimal suturing is possible, and to control oozing from cancellous bone. It should not, however, be used on bone surfaces to which prosthetic materials are to be attached with methylmethacrylate adhesives.

As a foreign protein, microfibrillar collagen hemostat may exacerbate infection, abscess formation, and dehiscence of cutaneous incisions. Use of this hemostatic is not recommended for skin incisions because healing of the wound edges is impaired. Despite its protein structure, allergic reactions have not been described.

Thrombin

Thrombin is a sterile protein derived from bovine prothrombin. It is applied topically as a powder or in a solution to control capillary oozing in operative procedures and to shorten effectively the duration of bleeding from puncture sites in heparinized patients. Thrombin may be combined with gelatin sponge but should not be used to moisten microfibrillar collagen hemostat. Thrombin alone does not control arterial bleeding.

When applied to denuded tissue, thrombin is inactivated by antithrombins and by absorption onto fibrin. A pH less than 5 also inactivates thrombin. Systemic absorption is unlikely, and direct intravenous injection is contraindicated because resulting thrombosis could be fatal. Allergic reactions are a theoretical possibility when thrombin is used.

BLOOD SUBSTITUTES

Blood substitutes are useful to restore intravascular fluid volume temporarily until definitive treatment can be established. Commonly used blood substitutes tend to be inexpensive, have prolonged storage times, and lack the risk of transmitting viral diseases. It must be recognized that blood substitutes lack coagulation activity.

Dextran

Dextran-70 is a water-soluble glucose polymer (polysaccharide) synthesized by certain bacteria from sucrose. The mean molecular weight of dextran-70 is about 70,000. This high–molecular-weight dextran is treated to yield low–molecular-weight dextran (dextran-40) with a molecular weight of about 40,000. The renal threshold for dextran is at a molecular weight of about 55,000. Therefore, more dextran-40 than dextran-70 is filtered by the glomeruli. Dextran-70 is ultimately degraded enzymatically to glucose.

Clinical Uses

High–molecular-weight dextrans remain in the intravascular space for 12 hours. For this reason, they may be suitable alternatives to blood or plasma for expansion of intravascular fluid volume. For replacement of intravascular fluid volume, the recommended maximum dose during the first 24 hours is 20 ml·kg^{-1} IV and then 10 ml·kg^{-1} IV on subsequent days. Therapy should not be continued for more than 5 days. Thirty-two percent dextran-70 is used in hysteroscopy to help distend and irrigate the uterine cavity and to reduce the likelihood of tubal adhesions after reconstructive tubal surgery for infertility. Because this dextran may be absorbed, adverse reactions are the same as those encountered after intravenous administration (Reisner, 1984). Dextran-40 remains intravascular for only 2 to 4 hours and is used most often to prevent thromboembolism by reducing blood viscosity.

Low–molecular-weight dextran injected concomitantly with epinephrine slows intravascular absorption of the catecholamine (Ueda et al, 1985). Likewise, intercostal nerve blocks performed with bupivacaine plus low–molecular-weight dextran provide postoperative analgesia lasting an average of 40 hours compared with less than 12 hours following bupivacaine alone (Kaplan et al, 1975). Presumably, dextran prolongs local anesthetic effects by delaying systemic absorption of the drug by an unknown mechanism.

Side Effects

The potential side effects of dextran must be considered before this blood substitute is selected in lieu of safer, although more expensive, products such as albumin or plasma protein fraction.

ALLERGIC REACTIONS. The incidence of allergic reactions following infusion of high– or low–molecular-weight dextrans appears to be approximately 1 in every 3300 administrations (Isbister and Fisher, 1980). Nevertheless, low–molecular-weight dextran probably has considerably less antigenic potential than high–molecular-weight dextran. Histamine release may manifest as urticaria, angioedema, hypotension, and bronchospasm. Discontinuation of the dextran infusion is usually sufficient treatment but, in rare cases, life-threatening allergic reactions require aggressive therapy. Indeed, fatal allergic reactions have occurred after intravenous administration of as little as 10 ml of dextran-70 (Isbister and Fisher, 1980).

INCREASED BLEEDING TIME. Increased bleeding time caused by decreased platelet adhesiveness occurs, especially when high–molecular-weight dextran is infused and the dose is greater than 1500 ml. This impairment of coagulation may not appear for 6 to 9 hours after the infusion. Plasma levels of fibrinogen and factors V, VIII, and IX may be decreased.

ROULEAUX FORMATION. Dextran solutions, regardless of their molecular weight, may induce rouleaux formation and, therefore, interfere with subsequent cross-matching of blood. For this reason, blood for cross-matching should be obtained prior to dextran infusion. Dextrans may also interfere with certain tests of renal and hepatic function and cause factitious elevations in blood glucose.

NONCARDIOGENIC PULMONARY EDEMA. Pulmonary edema in association with the use of 32% dextran-70 during hysteroscopy is probably a result of a direct toxic effect on the pulmonary capillaries following intravascular absorption (Mangar et al, 1989).

Hetastarch

Hetastarch (hydroxyethyl starch) is a synthetic colloid solution in which the molecular weight of at least 80% of the polymers ranges from 10,000 to 2,000,000. A 6% solution of hetastarch is as effective as 5% albumin as a plasma expander. The pH of hetastarch is about 5.5, and the osmolarity is near 310 mOsm·L^{-1}. The larger molecules (molecular weight greater than 50,000) are removed from the circulation and stored temporarily in tissues, principally the liver and spleen. These larger molecules are degraded enzymatically by amylase. The average elimination half-time of hetastarch is 17 days, with 90% being eliminated by the kidneys in about 42 days.

Clinical Uses

Hetastarch is used to expand intravascular fluid volume in the treatment of hypovolemia due to burns or hemorrhage (Puri et al, 1983). The usual total daily dose is 20 ml·kg^{-1} IV, but 40 to 60 ml·kg^{-1} IV has been administered to patients with severe hypovolemia.

Side Effects

The hemodynamic effects of hetastarch are similar to albumin. Hetastarch probably has the same risk as dextran for producing allergic reactions (Porter and Goldberg, 1986). Excessive doses of hetastarch decrease the hematocrit, dilute plasma proteins, and interfere with the normal coagulation mechanism by diluting platelets and procoagulants. Hetastarch does not cause rouleaux formation, and cross-matching of blood is not impaired. Hypervolemia is a potential danger, particularly in patients with impaired renal function, because hetastarch is excreted primarily by the kidneys.

Stroma-Free Hemoglobin

Stroma-free solutions of hemoglobin may be useful as plasma volume expanders with the potential capacity for delivering oxygen to tissues and carrying carbon dioxide away from these same tissues. The value of stroma-free solutions for expanding the intravascular fluid volume is related to the high molecular weight (68,000) of hemoglobin. There is no need for cross-matching, and prolonged storage is possible. Renal dysfunction does not accompany administration of stroma-free hemoglobin solutions.

REFERENCES

Alter HJ, Tabor E, Meryman HT, et al. Transmission of hepatitis B virus infection by transfusion of frozen-deglycerolized red blood cells. N Engl J Med 1978;298:637–42.

Barnette RE, Shupak RC, Pontius J, Rao AK. *In vitro* effect of fresh frozen plasma on the activated coagulation time in patients undergoing cardiopulmonary bypass. Anesth Analg 1988;67:57–60.

Bland JHL, Laver MB, Lowenstein E. Vasodilator effect of commercial 5% plasma protein fraction solutions. JAMA 1973;224:1721–4.

Bove JR. Fresh frozen plasma: Too few indications—Too much use (editorial). Anesth Analg 1985;64:849–50.

Chaplin H. Frozen red cells revisited. N Engl J Med 1984;311:1696–8.

Czer LS, Bateman TM, Gray RJ, et al. Treatment of severe platelet dysfunction and hemorrhage after cardiopulmonary bypass: Reduction in blood product usage with desmopressin. J Am Coll Cardiol 1987;9:1139–47.

D'Alauro F, Johns RA. Hypotension related to desmopressin administration following cardiopulmonary bypass. Anesthesiology 1988;69:962–3.

Ellison N. Diagnosis and management of bleeding disorders. Anesthesiology 1977;47:171–80.

Fuerth JH, Mahrer P. Myocardial infarction after factor IX therapy. JAMA 1981;245:1455–6.

Hackman T, Gascoyne RD, Naiman SC, et al. A trial of desmopressin (1-d vasopressin) to reduce blood loss in uncomplicated cardiac surgery. N Engl J Med 1989;321:1437–43.

Higby DJ, Burnett D. Granulocyte transfusions: Current status. Blood 1980;55:2–8.

Hoyer LW. Factor VIII complex: Structure and function. Blood 1981;58:1–13.

Isbister JP, Fisher MM. Adverse effects of plasma volume expanders. Anaesth Intensive Care 1980;8:145–51.

Kaplan JA, Miller ED, Gallagher EG. Postoperative analgesia for thoracotomy patients. Anesth Analg 1975;54:773–7.

Mangar D, Gerson JI, Constantine RM, Lenz V. Pulmonary edema and coagulopathy due to hyskon (32% dextran-70) administration. Anesth Analg 1989;68:686–7.

Milde LN. An anaphylactic reaction to fibrin glue. Anesth Analg 1989;69:684–6.

Murray DJ, Olson J, Strauss R, Tinker JH. Coagulation changes during packed red cell replacement of major blood loss. Anesthesiology 1988;69:839–45.

Porter SS, Goldberg RJ. Intraoperative allergic reactions to hydroxyethyl starch: A report of two cases. Can Anaesth Soc J 1986;33:394–8.

Prince AM. Use of hepatitis B immune globulin: Reassessment needed. N Engl J Med 1978;299:198–9.

Puri VK, Howard M, Paidipaty BB, Singh S. Resuscitation in hypovolemia and shock: A prospective study of hydroxyethyl starch and albumin. Crit Care Med 1983;11:518–23.

Rahilly GT, Berl T. Severe metabolic alkalosis caused by administration of plasma protein fraction in end-stage renal failure. N Engl J Med 1979;301:824–6.

Reisner LS. Anaphylaxis to intraperitoneal dextran. Anesthesiology 1984;60:259–60.

Salzman EW, Weinstein MJ, Weintraub RM, et al. Treatment with desmopressin acetate to reduce blood loss after cardiac surgery: A double-blind ramdomized trial. N Engl J Med 1986;314:1402–6.

Ueda W, Hirakawa M, Mori K. Inhibition of epinephrine absorption by dextran. Anesthesiology 1985;62:72–5.

Wright DG, Robichaud KJ, Rizzo PA, Deisseroth AB. Lethal pulmonary reactions associated with combined use of amphotericin B and leukocyte transfusion. N Engl J Med 1981;304:1185–9.

Hyperalimentation Solutions

INTRODUCTION

Hyperalimentation is designed to supply all the essential inorganic and organic nutritional elements necessary to maintain optimal body composition as well as positive nitrogen balance. Alimentation by the gastrointestinal tract (enteral nutrition) is preferred to intravenous alimentation (parenteral nutrition) so as to avoid catheter-induced sepsis and to maintain the absorptive activity of the small intestine.

Hyperalimentation is indicated to prevent malnutrition in patients with (1) intestinal obstruction, (2) major burns, (3) trauma, (4) prolonged hypermetabolic states as associated with infection and malabsorption syndromes, and (5) gastrointestinal dysfunction that occurs during chemotherapy or radiotherapy. It is recommended that debilitated patients who have lost more than 20% of their body weight be treated with supplemental nutrients before operation (Powell-Tuck and Goode, 1981).

Hyperalimentation increases survival and improves recovery from many diseases. Caloric needs should be individualized. Mildly catabolic patients usually gain weight with a daily provision of 35 to 45 calories·kg^{-1}, whereas patients in severe catabolic states may require up to 80 calories·kg^{-1}. Adequate caloric intake is essential for efficient utilization of amino acids.

ENTERAL NUTRITION

The ingredients and nutritional value of enteral alimentation solutions vary greatly. Some solutions contain minimally altered foods, and others provide nutrients in the form of processed or chemically isolated food derivatives. Carbohydrates are the source of up to 90% of the calories, emphasizing the increased osmolarity of these solutions. Fat has a higher caloric density than carbohydrates, does not increase the osmolarity of the formula as much as carbohydrates, and improves palatability. The amount of fat in enteral solutions varies. Unless the patient has maldigestion or malabsorption of fat, formulas with a normal range of fat content are preferred. In patients with hepatic cirrhosis or portacaval shunts, excessive plasma concentrations of fatty acids may act synergistically with high levels of ammonia and other toxins to exacerbate or cause hepatic encephalopathy. Selection of a formula that provides sufficient total nitrogen as protein or amino acids is essential for all patients. Low-protein formulations, however, are indicated for patients with severe renal dysfunction. Specialized crystalline amino acid supplements are available for nutritional deficiencies associated with liver or renal disease. Increased amounts of protein or amino acids are indicated when the nitrogen requirement is increased, as in patients with trauma, burns, or sepsis. The efficient use of amino acids for tissue synthesis depends on adequate caloric intake.

Enteral Tube Feeding

Enteral tube feeding may be necessary when patients are unable to consume nutritionally complete, liquefied food orally. Commercial formulations of natural foods can be so finely suspended that they pass through small-bore tubes. Defined-formula diets are necessary when luminal hydrolysis or absorption is impaired, as in malabsorption syndromes. The tip of the 4 to 8 French nasogastric tube used to deliver enteral nutrition must be properly positioned in the stomach, duodenum, or jejunum. Dislodgement of the tip can result in pulmonary aspiration. Surgical placement of an esophagostomy or gastrostomy tube may be indicated for long-term feeding. For slow-drip feeding, use of an automated infusion pump to control the rate of administration is useful. Indeed, absorption and tolerance are improved, and the incidence of side effects is reduced by slow, constant feeding over several hours. The rate of infusion is typically 100 to 120 ml·h^{-1}. This slow rate of infusion prevents the dumping syndrome, which may occur when hyperosmolar solutions are introduced rapidly into the small intestine.

Side Effects

Complications of enteral tube feedings are infrequent. Most side effects related to enteral nutrition are due to osmolar load. Too rapid administration of the more concentrated solutions may produce nausea and delayed gastric emptying as well as hypovolemia owing to osmotic diuresis induced by glycosuria. Hyperosmolar dehydration progressing to nonketotic coma results from administration of a high glucose load. Caution is necessary if enteral nutrition is administered to patients prone to develop hyperglycemia (as in diabetes mellitus, treatment with glucocorticoids, or adrenergic drugs). Excessive carbohydrates can also cause significant hypophosphatemia. Cutaneous rashes that occur after prolonged enteral nutrition are thought to be caused by fatty acid deficiency.

Pulmonary aspiration is always a danger when enteral tube feeding is used. Patients should be maintained in a semisitting position (the head of the bed elevated 30 degrees) during feeding and for 1 hour after feeding. Preparations containing large amounts of electrolytes should be given cautiously to patients with cardiovascular, renal, or hepatic disease. Many commercial formulas contain large amounts of sodium. Dry preparations mixed with water become excellent culture media unless they are kept sterile and refrigerated.

PARENTERAL NUTRITION

Parenteral nutrition is indicated for patients who are unable to ingest or digest nutrients or to absorb them from the gastrointestinal tract. Parenteral nutrition using isotonic solutions delivered through a peripheral vein is acceptable when the patient requires less than 2000 calories·day^{-1} and the anticipated need for nutritional support is brief. When caloric requirements are more than 2000 calories·day^{-1} or prolonged nutritional support is required, a catheter is placed in the central venous system to permit infusion of a hypertonic (1900 mOsm·L^{-1}) nutrition solution.

Short-Term Parenteral Therapy

Short-term parenteral therapy (3 to 5 days in patients without nutritional deficits) after uncomplicated surgical procedures is most often provided by a hypocaloric, non-nitrogen glucose-electrolyte solution. For example, glucose solutions, 5% to 10%, with supplemental sodium, chloride, and other electrolytes, are commonly administered for short-term therapy (Table 37-1). These solutions provide total fluid and electrolyte needs and sufficient calories to reduce protein catabolism and prevent ketosis. For example, daily infusion of approximately 150 g of glucose maintains brain and erythrocyte metabolism and decreases protein catabolism from skeletal muscle and viscera.

Amino acids may have a greater protein-sparing effect than glucose, but amino acids without glucose do not prevent negative nitrogen balance completely following major surgery. The higher cost of amino acid solutions relative to po-

Table 37–1
Contents of Various Crystalloid Solutions

	Glucose (mg·dl^{-1})	Sodium*	Chloride*	Potassium*	Magnesium*	Calcium*	Lactate*	pH	Osmolarity (mOsm·L^{-1})
5% Glucose in water	500	0	0	0	0	0	0	5.0	253
5% Glucose in 0.45% sodium chloride	500	77	77	0	0	0	0	4.2	407
5% Glucose in 0.9% sodium chloride	500	154	154	0	0	0	0	4.2	561
0.9% Sodium chloride	0	154	154	0	0	0	0	5.7	308
Lactated Ringer's solution	0	130	109	4.0	0	3.0	28	6.7	273
5% glucose in lactated Ringer's solution	500	130	109	4.0	0	3.0	28	5.3	527
Normosol-R	0	140	98	5.0	3.0	0	†	7.4	295

*mEq·L^{-1}.
†Contains 27 mEq·L^{-1} of acetate and 23 mEq·L^{-1} of gluconate.

tential benefit has prevented their popularity for use in place of glucose for short-term therapy.

Peripheral infusion of fat emulsions may be administered as a nonprotein source of calories to augment those supplied by glucose. Thrombosis of the peripheral vein used for infusion of the fat emulsion is a common problem.

Long-Term (Total) Parenteral Nutrition

Total parenteral nutrition (intravenous hyperalimentation) is the technique of providing total nutrition needs by intravenous infusion of amino acids combined with glucose and varying amounts of fat emulsion (Fleming et al, 1976). Lean body mass is preserved, wound healing may be enhanced, and there may even be improvement of an impaired immune response mechanism.

Total parenteral nutrition solutions contain a large proportion of calories from glucose and thus are hypertonic. For this reason, these solutions must be infused into a central vein with a high blood flow to provide rapid dilution. A catheter is often placed percutaneously into the subclavian vein and guided into the right atrium. The parenteral nutrition solution may be infused continuously or intermittently over a 12- to 16-hour period. When intermittent administration is used, the infusion must be reduced gradually during the 60 to 90 minutes preceding discontin-

uation to avoid hypoglycemia. The daily volume of infusion is about 40 ml·kg^{-1}.

The efficacy of nutritional support is reflected by body weight measurements that confirm a maintenance or increase of lean body mass. Daily weight gains greater than 0.5 kg, however, may signify fluid retention. Serum electrolytes, blood glucose concentration, and blood urea nitrogen should be measured frequently during total parenteral nutrition. Tests of hepatic and renal function are also recommended but can be performed at less frequent intervals.

Side Effects

The side effects of total parenteral nutrition are numerous and include catheter-related sepsis and metabolic abnormalities resulting from the administered nutrients (Table 37-2) (Michel et al, 1981).

SEPSIS. Total parenteral nutrition solutions infused through an intravenous catheter can support the growth of bacteria and fungi. Indeed, infection at the infusion site, as well as systemic infection, is a serious side effect of parenteral nutrition therapy.

A spiking temperature most likely reflects contamination via the delivery system or catheter. The catheter should be removed and the tip cultured to determine the appropriate antibiotic therapy. In view of the hazard of contamination, the use of a central venous hyperalimentation catheter for administration of medications, as during the perioperative period, or for sampling of blood, is not recommended.

FATTY ACID DEFICIENCY. Fatty acid deficiency may develop during prolonged total parenteral nutrition. Administering 3% of the total caloric input as linoleic acid prevents or corrects this deficiency.

HYPERGLYCEMIA. Blood glucose concentrations should be monitored until glucose tolerance is demonstrated, which usually occurs after 2 to 3 days of therapy as endogenous insulin production increases. In addition, blood glucose concentrations should be carefully monitored during the perioperative period. Persistent hyperglycemia may lead to osmotic diuresis with resulting hypovolemia. Nonketotic hyperosmolar hyperglycemic coma is a potential complication of total parenteral nutrition. For these reasons, it may be necessary to add insulin to total parenteral nutrition solutions.

HYPOGLYCEMIA. Accidental, sudden discontinuation of the infusion of total parenteral nutrition solution (catheter kink or disconnection) may cause hypoglycemia. Indeed, total parenteral nutrition infusion should be discontinued gradually over 60 to 90 minutes. Hypoglycemia occurs because the pancreatic insulin response does not always cease in unison with discontinuation of the parenteral nutrition solution. As a result, a high plasma concentration of insulin may persist in the absence of continued infusion of glucose. If total parenteral nutrition must be stopped suddenly, exogenous glucose should be infused for up to 90 minutes to prevent hypoglycemia.

METABOLIC ACIDOSIS. Hyperchloremic metabolic acidosis may occur because of the liberation of hydrochloric acid during the metabolism of amino acids in the parenteral nutrition solution.

HYPERCARBIA. Increased production of carbon dioxide resulting from the metabolism of large quantities of glucose may result in the need to initiate artificial ventilation of the lungs, or in failure to wean from long-term ventilation support (Askanazi et al, 1981).

Preparation of Total Parenteral Nutrition Solutions

Total parenteral nutrition solutions are prepared from commercially available solutions by mixing hypertonic glucose with an amino acid solution. Sodium, potassium, phosphorus, calcium, magnesium, and chloride ions are added to total parenteral nutrition solutions. Trace elements, including zinc, copper, manganese, and chromium, must also be added if the need for parenteral therapy is prolonged. Requirements for vitamins may be increased, emphasizing the need to add a multivitamin preparation to total parenteral nutrition solutions. Vitamin B_{12} and folic acid may be administered as components of a multivitamin preparation or separately. Vitamin D should be used sparingly because metabolic bone diseases may be associated with use of this vitamin in some patients on long-term total parenteral nutrition. Vitamin K is administered separately once every week. The serum albumin concentration will usually increase in patients receiving total parenteral nutrition if adequate amino acids and calories are given. Therefore, the routine administration of supplemental albumin is not necessary in the absence of signs or symptoms of hypoalbuminemia.

Fat emulsions are not mixed with the total parenteral nutrition solutions. Instead, these isotonic emulsions are administered intrave-

Table 37–2
Side Effects Associated with Total Parenteral Nutrition

Sepsis

Fatty acid deficiency

Hyperglycemia

Nonketotic hyperosmolar hyperglycemic coma

Hypoglycemia

Metabolic acidosis

Hypercarbia

Fluid overload

Renal dysfunction

Hepatic dysfunction

Thrombosis of central veins

nously through a separate peripheral vein or by a Y-connector into the same vein. Drugs should not be added to total parenteral nutrition solutions unless compatibility has been determined. To reduce the possibility of bacterial contamination, total parenteral nutrition solutions are prepared aseptically under a lamina air-flow hood, refrigerated, and administered within 24 to 48 hours.

Crystalline Amino Acid Solutions

Amino acid solutions contain a mixture of essential and nonessential amino acids but not peptides. Mild thrombophlebitis occurs infrequently during and after infusion of amino acid solutions. Flushing, fever, and nausea have been reported. Because amino acids increase the blood urea nitrogen concentration, they should be given cautiously to patients with impaired renal function. In patients with severe liver disease, hepatic coma may be precipitated by accumulation of nitrogenous substances in the blood.

Intralipid

Intralipid is a fat emulsion that is stabilized with egg yolk phospholipids and made isotonic by the addition of glycerol. The major component fatty acids are linoleic acid (50%), oleic acid, and palmitic acid. This emulsion is metabolized in the same manner as natural chylomicrons, and transient increases in the plasma concentrations of triglycerides often occur. These triglycerides are hydrolyzed to free fatty acids and glycerol.

Intralipid is used to prevent or correct essential fatty acid deficiency and to provide calories in high-density form on a regular basis during prolonged total parenteral nutrition. Because Intralipid is isotonic with plasma, it is suitable for peripheral infusion and, if sufficient calories can be provided by this method, the use of hypertonic glucose (more than 10%) by way of a central vein catheter may be avoided. Intralipid should account for no more than 60% of the total caloric intake, with the remainder supplied by glucose and amino acids.

Intralipid should not be mixed with other solutions, and electrolytes or vitamins are not added. The emulsion may be infused into the same vein as glucose–amino acid solutions by means of a Y-connector. The emulsion contains particles that are too large to pass through a bacterial or particulate filter.

Side Effects

Increased plasma concentrations of triglycerides occur predictably when Intralipid is infused too rapidly or the emulsion is administered to patients with impaired fat metabolism. Excessive accumulation of lipids can be recognized by visual inspection of the plasma 6 to 8 hours after the infusion is completed. Because free fatty acids compete with bilirubin for albumin binding sites, Intralipid may increase the risk of kernicterus in infants with hyperbilirubinemia and may interfere with estimation of serum bilirubin concentrations.

The fat particles in Intralipid do not aggregate, and there appears to be no risk of fat embolism. Hepatomegaly, altered liver function tests, decreased pulmonary diffusing capacity, thrombocytopenia, and anemia may occasionally occur. Indeed, periodic liver function tests and platelet counts should be performed during long-term total parenteral nutrition. Vomiting, chest pain, allergic reactions, and thrombophlebitis have occurred during the infusion of Intralipid.

Liposyn

Liposyn is an intravenous fat emulsion that is 77% linoleic acid. Osmolarity is 300 to 340 mOsm·L^{-1}. Liposyn, like Intralipid, is used to prevent essential fatty acid deficiency and as a source of calories during total parenteral nutrition.

Travamulsion

Travamulsion is an intravenous fat emulsion that is 56% linoleic acid. Osmolarity is about 270 mOsm·L^{-1}.

REFERENCES

Askanazi J, Nordenstrom J, Rosenbaum SH, et al. Nutrition for the patient with respiratory failure: Glucose vs. fat. Anesthesiology 1981;54:373–7.

Fleming CR, McGill DB, Hoffman HN, Nelson RA.

Total parenteral nutrition. Mayo Clin Proc 1976; 51:187–99.

Greenberg GR, Marliss EB, Anderson GH, et al. Protein-sparing therapy in postoperative patients: Effects of added hypocaloric glucose or lipid. N Engl J Med 1976;294:1411–6.

Michel L, Serrano A, Malt RA. Nutritional support of hospitalized patients. N Engl J Med 1981;304:1147–52.

Powell-Tuck J, Goode AW. Principles of enteral and parenteral nutrition. Br J Anaesth 1981;53:169–80.

Chapter

38

Antiseptics and Disinfectants

INTRODUCTION

Antiseptics and disinfectants are of obvious importance in the preoperative preparation of the patient and surgeon. Substances that are applied topically to living tissues to kill or prevent the growth of microorganisms are antiseptics. A disinfectant is an agent that is applied topically to an inanimate object to destroy pathogenic microorganisms and thus prevent transmission of infection. Antiseptics most often employed include (1) ethyl and isopropyl alcohols; (2) cationic surface-active quaternary ammonium compounds; (3) the biguanide, chlorhexidine; (4) iodine compounds; and (5) hexachlorophene. Disinfectants most often employed are (1) the aldehydes, formaldehyde and glutaraldehyde; (2) the phenolic compound, cresol; and (3) elemental chlorine.

Sterilization is the complete and total destruction of all microbial life, including vegetative bacteria, spores, fungi, and viruses. Ethylene oxide is the only chemical available that is approved for sterilization of objects that cannot be heated or sterilized by other physical methods such as radiation.

ALCOHOLS

Alcohols are applied topically to reduce local cutaneous bacterial flora prior to penetration of the skin with needles. Their antiseptic action can be enhanced by prior mechanical cleansing of the skin with water and a detergent and gentle rubbing with sterile gauze during application.

Ethyl alcohol is an antiseptic of low potency but moderate efficacy, being bactericidal to many bacteria. On the skin, 70% ethyl alcohol kills nearly 90% of the cutaneous bacteria within 2 minutes, provided the area is kept moist. Greater than a 75% reduction in cutaneous bacterial count is unlikely with a single wipe of an ethyl alcohol–wetted sponge followed by evaporation of the residual solution. Isopropyl alcohol has a slightly greater bactericidal activity than ethyl alcohol owing to its greater depression of surface tension. Neither of the alcohols, however, is fungicidal or virucidal.

QUATERNARY AMMONIUM COMPOUNDS

Quaternary ammonium compounds are bactericidal *in vitro* to a wide variety of gram-positive and gram-negative bacteria. Many fungi and viruses are also susceptible. *Mycobacterium tuberculosis,* however, is relatively resistant. Alcohol enhances the germicidal activity of quaternary ammonium compounds so that tinctures are more effective than aqueous solutions. The major site of action of quaternary ammonium compounds appears to be the cell membrane, where these solutions cause a change in permeability.

Benzalkonium and cetylpyridinium (mouthwash) are examples of quaternary ammonium compounds. These compounds may be used preoperatively to diminish the number of organisms on intact skin. There is a rapid onset of action, but the availability of superior agents has reduced their frequency of use. Quaternary ammonium compounds have been widely used for the sterilization of instruments. Endoscopes and other instruments made of polyethylene or polypropylene, however, absorb quaternary ammonium compounds, which may reduce the concentration of the active agent below the bactericidal concentration.

CHLORHEXIDINE

Chlorhexidine is a chlorophenyl biguanide that disrupts cell membranes of the bacterial cells and is effective against both gram-positive and gram-negative bacteria (Fig. 38-1). As a handwash or surgical scrub, 4% chlorhexidine causes a greater initial decrease in the number of normal cutaneous bacteria than does povidone-iodine or hexachlorophene, and it has a persistent effect equal to or greater than that of hexachlorophene. A 0.5% solution of chlorhexidine in 95% alcohol exerts a greater effect than 4% chlorhexidine alone.

Chlorhexidine is mainly used for the preoperative preparation of the surgeon and patient. It is also used to treat superficial infections caused by gram-positive bacteria and to disinfect wounds. As an antiseptic, chlorhexidine is rapid acting, has considerable residual adherence to the skin, has a low potential for producing contact sensitivity and photosensitivity, and is poorly absorbed even after many daily hand washings.

IODINE

Iodine is a rapid-acting antiseptic that, in the absence of organic material, kills bacteria, viruses, and spores. For example, on the skin, a 1% tincture of iodine will kill 90% of the bacteria in 90

seconds, whereas a 5% solution achieves this response in 60 seconds. In the presence of organic matter, some iodine is bound covalently, diminishing the immediate but not the eventual effect. Nevertheless, commercial preparations contain iodine in such excess that organic matter usually does not adversely influence immediate efficacy. The local toxicity of iodine is low, with cutaneous burns occurring only with concentrations greater than 7%. In rare instances, an individual may be allergic to iodine and react to topical application. Symptoms of an allergic reaction usually manifest as fever and generalized skin eruption.

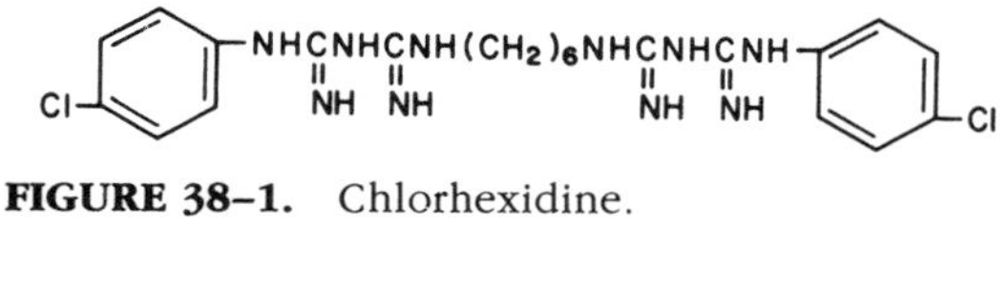

The most important use of iodine is disinfection of the skin, for which it is probably superior to any other antiseptic. For this use, it is best employed in the form of a tincture of iodine because the alcohol vehicle facilitates spreading and penetration. Iodine may also be used in the treatment of wounds and abrasions. Applied to abraded tissue, 0.5% to 1% iodine aqueous solutions are less irritating than the tincture.

Iodophors

An iodophor is a loose complex of elemental iodine with an organic carrier that not only increases the solubility of iodine but also provides a reservoir for sustained release. The most widely used iodophor is povidone-iodine, in which the carrier molecule is polyvinylpyrrolidone. A 10% solution contains 1% available iodine, but the free iodine concentration is less than 1 ppm. This is sufficiently low that little, if any, staining of the skin occurs. Because of the low concentration, the immediate bactericidal action is only moderate compared with that of iodine solutions.

Clinical Uses

The iodophors have a broad antimicrobial spectrum and are widely used as handwashes, including surgical scrubs, preparation of the skin prior to surgery or needle puncture, and treatment for minor cuts, abrasions, and burns. A standard surgical scrub with a 10% solution will decrease the usual cutaneous bacterial population by over 90%, with a return to normal in about 6 to 8 hours. As vaginal disinfectants, iodophors may be absorbed, introducing the risk of fetal hypothyroidism if used in a parturient (Vorherr et al, 1980). For the disinfection of endoscopes and other in-

FIGURE 38–1. Chlorhexidine.

struments, povidone-iodine is superior to 3% hexachlorophene.

HEXACHLOROPHENE

Hexachlorophene is a polychlorinated bis-phenol that exhibits bacteriostatic activity especially against gram-positive organisms (Fig. 38-2). Immediately after a hand scrub with hexa-chlorophene, the cutaneous bacterial population may be decreased by only 30% to 50% compared with over 90% following use of an iodophor. Nevertheless, 60 minutes later, the bacterial population surviving a hexachlorophene scrub will have decreased further to about 4%, whereas with the iodophor scrub, the bacterial population will have recovered to about 16% of normal.

Because most of the potentially pathogenic bacteria on the skin are gram-positive, hexachlorophene is commonly used by physicians and nurses to reduce spread of contaminants from hands. This antiseptic is also used to cleanse the skin of patients scheduled for certain surgical procedures. Daily bathing of neonates with hexachlorophene as a prophylactic measure against staphylococcal infections, however, has been associated with brain damage (Check, 1978). Indeed, hexachlorophene is absorbed through intact skin in amounts sufficient to produce neurotoxic effects, including cerebral irritability. In this regard, the routine use of hexachlorophene by health care providers who are pregnant may be questionable.

FORMALDEHYDE

Formaldehyde is a volatile, wide-spectrum disinfectant that kills bacteria, fungi, and viruses by precipitating proteins. A 0.5% concentration requires 6 to 12 hours to kill bacteria and 2 to 4 days to kill spores. A 2% to 8% concentration is used to disinfect inanimate objects such as surgical instruments.

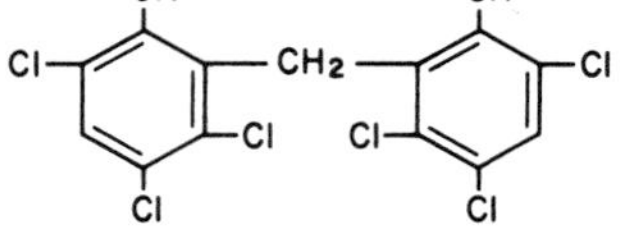

FIGURE 38–2.   Hexachlorophene.

GLUTARALDEHYDE

Glutaraldehyde is superior to formaldehyde as a disinfectant because it is rapidly effective against all microorganisms, including viruses and spores. This disinfectant also possesses tuberculocidal activity. Glutaraldehyde is less volatile than formaldehyde and hence causes minimal odor and irritant fumes. A period of 10 hours is necessary to sterilize dried spores, whereas an acid-stabilized solution kills dried spores in 20 minutes. Neither alkaline nor acidic solutions are damaging to most surgical instruments and endoscopes. As a sterilizing agent for endoscopes, glutaraldehyde is superior to iodophors and hexachlorophene.

CRESOL

Cresol is bactericidal against common pathogenic organisms including *Mycobacterium tuberculosis*. It is widely used for disinfecting inanimate objects. Cresol should not be used to disinfect materials that can absorb this agent because burns could result from subsequent tissue contact.

SILVER NITRATE

Silver nitrate is used as a caustic, antiseptic, and astringent. A solid form is used for cauterizing wounds and removing granulation tissue. It is conveniently dispensed in pencils that should be moistened before use. Solutions of silver nitrate are strongly bactericidal, especially for gonococci, accounting for its frequent use as prophylaxis of ophthalmia neonatorum.

Silver sulfadiazine or nitrate is used in the treatment of burns. In this regard, hypochloremia may occur, reflecting combination of the silver ion with chloride. Hyponatremia also may result because the cations are attracted by chloride ions into the exudate. Furthermore, absorbed nitrate can cause methemoglobinemia.

MERCURY

Organic mercurial compounds are nonirritating but lack bactericidal activity. In fact, these compounds possess only weak bacteriostatic activity and are less effective than ethyl alcohol. Serum and tissue proteins reduce antimicrobial activity, and skin sensitization is common.

ETHYLENE OXIDE

Ethylene oxide is readily diffusible, noncorrosive, and antimicrobial to all organisms at room temperature. This gaseous alkylating agent is widely used as an alternative to heat sterilization. It reacts with chloride and water to produce two additional active germicides, ethylene chlorohydrin and ethylene glycol. Special sterilizing chambers are required because the gas must remain in contact with the objects for several hours. Adequate airing of sterilized materials, such as tracheal tubes, is essential to ensure removal of residual ethylene oxide and thus minimize tissue irritation (Stetson et al, 1976). Ethylene oxide used to sterilize plastic components in disposable apheresis kits may evoke allergic reactions in plateletpheresis donors (Leitman et al, 1986).

REFERENCES

Check W. New study shows hexachlorophene is teratogenic in humans (editorial). JAMA 1978;240:513–4.

Leitman SF, Boltansky H, Alter HJ, Pearson FC, Kaliner MA. Allergic reactions in healthy plateletpheresis donors caused by sensitization to ethylene oxide gas. N Engl J Med 1986;315:1192–6.

Stetson JB, Whitboune BS, Eastman C. Ethylene oxide degassing of rubber and plastic materials. Anesthesiology 1976;44:174–80.

Vorherr H, Mehta P, Ulrich JA, Messer RH. Vaginal absorption of povidone-iodine. JAMA 1980;244:2628–9.

PHYSIOLOGY

Chapter

39

Cell Structure and Function

INTRODUCTION

The basic living unit of the body is the cell. It is estimated the entire body consists of 75 trillion cells, of which about 25 trillion are red blood cells (Guyton, 1986). Each organ is a mass of cells held together by intracellular supporting structures. A common characteristic of all cells is dependence on oxygen to combine with nutrients (carbohydrates, lipids, proteins) to release energy that is necessary for cellular function. Almost every cell is within 25 to 50 μ of a capillary, assuring prompt diffusion of oxygen to cells. All cells exist in nearly the same composition of extracellular fluid (milieu interieur), and the organs of the body (lungs, kidneys, gastrointestinal tract) function to maintain a constant composition (homeostasis) of extracellular fluid.

ANATOMY OF A CELL

Principal components of cells include the nucleus and the cytoplasm, which contains structures known as *organelles* (Fig. 39-1) (Junqueira et al, 1986). The nucleus is separated from the cytoplasm by a nuclear membrane, and the cytoplasm is separated from the surrounding fluids by a cell (plasma) membrane.

Cytoplasm

Cytoplasm consists of water; electrolytes; proteins, including enzymes; lipids; and carbohydrates. About 70% to 85% of the cell substance is water. Cellular chemicals are dissolved in the water, and these substances can diffuse to all parts of the cell in this fluid medium. Proteins are, next to water, the most abundant substance in most cells, accounting for 10% to 20% of the cell mass.

Cell Membrane

Each cell is surrounded by a cell membrane that acts as a permeability barrier, allowing the cell to maintain a cytoplasmic composition different from extracellular fluid. Proteins and phospholipids are the most abundant constituents of cell membranes (Table 39-1). A model of cell membrane structure envisions the membrane as a lipid bilayer (two molecules thick) that is interspersed with large globular proteins (Fig. 39-2)

Table 39–1
Cell Membrane Composition

Phospholipids
  Lecithins (phosphatidylcholines)
  Sphingomyelins
  Amino phospholipids (phosphatidylethanolamine)

Proteins
  Structural proteins (microtubules)
  Transport proteins (Na^+–K^+ ATPase)
  Channels
  Receptors
  Enzymes (adenylate cyclase)

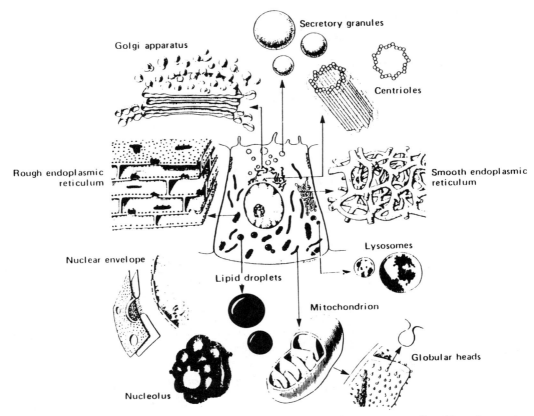

FIGURE 39–1.   Schematic diagram of a hypothetical cell (*center*) and its organelles. (From Junqueira LC, Carneiro J, Long JA. Basic Histology. 5th ed. Norwalk, CT: Appleton and Lange, 1986; with permission.)

(Lodish and Rothman, 1979). The lipid bilayer of cell membranes is nearly impermeable to water and water-soluble substances, such as ions and glucose. Conversely, fat-soluble substances, such as oxygen and carbon dioxide, readily cross plasma cell membranes.

There are several types of proteins in the plasma membrane (Table 39-1). In addition to structural proteins (microtubules), there are transport proteins (Na^+–K^+ ATPase) that function as pumps, actively transporting ions across the membrane. Other proteins function as passive channels for ions that can be opened or closed by changes in the conformation of the protein. There are proteins that function as receptors to bind ligands (hormones or neurotransmitters), thus initiating physiologic changes inside the cell. Another group of proteins function as enzymes (adenylate cyclase), catalyzing reactions at the surface of cell membranes. The protein structure of cell membranes, especially the enzyme content, varies from cell to cell.

Cell membranes are usually dynamic fluid structures reflecting the ability of the lipid bilayer to flow to other areas of the membrane and carry proteins or other dissolved substances with it. An example of membrane components that are not free to diffuse in the plane of the membrane is acetylcholine receptors that are sequestered at the motor endplate of skeletal muscle.

Nucleus

The nucleus is made up, in large part, of chromosomes that carry the blueprint for heritable char-

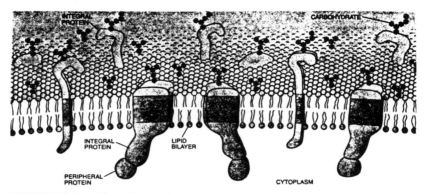

FIGURE 39–2. The cell membrane is a two-molecule–thick lipid bilayer containing protein molecules that extend through the bilayer. (From Lodish HF, Rothman JE. The assembly of cell membranes. Sci Am 1979; 246:48–63; with permission.)

acteristics of the cell. Each chromosome consists of a molecule of deoxyribonucleic acid (DNA) that is covered with proteins. The ultimate units of heredity are genes on the chromosomes, and each gene is a portion of the DNA molecule. The nucleus is surrounded by a membrane that separates its contents from the cytoplasm. This membrane consists of a bilayer of lipid molecules and protein channels through which dissolved or suspended substances, including ribonucleic acid (RNA), can pass from the nucleus to the cytoplasm.

During normal cell division by mitosis, the chromosomes duplicate themselves and then divide in such a way that each daughter cell receives a full complement (diploid number) of 46 chromosomes. Mature sperm and ova contain half the normal number (haploid number) of chromosomes. When a sperm and ovum unite, the resultant cell (zygote) has a full (diploid) complement of 46 chromosomes.

Structure and Function of Deoxyribonucleic Acid and Ribonucleic Acid

DNA consists of two nucleotide chains containing adenine, guanine, thymine, and cytosine (Fig. 39-3) (Murray et al, 1988). The genetic message is determined by the sequence of these amino acids in the nucleotide chains. DNA determines the type of RNA that is formed; it is RNA that is responsible for transferring the genetic message to the site of protein synthesis (ribosomes) in cytoplasm. Cell reproduction (mito-

sis) is determined by the DNA-genetic system. If there is an insufficient number of some types of cells in the body, these insufficient cells will grow and reproduce rapidly until appropriate numbers are again available. For example, nearly all the liver can be removed surgically and the remaining cells will reproduce until liver mass is returned to almost normal. Similar reproduction occurs for glandular cells, cells of the bone marrow, and gastrointestinal epithelium. Highly differentiated cells such as nerve and muscle cells, however, are not capable of reproduction to replace lost cells. Mutations occur when the amino acid sequence in the DNA structure is altered by mutagenic chemicals or radiation.

Regulation of Gene Expression

Genes may be activated by steroids and by proteins manufactured by other genes in the cell. Oncogenes are genes that, when activated, produce uncontrolled cell reproduction (tumors). These genes may alter receptors such that they are continuously stimulated by ligands or alter second messenger systems in the cell so that the response to normal stimulation is excessive. Still other genes may stimulate cells to produce growth factors that act on cells themselves.

TRANSFORMING GROWTH FACTOR-B. Transforming growth factor-B (TGF-B) is a mediator of normal cellular physiology, as emphasized by the fact that nearly all cells produce this factor and almost all cells have responsive receptors (Sporn and

Roberts, 1989). Its actions are widespread and include stimulation of proliferation of some cells, especially in connective tissues, while being a potent inhibitor of proliferation of other cells such as lymphocytes and most epithelial cells. Platelets are a concentrated source of TGF-B, which is released at sites of tissue injury. TGF-B is the most potent known chemotactic factor for macrophages. Excessive production of TGF-B may result in immunosuppression (glioblastomas secrete TGF-B) or fibrotic changes in target tissues (hepatic cirrhosis, rheumatoid arthritis).

Potential clinical applications of TGF-B include (1) stimulation of surgical wound healing; (2) acceleration of of bone fracture healing; (3) prevention of osteoporosis; (4) immunosuppression for organ transplants; and (5) chemoprevention of tumors that arise in epithelial cells. Tamoxifen is a potent stimulus for TGF-B secretion, which may explain its usefulness in enhancing bone formation, whereas usefulness in treating breast or skin cancer may reflect inhibition of epithelial cell proliferation.

Organelles

Organelles are structures in the cytoplasm that have specific roles in cellular function.

Mitochondria

Mitochondria are the power-generating units of cells containing the enzymes and substrates of the tricarboxylic acid cycle (Kreb's cycle). As a result, oxidative phosphorylation and synthesis of adenosine triphosphate (ATP) are localized to mitochondria. ATP leaves the mitochondria and diffuses throughout the cell, providing energy for cellular functions. Increased need for ATP in the cell leads to an increase in the number of mitochondria. In the absence of mitochondria, the cell is unable to extract sufficient energy from nutrients and oxygen, leading to cessation of cellular function.

Endoplasmic Reticulum

The endoplasmic reticulum is a complex series of tubules in the cytoplasm. Ribosomes, composed mainly of RNA, attach to the outer portions of many parts of the endoplasmic reticulum membranes, serving as the sites for protein synthesis (hormones, hemoglobin). The portion of the membrane containing these ribosomes is known as the rough endoplasmic reticulum. The part of the membrane that lacks ribosomes is the smooth endoplasmic reticulum. This smooth portion of the endoplasmic reticulum membrane functions in the synthesis of lipid substances and enzymatic processes.

Lysosomes

Lysosomes are scattered throughout the cytoplasm, providing an intracellular digestive system. Structurally, lysosomes are surrounded by bilayer lipid membranes and are filled with digestive (hydrolytic) enzymes. When cells are damaged or die, these digestive enzymes cause autolysis of the remnants. Bactericidal substances in the lysosome kill phagocytized bac-

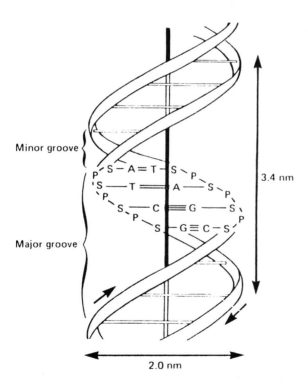

FIGURE 39–3. Double helical structure of deoxyribonucleic acid (*DNA*) with adenine (*A*) bonding to thymine (*T*) and cytosine (*C*) to guanine (*G*). (From Murray RK, Granner DK, Mayes PA, Rodwell VW. Harper's Biochemistry. 21st ed. Norwalk, CT: Appleton and Lange, 1988; with permission.)

teria before they can cause cellular damage. These bactericidal substances include (1) lysozyme, which dissolves the cell membranes of bacteria; (2) lysoferrin, which binds iron and other metals that are essential for bacterial growth; (3) acid that has a pH less than 4; and (4) hydrogen peroxide, which can disrupt some bacterial metabolic systems.

In gout, release of lysosomal enzymes may contribute to the inflammatory response in joints. Congenital absence of a lysosomal enzyme results in engorgement of the lysosome with the material normally degraded. This eventually disrupts the defective lysosome and is responsible for lysosomal storage diseases, such as Tay-Sachs disease.

Golgi Apparatus

The Golgi apparatus is a collection of membrane-enclosed sacs that are responsible for storing proteins to serve specific functions. Proteins synthesized in the endoplasmic reticulum are transported to the Golgi apparatus, where they are stored in highly concentrated packets (secretory vesicles) for subsequent release into the cell's cytoplasm. These vesicles may also diffuse to the surface of cell membranes and discharge their contents (often neurotransmitters) to the exterior by the process of exocytosis.

Specialized portions of the Golgi apparatus form lysosomes, and other portions form peroxisomes. Peroxisomes can both form and destroy hydrogen peroxide. Destruction of hydrogen peroxide, which is formed by many metabolic reactions, is essential, as accumulation of high concentrations has a toxic effect on important enzyme systems.

Nucleolus

This organelle contains granules rich in RNA and is the site of synthesis of ribosomes. RNA enters the cytoplasm and controls the formation of specific proteins, usually enzymes that control different cellular actions. The specific type of RNA formed and, thus, the protein synthesized is determined by DNA, which functions as a gene.

Centroles

These organelles are present in the cytoplasm near the nucleus and are concerned with the movement of chromosomes during cell division.

TRANSFER OF MOLECULES ACROSS CELL MEMBRANES

Endocytosis and exocytosis are examples of processes that transfer molecules such as nutrients across but not through cell membranes. The uptake of particulate matter (bacteria, damaged cells) by cells is phagocytosis, whereas uptake of materials in solution in the extracellular fluid is pinocytosis (Fig. 39-4) (Berne and Levy, 1988). The process of phagocytosis is initiated when antibodies attach to damaged tissue and foreign substances (opsonization) which results in acquirement of a positive charge. Typically, objects that have a negative charge are repelled by cell membranes and, thus, are not vulnerable to phagocytosis. Fusion of phagocytic or pinocytic vesicles with lysosomes allows intracellular digestion of materials to proceed. Molecules such as neurotransmitters are ejected from cells by exocytosis, a process that requires calcium ions (Ca^{2+}) and resembles endocytosis in reverse.

A Phagocytosis   B Pinocytosis

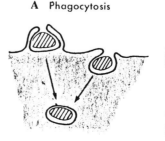 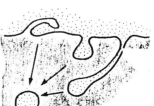

FIGURE 39-4. Schematic depiction of phagocytosis (ingestion of solid particles) and pinocytosis (ingestion of dissolved particles). (From Berne RM, Levy MN. Physiology. 2nd ed. St. Louis: CV Mosby, 1988; with permission.)

TRANSFER OF MOLECULES THROUGH CELL MEMBRANES

Some molecules (oxygen, carbon dioxide, nitrogen) move through cell membranes by diffusion among the molecules that make up the membrane, whereas the passage of other molecules (glucose, amino acids) requires the presence of specific transport proteins in cell membranes.

Diffusion

Diffusion is the process whereby molecules intermingle because of their random thermal motion. The diffusion rate across cell membranes is proportional to the area available for diffusion and the difference in concentration of the diffusing substances on the two sides of the membrane. Because of the slowness of diffusion over macroscopic distances, organisms have developed circulatory systems to deliver nutrients within reasonable diffusion ranges of cells (Table 39-2). Substances can diffuse through cell membranes by becoming dissolved in the lipid bilayer or by passing through protein channels.

Lipid Bilayer

The lipid bilayer of cell membranes is the principal barrier to substances that permeate membranes by simple diffusion. The positive correlation between lipid solubility and cell membrane permeability suggests that lipid-soluble molecules can dissolve in and diffuse across cell membranes. Highly lipid-soluble oxygen and carbon dioxide diffuse readily. Conversely, cell membranes are impermeable to charged water-soluble molecules, especially with molecular weights greater than 200.

Protein Channels

Because of their charge, most ions are relatively insoluble in cell membranes such that their passage across these membranes is thought to occur through protein channels. These channels are likely to be intermolecular spaces in proteins that extend through the entire cell membrane. Some channels are highly specific with respect to the ions allowed to pass (Na^+, K^+), whereas other channels allow all ions below a certain size to pass (Table 39-3). Tetrodotoxin is a specific blocker of Na^+ channels as a result of binding to the extracellular side of the channel, whereas tetraethylammonium blocks K^+ channels by attaching to the inside surface of the membrane.

Some channels are continuously open, whereas others are gated (gates open or close). Some channels are gated by alterations in membrane potential (voltage-gated Na^+ channels), whereas others are opened or closed when they bind a ligand such as a neurotransmitter or a hormone (chemically-gated acetylcholine receptors). For example, one end of the Na^+ channel may become blocked by the presence of a positive charge at its external opening. This charge is designated as a *gate* because it repels Na^+ and interferes with the passage of these ions through the channel.

Permeability of cell membranes to Na^+ and K^+ may change as much as 50- to 5000-fold during the course of nerve impulse transmission. These

Table 39-2
Predicted Relationship Between Diffusion Distance and Time

Diffusion Distance (mm)	Time Required for Diffusion
0.001	0.5 ms
0.01	50 ms
0.1	5 s
1	498 s
10	14 h

Table 39-3
Diameters of Ions, Molecules, and Channels

	Diameter (nm*)
Channel (average)	0.80
Water	0.30
Na^+ (hydrated)	0.51
K^+ (hydrated)	0.40
Cl^- (hydrated)	0.39
Glucose	0.86

*1 nm = 10 Å.

changes most likely reflect rapid alterations in the electrical charges lining the channels or guarding their entrances. Extracellular fluid concentrations of Ca^{2+} influence the permeability of channels. For example, decreased Ca^{2+} concentrations greatly increase channel permeability, manifesting as exaggerated activity of nerves throughout the body. Conversely, excess Ca^{2+} in extracellular fluid diminishes channel permeability and activity of nerves is greatly reduced. In the kidneys, the presence of antidiuretic hormone (ADH) enlarges pores in cells lining the collecting ducts, allowing water and other substances to diffuse from the renal tubules back into the peritubular capillaries.

Protein-Mediated Transport

Protein-mediated transport is responsible for movement of certain substances into or out of cells by way of specific carriers or channels that are intrinsic proteins of cell membranes. Transport across cell membranes may be facilitated (carrier-mediated diffusion) or active, with the principal distinction being that active transport is capable of moving a substance across cell membranes against a concentration gradient, whereas facilitated transport tends to equilibrate substances across the membrane.

Facilitated Diffusion

Poorly lipid-soluble substances, such as glucose and amino acids, may pass through lipid bilayers by facilitated diffusion. For example, glucose combines with a carrier to form a complex that is lipid soluble. This lipid-soluble complex can diffuse to the interior of the cell membrane where glucose is released into the cytoplasm, and the carrier moves back to the exterior of the cell membrane where it becomes available to transport more glucose from the extracellular fluid (Fig. 39-5) (Guyton, 1986). As such, the carrier renders glucose soluble in cell membranes that otherwise would prevent its passage. Insulin greatly speeds facilitated diffusion of glucose and some amino acids across cell membranes.

Active Transport

Active transport requires energy that is most often provided by hydrolysis of ATP. Indeed, car-

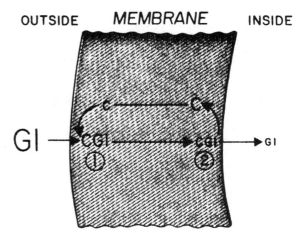

FIGURE 39–5. Glucose (*Gl*) can combine with a carrier substance (*C*) at the outside surface of the cell membrane to facilitate diffusion (carrier-mediated diffusion) of Gl across the cell membrane. At the inside surface of the cell membrane, Gl is released to the interior of the cell and the carrier becomes available for reuse. (From Guyton AC. Textbook of Medical Physiology. 7th ed. Philadelphia: WB Saunders, 1986; with permission.)

rier molecules are enzymes known as ATPases that catalyze the hydrolysis of ATP. The most important of the ATPases is Na^+–K^+ ATPase, which is also known as the Na^+ pump. There are H^+–K^+ ATPases in the gastric mucosa and renal tubules. Substances that are actively transported through cell membranes against a concentration gradient include Na^+, K^+, Ca^{2+}, H^+, Cl^-, Mg^{2+}, iodide (thyroid gland), carbohydrates, and amino acids.

Na^+–K^+ ATPase. This enzyme is present in all cells and is responsible for providing the energy (catalyzes conversion of ATP to adenosine diphosphate [ADP]) for extruding three Na^+ from the cell, while two K^+ enter the cell for each mole of ATP hydrolyzed to ADP (Fig. 39-6) (Guyton, 1986). As a result, there is net movement of positive charges out of the cell, which creates a potential (voltage) difference across cell membranes, with the interior of the cell being negative with respect to the exterior. Maintenance of this electrical potential difference is essential to nerve conduction and skeletal muscle contraction.

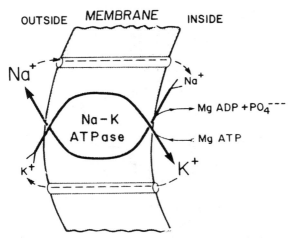

FIGURE 39-6. The active transport of Na^+ and K^+ ions across cell membranes (Na^+ inside to outside and K^+ outside to inside) uses a carrier mechanism that derives energy from the hydrolysis of adenosine triphosphate (*ATP*) to adenosine diphosphate (*ADP*). This hydrolysis of ATP is under the control of the enzyme, Na^+–K^+ ATPase. (From Guyton AC. Textbook of Medical Physiology. 7th ed. Philadelphia: WB Saunders, 1986; with permission.)

Na^+–K^+ ATPase opposes the tendency of cells to swell by continually transporting Na^+ to the exterior, which initiates an opposite osmotic tendency to move water out of the cell. This enzyme provides sufficient energy to transport Na^+ against concentration gradients as great as 20 to 1 and K^+ against concentration gradients as great as 30 to 1. When the metabolism of the cell ceases so that energy from ATP is not available to maintain enzyme activity, the cell begins to swell. Activity of Na^+–K^+ ATPase is also inhibited by cardiac glycosides, resulting in reduced intracellular extrusion of Ca^{2+}. The subsequent increase in intracellular Ca^{2+} concentration is consistent with the positive inotropic effect of cardiac glycosides.

Na^+ COTRANSPORT OF GLUCOSE. Despite the widespread presence of Na^+–K^+ ATPase, the active transport of Na^+ in some tissues is coupled to the transport of other substances. For example, a carrier system present in the gastrointestinal tract and renal tubules will transport Na^+ only in combination with a glucose molecule. As such, glucose is returned to the circulation, thus preventing its excretion. In the brain, transport by

Na^+–K^+ ATPase is coupled to the uptake of neurotransmitters back into nerve endings.

Na^+ COTRANSPORT OF AMINO ACIDS. Na^+ cotransport of amino acids is an active transport mechanism that supplements facilitated diffusion of amino acids into cells. Epithelial cells lining the gastrointestinal tract and renal tubules are able to reabsorb amino acids into the circulation by this mechanism, thus preventing their excretion. Other substances, including insulin, steroids, and growth hormone, influence amino acid transport by the Na^+ cotransport mechanism. For example, estradiol facilitates transport of amino acids into the musculature of the uterus, thus promoting development of this organ. The effect of steroids on skeletal muscle development is a widely publicized controversy as it relates to body-building.

Ca^{2+}-ATPase. This enzyme is present in cell membranes for the purpose of maintaining the large gradient between Ca^{2+} concentrations in the cytoplasm and extracellular fluid. This cell membrane ATPase is different from the Ca^{2+}-ATPase that is responsible for sequestering Ca^{2+} in the sarcoplasmic reticulum of skeletal muscles. In keeping with the vital role of Ca^{2+} as a controller of cellular processes, the activity of Ca^{2+}-ATPase is highly regulated by calmodulin, an intracellular regulatory protein that increases the affinity of this enzyme for Ca^{2+} at the inner surface of cell membranes.

ELECTRICAL POTENTIALS ACROSS CELL MEMBRANES

Electrical potentials exist in nearly all cell membranes, reflecting principally the difference in transmembrane concentrations of Na^+ and K^+. This unequal distribution of ions is created and maintained by the membrane-bound enzyme Na^+–K^+ ATPase, which causes a net transfer of positive charges out of the cell (three Na^+ out for two K^+ in), resulting in the establishment of a voltage difference across cell membranes known as the *resting membrane potential*. The cytoplasm is usually electrically negative (about -70 mv) relative to the extracellular fluid (Fig. 39-7) (Berne and Levy, 1988). The number of ions re-

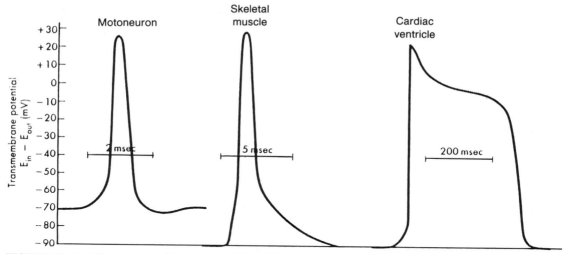

FIGURE 39-7. The transmembrane potential and duration of the action potential varies with the tissue site. (From Berne RM, Levy MN. Physiology. 2nd ed. St. Louis: CV Mosby, 1988; with permission.)

sponsible for the membrane potential is a minute fraction of the total number present.

Action Potential

An action potential is the rapid change in transmembrane potential followed by a return to the resting membrane potential. Propagation of the action potential along the entire length of a nerve axon or muscle cell is the basis of signal-carrying ability of nerve cells and allows muscle cells to contract simultaneously. The size and shape of the action potential varies among excitable tissues (Fig. 39-7) (Berne and Levy, 1988).

An action potential is triggered when successive conductance increases to Na^+ and K^+ cause a threshold potential (about -50 mv) to be reached. Acetylcholine, as an endogenous neurotransmitter, is the most important chemical substance that is capable of enlarging Na^+ channels and increasing permeability of cell membranes to Na^+ up to 5000-fold. The initial, sudden, inward rush of Na^+ leads to a positive charge inside the cell, corresponding to the phase of the action potential known as *depolarization*. Subsequent increased permeability of the cell membrane to K^+ allows loss of this positive ion, tending to return the electrical charge inside the cell toward the resting membrane potential. This phase of the action potential is known as *repolarization*.

Properties of Ion Channels

Ion channels may be voltage gated (regulated by membrane potential) or chemically gated (regulated by binding of a neurotransmitter). During an action potential, voltage-gated Na^+ channels open briefly, allowing a small quantity of extracellular Na^+ to flow into the cell, thus depolarizing the plasma membrane. A more slowly developing outward current, often of K^+ flowing through voltage-gated K^+ channels, helps to repolarize the membrane. Na^+ channels undergo transitions between ion-conducting states (open) and one of two nonconducting states known as the *resting* and *inactivated* form. Resting channels may activate to open channels, whereas inactivated channels must first undergo transition to the resting state.

MEASUREMENT OF CURRENT. Current flowing through individual ion channels can be measured by "patch clamping," which is a technique consisting of voltage clamping a small patch of excitable membrane containing only one or a few ion channels. Currents carried through different ion-selective channels can be separated by the use of specific inhibitors. For example, tetraethylammonium blocks many, but not all, types of K^+ channels, whereas tetrodotoxin blocks nearly all types of Na^+ channels.

Properties of Action Potentials

During much of the action potential, the membrane is completely refractory to further stimulation. This is called the *absolute refractory period* and is due to the presence of a large fraction of inactivated Na^+ channels. During the last portion of the action potential, a stronger than normal stimulus can evoke a second action potential. This relative refractory period reflects the need to activate a critical number of Na^+ channels to trigger an action potential.

A deficiency of Ca^{2+} in the extracellular fluid prevents the Na^+ channels from closing between action potentials. The resulting continuous leak of Na^+ contributes to sustained depolarization or repetitive firing of cell membranes (tetany). Conversely, high Ca^{2+} concentrations decrease cell membrane permeability to Na^+ and thus reduce excitability of nerve membranes. Low K^+ concentrations in extracellular fluid increase the negativity of the resting membrane potential, resulting in hyperpolarization and decreased membrane excitability. Skeletal muscle weakness that accompanies hypokalemia presumably reflects hyperpolarization of skeletal muscle membranes. Local anesthetics decrease permeability of nerve cell membranes to Na^+, preventing achievement of a threshold potential that is necessary for generation of an action potential. Blockage of cardiac Na^+ channels by local anesthetics may result in altered conduction of cardiac impulses and decreases in myocardial contractility.

Conduction of Action Potentials

Action potentials are conducted along nerve or muscle fibers by local current flow that produces depolarization of adjacent areas of the membrane

SPREAD OF DEPOLARIZATION

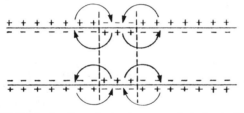

FIGURE 39–8. Depolarization spreads in both directions along cell membranes, resulting in propagation of an action potential.

(Fig. 39-8). These propagated action potentials travel in both directions along the entire extent of the fiber. The transmission of the depolarization process along nerve or muscle fibers is called a *nerve* or *muscle impulse*. The entire action potential usually occurs in less than 1 ms.

Conduction velocity is greatly increased by myelination, which decreases capacitance of the axon and permits action potentials to be generated only at the nodes of Ranvier. Myelination reflects wrapping of Schwann cell membranes around the axon, and nodes of Ranvier represent the lateral spaces (1 to 2 mm apart) between cells. Myelinated nerves are more efficient metabolically than nonmyelinated axons because ion exchange is restricted to the nodes of Ranvier and less ion pumping is thus required to maintain Na^+ and K^+ gradients. Another property of conduction in myelinated fibers that enhances conduction velocity is called *saltatory conduction* because the impulse jumps from one node of Ranvier to the next.

INTRACELLULAR COMMUNICATION

Cells communicate with each other via chemical messengers. Some messengers move from cell to cell without entering the extracellular fluid (gap junctions), whereas other cells are affected by chemical messengers secreted into the extracellular fluid that bind to receptors on cell membranes (Fig. 39-9) (Greenspan and Forsham, 1986). Chemical messengers (first messengers, ligands) generally exert their effects by increasing the concentrations of second messengers (cyclic adenosine monophosphate [cyclic AMP], Ca^{2+}) in target cells (Tables 39-4 and 39-5). Steroids and thyroid hormones are examples of chemical messengers that produce their effects by altering RNA in the cell's cytoplasm. Many of the chemical messengers are polypeptides to which antibodies can be produced, thus allowing measurement of messengers in body fluids or tissues by radioimmunoassay.

Receptors

Receptors on cell surfaces use a variety of membrane-signalling mechanisms to translate information encoded in neurotransmitters and hormones into cellular responses (Fig. 39-10)

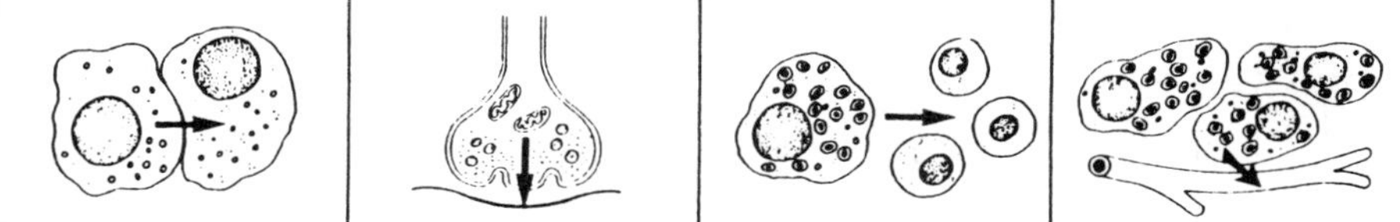

	GAP JUNCTIONS	SYNAPTIC	PARACRINE	ENDOCRINE
Message transmission	Directly from cell to cell	Across synaptic cleft	By diffusion in interstitial fluid	By circulating body fluids
Local or general	Local	Local	Locally diffuse	General
Specificity depends on	Anatomic location	Anatomic location and receptors	Receptors	Receptors

FIGURE 39-9. Intercellular communication by chemical mediators produces local to diffuse responses dependent on the anatomic location of the cell and/or specificity of receptors. (From Greenspan FS, Forsham PH. Basic and Clinical Endocrinology. 2nd ed. Norwalk, CT: Appleton and Lange, 1986; with permission.)

(Gelman, 1987; Maze, 1990). The resulting response is most often a change in transmembrane voltage and thus excitability.

One form of receptor is a protein-encompassed ion channel whose conductance is regulated by receptor activation. This is exemplified by the gamma-aminobutyric acid receptor, where Cl^- conductance through the associated ion channel is the effector mechanism (Fig. 39-10, *I*) (Maze, 1990). A second type of receptor involves the coupling of at least three separate components—a receptor protein, a guanine nucleotide binding protein (G protein), and an effector mechanism. Conceptually, the receptor protein functions as a recognition site that is stimulated or inhibited by a ligand. Stimulatory or inhibitory G proteins link the recognition site to the effector mechanism (catalytic site). These G proteins are the most prevalent proteins in the brain. The recognition site faces the exterior of the lipid cell membrane to facilitate access of water-soluble endogenous ligands and drugs, whereas the catalytic site faces the interior of the cell. In this type of receptor, a second messenger may or may not be generated. For example, when the muscarinic receptor is stimulated, the activated coupling G protein increases conductance of K^+ through a discrete ion channel (Fig. 39-10, *IIa*) (Maze, 1990). Alternatively, the activity of an enzyme may be changed to generate a second messenger. Such a receptor may regulate the activity of adenylate cyclase in a positive manner (beta-adrenergic receptor) through a stimulatory G protein or in a negative manner (alpha-2 adrenergic receptor) through an inhibitory G

Table 39-4

Ligands that Act by Altering Intracellular Cyclic Adenosine Monophosphate (cyclic AMP) Concentrations

Increase cyclic AMP
Adrenocorticotrophic hormone
Catecholamines (beta-1 and beta-2 receptors)
Glucagon
Parathyroid hormone
Thyroid-stimulating hormone
Follicle-stimulating hormone
Vasopressin

Decrease cyclic AMP
Catecholamines (alpha-2 receptors)
Dopamine (dopamine-2 receptors)
Somatostatin

Table 39-5

Ligands that Increase Intracellular Calcium Ion Concentration

Catecholamines (alpha-1 receptors)
Acetylcholine (muscarinic receptors)
Histamine (H-1 receptors)
Serotonin
Substance P
Vasopressin (V-1 receptors)
Oxytocin

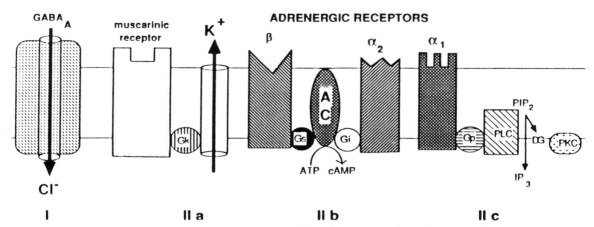

FIGURE 39-10. Schematic depiction of receptors on cell surfaces. Stimulation of the gamma-aminobutyric acid (GABA) receptor by an agonist (*GABA*) results in flow of Cl⁻ ions into the cell along the associated ion channel (*I*). Stimulation of the muscarinic receptor by an agonist (acetylcholine) causes the coupling G protein (*G_k*) to facilitate conductance of K⁺ ions to the exterior of the cell (*IIa*). Adenylate cyclase (*AC*) activity can be enhanced via a stimulatory G protein (*G_s*) on activation of a beta-adrenergic receptor by an agonist ligand, whereas this enzyme's activity can be attenuated via an inhibitory G protein (*G_i*) that is coupled to an alpha-2 adrenergic receptor, thus controlling the conversion of adenosine triphosphate (*ATP*) to cyclic adenosine monophosphate (*cAMP*) (*IIb*). On stimulation of the alpha-1 adrenergic receptor by an agonist ligand, the coupling protein (*G_p*) activates phospholipase C (*PLP*) to hydrolyze phosphatidylinositol biphosphate (*PIP_2*) into inositol triphosphate (*IP_3*) and diacylglycerol (*DG*), which then activates protein kinase C (*PKC*) (*IIc*). (From Maze M. Transmembrane signalling and the Holy Grail of anesthesia. Anesthesiology 1990; 72:959–61; with permission.)

protein, thereby controlling the intracellular concentration of cyclic AMP (Fig. 39-10, *IIb*) (Maze, 1990).

Another membrane-associated enzyme, similar to adenylate cyclase, is phospholipase C, which catalyzes reactions that result in production of second messengers (diacylglycerol and inositol triphosphate). Phospholipase C–coupled receptors (alpha-1 adrenergic receptors) are physiologically very important because the resulting second messengers activate protein kinase C and Ca²⁺ release from intracellular sites (Fig. 39-10, *IIc*) (Maze, 1990).

Receptors in cell membranes are not static components of the cell, but their numbers increase (up-regulation) and decrease (down-regulation) in response to various stimuli. For example, excess circulating concentrations of ligand (norepinephrine owing to a pheochromocytoma) results in down-regulation in an attempt to maintain a normal level of receptor-mediated activity. Conversely, chronic suppression of receptor activity, as with beta-antagonists, may result in up-regulation and unexpected hypersensitivity to

the endogenous ligand if the beta-antagonist is abruptly discontinued.

Receptor Diseases

Failure of parathyroid hormone and ADH to produce increases in cyclic AMP in target organs manifests as pseudohypoparathyroidism and nephrogenic diabetes insipidus, respectively. Grave's disease and myasthenia gravis reflect development of antibodies against thyroid-stimulating hormone and nicotinic acetylcholine receptors, respectively.

REFERENCES

Berne RM, Levy MN. Physiology. 2nd ed. St. Louis, CV Mosby, 1988.

Gelman AC. G proteins: Transducers of receptor-generated signals. Ann Rev Biochem 1987;56:615:–49.

Greenspan FS, Forsham PH. Basic and Clinical Endocrinology. 2nd ed. Norwalk, CT, Appleton and Lange, 1986.

Guyton AC. Textbook of Medical Physiology. 7th ed. Philadelphia, WB Saunders, 1986.

Junqueira LC, Carneiro J, Long JA. Basic Histology. 5th ed. Norwalk, CT, Appleton and Lange, 1986.

Lodish HF, Rothman JE. The assembly of cell membranes. Sci Am 1979;246:48–63.

Maze M. Transmembrane signalling and the Holy Grail of anesthesia. Anesthesiology 1990;72:959–61.

Murray RK, Granner DK, Mayes PA, Rodwell VW. Harper's Biochemistry. 21st ed. Norwalk, CT, Appleton and Lange, 1988.

Sporn MB, Roberts AB. Transforming growth factor-B: Multiple actions and potential clinical applications. JAMA 1989;262:938–41.

40

Body Fluids

INTRODUCTION

Total body fluid can be divided into intracellular and extracellular fluid depending on its location relative to the cell membrane (Fig. 40-1) (Gamble, 1954). About 25 L of the 40 L of total body fluid present in an adult weighing 70 kg are contained inside the estimated 75 trillion cells of the body. The fluid in these cells, despite individual differences in constituents, is collectively designated *intracellular fluid.* The 15 L of fluid outside the cells is collectively referred to as *extracellular fluid.* Extracellular fluid is divided into interstitial fluid and plasma (intravascular fluid) by the capillary membrane (Fig. 40-1) (Gamble, 1954).

Interstitial fluid is that fluid present in the spaces between cells. An estimated 99% of this fluid is held in the gel structure of the interstitial space. Plasma is the noncellular portion of blood. The average plasma volume is 3 L. Plasma communicates continually with the interstitial fluid through pores in the capillaries. Interstitial fluid is also in dynamic equilibrium with the plasma serving as an available reservoir from which water and electrolytes can be mobilized into the circulation. Loss of plasma from the intravascular space is minimized by colloid osmotic pressure exerted by the plasma proteins.

Other extracellular fluid that may be considered as part of the interstitial fluid includes cerebrospinal fluid, gastrointestinal fluid, and fluid in potential spaces (pleural space, pericardial space, peritoneal cavity, synovial cavities). Excess amounts of fluid in the interstitial space manifest as peripheral edema.

TOTAL BODY WATER

Water is the most abundant single constituent of the body and is the medium in which all metabolic reactions occur. The total amount of water in a male weighing 70 kg is about 40 L, accounting for nearly 60% of total body weight (Fig. 40-1) (Gamble, 1954). In a neonate, total body water may represent 70% of body weight. Total body water is less in females and in obese persons, reflecting the reduced water content of adipose tissue. For example, total body water represents about 50% of the body weight in females. Advanced age is also associated with increased fat content and decreased total body water (Table 40-1).

The normal daily intake of water by an adult averages 2 L, of which about 1.2 L is excreted as urine, 100 ml is lost in sweat, and 100 ml is present in feces. The remaining water intake is lost by evaporation from the respiratory tract and diffusion through the skin (insensible water loss, as this loss is not perceived by the individual). The cornified layer of the skin acts as a protector against greater insensible water loss through the skin. When the cornified layer becomes denuded, as after burn injury, the outward diffusion of water is greatly increased.

All gases that are inhaled become saturated with water vapor (47 mmHg at 37 C). This water vapor is subsequently exhaled, accounting for an average daily water loss through the lungs of 300 to 400 ml. The water content of inhaled gases decreases with decreases in environmental air temperature such that more endogenous water is required to achieve a saturated water vapor pressure at body temperature. As a result, insensible

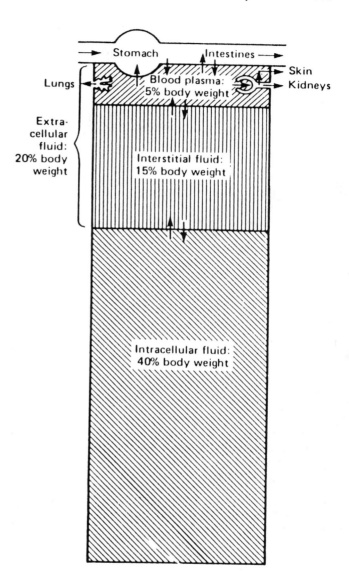

FIGURE 40–1. Body fluid compartments and the percentage of body weight represented by each compartment. The location relative to the capillary membrane divides extracellular fluid into plasma or interstitial fluid. Arrows represent fluid movement between compartments. (From Gamble JL. Chemical Anatomy, Physiology, and Pathology of Extracellular Fluid. 6th ed. Boston: Harvard University Press, 1954; with permission.)

water loss from the lungs is greatest in cold environments and least in warm temperatures. This is consistent with the dry feeling perceived in the respiratory passages in cold weather.

BLOOD VOLUME

Blood contains extracellular fluid, as represented by plasma, and intracellular fluid, as represented by the fluid in erythrocytes. The main

Table 40–1
Total Body Water, Age, and Sex

Age (years)	Total Body Water	
	Male (percent)	*Female (percent)*
18–40	61	51
40–60	55	47
Over 60	52	46

608   SECTION TWO: PHYSIOLOGY

priority of the body is to maintain intravascular fluid volume. Acute reductions in blood volume, as occur with (1) fluid deprivation in the perioperative period, (2) blood loss, or (3) surgical trauma that results in tissue edema, elicit the release of renin and antidiuretic hormone. These hormones evoke changes at the renal tubules that lead to restoration of intravascular fluid volume (see Chapter 53).

The average blood volume of an adult is 5 L, of which about 3 L is plasma and 2 L is erythrocytes. These volumes, however, vary greatly with age, weight, and sex. For example, in nonobese persons, the blood volume varies in direct proportion to body weight, averaging 70 ml·kg^{-1} for lean males and females. The greater the ratio of fat to body weight, however, the less is the blood volume in ml·kg^{-1} because adipose tissue has a reduced vascular supply.

Hematocrit

The true hematocrit is about 96% of the measured value because 3% to 8% of plasma remains entrapped among the erythrocytes even after centrifugation. The measured hematocrit is about 40% for males and 36% for females. The hematocrit of blood in arterioles and capillaries is less than that in large arteries and veins. This reflects axial streaming of erythrocytes in small vessels. Specifically, erythrocytes tend to migrate to the center of vessels, whereas a large portion of the plasma remains near the walls. In large vessels, the ratio of wall surface to total volume is slight so that the accumulation of plasma near the walls does not significantly affect the hematocrit. In small vessels, however, this ratio of wall surface to volume is great, causing the ratio of plasma to cells to be greater than in large vessels.

MEASUREMENT OF COMPARTMENTAL FLUID VOLUMES

The volume of a fluid compartment can be measured by the indicator dilution principle, in which a known amount of a substance is placed in the compartment and the resulting concentration of this material is then determined after complete mixing has occurred. Using this principle, blood volume, extracellular fluid volume, and total body water can be measured, whereas inter-

stitial fluid volume is calculated as extracellular fluid volume (15 L) minus plasma volume (3 L).

Blood Volume

Substances used for measuring blood volume must be capable of dispersing throughout the blood with ease and then must remain in the circulation long enough for measurements to be completed. Most often, a small amount of the patient's blood is removed and mixed with radioactive chromium. After determining the total content of chromium with a scintillation counter, the tagged blood sample is injected into the patient. After mixing in the systemic circulation for about 10 minutes, the chromium content of blood is determined. Using the dilution principle, the total blood volume is calculated.

CONSTITUENTS OF BODY FLUID COMPARTMENTS

The constituents of plasma, interstitial fluid, and intracellular fluid are identical, but the quantity of each substance varies greatly among the compartments (Fig. 40-2) (Leaf and Newburgh, 1955). The most striking differences are the low-protein content in interstitial fluid compared with intracellular fluid and plasma and the fact that sodium (Na$^+$) and chloride (Cl^{-1}) ions are largely extracellular, whereas most of the potassium ions (K$^+$) (about 90%) are intracellular. This unequal distribution of ions results in establishment of a potential (voltage) difference across cell membranes.

The constituents of the extracellular fluid are carefully regulated by the kidneys so that the cells remain bathed continually in a fluid containing the proper concentrations of electrolytes and nutrients for continued optimal function of the cells. The normal amount of Na$^+$ and K$^+$ in the body is about 58 mEq·kg^{-1} and 45 mEq·kg^{-1}, respectively. Trauma is associated with progressive loss of K$^+$ through the kidneys. For example, a patient undergoing surgery excretes about 100 mEq of K$^+$ in the first 48 hours and, after this period, about 25 mEq daily. Plasma K$^+$ is not a good indicator of total body K$^+$ because most K$^+$ is intracellular. There is a correlation, however, between the K$^+$ and hydrogen ion content of

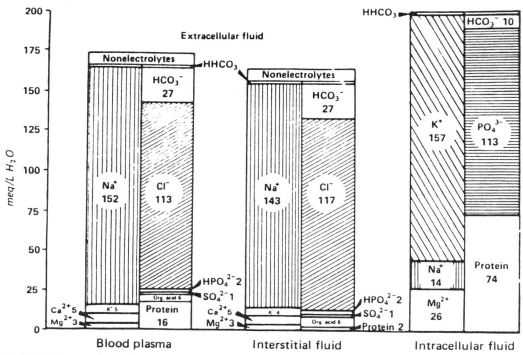

FIGURE 40–2. Electrolyte composition of body fluid compartments. (From Leaf A, Newburgh LH. Significance of the Body Fluids in Clinical Medicine. 2nd ed. Springfield, IL: Thomas, 1955; with permission.)

plasma, the two increasing and decreasing together.

OSMOSIS

Osmosis is the movement of water (solvent molecules) across a semipermeable membrane from a compartment in which the nondiffusible solute (ion) concentration is lower to one in which the solute concentration is higher (Fig. 40-3) (Ganong, 1987). A membrane is semipermeable when water can diffuse freely but Na^+ and K^+ cannot diffuse freely.

Osmotic Pressure

Osmotic pressure is the pressure on one side of the semipermeable membrane that is just sufficient to keep water from moving to a region of higher solute concentration (Fig. 40-3) (Ganong,

1987). The osmotic pressure exerted by nondiffusible particles in a solution is determined by the number of particles in solution (degree of ionization) and not the type of particles (molecular weight). Thus a 1 mol solution of glucose or albumin and a 0.5 mol solution of NaCl (dissociates into two ions) should exert the same osmotic pressure. Osmole is the unit used to express osmotic activity of solutes. Milliosmole (1/1000 Osm) is commonly used to express osmotic activity of solutes in the body.

The osmole concentration of a solution is called its *osmolality* when the concentration is expressed in osmole per kilogram of water. *Osmolarity* is the correct terminology when osmole concentration is expressed in liters. In the dilute solutions of the body, these terms are frequently used interchangeably. Furthermore, because it is much easier to express body fluids in liters rather than kilograms of water, almost all physiologic calculations are based on osmolarity rather than osmolality.

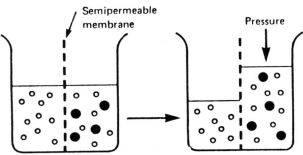

FIGURE 40–3. Diagrammatic representation of osmosis depicting water molecules (open circles) and solute molecules (solid circles) separated by a semipermeable membrane. Water molecules move across the semipermeable membrane to the area of greater concentration of solute molecules. Osmotic pressure is the pressure that would have to be applied to prevent continued movement of water molecules. (From Ganong WF. Review of Medical Physiology. 13th ed. Norwalk, CT: Appleton and Lange, 1987; with permission.)

Moles and Equivalents

A mole is the molecular weight of a substance in grams, and each mole contains about $6 \cdot 10^{23}$ molecules. A 1 molar solution of NaCl is 58.5 g and 1 mmol is 58.5 mg. An equivalent is 1 mol of an ionized substance divided by its valence. The mole is the standard unit for expressing concentrations in the Système International (SI) unit system.

Osmolarity of Body Fluids

The freezing point of plasma averages −0.54 C, which corresponds to a plasma osmolarity of about 290 mOsm·L^{-1}. All but about 20 mOsm of the 290 mOsm in each liter of normal plasma are contributed by Na^{+} and its accompanying anions, principally Cl^{-} and bicarbonate ions. Proteins normally contribute less than 1 mOsm·L^{-1}. The major nonelectrolytes of plasma are glucose and urea, and these substances can contribute significantly to plasma osmolarity when hyperglycemia or uremia is present (Table 40-2). Plasma osmolarity is important in evaluating dehydration, overhydration, and electrolyte abnormalities.

Table 40–2
Calculation of Plasma Osmolarity

Plasma osmolarity = 2(Na^{+}) + 0.055 (glucose) + 0.36 (blood urea nitrogen)

The transfer of water through cell membranes by osmosis occurs so rapidly that any lack of osmotic equilibrium between two fluid compartments in a given tissue is corrected usually within seconds.

Tonicity of Fluids

Tonicity is the term used to describe the osmolarity of a solution relative to plasma. Solutions that have the same osmolarity as plasma are said to be isotonic (no transfer of fluid into or out of cells), those with greater osmolarity are hypertonic (cells shrink), and those with lesser osmolarity are hypotonic (cells swell). This reflects the fact that plasma membranes of most cells are relatively impermeable to many solutes but are highly permeable to water. For example, packed erythrocytes must be suspended in isotonic solutions to avoid damage to the cells prior to infusion. A 0.9% solution of NaCl is isotonic and remains so because there is no net movement of the osmotically active particles in the solution into cells and the particles are not metabolized. A solution of 5% glucose in water is initially isotonic when infused, but glucose is metabolized, so the net effect is that of infusing a hypotonic solution. Lactated Ringer's solution plus 5% glucose is initially hypertonic (about 560 mOsm·L^{-1}), but as glucose is metabolized, the solution becomes less hypertonic. The maintenance of a normal cell volume and pressure depends on Na⁺–K⁺ ATPase, which, if absent, would permit Na⁺ and Cl⁻ to enter cells along their concentration gradients and water would follow along the osmotic gradient, causing the cells to swell.

CHANGES IN VOLUMES OF BODY FLUID COMPARTMENTS

Factors that may alter extracellular fluid or intracellular fluid volumes significantly include intravenous infusion of fluids and dehydration from gastrointestinal fluid loss, diaphoresis, and fluid loss by the kidneys. As a rule, chronic diseases are characterized by a decline in intracellular fluid volume and concomitant expansion of extracellular fluid volume.

Intravenous Fluids

Intravenous fluids that do not remain in the circulation can dilute extracellular fluid, causing it to become hypotonic with respect to intracellular fluid. When this occurs, osmosis begins instantly at cell membranes, with large amounts of water entering cells. Within a few minutes, this water becomes distributed almost evenly among all body fluid compartments. Increased intracellular fluid volume is particularly undesirable in pa-

tients with intracranial masses or elevated intracranial pressure.

Dehydration

Loss of water by gastrointestinal or renal routes or by diaphoresis is associated with an initial deficit in extracellular fluid volume. At the same instant, intracellular water passes to the extracellular fluid compartment by osmosis, thus keeping the osmolarities in both compartments equal despite reduced absolute volume (dehydration) of both compartments. The ratio of extracellular fluid to intracellular fluid is greater in infants than adults, but the absolute volume of extracellular fluid is obviously less, explaining why dehydration develops more rapidly and is often more severe in the very young.

REFERENCES

Gamble JL. Chemical Anatomy, Physiology, and Pathology of Extracellular Fluid. 6th ed. Boston, Harvard University Press, 1954.

Ganong WF. Review of Medical Physiology. 13th ed. Norwalk, CT, Appleton and Lange, 1987.

Leaf A, Newburgh LH. Significance of the Body Fluids in Clinical Medicine. 2nd ed. Springfield, IL, Thomas, 1955.

41

Central Nervous System

INTRODUCTION

The brain is a complex collection of neural systems that regulate their own and each other's activity. For example, activity of the central nervous system reflects a balance between excitatory and inhibitory influences that are normally maintained within relatively narrow limits. Anatomic divisions of the brain reflect the distribution of brain functions. The three principal components of the central nervous system are the cerebral hemispheres, brain stem, and spinal cord. The two cerebral hemispheres constitute the cerebral cortex, where sensory, motor, and associational information is processed. The limbic system lies beneath the cerebral cortex and integrates the emotional state with motor and visceral activities. The thalamus lies in the center of the brain beneath the cortex and basal ganglia and above the hypothalamus. The neurons of the thalamus are arranged in nuclei that act as relays between the incoming sensory pathways and the cerebral cortex, hypothalamus, and basal ganglia. The hypothalamus is the principal integrating region for the autonomic nervous system and regulates other functions, including blood pressure, body temperature, water balance, secretions of the pituitary gland, emotion, and sleep.

The brain stem connects the cerebral cortex to the spinal cord. These connecting portions of the central nervous system contain most of the nuclei of the cranial nerves and the reticular activating system. The reticular activating system is essential for regulation of sleep and wakefulness.

The cerebellum arises from the posterior pons and is responsible for maintenance of body posture.

The spinal cord extends from the medulla oblongata to the lower lumbar vertebrae. Ascending and descending tracts are located within the white matter of the spinal cord, whereas intersegmental connections and synaptic contacts are concentrated in the gray matter. Sensory information flows into the dorsal portion of the gray matter, and motor outflow exits from the ventral portion. Preganglionic neurons of the autonomic nervous system are found in the intermediolateral columns of the gray matter.

CEREBRAL HEMISPHERES

The two cerebral hemispheres, known as the cerebral cortex, constitute the largest division of the brain. Regions of the cerebral cortex are classified as sensory, motor, visual, auditory, and olfactory, depending on the type of information that is processed. *Frontal, temporal, parietal,* and *occipital* designate anatomic positions of the cerebral cortex. For each area of the cerebral cortex, there is a corresponding and connecting area to the thalamus such that stimulation of a small portion of the thalamus activates the corresponding and much larger portion of the cerebral cortex. Indeed, the cerebral cortex is actually an outgrowth of the lower regions of the nervous system, especially the thalamus. The functional part of the cerebral cortex is comprised mainly of a 2- to 5-mm layer of neurons covering the surface of all the convolutions. It is estimated that the cerebral cortex contains 50 to 100 billion neurons.

Anatomy of the Cerebral Cortex

The sensorimotor cortex is the area of the cerebral cortex that is responsible for receiving sensation from somatic sensory areas of the body and for controlling body movement (Fig. 41-1) (Guyton, 1986). The premotor cortex is important for controlling the functions of the motor cortex. The motor cortex lies anterior to the central sulcus. Its posterior portion is characterized by the presence of large, pyramid-shaped (pyramidal, or Betz) cells.

Topographic Areas

The area of the cerebral cortex to which the peripheral sensory signals are projected from the thalamus is designated the *somesthetic cortex* (Fig. 41-1) (Guyton, 1986). Each side of the cerebral cortex receives sensory information exclusively from the opposite side of the body. The size of these areas is directly proportional to the number of specialized sensory receptors in each respective area of the body. For example, a large

number of specialized nerve endings are present in the lips and thumbs, whereas only a few are present in the skin of the trunk.

In the motor cortex, there are various topographic areas from which skeletal muscles in different parts of the body can be activated. In general, the size of the area in the motor cortex is proportional to the preciseness of the skeletal muscle movement required. As such, the digits, lips, tongue, and vocal cords have large representations in humans. The various topographic areas in the motor cortex were originally determined by electrical stimulation of the brain during local anesthesia and observation of the evoked skeletal muscle response. Such stimulation can be used intraoperatively to identify the location of the motor cortex and avoid damage to this area. The motor cortex is commonly damaged by loss of blood supply, as occurs during a stroke. The spatial organization of the somatic sensory cortex is similar to the motor areas of the cerebral cortex.

Corpus Callosum

The two hemispheres of the cerebral cortex, with the exception of the anterior portions of the temporal lobes, are connected by fibers in the corpus callosum. The anterior portions of the temporal lobes, including the amygdala, are connected by fibers that pass through the anterior commissure. One of the functions of the corpus callosum and anterior commissure is to make information stored in one hemisphere available to the other hemisphere.

Dominant Versus Nondominant Hemisphere

Language function and interpretation depend more on one cerebral hemisphere (dominant hemisphere) than the other, whereas spatiotemporal relationships (ability to recognize faces) depend on the other nondominant hemisphere. Based on genetic determination, 90% of individuals are right-handed and the left hemisphere is dominant. Likewise, the left hemisphere is dominant in about 70% of persons who are left-handed. For reasons that are not clear, dyslexia is more common in left-handed persons. Destruction of the dominant cerebral hemisphere results

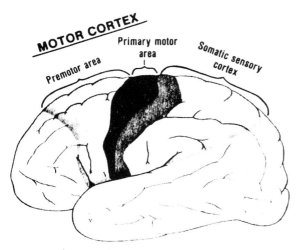

FIGURE 41–1. The sensorimotor cortex consists of the motor cortex, pyramidal (Betz) cells, and the somesthetic cortex. (From Guyton AC. Textbook of Medical Physiology. 7th ed. Philadelphia: WB Saunders, 1986; with permission.)

in loss of nearly all intellectual function, whereas destruction of the prefrontal areas of the frontal lobes is less harmful.

Failure to document an important role of prefrontal lobes in intellectual function is surprising because the main difference between the brains of monkeys and humans is the prominence of human prefrontal areas. It seems that the importance of the prefrontal areas in humans is to provide additional cortical area in which cerebration can occur. Furthermore, selection of behavior patterns for different situations may be an important role of the prefrontal areas that transmit signals to the limbic areas of the brain. Persons without prefrontal lobes may react precipitously in response to incoming signals, manifesting undue anger at slight provocations. Ability to maintain a sustained level of concentration is lost in the absence of the prefrontal lobes.

Memory

The cerebral cortex, especially the temporal lobes, serves as a storage site for information that is often characterized as memory. The mechanisms for short-term and long-term memory are not documented.

Short-Term Memory

Short-term memory may involve the presence of reverberating circuits. As the reverberating circuit fatigues or as new signals interfere with the reverberations, the short-term memory fades. Evidence in favor of a reverberating theory of short-term memory is the ability of a general disturbance of brain function (fright, loud noise) to erase short-term memory immediately.

An alternative explanation for short-term memory is the phenomenon of posttetanic potentiation. For example, tetanic stimulation of a synapse for a few seconds causes increased excitability of the synapse that lasts for seconds to hours. This change in excitability of the synapse could function as short-term memory. Another change that often occurs in neurons following a prolonged period of excitation is a sustained decrease in the resting transmembrane potential of the neuron. This change in excitability of the neuron could also result in short-term memory.

Long-Term Memory

Long-term memory does not depend on continued activity of the nervous system, as evidenced by total inactivation of the brain by hypothermia or anesthesia without detectable significant loss of long-term memory. For this reason, it is assumed that long-term memory results from physical or chemical alterations of the synapses. Anatomically, repeated use of a neuronal circuit may result in changes in the number of presynaptic terminals or alterations in the size and conductivities of the dendrites. These anatomic changes could cause permanent or semipermanent increases in the degree of facilitation of specific neuronal circuits. The entire facilitated circuit is called a *memory engram* or *memory trace*. If memory is to persist, these synapses must become permanently facilitated (consolidated). Maximum consolidation requires at least 1 hour. For example, if a strong sensory impression is made on the brain but is followed within a few seconds to minutes by a disruptive signal, such as an electrically induced convulsion or institution of deep general anesthesia, the sensory experience is erased. An obvious analogy is the lightly anesthetized patient who reacts purposefully to a painful stimulus but later has no recall if the depth of anesthesia is increased following the purposeful movement. Conversely, the same sensory stimulus allowed to persist for 5 to 10 minutes may result in at least partial establishment of the memory trace. If the sensory stimulus is unopposed for 60 minutes, it is likely the memory will have become fully consolidated. Indeed, intraoperative awareness with or without associated pain is a recognized phenomenon, especially when minimal amounts of anesthetic drugs are combined with neuromuscular blocking drugs (Bennett et al, 1985; Bogetz and Katz, 1984; Hilgenberg, 1981; Saucier et al, 1983).

Rehearsal of the same information accelerates and potentiates the process of consolidation, thus converting short-term to long-term memory. This explains why a person can remember small amounts of information studied in depth better than large amounts of information studied only superficially. Each time a memory is recalled, a more indelible memory trace develops that may last a lifetime. An important feature of consolidation is that long-term memory is encoded into different categories. Thus, during consolidation, new memories are not stored randomly in the brain but rather are stored in association with previously encoded and similar information. This form of storage is necessary to permit scanning of the memory store to retrieve desired information at a later date.

Pyramidal and Extrapyramidal Tracts

A major pathway for transmission of motor signals from the cerebral cortex to the anterior motor neurons of the spinal cord is through the pyramidal (corticospinal) tracts (Fig. 41-2) (Guyton, 1986). All pyramidal tract fibers pass downward through the brain stem and then cross to the opposite side to form the pyramids of the medulla. After crossing the midline at the level of the medulla, these fibers descend in the lateral corticospinal tracts of the spinal cord and terminate on motor neurons in the dorsal horn of the spinal cord. A few fibers do not cross to the opposite side of the medulla but rather descend in the ventral corticospinal tracts. In addition to these pyramidal fibers, a large number of collateral fibers pass from the motor cortex into the basal ganglia, forming the extrapyramidal tracts. Extrapyramidal tracts are all those tracts beside the pyramidal tracts that transmit motor impulses from the cerebral cortex to the spinal cord.

The pyramidal and extrapyramidal tracts have opposing effects on the tone of skeletal muscles. For example, the pyramidal tracts cause continuous facilitation and, therefore, a tendency to produce increases in skeletal muscle tone. Conversely, the extrapyramidal tracts transmit inhibitory signals through the basal ganglia with resultant inhibition of skeletal muscle tone. Selective or predominant damage to one of these tracts manifests as spasticity or flaccidity.

Babinski Sign

A positive Babinski sign is characterized by upward extension of the first toe and outward fanning of the other toes in response to a firm tactile stimulus applied to the dorsum of the foot. A normal response to the same tactile stimulus is downward motion of all the toes. A positive Babinski sign reflects damage to the pyramidal tracts. Damage to the extrapyramidal tracts does not cause a positive Babinski sign.

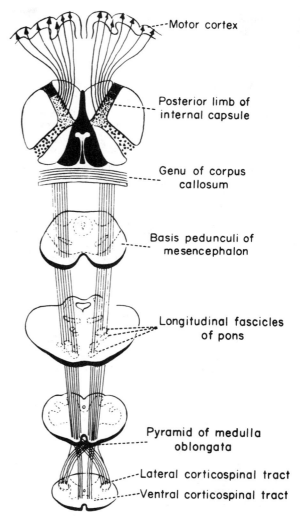

Motor cortex

Posterior limb of internal capsule

Genu of corpus callosum

Basis pedunculi of mesencephalon

Longitudinal fascicles of pons

Pyramid of medulla oblongata

Lateral corticospinal tract

Ventral corticospinal tract

FIGURE 41-2. The pyramidal tracts are major pathways for transmission of motor signals from the cerebral cortex to the spinal cord. (From Guyton AC. Textbook of Medical Physiology. 7th ed. Philadelphia: WB Saunders, 1986; with permission.)

Thalamocortical System

The thalamocortical system serves as the pathway for passage of nearly all afferent impulses from the cerebellum, basal ganglia, visual, auditory, taste, and pain receptors as they pass through the thalamus on the way to the cerebral cortex. Signals from olfactory receptors are the only peripheral sensory signals that do not pass through the thalamus. Overall, the thalamocortical system controls the activity level of the cerebral cortex.

BRAIN STEM

Subconscious activities of the body (intrinsic life processes) are controlled in the brain stem. The brain stem includes the medulla, pons, thalamus, limbic system, basal ganglia, reticular activating system, and cerebellum. Examples of subconscious activities of the body regulated by the brain stem include control of blood pressure and breathing in the medulla. The thalamus serves as a relay station for most afferent impulses before they are transmitted to the cerebral cortex. The hypothalamus receives fibers from the thalamus and is also closely associated with the cerebral cortex.

Limbic System and Hypothalamus

Behavior associated with emotions is primarily a function of structures known as the *limbic system* (hippocampus and basal ganglia) located in basal regions of the brain. The hypothalamus functions in many of the same roles as the limbic system and is considered by some to be a part of the limbic system rather than a separate structure. In addition, the hypothalamus controls many internal conditions of the body, such as core temperature, thirst, and appetite. These internal functions represent responses whose control is closely related to behavior. In addition, the hypothalamus indirectly affects cerebral function, and thus behavior, by activation or inhibition of the reticular activating system.

Basal Ganglia

Basal ganglia include the caudate nucleus, putamen, globus pallidus, substantia nigra, and the subthalamus. Many of the impulses from basal ganglia are inhibitory, and the inhibitory neurotransmitters are dopamine and gamma-aminobutyric acid (GABA). The balance between agonist and antagonist skeletal muscle contractions is an important role of the basal ganglia. A general effect of diffuse excitation of basal ganglia is inhibition of skeletal muscles, reflecting

transmission of inhibitory signals from the basal ganglia to both the motor cortex and the lower brain stem. Therefore, whenever destruction of the basal ganglia occurs, there is associated skeletal muscle rigidity. For example, damage to the caudate and putamen nuclei that normally secrete GABA results in random and continuous uncontrolled movements designated as *chorea.* Destruction of the substantia nigra and loss of dopamine result in a predominance of the excitatory neurotransmitter acetylcholine, manifesting as skeletal muscle rigidity that is characterized as Parkinson's disease. Indeed, dopamine precursors or anticholinergic drugs are used in treatment of Parkinson's disease in an attempt to restore the balance between excitatory and inhibitory impulses traveling from the basal ganglia.

Reticular Activating System

The reticular activating system is a polysynaptic pathway that is intimately concerned with electrical activity of the cerebral cortex. Neurons of the reticular activating system are both excitatory and inhibitory, and the presumed neurotransmitter is acetylcholine. The reticular activating system determines the overall level of central nervous system activity, including sleep and wakefulness. Selective activation of certain areas of the cerebral cortex by the reticular activating system is crucial for the direction of the attention of certain aspects of mental activity. It is likely that many of the clinically used injected and inhaled anesthetics exert depressant effects on the reticular activating system.

Sleep and Wakefulness

Sleep is a state of unconsciousness from which an individual can be aroused by sensory stimulation. Therefore, depression of the reticular activating system by anesthetics or as present in comatose individuals cannot be defined as sleep. Sleep can occur from decreased activity of the reticular activating system (slow-wave sleep) or it can result from abnormal channeling of signals in the brain even though activity of the reticular activating system may not be depressed (desynchronized sleep). Sleep deprivation is associated with the appearance in the blood and cerebrospinal fluid of a low–molecular-weight polypeptide that produces sleep when injected into the third ventricle of animals (Pappenheimer, 1976). The physiologic significance of this sleep factor is not established. Depletion of central nervous system catecholamine stores by antihypertensive drugs is associated with sedation and decreases in anesthetic requirements (MAC) for inhaled drugs (Miller et al, 1968).

SLOW-WAVE SLEEP. Most of the sleep that occurs each night is slow-wave sleep. The electroencephalogram (EEG) is characterized by the presence of high-voltage delta waves occurring at a frequency of less than 4 cycles·sec^{-1}. Presumably, decreased activity of the reticular activating system that accompanies sleep permits an unmasking of this inherent rhythm in the cerebral cortex. Slow-wave sleep is restful and devoid of dreams. During slow-wave sleep, sympathetic nervous system activity decreases, parasympathetic nervous system activity increases, and skeletal muscle tone is greatly reduced. As a result, there is a 10% to 30% decrease in blood pressure, heart rate, breathing frequency, and basal metabolic rate.

DESYNCHRONIZED SLEEP. Periods of desynchronized sleep typically occur for 5 to 20 minutes during each 90 minutes of sleep. These periods tend to be shortest when the person is extremely tired. This form of sleep is characterized by active dreaming, irregular heart rate and breathing, and a desynchronized pattern of low-voltage beta waves on the EEG similar to those that occur during wakefulness. This brain wave pattern emphasizes that desynchronized sleep is associated with an active cerebral cortex, but this activity is not channeled in a direction that permits persons to be aware of their surroundings and thus be awake. Despite the inhibition of skeletal muscle activity, the eyes are an exception, exhibiting rapid movements. For this reason, desynchronized sleep is also referred to as *paradoxical sleep* or *rapid eye movement sleep.*

Cerebellum

The cerebellum operates subconsciously to monitor and elicit corrective responses in motor activities caused by stimulation of other parts of the brain and spinal cord. Rapid skeletal muscle activities, such as typing, playing musical instruments, and running, require intact function of the cerebellum. Loss of function of the cerebellum causes incoordination of fine skeletal muscle activities even though paralysis of the muscles does not occur. The cerebellum is also important in maintenance of equilibrium and postural adjustments of the body. For example, sensory signals are transmitted to the cerebellum from receptors in muscle spindles, Golgi tendon organs, and receptors in skin joints. These spinocerebellar pathways can transmit impulses at velocities greater than 100 m·sec^{-1}, which is the most rapid conduction of any pathway in the central nervous system. This extremely rapid conduction is important for the instantaneous appraisal by the cerebellum of changes that take place in the positional status of the body.

Dysfunction of the Cerebellum

In the absence of cerebellar function, a person cannot predict prospectively how far movements will go, this results in overshoot of the intended mark (past pointing). This overshoot is known as *dysmetria,* and the resulting incoordinate movements are called *ataxia.* Dysarthria is present when rapid and orderly succession of skeletal muscle movements of the larynx, mouth, and chest do not occur. Failure of the cerebellum to dampen skeletal muscle movements results in intention tremor when a person performs a voluntary act. Cerebellar nystagmus is associated with loss of equilibrium, presumably because of dysfunction of the pathways that pass through the cerebellum from the semicircular canals. In the presence of cerebellar disease, a person is unable to activate antagonist muscles that will prevent a certain portion of the body from moving unexpectedly in an unwanted direction. For example, a person's arm that was previously contracted but restrained by another person will move back rapidly when it is released rather than automatically remain in place.

SPINAL CORD

The spinal cord extends from the medulla oblongata to the lower border of the first and, occasionally, the second lumbar vertebra. Below the spinal cord, the vertebral canal is filled by the roots of the lumbar and sacral nerves, which are collectively known as the *cauda equina.* The spinal cord is composed of gray and white matter, spinal nerves, and covering membranes.

Gray Matter

The gray matter of the spinal cord functions as the initial processor of incoming sensory signals from peripheral somatic receptors and as a relay station to send these signals to the brain. In addition, this area of the spinal cord is the site for final processing of motor signals that are being transmitted downward from the brain to skeletal muscles. Anatomically, the gray matter of the spinal cord is divided into anterior, lateral, and dorsal horns consisting of nine separate laminae that have the shape of the letter "H" when viewed in cross-section (Fig. 41-3). The anterior horn is the location of alpha- and gamma-motor neurons that give rise to nerve fibers that leave the spinal cord via the anterior (ventral) nerve roots and innervate skeletal muscles. Cells of Renshaw in the anterior horn are intermediary neurons, providing nerve fibers that synapse in the gray matter with anterior motor neurons. These cells inhibit

the action of anterior motor neurons to limit excessive activity. Cells of the preganglionic neurons of the sympathetic nervous system are located in the lateral horns of the thoracolumbar portions of the spinal cord. Cells of the intermediate neurons located in the portion of the dorsal horns of the spinal cord known as the *substantia gelatinosa* (laminae II–III) transmit afferent tactile, temperature, and pain impulses to the spinothalamic tract. The dorsal horn serves as a gate in which impulses in sensory nerve fibers are translated into impulses in ascending tracts (see Chapter 43).

White Matter

The white matter of the spinal cord is formed by the axons of intermediate neurons and their respective ascending and descending tracts. This area of the spinal cord is divided into dorsal, lateral, and ventral columns (Fig. 41-3). The dorsal column of the spinal cord is composed of spinothalamic tracts that transmit touch and pain impulses to the brain.

Spinal Nerve

A pair of spinal nerves arises from each of 31 segments of the spinal cord. Spinal nerves are made up of fibers of the anterior and dorsal (posterior) roots. Efferent motor fibers travel in the anterior nerve roots that originate from axons in the anterior and lateral horns of the spinal cord gray matter. Sensory fibers travel in the dorsal nerve roots that originate from axons that arise from cell bodies in the spinal cord ganglia. These cell bodies send branches to the spinal cord and to the periphery. The anterior and dorsal nerve roots leave the spinal cord through the intervertebral foramen enclosed in a common dural sheath that extends just past the spinal cord ganglia where the spinal nerve originates.

Dermatomes and Myotomes

Each spinal nerve innervates a segmental area of skin designated a *dermatome* and an area of skeletal muscle known as a *myotome.* A dermatome map is useful in determining the level of spinal cord injury or level of sensory anesthesia produced by a regional anesthetic (Fig. 41-4) (Guyton, 1986). Despite common depiction of

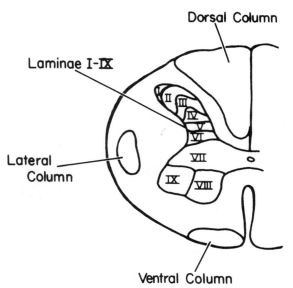

FIGURE 41–3. Schematic diagram of a cross-section of the spinal cord depicting anatomic laminae I to IX of the spinal cord gray matter and the ascending dorsal, lateral, and ventral sensory columns of the spinal cord white matter.

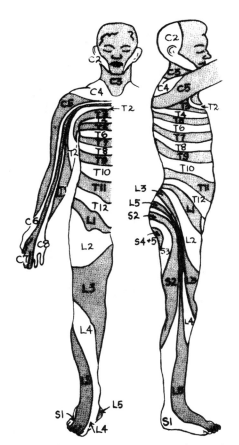

FIGURE 41-4. Dermatome map used to evaluate the level of sensory anesthesia produced by a regional anesthetic. (From Guyton AC. Textbook of Medical Physiology. 7th ed. Philadelphia: WB Saunders, 1986; with permission.)

causing emptying of the bladder and rectum. Segmental temperature reflexes allow localized cutaneous vasodilation or vasoconstriction in response to changes in skin temperature. The function of the spinal cord component of the nervous system and spinal cord reflexes is particularly apparent in patients with transection of the spinal cord.

Covering Membranes

The spinal cord is enveloped by membranes (dura, arachnoid, pia) that are direct continuations of the corresponding membranes surrounding the brain. The dura consists of an inner and an outer layer. The outer periosteal layer in the cranial cavity is the periosteum of the skull, whereas this layer in the spine is the periosteal lining of the spinal canal. The epidural space is located between the inner and outer layers of the dura. The fact that the inner layer of the dura adheres to the margin of the foramen magnum and blends with the periosteal layer means the epidural space does not extend beyond this point. As a result, drugs such as local anesthetics or opioids cannot travel cephalad in the epidural space beyond the foramen magnum. The inner layer of the dura extends as a dural cuff that blends with the perineurium of spinal nerves. The cerebral arachnoid extends as the spinal arachnoid, ending at the second sacral vertebra. The pia is in close contact with the spinal cord.

Computed tomography demonstrates the presence of a connective tissue band (dorsomedian connective tissue band or plica mediana dorsalis) that divides the epidural space at the dorsal midline (Savolaine et al, 1988). This band binds the dura mater and the ligamentum flavum at the midline, making it difficult to feel loss of resistance during attempted midline identification of the epidural space. This band may also explain the occasional occurrence of unilateral analgesia following injection of local anesthetic into the epidural space (Gallart et al, 1990).

PATHWAYS FOR PERIPHERAL SENSORY IMPULSES

Sensory information from somatic segments of the body enter the gray matter of the spinal cord via the dorsal nerve roots. After entering the spi-

dermatomes as having distinct borders, there is extensive overlap between segments. For example, three consecutive dorsal nerve roots need to be interrupted to produce complete denervation of a dermatome. Segmental innervation of myotomes is even less well defined than that of dermatomes, emphasizing that skeletal muscle groups receive innervation from several anterior nerve roots.

Sensory signals from the periphery are transmitted through spinal nerves into each segment of the spinal cord, resulting in automatic motor responses that occur instantly (muscle stretch reflex, withdrawal reflex) in response to sensory signals. Spinal cord reflexes are important in nal cord, these neurons give rise to long, ascending fiber tracts that transmit sensory information to the brain. These sensory signals are transmitted to the brain by the dorsal-lemniscal system, which includes dorsal column pathways and spinocervical tracts, and by anterolateral spinothalamic tracts (Figs. 41-5 and 41-6) (Guyton, 1986). Impulses in the dorsal column pathways cross in the spinal cord to the opposite side before passing upward to the thalamus. Synapses in the thalamus are followed by neurons that extend into the somatic sensory area of the cerebral cortex. Nerve fibers of the anterolateral spinothalamic system cross in the anterior commissure to the opposite side of the spinal cord, where they turn upward toward the brain as the ventral and lateral spinothalamic tracts. Sensory signals from the anterior lateral spinothalamic system are re-

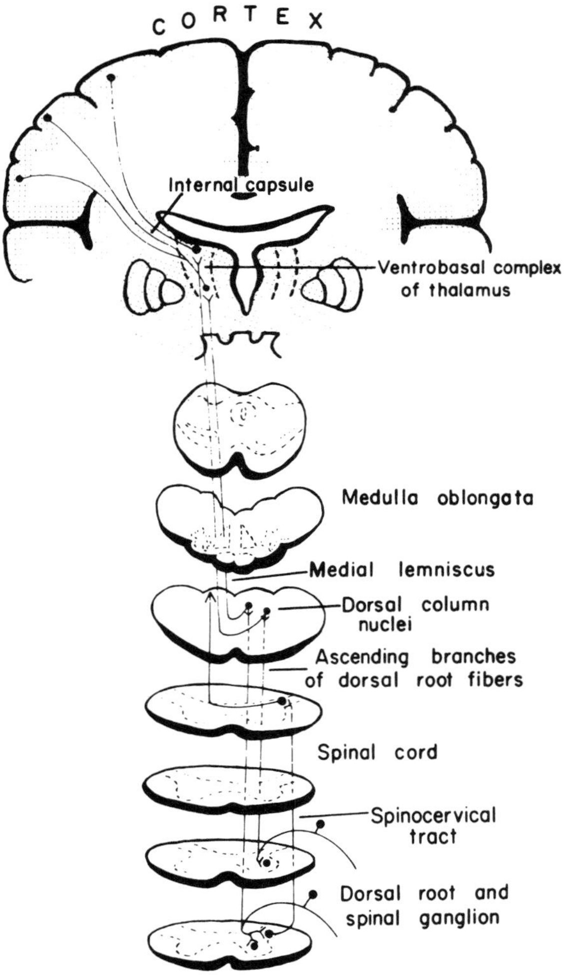

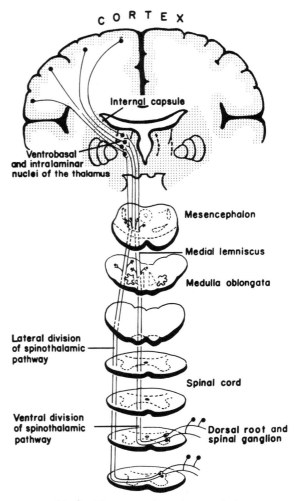

FIGURE 41–5. Sensory signals are transmitted to the brain by the dorsal column pathways and spinocervical tracts of the dorsal–lemniscal system. (From Guyton AC. Textbook of Medical Physiology. 7th ed. Philadelphia: WB Saunders, 1986; with permission.)

FIGURE 41–6. The anterolateral spinothalamic system fibers cross in the anterior commissure of the spinal cord before ascending to the brain. The fibers of this system transmit signals via ventral and lateral spinothalamic tracts. (From Guyton AC. Textbook of Medical Physiology. 7th ed. Philadelphia: WB Saunders, 1986; with permission.)

layed from the thalamus to the somatic sensory area of the cerebral cortex. All sensory information that enters the cerebral cortex, with the exception of the olfactory system, passes through the thalamus.

PATHWAYS FOR PERIPHERAL MOTOR RESPONSES

Sensory information is integrated at all levels of the nervous system and causes appropriate motor responses, beginning in the spinal cord with relatively simple reflex responses. Motor responses originating in the brain stem are more complex, while the most complicated and precise motor responses originate from the cerebral cortex.

Anterior motor neurons in the anterior horns of the spinal cord gray matter give rise to A-alpha fibers, which leave the spinal cord by way of anterior nerve roots and innervate skeletal muscles. Skeletal muscles and tendons contain muscle spindles and Golgi tendon organs that operate at a subconscious level to relay information to the spinal cord and brain relative to changes in length and tension of skeletal muscle fibers. The stretch reflex is reflex contraction of the skeletal muscle whenever stretch results in stimulation of the muscle spindle. Tapping the patellar tendon elicits a knee jerk, which is a stretch reflex of the quadriceps femoris muscle. The ankle jerk is due to reflex contraction of the gastrocnemius muscle. Transmission of large numbers of facilitatory impulses from upper regions of the central nervous system to the spinal cord results in exaggerated stretch reflex responses. For example, lesions in the contralateral motor areas of the cerebral cortex, as caused by a cerebral vascular accident or a brain tumor, cause greatly enhanced stretch reflexes. Clonus occurs when evoked muscle jerks oscillate. This phenomenon typically occurs when the stretch reflex is sensitized by facilitatory impulses from the brain, resulting in exaggerated facilitation of the spinal cord. When associated with recovery from general anesthesia, clonus as initiated by abrupt dorsiflexion of the foot can be eliminated by flexing the knees and keeping them in a flexed position (Azzam, 1987).

Transection of the brain stem at the level of the pons (isolates the spinal cord from the rest of the brain) results in spasticity known as *decere-*

brate rigidity. Decerebrate rigidity reflects diffuse facilitation of stretch reflexes.

The motor system is often divided into upper and lower motor neurons. Lower motor neurons are those from the spinal cord that directly innervate skeletal muscles. A lower motor neuron lesion is associated with flaccid paralysis, atrophy of skeletal muscles, and absence of stretch reflex responses. Spastic paralysis with accentuated stretch reflexes in the absence of skeletal muscle paralysis is due to destruction of upper motor neurons in the brain.

Withdrawal flexor reflexes are most often elicited by a painful stimulus. Associated with withdrawal of the stimulated limb is extension of the opposite limb (cross-extensor reflex) that occurs 0.2 to 0.5 second later and serves to push the body away from the object causing the painful stimulus. The delayed onset of the cross-extensor reflex is due to the time necessary for the signal to pass through the additional neurons to reach the opposite side of the spinal cord.

Spasm of skeletal muscles surrounding a broken bone seems to result from nociceptive impulses initiated from the broken edges of bone. Relief of pain and skeletal muscle spasm is provided by infiltration of a local anesthetic. In some instances, general anesthesia may be necessary to relieve skeletal muscle spasm and permit proper alignment of the two ends of the bone. Abdominal muscle spasm caused by irritation of the parietal peritoneum by peritonitis is an example of local skeletal muscle spasm caused by a spinal cord reflex. Similar spasm of the abdominal skeletal muscles occurs during surgical operations in which stimulation of the parietal peritoneum causes the abdominal muscles to contract and cause extrusion of intestines through the surgical wound. During surgical operations in the abdomen, this skeletal muscle spasm is attenuated by volatile anesthetics and abolished by regional anesthesia or neuromuscular blocking drugs.

Autonomic Reflexes

Segmental autonomic reflexes occur in the spinal cord and include changes in vascular tone, diaphoresis, and evacuation reflexes from the bladder and colon. Simultaneous excitation of all the segmental reflexes is the mass reflex (denervation hypersensitivity or autonomic hyperreflexia) (see Chapter 42). The mass reflex typically occurs in the presence of spinal cord transection when a painful stimulus to the skin below the level of spinal cord transection or distension of a hollow viscus, such as the bladder or gastrointestinal tract, occurs. This mass reflex is analogous to epileptic attacks that involve the central nervous system. The principal manifestation of the mass reflex is hypertension owing to intense peripheral vasoconstriction, reflecting an inability of vasodilating inhibitory impulses from the central nervous system to pass beyond the site of spinal cord transection. Carotid sinus baroreceptor-mediated reflex bradycardia accompanies the hypertension associated with the mass reflex.

Spinal Shock

Spinal shock is a manifestation of the abrupt loss of spinal cord reflexes that immediately follows transection of the spinal cord. This emphasizes the dependence of spinal cord reflexes on continual tonic discharges from higher centers. The immediate manifestations of spinal shock are hypotension owing to loss of vasoconstrictor tone and absence of all skeletal muscle reflexes. Within a few days to weeks, spinal cord neurons gradually regain their intrinsic excitability. Sacral reflexes for control of bladder and colon evacuation are completely suppressed for the first few weeks following spinal cord transection, but these spinal cord reflexes also eventually return.

ANATOMY OF NERVE FIBERS

Nerve fibers are afferent if they transmit impulses from peripheral receptors to the spinal cord and efferent if they relay signals from the spinal cord and central nervous system to the periphery.

Neurons

The principal function of neurons is to relay information between the periphery and the central nervous system. A neuron consists of a cell body, or soma; dendrites; and a nerve fiber, or axon (Fig. 41-7). Dendrites are extensions of the cell body. The axon of one neuron terminates (synapses) near the cell body or dendrites of another

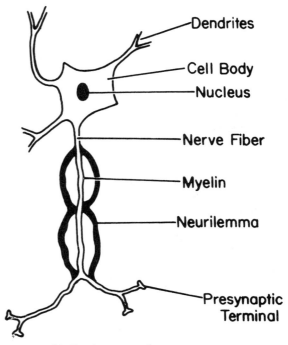

FIGURE 41-7. Anatomy of a neuron.

neuron. The end areas of an axon are called *presynaptic terminals.* The space between the presynaptic terminals and the cell body or dendrites of the next neuron is known as the *presynaptic cleft.* Transmission of impulses between responsive neurons at a synapse is mediated by presynaptic release of a chemical mediator (neurotransmitter), such as norepinephrine or acetylcholine. This chemically mediated response differs from electrical transmission of impulses along axons. Nerve membranes of postsynaptic neurons are speculated to contain receptors that bind neurotransmitters released from presynaptic nerve terminals.

Functionally, the nerve membrane is the most important part of the nerve fiber for impulse conduction. Indeed, removal of the axoplasm from the nerve fiber does not alter conduction of impulses. Nerve fibers derive their nutrition from the cell body. Interruption of a nerve fiber causes the peripheral portion to degenerate (Wallerian degeneration). The central part of the neuron, however, is able to regenerate, as does the myelin sheath. Nevertheless, lack of neurilemma prevents this type of regeneration from occurring in the brain or spinal cord.

Classification of Afferent Nerve Fibers

Afferent nerve fibers are classified as A, B, and C on the basis of fiber diameter and velocity of conduction of nerve impulses (Table 41-1). The largest-diameter A fibers are subdivided into alpha, beta, gamma, and delta. Type A-alpha fibers innervate skeletal muscles. Tactile sensory receptors (Meissner's corpuscles, hair receptors, Pacinian corpuscles) transmit signals in type A-beta fibers. Type A-gamma fibers are distributed to skeletal muscle spindles. Touch and fast pain are transmitted by type A-delta fibers (see Chapter 43). Type C fibers transmit slow pain, pruritus, and temperature impulses. Types A and B fibers are myelinated, whereas type C fibers are unmyelinated.

Myelin that surrounds type A and B nerve fibers acts as an insulator that prevents flow of ions across nerve membranes. The myelin sheath, however, is interrupted approximately every millimeter by nodes of Ranvier (Fig. 41-8) (Guyton, 1986). Ions can flow freely between nerve fibers and extracellular fluid at nodes of Ranvier. Action potentials are conducted from node to node by the myelinated nerve rather than continuously along the entire fiber as occurs in unmyelinated nerve fibers. This successive excitation of nodes of Ranvier by an impulse that jumps between successive nodes is termed *saltatory excitation* (Fig. 41-8) (Guyton, 1986). Saltatory conduction greatly increases velocity of nerve transmission in myelinated nerve fibers and also conserves energy because only the nodes of Ranvier depolarize, resulting in less loss of ions than would otherwise occur. Furthermore, because depolarization is limited to only the nodes of Ranvier, little additional metabolism for reestablishing sodium (Na^+) and potassium (K^+) ion concentra-

Table 41-1
Classification of Peripheral Nerve Fibers

	Myelinated	*Fiber Diameter (microns)*	*Conduction Velocity (m·sec⁻¹)*	*Function*	*Sensitivity to Local Anesthetic (subarachnoid, procaine) (percent)*
A					
A-alpha	Yes	12–20	70–120	Innervation of skeletal muscles Proprioception	1
A-beta	Yes	5–12	30–70	Touch Pressure	1
A-gamma	Yes	3–6	15–30	Skeletal muscle tone	1
A-delta	Yes	2–5	12–30	Fast pain Touch Temperature	0.5
B	Yes	3	3–15	Preganglionic autonomic fibers	0.25
C	No	0.4–1.2	0.5–2	Slow pain Touch Temperature Postganglionic sympathetic fibers	0.5

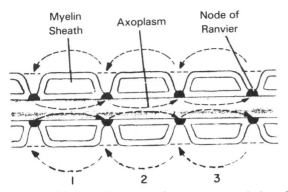

FIGURE 41–8. Saltatory conduction is transmission of nerve impulses that jump between successive nodes of Ranvier of myelinated nerves. (From Guyton AC. Textbook of Medical Physiology. 7th ed. Philadelphia: WB Saunders, 1986; with permission.)

tion differences across nerve membranes is necessary.

NEUROTRANSMITTERS

Neurotransmitters are chemical mediators that are released into the synaptic cleft in response to the arrival of an action potential at the nerve ending. Release of all neurotransmitters is voltage dependent and requires the influx of calcium ions (Ca^{2+}) into the presynaptic terminals. Synaptic vesicles on the cell body and dendrites of neurons are the sites for continuous synthesis and storage of neurotransmitters. These vesicles may contain and release more than one neurotransmitter simultaneously, so a single agonist or antagonist drug might not produce total reversal of the anticipated response. Neurotransmitters may be excitatory or inhibitory, depending on the configurational change produced in the protein receptor by its interaction with the neurotransmitter. Specifically, permeability to most ions is increased by interaction of an excitatory neurotransmitter and receptor, whereas inhibitory responses typically reflect increased permeability to chloride ions (Cl^-) and K^+. A postsynaptic receptor may be excited or inhibited, reflecting the existence of both types of receptors in the same postsynaptic neuron. Furthermore, the same neurotransmitter may be inhibitory at one site and cause excitation at another. Some neurotransmitters function as neuromodulators in that they influence the sensitivity of receptors to other neurotransmitters. General anesthetics depress excitable tissues at all levels of the nervous system by stabilizing neuronal membranes, resulting in a decreased release of neurotransmitter and transmission of impulses at synapses as well as a general depression of postsynaptic responsiveness and ion movement.

Types of Neurotransmitters

The list of chemical mediators functioning as excitatory or inhibitory neurotransmitters continues to increase (Table 41-2). Acetylcholine, dopamine, and norepinephrine are widely and unevenly distributed, suggesting these substances are important neurotransmitters in the central nervous system. Neuromodulators coexist in presynaptic terminals with neurotransmitters but do not themselves cause substantive voltage or conductance changes in postsynaptic cell membranes. They can, however, amplify, prolong, reduce, or shorten the postsynaptic response to selected neurotransmitters.

Acetylcholine

Acetylcholine is an excitatory neurotransmitter that interacts with muscarinic and nicotinic receptors in the central nervous system. This excitatory effect on the central nervous system contrasts with the inhibitory effects (increased K^+ permeability leading to hyperpolarization of

Table 41–2
Chemicals that Act at Synapses as Neurotransmitters

Acetylcholine	Serotonin
Dopamine	Histamine
Norepinephrine	Vasopressin
Epinephrine	Oxytocin
Glycine	Prolactin
Gamma-aminobutyric acid	Cholecystokinin
Glutamic acid	Vasoactive
Substance P	intestinal
Endorphins	peptide
	Gastrin
	Glucagon

postsynaptic membranes) of acetylcholine on the peripheral parasympathetic nervous system.

Dopamine

Dopamine represents more than 50% of the central nervous system content of catecholamines, with high concentrations especially in the basal ganglia. It is most likely that dopamine is an inhibitory neurotransmitter, perhaps by acting on dopamine-sensitive adenylate cyclase.

Norepinephrine

Norepinephrine is present in large amounts in the reticular activating system and the hypothalamus. Neurons responding to norepinephrine send predominantly inhibitory impulses to widespread areas of the brain, such as the cerebral cortex.

Epinephrine

Epinephrine-containing neurons are present in the reticular activating system, where its presumed effect is that of an inhibitory neurotransmitter.

Glycine

Glycine is the principal inhibitory neurotransmitter in the spinal cord acting to increase Cl^- conductance. Strychnine and tetanus toxin result in seizures because they antagonize the effects of glycine on postsynaptic inhibition. Visual disturbances following transurethral resection of the prostate in which glycine is the irrigating solution may reflect the role of this substance as an inhibitory neurotransmitter in the retina (Ovassapian et al, 1982). Amplitude and latency of visual evoked potentials are altered by intravenous infusions of glycine (Wang et al, 1989).

Gamma-Aminobutyric Acid

GABA is an inhibitory neurotransmitter present in diverse areas of the nervous system including the spinal cord, cerebellum, basal ganglia, and cerebral cortex. It is estimated that as many as one third of synapses in the brain are GABA-ergic. When two molecules of GABA bind to the receptor, the Cl^- channels open and allow Cl^- to flow into the neuron, causing it to become hyperpolarized. A hyperpolarized cell membrane

is more resistant to neuronal excitation, accounting for the inhibitory effects of GABA. The alpha- and beta-subunits of the GABA receptor constitute the Cl^- channel.

There is an increase in the amount of GABA released in the brain when the EEG manifests a slow-wave sleep pattern. Nonselective central nervous system stimulants may act as selective antagonists of GABA (see Chapter 33). Life cannot be sustained without GABA-ergic neurotransmission to counterbalance the influence of excitatory neurotransmitters.

Glutamic Acid

Glutamic acid is an excitatory neurotransmitter secreted by many sensory pathways in the central nervous system. This neurotransmitter causes depolarization of cell membranes primarily by increasing permeability to Na^+.

Substance P

Substance P is an excitatory neurotransmitter presumed to be released by terminals of pain fibers that synapse in the substantia gelatinosa of the spinal cord (see Chapter 43).

Endorphins

Endorphins are secreted by nerve terminals in the spinal cord, brain stem, thalamus, and hypothalamus, where they most likely act as excitatory neurotransmitters for descending pathways that inhibit the transmission of pain.

Serotonin

Serotonin is present in high concentrations in the brain, where it is believed to act as an inhibitory neurotransmitter exerting profound effects on mood and behavior. Lysergic acid diethylamide (LSD) is a serotonin antagonist. The similarities of the effects of ketamine and LSD on behavior suggest a common effect on serotonin.

Histamine

Histamine is present in high concentrations in the hypothalamus and the reticular activating system, where it is presumed to act as an inhibitory neurotransmitter. Cyclic adenosine monophosphate may serve as a second messenger to mediate the actions of histamine in the central nervous system.

ELECTRICAL EVENTS DURING NEURONAL EXCITATION

Resting transmembrane potentials of neurons in the central nervous system are about −70 mv, which is less than the −90 mv in large peripheral nerve fibers and skeletal muscles. This reduced magnitude of the resting transmembrane potential is important for controlling the responsiveness of neurons. At inhibitory synapses, a neurotransmitter increases the permeability of postsynaptic receptors to K^+ and Cl^-. Receptors responding to inhibitory neurotransmitters are associated with channels that are too small to allow passage of larger hydrated Na^+. The predominant outward diffusion of K^+ increases the negativity of the resting transmembrane potential, and the neuron is hyperpolarized (functions as an inhibitory neuron). Conversely, permeability changes evoked by an excitatory neurotransmitter decrease the negativity of the resting transmembrane potential, bringing it nearer threshold potential. As a result, these neurons function in the excitatory mode. In addition to postsynaptic inhibition caused by inhibitory synapses at neuron cell membranes, there is also presynaptic inhibition. GABA may be the presynaptic inhibitory neurotransmitter in the brain, whereas glycine may be the presynaptic inhibitory neurotransmitter in the spinal cord.

Synaptic Delay

Synaptic delay is the 0.3 to 0.5 seconds necessary for the transmission of an impulse from the synaptic varicosity to the postsynaptic neuron. This synaptic delay reflects the time for release of neurotransmitter from the synaptic varicosity, diffusion of neurotransmitter to the postsynaptic receptor, and the subsequent change in permeability of the postsynaptic membrane to various ions.

Synaptic Fatigue

Synaptic fatigue is a decrease in the number of discharges by the postsynaptic membrane when excitatory synapses are repetitively and rapidly stimulated. For example, synaptic fatigue decreases excessive excitability of the brain such as may accompany a seizure, thus acting as a protective mechanism against excessive neuronal activity. The mechanism of synaptic fatigue is presumed to be exhaustion of the stores of neurotransmitter in the synaptic varicosities.

Posttetanic Facilitation

Posttetanic facilitation is increased responsiveness of the postsynaptic neuron to stimulation after a rest period that was preceded by repetitive stimulation of an excitatory synapse. This phenomenon may reflect increased release of neurotransmitter owing to enhanced permeability of synaptic varicosities to Ca^{2+}. Posttetanic facilitation may be a mechanism for short-term memory.

Factors that Influence Neuron Responsiveness

Neurons are highly sensitive to changes in the pH of the surrounding interstitial fluids. For example, alkalosis enhances neuron excitability. Indeed, voluntary hyperventilation can evoke a seizure in a susceptible person. Conversely, acidosis depresses neuron excitability with a decrease in arterial pH to 7.0, causing coma. Lack of oxygen can cause total inexcitability of neurons within 3 to 5 seconds, as reflected by the onset of unconsciousness owing to cessation of cerebral blood flow.

Inhaled anesthetics may increase cell membrane threshold for excitation and thus decrease neuron activity throughout the body. This concept is based on the speculation that most lipid-soluble volatile anesthetics may change the permeability characteristics of cell membranes, making the neuron less responsive to excitatory neurotransmitters.

CEREBRAL BLOOD FLOW

Cerebral blood flow averages 50 ml·100 g^{-1}·min^{-1} of brain tissue. For an adult, this is equivalent to 750 ml·min^{-1}, or about 15% of the resting cardiac output, delivered to an organ that represents only about 2% of the body's mass. The gray matter of the brain has a higher cerebral blood flow (80 ml·100 g^{-1}·min^{-1}) than the white matter (20 ml·100 g^{-1}·min^{-1}). As in most other tissues of the body, cerebral blood flow parallels cerebral metabolic requirements for oxygen (3 to 5 ml oxygen·100 g^{-1}·min^{-1}). $PaCO_2$ and PaO_2 influence cerebral blood flow, whereas sympathetic and parasympathetic nerves play little or no role in the regulation of cerebral blood flow (Fig. 41-9). Changes in the $PaCO_2$ between about 20 and 80 mmHg produce corresponding changes in cerebral blood flow. For example, in this range, a 1-mmHg increase in the $PaCO_2$ evokes a 2-ml·100 g^{-1}·min^{-1} increase in cerebral blood flow. Carbon dioxide increases cerebral blood flow by combining with water in body fluids to form carbonic acid, with subsequent dissociation to form hydrogen ions (H^+). H^+ produce vasodilation of cerebral vessels that is proportional to the increase in H^+ concentration. Any other acid that increases H^+ concentration, such as lactic acid, also increases cerebral blood flow. Increased cerebral blood flow in response to elevations in $PaCO_2$ serves to carry away excess H^+ that would otherwise greatly depress neuronal activity.

Unlike the continuous response of cerebral blood flow to changes in $PaCO_2$, the response to PaO_2 is a threshold phenomenon (Fig. 41-9). If the $PaCO_2$ is maintained constant, cerebral blood flow begins to increase when the PaO_2 declines below 50 mmHg or the cerebral venous PO_2 decreases from its normal value of 35 mmHg to about 30 mmHg.

Autoregulation

Cerebral blood flow is closely autoregulated between mean arterial pressures of about 60 and 140 mmHg (Fig. 41-9). As a result, changes in blood pressure within this range will not significantly alter cerebral blood flow. Chronic hypertension shifts the autoregulation curve to the right such that reductions in cerebral blood flow may occur at mean arterial pressures greater than 60 mmHg. Autoregulation of cerebral blood flow is reduced or abolished by hypercapnia, arterial hypoxemia, and volatile anesthetics. Furthermore, autoregulation is often abolished in the area surrounding an acute cerebral infarction. For example, reactivity of blood vessels in areas surrounding cerebral infarcts and tumors is abolished. These blood vessels are maximally

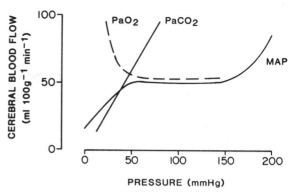

FIGURE 41-9. Cerebral blood flow is influenced by PaO_2, $PaCO_2$, and mean arterial pressure (*MAP*).

vasodilated, presumably reflecting accumulation of acidic metabolic products. As a result, cerebral blood flow to this area is already maximal (luxury perfusion) and changes in $PaCO_2$ will have no effect on its local blood flow. If $PaCO_2$ should increase, however, it is theoretically possible that resulting vasodilation in normal blood vessels would shunt blood flow away from the diseased area (intracerebral steal syndrome). Conversely, a decrease in $PaCO_2$ that constricts normal cerebral vessels could divert blood flow to diseased areas (Robin Hood phenomenon). Elevations in mean arterial pressure above the limits of autoregulation can cause leakage of intravascular fluid through capillary membranes, resulting in cerebral edema. Because the brain is enclosed in a solid vault, the accumulation of edema fluid increases intracranial pressure and compresses blood vessels, decreasing cerebral blood flow and leading to destruction of brain tissue.

Measurement of Cerebral Blood Flow

Cerebral blood flow can be measured by injecting a radioactive substance, usually xenon, into the carotid artery and measuring the rate of decay of the radioactivity in each tissue segment using scintillation detectors. Using this technique, it can be demonstrated that cerebral blood flow changes within seconds in response to changes in local neuronal activity. For example, clasping the hand can be shown to cause an immediate increase in blood flow in the motor cortex of the opposite cerebral hemisphere. Reading increases blood flow in the occipital cortex and the language areas of the temporal cortex. This measuring procedure can be used to localize the origin of epileptic attacks because blood flow increases acutely at the site of origin of the seizure.

ELECTROENCEPHALOGRAM

The EEG is a recording of the brain waves that result from the continuous electrical activity in the brain. The intensity of the electrical activity recorded from the surface of the scalp ranges from 0 to 300 μv, and the frequency may exceed 50 cycles·sec⁻¹. The character of the waves is greatly dependent on the level of activity of the cerebral cortex and the degree of wakefulness. There is a direct relationship between the degree of cerebral activity and the frequency of brain waves. Furthermore, during periods of increased mental activity, brain waves usually become asynchronous rather than synchronous, so the voltage decreases despite cortical activity.

Classification of Brain Waves

Brain waves are classified as alpha, beta, theta, and delta waves depending on their frequency and amplitude (Fig. 41-10). The classic EEG is a plot of voltage against time, usually recorded by 16 channels on paper running at 30 mm·sec⁻¹. One page of recording is 10 seconds of data.

Alpha Waves

Alpha waves occur at a frequency of 8 to 12 cycles·sec⁻¹ and a voltage of about 50 μv. These waves are typical of an awake, resting state of cerebration with the eyes closed. During sleep, alpha waves disappear. Because alpha waves do not occur when the cerebral cortex is not connected to the thalamus, it is assumed these waves result from spontaneous activity in the thalamocortical system.

Beta Waves

Beta waves occur at a frequency of 13 to 30 cycles·sec⁻¹ and a voltage usually less than 50 μv. These high-frequency and low-voltage asynchronous waves replace alpha waves in the presence of increased mental activity or visual stimulation.

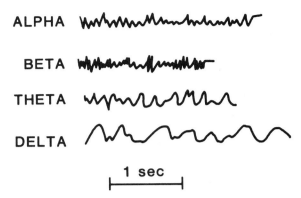

FIGURE 41–10. The electroencephalogram consists of alpha, beta, theta, and delta waves.

Theta Waves

Theta waves occur at a frequency of 4 to 7 cycles·sec⁻¹. These waves occur in healthy children during sleep and also during general anesthesia.

Delta Waves

Delta waves include all the brain waves with a frequency of less than 4 cycles·sec⁻¹. These waves occur (1) in deep sleep; (2) during general anesthesia; and (3) in the presence of organic brain disease. Delta waves occur even when the connections of the cerebral cortex to the reticular activating system are severed, indicating these waves originate in the cerebral cortex independently of lower brain structures. Occurrence of delta waves during sleep suggests that the cerebral cortex is released from the activating influences of the reticular activating system.

Clinical Uses

The EEG is useful in diagnosing different types of epilepsy and for determining the focus in the brain causing seizures. Brain tumors, which compress surrounding neurons and cause abnormal electrical activity, may be localized using the EEG. Monitoring the EEG during carotid endarterectomy, cardiopulmonary bypass, or deliberate hypotension may provide an early warning of inadequate cerebral blood flow. In this regard, the EEG may be influenced by anesthetic drugs, depth of anesthesia, and hyperventilation of the lungs (see Chapter 2).

Epilepsy

Epilepsy is characterized by excessive activity of either a part or all of the central nervous system. About 1 in 50 persons manifests a hereditary predisposition for epilepsy. In these individuals, alkalosis, fever, sudden loud noises, or flashing lights may precipitate an attack. Even in persons not genetically predisposed, traumatic lesions in the brain can cause excess excitability of local brain areas which can transmit signals to the reticular activating system to elicit grand mal seizures.

GRAND MAL EPILEPSY. Grand mal epilepsy is characterized by intense neuronal discharges in multiple areas of the cerebral cortex and reticular activating system. These impulses are transmitted to the spinal cord, resulting in alternating skeletal muscle contractions known as tonic-clonic seizures. Signals to the viscera often result in defecation or urination. The grand mal seizure lasts from a few seconds to several minutes and is followed by generalized depression of the entire central nervous system. The EEG during a grand mal seizure reveals high-voltage, synchronous brain wave discharges over the entire cerebral cortex. Synaptic fatigue is a likely mechanism that contributes to spontaneous cessation of a grand mal seizure and postictal depression.

Status epilepticus is present when grand mal seizure activity is sustained. Diazepam, administered intravenously, is an often recommended treatment to stop seizures and permit resumption of effective breathing. Drugs such as thiopental are also effective, but their depressant effect on the central nervous system is generalized, nonspecific, and may be associated with lingering sedative effects. In the rare instance where conventional drug therapy is ineffective, volatile anesthetics such as halothane or isoflurane may be administered to stop status epilepticus (Kofke et al, 1989). When volatile anesthetics are used for this purpose, it will usually be necessary to support blood pressure with intravenous administration of fluids and/or sympathomimetics. Evidence that volatile anesthetics do not reverse the underlying cause of seizures is the predictable reappearance of seizure activity when administration of the anesthetic is discontinued.

PETIT MAL EPILEPSY. Petit mal epilepsy is characterized by transient periods of unconsciousness (less than 30 seconds) and is associated with twitching contractions of some skeletal muscles, particularly in the face. The brain waves on the EEG manifest as a spike-and-dome pattern, which can be recorded over most of the cerebral cortex, confirming that the seizure activity usually involves the reticular activating system. Occasionally, petit mal seizures are more localized, suggesting an origin in focal regions of specific thalamic nuclei.

FOCAL EPILEPSY. Focal epilepsy can involve nearly any part of the brain and almost always results from a localized lesion such as (1) a scar that pulls on neuronal tissue, (2) a tumor that compresses an area of the brain, or (3) a congenital abnormality in neuronal circuitry. Lesions such as these can promote rapid discharges in local neurons that result in progressive spread (march) of skeletal muscle contractions, most often beginning in the mouth region and eventually spreading to the legs.

PSYCHOMOTOR EPILEPSY. Psychomotor epilepsy is a form of focal epilepsy characteristically involving the limbic portion of the brain that includes the temporal cortex. The EEG may be used to localize the site of origin of the abnormal activity. Anesthetic drugs, such as methohexital or etomidate, may be used to activate these seizure sites, thus facilitating their identification and subsequent surgical resection (Gancher et al, 1984; Rockoff and Goudsouzian, 1981).

EVOKED POTENTIALS

Evoked potentials are the electrophysiologic responses of the nervous system to sensory stimulation. The waveforms resulting from sensory stimulation reflect transmission of impulses through specific sensory pathways. Poststimulus latency is the time in milliseconds from application of the stimulus to a peak in the recorded waveform. The amplitude and latency of evoked potentials may be influenced by a number of events, especially volatile anesthetics. Evoked potentials are used to monitor (1) spinal cord function during operations near or on the spinal cord, and (2) auditory nerve and brain stem function, as during operations on pituitary tumors or other lesions that impinge on the optic nerves or optic chiasm. The modes of sensory stimulation used to produce evoked potentials in the operating room are somatosensory, auditory, and visual.

Somatosensory Evoked Potentials

Somatosensory evoked potentials are produced by application of a low-voltage electrical current that stimulates a peripheral nerve such as the median nerve at the wrist or posterior tibial nerve at the ankle. The resulting evoked potentials reflect the intactness of neural pathways from the peripheral nerve to the somatosensory cortex. Inhaled anesthetics, especially volatile anesthetics, produce dose-dependent depression of somatosensory evoked potentials (see Chapter 2). Although less so than volatile anesthetics, morphine and fentanyl also produce depressant effects on somatosensory evoked potentials, with a low-dose, continuous infusion of an opioid producing less depression than intermittent injections (Pathak et al, 1984). Ketamine or etomidate may increase the amplitude of somatosensory evoked potentials (see Chapter 4). Acute hyperventilation of the lungs to produce a $PaCO_2$ near 20 mmHg does not significantly alter amplitude or latencies of evoked potentials (Schubert and Drummond, 1986).

Auditory Evoked Potentials

Auditory evoked potentials arise from brain stem auditory pathways. Volatile anesthetics produce dose-dependent depression of auditory evoked potentials.

Visual Evoked Potentials

Visual evoked potentials are produced by flashes from light-emitting diodes that are mounted on goggles placed over the patient's closed eyes. During neurosurgical procedures involving visual pathways (transphenoidal or anterior fossa surgery), the monitoring of visual evoked potentials has been used. Volatile anesthetics produce dose-dependent depression of visual evoked potentials, especially above concentrations equivalent to about 0.8 MAC (Chi and Field, 1986).

CEREBROSPINAL FLUID

Cerebrospinal fluid is present in (1) the ventricles of the brain, (2) the cisterns around the brain, and (3) the subarachnoid space around the brain and spinal cord (Fig. 41-11). The total volume of cerebrospinal fluid is about 150 ml, and the specific gravity is 1.002 to 1.009. A major function of cerebrospinal fluid is to cushion the brain in the cranial cavity. A blow to the head moves the entire brain simultaneously, causing no one portion of the brain to be selectively contorted by the blow. When a blow to the head is particularly severe, it usually does not damage the brain on the ipsilateral side, but instead damage manifests on

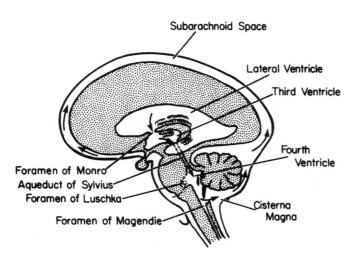

FIGURE 41-11. Circulation of cerebrospinal fluid.

the opposite side. This phenomenon is known as *contrecoup* and reflects the creation of a vacuum between the brain and skull opposite the blow caused by sudden movement of the brain at this site away from the skull. When the skull is no longer being accelerated by the blow, the vacuum suddenly collapses and the brain strikes the interior surface of the skull.

Formation

The choroid plexuses (cauliflower-like growths of blood vessels covered by a thin layer of epithelial cells) in the four cerebral ventricles are the major site of formation of cerebrospinal fluid, which continually exudes from the surface of the choroid plexus at a rate of about 30 ml·h^{-1}. The rate of cerebrospinal fluid production is increased by enflurane but not isoflurane, halothane, or fentanyl.

In comparison with other extracellular fluids, the concentrations of Na$^+$ and Cl$^-$ in the cerebrospinal fluid are 7% greater and the concentrations of glucose and K$^+$ are 30% and 40% less, respectively. This difference in composition from other extracellular fluids emphasizes that cerebrospinal fluid is a choroid secretion and not a simple filtrate from the capillaries. The pH of cerebrospinal fluid is closely regulated and maintained at 7.32. Changes in PaCO$_2$, but not arterial pH, promptly alter cerebrospinal fluid pH, reflecting the ability of carbon dioxide, but not H$^+$, to cross the blood-brain barrier easily. As a result, acute respiratory acidosis or alkalosis produces corresponding changes in cerebrospinal fluid pH. Active transport of bicarbonate ions eventually returns cerebrospinal fluid pH to 7.32, despite persistence of alterations in the arterial pH.

Reabsorption

Almost all the cerebrospinal fluid formed each day is reabsorbed into the venous circulation through special structures known as *arachnoid villi* or *granulations*. These villi project from the subarachnoid spaces into the venous sinuses of the brain and occasionally into the veins of the spinal cord. Arachnoid villi are actually trabeculae that protrude through the venous walls, resulting in highly permeable areas that permit relatively free flow of cerebrospinal fluid into the

circulation. The magnitude of reabsorption depends on the pressure gradient between cerebrospinal fluid and the venous circulation. Enflurane, but not isoflurane, increases resistance to the reabsorption of cerebrospinal fluid (see Chapter 2).

Circulation

Cerebrospinal fluid formed in the lateral cerebral ventricles passes into the third ventricle through the foramen of Monro (Fig 41-11). In the third ventricle, the cerebrospinal fluid mixes with that secreted in the lateral ventricle and then passes along the aqueduct of Sylvius into the fourth cerebral ventricle, where still more cerebrospinal fluid is formed. The cerebrospinal fluid then passes into the cisterna magna through the lateral foramen of Luschka and via a middle foramen of Magendie. From this point, cerebrospinal fluid flows through the subarachnoid spaces upward toward the cerebrum, where most of the arachnoid villi are located.

Hydrocephalus

Obstruction to free circulation of cerebrospinal fluid in the neonate results in hydrocephalus. For example, blockage of the aqueduct of Sylvius results in expansion of the lateral and third ventricles and compression of the brain (Fig. 41-11). This type of obstruction producing a noncommunicating type of hydrocephalus is treated by surgical creation of an artificial pathway for flow of cerebrospinal fluid between the ventricular system and the subarachnoid space.

Intracranial Pressure

Normal intracranial pressure is less than 15 mmHg. This pressure is regulated by the rate of cerebrospinal fluid formation and resistance to reabsorption through arachnoid villi as determined by venous pressure. In addition, increases in cerebral blood flow, as during inhalation of volatile anesthetics, can cause the intracranial pressure to rise because of the concomitant increase in cerebral blood flow and cerebral blood volume. Arterial blood pressure does not alter intracranial pressure within the range of normal autoregulation. Phasic variations in blood pressure, however, are transmitted as variations in intracranial pressure.

Papilledema

Anatomically, the dura of the brain extends as a sheath around the optic nerve and then connects with the sclera of the eye. When intracranial pressure increases, it is also reflected in the optic nerve sheath. Increased pressure in the optic sheath impedes blood flow in the retinal veins, leading to elevations in retinal capillary pressure and retinal edema. The tissues of the optic disc are more distensible than the rest of the retina, so the disc becomes more edematous than the remainder of the retina and swells into the cavity of the eye. This swelling of the optic disc is termed *papilledema.*

Blood-Brain Barrier

The blood-brain barrier reflects the lack of permeability of capillaries in the central nervous system, including the choroid plexuses, to circulat-

ing substances such as electrolytes and exogenous drugs or toxins. As a result, the internal consistency of the environment to which brain neurons are exposed is maintained over narrow limits. An anatomic explanation for the blood-brain barrier is the tight junction between endothelial cells of brain capillaries and envelopment of brain capillaries by glial cells, which further reduces their permeability. The blood-brain barrier is less developed in the neonate and tends to break down in areas of the brain that are irradiated or infected or are the site of tumors. The exception of the existence of a blood-brain barrier is the area around the posterior pituitary and the chemoreceptor trigger zone.

VISION

The eye is optically equivalent to a photographic camera in that it contains a lens system, a variable aperture system (pupil), and the retina that corresponds to the film (Fig. 41-12) (Ganong, 1987). The lens system of the eye focuses an image on the retina. Relaxation and contraction

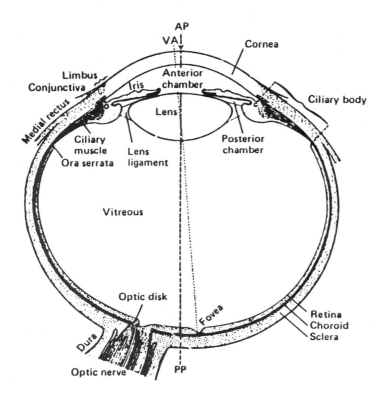

FIGURE 41–12. Schematic diagram of the eye. AP, anterior pole; PP, posterior pole; VA, visual axis. (From Ganong WF. Review of Medical Physiology. 13th ed. Norwalk, CT: Appleton and Lange, 1987; with permission.)

of the ciliary muscles are responsible for altering the tension of ligaments attached to the lens, causing its refractive power to change. One diopter is equivalent to the ability of a lens to converge parallel light rays to a focal point 1 m beyond the lens (59 diopters equal the total refractive power of the eye). Stimulation of parasympathetic nervous system fibers to the ciliary muscle causes this muscle to relax, which in turn relaxes the ligaments of the lens and increases its refractive power. This increased refractive power allows the eye to focus on objects that are nearby. Interference with this process of accommodation may be noted by patients in the postoperative period who have received an anticholinergic drug in the preoperative medication. The principal function of the pupil is to increase or decrease the amount of light that enters the eye. For example, the pupil may vary from 1.5 to 8 mm in diameter, permitting a 30-fold variation in the amount of light that enters the eye.

The lens loses its elastic nature with aging because of progressive denaturation of the lens's proteins. As a result, the ability to accommodate is almost totally absent by 45 to 50 years of age. This lack of ability of the lens to accommodate is known as *presbyopia*.

Progressive denaturation of the proteins in the lens leads to the formation of a cataract. In later stages, Ca^{2+} is often deposited in the coagulated proteins, thus further increasing the opacity. When the cataract impairs vision, the lens is surgically removed and replaced by an artificial convex lens that compensates for the loss of refractive power caused by removal of the lens.

Intraocular Fluid

Intraocular fluid consists of aqueous humor, which lies in front and at the sides of the lens, and vitreous humor, which lies between the lens and retina. Aqueous humor is freely flowing fluid that is continuously formed (2 to 3 ml·min^{-1}) and reabsorbed. This fluid is secreted by ciliary processes of the ciliary body in a manner similar to formation of cerebrospinal fluid by the choroid plexus. After flowing into the anterior chamber, aqueous humor enters Schlemm's canal, which is a thin vein that extends circumferentially around the eye. Vitreous humor is a gelatinous mass into which substances can diffuse slowly, but there is little flow of fluid.

Intraocular Pressure

Intraocular pressure is normally 15 to 25 mmHg. This pressure is measured clinically by tonometry, in which the amount of displacement of the tonometer is calibrated in terms of intraocular pressure. It is believed that intraocular pressure is regulated primarily by resistance to outflow of aqueous humor from the anterior chamber into Schlemm's canal. Glaucoma is associated with increased intraocular pressure sufficient to compress retinal artery inflow to the eye leading to ischemic pain and eventually blindness. When medical control of glaucoma fails, it may be necessary to surgically create an artificial outflow tract for aqueous humor.

Retina

The retina is the light-sensitive portion of the eye containing the cones, which are responsible for color vision, and the rods, which are mainly responsible for vision in the dark. When the cones and rods are stimulated, impulses are transmitted through successive neurons in the retina and optic nerve before reaching the cerebral cortex. The presence of melanin in the pigment layer of the retina prevents reflection of light throughout the globe. Without this pigment, light rays would be reflected in all directions within the globe, causing visual acuity to be impaired. Indeed, albinos, who lack melanin, have greatly decreased visual acuity.

The nutrient blood supply for the retina is largely derived from the central retinal artery, which accompanies the optic nerve. This independent retinal blood supply prevents rapid degeneration of the retina should it become detached from the pigment epithelium and allows time for surgical correction of a detached retina.

Photochemicals

The light-sensitive photochemical continuously synthesized in rods is rhodopsin. Cones contain photochemicals that resemble rhodopsin. Vitamin A is an important precursor of photochemicals, which explains the occurrence of night blindness when this vitamin becomes deficient. Photochemicals in rods and cones decompose on exposure to light and in the process stimulate fibers of the optic nerve. Decomposition of rhodopsin decreases conductance of the membranes of rods for Na^+. The resulting hyperpolarization in rods is opposite to the effect that occurs in almost all other sensory receptors. The intensity of the hyperpolarization signal is proportional to the logarithm of light energy, in contrast to the more linear response of most other receptors. This logarithmic response is important to vision because it allows the eyes to detect contrasts on the image even when light intensities vary several thousandfold.

If a person is in bright light for a prolonged period, large proportions of photochemicals in the rods and cones are depleted, resulting in decreased sensitivity of the eye to light (light adaptation). Conversely, during total darkness, the sensitivity of the retina is increased, reflecting conversion of photochemicals to rhodopsin (dark adaptation). The eye can also adapt to changes in light intensity by changing the size of the pupillary opening up to 30-fold.

Color Blindness

Red-green color blindness is present when red or green types of cones are absent. Color blindness is a sex-linked recessive trait that will not appear as long as one X chromosome carries the genes necessary for the development of color-receptor cones. Because males have only one X chromosome, all three color genes must be present in this single chromosome to prevent color blindness. In about 1 of every 50 times, the X chromosome lacks the gene from the red cone and, in about 1 in every 16 times, the gene for the green cone is absent. As a result, about 2% of males are color blind. Color blindness is rare in females because they possess two X chromosomes.

Visual Pathway

Impulses from the retina pass backward through the optic nerve (Fig. 41-13) (Ganong, 1987).

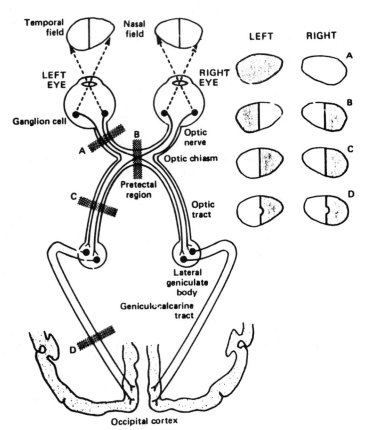

FIGURE 41-13. Visual impulses from the retina pass to the optic chiasm where fibers from the nasal halves of the retina cross to the opposite side to join temporal fibers and form the optic tract. These fibers synapse in the lateral geniculate body before passing to the visual (occipital) area of the cerebral cortex. Visual field defects reflect lesions at various sites (*A–D*) in the nerve pathways. (From Ganong WF. Review of Medical Physiology. 13th ed. Norwalk, CT, Appleton and Lange, 1987; with permission.)

The macula is a small area in the center of the retina that is composed mainly of cones to permit detailed vision. The fovea is the central portion of the macula and is the site of the most clear vision. At the optic chiasm, all the fibers from the nasal halves of the retina cross to the opposite side to join fibers from the opposite temporal retina to form the optic tracts. Fibers of the optic tract synapse in the lateral geniculate body before passing into the visual (occipital) area of the cerebral cortex. Specific points of the retina connect with specific points of the visual cortex, which results in the detection of lines, borders, and colors.

Field of Vision

Field of vision is the area seen by the eye at a given instant. The area seen to the nasal side is called the *nasal field of vision,* and the area seen to the lateral side is called the *temporal field of vision* (Fig. 41-13) (Ganong, 1987). Blind spots called *scotomata* are due to lack of rods and cones in the retina. An important use of visual fields is localization of lesions in the visual neural pathway. For example, anterior pituitary tumors may compress the optic chiasm, causing blindness in both temporal fields of vision (bitemporal hemianopia). Thrombosis of the posterior cerebral artery is a cause of infarction of the visual cortex.

Muscular Control of Eye Movements

The cerebral control system for directing the eyes toward the object to be viewed is as important as the cerebral system for interpretation of the visual signals. Movements of the eyes are controlled by three pairs of skeletal muscles designated as (1) the medial and lateral recti, (2) the superior and inferior recti, and (3) the superior and inferior obliques. The medial and lateral recti contract reciprocally to move the eyes from side to side; the superior and inferior recti move the eyes upward or downward; and rotation of the globe is accomplished by the superior and inferior obliques. Each of the three sets of eye muscles is reciprocally innervated by cranial nerves III, IV, and VI so that one muscle of the pair contracts while the other relaxes.

Simultaneous movement of both eyes in the same direction is called *conjugate movement* of the eyes. Occasionally, abnormalities occur in the control system for eye movements that cause continuous nystagmus. Nystagmus is likely to occur when one of the vestibular apparatuses is damaged or when deep nuclei in the cerebellum are damaged.

Innervation of the Eye

The eyes are innervated by the sympathetic and parasympathetic nervous system. The preganglionic fibers of the parasympathetic nervous system arise in the Edinger-Westphal nucleus of cranial nerve III and then pass to the ciliary ganglion, which gives rise to nerve fibers that innervate the ciliary muscle and sphincter of the iris. Sympathetic nervous system fibers innervate the radial fibers of the iris as well as several extraocular structures. Stimulation of the parasympathetic nervous system fibers to the eye excites the ciliary sphincter, causing miosis. Conversely, stimulation of sympathetic nervous system fibers to the eye excites the radial fibers of the iris and causes mydriasis.

Horner's Syndrome

Interruption in the superior cervical chain of the sympathetic nervous system innervation to the eye results in miosis, ptosis, and vasodilation with absence of sweating on the ipsilateral side. These findings are known as *Horner's syndrome* and characteristically occur following performance of a stellate ganglion block. Miosis occurs because of interruption of sympathetic nervous system innervation to the radial fibers of the iris. Ptosis reflects the normal innervation of the superior palpebral muscle by the sympathetic nervous system.

HEARING

Receptors for hearing and equilibrium are housed in the ear (Fig. 41-14) (Ganong, 1987). The external ear, middle ear, and cochlea of the inner ear are concerned with hearing based on mechanical vibrations of sound waves in air. Transmission of sound from the tympanic membrane to the cochlea utilizes an ossicle system.

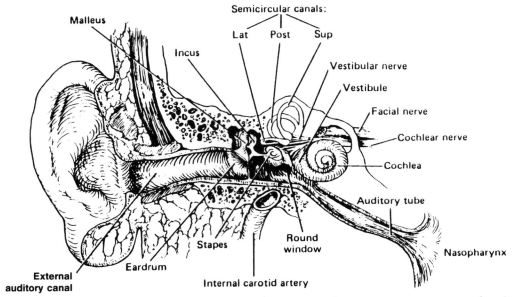

FIGURE 41–14.   Schematic diagram of the outer and inner ear. (From Ganong WF. Review of Medical Physiology. 13th ed. Norwalk, CT: Appleton and Lange, 1987; with permission.)

Ossicle System

The middle ear is an air-filled cavity containing the ossicle system that includes the malleus, incus, and stapes. The handle of the malleus is attached to the tympanic membrane, whereas the other end is bound by ligaments to the incus. The opposite end of the incus articulates with the stapes, which lies against the membranous labyrinth in the opening of the oval window where sound waves are transmitted to the cochlea. The handle of the malleus is constantly pulled inward by ligaments and by the tensor tympanic muscle, which keeps the tympanic membrane tensed. This allows vibrations on any portion of the tympanic membrane to be transmitted to the malleus. The eustachian tube allows pressures on both sides of the tympanic membrane to be equalized during swallowing or chewing. Nitrous oxide may increase middle ear pressure and even cause rupture of the tympanic membrane when inflammation or scarring of the eustachian tube opening into the nasopharynx prevents spontaneous decompression of middle ear pressures (Owens et al, 1978).

Cochlea

The cochlea is a system of coiled tubes embedded in a bony cavity in the temporal bone. The organ of Corti contains hair cells that function as end organs to generate nerve impulses in response to sound vibrations. These hair cells synapse with cochlear nerve endings, which enter the central nervous system for transmission to the auditory cerebral cortex.

Deafness

Nerve deafness is due to an abnormality of the cochlear or auditory nerve. Conversely, conduction deafness is present when an abnormality exists in the middle ear mechanisms for transmitting sounds into the cochlea. Certain drugs such as streptomycin, kanamycin, and chloramphenicol may damage the organ of Corti, causing nerve deafness. Conduction deafness is often caused by fibrosis of structures in the middle ear following repeated infections in the middle ear or by the hereditary disease known as *osteosclerosis.*

EQUILIBRIUM

Semicircular canals, the utricle and saccule of the inner ear, are concerned with equilibrium (Fig. 41-14) (Ganong, 1987). The utricle and saccule contain cilia that transmit nerve impulses to the brain necessary for maintaining orientation of the head in space. Endolymph present in the semicircular canals flows with changes in head position, causing signals to be transmitted via the vestibular nerve nuclei and the cerebellum. The semicircular canals predict ahead of time that loss of equilibrium is going to occur, leading to initiation of preventive responses.

A simple test of the integrity of the equilibrium mechanisms is to have the individual stand motionless with the eyes closed. In the absence of a functioning static equilibrium system of the utricles, the person will tend to fall to one side. Nevertheless, proprioceptive mechanisms (joint receptors) may be sufficiently developed to maintain balance even with the eyes closed. Separate testing of the semicircular canals is accomplished by placing ice water in the external auditory canal. The external semicircular canal is adjacent to the tympanic membrane such that selective cooling of the endolymph occurs. This cooling causes nystagmus in the presence of normally functioning semicircular canals.

CHEMICAL SENSES

Chemical senses are manifest as taste and smell.

Taste

Taste is mainly a function of taste buds located principally in the papillae of the tongue. Sweet, sour, salty, and bitter are the four primary sensations of taste. Sour taste is caused by acids, and the taste sensation is approximately proportional to the logarithm of the H^+ concentration. The bitter taste of alkaloids causes the individual to reject these substances. This is probably protective because many toxins in poisonous plants are alkaloids. Adaptation to taste sensations is almost complete within 1 to 5 minutes of continuous stimulation. Persons with upper respiratory tract infections complain of loss of taste sensation when, in fact, taste bud function is normal, emphasizing that most of what is considered taste is actually smell. Taste preference is presumed to be a central nervous system phenomenon.

Smell

Olfactory hairs, or cilia, are believed to sense odors in the air, causing stimulation of olfactory cells. It is presumed that olfactory cells initiate impulses in olfactory nerve fibers. A substance must be volatile and lipid soluble to stimulate olfactory cells. The importance of upward air movement in smell acuity is the reason sniffing improves the sense of smell, whereas holding one's breath prevents the sensation of an unpleasant smell. Olfactory receptors adapt rapidly such that smell sensation may become extinct in about 60 seconds. Compared with lower animals, the sense of smell in humans is almost rudimentary. Nevertheless, the threshold for smell is low as reflected by the detection of trace concentrations of methyl mercaptan that is mixed with odorless natural gas so as to alert one to a gas leak.

BODY TEMPERATURE

Heat is continually being produced in the body as a byproduct of metabolism. Metabolism refers to all the chemical reactions of the body, whereas metabolic rate is expressed in terms of the rate of heat liberation during these chemical reactions. As heat is produced, it is also continuously being lost to the environment. The net effect is regulation of body temperature within narrow limits, with a normal core body temperature range being 36.3 to 37.1 C (Ganong, 1987). Core temperature undergoes circadian fluctuations, being lowest in the morning and highest in the evening. This is consistent with a 10% to 15% decrease in basal metabolic rate during physiologic sleep, presumably reflecting decreased activity of skeletal muscles and the sympathetic nervous system.

An estimated 55% of the energy in nutrients becomes heat during the formation of adenosine triphosphate. The calorie is the unit for expressing the quantity of energy released from different nutrients. The average daily caloric requirement for basal function is about 2000 calories (Table 41-3).

Table 41-3
*Energy Expenditure for Various Forms of
Physical Activity*

Activity	Calories per Hour
Physiologic sleep	65
Awake at rest	77–100
Typing	140
Walking slowly (2.6 mph)	200
Swimming	500
Running (5.3 mph)	570
Walking up steps	1100

Heat Loss

Heat loss occurs as radiation, conduction, convection, evaporation, and diaphoresis. Most heat is lost by radiation in the form of infrared heat rays that pass from points of contact of the body with a cooler environment as represented by the skin and airways. Conduction of heat from the body to the air is self-limited unless new unheated air is continually brought into contact with the skin. After heat is conducted to air, this heat is carried away by air currents designated *convection*. The rate of heat loss to water is greater than the rate of heat loss to air because water has a greater specific heat (can absorb more heat) than air. Evaporation is the only mechanism by which the body can eliminate excess heat when the temperature of the surroundings is greater than that of the skin. Diaphoresis occurs in response to stimulation of the preoptic area in the hypothalamus. A normal unacclimatized person can produce maximally about 700 ml·h^{-1} of sweat, but with continued exposure to a warm environment, sweat production may increase to 1500 ml·h^{-1}. Evaporation of this much sweat can remove heat from the body at a rate more than 10 times the normal basal rate of heat production.

Regulation of Body Temperature

Regulation of body temperature is by nervous system feedback mechanisms that operate principally through the preoptic area in the hypothalamus. This area contains heat-sensitive neurons that function as temperature sensors for controlling body temperature. The overall heat-controlling mechanism of the hypothalamus is that of a hypothalamic thermostat. This thermostat detects body temperature changes and initiates heat-decreasing or heat-increasing responses. For example, the hypothalamic thermostat inhibits sympathetic nervous system centers in the hypothalamus that normally cause vasoconstriction. As a result, vasodilation is maximal and the rate of heat transfer to the skin is maximized. Conversely, body temperature is increased when the hypothalamic thermostat induces vasoconstriction of cutaneous blood vessels. Other heat-sensing areas in addition to the hypothalamus are located in the spinal cord, midbrain, brain stem, abdominal organs, and skeletal muscles (Imrie and Hall, 1990). Maintenance of body temperature at a value close to the optimum for enzyme activity assures a constant high rate of metabolism, rapid nervous system conduction, and skeletal muscle contraction. Protein denaturation begins at about 42 C, whereas ice crystals form in cells at about −1 C.

Chemical thermogenesis is an increase in the rate of cellular metabolism evoked by sympathetic nervous system stimulation or by circulating catecholamines. In adults, who have almost no brown fat, it is rare that chemical thermogenesis increases the rate of heat production more than 10% to 15%. In infants, however, chemical thermogenesis in brown fat located in the interscapular space and around large blood vessels can increase the rate of heat production as much as 100%. Brown fat contains large numbers of mitochondria, and these cells are innervated by the sympathetic nervous system. This is probably an important factor in maintaining normal body temperature in neonates. Shivering can increase body heat production when core temperature decreases. Indeed, the major source of metabolic heat is skeletal muscle activity.

Fever

Pyrogens are breakdown products of proteins and polysaccharide toxins secreted by bacteria that can cause the setpoint of the hypothalamic thermostat to rise. Presumably, pyrogens interact with polymorphonuclear leukocytes to form interleukins (endogenous pyrogens) that evoke the release of prostaglandins, leading to stimulation of heat-sensitive neurons in the hypothalamus. Dehydration can cause fever, which in part reflects the lack of available fluid for sweating. In addition, dehydration in some way stimulates the hypothalamus.

Chills

Sudden resetting of the hypothalamic thermostat to a higher level as a result of tissue destruction, pyrogens, or dehydration results in a lag between blood temperature and the resetting of the hypothalamus. During this period, the person experiences chills and feels cold even though body temperature may already be elevated. The skin is cold because of vasoconstriction of cutaneous blood vessels. Chills continue until the body temperature rises to the new setting of the hypothalamic thermostat. As long as the factor causing the hypothalamic thermostat to be set at a higher level is present, the body's core temperature remains elevated above normal. Sudden removal of the factor that is causing body temperature to remain elevated is accompanied by intense diaphoresis and a warm feeling of the skin because of generalized vasodilation of cutaneous blood vessels.

Cutaneous Blood Flow

Cutaneous blood flow is among the most variable in the body, reflecting its primary role in regulation of body temperature in response to alterations in the rate of metabolism and the temperature of the external surroundings. Nutritional requirements are so low for skin that this need does not significantly influence cutaneous blood flow. For example, at ordinary skin temperature, cutaneous blood flow is about ten times that needed to supply nutritive needs of the skin.

Cutaneous blood flow is largely regulated by the sympathetic nervous system and not local regulatory mechanisms that reflect tissue oxygen needs. Vascular structures concerned with heat loss from skin consist of subcutaneous venous plexuses that can hold large quantities of blood. Furthermore, in some areas of the skin, direct arteriovenous anastomoses facilitate heat loss. In an adult, cutaneous blood flow is about 400 ml·min⁻¹. This flow can decrease to as little as 50 ml·min⁻¹ in severe cold and to as much as 2800 ml·min⁻¹ in extreme heat. Indeed, patients with borderline cardiac function may become sympto-

matic in hot environments, emphasizing the increase in cardiac output necessitated by marked elevations in cutaneous blood flow. During acute hemorrhage, the sympathetic nervous system can produce sufficient vasoconstriction to transfer large amounts of blood into the central circulation. As such, the cutaneous veins act as an important blood reservoir that can supply 5% to 10% of the blood volume in times of need. Inhaled anesthetics increase cutaneous blood flow, perhaps by inhibiting the temperature-regulating center of the hypothalamus (Heistad and Abboud, 1974).

Skin Color

Skin color is principally due to the color of blood in the cutaneous capillaries and veins. The skin has a pinkish hue when arterial blood is flowing rapidly through these tissues. Conversely, when the skin is cold and blood is flowing slowly, the removal of oxygen for nutritive purposes gives the skin the bluish hue (cyanosis) of deoxygenated blood. Severe vasoconstriction of the skin forces most of the blood into the central circulation, and skin takes on the whitish hue (pallor) of underlying connective tissue, which is composed primarily of collagen fibers.

Perioperative Temperature Changes

Several events occur during surgery that contribute to reductions in body temperature (Table 41-4). Inhaled anesthetics interfere with hypothalamic temperature regulation, but after 1 to 2 hours a thermal steady state is reached and there

Table 41-4
Events that Contribute to Reductions in Body Temperature During Surgery

Environmental temperature less than 21 C

Administration of unwarmed intravenous solutions

Heat required to humidify inhaled gases

Body cavities exposed to environmental temperature

Basal metabolic rate decreased

Drug-induced vasodilation

Anesthetics interfere with hypothalamic thermostat

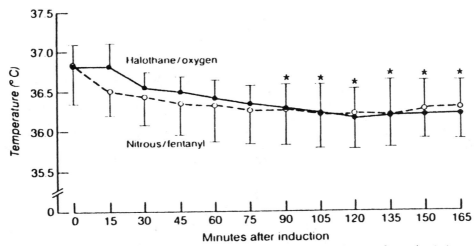

FIGURE 41–15. A thermal steady state is reached after about 2 hours of anesthesia in patients undergoing eye surgery. (From Sessler DI, Rubenstein EH, Eger EI. Core temperature changes during N_2O/fentanyl and halothane/O_2 anesthesia. Anesthesiology 1987; 67:137–9; with permission.)

is evidence of return of temperature regulation (Fig. 41-15) (Sessler et al 1987; Sessler et al, 1988). Isoflurane and enflurane produce dose-dependent reductions in body temperature but the magnitude of decrease is greater with iso-flurane (Smith et al, 1990). General anesthesia abolishes thermal sensation but does not alter sensitivity of thermoreceptors. Decreases in body temperature are associated with reductions in anesthetic requirements, prolongation of the elimination half-time of drugs dependent on hepatic or renal clearance, and an increase in blood viscosity. More than 50% of patients have body temperatures lower than 36 C when they are admitted to the postanesthesia recovery room (Vaughn et al, 1981). Pediatric patients and the elderly are particularly vulnerable to intraoperative decreases in body temperature. Loss of heat can be attenuated by adequate humidification of the inhaled gases, warming of solutions for intravenous infusions, and maintenance of a warmer operating room temperature (greater than 21 C). The major benefit of radiant heating is suppression of shivering. Likewise, a forced-air system (Bair Hugger system) is useful for warming hypothermic postoperative patients and decreasing the incidence of shivering (Lennon et al, 1990).

Measurement of Body Temperature

The lower 25% of the esophagus (about 24 cm beyond the corniculate cartilages or site of loudest heart sounds heard through an esophageal stethoscope) gives a reliable approximation of blood and cerebral temperature. Readings elsewhere in the esophagus are more likely to be influenced by the temperature of inhaled gases. A nasopharyngeal temperature probe positioned behind the soft palate gives a less reliable measure of cerebral temperature than a correctly positioned esophageal probe. Leakage of gases around the tracheal tube may also influence these measurements. Rectal temperature is influenced by heat-producing gut flora, blood returning from the lower limbs, and insulation of the probe by feces. Bladder temperature is subject to the same slow responsiveness as rectal temperature if urine flow is less than 270 ml·h^{-1} (Imrie and Hall, 1990). Tympanic membrane and aural canal temperatures provide a rapidly responsive and accurate estimate of hypothalamic temperature and correlate well with esophageal temperature. Potential damage to the tympanic membrane has limited the acceptance of tympanic membrane probes. Thermistors in pulmonary artery catheters provide the best continuous estimate of body temperature. Skin temperature gives no information other than the temperature of that area of skin.

NAUSEA AND VOMITING

Nausea is the conscious recognition of excitation of an area in the medulla that is associated with the vomiting center (Fig. 41-16) (Swenson and Orkin, 1983). Impulses are transmitted by afferent fibers of the parasympathetic and sympathetic nervous system to the vomiting center. Motor impulses transmitted via cranial nerves V, VII, IX, X, and XII to the gastrointestinal tract and through the spinal nerves to the diaphragm and abdominal muscles are required to cause the mechanical act of vomiting. Psychic stimuli, including unpleasant visual input or odors, most likely cause vomiting by stimulating the vomiting center.

Vomiting can also be caused by impulses that arise in areas of the brain outside the medullary vomiting center. For example, stimulation of the chemoreceptor trigger zone located in the floor of the fourth ventricle initiates vomiting. Motion can stimulate equilibrium receptors in the inner ear, which may also stimulate the chemoreceptor trigger zone. Blocking of impulses from the

chemoreceptor trigger zone does not prevent vomiting owing to irritative stimuli (ipecac) arising in the gastrointestinal tract.

REFERENCES

Azzam FJ. A simple and effective method for stopping post-anesthesia clonus. Anesthesiology 1987;66:98.

Bennett HL, Davis HS, Giannini JA. Non-verbal response to intraoperative conversation. Br J Anaesth 1985;57:174–9.

Bogetz MS, Katz JA. Recall of surgery for major trauma. Anesthesiology 1984;61:6–9.

Chi OZ, Field C. Effects of isoflurane on visual evoked potentials in humans. Anesthesiology 1986;65:328–30.

Gallart L, Blanco D, Samso E, Vidal F. Clinical and radiologic evidence of the epidural plica medina dorsalis. Anesth Analg 1990;71:698–701.

Gancher S, Laxer KD, Krieger W. Activation of epileptogenic activity by etomidate. Anesthesiology 1984;61:616–8.

Ganong WF. Review of Medical Physiology. 13th ed. Norwalk, CT, Appleton and Lange, 1987.

Guyton AC. Textbook of Medical Physiology. 7th ed. Philadelphia, WB Saunders, 1986.

Heistad DD, Abboud FM. Factors that influence blood flow in skeletal muscle and skin. Anesthesiology 1974;41:139–56.

Hilgenberg JC. Intraoperative awareness during high-dose fentanyl-oxygen anesthesia. Anesthesiology 1981;54:341–3.

Imrie MM, Hall GM. Body temperature and anaesthesia. Br J Anaesth 1990;64:346–54.

Koblin DD, Eger EI. Theories of narcosis. N Engl J Med 1979;301:1224–6.

Kofke WA, Young RSK, Davis P, et al. Isoflurane for refractory status epilepticus: A clinical series. Anesthesiology 1989;71:653–9.

Lennon RL, Hosking MP, Conover MA, Perkins WJ. Evaluation of a forced-air system for warming hypothermic postoperative patients. Anesth Analg 1990;70:424–7.

Miller RD, Way WL, Eger EI. The effects of alpha-methyldopa, reserpine, guanethidine, and iproniazid on minimal alveolar anesthetic requirement (MAC). Anesthesiology 1968;29:1153–8.

Ovassapian A, Joshi CW, Brunner EA. Visual disturbances: An unusual symptom of transurethral prostatic resection reaction. Anesthesiology 1982;57:332–4.

Owens WD, Gustave F, Schlaroff A. Tympanic membrane rupture with nitrous oxide anesthesia. Anesth Analg 1978;57:283–6.

Pappenheimer JR. The sleep factor. Sci Am 1976;235:24–9.

Pathak KS, Brown RH, Cascorbi HF, Nash CL. Effects of

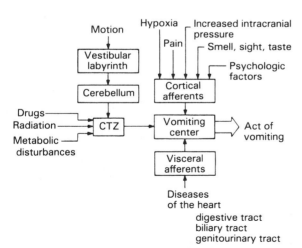

FIGURE 41–16. Schematic diagram of stimuli causing nausea and vomiting. CTZ, chemoreceptor trigger zone. (From Swenson EJ, Orkin FK. Postoperative nausea and vomitting. In Orkin FK, Cooperman LH, eds. Complications in Anesthesiology. Philadelphia: JB Lippincott, 1983; with permission.)

fentanyl and morphine on intraoperative somatosensory cortical-evoked potentials. Anesth Analg 1984; 63:833–7.

Rockoff MA, Goudsouzian NG. Seizures induced by methohexital. Anesthesiology 1981;54:333–5.

Saucier N, Walts LF, Moreland JR. Patient awareness during nitrous oxide, oxygen, and halothane anesthesia. Anesth Analg 1983;62:293–4.

Savolaine ER, Pandya JB, Greenblatt SH, Conover SR. Anatomy of the human lumbar epidural space. New insights using CT-epidurography. Anesthesiology 1988;68:217–20.

Schubert A, Drummond JC. The effect of acute hypocapnia on human median nerve somatosensory evoked responses. Anesth Analg 1986;65:240–4.

Sessler DI, Olofsson CI, Rubinstein EH, Beebe JJ. The thermoregulatory threshold in humans during halothane anesthesia. Anesthesiology 1988;68:836–42.

Sessler DI, Rubinstein EH, Eger EI. Core temperature changes during N_2O/fentanyl and halothane/O_2 anesthesia. Anesthesiology 1987;67:137–9.

Smith D, Wood M, Pearson J, Mehta RL, Carli F. Effects of enflurane and isoflurane in air-oxygen on changes in thermal balance during and after surgery. Br J Anaesth 1990;65:754-9.

Swenson EJ, Orkin FK. Postoperative nausea and vomiting. In Orkin FK, Cooperman LH, eds. Complications in Anesthesiology. Philadelphia, JB Lippincott, 1983:429.

Vaughn MS, Vaughn RW, Cork RC. Postoperative hypothermia in adults: Relationship of age, anesthesia, and shivering to rewarming. Anesth Analg 1981;60:746–51.

Wang JM-L, Creel DJ, Wong KC. Transurethral resection of the prostate: Serum glycine levels and ocular evoked potentials. Anesthesiology 1989;70:36–41.

Chapter

42

Autonomic Nervous System

INTRODUCTION

The autonomic nervous system controls the visceral functions of the body. In addition, the autonomic nervous system exerts partial control of blood pressure, gastrointestinal motility and secretion, urinary bladder emptying, and sweating and body temperature. Activation of the autonomic nervous system occurs principally via centers located in the hypothalamus, brain stem, and spinal cord (see Chapter 41). Impulses are conducted over the sympathetic and parasympathetic nervous system divisions of the autonomic nervous system.

The sympathetic and the parasympathetic nervous systems usually function as physiologic antagonists such that activity of organs innervated by both divisions of the autonomic nervous system represents a balance of the influence of each component (Table 42-1). An understanding of the anatomy and physiology of the autonomic nervous system is essential for predicting the pharmacologic effects of drugs that act on either the sympathetic nervous system or the parasympathetic nervous system (Table 42-2).

ANATOMY OF THE SYMPATHETIC NERVOUS SYSTEM

Nerves of the sympathetic nervous system arise from the thoracolumbar (T1 to L2) segments of the spinal cord (Fig. 42-1) (Guyton, 1986). These nerve fibers pass to the paravertebral sympathetic chains located lateral to the spinal cord. From the paravertebral chain, nerve fibers pass to tissues and organs that are innervated by the sympathetic nervous system.

Each nerve of the sympathetic nervous system consists of a preganglionic neuron and a postganglionic neuron (Fig. 42-2). Cell bodies of preganglionic neurons are located in the intermediolateral horn of the spinal cord. Fibers from these preganglionic cell bodies leave the spinal cord with anterior (ventral) nerve roots and pass via white rami into one of 22 pairs of ganglia composing the paravertebral sympathetic chain. Axons of preganglionic neurons are mostly myelinated, slow-conducting type B fibers (see Table 41-1). In the ganglia of the paravertebral sympathetic chain, the preganglionic fibers can synapse with cell bodies of postganglionic neurons or pass cephalad or caudad to synapse with postganglionic neurons (mostly unmyelinated type C fibers) in other paravertebral ganglia. Postganglionic neurons then exit from paravertebral ganglia to travel to various peripheral organs. Other postganglionic neurons return to spinal nerves by way of gray rami and subsequently travel with these nerves to influence vascular smooth muscle tone and activity of piloerector muscles and sweat glands.

Fibers of the sympathetic nervous system are not necessarily distributed to the same part of the body as the spinal nerve fibers from the same segments. For example, fibers from T1 usually ascend in the paravertebral sympathetic chain into the head, T2 into the neck, T3 to T6 into the

Table 42–1
Responses Evoked by Autonomic Nervous System Stimulation

	Sympathetic Nervous System Stimulation	*Parasympathetic Nervous System Stimulation*
Heart		
Sinoatrial node	Increase heart rate	Decrease heart rate
Atrioventricular node	Increase conduction velocity	Decrease conduction velocity
His-Purkinje system	Increase automaticity, conduction velocity	Minimal effect
Ventricles	Increase contractility, conduction velocity, automaticity	Minimal effects, slight decrease in contractility(?)
Bronchial smooth muscle	Relaxation	Contraction
Gastrointestinal Tract		
Motility	Decrease	Increase
Secretion	Decrease	Increase
Sphincters	Contraction	Relaxation
Gallbladder	Relaxation	Contraction
Urinary Bladder		
Smooth muscle	Relaxation	Contraction
Sphincter	Contraction	Relaxation
Eye		
Radial muscle	Mydriasis	
Sphincter muscle		Miosis
Ciliary muscle	Relaxation for far vision	Contraction for near vision
Liver	Glycogenolysis Gluconeogenesis	Glycogen synthesis
Pancreatic Beta Cell Secretion	Decrease	
Salivary Gland Secretion	Increase	Marked increase
Sweat Glands	Increase*	
Apocrine Glands	Increase	
Arterioles		
Coronary	Constriction (alpha) Relaxation (beta)	Relaxation(?)
Skin and mucosa	Constriction	Relaxation
Skeletal muscle	Constriction (alpha) Relaxation (beta)	Relaxation
Pulmonary	Constriction	Relaxation

*Postganglionic sympathetic fibers to sweat glands are cholinergic.

Table 42–2

Mechanisms of Action of Drugs that Act on the Autonomic Nervous System

Mechanism	Site	Drug
Inhibition of neuro-transmitter synthesis	SNS	Alpha-methyltyrosine
False neurotransmitter	SNS	Alpha-methyldopa
Inhibition of uptake of neurotransmitter	SNS	Tricyclic antidepressants, cocaine, ketamine(?)
Displacement of neuro-transmitter from storage sites	SNS	Amphetamine, guanethidine
	PNS	Carbachol
Prevention of neuro-transmitter release	SNS	Bretylium
	PNS	Botulinum toxin
Mimic action of neuro-transmitter at receptor	SNS	
	alpha-1	Phenylephrine, methoxamine
	alpha-2	Clonidine, dexmedetomidine
	beta-1	Dobutamine
	beta-2	Terbutaline, albuterol
Inhibition of action of neurotransmitter on postsynaptic receptor	SNS	
	alpha-1	Prazosin
	alpha-2	Yohimbine
	alpha-1, alpha-2	Phentolamine
	beta-1	Metoprolol, esmolol
	beta-1, beta-2	Propranolol
	PNS	
	M-1	Pirenzipine
	M-1, M-2	Atropine
	N-1	Hexamethonium
	N-2	d-Tubocurarine
Inhibition of metabolism of neurotransmitter	SNS	Monoamine oxidase inhibitors
	PNS	Neostigmine, pyridostigmine, edrophonium

SNS, sympathetic nervous system; PNS, parasympathetic nervous system.

chest, T7 to T11 into the abdomen, and T12 and L1 to L2 into the legs. The distribution of these sympathetic nervous system fibers to each organ is determined in part by the position in the embryo from which the organ originates. In this regard, the heart receives many sympathetic nervous system fibers from the neck portion of the paravertebral sympathetic chain because the heart originates in the neck of the embryo. Abdominal organs receive their sympathetic nervous system innervation from the lower thoracic segments, reflecting the origin of the gastrointestinal tract from this area.

ANATOMY OF THE PARASYMPATHETIC NERVOUS SYSTEM

Nerves of the parasympathetic nervous system leave the central nervous system through cranial nerves III, V, VII, IX, and X (vagus) and from the sacral portions of the spinal cord (Fig. 42-3) (Guyton, 1986). About 75% of all parasympathetic nervous system fibers are in the vagus nerves passing to the thoracic and abdominal regions of the body. As such, the vagus nerves supply parasympathetic nervous system innervation to the heart, lungs, esophagus, stomach, small intestine, liver, gallbladder, pancreas, and upper portions of the ureters. Fibers of the parasympathetic nervous system in cranial nerve III pass to the eye. The lacrimal, nasal, and submaxillary glands receive parasympathetic nervous system fibers via cranial nerve VII, whereas the parotid gland receives parasympathetic nervous system innervation via cranial nerve IX.

The sacral part of the parasympathetic nervous system consists of the second and third sacral nerves, and, occasionally, the first and fourth sacral nerves. Sacral nerves form the sacral plexus on each side of the spinal cord. These nerves distribute fibers to the distal colon, rectum, bladder, and lower portions of the ureters. In addition, parasympathetic nervous system fibers to the ex-

ternal genitalia transmit impulses that elicit various sexual responses.

In contrast to the sympathetic nervous system, preganglionic fibers of the parasympathetic nervous system pass uninterrupted to ganglia near or in the innervated organ (Fig. 42-3) (Guyton, 1986). Postganglionic neurons of the parasympathetic nervous system are short because of the location of the corresponding ganglia. This contrasts with the sympathetic nervous system in which postganglionic neurons are relatively long, reflecting their origin in the ganglia of the paravertebral sympathetic chain, which is often distant from the innervated organ.

PHYSIOLOGY OF THE AUTONOMIC NERVOUS SYSTEM

Postganglionic fibers of the sympathetic nervous system secrete norepinephrine as the neurotransmitter (Fig. 42-4). These norepinephrine-secreting neurons are classified as adrenergic fibers. Postganglionic fibers of the parasympathetic nervous system secrete acetylcholine as the neurotransmitter (Fig. 42-4). These acetylcholine-secreting neurons are classified as cholinergic fibers. In addition, innervation of sweat glands and some blood vessels is by postganglionic sympathetic nervous system fibers that release acetylcholine as the neurotransmitter. All preganglionic neurons of the sympathetic and parasympathetic nervous systems release acetylcholine as the neurotransmitter and are thus classified as cholinergic fibers. For this reason, acetylcholine released at preganglionic fibers will activate both sympathetic and parasympathetic postganglionic neurons.

Norepinephrine as a Neurotransmitter

Synthesis

Synthesis of norepinephrine involves a series of enzyme-controlled steps that begin in the cytoplasm of postganglionic sympathetic nerve endings (varicosities) and are completed in the synaptic vesicles (Fig. 42-5). For example, the initial enzyme-mediated steps leading to the formation of dopamine take place in the cytoplasm. Dopamine then enters the synaptic vesicle, where it is converted to norepinephrine by dopamine beta-hydroxylase. It is likely that the enzymes that participate in the synthesis of

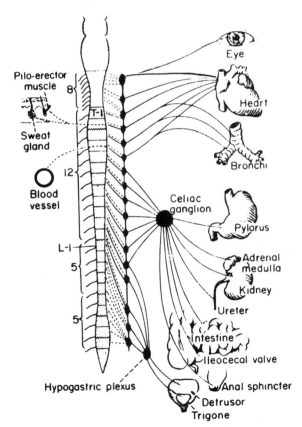

FIGURE 42–1. Anatomy of the sympathetic nervous system. Dashed lines represent postganglionic fibers in gray rami leading into spinal nerves for subsequent distribution to blood vessels and sweat glands. (From Guyton AC. Textbook of Medical Physiology. 7th ed. Philadelphia: WB Saunders, 1986; with permission.)

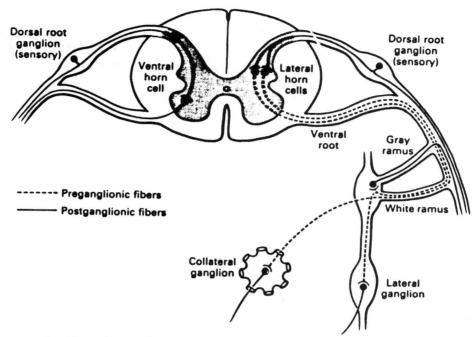

FIGURE 42–2. Anatomy of a sympathetic nervous system nerve. Preganglionic fibers pass through the white ramus to a paravertebral ganglia where they may synapse, course up the sympathetic chain to synapse at another level, or exit the chain without synapsing to pass to an outlying collateral ganglion.

norepinephrine are produced in postganglionic sympathetic nerve endings. These enzymes are not highly specific, and other endogenous substances, as well as certain drugs, may be acted on by the same enzyme. For example, dopa-decarboxylase can convert the antihypertensive drug, alpha-methyldopa, to alpha-methyldopa-mine, which is subsequently converted by dopamine beta-hydroxylase to the weakly active (false) neurotransmitter, alpha-methylnorepine-phrine (see Chapter 15).

Storage and Release

Norepinephrine is stored in synaptic vesicles for subsequent release in response to an action potential. Calcium ions (Ca^{2+}) are important in coupling the nerve impulse to the subsequent release of norepinephrine from postganglionic sympathetic nerve endings into the extracellular fluid. Evidence that exocytosis is the primary event in the release of norepinephrine from synaptic vesicles in the nerve terminals is the observation that increased activity of the sympathetic nervous system is accompanied by elevated circulating concentrations of dopamine beta-oxidase, and norepinephrine. This should occur only if the entire contents of the synaptic vesicles are released.

Adrenergic fibers can sustain output of norepinephrine during prolonged periods of stimulation. Tachyphylaxis, which may accompany administration of ephedrine and other indirect-acting sympathomimetics, may reflect depletion of the limited pool of neurotransmitter at these binding sites in contrast to the large total amount of norepinephrine stored in the sympathetic nerve ending.

Termination of Action

Termination of the action of norepinephrine is by (1) uptake (reuptake) back into postganglionic sympathetic nerve endings, (2) dilution by diffusion from receptors, and (3) metabolism by the enzymes, monoamine oxidase (MAO) and catechol-O-methyltransferase (COMT). Norepinephrine released in response to an action potential exerts its effects at receptors for only a brief period, reflecting the efficiency of these termination mechanisms.

UPTAKE. Uptake of previously released norepinephrine back into postganglionic sympathetic nerve endings is probably the most important mechanism for terminating the action of this neurotransmitter on receptors. Indeed, it is estimated that as much as 80% of released norepinephrine undergoes uptake. Furthermore, this uptake provides a source for reuse of norepinephrine in addition to synthesis.

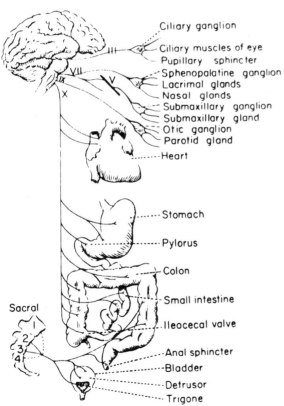

FIGURE 42-3. Anatomy of the parasympathetic nervous system. (From Guyton AC. Textbook of Medical Physiology. 7th ed. Philadelphia: WB Saunders, 1986; with permission.)

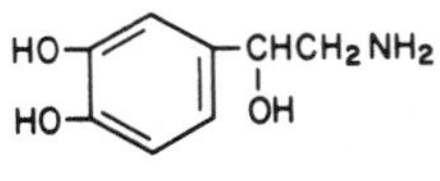

Norepinephrine

Acetylcholine

FIGURE 42-4. Neurotransmitters of the autonomic nervous system.

It is likely that two active transport systems are involved in uptake of norepinephrine, with one system responsible for uptake into the cytoplasm of the varicosity and a second system for passage of norepinephrine into the synaptic vesicle for storage and reuse. The active transport systems for norepinephrine uptake can concentrate the neurotransmitter 10,000-fold in the postganglionic sympathetic nerve endings. Magnesium and adenosine triphosphate are essential for function of the transport system necessary for the transfer of norepinephrine from the cytoplasm into the synaptic vesicle. The transport system for uptake of norepinephrine into cytoplasm is blocked by numerous drugs, including cocaine and tricyclic antidepressants.

Metabolism

Metabolism of norepinephrine is of relatively minor significance in terminating the actions of endogenously released norepinephrine. The exception may be at some blood vessels, where enzymatic breakdown and diffusion account for the termination of the action of norepinephrine. Norepinephrine that undergoes uptake is vulnerable to metabolism in the cytoplasm of the varicosity by MAO. Any neurotransmitter that escapes uptake is vulnerable to metabolism by COMT, principally in the liver. Inhibitors of MAO cause an increase in tissue levels of norepinephrine and are accompanied by a variety of pharmacologic effects (see Chapter 19). Conversely, no striking pharmacologic change accompanies inhibition of COMT.

The primary urinary metabolite resulting from metabolism of norepinephrine by MAO or

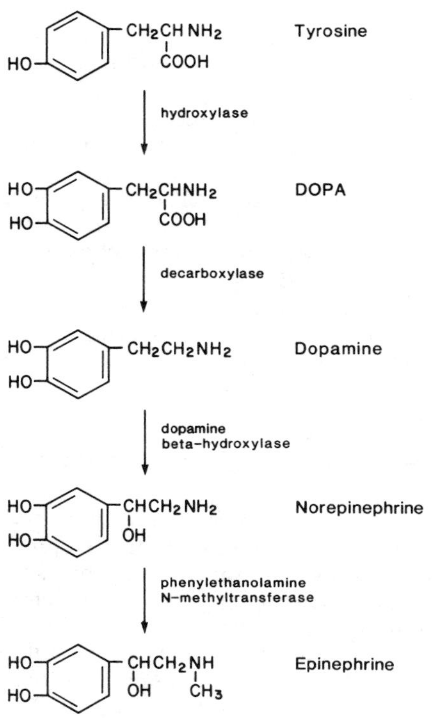

FIGURE 42-5. Steps in enzymatic synthesis of endogenous catecholamines and neurotransmitters.

COMT is 3-methyoxy-4-hydroxymandelic acid (Fig. 42-6). This metabolite is also referred to as *vanillylmandelic acid.* Normally, the 24-hour urinary excretion of 3-methoxy-4-hydroxyman-delic acid is 2 to 4 mg, representing primarily norepinephrine that is deaminated by MAO in the cytoplasm of the varicosity of postganglionic sympathetic nerve endings.

Acetylcholine as a Neurotransmitter

Synthesis

Synthesis of acetylcholine occurs in the cytoplasm of varicosities of the preganglionic and postganglionic parasympathetic nerve endings. The enzyme, choline acetyltransferase, is responsible for catalyzing the combination of choline with acetyl coenzyme A to form acetylcholine. Choline enters parasympathetic nerve endings from the extracellular fluid through an active transport system. Acetylcoenzyme A is synthesized in mitochondria present in high concentrations in parasympathetic nerve endings.

Storage and Release

Acetylcholine is stored in synaptic vesicles for release in response to an action potential. Arrival of

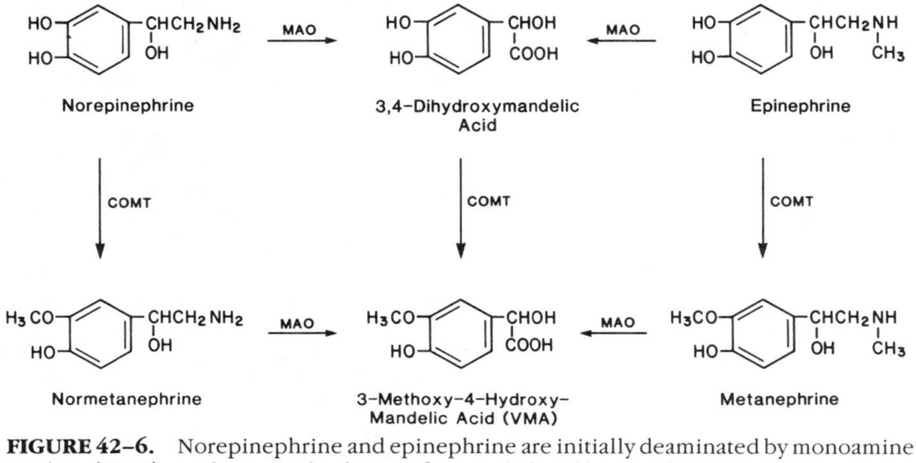

FIGURE 42-6. Norepinephrine and epinephrine are initially deaminated by monoamine oxidase (*MAO*) or, alternatively, they are first methylated by catechol-O-methyltransferase (COMT). The resulting metabolites are then further metabolized by the other enzyme to form the principal end-metabolite, 3-methoxy-4-hydroxymandelic acid (vanillylmandelic acid, or VMA).

an action potential at the parasympathetic nerve ending results in the release of 100 or more vesicles of acetylcholine. It is estimated that a single nerve ending contains 300,000 or more synaptic vesicles.

Preceding arrival of the action potential is the initial depolarization that permits the influx of Ca^{2+}. Conceptually, Ca^{2+} binds to sites on axonal and vesicular membranes, resulting in the extrusion of the contents of the synaptic vesicles. Thus, the presence of Ca^{2+} in the extracellular fluid is essential for the subsequent release of acetylcholine in response to an action potential. The effect of Ca^{2+} is antagonized by magnesium.

Metabolism

Acetylcholine has a brief effect at receptors (1 msec or less) because of its rapid hydrolysis by

Table 42–3
Responses Evoked by Selective Stimulation of Adrenergic Receptors

Alpha-1 (postsynaptic) Receptors
Vasoconstriction
Mydriasis
Relaxation of gastrointestinal tract
Contraction of gastrointestinal sphincters
Contraction of bladder sphincter

Alpha-2 (presynaptic) Receptors
Inhibition of norepinephrine release

Alpha-2 (postsynaptic) Receptors
Platelet aggregation
Hyperpolarization of cells in the central nervous system

Beta-1 (postsynaptic) Receptors
Increased conduction velocity
Increased automaticity
Increased contractility

Beta-2 (postsynaptic) Receptors
Vasodilation
Bronchodilation
Gastrointestinal relaxation
Uterine relaxation
Bladder relaxation
Glycogenolysis
Lipolysis

Dopamine-1 (postsynaptic) Receptors
Vasodilation

Dopamine-2 (presynaptic) Receptors
Inhibition of norepinephrine release

acetylcholinesterase (true cholinesterase) to choline and acetate. Choline is transported back into parasympathetic nerve endings, where it is used for synthesis of new acetylcholine.

Plasma cholinesterase (pseudocholinesterase) is an enzyme found in only low concentrations around receptors, being present in the greatest amounts in plasma. The physiologic significance of plasma cholinesterase is unknown. Indeed, the enzyme hydrolyzes acetylcholine too slowly to be physiologically important. Furthermore, absence of plasma cholinesterase produces no detectable signs or symptoms until a drug such as succinylcholine is administered.

INTERACTIONS OF NEUROTRANSMITTERS WITH RECEPTORS

Norepinephrine and acetylcholine, acting as neurotransmitters, interact with receptors (protein molecules) in lipid cell membranes (see Chapter 39). This receptor–neurotransmitter interaction most often activates or inhibits effector enzymes, such as adenylate cyclase, or alters flux of sodium (Na^+) and potassium (K^+) ions across ion channels. The net effect of these changes is transduction of external stimuli into intracellular signals.

Norepinephrine Receptors

The pharmacologic effects of catecholamines led to the original concept of alpha- and beta-adrenergic receptors (Ahlquist, 1948). Subdivision of these receptors into alpha-1 (postsynaptic), alpha-2 (presynaptic), beta-1 (cardiac), and beta-2 (noncardiac) allows an understanding of drugs that act as either agonists or antagonists at these sites (Table 42-3) (see Chapter 12). Dopamine receptors are also subdivided as dopamine-1 (postsynaptic) and dopamine-2 (presynaptic). Activation of dopamine-1 receptors is responsible for vasodilation in the splanchnic and renal circulations. Presynaptic alpha- and dopamine-2 receptors function as a negative feedback loop such that their activation inhibits subsequent release of neurotransmitter (Table 42-3). Postsynaptic alpha-2 receptors are also present on platelets, where they mediate platelet aggregation by influencing platelet adenylate cyclase concentrations. In the central nervous system, stimulation of postsynaptic alpha-2 receptors results in enhanced K^+ conductance and membrane hyperpolarization manifesting as marked reductions in anesthetic requirements (Segal et al, 1988) (see Chapter 1). Transmembrane signalling systems (receptors) consist of three components that are described as (1) recognition sites, (2) effectors or catalytic sites, and (3) transducing or coupling proteins (see Fig. 39-10).

Beta-1, beta-2, and dopamine-1 receptors result in formation of cyclic adenosine monophosphate (cyclic AMP) as the second messenger. The resulting increased intracellular concentration of cyclic AMP then initiates a series of intracellular events (cascading protein phosphorylation reactions; and stimulation of the Na^+–K^+ pump), resulting in the metabolic and pharmacologic effects considered typical of beta-adrenergic receptor stimulation by norepinephrine, epinephrine, or agonist drugs. In contrast to beta-receptors, alpha-1 receptors facilitate Ca^{2+} influx and stimulate hydrolysis of polyphosphoinositides. Alpha-2 and dopamine-2 receptors inhibit adenylate cyclase. Stimulatory or inhibitory G proteins are needed for this receptor-mediated activation or inhibition of adenylate cyclase or stimulation of phosphoinositide hydrolysis.

Acetylcholine Receptors

Cholinergic receptors are classified as nicotinic and muscarinic. There are at least two pharmacologically distinguishable subtypes for each receptor classification. Nicotinic receptors are designated *N-1* and *N-2*. N-1 receptors are present at autonomic ganglia and N-2 receptors are present at the neuromuscular junction. Hexamethonium produces blockade at N-1 receptors, whereas nondepolarizing neuromuscular blocking drugs produce blockade at N-2 receptors. Among the nondepolarizing neuromuscular blocking drugs, d-tubocurarine in high doses produces some degree of autonomic ganglia blockade, although the effects at N-2 receptors still predominate. Muscarinic receptor subtypes are designated *M-1* and *M-2*. M-1 receptors are present in autonomic ganglia and in the central nervous system, whereas M-2 receptors are present chiefly in the heart and salivary glands. Pirenzepine is an example of a drug that is a selective antagonist at M-1 receptors, whereas atropine is a nonselective antagonist at M-1 and M-2 receptors. A possible molecular basis for the difference between nicotinic and muscarinic receptors is a different distance between atoms of the receptors necessary to interact with acetylcholine or drugs.

Like norepinephrine, acetylcholine receptors are coupled by G proteins to a variety of effectors. The arrival of an electrical impulse at cholinergic nerve endings increases the permeability of the nerve membrane, and the resultant influx of Ca^{2+} causes the secretion of acetylcholine into synaptic clefts. Acetylcholine causes changes in the permeability of ion channels. For example, M-1 receptors probably mediate decreased K^+ conductance and are therefore excitatory. Conversely, M-2 receptors are thought to increase K^+ conductance, resulting in hyperpolarization of cell membranes that manifests as inhibitory effects.

RESIDUAL AUTONOMIC NERVOUS SYSTEM TONE

The sympathetic and parasympathetic nervous systems are continually active, and this basal rate of activity is referred to as *sympathetic* or *parasympathetic tone.* The value of this tone is that it permits alterations in sympathetic or parasympathetic nervous system activity to either increase or decrease responses at innervated organs. For example, sympathetic nervous system tone normally keeps blood vessels about 50% constricted. As a result, increased or decreased sympathetic activity produces corresponding changes in systemic vascular resistance. If sympathetic tone did not exist, the sympathetic nervous system could only cause vasoconstriction.

In addition to continual direct sympathetic nervous system stimulation, a portion of overall sympathetic tone reflects basal secretion of norepinephrine and epinephrine by the adrenal medulla. The normal resting rate of secretion of norepinephrine is about 0.05 $\mu g \cdot kg^{-1} \cdot min^{-1}$ and of epinephrine is about 0.2 $\mu g \cdot kg^{-1} \cdot min^{-1}$. These secretion rates are nearly sufficient to maintain blood pressure in a normal range even if all direct sympathetic nervous system innervation to the cardiovascular system is removed.

Acute Denervation

Acute removal of sympathetic nervous system tone, as produced by a regional anesthetic or spinal cord transection, results in immediate maximal vasodilation of blood vessels (spinal shock). Over several days, however, intrinsic tone of vascular smooth muscle increases, usually restoring almost normal vasoconstriction. Similar intrinsic parasympathetic nervous system compensation occurs, but return of an organ to basal function may require several months.

Denervation Hypersensitivity

Denervation hypersensitivity is the increased responsiveness (decreased threshold) of the innervated organ to norepinephrine or epinephrine that develops during the first week or so after acute interruption of autonomic nervous system innervation (see Chapter 41). The presumed mechanism for denervation hypersensitivity is the proliferation of receptors (up-regulation) on postsynaptic membranes that occurs when norepinephrine or acetylcholine is no longer released at synapses. As a result, more receptor sites become available to produce an exaggerated response when circulating neurotransmitter does become available.

ADRENAL MEDULLA

The adrenal medulla is innervated by preganglionic fibers that bypass the paravertebral ganglia. As a result, these fibers pass directly from the spinal cord to the adrenal medulla. Cells of the adrenal medulla are derived embryologically from neural tissue and are analogous to postganglionic neurons. Stimulation of the sympathetic nervous system causes release of epinephrine (80%) and norepinephrine from the adrenal medulla. Epinephrine and norepinephrine released by the adrenal medulla function as hormones and not neurotransmitters.

Synthesis

In the adrenal medulla, most of the formed norepinephrine is converted to the hormone epinephrine by the action of phenylethanolamine-N-methyltransferase (Fig. 42-5). Activity of this enzyme is enhanced by cortisol, which is carried by the intraadrenal portal vascular system directly to the adrenal medulla. For this reason, any stress that releases glucocorticoids also results in increased synthesis and release of epinephrine.

Release

The triggering event in the release of epinephrine and norepinephrine from the adrenal medulla is the liberation of acetylcholine by preganglionic cholinergic fibers. Acetylcholine acts on specific receptors, resulting in a change in permeability (localized depolarization) that permits entry of Ca^{2+}. Ca^{2+} results in extrusion, by exocytosis, of synaptic vesicles containing epinephrine.

Norepinephrine and epinephrine released from the adrenal medulla evoke responses similar to direct sympathetic stimulation. The difference, however, is that effects are greatly prolonged (10 to 30 seconds) compared with the brief duration of action on receptors that is produced by norepinephrine released as a neurotransmitter from postganglionic sympathetic nerve endings. The prolonged effect of circulating epinephrine and norepinephrine released by the adrenal medulla reflects the time necessary for metabolism of these substances by COMT.

Circulating norepinephrine from the adrenal medulla causes vasoconstriction of blood vessels, inhibition of the gastrointestinal tract, increased cardiac activity, and dilatation of the pupils (Table 42-1). Effects of circulating epinephrine differ from norepinephrine in that the cardiac and metabolic effects of epinephrine are greater, whereas relaxation of blood vessels in skeletal muscle reflects a predominance of beta- over alpha-effects at low concentrations of epinephrine. Circulating norepinephrine and epinephrine released by the adrenal medulla and acting as hormones can substitute for sympathetic innervation of an organ. Another important role of the adrenal medulla is the ability of circulating norepinephrine and epinephrine to stimulate areas of the body that are not directly innervated by the sympathetic nervous system. For example, the metabolic rate of all cells can be influenced by hormones released from the adrenal medulla, even though these cells are not directly innervated by the sympathetic nervous system.

REFERENCES

Ahlquist RP. A study of adrenotropic receptors. Am J Physiol 1948;53:586–606.

Guyton AC. Textbook of Medical Physiology. 7th ed. Philadelphia, WB Saunders, 1986.

Segal IS, Vickery RG, Walton JK, Doze VA, Maze M. Dexmedetomidine diminishes halothane anesthetic requirements in rats through a postsynaptic alpha-2 adrenergic receptor. Anesthesiology 1988; 69:818–23.

Chapter

43

Pain

INTRODUCTION

Pain (nociception) is a protective mechanism that occurs when tissues are being damaged and causes the individual to react to remove the painful stimulus (Abram, 1985; Liebeskind et al, 1985). For example, pressure on a certain part of the body during sitting results in painful ischemia, which causes the person unconsciously to shift the weight. Additionally, pain may promote healing by motivating the organism to avoid motion of an injured area.

TYPES OF PAIN

Two qualitatively different types of pain can be readily appreciated. Fast pain is a short, well-localized, stabbing sensation that is matched to the stimulus, such as a pinprick or surgical skin incision. This pain starts abruptly when the stimulus is applied and ends promptly when the stimulus is removed. Fast pain results from stimulation of small, myelinated type A-delta nerve fibers with conduction velocities of 12 to 30 m·sec^{-1}. The second type of sensation is categorized as slow pain and is characterized as a throbbing, burning, or aching sensation that is poorly localized and less specifically related to the stimulus. This pain may continue long after the removal of the stimulus. Slow pain results from stimulation of more primitive, unmyelinated type C nerve fibers with conduction velocities of 0.5 to 2 m·sec^{-1}. The farther from the brain the stimulus originates, the greater is the temporal distinction

of the two components. It is the immediate, stabbing pain that instantly tells the person that tissue damage is occurring, whereas burning pain becomes the source of continued discomfort.

Nerve fibers for temperature follow the same pathways as fibers for pain. Indeed, artificially applied pain in the form of a heat stimulus causes pain in almost all subjects when skin temperature exceeds 43 C (pain threshold). This is also the temperature that, if maintained, can produce tissue damage. Although pain threshold is fairly constant among individuals, different people, nevertheless, react very differently to the same intensity of painful stimulation, emphasizing the importance of personality and ethnic origin on pain tolerance and the description of pain.

PAIN RECEPTORS

Pain receptors (nociceptors) are naked, afferent nerve endings of myelinated A-delta and unmyelinated C fibers that encode the occurrence, intensity, duration, and location of noxious stimuli and signal pain sensation. These pain receptors are widespread in superficial layers of the skin and also certain internal tissues such as the periosteum, joint surfaces, skeletal muscle, and tooth pulp. Most of the other deep tissues are not richly supplied with pain receptors, although widespread tissue damage can summate to cause aching pain in these areas.

Three categories of pain receptors are described in skin (Abram, 1985). Pain receptors that are activated by mechanical stimulation and conduct impulses by way of A-delta fibers are termed *mechanosensitive pain receptors.* A second type of pain receptors is represented by *mechanothermal receptors* that are activated by mechanical and thermal (greater than 43 C) stimulation. These receptors also conduct impulses by way of A-delta fibers. A third category, known as *polynodal pain receptors,* responds to mechanical, thermal, and chemical stimuli and conduct impulses by way of unmyelinated C fibers. Chemicals capable of activating these receptors include acetylcholine, bradykinin, histamine, prostaglandins, and potassium ions.

In contrast to other sensory receptors, pain receptors do not adapt. Failure of pain receptors to adapt is protective because it allows the person to remain aware of continued tissue damage. After damage has occurred, pain is usually minimal. The onset of pain in a tissue rendered acutely ischemic is related to its rate of metabolism. For example, pain occurs in exercising ischemic muscle in 15 to 20 seconds but not for 20 to 30 minutes in ischemic skin.

Hyperalgesia

Hyperalgesia is a decrease in pain threshold in an area of inflammation such that even trivial stimuli cause pain. This hyperalgesia is most likely due to local release of chemical mediators from injured cells in the inflamed area, resulting in the sensitization of pain receptors. The metabolites of arachidonic acid and bradykinin appear to play an important role in sensitization of pain receptors.

Skeletal Muscle Spasm

Skeletal muscle spasm is a common cause of pain and may become the basis for a myofascial pain syndrome. This pain most likely reflects the direct effects of skeletal muscle spasm in stimulating mechanosensitive pain receptors, as well as an indirect effect of skeletal muscle spasm causing ischemia and thereby stimulating polynodal pain receptors. Skeletal muscle spasm compresses blood vessels and decreases blood flow but also simultaneously increases the rate of metabolism in skeletal muscles, thus making the relative ischemia even greater and creating conditions for the release of pain-inducing chemicals.

Autonomic Nervous System Responses

Painful stimulation may evoke reflex increases in sympathetic nervous system efferent activity. It is possible that associated vasoconstriction leads to acidosis, tissue ischemia, and release of chemicals that further activate pain receptors. Resulting sustained, painful stimulation produces further increases in sympathetic nervous system activity, and the vicious cycle termed *reflex sympathetic dystrophy* may develop.

Following certain types of nerve injury, pain may occur without activation of pain receptors. Spontaneous firing that occurs from injured peripheral nerves, especially in response to sympathetic stimulation, may reflect a proliferation of alpha-adrenergic receptors on the increased number of neuroma sprouts (Devor, 1983). Spontaneous firing may also occur from dorsal root ganglia whose peripheral projections have been interrupted, as follows nerve transection or limb amputation.

TRANSMISSION OF PAIN SIGNALS

Pain signals are transmitted from pain receptors along myelinated A-delta fibers (rapid conduction) and unmyelinated C fibers (slow conduction). These afferent fibers enter the spinal cord through the dorsal nerve roots and terminate on cells in the dorsal horn. Anatomically, A-delta fibers synapse with cells in laminae I and V (wide dynamic-range neurons) of the dorsal horn, whereas C fibers synapse with cells in laminae II and III, which are also known as the *substantia gelatinosa* (see Fig. 41-3).

The spinothalamic tracts as well as other ascending pathways are responsible for cephalad transmission of pain impulses after they have been processed in the dorsal horn of the spinal cord. Cells in laminae I and V are spinothalamic cells, and about 75% of fibers originating from these cells cross to the contralateral spinothalamic tract. The phylogenetically newer portion of the spinothalamic tract (neospinothalamic) projects to the posterior portions of the thalamus and is considered to be involved with the spatial and temporal aspects of pain perception. The phylogenetically older portion of the spinothalamic (paleospinothalamic) tract projects to the medial thalamus and is responsible for initiation of unpleasant aspects of pain as well as automatic nervous system responses to pain. Other pathways involved in cephalad transmission of pain impulses include the spinocervical tracts, spinoreticular tracts, and spinomesencephalic tracts. Pain impulses travel from the thalamus to the somatosensory areas of the cerebral cortex. Complete removal of these cortical areas does not destroy the person's ability to perceive pain, suggesting that the thalamus participates in the conscious perception of pain. It is speculated that the cerebral cortex is important for interpreting the intensity of pain even though perception of pain seems predominantly to be a function of lower brain centers. Localization of pain probably results from simultaneous activation of tactile receptors along with painful stimulation. Nevertheless, burning and aching types of pain are transmitted by C fibers, which is consistent with the diffuse projections of these fibers from the thalamus into the limbic and subcortical areas.

Afferent fibers conducting burning and aching types of pain terminate in the reticular area of the brain stem. This area transmits activating signals into most areas of the brain, especially through the thalamus to the cerebral cortex and hypothalamus. Stimulation of the reticular activating system by burning and aching pain awakens the person from sleep and produces generalized activation of the nervous system. These signals are poorly localized and only alert the person to continuing tissue damage. Even weak pain signals via this pathway may summate with time, converting initially tolerable discomfort into intolerable pain.

Conceptual Model of Pain Transmission

A conceptual model of pain transmission includes ascending excitatory afferent pain pathways, descending inhibitory pain pathways, and a variety of neuromodulators and neurotransmitters (Fig. 43-1) (Cousins and Mather, 1984). Pain impulses traveling via afferent nerves from pain receptors enter the dorsal horn of the spinal cord. At this site, release of excitatory neurotransmitters, such as glutamate or an 11-amino-acid peptide known as *substance P,* are necessary for further cephalad transmission of pain impulses (Yaksh and Hammond, 1982). Indeed, release of substance P into the cerebrospinal fluid is inhibited by concurrent administration of intrathecal

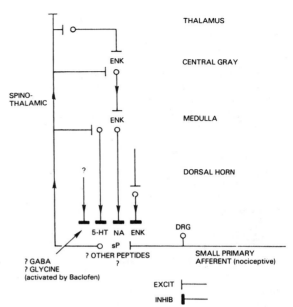

FIGURE 43–1. A conceptual model of pain transmission includes ascending excitatory and descending inhibitory pain pathways and a variety of neurotransmitters. Primary afferent pain (nociceptive) signals travel by the dorsal root ganglion (*DRG*) to cells in the dorsal horn of the spinal cord where substance P acts as the excitatory neurotransmitter. The endogenous endorphin (*ENK*) system is activated by pain signals that reach the thalamus. Activation of descending inhibitory pain pathways by ENK results in inhibition of dorsal horn neurons in the spinal cord through the release of inhibitory neurotransmitters that may include serotonin (*5-HT*), norepinephrine (*NA*), endorphins (*ENK*), gamma aminobutyric acid (*GABA*), and glycine (From Cousins MJ, Mather LE. Intrathecal and epideral administration of opioids. Anesthesiology 1984; 61: 276–310; with permission).

morphine, whereas depletion of substance P renders animals insensitive to noxious thermal stimuli (Yaksh and Hammond, 1982; Yaksh et al, 1980).

Transmission of pain impulses may be modulated by activation of descending inhibitory pain pathways that pass from the brain to the spinal cord. Activation of these inhibitory pathways blocks the release of substance P or other excitatory neurotransmitters and thus prevents the cephalad transmission of pain impulses (Fig. 43-1) (Cousins and Mather, 1984). It seems likely that a central nervous system substrate, possibly endorphins, is responsible for activating these descending inhibitory pathways. Opioid receptors in the substantia gelatinosa of the spinal cord are probably on substance P–containing terminals and produce analgesia by inhibiting release of substance P. Furthermore, opioid binding sites and endorphins are present in the periaqueductal gray area of the midbrain, where electrical stimulation-produced analgesia can be evoked. Thus endorphins and their receptors are well situated to function in an endogenous pain suppression system. Indeed, electrical stimulation–produced analgesia may evoke the release of endorphins. In addition to endorphins, other nonopioid inhibitory neurotransmitters released by descending pathway fibers may include serotonin, norepinephrine, and, possibly, glycine and gamma-aminobutyric acid (Fig. 43-1) (Cousins and Mather, 1984). Evidence for a role of norepinephrine as an inhibitory neurotransmitter is production of spinal analgesia by the alpha-1 adrenergic agonist, clonidine. The response to placebos may represent activation of descending pathways based on learning and experience with previous relief of pain. The net effect of activating these descending inhibitory pathways and releasing inhibitory neurotransmitters is to inhibit transmission of pain impulses from pain receptors via ascending afferent fibers. These inhibitory systems appear to produce additive effects, and pain seems to be blocked selectively, leaving sensory, motor, and sympathetic nervous system function intact.

Sites Amenable to Surgical Section of Pain Pathways

Multiple sites in the peripheral and central nervous systems are amenable to surgical ablative procedures to relieve pain (Fig. 43-2) (Ganong, 1987). Surgical section through the anterolateral quadrant of the spinal cord (cordotomy) at the thoracic level interrupts the anterolateral spinothalamic tract and relieves pain from the limb on the side opposite the cord transection. Cordotomy may be unsuccessful because some pain fibers do not cross to the opposite side of the spinal cord until they have reached the brain. Furthermore, pain that is more intense than the original pain may develop several months after the cordotomy.

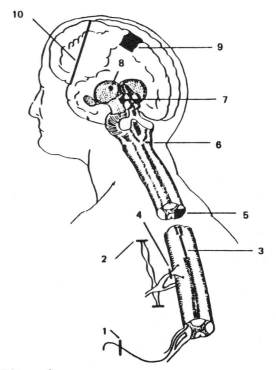

FIGURE 43–2. Diagram of various surgical procedures designed to interrupt pain pathways. *1*—nerve section; *2*—sympathectomy for visceral pain; *3*—myelotomy to section spinothalamic fibers in the anterior white commissure; *4*—posterior rhizotomy; *5*—anterolateral cordotomy; *6*—medullary tractotomy; *7*—mesencephalic tractotomy; *8*—thalamotomy; *9*—gyrectomy; *10*—prefrontal lobotomy (From Ganong WF. Review of Medical Physiology. 13th ed. Norwalk, CT: Appleton and Lange, 1987; with permission.)

Gate Control Theory

Conceptually, the dorsal horn of the spinal cord may function as a gate controlling the subsequent synaptic transmission of pain impulses via the spinothalamic tract (Melzack and Wall, 1965). Specifically, the activity of large afferent pain fibers can cause inhibition of smaller pain fibers by which pain impulses are being initiated. For example, rubbing activates these larger fibers so as to inhibit transmission of pain impulses. Stimulating electrodes, as represented by transcutaneous electrical nerve stimulation, take advantage of this counterirritant effect to reduce pain intensity. For the same reason, application of irritant ointments produces varying degrees of pain relief.

REACTION TO PAIN

Although pain threshold is similar, people's reactions to pain vary greatly. Pain causes both reflex motor and psychic reactions. Involuntary reflex withdrawal reactions occur in the spinal cord even before pain signals reach the brain. Psychic reactions to pain vary widely and include anxiety, depression, and skeletal muscle excitability. Pain and anxiety are interrelated such that anxiety makes pain less tolerable, while increases in pain enhance anxiety. Indeed, the preoperative level of anxiety is a useful predictor of the likely intensity of postoperative pain (Scott et al, 1983).

Surgical procedures that activate afferent pain pathways, especially in lightly anesthetized patients, produce changes in the central nervous system that subsequently lead to amplification and prolongation of postoperative pain. In this regard, it is logical to administer an opioid in the preoperative medication and/or with the induction of anesthesia so as to minimize release of substance P that could enhance postoperative pain. Indeed, the dose of opioid required to prevent C-fiber–induced excitability changes from occurring in the spinal cord is lower than that required to suppress these changes once they occur (Woolf and Wall, 1986; Woolf, 1989). The key to postoperative pain control is pain prevention.

VISCERAL PAIN

Pain receptors in viscera are similar to those in the skin but are more sparsely distributed than in somatic structures. Indeed, highly localized damage to a viscus, as produced by a surgical incision, is not associated with intense pain. Nevertheless, the liver capsule is highly sensitive to direct trauma and stretch and the bile ducts are sensitive to pain. Any event that causes stimulation of nerve endings throughout a viscus causes intense pain that is diffuse, poorly localized, and often associated with nausea and signs of autonomic nervous system activation. Visceral pain typically radiates and may be referred to surface areas of the body far removed from the painful viscus but with the same dermatome origin as the diseased viscus. Often visceral pain occurs as rhythmic contractions of smooth muscle. A cramping type of visceral pain frequently accompanies gastroenteritis, gallbladder disease, ureteral obstruction, menstruation, and distension of the uterus during the first stage of labor. Visceral pain, like deep somatic pain, initiates reflex contraction of nearby skeletal muscles, which makes the abdominal wall rigid when inflammatory processes involve the peritoneum.

Causes of viscus pain include ischemia, stretching of ligament attachments, spasm of smooth muscle, or distension of a hollow structure such as the gallbladder, common bile duct, or ureter. Distension of a hollow viscus results in pain due to stretch of the tissues and possibly ischemia due to compression of blood vessels by overdistension of the tissue.

Pain impulses from most of the abdominal and thoracic viscera are conducted through afferent fibers that travel with the sympathetic nervous system, whereas impulses from the esophagus, trachea, and pharynx are mediated via vagal and glossopharyngeal afferents, and impulses from structures deep in the pelvis are transmitted via the sacral parasympathetic nerves (Fig. 43-3) (Ganong 1987). Pain impulses from the heart are conducted through sympathetic nervous system nerves to the middle cervical ganglia, stellate ganglion, and the first four or five thoracic ganglia of the sympathetic chain. These impulses enter the spinal cord through the second, third, fourth, and fifth thoracic nerves. The cause of pain impulses from the heart is almost always myocardial ischemia. Parenchyma of the brain, liver, and alveoli of the lungs are devoid of pain receptors. Nevertheless, the bronchi and parietal pleura are very sensitive to pain.

SOMATIC PAIN

Somatic pain is sharp, stabbing, well-localized pain that typically arises from skin, skeletal muscles, and the peritoneum. Pain from a surgical incision, the second stage of labor, or peritoneal irritation is somatic pain. Disease of a viscus that spreads to the parietal wall elicits stabbing pain that is transmitted by spinal nerves. In this respect, the parietal wall resembles the skin in

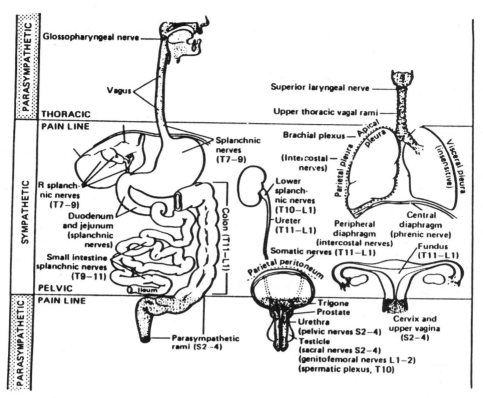

FIGURE 43-3.   Pain innervation of the viscera. Pain afferents from structures above the thoracic pain line and below the pelvic pain line traverse parasympathetic pathways (From Ganong WF. Review of Medical Physiology. 13th ed. Norwalk, CT: Appleton and Lange, 1987; with permission.)

being extensively innervated by spinal nerves. Indeed, a surgical incision through parietal peritoneum is exquisitely painful, whereas incision of visceral peritoneum is not painful. In contrast to diffuse and poorly localized visceral pain, parietal pain is usually localized directly over the damaged area.

The presence of both visceral and parietal pain pathways can result in localization of pain from viscera to dual surface areas of the body at the same time. For example, pain impulses from an inflamed appendix pass through the sympathetic nervous system visceral pain fibers into the sympathetic chain and then into the spinal cord at T10 to T11. This pain is referred to an area around the umbilicus and is aching or cramping in character. In addition, pain impulses originate in the parietal peritoneum where the inflamed

appendix touches the abdominal wall, and these impulses pass through the spinal nerves into the spinal cord at L1 to L2. This stabbing pain is localized directly over the irritated peritoneal surface in the right lower quadrant.

EMBRYOLOGIC ORIGIN AND LOCALIZATION OF PAIN

The position in the spinal cord to which visceral afferent fibers pass for each organ depends on the segment (dermatome) of the body from which the organ developed embryologically. This explains the phenomenon of referred pain to a site distal from the tissue causing the pain. For example, the heart originates in the neck and upper thorax such that visceral afferents enter the spinal cord at C3 to C5. As a result, the referred pain of myocardial ischemia is to the neck and arm. The gallbladder originates from the ninth thoracic segment, so visceral afferents from the gallbladder enter the spinal cord at T9. Skeletal muscle spasm caused by damage in adjacent tissues may also be a cause of referred pain. For example, pain from the ureter can cause reflex spasm of the lumbar muscles.

REFERENCES

Abram SE. Pain pathways and mechanisms. Semin Anesth 1985;4:267–74.

Cousins MJ, Mather LE. Intrathecal and epidural administration of opioids. Anesthesiology 1984;61:276–310.

Devor M. Nerve pathophysiology and mechanisms of pain in causalgia. J Auton Nerv Syst 1983;7:371–85.

Ganong WF. Review of Medical Physiology. 13th ed. Norwalk, CT, Appleton and Lange, 1987.

Liebeskind JC, Sherman JE, Cannol JT, Terman GW. Neural and neurochemical mechanisms of pain inhibition. Semin Anesth 1985;4:218–22.

Melzack R, Wall PD. Pain mechanisms: A new theory. Science 1965;150:971–9.

Scott LE, Clum GA, Peoples JB. Preoperative predictors of postoperative pain. Pain 1983;15:283–93.

Woolf CJ. Recent advances in the pathophysiology of acute pain. Br J Anaesth 1986;63:139–46.

Woolf CJ, Wall PD. Morphine-sensitive and morphine-insensitive actions of C-fiber input on the rat spinal cord. Neurosci Lett 1989;64:221–5.

Yaksh TL, Hammond DL. Peripheral and central substances involved in the rostrad transmission of nociceptive information. Pain 1982;13:1–86.

Yaksh TL, Jessell TM, Gamse R, Mudge AW, Leeman SE. Intrathecal morphine inhibits substances P release from mammalian spinal cord *in vivo*. Nature 1980;286:155–6.

44

Systemic Circulation

INTRODUCTION

The systemic circulation supplies blood to all the tissues of the body except the lungs. Important considerations in understanding the physiology of the systemic circulation include (1) components of the systemic circulation; (2) physical characteristics of the systemic circulation; (3) physical characteristics of blood; (4) determinants and control of tissue blood flow; (5) regulation of blood pressure; and (6) regulation of cardiac output and venous return. In addition, the fetal circulation possesses many unique features that distinguish it from the systemic circulation after birth.

COMPONENTS OF THE SYSTEMIC CIRCULATION

Components of the systemic circulation are the arteries, arterioles, capillaries, venules, and veins.

Arteries

The function of the arteries is to transport blood under high pressure to tissues. For this reason, arteries have strong vascular walls and blood flows rapidly.

Arterioles

Arterioles are the last small branches of the arterial system having diameters less than 200 μ. Arterioles have strong muscular walls that are capable of dilating or contracting and thus con-

trolling blood flow into the capillaries. Indeed, blood flow to each tissue is controlled almost entirely by resistance to flow in the arterioles. Metarterioles arise at right angles from arterioles and branch several times, forming 10 to 100 capillaries.

Capillaries

Capillaries serve as the sites for transfer of oxygen and nutrients to tissues and receipt of metabolic byproducts (see Chapter 45).

Venules and Veins

Venules collect blood from capillaries for delivery to veins, which act as conduits for transmitting blood to the right atrium. Because the pressure in the venous system is low, venous walls are thin. Nevertheless, walls of veins are muscular, which allows these vessels to contract or expand and thus store varying amounts of blood, depending on physiologic needs. As a result, veins serve an important function beyond being conduits to return blood to the right atrium. A venous pump mechanism is important for propelling blood forward to the heart.

PHYSICAL CHARACTERISTICS OF THE SYSTEMIC CIRCULATION

The systemic circulation contains about 80% of the blood volume, with the remainder present in the pulmonary circulation and heart (Fig. 44-1) (Guyton, 1986). Of the blood volume in the systemic circulation, about 64% is in veins and 7% is in the cardiac chambers. The heart ejects blood intermittently into the aorta such that blood pressure in the aorta fluctuates between a systolic level of about 120 mmHg and a diastolic level of about 80 mmHg (Table 44-1; Fig. 44-2) (Guyton, 1986).

Progressive Declines in Blood Pressure

As blood flows through the systemic circulation, its pressure falls progressively to nearly 0 mmHg by the time it reaches the right atrium (Fig. 44-2) (Guyton, 1986). The decrease in blood pressure in each portion of the systemic circulation is directly proportional to the resistance to flow in the vessel. Resistance to blood flow in the aorta and other large arteries is minimal, and mean arterial pressure decreases only 3 to 5 mmHg as blood travels into arteries as small as 3 mm in diameter. Resistance to blood flow begins to increase rapidly in small arteries, causing the mean arterial pressure to decrease to about 85 mmHg at the beginning of the arterioles. It is in the arterioles that resistance to blood flow is greatest, accounting for about 50% of the resistance in the entire systemic circulation. As a result, blood pressure decreases to about 30 mmHg at the point where blood enters the capillaries. At the venous end of the capillaries, the intravascular pressure has decreased to about 10 mmHg. The decrease in

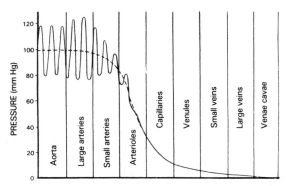

FIGURE 44-2.   Blood pressure decreases as blood travels from the aorta to large veins. (From Guyton AC. Textbook of Medical Physiology. 7th ed. Philadelphia, WB Saunders, 1986; with permission.)

blood pressure from 10 mmHg to nearly 0 mmHg as blood traverses veins indicates that these vessels impart far more resistance to blood flow than would be expected for vessels of their large sizes. This resistance to blood flow is caused by compression of the veins by external forces that keep many of them, especially the vena cavae, partially collapsed.

Pulse Pressure in Arteries

Pulse pressure reflects the intermittent ejection of blood into the aorta by the heart (Table 44-1).

Table 44–1
Normal Pressures in the Systemic Circulation

	Mean Value (mmHg)	Range (mmHg)
Systolic blood pressure*	120	90–140
Diastolic blood pressure*	80	70–90
Mean arterial pressure	92	77–97
Left ventricular end-diastolic pressure	6	0–12
Left atrium	8	2–12
a wave	10	4–16
v wave	13	6–20
Right atrium	5	3–8
a wave	6	2–10
c wave	5	2–10
v wave	3	0.8

*Measured in the radial artery.

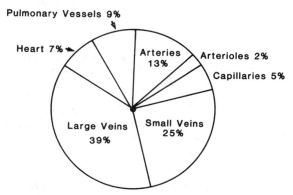

FIGURE 44-1.   Distribution of blood volume in the systemic and pulmonary circulation. (From Guyton AC. Textbook of Medical Physiology. 7th ed. Philadelphia: WB Saunders, 1986; with permission.)

The difference between systolic and diastolic blood pressure is the pulse pressure. A typical blood pressure curve recorded from a large artery is characterized by a rapid decline in pressure during ventricular systole followed by a maintained high level of blood pressure for 0.2 to 0.3 second (Fig. 44-3). This plateau is followed by the dicrotic notch (incisura) at the end of systole and a subsequent, more gradual decline of pressure back to the diastolic level. The dicrotic notch reflects a decline in the intraventricular pressure and a backflow of blood in the aorta that closes the aortic valve.

Factors that Alter Pulse Pressure

The principal factors that alter pulse pressure in the arteries are the left ventricular stroke volume, velocity of blood flow, and compliance of the arterial tree. The greater the stroke volume, the greater is the volume of blood that must be accommodated in the arterial vessels with each contraction, resulting in an increased pulse pressure. Pulse pressure also increases when systemic vascular resistance decreases and flow of blood from arteries to veins is accelerated. Indeed, pulse pressure is increased in the presence of patent ductus arteriosus and aortic regurgitation, reflecting rapid runoff of blood into the pulmonary circulation or left ventricle, respectively. In this regard, attempts have been made to predict systemic vascular resistance by the position of the dicrotic notch relative to the diastolic pressure. A controlled study, however, failed to con-

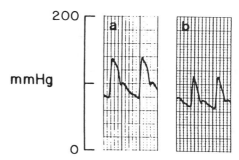

FIGURE 44-4. Despite a different height of the dicrotic notch (measured from baseline to the peak of the notch), the calculated systemic vascular resistance is similar for tracings *a* and *b*. (From Gerber MJ, Hines RL, Barash PG. Arterial waveforms and systemic vascular resistance: Is there a correlation? Anesthesiology 1987; 66:823–5; with permission.)

firm a correlation between the position of the dicrotic notch and the calculated systemic vascular resistance (Fig. 44-4) (Gerber et al, 1987). An increase in heart rate while the cardiac output remains constant causes the stroke volume and pulse pressure to decrease. Pulse pressure is inversely proportional to the compliance (distensibility) of the arterial system. For example, with aging, the distensibility of the arterial walls often decreases (elastic and muscular tissues are replaced by fibrous tissue) and pulse pressure increases.

Transmission of the Pulse Pressure

There is often enhancement of the pulse pressure as the pressure wave is transmitted peripherally (Fig. 44-5) (Guyton, 1986). Part of this augmentation results from a progressive decrease in compliance of the more distal portions of the large arteries. Second, pressure waves are reflected to some extent by the peripheral arteries. Specifically, when a pulsatile pressure wave enters the peripheral arteries and distends them, the pressure on these peripheral arteries causes the pulse wave to begin traveling backward. If the returning pulse wave strikes an oncoming wave, the two summate, causing a much higher pressure than would otherwise occur. These changes in the contour of the pulse wave are most pronounced in young patients, whereas in elderly patients

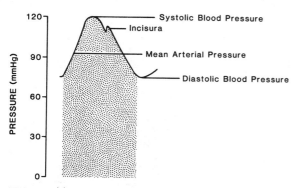

FIGURE 44-3. Schematic depiction of blood pressure recorded from a large systemic artery. Mean arterial pressure is equal to the area under the blood pressure curve divided by the duration of systole.

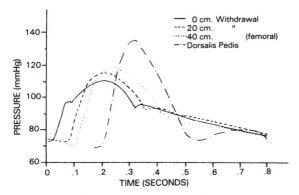

FIGURE 44-5. There is enhancement of the pulse pressure as the blood pressure is transmitted peripherally. (From Guyton AC. Textbook of Medical Physiology. 7th ed. Philadelphia: WB Saunders, 1986; with permission.)

with less compliant arteries, the pulse wave may be transmitted virtually unchanged from the aorta to peripheral arteries.

Augmentation of the peripheral pulse pressure must be recognized whenever blood pressure measurements are made in peripheral arteries. For example, systolic pressure in the radial artery is sometimes as much as 20% to 30% above that in the central aorta, and diastolic pressure is often reduced as much as 10% to 15%. Mean arterial pressures are similar regardless of the site of blood pressure measurement.

Reversal of the usual relationship between aortic and radial artery blood pressures can occur during the late period of hypothermic cardiopulmonary bypass and in the early period following termination of cardiopulmonary bypass (Fig. 44-6) (Pauca et al, 1989; Stern et al, 1985). The mechanism proposed for this unpredictable and transient disparity (usually persists for 10 to 60 minutes) is a high blood flow in the forearm and hand after rewarming on cardiopulmonary bypass, causing an increased pressure drop along the normal resistance provided by the arteries leading to the radial site. Failure to recognize this disparity may lead to an erroneous diagnosis and inappropriate treatment. Blood pressure measured in the brachial artery is more accurate and reliable during the periods surrounding cardiopulmonary bypass which are most likely to be associated with disparities between the aortic and radial artery blood pressures (Bazaral et al, 1990).

Pulse pressure becomes progressively less as blood passes through small arteries and arterioles until it becomes almost absent in capillaries (Fig. 44-2) (Guyton, 1986). This reflects the extreme distensibility of small vessels such that the small amount of blood that is caused to flow during a pulsatile pressure wave produces progressively less pressure rise in the more distal vessels. Furthermore, resistance to blood flow in these small vessels is such that the flow of blood and, consequently, the transmission of pressure are greatly impeded.

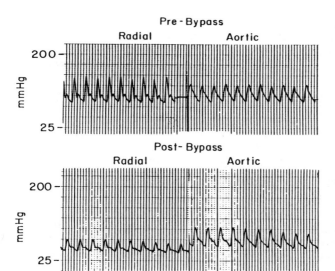

FIGURE 44-6. There may be a reversal of the usual relationship of simultaneous recordings of radial and aortic blood pressures (*Pre-Bypass*) in the early period following separation from cardiopulmonary bypass (*Post-Bypass*). (From Stern DH, Gerson JI, Allen FB, Parker FB. Can we trust the direct radial artery pressure immediately following cardiopulmonary bypass? Anesthesiology 1985; 62:557–61; with permission.)

Pulsus Paradoxus

Pulsus paradoxus is an exaggerated decrease in systolic blood pressure (greater than 10 mmHg) during inspiration in the presence of elevated intrapericardial pressures (cardiac tamponade).

Pulsus Alternans

Pulsus alternans is alternating weak and strong cardiac contractions causing a similar alteration in the strength of the peripheral pulse. Digitalis intoxication and varying degrees of atrioventricular heart block are commonly associated with pulsus alternans.

Pulse Deficit

In the presence of atrial fibrillation or ectopic ventricular beats, two beats of the heart may occur so close together that the ventricle does not fill adequately and the second cardiac contraction pumps insufficient blood to create a peripheral pulse. In this circumstance, a second heart beat is audible with a stethoscope applied on the chest directly over the heart, but a corresponding pulsation in the radial artery cannot be palpated. This phenomenon is called a *pulse deficit.*

Measurement of Blood Pressure by Auscultation

Measurement of blood pressure by auscultation uses the principle that blood flow in large arteries is laminar and not audible. If blood flow is arrested by an inflated cuff and the pressure in the cuff is released slowly, audible tapping sounds (Korotkoff sounds) can be heard when the pressure of the cuff falls just below systolic blood pressure and blood starts flowing in the brachial artery. These tapping sounds occur because flow velocity through the constricted portion of the blood vessel is increased, resulting in turbulence and vibrations that are heard through the stethoscope. Diastolic blood pressure correlates with the onset of muffled auscultatory sounds. The auscultatory method for determining systolic and diastolic blood pressure usually gives values within 10% of those determined by direct measurements from the arteries.

Right Atrial Pressure

Right atrial pressure is regulated by a balance between venous return and the ability of the right ventricle to eject blood. Normal right atrial pressure is about 5 mmHg, with a lower limit of about −5 mmHg, which corresponds to the pressure in the pericardial and intrapleural spaces that surround the heart. Right atrial pressure approaches these low values when right ventricular contractility is increased or venous return to the heart is decreased by hemorrhage. Poor right ventricular contractility or any event that increases venous return (hypervolemia, venoconstriction) will tend to elevate right atrial pressure. Pressure in the right atrium is commonly designated the *central venous pressure.*

Peripheral Venous Pressure

Large veins offer little resistance to blood flow when they are distended. Most large veins, however, are compressed at multiple extrathoracic sites. For example, pressure in the external jugular vein is often so low that atmospheric pressure on the outside of the neck causes it to collapse. Veins coursing through the abdomen are compressed by intraabdominal pressure, which may increase to 15 to 20 mmHg as a result of pregnancy or ascites. When this occurs, pressure in leg veins must increase above abdominal pressure. It is important to recognize that veins inside the thorax are not collapsed because of the distending effect of negative intrathoracic pressure.

Effect of Hydrostatic Pressure

Pressure in veins below the heart is increased and that in veins above the heart is decreased by the effect of gravity (Fig. 44-7) (Guyton, 1986). As a guideline, pressure changes about 0.77 mmHg for every centimeter the vessel is above or below the heart. For example, in a standing human, pressure in the veins of the feet is about 90 mmHg because of the distance from the heart to the feet. Conversely, veins above the heart tend to collapse, with the exception being veins inside the skull, which are held open by bone. As a result, negative pressure can exist in the dural sinuses and air can be entrained immediately if these sinuses are entered during surgery.

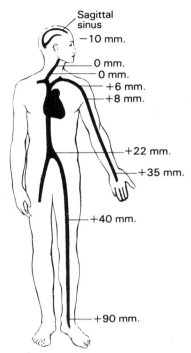

FIGURE 44–7.   Effect of hydrostatic pressure on venous pressures throughout the body. (From Guyton AC. Textbook of Medical Physiology. 7th ed. Philadelphia: WB Saunders, 1986; with permission.)

Hydrostatic pressure affects peripheral pressures in arteries and capillaries as well as veins. For example, a standing human who has a blood pressure of 100 mmHg at the level of the heart has a blood pressure of about 190 mmHg in the feet.

Venous Valves and the Pump Mechanism

Valves in veins are arranged so that the direction of blood flow can be only toward the heart. In a standing human, movement of the legs compresses skeletal muscles and veins so blood is directed toward the heart. This venous pump or skeletal muscle pump is usually sufficient to maintain venous pressure in a walking human below 25 mmHg. If an individual stands immobile, the venous pump does not function. As a result, pressures in the veins and capillaries of the leg can increase rapidly, resulting in leakage of fluid from the intravascular space. Indeed, as much as 15% of the blood volume can be lost from the intravascular space in the first 15 minutes of quiet standing.

Varicose Veins

Valves of the venous system can be destroyed when the veins are chronically distended by increased venous pressure as occurs during pregnancy or in a person who stands most of the day. The end result is varicose veins characterized by bulbous protrusions of the veins beneath the skin of the leg. Venous and capillary pressures remain elevated because of the incompetent venous pump, and this causes constant edema in the legs of these individuals. Edema interferes with diffusion of nutrients from capillaries to tissues, so there is often skeletal muscle discomfort and the skin may ulcerate.

Reference Level for Measuring Venous Pressures

Hydrostatic pressure does not alter venous or arterial pressures that are measured at the level of the tricuspid valve. As a result, the reference point for pressure measurement is considered to be the level of the tricuspid valve. External reference points for the level of the tricuspid valve are one third the distance from the anterior chest and about one fourth the distance above the lower end of the sternum. A precise hydrostatic point to which pressures are referenced is essential for accurate interpretation of venous pressure measurements. For example, each centimeter below the hydrostatic point adds 0.77 mmHg to the measured pressure, whereas 0.77 mmHg is subtracted for each centimeter above this point. The potential error introduced by measuring pressure above or below the tricuspid valve is greatest with venous pressures that are normally low. For example, an error introduced by 5 cm of hydrostatic pressure has a much greater influence on the clinical interpretation of central venous pressure than arterial pressure.

The reason for lack of hydrostatic effects at the tricuspid valve is the ability of the right ventricle to act as a regulator of pressure at this point. For example, if the pressure at the tricuspid valve increases, the right ventricle fills to a greater extent, thereby decreasing the pressure at the tricuspid valve toward normal. Conversely, if the pressure decreases at the tricuspid valve, the right ventricle does not fill optimally and blood pools in the veins until pressure at the tricuspid valve again increases to a normal value.

Measurement of right atrial pressure is accomplished by using a transducer or a fluid-filled manometer referenced to the level of the tricuspid valve. A venous pressure measurement in mmHg can be converted to cmH_2O by multiplying the pressure by 1.36, which adjusts for the density of mercury relative to water (10 mmHg equals 13.6 cmH_2O). Conversely, dividing the central venous pressure measurement in cmH_2O by 13.6 converts this value to an equivalent pressure in mmHg.

PHYSICAL CHARACTERISTICS OF BLOOD

Blood is a viscous fluid composed of cells and plasma. More than 99% of the cells in plasma are erythrocytes. As a result, leukocytes exert a minimal influence on the physical characteristics of blood. The percentage of blood comprising erythrocytes is the hematocrit, which to a large extent determines the viscosity of blood (Fig. 44-8) (Guyton, 1986). When the hematocrit increases to 60% to 70%, viscosity of blood is increased about tenfold compared with water and flow through blood vessels is greatly reduced.

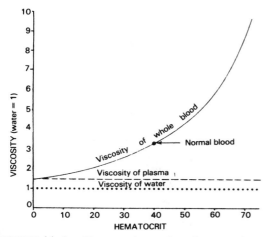

FIGURE 44-8. Hematocrit greatly influences the viscosity of blood. (From Guyton AC. Textbook of Medical Physiology. 7th ed. Philadelphia: WB Saunders, 1986; with permission.)

Plasma protein concentrations influence blood viscosity only minimally.

Viscosity exerts fewer effects on blood flow in capillaries than in larger vessels. This most likely reflects alignment of erythrocytes as they pass through small blood vessels rather than the random arrangement characteristic of flow through larger vessels. This alignment of erythrocytes, which greatly reduces the viscous resistance that occurs normally between cells, is largely offset by a reduced velocity of flow that greatly increases viscosity. The net effect may be that viscous effects in small blood vessels are similar to those that occur in large blood vessels.

Plasma is considered extracellular fluid that is identical to interstitial fluid except for the greater concentrations of proteins (albumin, globulin, and fibrinogen) in plasma. These greater concentrations reflect the inability of plasma proteins to pass easily through capillaries into the interstitial spaces. Indeed, the primary function of albumin is to create colloid osmotic pressure, which prevents fluid from leaving the capillaries.

DETERMINANTS OF TISSUE BLOOD FLOW

Tissue blood flow is directly proportional to the pressure difference between two points (not absolute pressure) and inversely proportional to resistance to flow through the vessel. This relationship between flow, pressure, and resistance can be expressed mathematically as a variant of Ohm's law in which blood flow (amperes) is directly proportional to the pressure drop across two points (voltage) and inversely proportional to resistance (Fig. 44-9). Rearrangement of this formula emphasizes that pressure is directly proportional to flow times resistance. Likewise, resistance is directly proportional to pressure and inversely proportional to flow. Furthermore, resistance is directly proportional to viscosity of blood and the length of the vessel and inversely proportional to the fourth power of the radius of the vessel (doubling the radius of the vessel or intravenous catheter size decreases resistance to flow 16-fold [Poiseuille's law]).

It is important to remember that resistance to blood flow cannot be measured, but rather is calculated based on measurement of driving pressures and the cardiac output. For example, systemic vascular resistance is calculated as the

$$\frac{\text{BLOOD FLOW}}{(Q)} = \frac{\text{PRESSURE DIFFERENCE BETWEEN}}{\text{RESISTANCE TO FLOW (R)}}$$

$$\Delta P = Q \times R$$

$$R = \Delta P / Q$$

FIGURE 44–9. The relationship between blood flow, pressure, and resistance to flow can be expressed as a variant of Ohm's law.

difference between mean arterial and right atrial pressures divided by cardiac output. Pulmonary vascular resistance is calculated as the difference between mean pulmonary artery and left atrial pressures divided by cardiac output. Resistance is expressed in units or dynes–sec·cm^{-5} if the calculated value is multiplied by 80. Conductance is the reciprocal of resistance and is a measure of the amount of blood flow that can pass through a blood vessel in a given time for a given pressure gradient.

Vascular Distensibility

Blood vessels are distensible such that increases in blood pressure cause the vascular diameter to increase, which in turn reduces resistance to blood flow. Conversely, reductions in intravascular pressure increase the resistance to blood flow. The ability of blood vessels to distend as intravascular pressure increases varies greatly in different parts of the circulation. Anatomically, walls of arteries are stronger than those of veins. As a result, veins are six to ten times as distensible as the arteries. Blood pressure can eventually decline to a level where the intravascular pressure is no longer capable of keeping the vessel open. This pressure averages 20 mmHg and is defined as the *critical closing pressure*. When the heart is abruptly stopped, the pressure in the entire circulatory system (mean circulatory pressure) equilibrates at about 7 mmHg.

Vascular Compliance

Vascular compliance is defined as the increase in volume (capacitance) of a vessel produced by an increase in intravascular pressure. The compliance of the entire circulatory system is estimated to be 100 ml for each mmHg increase in intravascular pressure (Guyton, 1986). Compli-

ance of veins is much greater than that of arteries. For example, the volume of blood normally present in all veins is about 2500 ml, whereas the arterial system contains only about 750 ml of blood when the mean arterial pressure is 100 mmHg. Sympathetic nervous system activity can greatly alter the distribution of blood volume. Enhancement of sympathetic nervous system activity to the blood vessels, especially the veins, reduces the dimensions of the circulatory system, and the circulation continues to function almost normally even when as much as 25% of the total blood volume has been lost. *Vasoconstriction* or *vasodilation* refers to resistance changes in arterioles, whereas changes in the caliber of veins are described as *venoconstriction* or *venodilation.*

CONTROL OF TISSUE BLOOD FLOW

Control of blood flow to different tissues includes (1) local mechanisms, (2) autonomic nervous system responses, and (3) release of hormones. Total tissue blood flow or cardiac output is about 5 L·min^{-1}, with large amounts being delivered to the heart, brain, liver, and kidneys (Table 44-2) (Guyton, 1986). A high cerebral blood flow limits excessive accumulation of hydrogen ions (H$^+$) and carbon dioxide in the brain. Hepatic blood flow parallels the high level of metabolic activity of this organ. In contrast, skeletal muscle represents 35% to 40% of body mass but receives only about 15% of the total cardiac output, reflecting the low metabolic rate of inactive skeletal muscles.

Local Control of Blood Flow

Local control of blood flow is most often based on the need for delivery of oxygen or other nutrients such as glucose or fatty acids to the tissues.

Table 44-2
Tissue Blood Flow

| | Approximate Blood Flow | | Cardiac Output |
	$(ml \cdot min^{-1})$	$(ml \cdot 100\ g^{-1} \cdot min^{-1})$	*(percent of total)*
Brain	750	50	15
Liver	1450	100	29
Portal vein	1100		
Hepatic artery	350		
Kidneys	1000	320	20
Heart	225	75	5
Skeletal muscles (at rest)	750	4	15
Skin	400	3	8
Other tissues	425	2	8
TOTAL	5000		100

(Adapted from Guyton AC. Textbook of Medical Physiology. 7th ed. Philadelphia: WB Saunders, 1986; with permission)

The response to decreased oxygen delivery may reflect the local release of vasodilatory substances (adenosine, lactic acid, carbon dioxide, potassium ions [K^+]), which results in increased tissue blood flow and oxygen delivery.

Autoregulation of Blood Flow

Autoregulation is a local mechanism of control of blood flow in which a specific tissue is able to maintain a relatively constant blood flow over a wide range of mean arterial pressure. Conceptually, when the mean arterial pressure increases, the associated increase in tissue blood flow will deliver too many nutrients or flush out vasodilator substances, either of which will cause the blood vessels to constrict. As a result, increased perfusion pressure will not increase blood flow because of the modifying effect of vasoconstriction. Conversely, reductions in mean arterial pressure result in decreased delivery of nutrients to tissues such that vasodilation occurs to maintain an unchanged tissue blood flow despite a decreased perfusion pressure. Autoregulatory responses to sudden changes in mean arterial pressure occur within 60 to 120 seconds. The ability of autoregulation to return local tissue blood flow to normal is incomplete.

Long-Term Local Control of Blood Flow

Long-term regulatory mechanisms that return local tissue blood flow to normal involve a change in vascularity of tissues. For example, sustained elevation of mean arterial pressure to specific tissues, as occurs with coarctation of the aorta, is accompanied by a decrease in the size and number of blood vessels. Likewise, if metabolism in a tissue becomes chronically elevated, vascularity increases; or, if metabolism is reduced, vascularity decreases. Indeed, inadequate delivery of oxygen to a tissue is the stimulus for the development of collateral vessels. Neonates exposed to excessive concentrations of oxygen may manifest cessation of new vascular growth in the retina. Subsequent removal of the neonate from a high oxygen environment causes an overgrowth of new vessels to offset the abrupt decrease in availability of oxygen. There may be so much overgrowth that the new vessels cause blindness (retrolental fibroplasia).

Autonomic Nervous System Control of Blood Flow

Autonomic nervous system control of blood flow is characterized by a rapid response time (within

1 second) and an ability to regulate blood flow to certain tissues at the expense of other tissues. The sympathetic nervous system is the most important component of the autonomic nervous system in the regulation of blood flow. Release of norepinephrine stimulates alpha-receptors to produce vasoconstriction characteristic of sympathetic nervous system stimulation. Constriction of small arteries influences resistance to blood flow through tissues, whereas venoconstriction alters vascular capacitance and distribution of blood in the peripheral circulation. Sympathetic nervous system innervation is prominent in the kidneys and skin and minimal in the cerebral circulation.

Vasomotor Center

The vasomotor center, which is located in the pons and medulla, transmits sympathetic nervous system impulses through the spinal cord to all blood vessels. Evidence for a continuous, sustained state of partial vasoconstriction (vasomotor tone) is the abrupt decrease in blood pressure that occurs when sympathetic nervous system innervation of the vasculature is suddenly interrupted, as by traumatic spinal cord transection or regional anesthesia. Activity of the vasomotor center can be influenced by impulses from a number of sites, including diffuse areas of the reticular activating system, hypothalamus, and cerebral cortex. Sympathetic nervous system impulses are transmitted to the adrenal medulla at the same time they are transmitted to the peripheral vasculature. These impulses stimulate the medulla to secrete epinephrine and norepinephrine into the circulation, where they act directly on adrenergic receptors in the walls of vascular smooth muscle.

The medial and lower portions of the vasomotor center do not participate in transmission of vasoconstrictor impulses but rather function as an inhibitor of sympathetic nervous system activity, which allows blood vessels to dilate. Conceptually, this portion of the vasomotor center is functioning as the parasympathetic nervous system.

MASS REFLEX. The mass reflex is characterized by stimulation of all portions of the vasomotor center, resulting in generalized vasoconstriction and an increase in cardiac activity in an attempt to maintain tissue blood flow. The alarm reaction resembles the mass reflex, but associated skeletal muscle vasodilation and psychic excitement are intended to prepare the individual to confront a threatening situation.

SYNCOPE. Emotional fainting (vasovagal syncope) may reflect profound skeletal muscle vasodilation such that blood pressure falls abruptly and syncope occurs. Associated vagal stimulation results in bradycardia. This phenomenon may occur in patients who have an intense fear of needles, resulting in syncope during placement of an intravenous catheter.

Hormone Control of Blood Flow

Vasoconstrictor hormones that may influence local tissue blood flow include epinephrine, norepinephrine, angiotensin, and antidiuretic hormone (ADH). Bradykinin, serotonin, histamine, prostaglandins, and low circulating concentrations of epinephrine are vasodilating substances. Local chemical factors, such as accumulation of K^+, H^+, and carbon dioxide, relax vascular smooth muscle and cause vasodilation. Carbon dioxide also has an indirect vasoconstrictor effect because it stimulates the outflow of sympathetic nervous system impulses from the vasomotor center.

REGULATION OF BLOOD PRESSURE

Blood pressure is maintained over a narrow range by reciprocal changes in cardiac output and systemic vascular resistance. The autonomic nervous system and baroreceptors play a key role in moment-to-moment regulation of blood pressure. Long-term regulation of blood pressure is dependent on control of fluid balance by the kidneys, adrenal cortex, and central nervous system so as to maintain a constant blood volume.

Systolic, diastolic, and mean arterial pressures tend to increase progressively with age. Because a greater portion of the cardiac cycle is nearer the diastolic blood pressure, it follows that mean arterial pressure is not the arithmetic average of the systolic and diastolic blood pressures. Mean arterial blood pressure is the important determinant of tissue blood flow because it is the average pressure tending to drive blood through the systemic circulation.

Rapid-Acting Mechanisms for the Regulation of Blood Pressure

Rapid-acting mechanisms for regulation of blood pressure involve nervous system responses as reflected by the (1) baroreceptor reflexes, (2) chemoreceptor reflexes, (3) atrial reflexes, and (4) the central nervous system ischemic reflex. These reflex mechanisms respond almost immediately to changes in blood pressure. Furthermore, within about 30 minutes, these nervous system reflex responses are further supplemented by activation of hormonal mechanisms and shift of fluid into the circulation to readjust the blood volume. These short-term mechanisms can return blood pressure toward but never en-

tirely back to normal. Indeed, the impact of many of the rapidly acting regulatory mechanisms, such as the baroreceptor reflexes, diminish with time as these mechanisms adapt to the new level of blood pressure.

Baroreceptor Reflexes

Baroreceptors are nerve endings in the walls of large arteries in the neck and thorax, especially in the internal carotid arteries just above the carotid bifurcation and the arch of the aorta (Fig. 44-10) (Ganong, 1987). These nerve endings respond rapidly to changes in blood pressure and are crucial for maintaining normal blood pressure when an individual changes from the supine to standing position. An increase in mean arterial pressure produces stretch of baroreceptor nerve endings, and increased numbers of nerve impulses are transmitted to the depressor portion of the vasomotor center, leading to a relative de-

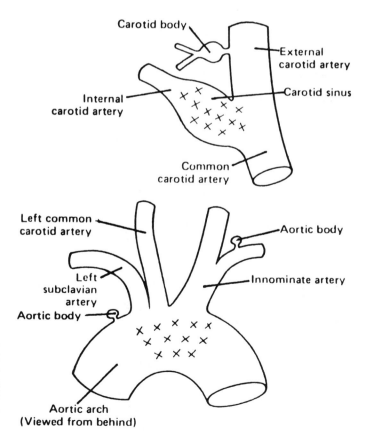

FIGURE 44–10. Baroreceptors are represented by the carotid sinus and receptors in the arch of the aorta. Chemoreceptors are located in the carotid and aortic bodies. (From Ganong WF. Review of Medical Physiology. 13th ed. Norwalk, CT: Appleton and Lange, 1987; with permission.)

cline in the central nervous system outflow of sympathetic nervous system (vasoconstrictive) impulses (Fig. 44-11) (Ganong, 1987). The net effects are vasodilation throughout the peripheral circulation, decreased heart rate, and reduced myocardial contractility, which all act to decrease blood pressure back toward normal. Conversely, decreases in blood pressure reflexly produce changes likely to elevate blood pressure. Baroreceptors adapt in 1 to 3 days to whatever blood pressure level they are exposed to, emphasizing that these reflexes are probably of no importance in long-term regulation of blood pressure. Volatile anesthetics, particularly halothane, inhibit the heart rate response portion of the baroreceptor reflex that occurs in response to changes in blood pressure (see Chapter 2).

Chemoreceptor Reflexes

Chemoreceptors are chemosensitive cells located in the carotid bodies and aortic body (Fig. 44-10) (Ganong, 1987). Each carotid or aortic body is supplied with an abundant blood flow through a nutrient artery so that the chemoreceptors are always exposed to oxygenated blood. Whenever the blood pressure, and thus the blood flow, decrease below a critical level, chemoreceptors are stimulated by decreased availability of oxygen and also because of excess carbon di-

oxide and H^+ that are not removed by the sluggish flow of blood. Impulses from the chemoreceptors are transmitted to the vasomotor center, which results in reflex changes that tend to elevate blood pressure back toward the normal level. Nevertheless, chemoreceptors do not respond strongly until blood pressure decreases below 80 mmHg. Instead, chemoreceptors are more important in stimulating breathing when the PaO_2 decreases below 60 mmHg (ventilatory response to arterial hypoxemia). The ventilatory response to arterial hypoxemia is inhibited by subanesthetic concentrations of volatile anesthetics (0.1 MAC) as well as injected drugs such as barbiturates and opioids (Knill et al, 1982).

Atrial Reflexes

The atria contain low-pressure stretch receptors similar to baroreceptors in large arteries. Stretching of the atria evokes reflex vasodilation and decreases the blood pressure back toward the normal level. An increase in atrial pressure also causes an acceleration in heart rate due to a direct effect of the increased atrial volume on stretch of the sinoatrial node, as well as to the Bainbridge reflex. The increase in heart rate evoked by stretching of the atria prevents accumulation of blood in the atria, veins, or pulmonary circulation.

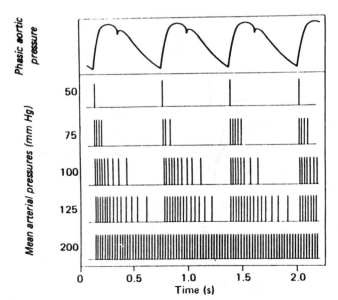

FIGURE 44–11. Discharges (*vertical lines*) in a single afferent nerve fiber from the carotid sinus at various arterial pressures, plotted against changes in aortic pressure with time. (From Ganong WF. Review of Medical Physiology. 13th ed. Norwalk, CT: Appleton and Lange, 1987; with permission.)

Central Nervous System Ischemic Reflex

The central nervous system ischemic reflex response occurs when blood flow to the medullary vasomotor center is reduced to the extent that ischemia of this vital center occurs. As a result of this ischemia, there is an intense outpouring of sympathetic nervous system activity, resulting in profound elevations in blood pressure. It is believed that this reflex response is caused by failure of slowly flowing blood to remove carbon dioxide from the vasomotor center. The central nervous system reflex response does not become highly active until mean arterial pressure decreases below 50 mmHg and reaches its greatest degree of stimulation at pressures of 15 to 20 mmHg. This reflex response is not useful for regulation of normal blood pressure but rather acts as an emergency control system to prevent further reductions in blood pressure when cerebral blood flow is dangerously reduced.

CUSHING REFLEX.   The Cushing reflex is a special type of central nervous system ischemic reflex response that results from increased intracranial pressure. When intracranial pressure increases to equal arterial pressure, the Cushing reflex acts to elevate blood pressure above intracranial pressure.

Respiratory Variations in Blood Pressure

Blood pressure usually increases and decreases 4 to 6 mmHg in a wavelike manner during quiet spontaneous breathing. Typically, blood pressure is increased during end-inspiration and the beginning of exhalation and decreased during the remainder of the breathing cycle. Positive-pressure ventilation of the lungs produces a different sequence because the initial positive pressure pushes more blood toward the left ventricle followed by impaired venous return. As a result, blood pressure becomes maximal during the early phases of the mechanically produced inspiration.

Blood Pressure Vasomotor Waves

Cyclic increases and decreases in blood pressure lasting 7 to 10 seconds are referred to as *vasomotor* or *Traube-Hering waves*. The presumed cause of vasomotor waves is oscillation in the reflex activity of baroreceptors. For example, increased blood pressure stimulates baroreceptors, which then inhibit the sympathetic nervous system, causing a decrease in blood pressure. Decreased blood pressure reduces baroreceptor activity and allows the vasomotor center to become active once again, increasing the blood pressure to a higher value.

Moderately Rapid-Acting Mechanisms for the Regulation of Blood Pressure

There are at least three hormonal mechanisms that provide either rapid or moderately rapid control of blood pressure. These hormonal mechanisms are (1) catecholamine-induced vasoconstriction, (2) renin-angiotensin–induced vasoconstriction, and (3) ADH-induced vasoconstriction, all of which increase blood pressure by increasing systemic vascular resistance. Circulating catecholamines may even reach parts of the circulation that are devoid of sympathetic nervous system innervation, such as metarterioles. Renin-angiotensin–induced vasoconstriction manifests to a greater degree on arterioles than veins and requires about 20 minutes to become fully active.

In addition to hormonal mechanisms, there are two intrinsic mechanisms: capillary fluid shift and stress relaxation of blood vessels, which begin to react within minutes of changes in blood pressure. For example, changes in blood pressure produce corresponding changes in capillary pressure, thus allowing fluid to enter or leave the capillaries to maintain a constant blood volume. Stress-relaxation is the gradual change in blood vessel size to adapt to changes in blood pressure and the amount of blood that is available. The stress-relaxation mechanism has definite limitations such that increases in blood volume greater than about 30% or decreases of more than about 15% cannot be corrected by this mechanism alone.

Long-Term Mechanisms for the Regulation of Blood Pressure

Long-term mechanisms for the regulation of blood pressure, unlike the short-term regulatory mechanisms, have a delayed onset but do not adapt, providing a sustained regulatory effect on blood pressure. The renal–body fluid system plays a predominant role in long-term control of blood pressure as it controls both the cardiac output and systemic vascular resistance. This crucial role is supplemented by accessory mechanisms, including the renin-angiotensin system, aldosterone, and ADH.

Renal–Body Fluid System

Increased blood pressure, as provoked by modest increases in blood volume, results in sodium ion (Na^+) and water excretion by the kidneys. The resultant decrease in blood volume leads to reductions in cardiac output and blood pressure. After several weeks, the cardiac output returns toward normal and systemic vascular resistance decreases to maintain the lower but more acceptable blood pressure. Conversely, a decrease in blood pressure stimulates the kidneys to retain fluid. A special feature of this regulatory mechanism is its ability to return blood pressure completely back to normal values. This contrasts with rapid-acting to moderately rapid-acting mechanisms, which cannot return blood pressure entirely back to normal.

Renin-Angiotensin System

Aldosterone secretion that results from the action of angiotensin II on the adrenal cortex exerts a long-term effect on blood pressure by stimulating the kidneys to retain Na^+ and water. The resulting increase in extracellular fluid volume causes cardiac output and subsequently blood pressure, to increase.

REGULATION OF CARDIAC OUTPUT AND VENOUS RETURN

Cardiac output is the amount of blood pumped by the left ventricle into the aorta each minute (product of stroke volume and heart rate), and venous return is the amount of blood flowing from the veins into the right atrium each minute. Because the circulation is a closed circuit, the cardiac output must equal venous return. Cardiac output for the average male weighing 70 kg and with a body surface area of 1.7 m^2 is about 5 L·min^{-1}. This value is about 10% less in females.

Determinants of Cardiac Output

Venous return is more important than myocardial contractility in determining cardiac output. In essence, the metabolic requirements of tissues control cardiac output through alterations in resistance to tissue blood flow. For example, increased local metabolic needs lead to regional vasodilation, with a resulting increase in tissue blood flow and thus venous return. Cardiac output is increased by an amount equivalent to the venous return.

Any factor that interferes with venous return can lead to decreased cardiac output. Hemorrhage reduces blood volume such that venous return decreases and cardiac output declines. Acute venodilation, such as that produced by spinal anesthesia and accompanying sympathetic nervous system blockade, can so increase the capacitance of peripheral vessels that venous return is reduced and cardiac output declines. Indeed, the optimal therapy for hypotension resulting from spinal anesthesia is appropriate positioning of the patient and intravenous infusion of fluids to improve venous return. Positive-pressure ventilation of the lungs, particularly in the presence of a reduced blood volume, causes a decrease in venous return and cardiac output.

Factors that increase cardiac output are associated with reductions in systemic vascular resistance. For example, anemia reduces the viscosity of blood, leading to a decrease in systemic vascular resistance and increase in venous return. An increased blood volume increases cardiac output by increasing the gradient for flow to the right atrium and by distending blood vessels, which reduces resistance to blood flow. Increased cardiac output caused by the increased blood volume lasts only 20 to 40 minutes because elevated capillary pressures cause fluid to enter tissues, thereby returning blood volume to normal. Furthermore, increased pressure in veins caused by the increased blood volume causes the veins to distend (stress-relaxation). Cardiac output increases during exercise, in hyperthyroidism, and in the presence of arteriovenous shunts associated with hemodialysis, reflecting reductions in systemic vascular resistance.

Sympathetic nervous system stimulation increases myocardial contractility and heart rate to increase cardiac output beyond that possible from venous return alone. Maximal stimulation by the sympathetic nervous system can double cardiac output. Nevertheless, this sympathetic nervous system–induced elevation of cardiac output is only transient despite sustained elevations in nervous system activity. A reason for this transient effect is autoregulation of tissue blood flow, which manifests as vasoconstriction to reduce venous return and cardiac output back toward normal. In addition, increased blood pressure associated with elevations in the cardiac output causes fluid to leave the capillaries, thereby decreasing blood volume, venous return, and cardiac output.

Ventricular Function Curves

Ventricular function curves (Frank-Starling curves) depict the cardiac output at different atrial (ventricular end-diastolic) filling pressures (Fig. 44-12). Improved cardiac function (sympathetic nervous system stimulation) is characterized by a shift of the cardiac output curve to the left of the normal curve (greater cardiac output as filling pressure increases), whereas a shift of the curve to the right of normal (myocardial infarction, valvular heart disease) reflects decreased cardiac function. A point is reached where further stretching of the cardiac muscle results in a decrease in cardiac output. Clinically, ventricular function curves are used to estimate myocardial contractility.

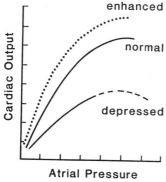

FIGURE 44–12. Ventricular function curves (Frank-Starling curves) depict the volume of forward ventricular ejection (cardiac output) at different atrial filling pressures and varying degrees of myocardial contractility.

Circulatory Shock

Circulatory shock is characterized by inadequate tissue blood flow and oxygen delivery to cells, resulting in generalized deterioration of organ function. The usual cause of inadequate tissue perfusion is inadequate cardiac output owing to decreased venous return or myocardial depression.

Hemorrhage is the most common cause of shock owing to decreased venous return. Any decrease in blood pressure initiates powerful baroreceptor-mediated increases in sympathetic nervous system activity manifesting as arterial constriction, venoconstriction, and direct myocardial stimulation. Venoconstriction is particularly important for maintaining venous return to the heart and cardiac output. Arterial constriction is responsible for initially maintaining blood pressure despite reductions in cardiac output. This maintenance of blood pressure sustains cerebral and coronary blood flow because significant vasoconstriction does not occur in these organs. In other organs, such as the kidneys, intense sympathetic nervous system–mediated vasoconstriction may reduce blood flow dramatically.

Loss of plasma from the circulation in the absence of blood loss can result in shock similar to that produced by hemorrhage. Intestinal obstruction results in extreme loss of plasma volume into the gastrointestinal tract. Severe burns may also be associated with sufficient plasma loss to result in shock. Hypovolemic shock that results from plasma loss has almost the same characteristics as hemorrhagic shock except that selective loss of plasma greatly increases viscosity of blood and exacerbates sluggishness of blood flow.

Neurogenic shock occurs in the absence of blood loss when vascular capacity increases so greatly that even a normal blood volume is not capable of maintaining venous return and cardiac output. A classic cause of loss of vasomotor tone and subsequent neurogenic shock is acute blockade of the peripheral sympathetic nervous system by spinal or epidural anesthesia.

Septic shock is characterized by profound peripheral vasodilation, elevated cardiac output secondary to decreased systemic vascular resistance, and development of disseminated intravascular coagulation. Causes of septic shock are most often release of endotoxins from ischemic portions of the gastrointestinal tract or bacteremia owing to extension of urinary tract infections. The end-stages of septic shock are not greatly different from the end-stages of hemorrhagic shock, even though the initiating factors are markedly different.

Decreased cardiac output associated with shock reduces tissue oxygen delivery, which in turn reduces the level of metabolism that can be maintained by different cells of the body. Skeletal muscle weakness is prominent, reflecting inadequate delivery of oxygen to this tissue. Metabolism is depressed, and the amount of heat liberated is reduced. As a result, body temperature tends to decrease, especially in the presence of a cold environment. In the early stages of shock, consciousness is usually maintained although mental clarity may be impaired. Consciousness is likely to be lost as shock progresses. Low cardiac output greatly diminishes urine output or even causes anuria because glomerular pressure decreases below the critical value required for filtration of fluid into Bowman's capsule. Furthermore, the kidney has such a high rate of metabolism and requires such large amounts of nutrients that decreased renal blood flow often causes acute tubular necrosis.

An important feature of persistent shock is eventual progressive deterioration of the heart. In addition to myocardial depression caused by decreased coronary blood flow, the myocardium can also be depressed by lactic acid, bacterial endotoxins, and myocardial depressant factor released from an ischemic pancreas.

Measurement of Cardiac Output

Indirect methods of cardiac output measurement are (1) the Fick method, (2) the indicator dilution method, and (3) the thermodilution method. Echocardiography uses pulses of ultrasonic waves to record movements of the ventricular wall, septum, and valves during the cardiac cycle.

Fick Method

Cardiac output is calculated as oxygen consumption divided by the arteriovenous difference for oxygen (Fig. 44-13) (Guyton, 1986). Oxygen consumption is usually measured by a respirometer containing a known oxygen mixture. The patient's exhaled gases are collected in a Douglas bag. The volume and oxygen concentra-

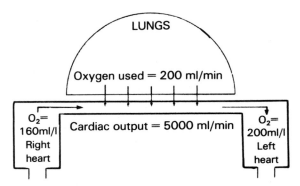

FIGURE 44-13. The Fick method calculates cardiac output as oxygen consumption divided by the arteriovenous difference for oxygen. (From Guyton AC. Textbook of Medical Physiology. 7th ed. Philadelphia: WB Saunders, 1986; with permission.)

tion of the exhaled gases allows calculation of oxygen consumption. Venous blood for calculation of oxygen content must be obtained from the right ventricle or, ideally, the pulmonary artery to ensure adequate mixing. Blood from the right atrium may not yet be adequately mixed to provide a true mixed venous sample. Blood used for determining the oxygen saturation in arterial blood can be obtained from any artery because all arterial blood is thoroughly mixed before it leaves the heart and, therefore, has the same concentration of oxygen.

Indicator Dilution Method

In measuring the cardiac output by the indicator dilution method, a nondiffusible dye (indocyanine green) is injected into the right atrium (or central venous circulation), and the concentration of dye is subsequently measured continuously in the arterial circulation by a spectrophotometer. The area under the resulting time-concentration curve before recirculation of the dye occurs, combined with knowing the amount of dye injected, allows calculation of the pulmonary blood flow, which is the same as the cardiac output. It is necessary to extrapolate the dye curve to zero because recirculation of the dye occurs before the downslope of the curve reaches baseline. Early recirculation of the dye may indicate the presence of a right-to-left intracardiac shunt (foramen ovale), permitting direct passage of a portion of the dye to the left side of the heart without passing through the lungs.

Thermodilution Method

A pulmonary artery catheter with ports in the right atrium and pulmonary artery and a temperature sensor on the distal port is used to measure thermodilution cardiac output. Thermodilution cardiac outputs are determined by measuring the change in blood temperature between two points (right atrium and pulmonary artery) following injection of a known volume of cold saline solution at the proximal right atrial port. The change in blood temperature as measured at the distal pulmonary artery port is inversely proportional to pulmonary blood flow (the extent to which the cold saline solution is diluted by blood), which is equivalent to cardiac output. A computer converts the area under the temperature-time curve

to its equivalent in cardiac output. Advantages of this technique compared with the indicator dilution method include dissipation of cold in tissues so recirculation is not a problem, and safety of repeated measurements because saline is innocuous.

FETAL CIRCULATION

Fetal circulation is considerably different than circulation after birth. For example, *in utero,* the placenta acts as the fetal lung, and oxygenated blood (saturation about 80%) from the placenta passes through a single umbilical vein to the fetus. This blood flows predominately through the ductus venosus and into the inferior vena

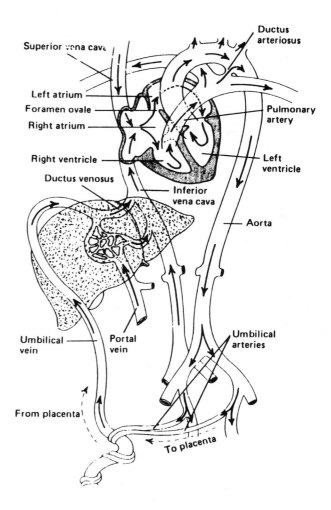

FIGURE 44–14. The placenta acts as the lung for the fetus. Most of the oxygenated blood reaching the fetal heart via the umbilical vein and inferior vena cava is diverted through the foramen ovale and pumped out the aorta to the head. Deoxygenated blood returned via the superior vena cava is mostly pumped through the pulmonary artery and ductus arteriosus to the feet and the umbilical arteries. (From Ganong WF. Review of Medical Physiology. 13th ed. Norwalk, CT: Appleton and Lange, 1987; with permission.)

cava, thus bypassing the liver (Fig. 44-14) (Ganong, 1987). Most of the oxygenated blood entering the right atrium from the inferior vena cava preferentially passes through the foramen ovale into the left atrium, thus bypassing the lungs. Passage of this oxygenated blood directly to the left atrium allows perfusion of the fetal brain with maximal available concentrations of oxygen. Fetal hemoglobin differs from adult hemoglobin in binding oxygen less avidly, thus maximizing oxygen transfer to tissues despite low hemoglobin saturations with oxygen.

Blood entering the right atrium from the superior vena cava is mainly deoxygenated blood from the fetal head regions. This blood enters the right ventricle for delivery into the pulmonary artery and then to the descending thoracic aorta by the ductus arteriosus. As a result, this deoxygenated blood is delivered distal to the blood vessels that supply the fetal brain. Blood is returned to the placenta for oxygenation by two umbilical arteries.

The principal changes in the fetal circulation at birth are increased systemic vascular resistance and blood pressure owing to cessation of blood flow through the placenta. In addition, pulmonary vascular resistance decreases dramatically with expansion of the lungs, leading to a marked increase in pulmonary blood flow. These alterations in pulmonary and systemic vascular resistances change the pressure gradient across the foramen ovale, causing the flaplike valve that is present on the left atrial septum to occlude the opening and prevent continued right-to-left shunting of blood at this site. In about two thirds of individuals, this valve becomes adherent over the foramen ovale in a few months. In the absence of permanent closure over the foramen ovale, events that increase right atrial pressure above left atrial pressure (positive-pressure ventilation of the lungs, especially with positive end-expiratory pressure, right ventricular failure, and pulmonary embolism) may introduce an unexpected right-to-left intracardiac shunt at this site. Arterial hypoxemia may be the initial manifestation of this intracardiac shunt when right atrial pressure is acutely and selectively increased.

Flow through the ductus arteriosus decreases after birth owing to constriction of the muscular wall of this vessel on exposure to higher concentrations of oxygen. Failure of the ductus arteriosus to close after birth results in reversal of flow compared with that present before birth. This reversal of flow occurs because pressure in the aorta exceeds pressure in the pulmonary artery following birth. The muscular wall of the ductus venosus also contracts following birth, diverting portal venous blood through the liver.

REFERENCES

Bazaral MG, Welch M, Golding LAR, Badhwar K. Comparison of brachial and radial arterial pressure monitoring in patients undergoing coronary artery bypass surgery. Anesthesiology 1990;73:38–45.

Guyton AC. Textbook of Medical Physiology. 7th ed. Philadelphia, WB Saunders, 1986.

Ganong WF. Review of Medical Physiology. 13th ed. Norwalk, CT, Appleton and Lange, 1987.

Gerber MJ, Hines RL, Barash PG. Arterial waveforms and systemic vascular resistance: Is there a correlation? Anesthesiology 1987;66:823–5.

Knill RL, Clement JL. Variable effects of anaesthetics on the ventilatory response to hypoxaemia in man. Can Anaesth Soc J 1982;29:93–9.

Pauca AL, Hudspeth AS, Wallenhaupt SL, et al. Radial artery-to-aorta pressure difference after discontinuation of cardiopulmonary bypass. Anesthesiology 1989;70:935–41.

Stern DH, Gerson JI, Allen FB, Parker FB. Can we trust the direct radial artery pressure immediately following cardiopulmonary bypass? Anesthesiology 1985;62:557–61.

Chapter

45

Capillaries and Lymph Vessels

CAPILLARIES

The circulation is designed to supply tissues with blood in amounts commensurate with their needs for oxygen and nutrients. Capillaries serve as the site for this transfer of oxygen and nutrients to tissues and receipt of metabolic byproducts. There are an estimated 10 billion capillaries providing a total surface area that exceeds 6300 m² for nutrient exchange. Capillary density varies from tissue to tissue. Capillaries are numerous in metabolically active tissues, such as cardiac and skeletal muscles, whereas in less active tissues, capillary density is low. Nevertheless, it is unlikely that any functional cell is more than 50 μ away from a capillary.

Anatomy of the Microcirculation

Arterioles give rise to metarterioles, which give rise to capillaries (Fig. 45-1) (Ganong, 1987). Other metarterioles serve as thoroughfare channels to the venules, bypassing the capillary bed. Capillaries drain via short collecting venules to the venules. Blood flow through capillaries is regulated by muscular precapillary sphincters present at the capillary opening. The arterioles, metarterioles, and venules contain smooth muscle. As a result, the arterioles serve as the major resistance vessels and regulate regional blood flow to the capillary beds, whereas the venules and veins serve primarily as collecting channels and storage or capacitance vessels.

Capillary walls are about 0.5 nm thick, consisting of a single layer of endothelial cells surrounded by a thin basement membrane on the outside (Fig. 45-2) (Ganong, 1987). The structure of the capillary wall varies from tissue to tissue, but in many organs, including those in skeletal, cardiac, and smooth muscle, the interdigitated junction between endothelial cells allows passage of molecules up to 10 nm in diameter. In addition, the cytoplasm of endothelial cells is attenuated to form gaps or pores that are 20 to 100 nm in diameter. These pores permit the passage of relatively large molecules. It also appears that plasma and its dissolved proteins are taken up by endocytosis, transported across endothelial cells, and discharged by exocytosis into the interstitial fluid. In the brain, the capillaries resemble those in skeletal muscles, except the interdigitated junctions between endothelial cells are tighter (blood-brain barrier), permitting passage of only small molecules.

The diameter of capillary pores is about 25 times the diameter of the water molecule (0.3 nm), which is the smallest molecule that normally passes through capillary channels. Plasma proteins have diameters that exceed the width of capillary pores. Other substances such as sodium (Na^+), potassium (K^+), and chloride (Cl^-) ions, and glucose have intermediate diameters (0.39 to 0.86 nm) such that permeability of capillary pores for different substances varies according to their molecular weights (Table 45-1) (Guyton, 1986). Oxygen and carbon dioxide are both lipid soluble and readily pass through endothelial cells.

679

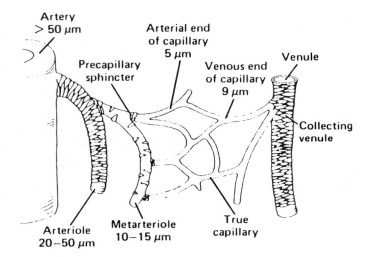

FIGURE 45–1. Anatomy of the microcirculation. (From Ganong WF. Review of Medical Physiology. 13th ed. Norwalk, CT: Appleton and Lange, 1987; with permission.)

True capillaries are devoid of smooth muscle and are therefore incapable of active constriction. Nevertheless, the endothelial cells that form the capillary wall contain actin and myosin and can alter their shape in response to certain chemical stimuli. The diameter of capillaries (7 to 9 μm) is just sufficient to permit erythrocytes to squeeze through in single file. The thin walls of capillaries are able to withstand high intraluminal pressures because their small diameter prevents excessive wall tension (Laplace's law).

Blood Flow in Capillaries

Blood flow in capillaries is intermittent rather than continuous. This intermittent blood flow reflects contraction and relaxation of metarterioles and precapillary sphincters in alternating cycles 6 to 12 times per minute. The phenomenon of alternating contraction and relaxation is known as *vasomotion*. Oxygen is the most important determinant of the degree of opening and closing of metarterioles and precapillary sphincters. A low

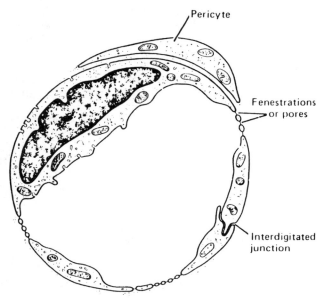

FIGURE 45–2. Capillaries include interdigitated junctions and pores to facilitate passage of lipid-insoluble ions and molecules. (From Ganong WF. Review of Medical Physiology. 13th ed. Norwalk, CT: Appleton and Lange, 1987; with permission.)

Table 45–1
Permeability of Capillary Membranes

	Molecular Weight	Relative Permeability
Water	18	1.0
Sodium chloride	58.5	0.96
Glucose	180	0.6
Hemoglobin	66,700	0.01
Albumin	69,000	0.0001

PO_2 allows more blood to flow through capillaries to supply tissues. In this regard, the impact of oxygen on capillary blood flow provides a form of autoregulation of tissue blood flow.

In addition to nutritive blood flow through tissues that is regulated by oxygen, there is also nonnutritive blood flow regulated by the automatic nervous system. This nonnutritive blood flow is characterized by direct vascular connections between arterioles and venules. Some of these arteriovenous connections have muscular coverings so blood flow can be altered over a wide range. In some parts of the skin, these arteriovenous anastomoses provide a mechanism to permit rapid inflow of arterial blood to warm the skin.

Fluid Movement Across Capillary Membranes

Solvent and solute movement across capillary endothelial cells occurs by filtration, diffusion, and pinocytosis via endothelial vesicles. It is important to distinguish between filtration and diffusion through capillary membranes. Filtration is the net outward movement of fluid at the arterial end of capillaries. Diffusion of fluid occurs in both directions across capillary membranes.

Filtration

The four pressures that determine whether fluid will move outward across capillary membranes (filtration) or inward across capillary membranes (reabsorption) are (1) capillary pressure, (2) interstitial fluid pressure, (3) plasma colloid osmotic pressure, and (4) interstitial fluid colloid osmotic pressure. The net effect of these four pressures is a positive filtration pressure at the arterial end of capillaries, causing fluid to move

outward across cell membranes into interstitial fluid spaces (Table 45-2). At the venous end of capillaries, the net effect of these four pressures is a positive reabsorption pressure causing fluid to move inward across capillary membranes into capillaries (Table 45-3). Overall, the mean values of the four pressures acting across capillary membranes are nearly identical such that the amount of fluid filtered nearly equals the amount reabsorbed (Table 45-4). Any fluid that is not reabsorbed enters the lymph vessels.

CAPILLARY PRESSURE. Capillary pressure tends to move fluid outward across the arterial ends of capillary membranes. It is estimated that capillary pressure at the arterial end of capillaries is 25 mmHg, whereas pressure at the venous end of capillaries is 10 mmHg, corresponding to the pressure in venules. The mean capillary pressure is about 17 mmHg. Changes in arterial pressure have little effect on capillary pressure and flow owing to adjustments of precapillary resistance vessels. *Autoregulation* describes the maintenance of unchanged tissue blood flow despite changes in perfusion pressure.

INTERSTITIAL FLUID PRESSURE. Interstitial fluid pressure tends to move fluid outward across capillary membranes. It is estimated that average interstitial fluid pressure is −6.3 mmHg. This negative pressure acts as a vacuum to hold tissues together and maintain a minimal distance for diffusion of nutrients. Under normal conditions, almost all of the interstitial fluid is held in a gel that fills the spaces between cells. This gel contains large quantities of mucopolysaccharides, the most abundant of which is hyaluronic acid.

Table 45–2
Filtration of Fluid at the Arterial Ends of Capillaries

Pressures favoring outward movement		
Capillary pressure	25	mmHg
Interstitial fluid pressure	−6.3	mmHg
Interstitial fluid colloid osmotic pressure	5	mmHg
Total	36.3	mmHg
Pressure favoring inward movement		
Plasma colloid osmotic pressure	28	mmHg
Net filtration pressure	8.3	mmHg

Table 45–3
Reabsorption of Fluid at the Venous Ends of Capillaries

Pressures favoring outward movement		
Capillary pressure	10	mmHg
Interstitial fluid pressure	– 6.3	mmHg
Interstitial fluid colloid osmotic		
pressure	5	mmHg
Total	21.3	mmHg
Pressure favoring inward movement		
Plasma colloid osmotic pressure	28	mmHg
Net reabsorption pressure	6.7	mmHg

Loss of negative interstitial fluid pressure allows fluid to accumulate in tissue spaces as edema.

PLASMA COLLOID OSMOTIC PRESSURE. Plasma proteins are principally responsible for the plasma colloid osmotic (oncotic) pressure that tends to cause movement of fluid inward through capillary membranes. Each gram of albumin exerts twice the colloid osmotic pressure of a gram of globulin. Because there is about twice as much albumin as globulin in the plasma, about 70% of the total colloid osmotic pressure results from albumin and only about 30% from globulin and fibrinogen.

A special phenomenon known as *Donnan equilibrium* causes the colloid osmotic pressure to be about 50% greater than that caused by proteins alone. This reflects the negative charge characteristic of proteins that necessitates the presence of an equal number of positively charged ions, mainly Na^+, on the same side of the

Table 45–4
Mean Values of Pressures Acting Across Capillary Membranes

Pressures favoring outward movement		
Capillary pressure	17	mmHg
Interstitial fluid pressure	–6.3	mmHg
Interstitial fluid colloid osmotic		
pressure	5	mmHg
Total	28.3	mmHg
Pressure favoring inward movement		
Plasma colloid osmotic pressure	28	mmHg
Net overall filtration pressure	0.3	mmHg

capillary membrane as the proteins. These extra positive ions increase the number of osmotically active substances and thus increase the colloid osmotic pressure. Indeed, about one third of the normal plasma colloid osmotic pressure of 28 mmHg is caused by positively charged ions held in the plasma by proteins. This is the reason that plasma proteins cannot be replaced by inert substances, such as dextran, without some decrease in plasma colloid osmotic pressure.

INTERSTITIAL FLUID COLLOID OSMOTIC PRESSURE. Proteins present in the interstitial fluid are principally responsible for the interstitial fluid colloid osmotic pressure of about 5 mmHg, which tends to cause movement of fluid outward across capillary membranes. Albumin, because of its smaller size, normally leaks 1.6 times as readily as globulins through capillaries, causing the proteins in interstitial fluids to have a disproportionately high albumin to globulin ratio. The total protein content of interstitial fluid is similar to the total protein content of plasma, but, because the volume of the interstitial fluid is four times the volume of plasma, the average interstitial fluid protein content is only one fourth that in plasma, or about 1.8 $g \cdot dl^{-1}$. Interstitial fluid protein content also remains low because proteins cannot readily diffuse across capillary membranes, and any that crosses is likely to be removed by lymph vessels.

Diffusion

Diffusion is the most important mechanism for transfer of nutrients between the plasma and the interstitial fluid. Oxygen, carbon dioxide, and anesthetic gases are examples of lipid-soluble molecules that can diffuse directly through capillary membranes independently of pores. Na^+, K^+, Cl^-, and glucose are insoluble in lipid capillary membranes and, therefore, must pass through pores to gain access to interstitial fluids. The diffusion rate of lipid-soluble molecules across capillary membranes in either direction is proportional to the concentration difference between the two sides of the membrane. For this reason, large amounts of oxygen move from capillaries toward tissues, whereas carbon dioxide moves in the opposite direction. Typically, only slight partial pressure differences suffice to maintain adequate transport of oxygen between the plasma and interstitial fluid.

Pinocytosis

Pinocytosis is the process by which capillary endothelial cells ingest small amounts of plasma or interstitial fluid followed by migration to the opposite surface where the fluid is released. Transport of high–molecular-weight substances such as plasma proteins, glycoproteins, and polysaccharides (dextran) most likely occurs principally by pinocytosis.

LYMPH VESSELS

Lymph vessels represent an alternate route by which excess fluids can flow from interstitial fluid spaces into the blood. The most important function of the lymphatic system is return of protein into the circulation and maintenance of a low-protein concentration in the interstitial fluid. The small amount of protein that escapes from the arterial end of the capillary cannot undergo reabsorption at the venous end of the capillary. If lymph vessels were not available, this protein would be progressively concentrated in the interstitial fluid, resulting in increases in interstitial fluid colloid osmotic pressure that, within a few hours, would produce life-threatening edema.

Anatomy

The terminal lymph vessels are the thoracic duct and the right lymphatic duct (Fig. 45-3). The thoracic duct is the larger of the two (2 mm in diameter), entering the venous system in the angle of the junction of the left internal jugular and subclavian veins. The right lymphatic duct is not always present and, if it is, rarely exists as such because the three vessels that occasionally unite to form it usually open separately into the right internal jugular, subclavian, and innominate veins. Avoidance of possible damage to the thoracic duct is often the reason to select the right side of the neck as the preferential site for percutaneous placement of venous catheters into the right internal jugular vein.

Lymph vessels contain flaplike valves between endothelial cells that open toward the interior, allowing the unimpeded entrance of interstitial fluid and proteins. Backflow out of the lymph vessel is not possible because any flow in this direction causes the flaplike vessels to close. The central nervous system is devoid of lymphatics.

Formation

Lymph is interstitial fluid that flows into lymphatic vessels. As such, the protein concentration of lymph is about 1.8 g·dl^{-1}, with the exception of lymph from the gastrointestinal tract and liver, which contains two to three times this concentration of protein. The lymphatic system is also one of the major channels for absorption of nutrients, especially fat, from the gastrointestinal tract. Bacteria that enter lymph vessels are removed and destroyed by lymph nodes.

Flow

Flow of lymph through the thoracic duct is about 100 ml·h^{-1}. A decrease in the negative value of interstitial fluid pressure increases the flow of interstitial fluid into terminal lymph vessels and consequently increases the rate of lymph flow. For example, at 0 mmHg interstitial fluid pressure, the rate of lymph flow is increased 10 to 50 times compared with flow at an average interstitial fluid pressure of −6.3 mmHg. Skeletal muscle contraction and passive movements of the extremities facilitate flow of lymph. For example, during exercise, lymph flow is increased up to 14 times that present at rest.

EDEMA

Edema is the presence of excess interstitial fluid in peripheral tissues that results in positive pressure in interstitial fluid spaces and exceeds the ability of lymph vessels to transport the excess fluid. When this occurs, external pressure in one area will displace fluid to another area, resulting in pitting edema. Also, fluid flows downward in tissues because of gravity, resulting in dependent edema. Coagulation of edema fluid may occur with infection or trauma and manifest as nonpitting or brawny edema.

Edema may also be accompanied by the presence of fluid in potential spaces such as the pleural cavity, pericardial space, peritoneal cavity, and synovial spaces. Fluid that collects in these spaces is called *transudate* if it is sterile and *exudate* if it contains bacteria. Excessive fluid in the peritoneal space, one of the spaces most prone to develop edema fluid, is called *ascites.* The peritoneal cavity is susceptible to the development of edema fluid because any increased

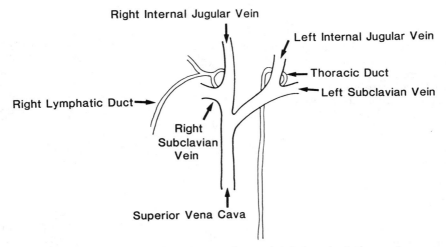

FIGURE 45–3. Depiction of the thoracic duct and right lymphatic duct as they enter the venous system.

pressure in the liver, as due to cirrhosis or cardiac failure, causes transudation of protein-containing fluids from the liver into the peritoneal cavity.

Causes of increased interstitial fluid volume that manifests as edema include (1) increased capillary pressure, (2) decreased plasma protein concentrations, (3) obstruction to lymph vessels, and (4) increased permeability of capillaries. Renal dysfunction leading to excessive retention of fluid is also a cause of edema.

Increased Capillary Pressure

Increased capillary pressure, as accompanies impaired venous return owing to cardiac failure, results in filtration of fluid from capillaries that exceeds reabsorption. Local edema, as associated with allergic reactions, reflects histamine-induced smooth muscle relaxation of arterioles and constriction of veins. Angioneurotic edema reflects activation of the complement cascade and release of vasoactive substances that increase capillary permeability.

Decreased Plasma Protein Concentrations

Decreased plasma protein concentrations lower the colloid osmotic pressure such that capillary pressure predominates and excess fluid leaves the circulation. It is estimated that edema begins to appear when the plasma colloid osmotic pressure declines below 11 mmHg. Albumin may be lost from the plasma in large quantities when the skin is burned. Renal disease may be associated with urinary loss of albumin sufficient to lower the plasma colloid osmotic pressure. Nutritional edema occurs when dietary intake is not adequate to support formation of sufficient amounts of protein.

Obstruction of Lymph Vessels

Obstruction of lymph vessels results in accumulation of protein in interstitial fluid. The subsequent rise in interstitial fluid colloid osmotic pressure causes excess fluid to collect in the interstitial fluid space. Obstruction of lymph vessels with associated edema may follow operations, such as radical mastectomy, in which it is necessary to remove lymph nodes as part of the procedure. Edema owing to this cause typically regresses over 2 to 3 months as new lymph vessels develop.

REFERENCES

Ganong WF. Review of Medical Physiology. 13th ed. Norwalk, CT, Appleton and Lange, 1987.

Guyton AC. Textbook of Medical Physiology. 7th ed. Philadelphia, WB Saunders, 1986.

Chapter

46

Pulmonary Circulation

INTRODUCTION

The pulmonary circulation is a low-pressure, low-resistance system in series with the systemic circulation. The volume of blood flowing through the lungs and systemic circulation is essentially identical. Blood passes through pulmonary capillaries in about 1 second, during which time it is oxygenated and excess carbon dioxide is removed. Increasing the cardiac output may shorten capillary transit time to less than 0.5 second.

ANATOMY

Anatomically, the right ventricle is wrapped halfway around the left ventricle. The semilunar shape of the right ventricle allows it to pump with minimal shortening of its muscle fibers. The thickness of the right ventricle is one third that of the left ventricle, reflecting the difference in pressures between the two ventricles. The wall of the right ventricle is only about three times as thick as the atrial walls.

The pulmonary artery extends only about 4 cm beyond the apex of the right ventricle and then divides into the right and left main pulmonary arteries. The pulmonary artery is also a thin structure with a wall thickness about twice that of the vena cavae and one third that of the aorta. The large diameter and distensibility of the pulmonary arteries allows the pulmonary circulation to easily accommodate the stroke volume of the right ventricle. Pulmonary veins, like pulmonary arteries, are large in diameter and highly distensible. Pulmonary capillaries supply the estimated 300 million alveoli, providing a gas-exchange surface of about 70 m^2.

Pulmonary blood vessels are innervated by the sympathetic nervous system, but the density of these fibers is less than in systemic vessels. Alpha-adrenergic stimulation from norepinephrine produces vasoconstriction of the pulmonary vessels, whereas beta-adrenergic stimulation, as produced by isoproterenol, results in vasodilation. Parasympathetic nervous system fibers from the vagus nerves release acetylcholine, which produces vasodilation of pulmonary vessels. Despite the presence of autonomic nervous system innervation, the resting vasomotor tone is minimal and pulmonary vessels are almost maximally dilated in the normal resting state. Indeed, overall regulation of pulmonary blood flow is passive, with local adjustments of perfusion relative to ventilation being determined by local effects of oxygen or its lack.

The diameter of thin-walled pulmonary vessels changes in response to alterations in the transmural pressure (intravascular pressure minus alveolar pressure). If alveolar pressure exceeds intravascular pressure as during positive-pressure ventilation of the lungs, pulmonary capillaries collapse and flow ceases. The size of larger vessels embedded in the lung parenchyma is largely dependent on lung volume. For example, resistance to flow through these vessels decreases as lung volumes increase. The largest pulmonary vessels in the hilum of the lung vary in size with changes in intrapleural pressure.

Bronchial Circulation

Bronchial arteries from the thoracic aorta supply oxygenated nutrient blood to supporting tissues of the lungs, including connective tissue and airways. After bronchial arterial blood has passed through supporting tissues, it empties into pulmonary veins and enters the left atrium rather than passing back to the right atrium. The entrance of deoxygenated blood into the left atrium dilutes oxygenated blood and accounts for an anatomic shunt that is equivalent to 1% to 2% of the cardiac output. This anatomic shunt is the reason that the cardiac output of the left ventricle exceeds that of the right ventricle by an amount equal to the bronchial blood flow.

Pulmonary Lymph Vessels

Pulmonary lymph vessels extend from all the supportive tissues of the lung to the hilum of the lung and then to the thoracic duct. Particulate matter entering the alveoli is usually removed rapidly by lymph vessels. In addition, protein is also removed from lung tissues to prevent formation of interstitial pulmonary edema.

INTRAVASCULAR PRESSURES

Pressures in the pulmonary circulation are about one fifth those present in the systemic circulation (Fig. 46-1) (Guyton, 1986). The normal pressure in the pulmonary artery is about 22/8 mmHg, with a mean pulmonary artery pressure of 13 mmHg. The mean pulmonary capillary pressure is about 10 mmHg, and the mean pressure in the pulmonary veins is about 4 mmHg, such that the pressure gradient across the pulmonary circulation is 9 mmHg.

Approximately 0.16 second prior to ventricular contraction, the atria contract, delivering blood into the ventricles. Immediately following this priming by the right atrium, the right ventricle contracts and the right ventricular pressure rises rapidly until it equals the pressure in the pulmonary artery. At this time, the pulmonary valve opens and blood flows from the right ventri-

cle into the pulmonary artery. When the right ventricular pressure begins to decline, the pulmonary valve closes and the right ventricular pressure continues to fall to a diastolic pressure near 0 mmHg.

At low pulmonary artery pressures, the resistance to blood flow is increased due to compression of vessels by extravascular structures. Once pressure in the vessels is sufficient to overcome this compression, pulmonary vessels distend and resistance to blood flow decreases to low values. Overall, the resistance to blood flow in the pulmonary circulation is about one tenth the resistance in the systemic circulation.

Pulmonary artery pressure is not influenced by left atrial pressures below 7 mmHg. When left atrial pressure exceeds about 7 mmHg, previously collapsed pulmonary veins have all been reexpanded, and pulmonary artery pressure increases in parallel with increases in left atrial pressure. In the absence of left ventricular failure, even marked increases in systemic vascular resistance do not cause the left atrial pressure to increase above this level. Consequently, the right ventricle continues to eject its stroke volume against a normal pulmonary artery pressure de-

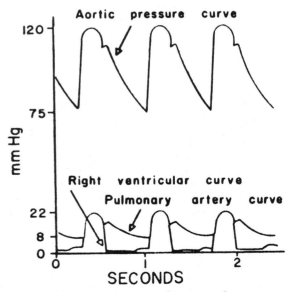

FIGURE 46-1. Comparison of intravascular pressures in the systemic and pulmonary circulations. (From Guyton AC. Textbook of Medical Physiology. 7th ed. Philadelphia: WB Saunders, 1986; with permission.)

spite this increased work load imposed on the left ventricle. This means, also, that the right ventricular stroke volume is not measurably altered by changes in systemic vascular resistance unless the left ventricle fails.

When the left ventricle fails, left atrial pressures can increase above 15 mmHg. Mean pulmonary artery pressures also increase, placing an increased work load on the right ventricle. Up to a mean pulmonary artery pressure of 30 to 40 mmHg, however, the right ventricle continues to eject its normal stroke volume with only a slight elevation in right atrial pressure. Above this pulmonary artery pressure, the right ventricle begins to fail, so that further increases in pulmonary artery pressure cause exaggerated increases in right atrial pressure with associated reductions in stroke volume.

Measurement of Left Atrial Pressure

The left atrial pressure can be estimated by inserting a balloon-tip catheter into a small pulmonary artery and inflating the balloon such that flow does not occur around the catheter. As a result, pressure equilibrates with that in the pulmonary veins. The resulting pulmonary artery occlusion pressure (wedge pressure) is usually 2 to 3 mmHg greater than left atrial pressure. In the absence of pulmonary hypertension, the pulmonary artery end-diastolic pressure correlates with the pulmonary artery occlusion pressure.

INTERSTITIAL FLUID SPACE

The interstitial fluid space in the lung is minimal, and a continual negative pulmonary interstitial pressure of about −8 mmHg dehydrates interstitial fluid spaces of the lungs and pulls alveolar epithelial membranes toward capillary membranes. As a result, the distance between gas in the alveoli and the capillary blood is minimal, averaging a distance of about 0.4 μ. Another consequence of negative pressure in pulmonary interstitial spaces is that it pulls fluid from alveoli through alveolar membranes and into interstitial fluid spaces, thus keeping the alveoli dry. Furthermore, mean pulmonary capillary pressure is about 10 mmHg, whereas plasma colloid osmotic pressure is 28 mmHg. This net pressure gradient of about 18 mmHg encourages movement of fluids into capillaries, thus reducing the likelihood of pulmonary edema.

PULMONARY BLOOD VOLUME

Blood volume in the lungs is about 450 ml. Of this amount, about 70 ml is in capillaries and the remainder is divided equally between pulmonary arteries and veins. Cardiac failure or increased resistance to flow through the mitral valve causes pulmonary blood volume to increase.

Cardiac output can increase nearly four times before pulmonary artery pressure becomes elevated (Fig. 46-2) (Guyton, 1986). This reflects the distensibility of the pulmonary arteries and opening of previously collapsed pulmonary capillaries. The ability of the lungs to accept greatly increased amounts of pulmonary blood flow, as during exercise, without excessive elevations in pulmonary artery pressures is important in preventing development of pulmonary edema or right-ventricular heart failure.

Pulmonary blood volume can increase up to 40% when an individual changes from the standing to the supine position. This sudden shift of blood from the systemic circulation to pulmonary circulation is responsible for the decrease in vital capacity in the supine position and the occurrence of orthopnea in the presence of left ventricular failure.

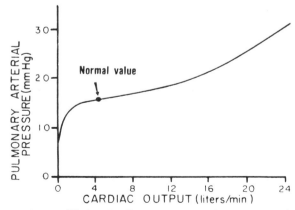

FIGURE 46-2. Cardiac output can increase nearly fourfold without greatly increasing the pulmonary arterial pressure. (From Guyton AC. Textbook of Medical Physiology. 7th ed. Philadelphia: WB Saunders, 1986; with permission.)

PULMONARY BLOOD FLOW AND DISTRIBUTION

Optimal oxygenation is dependent on matching ventilation to pulmonary blood flow. Shunt occurs in lung areas that are partially but inadequately perfused, whereas dead space applies to lung areas that are ventilated but inadequately perfused (Fig. 46-3). Although the lungs are innervated by the autonomic nervous system, it is doubtful that neural influences exert a major effect in the normal control of pulmonary blood flow. There is no doubt, however, that decreases in PaO_2 cause increases in pulmonary artery and right ventricular pressures. Clinically, segmental pulmonary blood flow can be studied by intravenous injection of radioactive xenon while monitoring is performed externally over the chest with radiation detectors. Xenon rapidly diffuses into alveoli, and in well-perfused regions of the lung, radioactivity is detected early.

Hypoxic Pulmonary Vasoconstriction

Alveolar hypoxia (PAO_2 below about 70 mmHg) evokes vasoconstriction in the pulmonary arterioles supplying these alveoli. The net effect is to divert blood flow away from poorly ventilated alveoli. As a result, the shunt effect is minimized and the resulting PaO_2 is maximized. The mechanism for hypoxic pulmonary vasoconstriction is presumed to be locally mediated, as this response occurs in isolated and denervated lungs as well as intact lungs. It is possible that local release of a vasoconstrictor substance by the periarterial mast cells in response to alveolar

hypoxia acts on alpha-adrenergic receptors, causing localized vasoconstriction.

Drug-induced inhibition of hypoxic pulmonary vasoconstriction could result in unexpected decreases in PaO_2. Indeed, potent vasodilating drugs, such as nitroprusside and nitroglycerin, may be accompanied by reductions in PaO_2 that have been attributed to inhibition of hypoxic pulmonary vasoconstriction (Colley et al, 1979). Animal models suggesting that inhaled but not injected anesthetics inhibit hypoxic pulmonary vasoconstriction have not been supported by measurements in patients (Fig. 46-4) (Rogers and Benumof, 1985; Carlsson et al, 1987). Indeed, the present consensus is that potent volatile anesthetics are acceptable choices for thoracic surgery requiring one-lung ventilation, particularly in view of the salutory effects of these drugs on bronchomotor tone and high potency that allows delivery of maximal concentrations of oxygen (Eisenkraft, 1990).

Effect of Breathing

Inspiration increases venous return to the heart due to contraction of the diaphragm and abdominal muscles, which increases the gradient from the intraabdominal portion of the inferior vena cava to its intrathoracic portion. In addition, decreases in intrapleural pressure associated with inspiration serve to distend the intrathoracic portion of the vena cava further, facilitating venous return. The resulting augmented blood flow to the right atrium increases right ventricular stroke volume. In contrast to spontaneous breathing, a mechanically delivered inspiration impedes ve-

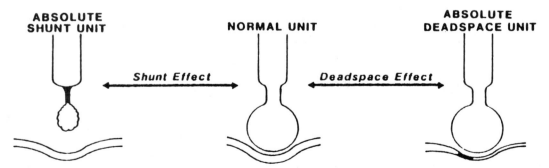

FIGURE 46–3. Gas exchange is maximally effective in normal lung units with optional ventilation to perfusion (V/Q) relationships. The continuum of V/Q relationships is depicted by the ratios between normal and absolute shunt or dead space units.

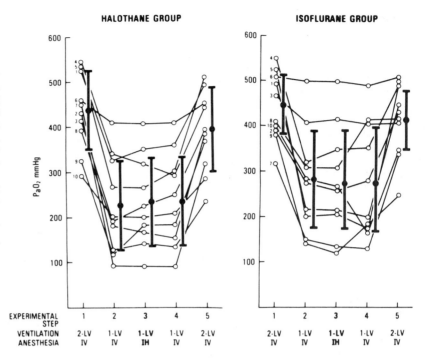

FIGURE 46–4. PaO$_2$ was measured during two-lung ventilation (*2-LV*) and then during one-lung ventilation (*1-LV*) in patients anesthetized with fentanyl and diazepam without (experimental steps 2 and 4) and with halothane or isoflurane (experimental step 3). Addition of halothane or isoflurane (about 1.2 MAC) does not alter the PaO$_2$, suggesting these drugs do not inhibit hypoxic pulmonary vasoconstriction. Clear circles are individual patient data and closed circles are mean ± SD for each group. (From Rogers SN, Benumof JL. Halothane and isoflurane do not decrease PaO$_2$ during one-lung ventilation in intravenously anesthetized patients. Anesth Analg 1985; 64: 946–54; with permission.)

nous return to the heart and reduces right ventricular stroke volume.

Hydrostatic Pressure Gradients

Blood flow to the lungs in the upright position is mainly gravity dependent. Lateral wall pressure in the pulmonary artery decreases by about 1.25 mmHg·cm^{-1} of vertical distance up the lung. The amount of blood flow to the various areas of the lung along this vertical axis depends on the relationship between pulmonary artery pressure, alveolar pressure, and pulmonary venous pressure. Traditionally, the lung is divided into three blood flow zones, reflecting the impact of alveolar pressure, pulmonary artery pressure, and pulmonary venous pressure on the caliber of pulmonary blood vessels (Fig. 46-5) (West et al, 1964). The limits of these zones are not fixed but vary with physiologic or pathologic changes.

Zone 1

Zone 1 is the upper part of the lung, where alveolar pressure exceeds pulmonary artery pressure,

leading to collapse of the pulmonary capillaries. The absence of pulmonary blood flow to this area means that ventilation to corresponding alveoli represents dead space or wasted ventilation. Normally, zone 1 is of limited extent, but when pulmonary artery pressure decreases (hypovolemia, decreased cardiac output) or alveolar pressure increases (positive-pressure ventilation of the lungs, positive end-expiratory pressure), zone 1 may extend, causing a wide discrepancy between PaCO$_2$ and PetCO$_2$. Indeed, it is not uncommon for the gradient between arterial and exhaled PCO$_2$ to increase during general anesthesia, presumably reflecting changes in perfusion pressures, effects of positive-pressure ventilation, or both.

Zone 2

Zone 2 is an intermittent pulmonary blood flow zone because pulmonary artery pressure exceeds alveolar pressure during systole but not diastole. In a standing patient, zone 2 begins 7 to 10 cm above the level of the heart and extends to the uppermost portions of the lungs. This zone is referred to as a *Starling resistor* or *waterfall zone* by analogy to a waterfall over a dam.

Zone 3

Zone 3 is termed the *distension zone* because pulmonary artery pressure always exceeds alveolar pressure and pulmonary blood flow is continuous. This zone extends from about 7 to 10 cm above the heart to the lowermost portions of the lung. In the supine position, all portions of the lung become zone 3, with pulmonary blood flow being more evenly distributed. Increases in pulmonary artery pressure, as with exercise, recruit previously underperfused capillaries, converting most of the lung to a zone 3 pattern of pulmonary blood flow.

PULMONARY EDEMA

Pulmonary edema is present when there are excessive quantities of fluid either in pulmonary interstitial spaces or in alveoli. Mild degrees of pulmonary edema may be limited to only an increase in the interstitial fluid volume. The alveolar epithelium, however, is not able to withstand more than a modest increase in interstitial fluid pressure before fluid spills into alveoli. Dehydrating forces of the colloid osmotic pressure of the blood in the lungs provide a large safety factor against development of pulmonary edema. In humans, plasma colloid osmotic pressure is about 28 mmHg, so pulmonary edema will rarely develop below a pulmonary capillary pressure of 30 mmHg. The most common cause of acute pulmonary edema is greatly elevated pulmonary capillary pressure resulting from left ventricular failure and pooling of blood in the lungs.

During chronic elevations of left atrial pressure, pulmonary edema may not occur despite pulmonary capillary pressures as high as 45 mmHg. Enlargement of the pulmonary lymph vessels allowing lymph flow to increase up to 20 times is the most likely reason pulmonary edema does not occur in the presence of chronically elevated left atrial pressures.

Pulmonary edema can also result from the local capillary damage that occurs with inhalation of acidic gastric fluid or irritant gases, such as smoke. The result is rapid transudation of fluid and proteins into alveoli and interstitial spaces.

EVENTS THAT OBSTRUCT PULMONARY BLOOD FLOW

Causes of obstruction to pulmonary blood flow most often reflect emboli represented by gases or particulate matter. Less dramatic increases in re-

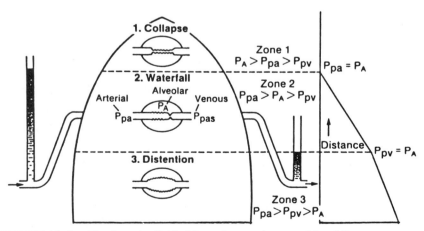

FIGURE 46–5. The lung is divided into three pulmonary blood flow zones reflecting the impact of alveolar pressure (P_A), pulmonary artery pressure (P_{pa}) and pulmonary venous pressure (P_{pv}) on the caliber of pulmonary blood vessels. (From West JB, Dollery CT, Naimark A. Distribution of blood flow in isolated lung: Relation to vascular and alveolar pressures. J Appl Physiol 1964;19:713–8; with permission.)

sistance to pulmonary blood flow occur with conditions such as pulmonary emphysema, anthracosis, and atelectasis in which there is loss of functioning lung tissues or surface area.

Pulmonary Embolism

Total blockage of one of the major branches of the pulmonary artery by an embolus is usually not immediately fatal because the opposite lung can accommodate all the pulmonary blood flow. As the blood clot extends, however, death ensues because of right ventricular failure due to excessive elevations in pulmonary artery pressure. Tachypnea and dyspnea are characteristic responses in awake patients experiencing pulmonary embolism. Tachypnea may reflect stimulation of pulmonary deflation receptors that are innervated by the vagus. Anticoagulation is recommended to prevent extension of the clot and, in occasional patients, surgical removal of the embolus may be lifesaving.

Diffuse pulmonary emboli, as occur with fat or air, produce increased pulmonary artery pressures similar to that which occur with an isolated embolus. In addition, reflex-mediated pulmonary vasospasm initiated by pulmonary emboli further increases resistance to blood flow. This vasospasm may reflect reflex sympathetic nervous system stimulation or local release of chemical mediators, such as histamine or serotonin.

Pulmonary Emphysema

Destruction of alveoli that characterizes pulmonary emphysema is accompanied by a concomitant loss of pulmonary vasculature and elevation in pulmonary artery pressures. Pulmonary hypertension is further exaggerated by arterial hypoxemia, which increases the cardiac output and thus enhances blood flow into the pulmonary circulation. Modest increases in the inhaled concentrations of oxygen may be sufficient to lower pulmonary artery pressures in these patients.

Anthracosis

Anthracosis is an example of a condition in which there is fibrosis of the supportive tissues in the lungs. Pulmonary artery pressures may remain normal at rest. Conversely, even modest activity may evoke dramatic increases in pulmonary artery pressures because vessels surrounded by fibrous tissue cannot expand with increases in pulmonary blood flow. In chronic situations, pulmonary artery pressures remain elevated and right ventricular failure eventually occurs.

Atelectasis

Atelectasis most commonly occurs when pulmonary blood flow absorbs air from unventilated alveoli, as occurs when secretions plug bronchi. Subsequent collapse of these alveoli increases resistance to pulmonary blood flow and thus diverts blood flow to better perfused alveoli. In addition, the hypoxic pulmonary vasoconstriction reflex response diverts pulmonary blood flow to better ventilated alveoli.

REFERENCES

Carlsson AJ, Bindslev L, Hedenstierna G. Hypoxia-induced pulmonary vasoconstriction in the human lung: The effect of isoflurane anesthesia. Anesthesiology 1987;66:312–6.

Colley PS, Cheney FW, Hlastala MP. Ventilation-perfusion and gas exchange effects of sodium nitroprusside in dogs with normal and edematous lungs. Anesthesiology 1979;50:489–95.

Eisenkraft JB. Effects of anaesthetics on the pulmonary circulation. Br J Anaesth 1990;65:63–78.

Guyton AC. Textbook of Medical Physiology. 7th ed. Philadelphia, WB Saunders, 1986.

Rogers SN, Benumof JL. Halothane and isoflurane do not decrease PaO_2 during one-lung ventilation in intravenously anesthetized patients. Anesth Analg 1985;64:946–54.

West JB. Blood flow to the lung and gas exchange. Anesthesiology 1974;41:124–38.

West JB, Dollery CT, Naimark A. Distribution of blood flow in isolated lung: Relation to vascular and alveolar pressures. J Appl Physiol 1964;19:713–8.

Chapter

47

Heart

CARDIAC PHYSIOLOGY

The heart can be characterized as a pulsatile four-chamber pump composed of two atria and two ventricles. The atria function primarily as conduits (primer pumps) to the ventricles, but they also contract weakly to facilitate movement of blood into the ventricles. The ventricles serve as power pumps to supply the main force that propels blood through the systemic and pulmonary circulations. *Systole* means contraction and is the time interval between closure of the tricuspid and mitral valves and closure of the pulmonary and aortic valves. *Diastole* is a period of relaxation corresponding to the interval between closure of the pulmonary and aortic valves and closure of the tricuspid and mitral valves. Special mechanisms in the heart maintain cardiac rhythm and transmit action potentials through cardiac muscle to initiate contraction.

Cardiac Muscle

Cardiac muscle is a syncytium in which the cells are so tightly bound together that when one of these cells becomes excited, the action potential spreads to all of them. As a result, stimulation of a single atrial or ventricular cell causes the action potential to travel over the entire muscle mass such that the atria or ventricles contract as a single unit. The atrial syncytium is separated from the ventricular syncytium by the fibrous tissue surrounding the valvular rings. The cardiac action potential is conducted from the atrial syncytium into the ventricular syncytium by a specialized conduction pathway known as the *atrioventricular bundle*. Cardiac muscle, like skeletal muscle, is striated and contains actin and myosin filaments. These filaments interdigitate and slide along each other during contraction in the same manner as occurs in skeletal muscle.

Cardiac Action Potential

The normal cardiac action potential results from time-dependent changes in the permeability of the cardiac muscle cell membranes to sodium (Na^+), potassium (K^+), calcium (Ca^{2+}), and chloride (Cl^-) ions during phases 0 to 4 of the action potential (Fig. 47-1; Table 47-1). The resting transmembrane potential of normal cardiac muscle cell membranes is about −90 mv and is designated phase 4. Depolarization and reversal of the transmembrane potential is designated phase 0, whereas the three phases of repolarization are labeled 1, 2, and 3. In nonpacemaker contractile atrial and ventricular cardiac cells, phase 4 is constant during diastole, and these cells remain at rest until activated by a propagated cardiac impulse or an external stimulus. In contrast, pacemaker cardiac cells exhibit spontaneous phase 4 depolarization until threshold potential is reached (about −70 mv), resulting in self-excitation and propagation of an action potential. Indeed, the principal distinguishing feature of pacemaker cells is the presence of spontaneous phase 4 depolarization in the absence of external stimulation. Compared with the transmembrane potential recorded from a ventricular myocardial cell, the resting potential of a sinoatrial node pacemaker cell is usually less (about −60 mv), the upstroke of phase 0 has a slower velocity, a

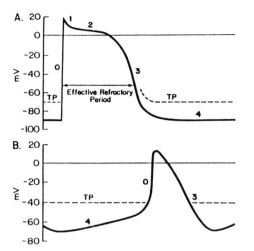

FIGURE 47–1. Cardiac action potential recorded from a ventricular contractile cell (*A*) or atrial pacemaker cell (*B*). TP, threshold potential.

plateau is absent, and repolarization (phase 3) is more gradual (Fig. 47-1).

Phase 0 of the cardiac action potential is generated by the brief but intense inward movement of Na⁺ through specific channels that are activated when spontaneous phase 4 depolarization reaches threshold potential. The rate of depolarization during phase 0 is referred to as *Vmax*. Vmax is a reflection of myocardial contractility. During phase 0, the resting transmembrane potential across cardiac cells relative to extracellular fluid changes from about −90 mv to a peak spike potential of about 20 mv (Fig. 47-1). Repolarization that follows phase 0 includes a brief phase 1 followed by a plateau lasting up to 150

msec. Phase 2 reflects closure of Na⁺ channels and inward flux of Ca²⁺ through specific slow Ca²⁺ channels. The plateau characterizing phase 2 of the cardiac action potential of ventricular contractile cells provides the sustained contraction of ventricular fibers necessary to eject blood and distinguishes cardiac action potentials from those developed by skeletal muscle cells. Phase 3 is due principally to a return to normal of cardiac cell membrane permeability to Na⁺ and a sudden increase in permeability to K⁺, allowing a rapid loss of this ion so as to restore the transmembrane potential to −90 mv.

The frequency of discharge of cardiac pacemaker cells is determined by the rate of phase 4 depolarization, the threshold potential, and the resting transmembrane potential (Fig. 47-2). When the rate of spontaneous phase 4 depolarization increases, the threshold potential is reached sooner and the heart rate increases. A similar response occurs when the rate of spontaneous phase 4 depolarization remains constant but the threshold potential becomes more negative or the resting transmembrane potential becomes less negative. Norepinephrine increases heart rate by increasing the rate of spontaneous phase 4 depolarization. Conversely, vagal stimulation through the release of acetylcholine diminishes the heart rate by hyperpolarizing cardiac pacemaker cells and reducing the slope of spontaneous phase 4 depolarization.

Cardiac muscle, like other excitable tissue, is refractory to stimulation during the action potential. The absolute refractory period extends through phases 1, 2, and part of phase 3 of the cardiac action potential. During the remainder of phase 3, the cardiac cells respond to stimuli of greater than normal intensity (relative refractory period). The absolute refractory period of atrial

Table 47–1
Ion Movement During Phases of the Cardiac Action Potential

Phase	Ion	Movement Across Cell Membrane
0	Na⁺	In
1	K⁺	Out
	Cl⁻	In
2	Ca²⁺	In
	K⁺	Out
3	K⁺	Out
4	Na⁺	In

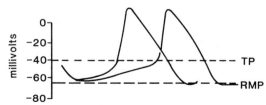

FIGURE 47–2. The rate of pacemaker discharge is dependent on the slope of spontaneous phase 4 depolarization, negativity of the threshold potential (*TP*), and negativity of the resting transmembrane potential (*RMP*).

muscle is shorter than that of ventricular muscle such that the rhythmic rate of contraction of the atria can be much faster than that of the ventricles.

Cardiac Cycle

The cardiac cycle consists of a period of relaxation (diastole) followed by a period of contraction (systole) (Fig. 47-3) (Guyton, 1986). Each cardiac cycle is initiated by the spontaneous generation of an action potential in the sinoatrial node. Delay of transmission of this action potential for 0.1 second in the atrioventricular node allows the atria to contract before the ventricles, thereby pumping blood into the ventricles prior to forceful ventricular contraction. As such, the atria act as primer pumps for the ventricles, and the ventricles then provide the major source of power for forcing blood through the systemic and pulmonary circulations. Excessive increases in heart rate may so shorten diastole that insufficient time is available for complete filling of the cardiac chambers prior to systole.

Atrial Pressure Curves

Atrial pressure curves consist of a, c, and v waves (Fig. 47-3) (Guyton, 1986). Ordinarily, right atrial pressure is 4 to 6 mmHg, and left atrial pressure is 6 to 8 mmHg during atrial contraction.

The c wave occurs when the ventricles begin to contract and is caused by bulging of the tricuspid and mitral valves backward toward the aorta because of increasing pressure in the ventricles. In addition, pulling on atrial muscle by the contracting ventricles contributes to the c wave. Atrial contraction is responsible for the a wave, explaining the absence of this wave in the presence of atrial fibrillation. The v wave occurs toward the end of ventricular contraction and is due to accumulation of blood in the atria. Retrograde flow into the atria through an incompetent tricuspid or mitral valve will manifest as a large v wave. Likewise, acute mitral regurgitation secondary to papillary muscle ischemia owing to coronary artery disease may be first recognized by the appearance of a large v wave on the recording of left atrial pressure from a pulmonary artery catheter.

Atria as Pumps

During ventricular systole, large amounts of blood accumulate in the atria because of the closed tricuspid and mitral valves. At the conclusion of ventricular systole and when ventricular pressures fall rapidly, the higher pressures in the atria force the valves open and allow blood to flow rapidly into the ventricles. This period of rapid ventricular filling lasts for the first one third of diastole and accounts for about 70% of the blood that enters the ventricles. During the latter portion of diastole, the atria contract to deliver

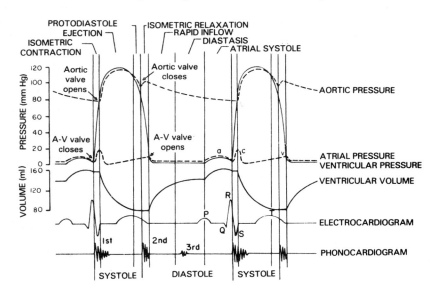

FIGURE 47–3. Events of the cardiac cycle, including changes in intravascular pressures, ventricular volume, electrocardiogram, and phonocardiogram. (From Guyton AC. Textbook of Medical Physiology. 7th ed. Philadelphia: WB Saunders, 1986; with permission.)

about 30% of the blood that normally enters the ventricle during each cardiac cycle. This component of ventricular filling is lost during atrial fibrillation and contributes to the reduction in stroke volume that accompanies this cardiac dysrhythmia.

Ventricles as Pumps

The start of ventricular systole causes an abrupt increase in intraventricular pressure, resulting in closure of the tricuspid and mitral valves (Fig. 47-3) (Guyton, 1986). An additional 0.02 to 0.03 second is required for each ventricle to develop sufficient pressure to open the pulmonary and aortic valves, which are kept closed by the back pressure of blood in the pulmonary artery and aorta. During this brief period of isovolemic contraction, there is no blood ejection from the ventricles. When intraventricular pressures are sufficient, the pulmonary and aortic valves open and about 60% of the total ventricular ejection of blood occurs during the first one fourth of systole. At the end of systole, intraventricular pressures decline rapidly, allowing higher pressures in the arteries to close the pulmonary and aortic valves.

During diastole, filling of the ventricles with blood from the atria normally increases the volume of blood in each ventricle to about 130 ml. This volume is known as the end-diastolic volume. Subsequent ventricular ejection creates a stroke volume of about 70 ml. The remaining volume in the ventricle is called the end-systolic volume. The ejection fraction (ratio of stroke volume to end-diastolic volume) is a clinically useful measurement of left ventricular function (Robotham et al, 1991). For example, ejection fraction is decreased (less than 0.4) in patients with left ventricular dysfunction as due to myocardial ischemia or myocardial infarction. Conversely, an ejection fraction greater than 0.8 may accompany intense sympathetic nervous system stimulation or the presence of hypertrophic cardiomyopathy. Angiographic techniques and echocardiography are used to measure the ejection fraction.

Function of the Heart Valves

Heart valves open passively along a pressure gradient and close when a backward pressure gradient develops owing to a high pressure in the pulmonary artery and aorta. Papillary muscles are attached to the tricuspid and mitral valves by chordae tendineae. These papillary muscles prevent the valves from bulging too far backward into the atria during ventricular systole. Rupture of a chorda tendinea or dysfunction of a papillary muscle, as may accompany myocardial ischemia or acute myocardial infarction, results in an incompetent valve and appearance of large v waves during ventricular contraction.

High pressures in the arteries at the conclusion of systole cause the pulmonary and aortic valves to snap to a closed position in contrast to the softer closure of the tricuspid and mitral valves. Because of the rapid closure and rapid velocity of blood ejection, the edges of the pulmonary and aortic valves are subjected to much greater mechanical trauma than the tricuspid and mitral valves.

Work of the Heart

The work of the heart is the amount of energy that the heart converts to work while pumping blood into the arteries. The heart accounts for 12% of total body heat production even though it represents only 0.5% of the body weight. Work required to raise the pressure for ejection of blood is calculated as stroke volume times ejection pressure. Right ventricular work output is usually about one seventh the work output of the left ventricle because of the difference in systolic pressure against which the two ventricles must pump. The energy required for the work of the heart is derived mainly from metabolism of fatty acids and, to a lesser extent, of other nutrients, especially lactate and glucose.

Intrinsic Autoregulation of Cardiac Function

The intrinsic ability of the heart to adapt to changing venous return (preload) reflects the increased stretch of cardiac muscle produced by increased filling of the ventricles from the atria and is called the *Frank-Starling law of the heart.* Indeed, the most important factor determining cardiac output is the atrial pressure created by venous return. When cardiac muscle becomes stretched, it contracts with greater force (analogous to increased stretch of a rubber band), thereby pumping additional blood into the arteries. The ability of stretched cardiac muscle to contract with increased force is characteristic of all striated muscle, not just cardiac muscle. The increased force of contraction is probably caused by the fact that actin and myosin filaments are brought to a more nearly optimal degree of interdigitation for achieving contraction. A plot of cardiac output with changes in atrial filling pressures (ventricular function curves) (see Fig. 44-12) reflects the degree of stretch applied to cardiac muscle. In the presence of ventricular dysfunction, the heart may not be able to pump all the blood it receives and filling pressures increase.

Neural Control of the Heart

The atria are abundantly innervated by the sympathetic and parasympathetic nervous system, but the ventricles are supplied principally by the sympathetic nervous system (Fig. 47-4) (Guyton,

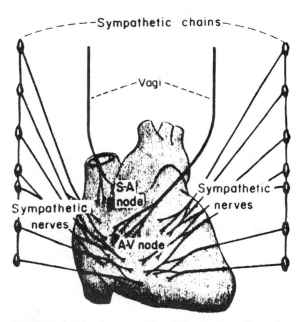

FIGURE 47–4. Innervation of the atria is from the sympathetic and parasympathetic (*vagi*) nervous systems, whereas the ventricles are supplied principally by the sympathetic nervous system. (From Guyton AC. Textbook of Medical Physiology. 7th ed. Philadelphia: WB Saunders, 1986; with permission.)

1986). These nerves affect cardiac output by changing the heart rate and strength of myocardial contraction. Sympathetic nervous system fibers to the heart continually discharge at a slow rate that maintains a strength of ventricular contraction about 20% to 25% above its strength in the absence of sympathetic stimulation. Maximal sympathetic stimulation can increase cardiac output by about 100% above normal. Conversely, maximal parasympathetic nervous system stimulation decreases ventricular contractile strength and subsequent cardiac output only about 30%, emphasizing that parasympathetic nervous system stimulation of the heart is small compared with the effect of sympathetic nervous system stimulation. Increased myocardial contractility associated with sympathetic nervous system stimulation of the heart is most likely due to norepinephrine-induced increases in the permeability of cardiac muscle cell membranes to Ca^{2+}.

CORONARY BLOOD FLOW

Unique features of coronary blood flow include interruption of blood flow during systole due to mechanical compression of vessels by myocardial contraction and absence of anastomosis between the left and right coronary arteries. Another characteristic of the coronary circulation is the maximal oxygen extraction (about 70%) that occurs, resulting in a coronary venous oxygen saturation of about 30%.

Anatomy of the Coronary Circulation

The two coronary arteries that supply the myocardium arise from the sinuses of Valsalva located behind the cusps of the aortic valve at the root of the aorta (Fig. 47-5). Resting coronary blood flow is 225 to 250 ml·min^{-1}, or 4% to 5% of the cardiac output. Assuming the normal adult heart weighs about 280 g, this is equivalent to a flow of 75 ml·100 g^{-1}·min^{-1}. Resting myocardial oxygen consumption is 8 to 10 ml·100 g^{-1}·min^{-1}, or about 10% of the total body consumption of oxygen.

The left coronary artery divides shortly after its origin into the left anterior descending and circumflex arteries, which supply the anterior part of the left ventricle. The right coronary artery supplies the right ventricle and the posterior portion of the left ventricle. In about 50% of individ-

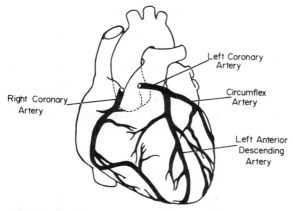

FIGURE 47–5. Anatomy of the coronary circulation.

uals, more blood flows through the right coronary artery than the left, in about 30% the flow in both arteries is similar, and in about 20% the left coronary artery is dominant. These large coronary arteries lie predominantly on the epicardial surface of the heart and serve principally as conductance vessels that offer little resistance to coronary blood flow. The second type of vessels are small coronary arterioles that ramify throughout cardiac muscle. These arterioles impose a highly variable resistance and regulate distribution of blood flow in the myocardium. Atherosclerosis characterized as coronary artery disease involves the epicardial coronary arteries and not the coronary arterioles.

Coronary blood flow, especially to the left ventricle, occurs predominantly during diastole when cardiac muscle relaxes and no longer obstructs blood flow through ventricular capillaries (Fig. 47-6) (Berne and Levy, 1987). It is estimated that at least 75% of total coronary blood flow occurs during diastole. During systole, blood flow through subendocardial arteries of the left ventricle falls almost to zero and is consistent with the observation that the subendocardial region of the left ventricle is the most common site for myocardial infarction. Tachycardia, with an associated decrease in the time for coronary blood flow to occur during diastole, further jeopardizes the adequacy of myocardial oxygen delivery, particularly if coronary arteries are narrowed by atherosclerosis. The impact of systole on coronary blood flow through the right ventricle is minimal. This reflects the fact that pressure in the coronary arteries is greater than the pressure developed in the right ventricle.

Most of the venous blood that has perfused the left ventricle enters the right atrium via the coronary sinus. This accounts for about 75% of the total coronary blood flow. Most of the coronary blood flow to the right ventricle enters anterior cardiac veins that empty into the right atrium independently of the coronary sinus. A small amount of coronary blood flows back into the heart through Thebesian veins that can empty into any cardiac chamber. Thebesian veins that empty into the left side of the heart contribute to the inherent anatomic shunt.

Determinants of Coronary Blood Flow

A striking feature of coronary blood flow is the parallelism between the local metabolic needs of

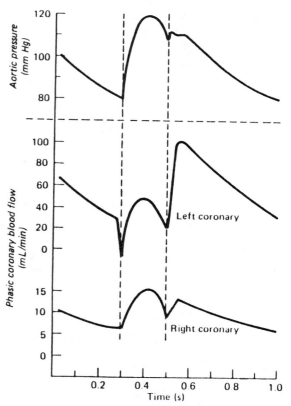

FIGURE 47–6. Phasic left and right coronary artery blood flow in relation to aortic pressure. (From Berne RM, Levy MD. Review of Medical Physiology. 13th ed. Norwalk, CT: Appleton and Lange, 1987; with permission.)

cardiac muscle for nutrients, especially oxygen, and the magnitude of coronary blood flow. This parallelism is present in the denervated heart and presumably reflects the local release of vasodilator substances that dilate coronary arterioles and thus increase oxygen delivery through increased coronary blood flow. The most potent local vasodilator substance released by cardiac cells is adenosine. Increased extraction of oxygen is not likely to offset local increases in oxygen needs because, even in the normal resting state, oxygen extraction by cardiac cells is nearly maximal. Therefore, little additional oxygen can be made available in the absence of increased coronary blood flow.

Arterial blood pressure acts as the perfusion pressure to drive blood through coronary arteries. For example, an increase in perfusion pressure will increase coronary blood flow. This increased flow, however, is transient, as autoregulation of coronary artery tone acts to return blood flow toward normal. Perfusion pressure is particularly important in maintaining coronary blood flow through atherosclerotic arteries that cannot dilate in response to autoregulatory mechanisms (pressure-dependent perfusion).

Myocardial Oxygen Consumption

Sympathetic nervous system stimulation with associated increases in heart rate, blood pressure, and myocardial contractility results in increased myocardial oxygen consumption. Elevations in heart rate that shorten diastolic time for coronary blood flow are likely to increase myocardial oxygen consumption more than elevations in blood pressure, which are likely to offset increased oxygen demands by enhanced pressure-dependent coronary blood flow. This is the reason that the absolute value of the rate-pressure product (product of heart rate and systolic blood pressure) is less important as an estimation of myocardial oxygen consumption than the absolute value of the individual components used to calculate the product. Furthermore, the validity of maintaining the rate-pressure product below a certain value (usually 12,000) has not been documented to be efficacious in anesthetized patients.

Increasing venous return (volume work) is the least costly means of increasing cardiac output in terms of myocardial oxygen consumption. This emphasizes that the most important aspect of hemodynamic management is to first optimize venous return by appropriate adjustments in the intravascular fluid volume. Usually, increases in myocardial oxygen consumption are paralleled by increases in coronary blood flow, resulting in a remarkably constant coronary sinus oxygen saturation of about 30% (PO_2 18 to 20 mmHg). When myocardial oxygenation is jeopardized, the heart produces lactate, with increases in coronary sinus lactate concentration being considered a conclusive indicator of global myocardial ischemia.

Nervous System Innervation

Coronary arteries contain alpha-, beta-, and histamine receptors. In general, epicardial coronary arteries have a preponderance of vasoconstricting alpha-receptors, whereas intramuscular arteries have a preponderance of vasodilating beta-receptors. Indeed, beta-antagonists are likely to increase coronary vascular resistance, but reductions in myocardial oxygen requirements occur because of drug-induced decreases in heart rate and myocardial contractility. H-1 receptors mediate coronary artery vasoconstriction, whereas H-2 receptors are responsible for coronary artery vasodilation. It is conceivable that H-2 antagonists administered preoperatively could allow H-1 vasoconstrictor effects to become predominant in the coronary arteries in the same manner as described for changes in bronchomotor tone. In some individuals, alpha-vasoconstrictor effects seem to be excessive, resulting in vasospastic myocardial ischemia (Prinzmetal's angina). Venous smooth muscle contains alpha-receptors, emphasizing the potential for venoconstriction following coronary artery bypass operations using venous grafts. This venoconstriction is readily offset by nitroglycerin. The distribution of parasympathetic nervous system fibers to the coronary arteries in the ventricles is sparse, and any direct effect on coronary blood flow as a result of vagal-induced vasodilation is likely to be modest.

Coronary Artery Steal

Coronary artery steal is an absolute decrease in collateral-dependent myocardial perfusion at the expense of an increase in blood flow to a normally perfused area of myocardium, as may follow drug-induced vasodilation of coronary arterioles (Fig. 47-7) (Becker, 1978; Cason et al, 1987). Conceptually, abnormal coronary arterioles

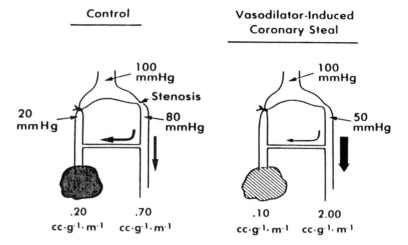

FIGURE 47-7. Schematic depiction of vasodilator-induced coronary steal. Following distal coronary artery vasodilation, flow increases to the normally perfused area and there is a significant pressure drop across the stenosis that reduces the pressure gradient across the collateral bed. (From Cason BA, Verrier ED, London MJ, Mangano DT, Hickey RF. Effects of isoflurane and halothane on coronary vascular resistance and collateral myocardial blood flow: Their capacity to induce coronary steal. Anesthesiology 1987; 67:665–75; with permission.)

might be fully dilated to compensate for the increased resistance imposed by narrowed atherosclerotic vessels. Drug-induced vasodilation of normal coronary arterioles might then divert (steal) blood flow from potentially ischemia areas of myocardium being perfused by atherosclerotic vessels. There is evidence that drugs that produce arteriolar vasodilation (nitroprusside, isoflurane) can redistribute coronary blood flow under certain conditions, leading to myocardial ischemia in patients with coronary artery disease (see Chapter 2) (Priebe, 1989). Coronary artery steal is most likely to occur in those patients with steal-prone anatomy. Steal-prone anatomy is characterized by one or more total occlusions of a coronary artery and a concomitant, hemodynamically significant stenosis (greater than 90%) of the collateral supplying vessel. An estimated 23% of patients with coronary artery disease have a zone of collateral-dependent myocardium that is supplied by a vessel with a proximal stenosis (steal-prone anatomy) (Fig. 47-8) (Buffington et al, 1988).

DYNAMICS OF HEART SOUNDS

Closure of the heart valves creates sudden pressure differentials such that blood vibrates, creating a sound that travels in all directions through the chest. In contrast, opening of heart valves is a relatively slowly-developing process that makes no audible sound.

First and Second Heart Sounds

Closure of the mitral and tricuspid valves produces the first heart sound, whereas the second heart sound is due to closure of the aortic and pulmonary valves (Fig. 47-3) (Guyton, 1986). An audible sound is produced by vibration of the taut valves immediately after closure as well as vibration of the adjacent blood, walls of the heart, and major vessels around the heart. These vibra-

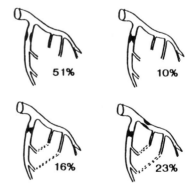

FIGURE 47-8. Anatomic variants of coronary artery disease and incidence on coronary angiograms. Steal-prone anatomy is present in 23% (*lower right*) because arteriolar dilation decreases pressure distal to the stenosis and reduces flow through the high-resistance collaterals. (Buffington CW, Davis KB, Gillispie S, Pettinger M. The prevalence of steal-prone coronary anatomy in patients with coronary artery disease: An analysis of the coronary artery surgery registry. Anesthesiology 1988; 69:721–7; with permission.)

tions then travel to the chest wall, where they can be heard as sound by a stethoscope (Fig. 47-9) (Guyton, 1986). The optimal areas for auscultation of heart sounds on the chest are not directly over the specific valve, emphasizing that sounds caused by closure of the mitral and tricuspid valves are transmitted to the chest wall through each respective ventricle and sounds from the aortic and pulmonary valves are transmitted along the courses of the respective vessels leading from the heart.

The loudness of the first heart sound is almost directly proportional to the rate of development of pressure differences across the mitral and tricuspid valves. For example, when the force of ventricular contraction is enhanced, the first heart sound is accentuated. Conversely, in a weakened heart in which the onset of contraction is sluggish, the intensity of the first heart sound is diminished. The loudness of the second heart sound is determined by the rate of ventricular pressure decrease at the end of systole. For this reason, the intensity of the second heart sound is accentuated in the presence of systemic or pulmonary hypertension. Conversely, when blood pressure is low, as in shock or cardiac failure, the second heart sound as heard through a stethoscope is diminished in intensity.

Third Heart Sound

Occasionally, a third heart sound is heard at the beginning of the middle third of diastole. This sound is of such low frequency that it usually cannot be detected with a stethoscope but can be recorded on the phonocardiogram (Fig. 47-3) (Guyton, 1986). This third heart sound is presumed to reflect the flaccid and inelastic condition of the heart during diastole.

Fourth Heart Sound

The fourth heart sound is caused by rapid inflow of blood into the ventricles due to atrial contraction. The frequency of this heart sound is so low that it rarely can be heard using a stethoscope.

Abnormal Heart Sounds

Abnormal heart sounds known as murmurs occur in the presence of abnormalities of the cardiac valves or congenital anomalies (Table 47-2).

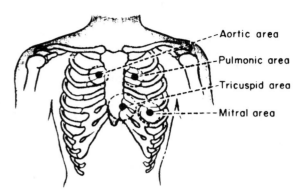

FIGURE 47–9.   Optimal sites for auscultation of heart sounds due to opening or closure of specific cardiac valves. (From Guyton AC. Textbook of Medical Physiology. 7th ed. Philadelphia: WB Saunders, 1986; with permission.)

Murmur of Aortic Stenosis

Resistance to ejection of blood through a stenotic aortic valve causes pressure in the left ventricle to increase to values as great as 350 mmHg while pressure in the aorta remains normal. Thus, a nozzle effect is created during systole, with blood jetting at a high velocity through the small opening of the aortic valve. This turbulent flow causes vibrations, and a systolic murmur is transmitted throughout the upper aorta and even into the carotid arteries.

Murmur of Aortic Regurgitation

Turbulence created by blood jetting backward into blood already in the left ventricle produces

Table 47–2
Heart Murmurs

	Timing of Murmur*
Aortic stenosis	Systole
Aortic regurgitation	Diastole
Mitral stenosis	Diastole
Mitral regurgitation	Systole
Patent ductus arteriosus	Continuous
Atrial septal defect	Systole
Ventricular septic defect	Systole

*Pulmonary and tricuspid stenosis or regurgitation produce murmurs during the cardiac cycle corresponding to the similar aortic or mitral valve abnormality.

the diastolic murmur characteristic of aortic regurgitation. This murmur is not as loud as that of aortic stenosis because the pressure differential between the aorta and left ventricle is not nearly as great as it is in aortic stenosis.

Murmur of Mitral Stenosis

In the presence of mitral stenosis, a low-intensity murmur occurs in diastole. The abnormal sounds present in mitral stenosis are of low intensity because, except for brief periods, the pressure differential forcing blood from the left atrium into the left ventricle rarely exceeds 35 mmHg.

Murmur of Mitral Regurgitation

Backward flow of blood through an incompetent mitral valve during left ventricular contraction produces a loud, swishing systolic murmur. The left atrium is located so deeply in the chest that it is difficult to hear the murmur directly over the atrium. As a result, the sound of mitral regurgitation is transmitted to the chest wall mainly through the left ventricle and typically is heard best at the apex of the heart. Presumably, the murmur of mitral regurgitation is caused by vibrations from the turbulence of blood ejected backward through the mitral valve against the atrial wall or into blood already in the atrium. The quality of the murmur of mitral regurgitation is similar to that of aortic regurgitation, but it occurs during systole rather than diastole.

Murmur of Patent Ductus Arteriosus

In the presence of a patent ductus arteriosus, blood flows backward from the aorta into the pulmonary artery, producing a continuous (machinery) murmur. This murmur is most audible in the pulmonic area, being more intense during systole when pressure in the aorta is elevated and less intense during the low-pressure phase of diastole. This accounts for a murmur that waxes and wanes with each heart beat. At birth, the amount of reversed blood flow may be inadequate to cause a murmur.

Murmur of Atrial Septal Defect

Increased flow through the pulmonary valve in the presence of an atrial septal defect produces a characteristic pulmonary systolic ejection murmur. The pulmonary valve closes late, causing a wide splitting of the second heart sound.

Murmur of Ventricular Septal Defect

A ventricular septal defect is characterized by blood flow from the systemic to pulmonary circulation resulting in a systolic murmur in contrast to the continuous murmur of patent ductus arteriosus.

CONDUCTION OF CARDIAC IMPULSES

Cardiac impulses are transmitted over a specialized conduction system in the heart, with normal impulses being spontaneously generated at the sinoatrial node so as to maintain resting heart rate at about 70 beats·min^{-1} (Fig. 47-10). The self-excitatory impulse travels from the sinoatrial node to the atrioventricular node, where it is delayed before passing into the ventricles. In the ventricles, the cardiac impulse travels via the atrioventricular bundle (bundle of His), which divides initially into the left and right bundle branches.

Bundle branches then divide into a complex network of conducting fibers known as *Purkinje fibers,* which ramify over the subendocardial surfaces of both ventricles.

Sinoatrial Node

The sinoatrial node is a specialized cardiac muscle (15 mm long, 5 mm wide, and 2 mm thick) located on the posterior surface of the heart at the site where the superior vena cava joins the right atrium. The fibers of the sinoatrial node are continuous with atrial fibers such that an action potential that begins in the sinoatrial node spreads immediately into the atria. Sinoatrial fibers exhibit a resting transmembrane potential of only about −60 mv in comparison with −90 mv in most other cardiac fibers (Fig. 47-1). This lower resting transmembrane potential is caused by increased leakiness of the membranes of sinoatrial fibers to Na$^+$ and is responsible for the self-excitation and rhythmic repetitiveness of the action potentials from the sinoatrial node. Immediately after the action potential is over, the sinoatrial transmembrane potential reaches its greatest degree of negativity (hyperpolariza-

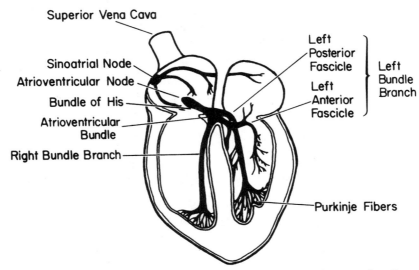

FIGURE 47–10. Anatomy of the conduction system for conduction of cardiac impulses.

tion), reflecting diffusion of K^+ (positive charges) from the interior of the cells. As the sinoatrial membrane becomes less permeable to K^+ and the natural leakiness of the membrane of Na^+ returns, the transmembrane potential slowly drifts back toward a less negative value (spontaneous phase 4 depolarization) until it reaches the threshold potential for self-excitation of the fiber.

Internodal Pathways

Action potentials originating in the sinoatrial node spread through the entire atrial muscle mass on their way to the atrioventricular node. There are, however, internodal pathways that conduct cardiac impulses from the sinoatrial to atrioventricular node more rapidly than in the general mass of atrial muscle.

Atrioventricular Node

The atrioventricular node is a specialized cardiac muscle (20 mm long, 10 mm wide, and 3 mm thick) located on the right side of the interatrial septum near the opening of the coronary sinus. There is a delay of transmission of cardiac im-

pulses in the atrioventricular node which allows the atria to empty blood into the ventricles before ventricular systole is initiated. Cardiac impulses originating in the sinoatrial node typically reach the atrioventricular node in about 0.04 second. Between this time and the time each impulse emerges from the atrioventricular node, another 0.11 second elapses. Slow conduction of cardiac impulses through the atrioventricular node is related to the small size of the conducting fibers and the presence of fewer points of tight fusion between cardiac muscle cells in this node.

Purkinje Fibers

Purkinje fibers originating in the atrioventricular node form the atrioventricular bundle (bundle of His), which passes subendocardially between the valves of the heart into ventricular muscle. This bundle divides almost immediately into left and right bundle branches, with the left bundle dividing into the left anterior and left posterior fascicle. These branches descend toward the apex of each ventricle, dividing into smaller branches that spread around each ventricle. Purkinje fibers that pass from the atrioventricular node through the atrioventricular bundle and into the ventricles are large fibers that transmit cardiac impulses so rapidly that both ventricles contract at almost exactly the same time. Any delay in transmission of cardiac impulses through the ventricle can make it possible for impulses from the last excited ventricular muscle fiber to reenter the first muscle fiber and produce ventricular fibrillation. Ordinarily, rapid transmission of cardiac impulses means the first stimulated fibers are still refractory at the time the last fibers are stimulated.

Cardiac Pacemakers

A cardiac pacemaker cell is one that undergoes spontaneous phase 4 depolarization to reach threshold potential and thus undergoes self-excitation. The role of the sinoatrial node as the normal cardiac pacemaker reflects the higher intrinsic discharge rate of this node relative to other potential cardiac pacemakers. For example, atrioventricular nodal fibers discharge at an intrinsic rate of 40 to 60 beats·min^{-1}, and Purkinje fibers discharge at a rate of 15 to 40 beats·min^{-1} compared with an intrinsic sinoatrial node rate of 70 to 80 beats·min^{-1}. A cardiac pacemaker other than the sinoatrial node is called an *ectopic pacemaker.*

Stimulation of the parasympathetic nervous system results in the release of acetylcholine, which depresses the intrinsic discharge rate of the sinoatrial node and slows the transmission rate of cardiac impulses through atrial internodal pathways to the atrioventricular node. Acetylcholine also depresses the activity of the atrioventricular node. The mechanism of these effects is the ability of acetylcholine to hyperpolarize cell membranes, rendering excitable tissue less excitable. Intense stimulation of the parasympathetic nervous system can totally suppress cardiac pacemaker activity, making the patient dependent on a ventricular escape pacemaker to survive.

Stimulation of the sympathetic nervous system results in the release of norepinephrine, which speeds the rate of spontaneous phase 4 depolarization and thus increases the intrinsic rate of discharge of the sinoatrial node. It is likely that norepinephrine results in increased permeability of cardiac muscle cell membranes to Na$^+$ and Ca^{2+}. A similar increase in permeability to Na$^+$ in the atrioventricular node decreases conduction time for cardiac impulses to travel to the ventricles.

CIRCULATORY EFFECTS OF HEART DISEASE

Valvular heart disease produces circulatory effects related to volume overload (regurgitant lesions) or pressure overload (stenotic lesions) of the atria or ventricles. Exercise tolerance is a valuable clinical indicator of both the presence and severity of valvular heart disease. During exercise, large quantities of venous blood are returned to the heart from the peripheral circulation, resulting in exacerbation of all the circulatory abnormalities associated with valvular heart disease.

Congenital heart disease produces circulatory effects predominantly due to the presence of a left-to-right or right-to-left intracardiac shunt. Pulmonary blood flow is greatly increased in the presence of a left-to-right intracardiac shunt, necessitating an increased cardiac output that often leads to cardiac failure. Right-to-left intracardiac shunts are characterized by decreased pulmonary blood flow, direct return of venous blood to the systemic circulation, and chronic arterial hypoxemia. Congenital heart defects are often associated with other congenital defects elsewhere in the body.

Aortic Valve Disease

Aortic stenosis or aortic regurgitation results in a decrease in forward left ventricular stroke volume. Compensatory responses to offset this decreased cardiac output include left ventricular hypertrophy (four to five times normal size) and an increased circulating blood volume that facilitates venous return. Myocardial ischemia is often present, reflecting impaired coronary blood flow owing to high intraventricular pressures (aortic stenosis) or low diastolic pressures (aortic regurgitation). Another cause of myocardial ischemia is failure of collateral coronary vessels to develop to the same degree as ventricular hypertrophy. Many patients with aortic valve disease are asymptomatic, emphasizing the importance of seeking the presence of cardiac murmurs during the preoperative physical examination.

Mitral Valve Disease

Mitral stenosis or mitral regurgitation results in accumulation of blood in the left atrium and accompanying increases in left atrial pressure. Pulmonary edema is likely when left atrial pressure exceeds 30 mmHg, although pulmonary lymphatics may efficiently remove excess fluid at even greater pressures. Elevated left atrial pressure predisposes to atrial fibrillation because the associated enlargement of the left atrium increases the distance cardiac impulses must travel, thus increasing the likelihood of reentry. There is intense constriction of pulmonary arterioles with resulting pulmonary hypertension and right ventricular hypertrophy.

Patent Ductus Arteriosus

The ductus arteriosus remains patent in about 1 of every 5500 neonates, resulting in backward flow of blood from the aorta into the pulmonary artery. As the child grows, the pulmonary blood flow may become two to three times systemic blood flow. Because cardiac output is elevated at rest, these patients exhibit reduced exercise tolerance. Increased pulmonary blood flow results in elevated pulmonary artery pressures and right ventricular hypertrophy. Cyanosis does not occur unless cardiac failure develops.

Atrial Septal Defect

Increased pulmonary blood flow owing to an atrial septal defect via a potent foramen ovale or a defect in the atrial septum eventually results in pulmonary hypertension, right ventricular hypertrophy, and right ventricular failure. In about one third of patients, the flaplike opening covering the foramen ovale does not adhere to the atrial septum such that events that selectively increase right atrial pressure over left atrial pressure (positive-pressure ventilation of the lungs with or without positive end-expiratory pressure) can produce an unexpected right-to-left intracardiac shunt and arterial hypoxemia (Moorthy and LoSasso, 1974).

Ventricular Septal Defect

A ventricular septal defect produces a left-to-right intracardiac shunt, reflecting the fact that pressure in the left ventricle is about six times that in the right ventricle. Blood flow through the intracardiac shunt elevates right ventricular pressure and pulmonary blood flow, leading to right ventricular hypertrophy and, ultimately, pulmonary hypertension. The presence of oxygenated blood in the right ventricle is consistent with the presence of this congenital defect.

Tetralogy of Fallot

Tetralogy of Fallot is the classic cause of right-to-left intracardiac shunt. Abnormalities associated with tetralogy of Fallot include an aorta that overrides the interventricular septum, pulmonary artery narrowing, a ventricular septal defect, and right ventricular hypertrophy. The major physiologic derangement caused by tetralogy of Fallot is shunting of as much as 75% of returning venous blood through the ventricular septal defect directly to the aorta, resulting in poor pulmonary blood flow and profound arterial hypoxemia, even at birth.

MYOCARDIAL INFARCTION

Humans with coronary artery disease have few collateral communications between the larger epicardial coronary arteries. Consequently, acute occlusion of an epicardial coronary artery leads rapidly to transmural infarction. Within 1 hour after an acute myocardial infarction, the muscle fibers in the center of the ischemic area die. During the next few days, collateral channels growing into the outer rim of the infarcted area cause the nonfunctional area of cardiac muscle to become smaller. Maximal collateral conductance following an infarct may be present within 1 month. Fibrous tissue develops among the infarcted fibers, and the resulting scarring contracts the size of the infarcted area and usually prevents any aneurysmal effect. Technetium-99m pyrophosphate is taken up selectively by areas of recent myocardial necrosis, providing a so-called "hot spot." The ability of the heart to increase its cardiac output following recovery from a myocardial infarction is commonly less than in a normal, undamaged heart.

The magnitude of cardiac cell death is determined by the product of the degree of ischemia and metabolism of the heart muscle. This emphasizes the need to avoid sympathetic nervous system stimulation following an acute myocardial infarction. The four major causes of mortality following a myocardial infarction are (1) decreased cardiac output; (2) pulmonary edema; (3) ventricular fibrillation; and, rarely, (4) rupture of the heart.

Decreased Cardiac Output

Decreased cardiac output occurs immediately after a myocardial infarction, reflecting the impaired contractility associated with ischemic or infarcted fibers. Cardiogenic shock is likely when more than 40% of the left ventricular muscle is infarcted. In some instances, when normal portions of the ventricle contract, the damaged muscle is forced outward (aneurysmal) by the intracavitary pressure (Fig. 47-11) (Guyton, 1986). As a result, much of the pumping force is dissipated into the area of the ventricular aneurysm.

Pulmonary Edema

Decreased cardiac output leads to pooling of blood in pulmonary capillaries with associated increases in capillary pressure. Furthermore, decreased cardiac output causes reduced renal blood flow with subsequent retention of fluid. Often, pulmonary edema develops suddenly several days following myocardial infarction in patients who previously had been recovering without complications.

Ventricular Fibrillation

Ventricular fibrillation is a common cause of sudden death related to acute myocardial infarction, especially in the first few minutes following the infarction. This potentially fatal cardiac dysrhythmia may reflect increased irritability owing to depletion of K[+] from damaged cardiac muscle or altered pathways for conduction of cardiac impulses necessitated by infarcted tissue.

Rupture of the Infarcted Area

Rupture of an area of acute myocardial infarction is unlikely in the first day. Several days later, however, the infarcted cardiac muscle may be degenerate and increase the likelihood of cardiac

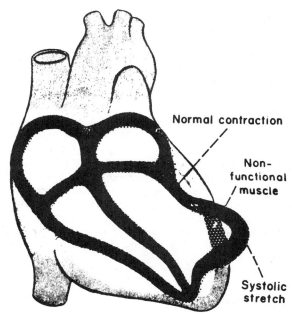

FIGURE 47–11. Aneurysmal dilatation of ischemic left ventricular muscle may follow a myocardial infarction, leading to reductions in cardiac output. (From Guyton AC. Textbook of Medical Physiology. 7th ed. Philadelphia: WB Saunders, 1986; with permission.)

rupture with subsequent acute cardiac tamponade.

ANGINA PECTORIS

Angina pectoris occurs when myocardial oxygen requirements exceed delivery, as may occur during exercise or an event associated with stimulation of the sympathetic nervous system. Distribution of pain into the arms and neck reflects the embryonic origin of the heart and arm in the neck such that both these structures receive pain fibers from the same spinal cord segments (T2 to T5). Stimulation of nerve endings in cardiac muscle by release of lactic acid, histamine, or kinins from ischemic muscle is the most likely cause of angina pectoris.

CARDIAC FAILURE

Cardiac failure manifests as decreased cardiac output or pulmonary edema, with selective left ventricular failure occurring 30 times more often than selective right ventricular failure. The weakened ventricle is unable to pump the blood delivered to it such that venous pressure is elevated and ventricular end-diastolic pressure rises. Dyspnea reflects increased left atrial pressure and accumulation of fluid in the lungs, whereas selective elevations in right atrial pressure manifest as hepatomegaly, ascites, and peripheral edema. Chronic reductions in cardiac output result in renal-induced retention of fluid in an effort to improve venous return to the heart. Any increased stress, such as exercise, sepsis, or trauma, may unmask reduced cardiac reserve in patients vulnerable to cardiac failure. Inhaled anesthetics produce exaggerated reductions in myocardial contractility when administered in the presence of cardiac failure (Kemmotsu et al, 1973).

REFERENCES

Becker L. Conditions for vasodilator-induced coronary steal in experimental myocardial ischemia. Circulation 1978;57:1103–10.

Berne RM, Levy MD. Review of Medical Physiology. 13th ed. Norwalk, CT, Appleton and Lange, 1987.

Buffington CW, Davis KB, Gillispie S, Pettinger M. The prevalence of steal-prone coronary anatomy in patients with coronary artery disease: An analysis of the coronary artery surgery registry. Anesthesiology 1988;69:721–7.

Cason BA, Verrier ED, London MJ, Mangano DT, Hickey RF. Effects of isoflurane and halothane on coronary vascular resistance and collateral myocardial blood flow: Their capacity to induce coronary steal. Anesthesiology 1987;67:665–75.

Guyton AC. Textbook of Medical Physiology. 7th ed. Philadelphia, WB Saunders, 1986.

Kemmotsu O, Hashimoto Y, Shimosati S. Inotropic effects of isoflurane on mechanics of contraction in isolated cat papillary muscles from normal and failing hearts. Anesthesiology 1973;39:470–7.

Moorthy SS, LoSasso AM. Patency of the foramen ovale in the critically ill patient. Anesthesiology 1974; 41:405–7.

Priebe H-J. Isoflurane and coronary hemodynamics. Anesthesiology 1989;71:960–76.

Robotham JL, Takata M, Berman M, Harasawa Y. Ejection fraction revisited. Anesthesiology 1991:74:172–83.

Chapter

48

The Electrocardiogram and Analysis of Cardiac Dysrhythmias

ELECTROCARDIOGRAM

Body fluids are good conductors, making it possible to record the sum of the action potentials of myocardial fibers on the surface of the body as the electrocardiogram (ECG). The normal ECG consists of a P-wave (atrial depolarization), a QRS complex (ventricular depolarization), and a T-wave (ventricular repolarization) (Fig. 48-1). Ventricular repolarization is prolonged, explaining the low voltage of the T-wave compared with the QRS complex. The atrial T-wave, which reflects repolarization of the atria, is obscured on the ECG by the larger QRS complex. A U-wave, if present, may reflect slow repolarization of the papillary muscles.

Recording the Electrocardiogram

Paper used for recording the ECG is designed such that each horizontal line corresponds to 0.1 mv and each vertical line corresponds to 0.04 second, assuming proper calibration and paper speed of the recording device (Fig. 48-1). Electric currents generated by cardiac muscle during each cardiac cycle can change potentials and polarity in less than 0.01 second. An oscilloscope display of the ECG, with or without the ability to provide a paper recording, is commonly used for clinical monitoring. Indeed, continuous monitoring of the ECG during anesthesia is considered to be a standard of monitoring for all patients under the anesthesiologist's care.

The duration of events during conduction of the cardiac impulse can be calculated from a recording of the ECG (Table 48-1). The interval between the beginning of atrial contraction and the beginning of ventricular contraction is the P-R interval (actually the P-Q interval, but the Q-wave is frequently absent). The P-R interval is dependent on heart rate averaging 0.18 second at a rate of 70 beats·min^{-1} and 0.14 second at a rate of 130 beats·min^{-1}. The QRS complex reflects ventricular depolarization, whereas the Q-T interval represents the time necessary for complete depolarization and repolarization of the ventricle. Like the P-R interval, the Q-T interval depends on heart rate. Using a small portable tape recorder (Holter monitor), it is possible to record the ECG for prolonged periods in ambulatory individuals.

Electrocardiogram Leads

The ECG is recorded using a unipolar lead (an exploring electrode connected to an indifferent electrode at zero potential) or bipolar leads (two active electrodes). Depolarization moving toward an active electrode produces a positive deflection, while depolarization moving in the

Table 48–1
Intervals and Corresponding Events on the Electrocardiogram

	Average	*Range*	*Event in Heart*
P-R interval*	0.18 sec	0.12–0.20 sec	Atrial depolarization and conduction through the atrioventricular node
QRS duration	0.08 sec	0.05–0.1 sec	Ventricular depolarization
Q-T interval*	0.40 sec	0.26–0.45 sec	Ventricular depolarization plus repolarization
S-T segment	0.32 sec		Ventricular repolarization

*Dependent on heart rate.

opposite direction produces a negative deflection. Electric current flow is normally from the base of the heart toward the apex during most of the depolarization phase with the exception being at the extreme end of the wave. Therefore, an electrode nearer the base of the heart will record a negative potential with respect to an electrode placed nearer the apex of the heart. The usual 12-lead ECG consists of three bipolar standard limb leads, six unipolar chest leads, and three unipolar augmented limb leads.

Standard Limb Leads

Standard limb leads are placed on the left and right arms and the left leg (Fig. 48-2). These leads record the potential difference between two points on the body. Polarity is positive for the ECG recorded from these standard limb leads. The legs of the three standard limb leads form the arms of an equilateral (Einthoven's) triangle. The direction of depolarization of the atria parallels lead II. For this reason, P-waves are prominent in this lead.

Chest Leads

Precordial unipolar leads (V_1 through V_6) are recorded by placing an electrode on the anterior surface of the chest over one of six separate points (Table 48-2). Each chest lead records

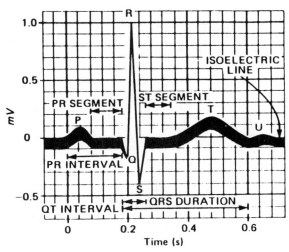

FIGURE 48–1. The normal waves and intervals on the electrocardiogram.

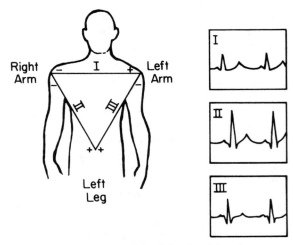

FIGURE 48–2. Standard limb leads of the electrocardiogram and typical recordings.

Table 48-2
Placement of Precordial Leads

V_1	Fourth intercostal space at the right sternal border
V_2	Fourth intercostal space at the left sternal border
V_3	Equidistant between V_2 and V_4
V_4	Fifth intercostal space in the left midclavicular line
V_5	Fifth intercostal space in the left anterior axillary line
V_6	Fifth intercostal space in the left midaxillary line

mainly the electrical potential of the cardiac muscle immediately beneath the electrode. The nearness of the heart surface to the electrode means that relatively minute abnormalities in the ventricles, particularly in the anterior ventricular wall, can produce marked changes in the corresponding ECG. In leads V_1 and V_2, the normal QRS recordings are mainly negative because the chest electrode in these leads is nearer the base of the heart than the apex. Conversely, the QRS complexes in V_4 through V_6 are mainly positive because the chest electrode in these leads is nearer the apex of the heart, which is the direction of electropositivity during depolarization.

Augmented Limb Leads

Augmented unipolar limb leads are similar to the standard limb lead recordings except that the recording from the right-arm lead (aVR) is inverted. When the positive terminal is on the right arm, the lead is aVR; when on the left arm, the lead is aVL; and when on the left leg, the lead is a aVF.

Interpretation of the Electrocardiogram

Abnormalities of the heart can be detected by analyzing the contours of the different waves in the various ECG leads. The electrical axis of the heart can be determined from the standard limb leads of Einthoven's triangle. In a normal heart, the average direction of the vector during spread of the depolarization wave is approximately 59 degrees (Fig. 48-3). When one ventricle of the heart hypertrophies, the axis of the heart shifts toward the enlarged ventricle. The predominant direction of the vector through the heart during depolarization and repolarization of the ventricles is from base to apex. As a result, the T-waves and most of the QRS complexes in the normal ECG

are positive. The vector of current flow during depolarization in the atria is similar to that in the ventricles. As a result, the P-waves recorded from the three standard limb leads are positive.

Abnormalities of the QRS Complex

The QRS complex is considered to be prolonged when it lasts more than 0.1 second. Hypertrophy of the ventricles prolongs the duration of the QRS complex, reflecting the longer pathway the ventricular depolarization wave must travel. Blockade of the Purkinje fibers necessary for conduction of the cardiac impulse greatly slows conduction and prolongs the duration of the QRS complex. Multiple peaks in an abnormally prolonged QRS complex most often reflect multiple local blocks in conduction of the cardiac impulse along Purkinje fibers as may occur from scar tissue formed at sites of myocardial infarction.

Voltage of the QRS interval in the standard limb leads of the ECG varies between 0.5 and 2 mv, with lead III usually recording the lowest voltage and lead II the greatest. High-voltage QRS complexes are considered to be present when the sum of the voltages of all the QRS complexes of the three standard limb leads is more than 4 mv. The most frequent cause of high-voltage QRS complexes is ventricular hypertrophy.

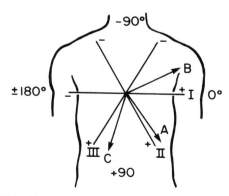

FIGURE 48-3. Electrical axis of the heart as determined from the standard limb leads of the electrocardiogram. In the normal heart, the electrical axis is approximately 59 degrees (A). Left axis deviation shifts the electrical axis to less than 0 degrees (B); right axis deviation is associated with an electrical axis greater than 100 degrees.

Decreased Voltage in the Standard Limb Leads

Causes of decreased voltage on the ECG recorded from standard limb leads are (1) multiple small myocardial infarctions that prevent generation of large quantities of electrical currents, (2) rotation of the apex of the heart toward the anterior chest wall, and (3) abnormal conditions around the heart so electric currents cannot be easily conducted from the heart to the surface of the body. For example, pericardial fluid diminishes voltage recorded from standard limb leads due to the ability of this fluid to rapidly conduct electric currents to multiple sites. Pulmonary emphysema is associated with reduced conduction of electric current through the lungs caused by the effects of excessive amounts of air in the lungs.

Current of Injury

A current of injury is due to the inability of damaged areas of the heart to undergo repolarization during diastole. The current of injury results when current flows between the pathologically depolarized (negative) and normally polarized (positive) areas. The most common cause of a current of injury is myocardial ischemia or infarction. Mechanical trauma to the heart and infectious processes that damage cardiac muscle membranes (pericarditis or myocarditis) may also be responsible for a current of injury. In these conditions, a current of injury occurs when the depolarization period of some cardiac muscle is so long that the muscle fails to repolarize completely before the next cardiac cycle begins.

Specific leads of the ECG are more likely than other leads to reflect myocardial ischemia that develops in areas of the myocardium supplied by an individual coronary artery (Table 48-3). An estimated 80% to 90% of S-T segment information contained in a conventional 12-lead ECG is present on lead V_5. Lead II has special value in diagnosis of inferior wall myocardial ischemia and the origin of cardiac dysrhythmias. Complete interruption of a coronary artery with infarction of the cardiac muscle results in a deep Q-wave in the ECG leads recording from the infarcted area. The Q-wave occurs because there is no electrical activity in the infarcted area. A Q-wave whose amplitude is more than one third of the corresponding R-wave and whose duration is more than 0.04 second is diagnostic of myocardial infarction. In the presence of an old anterior myocardial infarction, a Q-wave develops in lead I because of loss of muscle mass in the anterior left wall of the left ventricle. Conversely, in pos-

Table 48–3

Relationship of Electrocardiogram Lead Reflecting Myocardial Ischemia to Area of Myocardium Involved

Electrocardiogram Lead	Coronary Artery Responsible for Ischemia	Area of Myocardium Supplied by Coronary Artery
II, III, aVF	Right coronary artery	Right atrium Interatrial septum Right ventricle Sinoatrial node Atrioventricular node Inferior wall of left ventricle
V_3–V_5	Left anterior descending coronary artery	Anterior and lateral wall of left ventricle
I, aVL	Circumflex coronary artery	Lateral wall of left ventricle Sinoatrial node Atrioventricular node

terior myocardial infarction, a Q-wave develops in lead III because of loss of cardiac muscle in the posterior apical part of the ventricle.

Abnormalities of the T-wave

The T-wave is normally positive in the standard limb leads, reflecting repolarization of the apex of the heart before the endocardial surfaces of the ventricles. The direction in which repolarization spreads over the heart is backward to the direction in which depolarization occurs. The T-wave becomes abnormal when the normal sequence of repolarization does not occur. For example, delay of conduction of the cardiac impulse through the ventricles (prolonged depolarization), as occurs with left or right bundle branch block or ventricular premature contractions, results in a T-wave with a polarity opposite the QRS complex.

Myocardial ischemia is the most common cause of prolonged depolarization of cardiac muscle. When myocardial ischemia occurs in only one area of the heart, the duration of depolarization of this area increases disproportionately to that in other areas, resulting in abnormalities (inversion or biphasic) of the T-wave. Myocardial ischemia also leads to elevation of the S-T segment on the ECG. To be clinically significant, the S-T elevation should be at least 1 mm above the base line. Artifactual S-T elevation or depression may be introduced by filters incorporated in some ECG monitors to eliminate baseline drift due to movement such as that produced by breathing. For this reason, it is important to verify that the monitor is in the diagnostic mode before concluding that S-T changes represent myocardial ischemia. During exercise, the development of any change in T-waves or S-T segments is evidence that some portion of ventricular muscle has become ischemic and is manifesting an increased period of depolarization out of proportion to the rest of the heart.

His Bundle Electrogram

The His bundle electrogram is recorded from an electrode inserted through a vein and positioned near the tricuspid valve (Fig. 48-4) (Ganong, 1987). The A deflection reflects activation of the atrioventricular node, the H spike is transmission through the His bundle, and the V deflection oc-

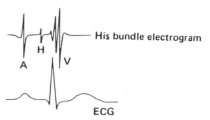

FIGURE 48–4. A normal His bundle electrogram and the corresponding electrocardiogram (ECG). (From Ganong WF. Review of Medical Physiology. 13th ed. Norwalk, CT. Appleton and Lange. 1987; with permission.)

curs during ventricular depolarization. Using the standard ECG and His bundle electrogram, it is possible to accurately measure conduction time from the sinus node to the atrioventricular node (AH interval), conduction time through the atrioventricular node, and conduction time through the bundle of His and bundle branches (HV interval) (Fig. 48-4) (Ganong, 1987). As such, the His bundle electrogram permits detailed analysis of the block site when there is a defect in the system for conduction of cardiac impulses through the heart.

CARDIAC DYSRHYTHMIAS

Mechanisms

Cardiac dysrhythmias may be caused by altered automaticity of pacemaker cardiac cells, altered excitability of myocardial cells, and altered conduction of cardiac impulses through the specialized conduction systems of the heart. Manifestations of these alterations may be the appearance of an ectopic cardiac pacemaker, development of heart block, or appearance of a reentry circuit. Cardiac dysrhythmias are observed to occur in 60% or more of patients undergoing anesthesia and surgery when continuous methods of monitoring are used (Atlee and Bosnjak, 1990).

Automaticity

Automaticity depicts the ability of pacemaker cardiac cells to undergo spontaneous phase 4 depolarization. Under normal circumstances, automaticity is exhibited by cells in the sinoatrial node, atrioventricular node, and specialized conducting fibers of the atria and ventricles.

Activation of the sympathetic nervous system by events such as arterial hypoxemia, acidosis, or release of catecholamines is the most common cause of enhanced automaticity. In addition, enhanced automaticity occurs when the threshold potential becomes more negative such that the difference between the threshold potential and resting transmembrane potential is less.

Decreased automaticity is produced by increased parasympathetic nervous system activity, which reduces responsiveness of sinoatrial and atrioventricular node cells by increasing outward flux of potassium ions (K^+). This increased outward movement of K^+ evoked by acetylcholine hyperpolarizes cardiac cell membranes and prevents them from depolarizing. Vagal stimulation may decrease the vulnerability of the heart to develop ventricular fibrillation, especially in the presence of sympathetic nervous system stimulation. Carotid sinus stimulation decreases the frequency of premature ventricular contractions and can abolish ventricular tachycardia.

ECTOPIC PACEMAKER. An ectopic cardiac pacemaker (focus) manifests as a premature contraction of the heart that occurs between normal beats. A depolarization wave spreads outward from the ectopic pacemaker and initiates the premature contraction. The usual cause of an ectopic pacemaker is an irritable area of cardiac muscle resulting from a local area of myocardial ischemia or use of stimulants such as caffeine or nicotine. Sometimes an ectopic pacemaker becomes persistent and assumes the role of pacemaker in place of the sinoatrial node. The most common point for development of an ectopic pacemaker is the atrioventricular node or atrioventricular bundle.

Excitability

Excitability is the ability of a cardiac cell to respond to a stimulus by depolarizing. A measure of excitability is the difference between the resting transmembrane potential and threshold potential of the cardiac cell membrane. The smaller the difference between these potentials, the more excitable, or irritable, is the cell. Although epinephrine enhances excitability, this is somewhat offset by a concomitant small increase in the negativity of the resting transmembrane poten-

tial. Once a cell depolarizes, it is no longer excitable, being refractory to all stimuli. After this absolute refractory period, cardiac cells enter a relative refractory period during which greater than normal stimuli can cause cardiac cell membranes to depolarize.

Conduction

Conduction of cardiac impulses proceeds through specialized conduction systems of the heart such that coordinated contractions occur (see Fig. 47-10). Abnormalities of conduction of cardiac impulses manifest as development of heart block, reentry circuits, or preexcitation syndromes.

HEART BLOCK. The most frequent sites of heart block are the atrioventricular bundle or one of the bundle branches. Causes of heart block at these sites include (1) excessive parasympathetic nervous system stimulation, (2) drug-induced (digitalis or propranolol) depression of impulse conduction, (3) myocardial infarction, (4) pressure on the conduction system by atherosclerotic plaques, and (5) age-related degenerative process of the conduction system.

REENTRY. Reentry (circus movements) implies re-excitation of cardiac tissue by return of the same cardiac impulse using a circuitous pathway (Fig. 48-5) (Akhtar, 1982). This contrasts with automaticity, in which a new cardiac impulse is generated each time to excite the heart. Reentry circuits can develop at any place in the heart where there is an imbalance between conduction and refractoriness. Causes of this imbalance include (1) elongation of the conduction pathway such as occurs in dilated hearts (especially a dilated left atrium associated with mitral stenosis); (2) decreased velocity of conduction of cardiac impulses as occurs with myocardial ischemia or hyperkalemia; and (3) a shortened refractory period of cardiac muscle as produced by epinephrine or electric shock from an alternating current. Each of these conditions creates a situation in which the cardiac impulse conducted by a normal Purkinje fiber can return retrograde through the abnormal Purkinje fiber, which is not in a refractory state (a reentry circuit). A reentry circuit is the most likely mechanism for supraventricular tachycardia, atrial flutter, atrial fibrillation, premature ventricular contractions, ventricular tach-

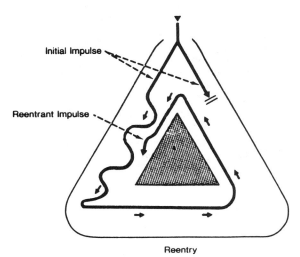

Reentry

FIGURE 48–5. The essential requirement for initiation of a reentry circuit is a unilateral block that prevents uniform anterograde propagation of the initial cardiac impulse. This same cardiac impulse, under appropriate conditions, can traverse the area of block in a retrograde direction and become a reentrant cardiac impulse. (From Akhtar M. Management of ventricular tachyarrhythmias. JAMA 1982;247:671–4; with permission.)

ycardia, and ventricular fibrillation. Reentry circuits can be eliminated by speeding conduction through normal tissue so the cardiac impulse reaches its initial site of origin when the fiber is still refractory, or by prolonging the refractory period of normal cells so the returning impulse cannot reenter.

PREEXCITATION SYNDROMES. A preexcitation syndrome is present when the atrial impulse bypasses the atrioventricular node to produce early excitation of the ventricle. The most common accessory conduction pathway providing a direct connection of the atrium to the ventricle is known as *Kent's bundle* (usually left atrium to left ventricle) (Table 48-4) (Wellens et al, 1987). Conduction via this accessory pathway produces the Wolff-Parkinson-White syndrome (P-R interval less than 0.12 second, QRS complex more than 0.12 second, delta wave) most often manifesting as intermittent bouts of supraventricular tachydysrhythmias. Normally, the ventricles are protected from rapid atrial rhythms by the refractory period of the atrioventricular node. Propra-

nolol has no specific effect on the accessory pathways, while digitalis preparations and verapamil may enhance conduction through these pathways.

Anesthesia

The ability of halogenated anesthetics to evoke nodal rhythms and/or increase ventricular automaticity may be related to altered K^+, and Ca^{2+} translocation dynamics across cell membranes (Atlee and Bosnjak, 1990). Halothane, enflurane, and isoflurane slow the rate of sinoatrial node discharge and prolong His–Purkinje and ventricular conduction times. Changes in $PaCO_2$ dramatically alter autonomic nervous system effects on the sinoatrial and atrioventricular node depolarization as well as reentry. Autonomic nervous system imbalance owing to drugs (anticholinergics, anticholinesterases, exogenous catecholamines, or beta-antagonists) or light anesthesia may be responsible for the initiation of cardiac dysrhythmias during anesthesia and surgery.

Types of Cardiac Dysrhythmias

Sinus Tachycardia

Sinus tachycardia is usually defined as a heart rate more than 100 beats·min^{-1}. A common cause of sinus tachycardia is sympathetic nervous system stimulation such as may occur during a noxious stimulus in the presence of low concentrations of anesthetic. Increased body temperature elevates heart rate approximately 18 beats·min^{-1} for every degree Celsius elevation. Fever causes tachycardia because increased temperature elevates the rate of metabolism in the sinoatrial node. Carotid sinus mediated reflex stimulation of the heart rate accompanies decreases in blood

Table 48–4
Accessory Pathways and Preexcitation Syndromes

	Connections
Kent's bundle	Atrium to ventricle
Mahaim bundle	Atrioventricular node to ventricle
Atrio-Hissian fiber	Atrium to His bundle
James fiber	Atrium to atrioventricular node

pressure as produced by vasodilator drugs or acute hemorrhage.

Sinus Bradycardia

Sinus bradycardia is usually defined as a heart rate less than 60 beats·min^{-1}. Heart-rate slowing accompanies parasympathetic nervous system stimulation of the heart. Bradycardia that occurs in physically conditioned athletes reflects the ability of their hearts to eject a greater stroke volume with each contraction compared with the less conditioned heart.

Sinus Arrhythmia

Sinus arrhythmia is present during normal breathing with heart rate varying approximately 5% during various phases of the quiet breathing cycle (Fig. 48-6). This variation may increase to 30% during deep breathing. These variations in heart rate with breathing most likely reflect baroreceptor reflex activity and changes in the negative intrapleural pressures that elicit a waxing and waning Bainbridge reflex

Atrioventricular Heart Block

First-degree atrioventricular heart block is considered to be present when the P-R interval is more than 0.2 second at a normal heart rate. Second-degree atrioventricular heart block is classified as the Wenckebach phenomenon (Type I) or Mobitz (Type II) heart block. Wenckebach phenomenon is characterized by a progressive prolongation of the P-R interval until conduction of the cardiac impulse is completely interrupted and a P-wave is recorded without a subsequent QRS complex. After this dropped beat, the cycle is repeated. Mobitz Type II heart block is the oc-

currence of a nonconducted atrial impulse without a prior change in the P-R interval.

Third-degree atrioventricular heart block occurs during complete block of the transmission of cardiac impulses from the atria to the ventricles. The P-waves are dissociated from the QRS complexes and the heart rate depends on the intrinsic discharge of the ectopic pacemaker beyond the site of conduction block. If the ectopic pacemaker is near the atrioventricular node, the QRS complexes appear normal and the heart rate is typically 40 to 60 beats·min^{-1} (Fig. 48-7). When the site of block is infranodal, the escape ventricular pacemaker often has a discharge rate less than 40 beats·min^{-1} and the QRS complexes are wide, resembling a bundle branch block (Fig.48-8). Patients may experience syncope (Stokes-Adams syndrome) at the onset of third-degree heart block, reflecting the 5- to 10-second period of asystole that may precede ventricular escape and appearance of an ectopic ventricular pacemaker. Occasionally, the interval of ventricular standstill at the onset of third-degree heart block is so long that death occurs. Treatment of patients with third-degree heart block is by insertion of a permanent artificial cardiac pacemaker. Temporary cardiac pacing may be provided with intravenous infusion of isoproterenol or a transvenous artificial cardiac pacemaker.

Premature Atrial Contractions

Premature atrial contractions are recognized by an abnormal P-wave and a shortened P-R interval (Fig. 48-9). The QRS complex of the premature atrial contraction has a normal configuration. Also, the interval between the premature atrial contraction and the next succeeding contraction is usually not prolonged. Premature atrial contractions are usually benign and often occur in persons without heart disease.

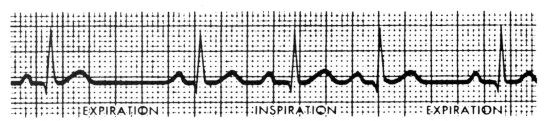

FIGURE 48–6. Sinus arrhythmia reflecting changes in sinoatrial pacemaker activity with the breathing cycle.

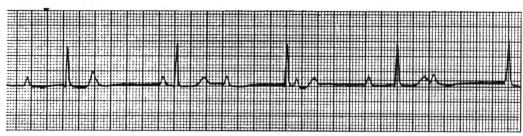

FIGURE 48–7. Third-degree atrioventricular heart block occurring at the level of the atrioventricular node (QRS complexes are narrow). There is no relation between P-waves and QRS complexes.

Premature Nodal Contractions

Premature nodal contractions are characterized by the absence of a P-wave preceding the QRS complex. The P-wave is obscured by the QRS complex of the premature contraction because the cardiac impulse travels retrograde into the atria at the same time it travels forward into the ventricles.

Premature Ventricular Contractions

Premature ventricular contractions result from an ectopic pacemaker in the ventricles. The QRS complex of the ECG is typically prolonged because the cardiac impulse is conducted mainly through the slowly conducting muscle of the ventricle rather than Purkinje fibers (Fig. 48-10). The voltage of the QRS complex of the premature ventricular contraction is increased, reflecting the absence of the usual neutralization that occurs when a normal cardiac impulse passes through both ventricles simultaneously. Following almost all premature ventricular contractions, the T-wave has an electric potential opposite to that of the QRS complex. A compensatory pause following a premature ventricular contraction occurs because the first impulse from the sinoatrial node reaches the ventricle during its refractory period. When a premature ventricular contraction occurs, the ventricle may not have filled adequately with blood and the stroke volume resulting from this contraction fails to produce a detectable pulse. The subsequent stroke volume, however, may be increased due to added ventricular filling that occurs during the compensatory pause that typically follows a premature ventricular contraction.

Premature ventricular contractions often reflect significant cardiac disease. For example, myocardial ischemia may be responsible for initiation of a premature contraction from an irritable site in poorly oxygenated ventricular muscle. Treatment of premature ventricular contractions includes supplemental oxygen and intravenous administration of lidocaine.

Atrial Paroxysmal Tachycardia

Atrial paroxysmal tachycardia, which often occurs in otherwise healthy young persons, is caused by

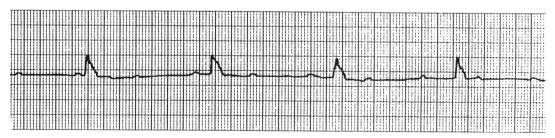

FIGURE 48–8. Third-degree atrioventricular heart block occurring at an infranodal level (QRS complexes are wide).

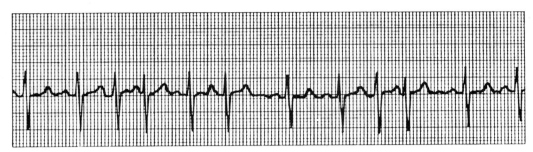

FIGURE 48–9.   Premature atrial contractions resulting in an irregular rhythm.

rapid rhythmic discharges of impulses from an ectopic atrial pacemaker. The rhythm on the ECG is perfectly regular and the P-waves are abnormal, often inverted, indicating a site of origin other than the sinoatrial node. The rapid discharge rate of this ectopic focus causes it to become the pacemaker. Typically, the onset of atrial paroxysmal tachycardia is abrupt (a single beat) and may end just as suddenly with the pacemaker shifting back to the sinoatrial node. Atrial paroxysmal tachycardia can be terminated by producing parasympathetic nervous system stimulation at the heart with drugs or by unilateral external pressure applied to the carotid sinus.

Nodal Paroxysmal Tachycardia

Nodal paroxysmal tachycardia resembles atrial paroxysmal tachycardia except P-waves are not identifiable on the ECG. P-waves are obscured by QRS complexes because the atrial impulse travels backward from the atrioventricular node at the same time the ventricular impulse travels through the ventricles.

Ventricular Tachycardia

Ventricular tachycardia on the ECG resembles a series of ventricular premature contractions that occur at a rapid and regular rate without any normal supraventricular beats interspersed (Fig. 48-11). Stroke volume is often severely depressed during ventricular tachycardia because the ventricles have insufficient time for cardiac filling. Sustained ventricular tachycardia may necessitate termination with electrical cardioversion. This cardiac dysrhythmia predisposes to ventricular fibrillation.

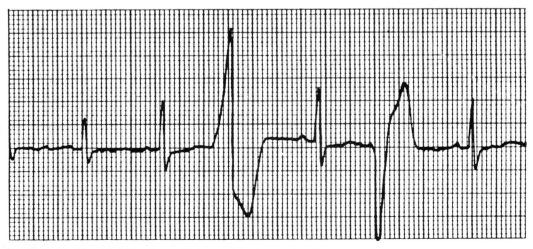

FIGURE 48–10.   Multifocal premature ventricular contractions.

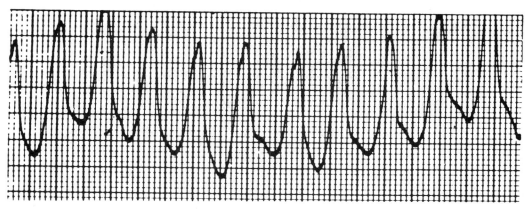

FIGURE 48–11. Ventricular tachycardia.

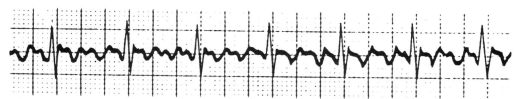

FIGURE 48–12. Atrial flutter.

Atrial Flutter

Atrial flutter on the ECG is characterized by 2:1, 3:1, or 4:1 conduction of atrial impulses to the ventricle (Fig. 48-12). This occurs because the functional refractory period of Purkinje fibers and ventricular muscle is such that no more than 200 impulses·min^{-1} can be transmitted to the ventricles. P-waves have a characteristic saw-toothed appearance, especially in lead II.

Atrial Fibrillation

Atrial fibrillation is characterized by normal QRS complexes occurring at a rapid and irregular rate in the absence of identifiable P-waves (Fig. 48-13). The irregular ventricular response reflects arrival of atrial impulses at the atrioventricular node at times that may or may not correspond to the refractory period of the node from a previous discharge. Stroke volume is reduced during atrial fibrillation because the ventricles do not have sufficient time to fill optimally between cardiac cycles. A pulse deficit (heart rate by palpation less than that calculated from the ECG) reflects the inability of each ventricular contraction to eject a sufficient stroke volume to produce a detectable peripheral pulse. Treatment of atrial fibrillation is classically with digitalis, which

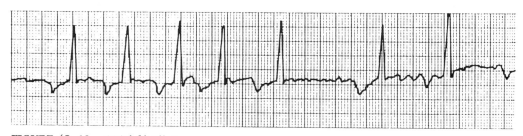

FIGURE 48–13. Atrial fibrillation.

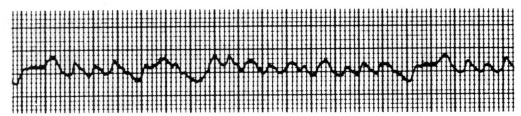

FIGURE 48–14.   Ventricular fibrillation.

prolongs the refractory period of the atrioventricular node. This prolongation decreases the ventricular response, which improves stroke volume by permitting additional time for filling the ventricles between cardiac cycles.

Ventricular Fibrillation

Ventricular fibrillation on the ECG is characterized by an irregular wavy line with voltages that range from 0.25 to 0.5 mv (Fig. 48-14). There is total incoordination of contraction with cessation of any effective pumping activity and disappearance of detectable blood pressure. Flutter or fibrillation is usually confined to either the atria or ventricles because the two masses of muscle are electrically insulated from each other by the rings of fibrous tissue around the heart valves. Most instances of atrial or ventricular fibrillation are due to a reentry mechanism. The only effective treatment of ventricular fibrillation is the delivery of a direct electric current through the ventricles (defibrillation), which simultaneously depolarizes all ventricular muscle. This depolarization allows the reestablishment of a cardiac pacemaker at a site other than the irritable focus that was responsible for ventricular fibrillation.

REFERENCES

Akhtar M. Management of ventricular tachyarrhythmias. JAMA 1982;247:671–4.

Atlee JL, Bosnjak ZJ. Mechanisms for cardiac dysrhythmias during anesthesia. Anesthesiology 1990;72:347–74.

Ganong WF. Review of Medical Physiology. 13th ed. Norwalk, CT. Appleton and Lange. 1987.

Wellens HJJ, Brugada P, Penn OC. The management of preexcitation syndromes. JAMA 1987;257:2325–33.

Chapter

49

Lungs

ANATOMY

The human thorax is composed of 12 thoracic vertebral bodies, 12 pairs of ribs, and the sternum, which are sufficiently rigid to protect the organ systems contained within but pliable enough to allow the lungs to act as a bellows. The ribs must be capable of movement and therefore cannot be rigidly attached to their points of articulation on the vertebral bodies. The sternum, consisting of the manubrium, body, and xiphoid process, is the most important anterior supporting skeletal chest wall structure. The suprasternal notch (the upper border of the manubrium between the sternoclavicular joints) is in the same horizontal plane as the midportion of the second thoracic vertebra. The second thoracic vertebra is a useful radiologic landmark because it corresponds to the midportion of the trachea, which is a desirable location for the distal tip of a trachea tube. External palpation of tracheal tube cuff inflation in the suprasternal notch is an indirect method for confirming that the distal end of the tracheal tube is properly positioned above the carina.

The trachea is a fibromuscular tube approximately 10 to 12 cm in length with a diameter of approximately 20 mm and a capacity of approximately 30 ml. The trachea begins at the level of the sixth cervical vertebra corresponding to the cricoid cartilage and extends downward until it bifurcates at the carina opposite the fifth thoracic vertebra. The mucosal lining of the trachea consists of ciliated columnar epithelium and mucus-secreting cells. Each ciliated cell has approximately 200 cilia beating 12 to 20 times·min^{-1} and

moving mucus toward the pharynx at a rate of 0.5 to 1.5 cm·min^{-1}.

The bifurcation of the trachea at the carina gives rise to the right and left main stem bronchi. The right main stem bronchus extends approximately 2.5 cm prior to its initial division into the bronchus to the right upper and middle lobes with a continuation as the right lower lobe bronchus. The left main stem bronchus extends approximately 5 cm prior to its initial division into branches to the left upper lobe and lingula and continuation as the bronchus to the left lower lobe. The takeoff of the right bronchus from the long vertical axis of the trachea is approximately 25 degrees in adults, whereas the angle for the left bronchus is approximately 45 degrees. Thus, in the adult, accidental endobronchial intubation or aspiration of foreign material is likely to enter the right main stem bronchus. The short length of the right main stem bronchus increases the technical difficulty in placing a right endobronchial tube without obstructing the orifice to the right upper lobe. For this reason, it is a common recommendation to routinely use left endobronchial tubes when a double-lumen tube is selected. In children younger than 3 years of age, the bifurcations of both the right and left bronchi are approximately equal, with takeoff angles of approximately 55 degrees.

Continued division of the right and left main stem bronchi give rise to bronchioles, characterized by absence of cartilage, and ultimately to respiratory bronchioles, which are the transitional zones between the bronchioles and alveolar ducts. Alveoli arise from alveolar ducts as well as alveolar sacs. Collateral ventilation may occur via pores of Kohn located in the interspaces between alveolar capillary networks as well as pathways directly communicating between terminal respiratory bronchioles and neighboring alveoli.

The lungs fill the chest cavity so the visceral pleura of the lungs is in contact with the parietal pleura of the chest cage. The two pleural surfaces are separated by only a thin liquid film that provides an adhesive bond holding the lung and chest wall together. The opposing lung and chest wall recoil forces produce a subatmospheric pressure of approximately −4 mmHg in the potential space between the visceral and parietal pleura during quiet breathing. Measurement of pressure in the lumen of the flaccid esophagus approximates the pleural pressure.

Respiratory Passageways

Airway smooth muscle is principally under the neural influence of the parasympathetic nervous system via the vagus nerve. Release of acetylcholine from efferent vagus nerve endings evokes bronchoconstriction, explaining the bronchodilating effects of inhaled anticholinergics. There are few if any sympathetic nervous system fibers present in airway smooth muscle, but beta receptors present in this smooth muscle can be stimulated by circulating catecholamines. Histamine stimulates H-1 receptors (bronchoconstriction) and H-2 receptors (bronchodilation) but the predominant effect is bronchoconstriction.

Inhaled gases are warmed, filtered, and humidified by the extensive vascular surfaces of the nasal turbinates and septum. Bypassing the nasal passageways as with a translaryngeal tracheal tube or tracheostomy can lead to an undesirable drying effect in the lungs. The filtering function of the nose is due to the mucous covering of the main respiratory passageways, which is sufficiently efficient to remove almost all particles more than 4 μ in diameter before they reach the lungs. Cilia move mucus-containing foreign particles and dust toward the pharynx where it is swallowed. Anesthetic drugs may depress the velocity of mucous flow by diminishing ciliary activity. For example, mucus flow decreases from 20 mm·min^{-1} to 7 mm·min^{-1} during halothane anesthesia (Lichtiger et al, 1975).

Inhaled particles that can reach the airways often accumulate in smaller bronchioles as a result of gravitational precipitation. For example,

bronchiolar disease is common in coal miners, reflecting the presence of settled dust particles. Even smaller particles (less than 0.5 μ), as are present in cigarette smoke, may be precipitated in the alveoli. Particles that are trapped in alveoli eventually cause fibrous tissue growth in alveolar septa, leading to irreversible damage.

Innervation of the Larynx

A knowledge of the innervation of the larynx is important when performing topical laryngeal anesthesia. The sensory innervation of the larynx is derived from the branches of the glossopharyngeal nerve (posterior tongue, pharynx, and tonsils) and the superior laryngeal nerve branch of the vagus nerve (epiglottis and mucous membranes of the larynx to the level of the false vocal cords.) The vocal cords and upper trachea receive sensory innervation from the recurrent laryngeal nerve branch of the vagus nerve. Motor innervation of the laryngeal muscles is from the recurrent laryngeal nerve with the exception of the cricothyroid muscle, a vocal cord tensor, which is innervated by the superior laryngeal nerve.

Cough Reflex

Cough is the mechanism by which passageways of the lungs are maintained free of foreign particles. The larynx and carina are particularly sensitive to stimulation, which results in the transmission of afferent impulses via the vagus nerves to the medulla. The medulla initiates a series of responses characterized by inhalation followed by closure of the glottis and contraction of abdominal muscles. The result is an increase in intrapulmonary pressure such that air is forced outward when the glottis suddenly opens. This rapidly moving air usually carries with it any foreign matter that is present in the larger passageways below the glottis. Depressant drugs such as opioids and volatile anesthetics as well as increasing age are associated with depression of the cough reflex (Fig. 49-1) (Pontoppidan and Beecher, 1960).

Sneeze Reflex

The sneeze reflex is similar to the cough reflex except that it facilitates clearance of secretions from the nasal passageways rather than passage-

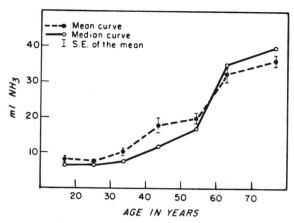

FIGURE 49–1. Volume of inhaled ammonia necessary to cause breath holding increases noticeably after 60 years of age, suggesting a decline in the sensitivity of protective airway reflexes with increasing age. (From Pontoppidan H, Beecher HK. Progressive loss of protective reflexes in the airway with the advance of age. JAMA 1960; 174: 2209–13; with permission.)

ways below the nose. The initiating stimulus for the sneeze reflex is stimulation of the nasal passageways.

MECHANICS OF BREATHING

The diaphragm is the principal muscle of breathing, accounting for approximately 75% of the air that enters the lungs during spontaneous inspiration. Contraction of the diaphragm during inspiration moves abdominal contents downward and forward, creating a potential space, which is filled by expansion of the lungs. This lung expansion causes pressure within alveoli to become slightly negative with respect to atmospheric pressure, and gases thus flow inward through the respiratory passages. It is estimated that the diaphragm moves 10 to 12 cm vertically during each inspiration. Two thirds of the diaphragm's fibers are slow twitch, being resistant to fatigue. The diaphragm is innervated by the phrenic nerve, which arises from the third, fourth, and fifth cervical nerves. During quiet breathing, the contribution of intercostal muscle contraction to inspiration is small. Overall, the oxygen cost of breathing is usually less than 5% of minute oxygen consumption. More than two thirds of the work of quiet breathing is spent in overcoming

the elastic recoil of the lungs and thorax. When the rate of breathing increases or airways are narrowed, a large proportion of work is spent in overcoming the resistance to gas flow.

In contrast to inspiration, the diaphragm relaxes during exhalation and the elastic recoil of the lungs, chest wall, and abdominal structures compresses the lungs. The inherent tendency for the lungs to collapse (recoil away from the chest wall) is due to elastic fibers that are stretched by lung inflation and, therefore, attempt to shorten. Even more important, surface tension of the fluid lining the alveoli causes a continual elastic tendency for alveoli to collapse (see the section entitled "Surface Tension and Pulmonary Surfactant"). Elastic fibers in the lungs normally account for approximately one third of the recoil tendency, and surface tension accounts for the remainder. These elastic recoil properties of stretched tissues lead to a rise in the alveolar pressure to above atmospheric and gas is forced outward. Abdominal muscles are the most important muscles for exhalation. These muscles of exhalation are active only during forced exhalation maneuvers (cough to clear secretions) or obstruction to the flow of gas. Indeed, paralysis of abdominal muscles produced by regional anesthesia does not influence alveolar ventilation, but the patient's ability to cough and clear secretions may be compromised.

Elastic recoil of the lungs is responsible for the negative intrapleural pressure of approximately -4 mmHg. This negative intrapleural pressure helps keep the lungs expanded to normal size. Expansion of the lungs during maximum inspiration creates an intrapleural pressure of -12 mmHg or greater.

Alveolar Volume and Distribution of Ventilation

Alveolar volume is not uniform throughout the lungs because of differences in distending pressures to which alveoli are subjected. Pleural pressure is most negative at the apex of the lung and becomes progressively less negative toward the lung base. These regional differences in transalveolar pressure (alveolar pressure minus pleural pressure) mean that alveoli in lung apices are more expanded than those at the lung bases.

Distribution of ventilation in the lungs and the volume at which airways in lung bases begin to close can be assessed by the single breath nitrogen washout test. The subject first takes a single breath of oxygen from residual volume to total lung capacity. During the subsequent slow exhalation from total lung capacity to residual volume, the concentration of nitrogen in the exhaled air is plotted against the exhaled volume (Fig. 49-2). The first gases exhaled from large airways are considered to represent dead space gases (see the section entitled "Dead Space"). The beginning of alveolar gas exhalation is reflected by an increase in the exhaled nitrogen concentration (Phase II) followed by a plateau (Phase III) if ventilation is distributed fairly evenly. If the nitrogen concentration continues to rise during Phase III, it can be assumed that alveoli are filling and emptying at different rates. Phase IV reflects higher nitrogen concentrations in alveoli of the lung spaces that continue to empty at low lung volumes that cause airways at lung bases to close.

Pneumothorax

When air enters the pleural space via a rupture in the lung or a hole in the chest wall, the lung on the affected side collapses because of its elastic recoil. Because the intrapleural pressure on the affected side is atmospheric, the mediastinum shifts toward the normal side, tending to kink the great vessels. If the communication between the pleural space and the atmosphere remains open (open pneumothorax), the resistance to air flow into the pleural cavity is less than resistance to air flow into the intact lung, and little air enters the intact lung during inspiration. There is marked stimulation of breathing owing to hypoxemia,

hypercarbia, and activation of pulmonary deflation receptors. Dyspnea is severe.

If there is a flap of tissue over the rupture in the lung or chest wall that acts as a flutter valve, permitting air to enter during inspiration but preventing its exit during exhalation, the pressure in the pleural space increases above atmospheric (tension pneumothorax). As with an open pneumothorax, there is a shift of the mediastinum toward the intact lung with kinking of the great vessels and development of hypoxemia. Life-saving treatment is decompression of the pneumothorax by removing the air. Spontaneous pneumothorax is due to rupture of the blebs on the surface of the visceral pleura. Air from a closed pneumothorax diffuses along a partial pressure gradient into venous blood, being completely absorbed in 1 to 2 weeks.

SURFACE TENSION AND PULMONARY SURFACTANT

Surface tension results from attraction of molecules in the fluid lining the alveoli. Furthermore, surface tension changes with the size of the alveoli in accordance with Laplace's law, which states that the pressure inside a bubble (an alveolus) necessary to keep it expanded is directly proportional to the tension on the wall of the bubble, which tends to collapse it, divided by the radius of the bubble. If surface tension is maintained constant and the radius of the alveolus is diminished, then the pressure of the alveolus will rise, thus emptying its content into a bigger alveolus. Surface tension, in addition to causing collapse of alveoli, acts to pull fluid into alveoli.

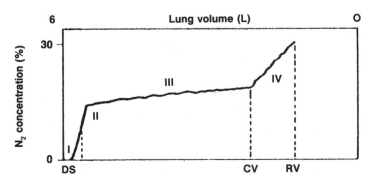

FIGURE 49-2. Single-breath nitrogen washout curve reflecting dead space volume (Phase I), exhalation of alveolar gas (Phases II and III), and airway closure in the lung bases (Phase IV).

Pulmonary surfactant is a lipoprotein secreted by Type II alveolar cells (pneumocytes) lining the alveoli. These cells begin to appear at approximately 21 weeks of gestation and surfactant is first produced between 28 to 32 weeks. Formation of pulmonary surfactant may be hastened by administration of corticosteroids to the parturient. The phospholipid component of pulmonary surfactant, dipalmitoyl lecithin, decreases surface tension of fluids lining the alveoli. For example, as an alveolus decreases in size, the pulmonary surfactant becomes more concentrated at the surface of the alveolar lining fluid, and surface tension is reduced. This prevents the development of high transalveolar pressures (according to Laplace's law) that can collapse alveoli as they become smaller. Conversely, as alveoli become larger and the surfactant is spread more thinly on the fluid surface, the surface tension becomes greater. Thus, pulmonary surfactant helps to stabilize the sizes of alveoli, causing larger alveoli to contract more and smaller ones to contract less. The net effect is the maintenance of alveoli in any area of the lung at about the same size.

Absence or inadequate amounts of pulmonary surfactant is characteristic of respiratory distress syndrome of the neonate in which a large number of alveoli are filled with fluid. In the absence of surfactant, lung expansion is difficult, requiring intrapleural pressures often approaching -30 mmHg to overcome the collapse tendency of the alveoli. Pulmonary surfactant may be diminished after cardiopulmonary bypass, following prolonged inhalation of 100% oxygen, and in persons who inhale tobacco smoke. When the surface area of the surfactant film is kept small, a rearrangement of molecules occurs, causing surface tension to increase with time. Therefore, peripheral alveoli tend to collapse during prolonged periods of shallow breathing. A single large breath or sigh opens these alveoli and expands their surface area, thus lowering surface tension.

COMPLIANCE

Compliance is expressed as the increase in the gas volume of the lungs for each unit increase of alveolar pressure. The combined compliance of normal lungs and thorax is 0.13 L·cm H_2O^{-1}. This means that the lungs expand 130 ml for every 1 cm H_2O increase in the alveoli. Any condition that destroys lung tissue or blocks bronchioles causes decreased pulmonary compliance. Deformities of the thoracic cage such as kyphosis or scoliosis reduce thoracic compliance.

LUNG VOLUMES AND CAPACITIES

The amount of gas in the lungs has been subdivided into four different volumes and capacities (Table 49-1; Fig. 49-3). A lung capacity is the sum of two or more lung volumes (Fig. 49-3). In normal persons, the volume of gas in the lungs depends primarily on body size and build. For example, large and athletic persons have larger lung volumes than small and asthenic individuals. Lung volumes and capacities are approximately 25% less in females than in males. Lung volumes and capacities also change with body position, most of them decreasing when the patient is supine and increasing when the patient is standing. Decreases in lung volumes in the recumbent position reflect the tendency for abdominal contents to press upward against the diaphragm plus an increase in pulmonary blood volume, both of which decrease space available in the lungs for gas.

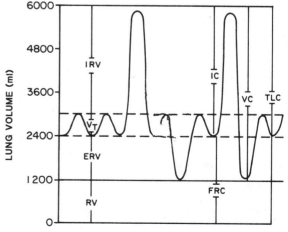

FIGURE 49–3. Schematic diagram of breathing excursions at rest and during maximal inhalation and/or exhalation (see Table 49–1 for definition of abbreviations). Lung capacities are the sum of two or more lung volumes.

Table 49-1
Lung Volumes and Capacities

	Abbreviation	Normal Adult Value
Tidal volume	V_T	500 ml (6–8 ml·kg^{-1})
Inspiratory reserve volume	IRV	3000 ml
Expiratory reserve volume	ERV	1200 ml
Residual volume	RV	1200 ml
Inspiratory capacity	IC	3500 ml
Functional residual capacity	FRC	2400 ml
Vital capacity	VC	4500 ml (60–70 ml·kg^{-1})
Forced exhaled volume in 1 sec	FEV$_1$	80%
Total lung capacity	TLC	5900 ml

In diseases associated with airway obstruction, such as asthma and emphysema, it is usually much more difficult to exhale than to inhale because the expiratory closing tendency of the airways is greatly increased, while the negative intrapleural pressure of inspiration actually pulls the airways open. As a result, gas tends to enter the lungs easily and become trapped in the lungs, leading to an increased residual volume and total lung capacity.

Functional Residual Capacity

Functional residual capacity (FRC) and residual volume provide a buffer in the alveoli such that abrupt alterations in PaO_2 and $PaCO_2$ do not occur. In the presence of a reduced FRC, transient interruptions in breathing as during direct laryngoscopy may result in rapid changes in PaO_2. Breathing 100% oxygen offsets the effect of apnea on PaO_2, especially when the FRC is reduced in volume as in the parturient.

Effects of Anesthesia

Following induction of anesthesia and placement of a tracheal tube, there is a decrease in the FRC of approximately 450 ml that is similar whether or not skeletal muscle paralysis is present (Nunn, 1990). Possible causes of this decrease in FRC include cephalad movement of the diaphragm, decrease in the cross-sectional area of the rib cage, and movement of blood into or out of the thorax. The impact of decreased FRC manifests on airway

caliber, airway closure, pulmonary collapse, and gas exchange. For example, changes in lung volume decrease airway caliber especially in dependent parts of the lungs. This effect is largely offset by the bronchodilator effect of inhaled anesthetics such that airway resistance does not usually change following induction of anesthesia. Airway closure, especially in elderly patients, is likely if FRC decreases below closing capacity. It seems likely that decreases in lung volumes and associated collapse of alveoli are responsible for the increase in right-to-left shunt equivalent to approximately 10% of the cardiac output that typically accompanies general anesthesia. Although positive end-expiratory pressure reduces this shunt, the beneficial effect on PaO_2 may be offset by decreases in cardiac output.

Vital Capacity

Other than the anatomical build of an individual, the major factors that determine vital capacity (VC) are the strength of the breathing muscles and the compliance of the lungs and chest. A tall, thin person usually has a larger VC than an obese person. A well-conditioned athlete may have a VC 30% to 40% above normal. Fibrotic changes in the lungs produced by chronic bronchial asthma or chronic bronchitis reduce pulmonary compliance and thus decrease VC. Any excess fluid in the lungs, such as may occur with heart failure, decreases pulmonary compliance and thus the VC. Indeed, an improvement in VC may reflect a decrease in pulmonary edema as associated with left ventricular dysfunction.

Forced Exhaled Vital Capacity

The forced exhaled VC is the volume of gas that can be rapidly and maximally exhaled starting from total lung capacity. It is customary to measure the volume of exhaled gases after 1 second (FEV_1) and 3 seconds (FEV_3). The FEV_1 and FEV_3 are also expressed as a percentage of the VC. In the normal person, the FEV_3 is more than 80% of the VC (Fig. 49-4). In the presence of obstructive airway disease, this value is less than 50%.

Measurement of the mean air flow rate over the middle half of the forced VC is the forced midexpiratory flow rate ($MEFR_{25\%-75\%}$). Reduction in this flow rate is a sensitive index of airway obstruction.

MINUTE VENTILATION

Minute ventilation is the total amount of gas moved into the lungs each minute (tidal volume times breathing frequency). The average minute ventilation is approximately 6 $L \cdot min^{-1}$.

Alveolar Ventilation

Alveolar ventilation is the volume of gas each minute that enters areas of the lung capable of participating in gas exchange with pulmonary capillary blood. Alveolar ventilation is less than minute ventilation because a portion of inhaled gases fill respiratory passageways that do not participate in gaseous exchange with the pulmonary capillary blood (see the section entitled "Dead Space"). As such, alveolar ventilation is equal to tidal volume from which dead space volume is subtracted (estimate 150 ml) times the frequency of breathing. The average alveolar ventilation is approximately 4.2 $L \cdot min^{-1}$. The $PaCO_2$, and to a lesser extent the PaO_2, are determined by alveolar ventilation. The frequency of breathing and tidal volume are important only insofar as they influence alveolar ventilation.

Dead Space

Anatomic dead space includes those areas of the respiratory tract (nasal passageways, pharynx, tra-

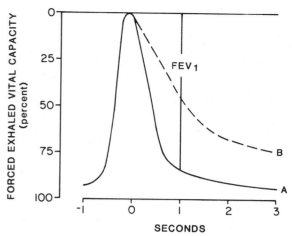

FIGURE 49–4. Schematic diagram of forced exhaled volume in normal patients (A) and in individuals with obstructive airway disease (B). A normal patient can exhale approximately 80% of the vital capacity in 1 sec (FEV_1) compared with approximately 50% in 1 sec in patients with obstructive airway disease.

chea, and bronchi) that do not normally participate in gas exchange with pulmonary capillary blood. Physiologic dead space is the gas volume of alveoli that are not functional or only partially functional because of absent or poor blood flow through corresponding pulmonary capillaries (wasted ventilation). The volume of dead space is determined by measuring the exhaled concentration of nitrogen following a single breath of oxygen. Gas being exhaled from dead space (2 $ml \cdot kg^{-1}$ or approximately 150 ml in an adult) contains no nitrogen (see Fig. 49-2). Normally, the contributions of anatomic and physiologic dead space are nearly equal. Chronic lung disease, however, accentuates the maldistribution of ventilation relative to pulmonary capillary blood flow, which tends to selectively increase physiologic dead space.

During exhalation, gas in dead space is exhaled before gas coming from the alveoli. This is why anesthetic breathing systems are designed to preferentially conserve dead space gas (oxygen and anesthetic not removed and devoid of carbon dioxide) and to eliminate alveolar gas (depleted of oxygen and anesthetic and carbon dioxide added). Conceptually, rebreathing dead space gas is similar to delivering fresh gases from the anesthesia machine.

CONTROL OF VENTILATION

Control of ventilation is designed to make adjustments in alveolar ventilation so as to maintain an optimal and unchanging PaO_2, $PaCO_2$, and concentration of hydrogen ions (H^+). Fine control of ventilation is provided by the respiratory center under the influence of chemical stimuli and peripheral chemoreceptors. The major factor in regulation of alveolar ventilation is the $PaCO_2$ and not the PaO_2. For example, a 50% increase in $PaCO_2$ evokes a tenfold increase in alveolar ventilation and a PaO_2 of 40 mmHg evokes a 1.5-fold increase in alveolar ventilation. An increase in alveolar ventilation occurs simultaneously with the onset of exercise due to direct stimulation of the respiratory center by the cerebral cortex (anticipatory stimulation) and indirect stimulation of the respiratory center by proprioceptors that are activated by joint movement. The respiratory center is depressed by inhaled anesthetics and other centrally acting depressant drugs such as barbiturates and opioids. Acute cerebral edema may lead to increases in intracranial pressure that compresses blood vessels supplying the respiratory center. Cerebrovascular accidents may damage the respiratory center, leading to abnormalities of the breathing pattern (see the section entitled "Periodic Breathing"). Stimulation of the medullary vasomotor center is associated with spillover of impulses to the nearby respiratory center. As a result, decreases in blood pressure that evoke increases in sympathetic nervous system activity from the vasomotor center also evoke increases in alveolar ventilation owing to increased activity of the respiratory center. Increased body temperature directly stimulates the respiratory center in addition to the indirect stimulation provided by increased carbon dioxide production. Voluntary control of alveolar ventilation is mediated through the cerebral cortex rather than the respiratory center.

Respiratory Center

The respiratory center is a widely dispersed group of neurons located bilaterally in the reticular substance of the medulla oblongata and pons (Fig. 49-5) (Guyton, 1986). This center is divided into three areas: (1) inspiratory area, (2) pneumotaxic area, and (3) expiratory area.

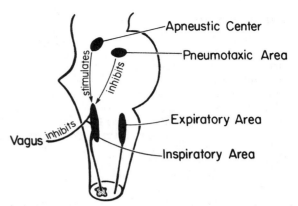

FIGURE 49–5. The respiratory center is located bilaterally in the reticular substance of the medulla oblongata and pons. (Redrawn from Guyton, AC. Textbook of Medical Physiology. 7th ed. Philadelphia: WB Saunders, 1986; with permission.)

Inspiratory Area

Rhythmic inspiratory cycles are generated in the inspiratory area located bilaterally in the dorsal portion of the medulla. Following contraction of the diaphragm, the neurons of the inspiratory area become dormant until intrinsic rhythmic activity again occurs. The vagus and glossopharyngeal nerves transmit signals from peripheral chemoreceptors to the inspiratory area. In addition, the vagus nerves transmit sensory signals from the lungs that help to control lung inflation and the frequency of breathing.

Pneumotaxic Area

Signals from the pneumotaxic area located in the pons are continuously transmitted to the inspiratory area for the purpose of inhibiting inspiration before the lungs become overinflated. Indirectly, this influences the rate of breathing. For example, a strong pneumotaxic signal limits the duration of inspiration, but the cycle may begin sooner so the net effect is a more rapid rate of breathing. A weak pneumotaxic signal results in a slow rate of breathing.

INFLATION REFLEX. Stretch receptors in the walls of bronchi transmit signals over the vagus nerves to the inspiratory area when overinflation of the lungs occur. These signals limit the duration of inspiration in the same way as do signals from the pneumotaxic area. This mechanism to limit inspiration is designated the *inflation reflex* or *Hering-Breuer reflex*. It seems unlikely that the inflation reflex is important in controlling normal lung inflation because it becomes activated only when the tidal volume is more than 1.5 L (Guyton, 1986). Rapid shallow breathing during inhalation of volatile anesthetics is not likely to be related to the inflation reflex (Paskin et al, 1968). Conversely, in situations of decreased pulmonary compliance, such as pulmonary fibrosis, the pattern of breathing becomes shallow and rapid to minimize elastic work presumably by stimulating these inflation receptors.

DEFLATION REFLEX. Deflation receptors are believed to be involved in tachypnea associated with pulmonary edema and pulmonary embolism. Tachypnea associated with inhalation of halothane may reflect stimulation of deflation receptors (Paintal, 1973). These deflation receptors are occasionally referred to as J receptors because of their juxtacapillary position.

APNEUSTIC CENTER. The apneustic center located in the pons transmits signals to the inspiratory center that, in the absence of pneumotaxic area activity, prevents cessation of inspiration. When apneustic center activity is unmasked because of damage to the pneumotaxic area, the pattern of breathing is maximal lung inflation with occasional expiratory gasps.

Expiratory Area

The expiratory area in the ventral portion of the medulla is normally dormant because exhalation results from passive recoil of the elastic structure of the lungs and surrounding chest wall. When the need for increased alveolar ventilation is enhanced, however, the expiratory area becomes active, providing signals that evoke forceful and frequent contraction of the diaphragm.

Chemical Control

Chemical control of breathing is influenced by the effect of changes in $PaCO_2$, PaO_2, and changes in H^+ concentration as sensed by a chemosensitive area in the medulla or by peripheral chemoreceptors. Signals from these sensory areas are transmitted to the respiratory center.

Chemosensitive Area

The chemosensitive area (also known as the medullary chemoreceptor) is located a few microns below the surface of the medulla (Fig. 49-6) (Guyton, 1986). H^+ are the most important stimulus of the chemosensitive area, but these ions do not easily cross the blood-brain barrier to enter the cerebrospinal fluid. For this reason, changes in blood pH have less effect on stimulating the chemosensitive area than does carbon dioxide, which readily crosses the blood-brain barrier. Carbon dioxide stimulates the chemosensitive area through its reaction with water in the cerebrospinal fluid to form carbonic acid, which subsequently dissociates to provide H^+ necessary for stimulation (Fig. 49-6) (Guyton, 1986). In normal individuals, the average ventilatory response to inhaled carbon dioxide is approximately 2.5 $L \cdot min^{-1}$ for every mmHg increase in $PaCO_2$. It is estimated that 70% to 80% of the ventilatory response to carbon dioxide reflects activation of the chemosensitive area and a subsequent increase in transmission of signals to the inspiratory area of the respiratory center. The remainder of the ventilatory response to carbon dioxide is mediated via the peripheral chemoreceptors.

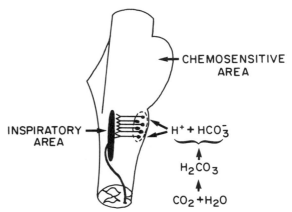

FIGURE 49-6. The chemosensitive area, located a few microns below the ventral surface of the medulla, transmits stimulatory impulses to the inspiratory area. This chemosensitive area is highly responsive to hydrogen ions (H^+) in the cerebrospinal fluid that results from hydration of carbon dioxide. (From Guyton AC. Textbook of Medical Physiology. 7th ed. Philadelphia: WB Saunders, 1986; with permission.)

An advantage of a cerebrospinal fluid system in the control of ventilation is the rapidity with which changes in $PaCO_2$ are reflected in the cerebrospinal fluid. This change occurs within seconds compared with at least 1 minute required for changes in the $PaCO_2$ to be reflected in interstitial fluid. This reflects rapid diffusion of H^+ formed in the cerebrospinal fluid to the chemosensitive area neurons located only a few microns below the surface of the medulla. In contrast to the limited buffering capacity of cerebrospinal fluid, the protein-rich interstitial fluid buffer changes in H^+ concentration.

The effect of increased $PaCO_2$ on alveolar ventilation peaks within 1 minute. After several hours, however, the stimulant effect wanes, reflecting active transport (ion pump) of bicarbonate ions (HCO_3^-) into the cerebrospinal fluid from the blood to return the cerebrospinal fluid pH to a normal value of 7.32 (Mitchell and Berger, 1975). These HCO_3^- combine with excess H^+ in the cerebrospinal fluid and, thus, stimulation of the chemosensitive area decreases with time. Therefore, a change in $PaCO_2$ has an intense initial effect on the control of ventilation but only a weak effect after several hours during which time adaptation occurs (cerebrospinal fluid pH returns to 7.32) by active transport of HCO_3^-.

Chemoreceptors

Carotid and aortic bodies are chemoreceptors located outside the central nervous system that are responsive to changes in the PO_2, PCO_2, and concentration of H^+ (see Fig. 44-10). These chemoreceptors transmit signals via the glossopharyngeal nerves (carotid bodies) and vagus nerves (aortic bodies) to the respiratory center in the medulla. Blood flow through the peripheral chemoreceptors is the highest of any tissue in the body, which means that needs of chemoreceptor tissue can be met almost entirely by dissolved oxygen. Therefore, it is the PaO_2 and not the arterial blood saturation with oxygen (SaO_2) that determines the stimulation level of the peripheral chemoreceptors. This is the reason that anemia or carbon monoxide poisoning, in which the amount of dissolved oxygen and thus PO_2 remain normal, do not stimulate alveolar ventilation via the chemoreceptors. Nevertheless, when mean arterial pressure declines below 60 mmHg, blood flow through chemoreceptors may decrease suf-

ficiently to lower tissue PO_2 and stimulate alveolar ventilation as well as evoke peripheral vasoconstriction in an attempt to restore perfusion pressure.

The carotid bodies are more involved with ventilatory responses than are the aortic bodies. Conversely, aortic bodies are more prominent than carotid bodies in influencing cardiovascular responses. Removal or denervation of the carotid bodies as may occur during carotid endarterectomy results in loss of the ventilatory response to hypoxemia and approximately a 30% reduction in the ventilatory response to carbon dioxide. Normally, peripheral chemoreceptors become strongly stimulated when PaO_2 decreases below approximately 60 mmHg. Conversely, the stimulating effect of increased $PaCO_2$ or H^+ concentrations on the peripheral chemoreceptors is much less than the effect of these changes on the respiratory center via changes in the pH of the cerebrospinal fluid.

The ventilatory response of peripheral chemoreceptors to arterial hypoxemia, metabolic acidosis, or both is greatly attenuated by injected and inhaled anesthetics including even subanesthetic concentrations (0.1 MAC) of volatile anesthetics (Fig. 49-7) (Knill and Clement, 1985). For this reason, arterial hypoxemia that might occur in the early postanesthetic period is unlikely to increase alveolar ventilation.

EFFECTS OF SLEEP ON BREATHING

In alert, conscious humans, stimuli from the environment act reflexively via brain centers to sustain breathing even at low levels of chemical drive. Reductions in the level of environmental stimulation as occur during sleep are associated with modest increases in $PaCO_2$, and the ventilatory response to carbon dioxide is decreased as reflected by rightward displacement of the carbon dioxide response curve. The ventilatory response to hypoxia is better maintained during sleep than are responses to carbon dioxide. Persons with depressed ventilatory responses to hypercapnia and hypoxia while awake breathe even less during sleep than do those who show normal awake responses.

Phasic and tonic activity of skeletal muscles decreases during sleep. Loss of activity in upper airway muscles during sleep is far greater than that of the diaphragm. Because of the relative loss

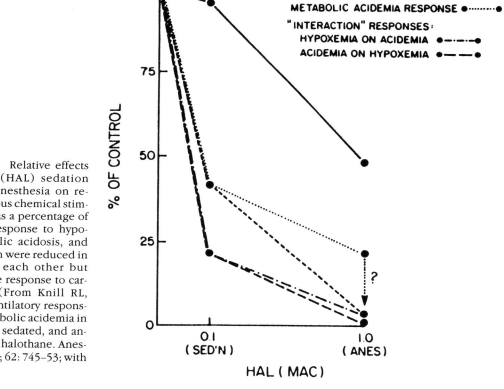

FIGURE 49–7. Relative effects of halothane (HAL) sedation SED'N), and anesthesia on responses to various chemical stimuli, expressed as a percentage of control. The response to hypoxemia, metabolic acidosis, and their interaction were reduced in proportion to each other but greater than the response to carbon dioxide. (From Knill RL, Clement JL. Ventilatory responses to acute metabolic acidemia in humans awake, sedated, and anesthetized with halothane. Anesthesiology 1985; 62: 745–53; with permission.)

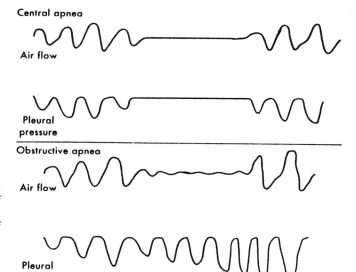

FIGURE 49–8. Central sleep apnea is characterized by cessation of air flow as a result of suspension of all respiratory effects. Obstructive sleep apnea is characterized by cessation of air flow despite persistent respiratory efforts as reflected by pleural pressure changes. (From Berne RM, Levy MN. Physiology. 2nd ed. St. Louis: CV Mosby, 1988; with permission.)

of tone in the upper airway, the negative airway pressure created by the diaphragm during inspiration may be sufficient to occlude the upper airway. Indeed, brief periods of upper airway obstruction occur even in normal people during sleep.

APNEIC PERIODS DURING SLEEP

Apneic periods occur during sleep in approximately one third of normal individuals and are particularly common among elderly men. Apnea may last for more than 10 seconds and may be associated with decreases in SaO_2 to 75% or less. Apneic spells are also common in premature infants.

Sleep apneas are classified as central (cessation of respiratory efforts) or obstructive (despite respiratory efforts, air flow ceases because of total upper airway obstruction) (Fig. 49-8) (Berne and Levy, 1988). Snoring is a manifestation of partial obstruction of the upper airway at sites including the pharynx and oropharynx. This may reflect failure of the genioglossus muscles to contract during inspiration, thus permitting the tongue to fall back and obstruct the upper airway. Arousal is evoked by chemoreceptor activation by hypoxemia. Hypercarbia may also be an important factor in terminating sleep apnea. Recurrent episodes of hypoxemia and hypercarbia may lead to polycythemia and pulmonary hypertension.

PERIODIC BREATHING

Cheyne-Stokes respiration, which is characterized by a waxing and waning pattern of ventilation, is the most common form of periodic breathing. Cyclic increases and decreases in $PaCO_2$ are the presumed mechanism for this form of periodic breathing. The normal absence of Cheyne-Stokes respiration reflects the damping effect provided by large tissue stores of carbon dioxide. When there is a delay in blood flow from the lungs to the brain as in congestive heart failure, however, the respiratory center may lag behind the $PaCO_2$, causing cyclic variations in the alveolar ventilation. Brain stem damage may increase the feedback gain control of the respiratory center such that a small change in $PaCO_2$ causes a large change in alveolar ventilation.

NONVENTILATORY FUNCTIONS OF THE LUNGS

Nonventilatory functions of the lungs include a number of metabolic functions as reflected by both synthesis, release, and removal of biologically active substances (Table 49-2) (Bakhle, 1990). For example, prostaglandins are removed from the circulation but they are also synthesized in the lungs and released into the blood when the lung tissue is stretched. Inhaled anesthetics may interfere with the removal of norepinephrine from the blood by the lungs (Bakhle, 1990). Endothelial cells of the pulmonary capillaries contain the converting enzyme responsible for conversion of angiotensin I to angiotensin II.

Table 49-2
Metabolic Functions of the Lung

Synthesized and used in the lung
  Surfactant

Synthesized and released into the blood
  Prostaglandins
  Histamine
  Kallikrein
  Von Willebrand factor
  Tissue plasminogen activator

Partially removed from the blood
  Prostaglandins
  Bradykinin
  Serotonin
  Norepinephrine
  Acetylcholine
  Fentanyl
  Propranolol
  Lidocaine
  Atrial natriuretic factor
  Adenosine
  Imipramine

Not removed from the blood
  Epinephrine
  Dopamine
  Prostacyclin
  Morphine
  Histamine
  Angiotensin II
  Vasopressin

Activated in the lung
  Angiotensin I
  Arachidonic acid

Methoxyflurane and halothane, but not enflurane, undergo metabolism in the lungs (Blitt et al, 1981). The lungs contain a fibrinolytic system that lyses clots in the pulmonary vessels. Indeed, the pulmonary capillaries, by receiving the entire cardiac output, act as filters for emboli and air. This filter effect is lost in the presence of a right-to-left intracardiac shunt or during cardiopulmonary bypass.

The majority of exogenous substances removed by passage through the pulmonary circulation are not metabolized but instead are bound to components of lung tissue. Drugs most effectively bound to lung tissue are lipid soluble with pK values more than 8.0. Drug extraction by metabolism or binding to tissues may prevent delivery of toxic concentrations of local anesthetics to the systemic circulation. Conversely, first-pass pulmonary uptake of some injected drugs is sufficiently great to influence the peak arterial concentration of these drugs (see Chapter 1).

REFERENCES

Bakhle YS. Pharmacokinetic and metabolic properties of the lung. Br J Anaesth 1990;65:79–93.

Berne RM, Levy MN. Physiology. 2nd ed. St. Louis. CV Mosby. 1988.

Blitt CD, Gandolfi AJ, Soltis JJ, Brown BR. Extrahepatic biotransformation of halothane and enflurane. Anesth Analg 1981;60:129–32.

Guyton AC. Textbook of Medical Physiology. 7th ed. Philadelphia. WB Saunders. 1986.

Knill RL, Clement JL. Ventilatory responses to acute metabolic acidemia in humans awake, sedated, and anesthetized with halothane. Anesthesiology 1985;62:745–53.

Lichtiger M, Landa JF, Hirsch MA. Velocity of tracheal mucous in anesthetized women undergoing gynecologic surgery. Anesthesiology 1975;42:753–6.

Mitchell RA, Berger AJ. Neural regulation of respiration. Am Rev Respir Dis 1975;111:206–24.

Nunn JF. Effects of anaesthesia on respiration. Br J Anaesth 1990;65:54–62.

Paintal AS. Vagal sensory receptors and their reflex effects. Physiol Rev 1973;53:159–227.

Paskin S, Skovsted P, Smith TC. Failure of the Hering-Breuer reflex to account for tachypnea in anesthetized man. A survey of halothane, fluroxene, methoxyflurane, and cyclopropane. Anesthesiology 1968;29:550–8.

Pontoppidan H, Beecher HK. Progressive loss of protective reflexes in the airway with the advance of age. JAMA 1960;174:2209–13.

50

Pulmonary Gas Exchange and Blood Transport of Gases

PULMONARY GAS EXCHANGE

The primary function of the lungs is to provide for the optimal exchange of oxygen and carbon dioxide between the ambient environment and pulmonary capillaries. This gas exchange process is termed *external respiration*. Pulmonary gas transport consists of (1) convection (initial bulk flow of gases in the same direction in the airways); (2) diffusion (random molecular motion leading to complete mixing of all gases beginning at the terminal bronchioles); and (3) gas exchange, which is greatly dependent on the matching of regional alveolar ventilation with pulmonary capillary perfusion ($\dot{V}/\dot{Q}$). Oxygen leaves alveoli to enter pulmonary capillary blood and carbon dioxide enters alveoli from pulmonary capillary blood by the process of diffusion. There is always a net diffusion of molecules from areas of high partial pressure to areas of low partial pressure.

Partial Pressure

The partial pressure (P) that a gas exerts is due to the constant impact of molecules in motion against a surface. The greater the concentration of gas molecules or the higher the temperature, the greater is the sum of the forces of all the molecules striking the surface at any instant. As a re-

sult, the partial pressure of a gas is directly proportional to its concentration and the surrounding temperature.

In a mixture of gases, the partial pressure that each gas contributes to the total partial pressure is directly proportional to its relative concentration (Table 50-1). For example, at sea level, 79% of the total atmospheric pressure (P_B) of 760 mmHg is due to nitrogen (PN_2 597 mmHg) and 21% is due to oxygen (PO_2, 159 mmHg). The P_B is the sum of all the individual partial pressures. Partial pressure may also be expressed in kilopascals (1 kp equals 7.6 mmHg or 10 cm H_2O).

When a gas-liquid or gas-tissue interface exists, gas molecules dissolve in the liquid or tissue until equilibrium is achieved. Equilibrium is present when the number of molecules leaving the gas phase equals the number returning to the gas phase. At equilibrium, the partial pressure of the gas dissolved in the liquid phase is equal to the partial pressure of the gas in the gas phase, each pushing against each other at the interface with equal force.

The concentration of a gas in liquid is determined not only by the partial pressure the gas exerts but also by the solubility coefficient of the gas. For example, some molecules (carbon dioxide) are physically or chemically attracted to water, while others are repelled. Molecules that are attracted to water dissolve in water without

Table 50-1
Partial Pressures of Respiratory Gases at Sea Level (760 mmHg)

Respiratory Gas	Inhaled Air (mmHg)	Alveolar Gases (mmHg)	Exhaled Gases (mmHg)
Oxygen	159	104	120
Carbon dioxide	0.3	40	27
Nitrogen	597	569	566
Water	3.7	47	47

building up excess partial pressure in the solution. Conversely, molecules that are repelled will develop high partial pressure for minimal solubility in a solution. Henry's law states that the concentration of a dissolved gas is equal to the partial pressure of that gas times its solubility coefficient.

Vapor Pressure of Water

Water in tissues has a tendency to escape into an adjoining gas phase just as molecules in the gas phase pass into the water. The pressure that water molecules exert to escape to the surface is the vapor pressure of water (P_{H_2O}). At normal body temperature (37°C), the P_{H_2O} is 47 mmHg. The greater the temperature, the greater the kinetic activity of the molecules and thus the greater the likelihood that water molecules will escape from the surface into the gas phase (P_{H_2O} more than 47 mmHg).

Composition of Alveolar Gases

Composition of alveolar gases is different from the composition of inhaled (atmospheric) gases because (1) oxygen is constantly being absorbed from the alveoli, (2) carbon dioxide is constantly being added to the alveoli, and (3) dry inhaled gases are humidified by the addition of water vapor (Table 50-1). Because the total partial pressure of gases in the alveoli remains unchanged, the addition of water vapor and carbon dioxide to the inhaled gases dilutes the delivered PO_2 from 159 mmHg to 104 mmHg and the PN_2 from 597 mmHg to 569 mmHg.

Alveolar Partial Pressure of Oxygen

The partial pressure of oxygen in the alveoli ($PACO_2$) is determined by the rate of delivery of new oxygen by alveolar ventilation and the rate of absorption of oxygen into pulmonary capillary blood. The normal rate of oxygen absorption in the resting state is 250 ml·min^{-1}. Exercise increases and drug-induced unconsciousness (anesthesia) reduce the need for oxygen absorption (Fig. 50-1).

The inspired partial pressure of oxygen (PIO_2) is diluted by the $PACO_2$ (40 mmHg) and P_{H_2O} (47 mmHg), both of which are independent of P_B. Thus, the impact of this dilution on the PAO_2 is greater when the PIO_2 is already reduced by decreased P_B as associated with altitude. Breathing supplemental oxygen offsets the dilutional effect of carbon dioxide and water vapor.

Alveolar Partial Pressure of Carbon Dioxide

The $PACO_2$ is determined by the rate of carbon dioxide delivery to the alveoli from pulmonary capillary blood and the rate of removal of this carbon dioxide from the alveoli by alveolar ventilation. The normal rate of delivery of carbon dioxide to alveoli by blood is 200 ml·min^{-1}. In the presence of a constant delivery of carbon dioxide to alveoli, the $PACO_2$ is directly proportional to alveolar ventilation.

Composition of Exhaled Gases

The composition of exhaled gases is determined by the proportion that is alveolar gas and the proportion that is dead space gases. The first portion of exhaled gas is from the large conducting airways (no gas exchange occurs) and is designated *dead space gas*. Because gas exchange does not occur in conducting airways, the composition of dead space gas resembles the composition of inhaled gas. Progressively, more and more alveolar gas becomes mixed with dead space gas until all the dead space gas has been exhaled and only alveolar gas remains. For this reason, collection of the last portion of exhaled alveolar gas (end-tidal sample) is a method for analyzing the composition of alveolar gas including anesthetic concentrations. Indeed, minimum alveolar concentration (MAC) uses the alveolar concentration of the inhaled anesthetic as an index of anesthetic depth and to compare equal potent concentrations of inhaled anesthetics. Contamination of end-tidal sample with inhaled gases invalidates the interpretation of the obtained values. Pure end-tidal samples are most reliably obtained from the tracheas of intubated patients.

Gas Diffusion from Alveoli to Blood

At birth, there are an estimated 12 million alveoli in each lung, and this number increases to approximately 150 million in each lung by age 8 to 9 years of age. Each alveolus has a diameter of approximately 0.25 mm. Alveolar walls are extremely thin (0.5 μ) and contain a network of interconnecting capillaries. The average diameter of the pulmonary capillaries is only 8 μ, which means that erythrocytes must squeeze through the vessels in single file such that the distance for diffusion of oxygen and carbon dioxide is minimized. The total surface area available for gas exchange is an estimated 70 m^2 over which 60 to 140 ml of blood are spread as a thin sheet.

In addition to the thickness of the membrane and its surface area, the rate of gas diffusion across the alveolar-capillary membrane is determined by the solubility of the gas in the constituents of the membrane and the partial pressure difference across the membrane. Carbon dioxide diffuses across the membrane approximately 20 times as rapidly as oxygen, and oxygen diffuses about twice as rapidly as nitrogen. The partial pressure difference for gases in blood and alveoli determines the direction of diffusion (oxygen into blood from alveoli and carbon dioxide into alveoli from blood). Any factor that increases the thickness of the membrane two to three times (pulmonary edema) interferes with the diffusion of oxygen more than with that of carbon dioxide. When the total surface area of the membrane is decreased to approximately one fourth normal as by emphysema (in which alveoli coalesce into large sacs), exchange of gases through the respiratory membrane is inadequate even under resting conditions.

O₂ Consumption (ml/min)

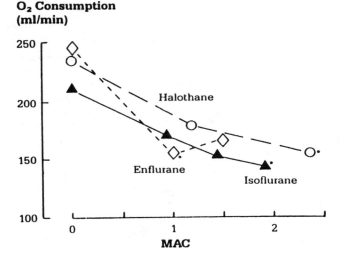

FIGURE 50–1. Potent inhaled anesthetics decrease oxygen consumption with the greatest change occurring in the transition from wakefulness to sleep. (From Eger EI. Isoflurane (Forane). A compendium and reference. Madison, WI. Ohio Medical Products, 1984; with permission.)

Ventilation-to-Perfusion Ratio

The $\dot{V}/\dot{Q}$ ratio determines the composition of the alveolar gas and the effectiveness of gas exchange especially for oxygen across the alveolar-capillary membrane. In the presence of an optimal $\dot{V}/\dot{Q}$ ratio, the PaO_2 is approximately 104 mmHg and the $PaCO_2$ is 40 mmHg. A $\dot{V}/\dot{Q}$ ratio of 0 is present when there is no ventilation to an alveolus that continues to be perfused by pulmonary capillary blood (shunt). A $\dot{V}/\dot{Q}$ ratio equal to infinity means that there is ventilation but no pulmonary capillary blood flow to the alveolus (wasted ventilation).

Physiologic Shunt

Physiologic shunt designates the 2% to 5% of the cardiac output that normally bypasses the lungs by flowing through bronchial veins into pulmonary veins or through Thebesian and anterior cardiac veins into the left side of the heart. Obstructive airway disease as associated with cigarette smoking is a common cause of physiologic shunt. Physiologic shunt is calculated from measurements of the oxygen concentration of mixed venous and arterial blood (Table 50-2).

Physiologic Dead Space

Conducting airways that do not participate in gas exchange as well as ventilation of alveoli in excess of pulmonary capillary blood flow is designated *physiologic dead space*. The ratio of physiologic dead space to tidal volume is calculated by measuring the tidal volume, the $PaCO_2$, and the $P_{ET}CO_2$ (Table 50-3).

Table 50-2
Calculation of Physiologic Shunt Fraction

$$Q_s/Q_T = \frac{Cc'O_2 - CaO_2}{Cc'O_2 - CvO_2}$$

Q_s = amount of pulmonary blood flow not exposed to ventilated alveoli

Q_T = total pulmonary blood flow

$Cc'O_2$ = O_2 content of pulmonary capillary blood, ml·dl^{-1}

CaO_2 = O_2 content of arterial blood, ml·dl^{-1}

CvO_2 = O_2 content of mixed venous blood, ml·dl^{-1}

Table 50-3
Calculation of the Physiologic Dead Space to Tidal Volume Ratio

$$V_D/V_T = \frac{PaCO_2 - P_{ET}CO_2}{PaCO_2}$$

V_D/V_T = ratio of physiologic dead space to V_T

$PaCO_2$ = arterial partial pressure of CO_2, mmHg

$P_{ET}CO_2$ = mixed exhaled partial pressure of CO_2, mmHg

BLOOD TRANSPORT OF OXYGEN AND CARBON DIOXIDE

After diffusion from alveoli into pulmonary capillary blood, oxygen is transported principally in combination with hemoglobin to tissue capillaries where it is released along a partial pressure gradient for use by cells. Carbon dioxide, formed in the cells from oxygen-dependent metabolic pathways, enters tissue capillaries along a partial pressure gradient for transport back to alveoli.

Oxygen Uptake into the Blood

The PvO_2 is approximately 40 mmHg, reflecting the large amount of oxygen that has been removed from the blood as it passes through various tissues (Fig. 50-2) (Guyton, 1986). This

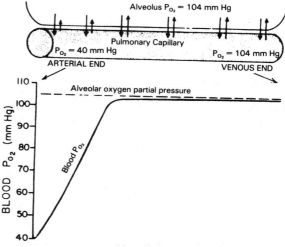

FIGURE 50–2. Schematic depiction of the uptake of oxygen by pulmonary capillary blood. (From Guyton AC. Textbook of Medical Physiology. 7th ed. Philadelphia: WB Saunders, 1986; with permission.)

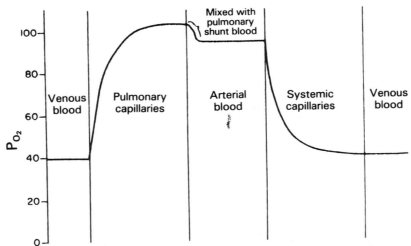

FIGURE 50-3.   Changes in the PO_2 as blood traverses the systemic and pulmonary circulations. (From Guyton AC. Textbook of Medical Physiology. 7th ed. Philadelphia: WB Saunders, 1986; with permission.)

mixed venous blood is exposed to a PAO_2 of approximately 104 mmHg, leading to a rapid diffusion of oxygen along this partial pressure gradient into pulmonary capillary blood. Indeed, the PO_2 of pulmonary capillary blood is nearly equal to the PAO_2 after passing through only the first one third of the capillary (Fig. 50-2) (Guyton, 1986). This rapid equilibration of pulmonary capillary blood with the PAO_2 provides an important safety factor for transfer of oxygen when blood flow through the lungs is accelerated as during exercise. Blood leaving the pulmonary capillaries has a PO_2 of approximately 104 mmHg, whereas the arterial blood, which contains bronchial blood flow has a PaO_2 of approximately 95 mmHg (Fig. 50-3) (Guyton, 1986). This is due to the diluent effect produced by the low PO_2 in the bronchial blood.

Diffusion of Oxygen from the Capillaries

Interstitial fluid PO_2 averages approximately 40 mmHg, providing a large initial partial pressure gradient for diffusion of oxygen from tissue capillaries with a PaO_2 near 95 mmHg (Fig. 50-4) (Guyton, 1986). At the end of the capillary, the PO_2 in blood and the interstitial fluid have nearly equilibrated such that the PvO_2 is also approximately 40 mmHg. Because approximately 97% of the oxygen transported in blood is carried by hemoglobin, a decrease in the concentration of hemoglobin has the same effect on interstitial fluid PO_2 as does a decrease in tissue blood flow.

Diffusion of Carbon Dioxide from the Cells

Continuous formation of carbon dioxide in cells maintains a partial pressure gradient for its diffusion into capillary blood (Fig. 50-5) (Guyton, 1986). Diffusion of carbon dioxide from cells into capillaries is rapid despite a partial pressure gradient of only 1 to 6 mmHg compared with approximately 64 mmHg for oxygen. On arrival at alveoli, the $PvCO_2$ is only 5 to 6 mmHg greater

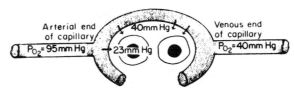

FIGURE 50-4.   Schematic depiction of the diffusion of oxygen from tissue capillaries into the interstitial fluid. (From Guyton AC. Textbook of Medical Physiology. 7th ed. Philadelphia: WB Saunders, 1986; with permission.)

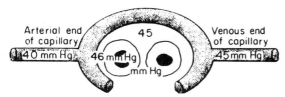

FIGURE 50–5. Schematic depiction of uptake of carbon dioxide by capillary blood. (From Guyton AC. Textbook of Medical Physiology. 7th ed. Philadelphia: WB Saunders, 1986; with permission.)

than the $PACO_2$. Nevertheless, passage from the capillaries to blood, like that from tissues into capillaries is rapid, reflecting the fact that the diffusion coefficient for carbon dioxide is 20 times that for oxygen.

Blood Transport of Oxygen

Approximately 97% of oxygen transported from alveoli to tissues is carried to tissues in chemical combination with hemoglobin, while approximately 3% of oxygen is transported in the dissolved state in plasma. A single molecule of hemoglobin can combine with four molecules of oxygen. When the PO_2 in pulmonary capillaries is elevated, oxygen binds with hemoglobin, but when the PO_2 is low as in tissue capillaries, oxygen is released from hemoglobin. This reaction occurs independently of any enzyme action or change in the ferrous state of iron in the hemoglobin molecule. Therefore, this uptake of oxygen by hemoglobin is termed oxygenation rather than oxidation.

Each gram of hemoglobin can combine with approximately 1.34 ml of oxygen (1.39 ml when hemoglobin is chemically pure). This combination is rapid, requiring approximately 10 ms. In the presence of a normal hemoglobin concentration of 15 $g \cdot dl^{-1}$, blood will carry approximately 20 ml of oxygen when the hemoglobin is 100% saturated. Approximately 5 ml of this 20 ml passes to tissues, reducing the hemoglobin saturation with oxygen to approximately 75%, corresponding to a PvO_2 of approximately 40 mmHg.

The amount of oxygen dissolved in plasma is a linear function of the PO_2 (0.003 $ml \cdot mmHg^{-1}$ or 0.3 ml·100 dl^{-1} when the PO_2 is 100 mmHg). Approximately 0.29 ml of oxygen is dissolved in 100 dl of blood when the PO_2 is 95 mmHg. When the

PO_2 of blood declines to 40 mmHg in tissue capillaries, approximately 0.12 ml of oxygen remains dissolved. This means that approximately 0.17 ml of oxygen is delivered to tissues in the dissolved state in 100 dl of blood compared with approximately 5 ml of oxygen attached to hemoglobin in the same amount of blood. Under resting conditions, approximately 5 ml of oxygen is released to the tissues for every 100 dl of blood, resulting in a total delivery of oxygen to tissues of 250 $ml \cdot min^{-1}$ when the cardiac output is 5 $L \cdot min^{-1}$. Ultimately, the amount of oxygen available each minute for use in any given tissue is determined by the content of oxygen in blood and the tissue blood flow.

Hemoglobin

Hemoglobin is a conjugated protein with a molecular weight of 66,700. The four heme molecules, each with a central iron atom, combine with *globin,* a globular protein synthesized in the ribosomes of the endoplasmic reticulum to form hemoglobin. The globin portion of the hemoglobin molecule comprises four polypeptide chains of more than 700 amino acids. The sequence of these amino acids, which is determined genetically, influences the binding affinity of hemoglobin for oxygen.

TYPES OF HEMOGLOBIN. Hemoglobin types are designated as A through S, depending on the sequence of amino acids in the polypeptide chains. Normal adult hemoglobin A consists of two identical alpha and beta polypeptide chains. Fetal erythrocytes contain hemoglobin F, which has a low concentration of 2,3 diphosphoglycerate (2,3-DPG) and a resulting high affinity for oxygen, which facilitates transfer of oxygen from the placenta to the fetus. Indeed, at a normal umbilical vein PO_2 of 28 mmHg, hemoglobin F is 80% saturated with oxygen (oxyhemoglobin dissociation curve shifted to the left), while hemoglobin A would only be approximately 50% saturated with oxygen at this same PO_2 (Fig. 50-6). After birth, the presence of hemoglobin F impairs release of oxygen to tissues accounting for the disappearance of hemoglobin F by 4 to 6 months of age.

With the exception of hemoglobin A and hemoglobin F, all other forms of hemoglobin are considered abnormal. The oxyhemoglobin dissociation curve for abnormal hemoglobin is shifted to the right, which interferes with transfer of oxy-

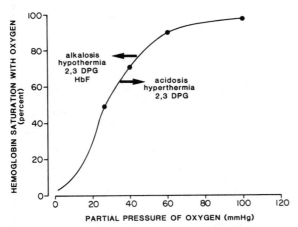

FIGURE 50-6. Oxyhemoglobin dissociation curve for hemoglobin A at pH 7.4 and 37°C. Changes in pH, body temperature, concentration of 2,3-diphosphyglycerate (2,3 DPG) and presence of different types of hemoglobin F shift the oxyhemoglobin dissociation curve to the left or right of its normal position.

gen from alveoli to hemoglobin. Abnormal hemoglobin results from changes in the amino acid sequences of the polypeptide chains of globin. For example, substitution of valene for glutamic acid in two of the four polypeptide chains of hemoglobin A results in hemoglobin S. Erythrocytes containing hemoglobin S become elongated when exposed to low concentrations of oxygen and are known as *sickle cells.*

MYOGLOBIN. *Myoglobin* is an iron-containing pigment resembling hemoglobin which is present in skeletal muscle. Unlike hemoglobin, myoglobin binds only one molecule of oxygen and this oxygen cannot be released until the PO_2 has decreased to very low values.

Oxyhemoglobin Dissociation Curve

The percentage of hemoglobin saturation with oxygen at different partial pressures of oxygen in the blood is described by the oxyhemoglobin dissociation curve (Fig. 50-6). The *S*-shape of the oxyhemoglobin dissociation curve explains important properties of hemoglobin. For example, increasing PaO_2 above 100 mmHg increases the concentration of oxygen in the blood only slightly. This reflects the fact that hemoglobin is already at least 97% saturated with oxygen when the PaO_2 is 100 mmHg. Likewise, reducing the PaO_2 to 60 mmHg maintains at least 90% saturation of hemoglobin with oxygen, reflecting the flat aspect of the oxyhemoglobin dissociation curve over this range. At tissue capillaries where the PO_2 is 20 to 40 mmHg, the oxyhemoglobin dissociation curve is steep such that small changes in the PaO_2 result in transfer of large amounts of oxygen from hemoglobin to tissues.

Shift of the Oxyhemoglobin Dissociation Curve

Factors that influence the position of the oxyhemoglobin dissociation curve include (1) hydrogen ion (H^+) concentration of the blood, (2) body temperature, (3) concentration of 2,3-DPG, and (4) type of hemoglobin (Fig. 50-6). For unknown reasons, inhaled anesthetics produce a modest rightward shift of the oxyhemoglobin dissociation curve (Gillies et al, 1970, Kambam, 1982). A convenient indicator of the position of the oxyhemoglobin dissociation curve is the PO_2 that produces 50% saturation of hemoglobin with oxygen. The PO_2 that produces this degree of hemoglobin saturation with oxygen is designated the P_{50}. In the normal adult at a pH of 7.4 and body temperature of 37°C, the P_{50} is approximately 26 mmHg (Fig. 50-6). A shift of the oxyhemoglobin dissociation curve to the right is reflected by an increase in the P_{50} to more than 26 mmHg, whereas the P_{50} is less than 26 mmHg when the oxyhemoglobin dissociation curve is shifted to the left. A shift of the oxyhemoglobin dissociation curve to the left means the PO_2 must decline further before oxygen is released from hemoglobin to tissues.

BOHR EFFECT. The shift in the position of the oxyhemoglobin dissociation curve caused by carbon dioxide entering or leaving the blood is the *Bohr effect.* For example, at tissues, carbon dioxide enters blood, causing the pH to decrease (acidosis), and the oxyhemoglobin dissociation curve shifts to the right, facilitating the release of oxygen from hemoglobin. The reverse change at the lungs results in alkalosis with a leftward shift of the oxyhemoglobin dissociation curve, thus enhancing the affinity of hemoglobin for oxygen.

2,3-DIPHOSPHOGLYCERATE. The effect of 2,3-DPG is to decrease the affinity of hemoglobin for oxygen (by shifting the oxyhemoglobin dissociation curve to the right), causing oxygen to be released to tissues at a higher PaO_2 than in the absence of this substance. Increases in the erythrocyte content of 2,3-DPG are evoked by anemia and arterial hypoxemia as produced by ascent to altitude. Storage of whole blood is associated with a progressive decline in erythrocyte content of 2,3-DPG. This decline is less in blood preserved in citrate-phosphate-dextrose than in acid-citrate-dextrose.

EXERCISE. During exercise, the oxyhemoglobin dissociation curve for skeletal muscle is shifted to the right, reflecting release of carbon dioxide by exercising muscle. In addition, temperature of exercising muscle may increase $3°C$ to $4°C$. These changes permit hemoglobin to continue to release oxygen to skeletal muscles even when the PO_2 in the blood has decreased to as low as 40 mmHg.

Carbon Monoxide

Carbon monoxide combines with hemoglobin at the same point on the hemoglobin molecule as does oxygen. Furthermore, the strength of this bonding is approximately 230 times greater than that exhibited by oxygen. Therefore, a carbon monoxide partial pressure of 0.4 mmHg is equivalent to a PO_2 of 92 mmHg. At this partial pressure of carbon monoxide, approximately half the hemoglobin is bound with this gas rather than oxygen. A carbon monoxide partial pressure of 0.7 mmHg can bind nearly all the hemoglobin sites normally occupied by oxygen. The PaO_2 remains normal despite the absence of oxyhemoglobin, reflecting the fact that dissolved oxygen and not that attached to hemoglobin determines the PO_2. Chemoreceptors that increase alveolar ventilation are not stimulated because the PaO_2 remains normal. The only treatment of carbon monoxide poisoning is administration of oxygen that produces a high PaO_2 to displace carbon monoxide from hemoglobin. This is the reason for considering the use of a hyperbaric oxygen chamber in the treatment of severe carbon monoxide poisoning.

Carbon monoxide results from incomplete combustion of organic matter and is the most abundant pollutant in the lower atmosphere. The automobile is the greatest source of carbon mon-

oxide. Another source of carboxyhemoglobin is cigarette smoking. Most victims of fires die from acute carbon monoxide poisoning. There is no excretion of carbon monoxide without alveolar ventilation. Therefore, valid measurements of carboxyhemoglobin concentrations can be obtained long after death.

Cyanosis

Blueness of the skin caused by excessive amounts of reduced hemoglobin in cutaneous capillaries is designated *cyanosis*. More than 5 g of reduced hemoglobin causes cyanosis regardless of the overall concentration of oxyhemoglobin. Therefore, patients with polycythemia may appear cyanotic despite adequate arterial concentrations of oxygen, whereas the anemic patient may lack sufficient hemoglobin to produce enough reduced hemoglobin to cause cyanosis even in the presence of profound tissue hypoxia. The degree of cyanosis is influenced by the rate of blood flow through the skin. If cutaneous blood flow is sluggish, even low skin metabolism may result in production of sufficient reduced hemoglobin to cause cyanosis. This explains the occurrence of peripheral cyanosis in cold weather particularly when the skin permits transmission of the color of reduced hemoglobin from the deeper vascular structures.

Blood Transport of Carbon Dioxide

Carbon dioxide formed as a result of metabolic processes in cells readily diffuses across cell membranes into capillary blood. Despite a small partial pressure difference between tissues and blood (1 to 6 mmHg), the high solubility of carbon dioxide (20 times more soluble than oxygen) permits rapid transfer. An average of 4 ml carbon dioxide in each $100 \ dl^{-1}$ of blood is transported to the lungs as (1) dissolved carbon dioxide, (2) bicarbonate ions (HCO_3^-), and (3) carbaminohemoglobin (Fig. 50-7) (Guyton, 1986).

Approximately 0.3 ml of the 4 ml carbon dioxide in every 100 dl of blood is transported to the lungs in the dissolved state. The $PvCO_2$ is increased approximately 5 mmHg compared with the $PaCO_2$, reflecting the addition of carbon dioxide from the tissues. This increase in the $PvCO_2$

lowers the venous blood pH to 7.36 compared with a pH of 7.4 in arterial blood and a $PaCO_2$ of 40 mmHg. The ratio of dissolved carbon dioxide to HCO_3^- is normally 20:1.

Approximately 2.8 ml of the 4 ml of carbon dioxide in every 100 dl of blood enters erythrocytes, where it reacts with water to form carbonic acid (Fig. 50-7) (Guyton, 1986). This reaction in erythrocytes is almost instantaneous due to the accelerating effects of the enzyme carbonic anhydrase. Carbonic anhydrase is essentially absent in the plasma. Immediately following the formation of carbonic acid, there is dissociation into H^+ and HCO_3^-. Most of the H^+ combines with reduced hemoglobin, which acts as a powerful acid-base buffer. HCO_3^- diffuses from erythrocytes into plasma and chloride ions (Cl^-) enter the cell to maintain electrochemical neutrality (chloride shift). The increase in osmotically active ions such as Cl^- and HCO_3^- in venous erythrocytes causes water retention by these cells, leading to an increase in their size. This is the reason a venous hematocrit is approximately 3% greater than the arterial hematocrit.

Haldane Effect

At the lungs, the combination of oxygen with hemoglobin causes hemoglobin to become a stronger acid. As a result, carbaminohemoglobin dissociates and the increased acidity provides H^+ to combine with HCO_3^- to form carbonic acid. Carbonic acid rapidly dissociates into water and carbon dioxide with the carbon dioxide instantly diffusing from pulmonary capillary blood into alveoli. This displacement of carbon dioxide from hemoglobin by oxygen that occurs at the lungs is known as the *Haldane effect.* The Haldane effect at the tissues facilitates the passage of carbon dioxide into the blood.

Body Stores of Carbon Dioxide

In contrast to total body oxygen stores of approximately 1.5 L (approximately 1 L in arterial blood), there are an estimated 120 L of carbon dioxide dissolved in the body. In the presence of apnea but provision of oxygen (apneic oxygenation), the rate at which the $PaCO_2$ rises during the first minute of apnea is approximately 5 to 10 mmHg (Eger and Severinghaus, 1961). This initial rapid rise in the $PaCO_2$ represents equilibration of the alveolar gas with the $PvCO_2$. Following the first minute of apnea, the $PaCO_2$ increases approximately 3 mmHg·min⁻¹, reflecting metabolic production of carbon dioxide.

Respiratory Quotient

The ratio of carbon dioxide output to oxygen uptake is the *respiratory quotient.* During resting conditions, the amount of oxygen added to blood (5 ml·dl⁻¹) exceeds the amounts of carbon dioxide that is removed from the blood (4 ml·dl⁻¹), resulting in a respiratory quotient of 0.8. The respiratory quotient varies with different metabolic conditions, being 1 when carbohydrates are being used exclusively for metabolism and decreasing to 0.7 when fat is the primary source of metabolic energy. The reason for this difference is the formation of one molecule of carbon dioxide for every molecule of oxygen consumed when carbohydrates are metabolized. When oxygen reacts with fats, a substantial amount of oxygen combines with H^+ to form water instead of carbon dioxide, thus reducing the respiratory quotient to near 0.7. Consumption of a normal diet consisting of carbohydrates, fats, and proteins results in a respiratory quotient of approximately 0.83.

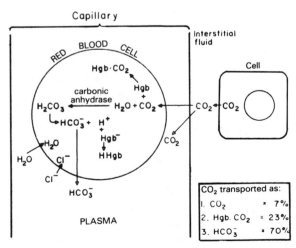

FIGURE 50–7. Schematic depiction of transport of carbon dioxide in blood. (From Guyton AC. Textbook of Medical Physiology. 7th ed. Philadelphia: WB Saunders, 1986; with permission.)

Table 50-4

Effects of Altitude on Respiratory Gases While Breathing Air

Altitude (m/feet)	P_B (mmHg)	PIO_2 (mmHg)	PAO_2 (mmHg)	$PACO_2$ (mmHg)	SaO_2 (percent)
Sea level	760	159	104	40	97
3300/10,000	523	110 (436)*	67	36	90
6600/20,000	349	73	40	24	70
9900/30,000	226	47	21	24	20

*Breathing 100% oxygen.

CHANGES ASSOCIATED WITH HIGH ALTITUDE

The total partial pressure of all gases in the atmosphere (P_B) decreases progressively as distance above sea level increases (Table 50-4; Fig. 50-8) (Ganong, 1987). For example, the P_B is 760 mmHg at sea level and 523 mmHg at 3300 m (10,000 ft) above sea level. Because the concentration of oxygen remains constant at approximately 21%, the decrease in the P_B above sea level is associated with a progressive decrease in the PO_2. For example, the PO_2 at sea level is 159 mmHg (21% × 760 mmHg) and 110 mmHg at 3300 m (21% × 523 mmHg). The decrease in the P_B with increasing altitude is not linear because air is compressible (Fig. 50-8) (Ganong, 1987).

The pharmacologic effect of inhaled anesthetics is reduced by decreased P_B. For example, 60% inhaled nitrous oxide produces a P_{N_2O} of 456 mmHg at sea level compared with a P_{N_2O} of 314 mmHg at 3300 m. The inhaled concentration of nitrous oxide at 3300 m elevation would have to be 87% to produce the same partial pressure produced by breathing 60% nitrous oxide at sea level. Likewise, 1% inhaled isoflurane producing 7.6 mmHg at sea level would have to be increased to nearly 1.5% to produce the same partial pressure at 3300 m.

Mental function remains intact up to 2700 to

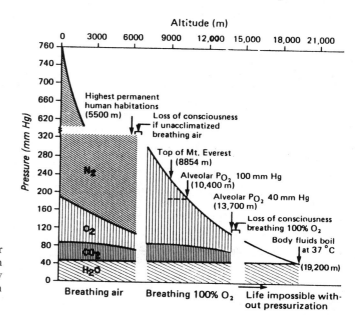

FIGURE 50-8. Composition of alveolar air breathing air (0–6100 m) and 100% oxygen (6100–13,700 m). (From Ganong WF. Review of Medical Physiology. Norwalk, CT: Appleton and Lange, 1987; with permission.)

3300 m above sea level. The frequency of breathing ordinarily does not increase until one ascends above 2400 m, at which point the peripheral chemoreceptors are stimulated.

Acclimatization to Altitude

Acclimatization to altitude occurs because of several compensatory responses (Table 50-5). The initial increase in alveolar ventilation lowers the $PaCO_2$, which blunts the magnitude of this compensatory response. Within a few days, however, active transport of HCO_3^- returns the cerebrospinal fluid pH to normal and alveolar ventilation again increases despite a low $PaCO_2$. Increased production of hemoglobin requires several months to reach its maximal effect, during which time the hemoglobin concentration may increase to more than 20 g·dl^{-1}. In addition, the plasma volume may increase as much as 30%. Cardiac output often increases as much as 30% immediately after ascent to altitude, but this increase is transient, returning to normal in a few days. Chronic exposure to altitude is associated with increased numbers of mitochondria and certain cellular oxidative systems, presumably reflecting improved ability to use available oxygen.

Acute Mountain Sickness

Acute mountain sickness is a syndrome of headache, insomnia, dyspnea, anorexia, and fatigue that has been described on rapid ascent to even intermediate altitude (2000 m) (Montgomery et al, 1989). Symptoms usually develop 8 to 24 hours after arrival at altitude and last 4 to 8 days. It is speculated that the low PO_2 at high altitude causes arteriolar dilation, and if cerebral autoregulation does not compensate, there is an in-

Table 50–5
Compensatory Responses Evoked by Ascent to Altitude

Increased alveolar ventilation

Increased hemoglobin production

Increased 2, 3-diphosphoglycerate concentrations

Increased diffusing capacity of the lungs

Increased vascularity of the tissues

Increased cellular use of oxygen

lary pressure that favors increased transudation of fluid into brain tissue. Alkalosis produced by treatment with acetazolamide is effective in reducing symptoms.

High-altitude pulmonary edema and cerebral edema are serious forms of acute mountain sickness. Pulmonary edema is apt to occur in individuals who ascent to altitudes above 2500 m and engage in strenuous physical activity during the first 3 days after arrival. Pulmonary hypertension is prominent and the protein content of edema fluid is high.

Chronic Mountain Sickness

An occasional sea level native who remains for prolonged periods at high altitude may develop chronic mountain sickness characterized by polycythemia, pulmonary hypertension, and right ventricular failure. Presumably, the increased hemoglobin concentration so increases the viscosity of blood that tissue blood flow becomes inadequate; at the same time, chronic arterial hypoxemia causes vasospasm of pulmonary vessels. Recovery is usually prompt when these individuals return to sea level.

CHANGES ASSOCIATED WITH EXCESSIVE BAROMETRIC PRESSURE

The P_B increases the equivalent of 1 atmosphere for every 10 m below the surface of sea water (10.4 m for fresh water). For example, a person 10 m beneath the water surface is exposed to 2 atm, reflecting the 1 atmosphere of pressure caused by the weight of air above the water and the second atmosphere by the weight of water. At 20 m below the water surface, the P_B is equivalent to 3 atm.

Another important effect of increased P_B below the surface of the water is compression of gases in the lungs to smaller volumes. High P_B produces nitrogen narcosis when the inhaled gases are air. Presumably, the PN_2 at an elevated P_B causes sufficient absorption and deposition of nitrogen molecules in lipid membranes to produce an anesthetic effect. Helium can be substituted for nitrogen to avoid narcosis associated with absorption of nitrogen. In addition to a lesser sedative effect, helium is less soluble, thus reducing the quantity of bubbles that result with return to normal P_B.

Nitrogen that is absorbed at high P_B remains dissolved in the tissues until the PN_2 of nitrogen decreases. Decompression sickness (caisson disease) occurs when sudden decreases in the P_B allow nitrogen bubbles to develop in body tissues and fluid. Nitrogen bubbles develop because pressure on the outside of the body is no longer able to keep the excess gas absorbed during high P_B in solution. As a result, nitrogen can escape from the dissolved state and form bubbles in the tissues. The most frequent sign of nitrogen bubble formation is pain in the extremities; the most serious sequelae are seizures and cerebral ischemia that occur as a result of bubble formation in the central nervous system. Nitrogen bubbles that form in the blood block pulmonary blood flow manifesting as dyspnea ("cho kes"). Symptoms of decompression sickness usually appear within minutes but may also be delayed for as long as 6 hours or more after decompression. The period during which a diver must be decompressed depends on the depth of submersion and duration of exposure. For example, submersion at 60 m for 1 hour requires approximately 3 hours for decompression.

Hyperbaric Oxygen Therapy

Hyperbaric oxygen therapy involves intermittent inhalation of 100% oxygen. Indications for hyperbaric oxygen therapy are evolving with primary treatment for decompression sickness and massive air embolism being a widely accepted use (Table 50-6) (Grim et al, 1990). Patients with carbon monoxide poisoning improve rapidly following treatment with hyperbaric oxygen. For example, the elimination half-time of carboxyhemoglobin is decreased from 320 minutes breathing room air to 80 minutes with 100% oxygen and 23 minutes with 100% oxygen at 3 atmospheres.

Table 50–6
Indications for Hyperbaric Oxygen Therapy

Decompression sickness

Air embolism

Carbon monoxide poisoning

Clostridial gangrene

Refractory osteomyelitis

Radiation necrosis

Profound anemia

Table 50–7
Complications of Hyperbaric Oxygen Therapy

Tympanic membrane rupture

Nasal sinus trauma

Pneumothorax

Air embolism

Central nervous system toxicity

Oxygen toxicity

Most hyperbaric oxygen treatments are performed at 2 to 3 atm. In treatment of decompression sickness and air embolism, where a mechanical reduction in bubble size by an increase in ambient pressure is crucial to therapeutic effect, treatments often are initiated at 6 atmosheres. For example, at 6 atmospheres, a bubble is reduced to 20% of its original volume and 60% of its original diameter.

Complications of hyperbaric oxygen therapy reflect barometric pressure changes or oxygen toxicity (Table 50-7) (Grim et al, 1990). The most common complications involve cavity trauma owing to changes in pressure. Any air-filled cavity that cannot equilibrate with ambient pressure, such as the middle ear when the eustachian tube is blocked, is subject to barotrauma during hyperbaric oxygen therapy. Almost all patients show oxygen toxicity after 6 continuous hours of 100% oxygen at 2 atmospheres. No hyperbaric oxygen therapy protocol requires this length of continuous exposure. Even 80% to 100% oxygen inhaled at 1 atmosphere for 8 hours or more causes the respiratory passageways to become irritated, manifesting as substernal distress, nasal congestion, sore throat, and coughing. Exposure for 24 to 48 hours at 1 atmosphere may cause damage to capillary endothelium with exudation of fluid into the interstitial spaces of the lung and development of pulmonary edema.

REFERENCES

Eger EI. Isoflurane (Forane). A compendium and reference. Madison WI. Ohio Medical Products. 1984.

Eger EI, Severinghaus JW. The rate of rise of $PaCO_2$ in the apneic anesthetized patient. Anesthesiology 1961;44:419–25.

Ganong WF. Review of Medical Physiology. Norwalk CT. Appleton and Lange. 1987.

Gillies IDS, Bird BD, Normal J, Gordon-Smith EC,

Whitwam JG. The effect of anaesthesia on the oxyhaemoglobin dissociation curve. Br J Anaesth 1970;42–561.

Grim PS, Gottlieb LJ, Boddie A, Batson E. Hyperbaric oxygen therapy. JAMA 1990;263:2216–20.

Guyton AC. Textbook of Medical Physiology. 7th ed. Philadelphia. WB Saunders. 1986.

Kamban JR. Isoflurane and oxy-hemoglobin dissociation. Anesthesiology 1982;57:A496.

Montgomery AB, Mills J, Lee JM. Incidence of acute mountain sickness at intermediate altitude. JAMA 1989;261:732–4.

Chapter

51

Acid-Base Balance

The concentrations of hydrogen (H^+) and bicarbonate (HCO_3^-) ions in plasma must be precisely regulated in the face of enormous variations in dietary intake, metabolic production, and normal excretory losses of these ions. Small changes in H^+ concentration from the normal value can cause marked alterations in enzyme activity and the rates of chemical reactions in the cells. H^+ are continuously produced as substrates are oxidized in the production of adenosine triphosphate. The largest contribution of metabolic acids arises from the oxidation of carbohydrates, principally glucose. The net production of H^+ by an individual consuming a mixed diet is approximately 60 mEq·day^{-1}.

The H^+ concentration is regulated to maintain the arterial pH between 7.35 and 7.45. The pH is equivalent to the negative logarithm of the H^+ concentration, which is most often expressed in nmol·L^{-1}. The pH notation is useful for expressing H^+ concentrations in the body because H^+ concentrations are low relative to other cations. For example, a normal pH of 7.4 is equivalent to an H^+ concentration of 40 nmol·L^{-1}, whereas a normal plasma concentration of sodium ions (Na^+) is 1 million times greater (140,000,000 nmol·L^{-1} or 140 mEq·L^{-1}). Compared with the osmotic effect of Na^+, the osmotic effect of H^+ is negligible. Expression of H^+ concentration as pH conceptually masks large variations in H^+ concentration despite small changes in pH. For example, a pH range of 7.1 to 7.7 is associated with a five-fold change (100 nmol·L^{-1} to 20 nmol·L^{-1}) in H^+ concentration (Table 51-1).

The pH of venous blood and interstitial fluids is approximately 7.35, reflecting the impact of additional carbon dioxide that forms carbonic acid. Intracellular pH is 6 to 7.4 in different cells, averaging approximately 7.0. A rapid rate of metabolism in cells increases carbon dioxide production and consequently decreases intracellular pH. Poor tissue blood flow also causes accumulation of carbon dioxide and a decrease in intracellular pH.

MECHANISMS FOR REGULATION OF HYDROGEN ION CONCENTRATION

Regulation of pH over a narrow range is a complex physiologic process that depends on (1) buffer systems, (2) ventilatory responses, and (3) renal responses. The buffer system mechanism is rapid but incomplete. Ventilatory and renal responses develop less rapidly but often produce nearly complete correction of the pH.

Table 51–1
Relation of Hydrogen Ion (H^+) Concentration to pH

H^+ (nmol·L^{-1})	pH
80	7.10
63	7.20
50	7.30
42	7.38
40	7.40
38	7.42
32	7.50
25	7.60
20	7.70

Buffer Systems

All body fluids contain acid-base buffer systems that instantly combine with any acid or alkali to prevent excessive changes in the H⁺ concentration, thus maintaining the pH near 7.4 (Fig. 51-1). By convention, an acid is any substance that increases the H⁺ concentration (a proton donor) and an alkali decreases the H⁺ concentration (a proton acceptor). A strong acid such as hydrochloric acid is fully dissociated to H⁺ and Cl⁻, whereas carbonic acid, which is a weaker acid, dissociates only partially to H⁺ and HCO_3^-.

Hemoglobin Buffering System

Hemoglobin, because of its higher concentration, is a more effective buffer than plasma proteins. The buffering capacity of hemoglobin varies with oxygenation with reduced hemoglobin being a weaker acid than oxyhemoglobin. As a result, at the capillaries, dissociation of oxyhemoglobin makes more base available to combine with H⁺ produced by the dissociation of carbonic acid in the tissues.

Protein Buffering System

The protein buffering system, because of the high intracellular concentration of proteins, is the most potent buffering system in the body. It is estimated that approximately 75% of all the buffering of body fluids occurs intracellularly and most of this results from intracellular proteins. For example, H⁺ produced in the mitochondria are buffered by local proteins. In the plasma, the low concentration of proteins limits their role as buffers in extracellular fluid.

Phosphate Buffering System

The phosphate buffering system is especially important in renal tubules where phosphate is greatly concentrated because of its poor reab-

sorption and concomitant reabsorption of water. Furthermore, renal tubular fluid is more acidic than extracellular fluid, bringing the pH of renal tubular fluid closer to the pK (6.8) of the phosphate buffering system. The phosphate buffering system is also important in intracellular fluids because the concentration of phosphate in these fluids is much greater than the concentration in extracellular fluid. Furthermore, like the renal tubular fluid, the more acidic pH of intracellular fluid is closer to the pK of the phosphate buffering system than is the pH of extracellular fluid.

Bicarbonate Buffering System

The HCO_3^- buffering system accounts for greater than 50% of the total buffering capacity of blood. HCO_3^- diffuse relatively easily into erythrocytes such that approximately one third of the HCO_3^- buffering capacity of blood occurs in erythrocytes. In contrast, the electrical charge of HCO_3^- limits diffusion of these ions into cells other than erythrocytes. The HCO_3^- buffering system is not a powerful buffer because its pK of 6.1 differs greatly from the normal pH of 7.4. This difference in pK and pH means that the ratio of HCO_3^- is 20:1. The Henderson-Hasselbalch equation can be used to calculate the pH of a solution if the concentration of HCO_3^- and dissolved carbon dioxide are known (Fig. 51-2).

The HCO_3^- buffering system consists of carbonic acid and sodium bicarbonate. Carbonic acid is a weak acid because of its limited degree of dissociation (estimated to be less than 5%) into H⁺ and HCO_3^- compared with that of other acids (Fig. 51-3). Furthermore, 99% of carbonic acid in solution almost immediately dissociates into carbon dioxide and water, with the net result being a high concentration of dissolved carbon dioxide but only a weak concentration of acid. Ordinarily, the amount of dissolved carbon dioxide is approximately 1000 times the concentration of the undissociated acid. The addition of a strong acid such as hydrochloric acid to the HCO_3^- buffer system results in conversion of the strong acid to weak carbonic acid (Fig. 51-4). Therefore, a strong acid

$$HHb \rightleftharpoons H^+ + Hb^-$$

$$HProt \rightleftharpoons H^+ + Prot^-$$

$$H_2PO_4^- \rightleftharpoons H^+ + HPO_4^{2-}$$

$$H_2CO_3 \rightleftharpoons H^+ + HCO_3^-$$

FIGURE 51-1.   Buffering systems present in the body.

$$pH = 6.10 + \log \frac{HCO_3^-}{PaCO_2 \ (0.03)}$$

FIGURE 51-2.   The Henderson-Hasselbalch equation can be used to calculate the pH of a solution.

$$CO_2 + H_2O \rightleftharpoons H_2CO_3 \rightleftharpoons HCO_3^- + H^+$$

FIGURE 51–3. Hydration of carbon dioxide results in carbonic acid (H_2CO_3), which can subsequently dissociate into bicarbonate (HCO_3^-) and hydrogen (H^+) ions.

lowers the pH of body fluids only slightly. The addition of a strong base, such as KOH to the HCO_3^- buffering system results in the formation of a weak base and water. The importance of the HCO_3^- buffering system, however, is enhanced by the fact that the concentration of its elements can be regulated by the lungs and kidneys.

Ventilatory Responses

Ventilatory responses for regulation of pH manifest as alterations in activity of the respiratory center within 1 to 5 minutes of the change in H^+ concentration. As a result, alveolar ventilation increases or decreases to produce appropriate changes in the concentration of carbon dioxide in tissues and body fluids. In the presence of a constant carbon dioxide production, the dissolved concentration of carbon dioxide is inversely proportional to alveolar ventilation.

Doubling alveolar ventilation eliminates sufficient carbon dioxide to increase pH to approximately 7.60. Conversely, reducing alveolar ventilation to one fourth of normal results in retention of carbon dioxide sufficient to reduce the pH to approximately 7.0.

Degree of Ventilatory Response

Ventilatory responses cannot return pH to 7.4 when a metabolic abnormality is responsible for the acid-base disturbance. This reflects the fact that the intensity of the stimulus responsible for increases or decreases in alveolar ventilation will begin to diminish as pH returns toward 7.4. As a buffer, ventilatory responses are able to buffer up to twice the amounts of acid or base as all the chemical buffers combined.

$$HCL + NaHCO_3 \rightarrow H_2CO_3 + NaCl$$

FIGURE 51–4. The addition of a strong acid (hydrochloric acid, HCl) to the bicarbonate buffering system results in the formation of weak acid (carbonic acid, H_2CO_3).

Renal Responses

Renal responses that regulate H^+ concentration do so by acidification or alkalinization of the urine. This is achieved by complex responses occurring principally in the proximal renal tubules in which there is incomplete titration of H^+ against HCO_3^-, leaving one or the other of these ions to enter the urine and, therefore, to be removed from extracellular fluid. In the presence of acidosis, the rate of H^+ secretion exceeds the rate of HCO_3^- filtration into the renal tubules. As a result, an excess of H^+ are excreted into the urine. In the presence of alkalosis, the effect of the titration process in the renal tubules is to increase the number of HCO_3^- filtered into the renal tubules relative to H^+ secretion. Excess HCO_3^- is excreted into the urine with another positive ion, most often Na^+.

Renal Tubular Secretion of Hydrogen Ions

H^+ are actively secreted into renal tubules by epithelial cells lining proximal renal tubules, distal renal tubules, and collecting ducts (Fig. 51-5). At the same time, Na^+ are reabsorbed in place of the secreted H^+, and HCO_3^- formed in the renal tubular epithelial cells enters peritubular capillaries to combine with Na^+. As a result, the amount of sodium bicarbonate in the plasma is increased during the secretion of H^+ into renal tubules.

The greater the concentration of carbon dioxide in the blood, the more rapidly are H^+ formed for secretion into renal tubules. Conversely, an event that decreases $PaCO_2$, such as hyperventilation of the lungs or reduced carbon dioxide production, also decreases the rate of H^+ secretion into renal tubules.

H^+ must combine with buffers in the lumens of renal tubules to prevent tubular fluid pH from declining below the pH that allows continued secretion of H^+ by the renal tubular epithelial cells. An important buffer mechanism for H^+ in renal tubular fluid is provided by ammonia, which is synthesized in the lumens of renal tubules (Fig. 51-6). Ammonia combines with H^+ to form ammonium (NH_4^+), which is secreted in the urine in combination with chloride ions (Cl^-) as the weak acid NH_4Cl.

Regulation of Chloride

In the process of altering the plasma concentration of HCO_3^-, it is mandatory to remove some other anion each time the concentration of HCO_3^- is increased or to increase some other anion when the HCO_3^- concentration is decreased. Typically, the anion that follows changes in the concentration of HCO_3^- is Cl^-. Thus, in controlling the pH of body fluids, the renal acid-base regulating system also regulates the ratio of Cl^- to HCO_3^- in extracellular fluid.

Degree of Renal Compensation

Renal responses for regulation of acid-base balance are slow to act (hours) but continue until

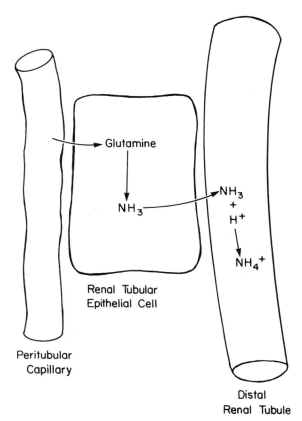

FIGURE 51–6. Ammonia (NH_3) formed in renal tubular epithelial cells combines with hydrogen ions (H^+) in the renal tubules to form ammonium (NH_4^+).

the pH returns to almost to 7.4. Thus, unlike ventilatory responses that are rapid but incomplete, the value of renal regulation of H^+ concentration is not its rapidity but instead its ability to nearly completely neutralize any excess acid or alkali that enters the body fluids. Ordinarily, the kidneys can remove up to 500 mM of acid or alkali each day. If greater quantities than this enter body fluids, the kidneys are unable to maintain normal acid-base balance, and acidosis or alkalosis occurs. Even when the plasma pH is 7.4, a small amount of acid is still lost each minute. This reflects the daily production of 50 to 80 mM more of acid than alkali. Indeed, the normal urine pH of approximately 6.4 rather than 7.4 is due to the presence of this excess acid in the urine.

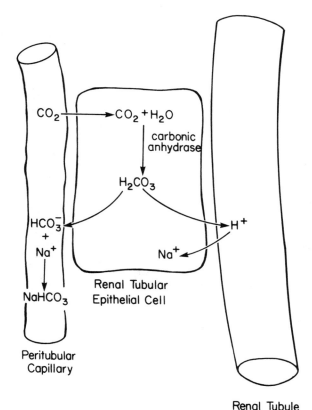

FIGURE 51–5. Schematic depiction of the renal tubular secretion of hydrogen ions (H^+), which are formed from the dissociation of carbonic acid (H_2CO_3) in renal tubular epithelial cells.

ACID-BASE DISTURBANCES

Acid-base disturbances are categorized as respiratory or metabolic acidosis (pH below 7.35) or alkalosis (pH above 7.45) (Table 51-2). An acid-base disturbance that results primarily from changes in alveolar ventilation is described as respiratory acidosis or alkalosis. An acid-base disturbance unrelated to changes in alveolar ventilation is designated as *metabolic acidosis* or *alkalosis. Compensation* describes the secondary renal or ventilatory responses that occur as a result of the primary acid-base disturbance. These compensatory changes tend to return the pH toward a normal value.

The principal manifestation of respiratory or metabolic acidosis is depression of the central nervous system. For example, coma is a characteristic of severe diabetic acidosis or uremia. The principal manifestation of respiratory or metabolic alkalosis is increased excitability of the peripheral nervous system and central nervous system. As a result, there may be repetitive stimulation, causing skeletal muscles to undergo sustained contraction, known as *tetany.* Tetany of respiratory muscles may interfere with adequate ventilation of the lungs. Central nervous system excitability may manifest as seizures.

Respiratory Acidosis

Any event (drugs or disease) that decreases alveolar ventilation results in an increased concentration of dissolved carbon dioxide in the plasma (increased $PaCO_2$), which in turn leads to formation of carbonic acid and H^+ (Fig. 51-3). By convention, carbonic acid resulting from dissolved carbon dioxide is considered a respiratory acid, and respiratory acidosis is present when the pH is less than 7.35.

Respiratory Alkalosis

Respiratory alkalosis is present when increased alveolar ventilation removes sufficient carbon dioxide from the body to reduce the H^+ concentration to the extent that pH becomes more than 7.45. A physiologic cause of respiratory alkalosis is stimulation of chemoreceptors by a low PO_2 associated with ascent to altitude. Kidneys compensate with time for this loss of carbon dioxide by excreting HCO_3^- in association with Na^+ and K^+. This renal compensation is evident in individuals residing at altitude who have a nearly normal pH despite a low $PaCO_2$. A frequent cause of acute respiratory alkalosis is iatrogenic hyperventilation of the lungs as during anesthesia. Tetany that accompanies alkalosis reflects hypocalcemia owing to the greater affinity of plasma proteins for calcium ions in an alkaline, compared with an acidic, solution.

Metabolic Acidosis

Any acid formed in the body other than carbon dioxide is considered a metabolic acid and its accumulation results in metabolic acidosis. Renal failure prevents excretion of acids formed by normal metabolic processes, and metabolic acidosis occurs. Inadequate tissue oxygenation results in anaerobic metabolism and accumulation of lactic acid that manifests as metabolic acidosis. Severe diarrhea and associated loss of sodium bicarbonate also rapidly leads to metabolic acidosis, especially in the pediatric age group. Lack of insulin secretion or starvation prevents use of glucose, forcing tissues to metabolize fat to meet energy needs. As a result, the plasma concentration of acetoacetic acid often increases sufficiently to cause metabolic acidosis. Excess K^+ compete with H^+ for renal secretion such that fewer H^+ are eliminated in the urine, and metabolic acidosis occurs. Inhibition of carbonic anhydrase by acetazolamide results in metabolic acidosis owing to interference with the reabsorption of HCO_3^- from renal tubular fluid. As a result, excess HCO_3^- are lost in the urine and the plasma concentration of HCO_3^- is decreased.

Metabolic acidosis impairs myocardial contractility and the responses to endogenous or exogenous catecholamines (Hindman, 1990). Hemodynamic deterioration is usually minimal when the pH remains above 7.2 owing to compensatory increases in sympathetic nervous system activity. Of great clinical importance is the accentuated detrimental effects of metabolic acidosis in persons with underlying left ventricular dysfunction or myocardial ischemia or in those in whom sympathetic nervous system activity may be impaired, as by beta blockade or general anesthesia. Respiratory acidosis may produce more

Table 51-2
Classification of Acid-Base Disturbances

	pH	PaCO$_2$	HCO$_3^-$
Respiratory Acidosis			
Acute	↑↑	↑↑↑	↑
Chronic	↓	↑↑↑	↑↑
Respiratory Alkalosis			
Acute	↑↑	↓↓↓	↓
Chronic	↓/NC	↓↓↓	↓↓
Metabolic Acidosis			
Acute	↓↓↓	↓	↓↓↓
Chronic	↓	↓↓↓	↓↓↓
Metabolic Alkalosis			
Acute	↑↑↑	↑	↑↑↑
Chronic	↑↑	↑↑	↑↑↑

NC, no change

rapid and profound myocardial dysfunction than does metabolic acidosis, reflecting the ability of carbon dioxide to freely diffuse across cell membranes and exacerbate intracellular acidosis to a greater extent than metabolic acids.

It has been standard practice to treat acute metabolic acidosis with intravenous administration of an exogenous buffer, usually sodium bicarbonate, in the hope that normalizing pH will attenuate the detrimental effects of acidosis. Nevertheless, use of sodium bicarbonate to treat metabolic acidosis has been challenged (Graf et al, 1985; Hindman, 1990). For example, sodium bicarbonate administration increases the carbon dioxide load to the lungs, leading to further increases in arterial and intracellular PCO$_2$ if alveolar ventilation is not concomitantly increased. It is estimated that sodium bicarbonate, 1 mEq·kg^{-1} administered intravenously, will produce approximately 180 ml of carbon dioxide and necessitate a transient doubling of alveolar ventilation to prevent hypercarbia. In the presence of increased dead space ventilation, even greater increases in alveolar ventilation are required for carbon dioxide elimination to equal production. Even if PaCO$_2$ is maintained normal, current data suggest that tissue (intracellular) pH and the likelihood of ventricular defibrillation will probably not be altered by administration of sodium bicarbonate during cardiopulmonary resuscitation.

Metabolic Alkalosis

Causes of metabolic alkalosis include vomiting with excess loss of hydrochloric acid, nasogastric suction, chronic administration of thiazide diuretics, and excess secretion of aldosterone. Excessive administration of sodium bicarbonate as during cardiopulmonary resuscitation may be an iatrogenic cause of metabolic alkalosis.

Compensation for Acid-Base Disturbances

Respiratory acidosis is compensated for within 6 to 12 hours by increased renal secretion of H$^+$ with a resulting increase in the plasma HCO$_3^-$ concentration. After a few days, the pH will be normal despite persistence of an increased PaCO$_2$. Sudden correction of chronic respiratory acidosis as may be produced by iatrogenic hyperventilation of the lungs may produce acute metabolic alkalosis because increased amounts of HCO$_3^-$ in the plasma cannot be promptly eliminated by the kidneys.

Respiratory alkalosis is compensated for by decreased reabsorption of HCO$_3^-$ from the renal tubules. As a result, more HCO$_3^-$ are excreted in the urine, thus decreasing the plasma concentration of HCO$_3^-$ and returning pH toward normal despite persistence of a decreased PaCO$_2$.

Metabolic acidosis stimulates alveolar ventilation and thus causes rapid removal of carbon dioxide from the body, which reduces the H^+ concentration toward normal. This respiratory compensation for metabolic acidosis, however, is only partial because pH remains somewhat below normal.

Metabolic alkalosis diminishes alveolar ventilation, which in turn causes accumulation of carbon dioxide and a subsequent increase in H^+ concentration. As with metabolic acidosis, the respiratory compensation for metabolic alkalosis is only partial. Renal compensation for metabolic alkalosis is by increased reabsorption of H^+. This metabolic compensation is limited by the availability of Na^+, K^+, and Cl^-. During prolonged vomiting, there may be excessive loss of Cl^- along with Na^+ and K^+. When this occurs, the kidneys preferentially conserve Na^+ and K^+ and the urine becomes paradoxically acid. Indeed the presence of paradoxical aciduria indicates electrolyte depletion.

REFERENCES

Graf H, Leach W, Arieff AI. Metabolic effects of sodium bicarbonate in hypoxic lactic acidosis in dogs. Am J Physiol 1985; 249:F630–5.

Hindman BJ. Sodium bicarbonate in the treatment of subtypes of acute lactic acidosis: Physiologic considerations. Anesthesiology 1990;72:1064–6.

Chapter

52

Endocrine System

Functions of the body are regulated by the nervous system and endocrine system. Glands of the endocrine system are primarily concerned with regulating different metabolic functions of the body. Endocrine glands secrete hormones into the blood for delivery to distant sites where a response is evoked. Hormone output is typically regulated by a negative feedback system in which increased circulating plasma concentrations of the hormone reduce its subsequent release from the parent gland. Tumors that secrete hormones, however, usually escape from this negative feedback control, and excess plasma concentrations of the hormone occur. Unrecognized endocrine dysfunction is unlikely if it can be established preoperatively that (1) body weight is unchanged, (2) heart rate and blood pressure are normal, (3) glycosuria is absent, (4) sexual function is normal, and (5) there is no history of recent medication.

MECHANISM OF HORMONE ACTION

Hormones typically exert their physiologic effects by attaching to specific receptors on plasma cell membranes. The combination of hormone and receptor activates adenylate cyclase, leading to conversion of adenosine triphosphate (ATP) to cyclic adenosine monophosphate (cyclic AMP). The resulting increased intracellular concentration of cyclic AMP is responsible for initiating cellular responses attributed to the effects of hormones. Examples of hormones that lead to production of cyclic AMP are anterior pituitary and posterior pituitary hormones and hypothalamic-releasing hormones. An alternative mechanism

of action for hormones is illustrated by corticosteroids that stimulate genes in cells to form specific intracellular proteins. These proteins then function as enzymes or carrier proteins, which in turn, activate other functions of cells.

PITUITARY GLAND

The pituitary gland lies in the sella turcica at the base of the brain and is connected to the hypothalamus by the pituitary stalk. Physiologically, the gland is outside the blood-brain barrier and is divided into the anterior pituitary (adenohypophysis) and posterior pituitary (neurohypophysis). The anterior pituitary synthesizes, stores, and secretes six tropic hormones. Adrenocorticotropic hormone (ACTH), prolactin, and human growth hormone (HGH) are polypeptides, whereas thyroid-stimulating hormone (TSH), luteinizing hormone (LH), and follicle-stimulating hormone (FSH) are glycoproteins. In addition, the anterior pituitary secretes beta-lipotropin, which contains the amino acid sequences of several endorphins that bind to opioid receptors. The posterior pituitary stores and secretes two hormones (antidiuretic hormone [ADH] and oxytocin), which are initially synthesized in the hypothalamus and subsequently transported to the posterior pituitary (Table 52-1).

Hormones designated as hypothalamic-releasing hormones and hypothalamic-inhibitory hormones originating in the hypothalamus control secretions from the anterior pituitary (Table 52-2). These hormones travel via hypothalamic-hypophyseal portal vessels to react with cell

Table 52–1
Pituitary Hormones

Hormone	Cell Type	Principal Action
Anterior Pituitary		
Human growth hormone (HGH, somatotropin)	Somatropes	Accelerates body growth
Prolactin	Mammotropes	Stimulates secretion of milk and maternal behavior, inhibits ovulation
Luteinizing hormone (LH)	Gonadotropes	Stimulates ovulation in females and testosterone secretion in males
Follicle-stimulating hormone (FSH)	Gonadotropes	Stimulates ovarian follicle growth in females and spermatogenesis in males
Adrenocorticotrophic hormone (ACTH)	Corticotropes	Stimulates adrenal cortex secretion and growth
Thyroid-stimulating hormone (TSH)	Thyrotropes	Stimulates thyroid secretion and growth
Beta-lipotropin	Corticotropes	Precursor of endorphins?
Posterior Pituitary		
Antidiuretic hormone (ADH, vasopressin)	Supraoptic nuclei	Promotes water retention and regulates plasma osmolarity
Oxytocin	Paraventricular nuclei	Causes ejection of milk and uterine contraction

Table 52–2
Hypothalamic Hormones

Hormone	Target Anterior Pituitary Hormone
Human growth hormone–releasing hormone	HGH*
Human growth hormone–inhibiting hormone (somatostatin)	HGH, prolactin, TSH
Prolactin-releasing factor	Prolactin
Prolactin-inhibiting factor	Prolactin
Luteinizing hormone-releasing hormone	LH, FSH
Corticotropin-releasing hormone	ACTH, beta-lipotropin, endorphins
Thyrotropin-releasing hormone	TSH

*See Table 52-1 for definition of abbreviations.

membrane receptors in the anterior pituitary, leading to increases in the intracellular concentrations of calcium ions (Ca^{2+}) and cyclic AMP. Synthesis and release of releasing and inhibitory hormones is controlled by many factors including adrenergic and dopaminergic receptors, pain signals, emotions, and olfactory sensations. As such, the hypothalamus is a collecting center for information and provides a link between the central nervous system and endocrine system and the response to the environment.

Anterior Pituitary

Anterior pituitary cells have been traditionally classified on the basis of their staining characteristics as agranular chromophobes and granular chromophils. Chromophils are subdivided into acidophils and basophils depending upon their staining response to acidic or basic dyes. With more modern techniques, including electron microscopy and immunochemistry, it is possible to identify at least five types of cells, some of which secrete more than one tropic hormone (Table 52-1).

Human Growth Hormone

HGH stimulates growth of all tissues in the body and evokes intense metabolic effects (Fig. 52-1) (Ganong, 1987). The most striking and specific effect is stimulation of linear bone growth that results from HGH action on the epiphyseal cartilage plates of long bones. Excess secretion of HGH before epiphyseal closure occurs results in giantism. Acromegaly occurs when excess HGH secretion is secreted after epiphyseal closure, because long bones can no longer increase in length but can increase in thickness. Metabolic effects of HGH include increased rates of protein synthesis (anabolic effect); increased mobilization of free fatty acids (ketogenic effect); and decreased rate of glucose use (diabetogenic effect). Many of the activities of HGH require the prior generation of a family of peptides known as *somatomedins.*

Secretion of HGH is regulated by releasing and inhibitory (somatostatin) hormones secreted by the hypothalamus as well as physiologic and pharmacologic events (Table 52-3). For example, anxiety and stress as associated with anesthesia evoke the release of HGH. Plasma concentrations of HGH characteristically increase during physiologic sleep. Drugs may influence the secretion of HGH presumably via effects on the hypothalamus. In this regard, large doses of corticosteroids suppress secretion of HGH, which may be responsible for inhibitory effects on growth observed in children receiving high doses of these drugs for prolonged periods as required for immunosuppression following organ transplantation. Conversely, dopaminergic agonists acutely increase the secretion of HGH.

Prolactin

Prolactin is responsible for growth and development of the breast in preparation for breast-feeding. Pregnancy is the principal event responsible for stimulating the release of prolactin; dopamine inhibits release of this hormone (Table 52-4). Preoperative anxiety is often accompanied by increased plasma concentrations of prolactin. Prolactin secretion in response to suckling is a potent inhibitor of ovarian function, explaining the usual lack of ovulation and the infertility during breast-feeding.

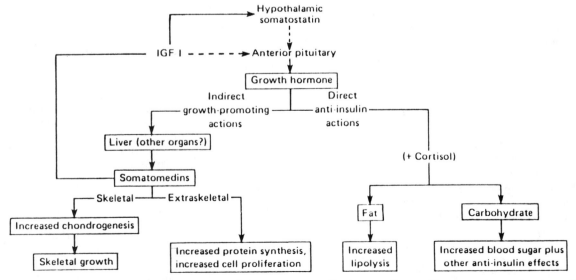

FIGURE 52–1.   Effects of human growth hormone manifesting as direct effects or via production of somatomedins in the liver. (From Ganong WF. Review of Medical Physiology. 13th ed. Norwalk, CT. Appleton and Lange. 1987; with permission.)

Table 52–3
Regulation of Human Growth Hormone (HGH) Secretion

Stimulation	Inhibition
HGH-releasing hormone	HGH-inhibiting hormone
Stress	HGH
Physiologic sleep	Pregnancy
Hypoglycemia	Hyperglycemia
Free fatty acid decrease	Free fatty acid increase
Amino acid increase	Cortisol
Fasting	Obesity
Estrogens	
Dopamine	
Alpha-agonists	

Gonadotropins

LH and FSH are gonadotropins responsible for pubertal maturation and secretion of steroid sex hormones by the gonads of either sex. These hormones presumably bind to plasma membrane receptors in the ovaries or testes to stimulate the synthesis of cyclic AMP.

Adrenocorticotropic Hormone

ACTH is principally responsible for regulating secretions of the adrenal cortex, especially cortisol. In addition, ACTH stimulates the formation of cholesterol in the adrenal cortex. Cholesterol is the initial building block for the synthesis of corticosteroids. Secretion of ACTH responds most dramatically to stress and is under the control of corticotropin-releasing hormone from the hypothalamus, as well as a negative feedback mechanism that depends on the circulating concentration of cortisol (Table 52-5) (Taylor and Fishman, 1988). Endorphin levels in the plasma parallel the release of ACTH in response to stress (apprehension before surgery) or lack of cortisol (Fig. 52-2) (Walsh et al, 1987). Secretory rates of corticotropin-releasing hormone and ACTH are high in the morning and low in the evening. This diurnal variation results in high plasma cortisol concentrations in the morning (approximately 20 $\mu g \cdot dl^{-1}$) and low levels (approximately 5 $\mu g \cdot dl^{-1}$) around midnight. For this reason, plasma concentrations of cortisol must be interpreted in terms of the time of day the measurement represents.

In the absence of ACTH, the adrenal cortex undergoes atrophy, but the zona glomerulosa, which secretes aldosterone, is least affected. Indeed, hypophysectomy has minimal effects on electrolyte balance, reflecting the continued release of aldosterone from the adrenal cortex. Pigmentary changes that may accompany certain endocrine diseases most likely reflect changes in plasma concentrations of ACTH, emphasizing the melanocyte-stimulating effects of this hormone. For example, pallor is a hallmark of hypopituitarism. Conversely, hyperpigmentation occurs in patients with adrenal insufficiency owing to primary adrenal gland disease, reflecting increased circulating concentrations of ACTH as the anterior pituitary attempts to stimulate corticosteroid secretion.

Table 52–4
Regulation of Prolactin Secretion

Stimulation	Inhibition
Prolactin-releasing factor	Prolactin-inhibiting factor
Pregnancy	Prolactin
Suckling	Dopamine
Stress	L-dopa
Physiologic sleep	
Metoclopramide	
Cimetidine	
Opioids	
Alpha-methyldopa	

Table 52–5
Regulation of Adrenocorticotrophic Hormone (ACTH) Secretion

Stimulation	Inhibition
Corticotropin-releasing hormone	ACTH
Cortisol decrease	Cortisol increase
Stress	Opioids
Sleep–wake transition	
Hypoglycemia	
Sepsis	
Trauma	
Alpha-agonists	
Beta-antagonists	

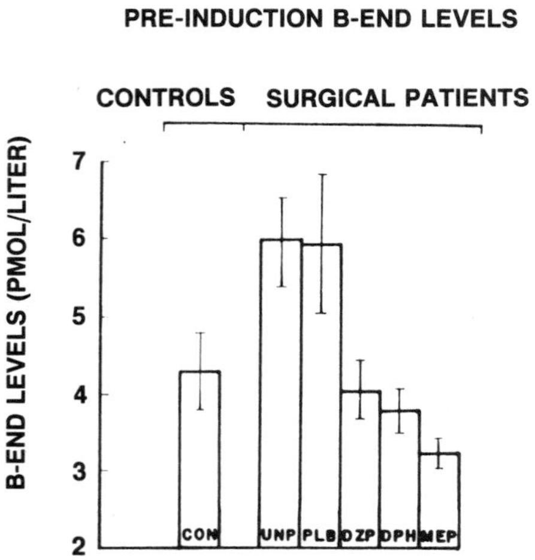

PRE-INDUCTION B-END LEVELS

CONTROLS   SURGICAL PATIENTS

FIGURE 52–2.   Beta-endorphin levels (mean ± SEM) in control (CON) and presurgical patients receiving no premedication (UNP), placebo (PLB), diazepam (DZP), diphenhydramine (DPH) or meperidine (MEP). (From Walsh J, Puig MM, Lovitz MA, Turndorf H. Premedication abolishes the increase in plasma beta-endorphin observed in the immediate preoperative period. Anesthesiology 1987; 66:402–5; with permission.)

Chronic administration of corticosteroids leads to functional atrophy of the hypothalamic–pituitary axis. Several months may be required for recovery of this axis after removal of the suppressive influence. In such patients, it is conceivable that stressful events during the perioperative period might evoke life-threatening hypotension. For this reason, it is a common practice to administer supplemental exogenous corticosteroids to patients considered at risk based on suppression of the hypothalamic–pituitary axis. Nevertheless, there are no controlled data to support this practice (Symreng et al, 1981).

Thyroid-Stimulating Hormone

TSH accelerates all the steps involved in the formation of thyroid hormone, including initial uptake of iodide into the thyroid gland. In addition, TSH causes proteolysis of thyroglobulin in the follicles of thyroid cells, with the resultant release of thyroid hormones into the circulation. Secretion of TSH from the anterior pituitary is under the control of thyrotropin-releasing hormone from the hypothalamus as well as a nega-

tive feedback mechanism, depending on the circulating concentration of thyroid hormones. Likewise, sympathetic nervous system stimulation and corticosteroids also suppress the secretion of TSH and thus diminish activity of the thyroid gland. Thyrotropin-releasing hormone is widely distributed in the central nervous system and is a potent analeptic. Furthermore, it is effective in reversing experimental hypovolemic shock and septic shock (Faden, 1984).

A long-acting thyroid stimulator is an immunoglobulin A antibody that can bind to receptor sites on thyroid cells. Presumably, the binding of these antibodies can mimic the effects of TSH and account for hyperthyroidism. Indeed, patients with hyperthyroidism often have detectable circulating concentrations of these proteins. Hypothyroidism with elevated plasma concentrations of TSH indicates a primary defect at the thyroid gland and an attempt by the anterior pituitary to stimulate hormonal output by releasing TSH. A defect at the hypothalamus or anterior pituitary is indicated by low circulating concentrations of both TSH and thyroid hormones.

Posterior Pituitary

The posterior pituitary is composed of cells that act as supporting structures for terminal nerve endings of fibers from the supraoptic and paraventricular nucleic of the hypothalamus. ADH is synthesized in the supraoptic nucleic and oxytocin in the paraventricular nucleic. These hormones are transported in secretory granules along axons from corresponding nuclei in the hypothalamus to the posterior pituitary for subsequent release in response to appropriate stimuli.

Antidiuretic Hormone

ADH is responsible for conserving body water and regulating the osmolarity of body fluids. Release of ADH is influenced by a number of factors, especially reductions in blood volume (Table 52-6). Painful stimulation and hemorrhage as associated with surgery are potent events for evoking the release of ADH (Fig. 52-3) (Philbin and Coggins, 1978). Hydration and establishment of an adequate blood volume before induction of anesthesia serves to maintain urine output presumably by blunting the release of

Table 52–6
Regulation of Antidiuretic Hormone (ADH) Secretion

Stimulation	Inhibition
Increased plasma osmolarity	Decreased plasma osmolarity
Hypovolemia	Ethanol
Pain	Alpha-agonists
Hypotension	Cortisol
Stress	Hypothermia
Hyperthermia	
Nausea and vomiting	
Opioids (?)	

ADH associated with painful stimulation or fluid deprivation prior to surgery (Mazze et al, 1963). Increased concentrations of ADH in the plasma in response to acute reductions of extracellular fluid volume may be sufficient to exert direct pressor effects on arterioles and thus contribute to maintenance of blood pressure. Administration of morphine, and presumably other opioids, in the absence of painful stimulation does not evoke the release of ADH (Philbin and Coggins, 1978). Ethanol inhibits the secretion of ADH. Decreased urine output and fluid retention previously attributed to release of ADH during positive pressure ventilation of the lungs is more likely due to changes in cardiac filling pressures that impair the release of atrial naturietic hormone (see Chapter 53).

ADH is transported in the blood to the kidneys, where it attaches to receptors on the capillary side of epithelial cells lining the distal convoluted renal tubules and collecting ducts of the renal medulla. This receptor-hormone interaction results in the formation of large amounts of cyclic AMP, which causes pores on the cell membranes to open and allow free permeability to water. Fluoride resulting from the metabolism of methoxyflurane and, to a lesser extent, enflurane, interferes with normal receptor responses to ADH, resulting in high volume output of dilute urine. Hypokalemia, hypercalcemia, cortisol, and lithium also interfere with renal responsiveness to ADH.

Diabetes insipidus results when there is destruction of neurons in or near the supraoptic and paraventricular nuclei of the hypothalamus. It will not occur when the posterior pituitary alone is damaged because the cut fibers of the pituitary stalk can still continue to secrete ADH. Diabetes insipidus, which develops in association with pituitary surgery, typically is due to trauma to the posterior pituitary and is usually transient.

Oxytocin

The primary role of oxytocin is to eject milk from the lactating mammary gland. In this regard, oxytocin causes contraction of the myoepithelial cells that surround the alveoli of the mammary glands, making milk available in response to suckling. In addition, oxytocin exerts a contracting effect on the pregnant uterus by lowering the threshold for depolarization of uterine smooth muscle. Large amounts of oxytocin cause sustained uterine contraction as necessary for postpartum hemostasis. Oxytocin has only 0.5% to 1% the antidiuretic activity of ADH and can be released abruptly and independently of ADH.

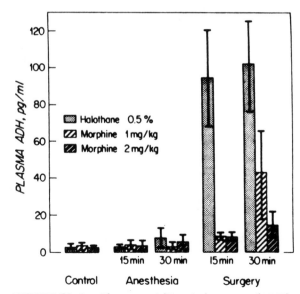

FIGURE 52–3. Plasma antidiuretic hormone (ADH) levels in adult patients are not altered by anesthesia in the absence of surgical stimulation. (From Philbin DM, Coggins CH. Plasma antidiuretic hormone levels in cardiac surgical patients during morphine and halothane anesthesia. Anesthesiology 1978; 49: 95–8; with permission.)

THYROID GLAND

The thyroid gland is responsible for maintaining the level of metabolism in tissues that is optimal for their normal function. The principal hormonal secretions of the thyroid gland are thyroxine (T_4) and triiodothyronine (T_3) (Fig. 52-4). In addition, the gland secretes reverse T_3 (RT_3), which is inert, and calcitonin, which is important for Ca^{2+} utilization. T_4 accounts for over 90% of the daily thyroid hormone secretion (approximately 80 μg), but T_3 is three to five times more potent than T_4. There is substantial conversion of T_4 to T_3 in the circulation, accounting for approximately 80% of the circulating T_3. It is of interest that iodine present in thyroid hormones is not necessary for biologic activity (Fig. 52-4).

The most obvious effect of thyroid hormones is to increase minute oxygen consumption in nearly all tissues, with the brain being an important exception. Failure of thyroid hormones to greatly alter the minute oxygen consumption of the brain is consistent with the minimal changes in anesthetic requirements (MAC) that accompany hyperthyroidism or hypothyroidism (Babad and Eger, 1968). Absence of thyroid gland hormones causes minute oxygen consumption to decrease to approximately 40% below normal, whereas excesses of these hormones can elevate minute oxygen consumption as much as 100% above normal. Thyroid hormones stimulate all aspects of carbohydrate metabolism and facilitate the mobilization of free fatty acids. Despite the latter effect, plasma concentrations of cholesterol usually decline, reflecting stimulation of low-

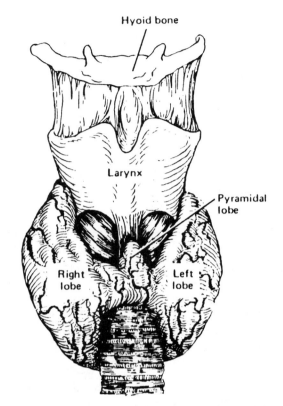

FIGURE 52-5. The two lobes of the thyroid and their relationship to the larynx and thyroid.

density lipoprotein receptor synthesis by thyroid hormones.

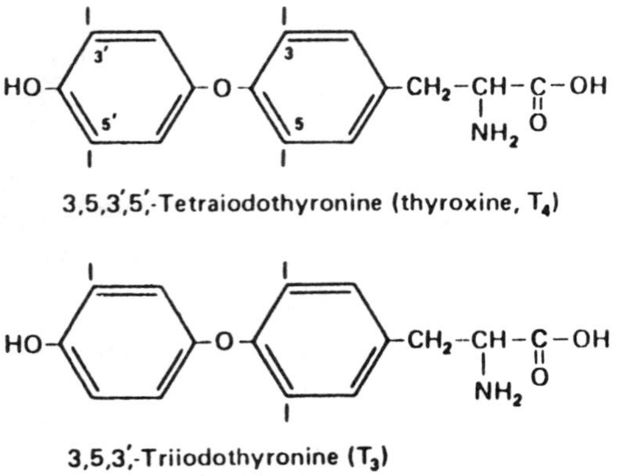

Anatomically, the thyroid gland consists of two lobes connected by a bridge of tissues known as the *thyroid isthmus* (Fig. 52-5). The gland is highly vascularized and receives innervation from the autonomic nervous system. Structurally, the gland consists of multiple follicles (acini) that are filled with colloid, which consists principally of thyroglobulin. Thyroid hormones are stored in combination with thyroglobulin. Stimulation of proteases by TSH results in cleavage of hormones from thyroglobulin, and their release into the circulation. In the circulation, T_4 and T_3 are bound to protein, primarily thyroxine-binding globulin with an estimated 0.03% of the total plasma T_4 concentration and 0.3% of the total plasma T_3 concentration in the free biologically active fraction. Pregnancy or administration

3,5,3',5'-Tetraiodothyronine (thyroxine, T_4)

3,5,3'-Triiodothyronine (T_3)

FIGURE 52-4. Chemical structure of thyroid hormones.

of estrogens results in increased circulating concentrations of thyroxine-binding globulin. Protein binding of thyroid hormones protects them from metabolism and excretion, resulting in elimination half-times of 6 to 7 days for T_4 and approximately 2 days for T_3. The plasma concentration of T_4 is the standard screening test for thyroid gland function.

Mechanism of Action

Thyroid hormones enter cells and T_3 binds to nuclear receptors. T_4 can also bind to these receptors but not as avidly. Indeed, T_4 serves principally as a prohormone for T_3, emphasizing that biologic effects of T_4 are largely a result of its intracellular conversion to T_3.

It is generally believed that thyroid hormones exert most, if not all, of their effects through control of protein synthesis. This most likely reflects the ability of thyroid hormones to activate the deoxyribonucleic acid (DNA) transcription process in the cell nucleus with resulting formation of new cell proteins including enzymes. Sympathomimetic effects that accompany thyroid hormone stimulation most likely reflect an increased number and sensitivity of beta receptors in response to release of T_4 and T_3. It has been proposed that thyroid hormones modulate conversion of alpha to beta receptors (Williams et al, 1977). Cardiac cholinergic receptor numbers are decreased by thyroid hormone, which is consistent with an increase in heart rate that is out of proportion to the elevation in cardiac output.

Increased metabolism produced by thyroid hormones causes vasodilation in tissues to provide the required blood flow to deliver necessary oxygen and carry away metabolites and heat. As a result, cardiac output often increases but blood pressure is unchanged as peripheral vasodilation offsets the impact of increased blood flow. Excess protein catabolism associated with increased secretion of thyroid hormones is the presumed mechanism of skeletal muscle weakness characteristic of hyperthyroidism. The fine muscle tremor that accompanies hyperthyroidism is probably due to increased sensitivity of neuronal synapses in the area of the spinal cord that controls skeletal muscle tone. Diarrhea reflects increased gastrointestinal tract motility that accompanies excess thyroid gland activity.

Calcitonin

Calcitonin, a polypeptide hormone secreted by the thyroid gland, causes a reduction in the plasma concentration of Ca^{2+}. This effect is due to a decrease in the activity of osteoclasts and an increase in osteoblastic activity. Calcitonin is most important in the early moments following ingestion of a high Ca^{2+} meal. Nevertheless, a total thyroidectomy and subsequent absence of calcitonin does not measurably influence regulation of the plasma concentration of Ca^{2+}, emphasizing the predominant role of parathyroid hormone.

PARATHYROID GLANDS

The four parathyroid glands secrete an amino acid polypeptide that constitutes parathyroid hormone, which is responsible for regulating the plasma concentration of Ca^{2+}. Secretion of parathyroid hormone is inversely related to the plasma ionized Ca^{2+} concentration. Slight decreases in the plasma concentration of Ca^{2+} are potent stimulants for the release of parathyroid hormone. Overall, the effect of parathyroid hormone is to increase the plasma concentration of Ca^{2+} and to decrease the plasma concentration of phosphate by acting on bone, the kidneys, and the gastrointestinal tract. The most prominent effect of parathyroid hormone is to promote mobilization of Ca^{2+} from bone, reflecting stimulation of osteoclastic activity. At the kidneys, parathyroid hormone increases renal tubular reabsorption of Ca^{2+} and inhibits renal tubular reabsorption of phosphate.

Parathyroid hormone is likely to exert its effect on target cells in bone, renal tubules, and the gastrointestinal tract by stimulating the formation of cyclic AMP. Indeed, a portion of cyclic AMP synthesized in the kidneys escapes into the urine, and its assay serves as a measure of parathyroid gland activity. It is likely that parathyroid hormone functions in bone in the same way that it works on the kidneys and gastrointestinal tract: by causing the conversion of vitamin D to its active form, 1,25-dihydroxycholecalciferol.

ADRENAL CORTEX

The two major classes of corticosteriods are mineralocorticoids and glucocorticoids. In addi-

Table 52–7
Physiologic Effects of Endogenous Corticosteroids (mg)

	Daily Secretion	Sodium Retention*	Gluco-corticoid Effect*	Anti-inflammatory Effect*
Aldosterone	0.125	3000	0.3	Insignificant
Desoxycorticosterone		100	0	0
Cortisol	20	1	1	1
Corticosterone	minimal	15	0.35	0.3
Cortisone	minimal	0.8	0.8	0.8

*Relative to cortisol.

tion, the adrenal cortex secretes sex steroids. The precursor of all corticosteroids is cholesterol. Mineralocorticoids affect the plasma concentrations of Na^+ and K^+, whereas glucocorticoids influence carbohydrate, fat, and protein metabolism as well as exhibiting anti-inflammatory effects. More than 30 different corticosteroids have been isolated from the adrenal cortex, but only two are of major importance: aldosterone, a mineralocorticoid, and cortisol, the principal glucocorticoid (Table 52-7). These corticosteroids are not stored in the adrenal cortex, emphasizing that the rate of synthesis determines the subsequent plasma concentration. Anatomically, the adrenal cortex is divided into three zones: the zona glomerulosa secretes mineralocorticoids, the zona fasciculata secretes glucocorticoids, and the zona reticularis produces androgens and estrogens.

Mineralocorticoids

Aldosterone accounts for approximately 95% of the mineralocorticoid activity produced by corticosteroids. Desoxycorticosterone is the other naturally occurring mineralocorticoid, but it has only 3% of the Na^+-retaining potency of aldosterone. Cortisol induces Na^+ retention and K^+ secretion, but much less effectively than does aldosterone.

Physiologic Effects

The principal functions of aldosterone are to sustain extracellular fluid volume by conserving Na^+ and to maintain a normal plasma concentration of

K^+. In this regard, aldosterone causes absorption of Na^+ and simultaneous secretion of K^+ by the lining renal tubular epithelial cells of the distal renal tubules and collecting ducts. As a result, aldosterone causes Na^+ to be conserved in the extracellular fluid while K^+ is excreted in the urine. Water follows Na^+ such that extracellular fluid volume tends to change in proportion to the rate of aldosterone secretion. Indeed, in the presence of excess aldosterone secretion, the extracellular fluid volume, cardiac output, and blood pressure are increased. When the plasma concentration of K^+ is reduced approximately 50% owing to excess secretion of aldosterone, skeletal muscle weakness or even paralysis occurs, reflecting hyperpolarization of nerve and muscle membranes, which prevents transmission of action potentials.

Aldosterone has effects on sweat glands and salivary glands that are similar to its effects on the renal tubules. For example, aldosterone increases the reabsorption of Na^+ and secretion of K^+ by sweat glands. This effect is important to conserve Na^+ in hot environments or when excess salivation occurs. Aldosterone also enhances Na^+ reabsorption by the gastrointestinal tract.

Mechanism of Action

Aldosterone diffuses to the interior of the renal tubular epithelial cells when it induces DNA to form messenger ribonucleic acid (mRNA) necessary for the transport of Na^+ and K^+. It is speculated that this mRNA is a specific ATPase that catalyzes energy transfer from cytoplasmic ATP to the Na^+ transport mechanism of cell membranes. It takes up to 30 minutes before the new mRNA appears and approximately 45 minutes before the rate of Na$^+$ transport begins to increase.

Regulation of Secretion

The most important stimulus of aldosterone secretion is an increase in the plasma K$^+$ concentration. For example, an increase in plasma K$^+$ concentration of less than 1 mEq·L^{-1} will triple the rate of aldosterone secretion. This establishes a powerful negative feedback system that maintains the plasma concentration of K$^+$ in a normal range. The renin–angiotensin system is also an important determinant of aldosterone secretion (see Chapter 22). The elimination half-time of aldosterone is approximately 20 minutes, with nearly 90% of the hormone being cleared by the liver in a single passage. Mineralocorticoid secretion is not under the primary control of ACTH. For this reason, hypoaldosteronism does not accompany loss of ACTH secretion from the anterior pituitary.

Glucocorticoids

At least 95% of the glucocorticoid activity results from the secretion of cortisol. In addition, a small amount of glucocorticoid activity is provided by corticosterone and an even smaller amount by cortisone. Cortisol is one of the few hormones essential for life.

Physiologic Effects

The most important physiologic effects of cortisol are (1) increased gluconeogenesis, (2) protein catabolism, (3) fatty acid mobilization, and (4) anti-inflammatory effects. Cortisol may improve cardiac function by increasing the number or responsiveness of cardiac beta-adrenergic receptors. Beside sustaining cardiac function and maintaining blood pressure, cortisol permits normal responsiveness of arterioles to the constrictive action of catecholamines. Cortisol inhibits bone formation.

GLUCONEOGENESIS. Cortisol stimulates gluconeogenesis by the liver as much as tenfold, reflecting principally mobilization of amino acids from extrahepatic sites and transfer to the liver for conversion to glucose. This increased rate of gluconeogenesis, in addition to a moderate re-duction in the rate of glucose use, also produced by cortisol causes the blood glucose concentration to increase. The resulting adrenal diabetes is responsive to the administration of insulin.

PROTEIN CATABOLISM. Cortisol decreases protein stores in nearly all cells except hepatocytes, reflecting mobilization of amino acids for gluconeogenesis. In the presence of sustained excesses of cortisol, skeletal muscle weakness may become profound.

FATTY ACID MOBILIZATION. Cortisol promotes mobilization of fatty acids from adipose tissue and enhances oxidation of fatty acids in cells. Despite these effects, excess amounts of cortisol cause deposition of fat in the head and chest regions, giving rise to a buffalo-like torso. This peculiar distribution of fat reflects deposition of fat at these sites at a rate that exceeds its mobilization.

ANTI-INFLAMMATORY EFFECTS. Cortisol in large amounts has anti-inflammatory effects, reflecting its ability to stabilize lysosomal membranes and to reduce migration of leukocytes into the inflamed area. Stabilization of lysosomal membranes reduces release of inflammation-causing lysosomes. Other anti-inflammatory effects of cortisol reflect decreased capillary permeability, which prevents loss of plasma into tissues. Even after inflammation has become well established, administration of cortisol can reduce its manifestations. This effect of cortisol is important in attenuating inflammation associated with disease states such as rheumatoid arthritis and acute glomerulonephritis.

Cortisol decreases the number of eosinophils and lymphocytes in the blood within a few minutes of its injection. In addition, there is atrophy of lymphoid tissue throughout the body, which results in decreased production of antibodies. As a result, the level of immunity against bacterial or viral infection is decreased, and fulminating infection can occur. Conversely, this ability of cortisol to suppress immunity is useful in reducing the likelihood of immunologic rejection of transplanted tissues.

The beneficial effect of cortisol in the treatment of allergic reactions reflects prevention of inflammatory responses that are responsible for many of the life-threatening effects of an allergic reaction such as laryngeal edema. Cortisol may also interfere with complement pathway activation and formation of chemical mediators derived from arachidonic acid such as leukotrienes. Cortisol does not, however, alter the antigen-antibody interaction or histamine release associated with allergic reactions.

Mechanism of Action

Cortisol stimulates DNA-dependent synthesis of mRNA in the nuclei of responsive cells, leading to the synthesis of appropriate enzymes.

Regulation of Secretion

The most important stimulus for the secretion of cortisol is the release of ACTH from the anterior pituitary (Table 52-5). Conversely, circulating cortisol exerts a direct negative feedback effect on the hypothalamus and anterior pituitary to reduce the release of corticotropin-releasing hormone and ACTH from these respective sites. Stress as associated with the intraoperative period can override the normal negative feedback control mechanisms, and plasma concentrations of cortisol are elevated. The beneficial effect of increased plasma concentrations of cortisol and other hormones in response to stressful stimuli may be the acute mobilization of cellular protein and fat stores for energy and synthesis of other compounds, including glucose. Large doses of opioids may attenuate the cortisol response to surgical stimulation (Bovill et al, 1983; Sebel et al, 1981). Volatile anesthetics provide less suppression to this stress-induced endocrine response. Etomidate is unique among drugs administered to induce anesthesia with respect to its ability to inhibit cortisol synthesis even in the absence of surgical stimulation (see Chapter 6). Suppression of the hypothalamic–pituitary axis as produced by chronic administration of corticosteroids also prevents the release of cortisol in response to stressful stimuli.

Cortisol is secreted and released by the adrenal cortex at a basal rate of approximately 20 mg daily. In response to maximal stressful stimuli (sepsis or burns), the output of cortisol is increased to approximately 150 mg daily (Hume et al, 1962). Therefore, this amount should be sufficient when provided to patients who lack adrenal function and are acutely ill or undergoing major surgery. The peak plasma concentration of 8 to 25 $\mu g \cdot dl^{-1}$ occurs shortly after awakening. In the cir-

culation, 80% to 90% of cortisol is bound to a specific globulin known as *transcortin*. It is the relatively small amount of unbound cortisol that exerts a biologic effect. The elimination half-time of cortisol is approximately 70 minutes. Degradation of cortisol occurs mainly in the liver with the formation of inactive 17-hydroxycorticosteroids that appear in the urine. Cortisol is also filtered at the glomerulus and may be excreted unchanged in the urine.

REPRODUCTIVE GLANDS

In both sexes, the reproductive glands (testes and ovaries) are responsible for production of germ cells and steroid sex hormones.

Testes

The testes secrete male sex hormones, which are collectively designated *androgens*. All androgens are steroid compounds that can be synthesized from cholesterol. Testosterone is the most potent and abundant of the androgens, being responsible for the development and maintenance of male sex characteristics. Skeletal muscle growth is an anabolic effect of testosterone in the male. Testosterone is produced in the testes only when stimulation occurs from LH, and FSH is necessary for spermatogenesis. Puberty occurs when the production of testosterone increases rapidly in response to hypothalamic-releasing hormones that evoke the release of LH and FSH. Hypertrophy of the laryngeal mucosa accompanies secretion of testosterone, leading to the characteristic change in voice at puberty. Testosterone increases secretion of sebaceous glands, leading to acne. Beard growth is the last manifestation of puberty. Testosterone production continues throughout life, although the amount produced decreases beyond the age of 40 years to become approximately one fifth the peak value at 80 years of age.

At most sites of action, testosterone is not the active form of the hormone being converted in target tissues to the more active dihydrotestosterone by a reductase enzyme. Dihydrotestosterone binds to a cytoplasmic protein receptor that results in increased synthesis of specific mRNA protein. In the absence of sufficient reductase enzyme, external genitalia fail to develop (pseudohermaphroditism) despite secretion of adequate amounts of testosterone. Not all target tissues, however, require the conversion of testosterone to dihydrotestosterone for activity. For example, effects of testosterone on skeletal muscle and bone marrow are mediated by the hormone or a metabolite other than dihydrotestosterone.

The adrenal cortex also secretes androgens but the effects of these hormones are usually inconsequential unless a hormone-secreting tumor develops. For example, in males, approximately 10% of androgens are produced in the adrenal cortex. This is an insufficient amount to maintain spermatogenesis or secondary sexual features in an adult male. In abnormal conditions, such as the adrenogenital syndrome, the adrenal cortex can secrete large quantities of steroids and androgenic precursors.

Ovaries

The two ovarian hormones, estrogen and progesterone, are secreted in response to LH and FSH, which are released from the anterior pituitary in response to hypothalamic-releasing hormones. In postpubertal females, an orderly secretion of LH and FSH is necessary for the occurrence of menstruation, pregnancy, and lactation. The Stein-Leventhal syndrome is characterized by virilization resulting from excessive ovarian secretion of androgens.

Estrogens

Estrogens are responsible for the development of female sexual characteristics. In the nonpregnant female, most of the estrogen comes from the ovaries although small amounts are also secreted by the adrenal cortex. The three most important estrogens are beta-estradiol, estrone, and estriol. These estrogens are conjugated in the liver to inactive metabolites that appear in the urine.

Progesterone

Progesterone is necessary for preparation of the uterus for pregnancy and the breast for lactation. Almost all of the progesterone in the nonpregnant female is secreted by the corpus luteum during the luteal phase of the menstrual cycle. The adrenal cortex forms small amounts of proge-

sterone. Progesterone is metabolized to pregnanediol in the liver. Pregnanediol appears in the urine, providing a valuable index of the secretion or metabolism of the hormone.

Menstruation

The overall duration of a normal menstrual cycle is 21 to 35 days and consists of three phases: the follicular, ovulatory, and luteal phases. The follicular phase begins with the onset of menstrual bleeding, reflecting a decrease in the plasma concentration of progesterone. After a variable length, the follicular phase is followed by the ovulatory phase lasting 1 to 3 days and culminating in ovulation. The rise in body temperature (approximately 0.5°C) that accompanies ovulation most likely reflects a thermogenic effect of progesterone. The luteal phase follows ovulation and is characterized by the development of a corpus luteum that secretes progesterone and estrogen. The corpus luteum degenerates after a fairly constant period of 13 to 14 days and the menstrual cycle repeats.

Pregnancy

During pregnancy, the placenta forms large amounts of estrogen, progesterone, chorionic gonadotropin, and chorionic somatomammotropin. Chorionic gonadotropin prevents the usual involution of the corpus luteum, which would lead to onset of menstrual bleeding. This placental hormone is the first key hormone of pregnancy and can be detected in the maternal plasma and urine within 9 days of conception, thus providing the basis for pregnancy tests. After approximately 12 weeks, the placenta secretes sufficient amounts of progesterone and estrogens to maintain pregnancy and the corpus luteum involutes. Chorionic somatomammotropin has important metabolic effects, including decreased insulin activity, making more glucose available to the fetus.

Increased circulating concentrations of estrogen cause enlargement of the breasts and uterus, while progesterone is necessary for development of decidual cells in the uterine endometrium and for suppression of uterine contractions that could result in abortion. Increased plasma concentrations of progesterone and associated sedative effects during pregnancy have been proposed as the explanation for reductions in anesthetic requirements (MAC) for volatile anesthetics in gravid animals (Palahniuk et al, 1974). Nevertheless, anesthetic requirements in animals return to nonpregnant values within 5 days postpartum, while the plasma concentration of progesterone remains elevated, suggesting that the reduction in MAC cannot be attributed entirely to progesterone (Strout and Nahrwold, 1981). Increased plasma concentrations of progesterone are presumed to be the stimulus for increased alveolar ventilation that accompanies pregnancy. Near term, the ovaries secrete a hormone designated as relaxin, which relaxes pelvic ligaments so the sacroiliac joints become limber and the symphysis pubis becomes elastic.

The parturient with asthma may experience unpredictable changes in airway reactivity. Exacerbation of asthma may reflect bronchoconstriction evoked by prostaglandins of the F series, which are present in all trimesters of pregnancy but especially during labor (see Chapter 20). Conversely, prostaglandins of the E series are bronchodilators and predominate during the third trimester. A role of corticosteroids in altered airway responsiveness is questionable, because increased plasma concentrations of cotisol associated with pregnancy are offset by concomitant increases in the carrier protein transcortin, with the net effect being an unchanged level of available cortisol.

Menopause

The ovaries gradually become unresponsive to the stimulatory effects of LH and FSH, resulting in the disappearance of sexual cycles between the ages of 45 and 55 years. Because the negative feedback effect of estrogen and progesterone on the anterior pituitary is reduced, there is increased output of LH and FSH manifesting as increased plasma concentrations of these gonadotropins. Sensations of warmth spreading from the trunk to the face (hot flashes) coincide with surges of LH secretion and are prevented by exogenous administration of estrogens.

PANCREAS

The pancreas secretes digestive substances into the duodenum as well as four hormones—insulin, glucagon, somatostatin, and pancreatic peptide—that are secreted by the islets of Langerhans and released into the circulation. Somatostatin regulates islet cell secretion, acting as a profound inhibitor of both insulin and glucagon release. This peptide hormone is the same as growth hormone-releasing inhibitory hormone that is secreted by the hypothalamus. The role of pancreatic peptide hormone is not known.

The pancreas contains 1 to 2 million islets, which, based on staining characteristics and morphology, are classified as alpha, beta, and delta cells. Beta cells account for 60% of the islet cells and are the site of insulin production as part of a larger preprohormone. Alpha cells account for 25% of the islet cells and are the site of glucagon production. Each islet receives a generous blood supply, which, like the gastrointestinal tract but unlike any other endocrine organ, drains into the portal vein.

Insulin

Insulin is an anabolic hormone promoting the storage of glucose, fatty acids, and amino acids (Fig. 52-6) (Berne and Levy, 1988). The amount of insulin secreted daily is equivalent to approximately 40 units. In the circulation, insulin has an elimination half-time of approximately 5 minutes, with more than 80% being degraded in the liver and kidneys. Insulin binds to receptor proteins in cell membranes, leading to activation of the glucose transport system (Fig. 52-7) (Ganong, 1987). Activation of Na^+–K^+ ATPase in cell membranes by insulin results in movement of K^+ into cells and a decrease in the plasma concentration of K^+.

Regulation of Secretion

The principal control of insulin secretion is via a negative feedback effect of the blood glucose concentration on the pancreas (Table 52-8). Virtually no insulin is secreted by the pancreas when blood glucose concentrations are less than 50 mg·dl^{-1}, and maximum stimulation for release of insulin occurs when blood glucose concentrations are more than 300 mg·dl^{-1}. This feedback system provides prompt responses that maintain blood glucose concentrations within a narrow range. The pancreas is richly innervated by the autonomic nervous system, with insulin release

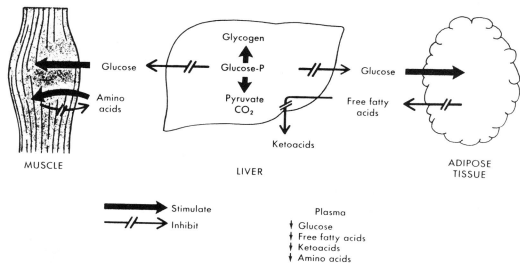

FIGURE 52–6. Insulin stimulates tissue uptake of glucose and amino acids, whereas release of fatty acids is inhibited. As a result, the plasma concentrations of glucose, free fatty acids, amino acids, and ketoacids decrease. (From Berne RM, Levy MN. Physiology. 2nd ed. St. Louis: CV Mosby, 1988; with permission.)

occurring in response to beta stimulation or release of acetylcholine. Conversely, alpha stimulation or beta blockade results in inhibition of insulin release. Oral glucose is more effective than glucose administered intravenously in evoking the release of insulin, suggesting the presence of an anticipatory signal from the gastrointestinal tract to the pancreas. Consistent with this is the more likely occurrence of glycosuria following intravenous rather than oral glucose administration. This observation has obvious implications for the intravenous infusion of fluids containing glucose during the perioperative period. Volatile anesthetics studied in isolated pancreas preparations inhibit the release of insulin but there is no evidence to support selecting a specific inhaled anesthetic based on its effects on insulin release (Gingerich et al, 1974).

Glucagon, HGH, and corticosteroids can potentiate glucose-induced stimulation of insulin secretion. Prolonged secretion of these hormones or their exogenous administration can lead to the exhaustion of pancreatic beta cells and the development of diabetes mellitus. Indeed, diabetes mellitus often occurs in patients who develop acromegaly or in those persons with a diabetic tendency who are treated with corticosteroids.

Physiologic Effects

Insulin promotes the use of carbohydrates for energy while depressing the use of fats and amino acids. For example, insulin facilitates storage of fat in adipose cells by inhibiting lipase enzyme, which normally causes hydrolysis of triglycerides in fat cells. In the liver, insulin inhibits enzymes necessary for gluconeogenesis, thus conserving amino acid stores.

Insulin facilitates glucose uptake and storage in the liver by its effects on specific enzymes. Enhanced uptake of glucose into liver cells reflects insulin-induced increases in the activity of glucokinase. Glucokinase is the enzyme that causes initial phosphorylation of glucose after it diffuses into hepatocytes. Once phosphorylated, glucose is trapped, being unable to diffuse back through cell membranes. Storage is further enhanced by insulin-induced inhibition of phosphorylase enzyme, which normally causes liver glycogen to split into glucose. The net effects of these actions of insulin on enzymes is to increase hepatic stores of glycogen up to a maximum of approximately 100 g. Ordinarily, approximately 60% of the glucose in a meal is stored in the liver as glycogen.

Resting skeletal muscles are almost impermeable to glucose except in the presence of insu-

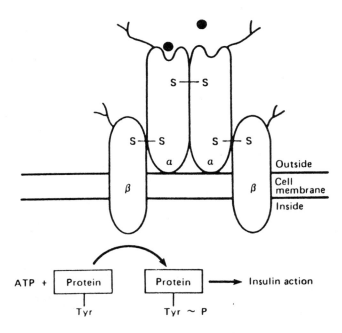

ATP + Protein — Tyr → Protein — Tyr ~ P → Insulin action

FIGURE 52–7.   The insulin receptor consists of two alpha and two beta subunits. Insulin attaches to the extracellular subunits. (From Ganong WF. Review of Medical Physiology. 13th ed. Norwalk, CT. Appleton and Lange. 1987; with permission.)

lin. Glucose that enters resting skeletal muscles under the influence of insulin is stored as glycogen for subsequent use as energy. The amount of glycogen that can be stored in skeletal muscles, however, is much less than the amount that can be stored in the liver. Furthermore, glycogen in skeletal muscles, in contrast to that stored in the liver, cannot be reconverted to glucose and released into the circulation. This occurs because skeletal muscles lack glucose phosphatase enzyme, which is necessary for splitting glycogen. Exercise increases the permeability of skeletal muscle membranes to glucose, perhaps reflect-

ing the release of insulin from within the skeletal muscle itself or its vasculature.

Brain cells are unique in that permeability of these membranes to glucose is not dependent on the presence of insulin. This characteristic is crucial because brain cells use only glucose for energy, and it emphasizes the importance of maintaining the blood glucose concentration above a critical level of approximately 50 mg·dl^{-1}. Indeed, lack of insulin causes use of mainly fat to the exclusion of glucose except by brain cells.

Diabetes Mellitus

An estimated 5% of the population suffers from either an absolute (juvenile-onset) or relative (maturity-onset) lack of insulin. Even in the absence of overt diabetes, patients with latent disease release less insulin in response to glucose stimulation.

In the absence of sufficient insulin, there is a marked reduction in the rate of transport of glucose across certain cell membranes, resulting in hyperglycemia. The formation of glucose from protein accounts for the observation that glucose lost in the urine may exceed oral intake. Much of the protein for glucose formation comes from skeletal muscles; glucose loss may manifest in ex-

Table 52–8
Regulation of Insulin Secretion

Stimulation	Inhibition
Hyperglycemia	Hypoglycemia
Beta-agonists	Beta-antagonists
Acetylcholine	Alpha-agonists
Glucagon	Somatostatin
	Diazoxide
	Thiazide diuretics
	Volatile anesthetics
	Insulin

treme cases as skeletal muscle wasting. Increased free fatty acid concentrations in the plasma of diabetic patients reflects loss of insulin-induced inhibition of the lipase enzyme system such that mobilization of fatty acids proceeds unopposed. The insulin-deficient liver is likely to use fatty acids to produce ketones, which can serve as an energy source for skeletal muscle and cardiac muscles. Production of ketones can lead to ketoacidosis whereas urinary excretion of these anions contributes to the depletion of electrolytes, especially K^+. Hypokalemia, however, may not be apparent, because intracellular K^+ is exchanged for extracellular K^+ to compensate for the acidosis.

Low plasma concentrations of insulin, although inadequate to prevent hyperglycemia, may be quite effective in blocking lipolysis. This differential effect of insulin explains the frequent observation in patients with diabetes mellitus that hyperglycemia can exist without the presence of ketone bodies. Ketosis can be reliably prevented by continuously providing all diabetic patients with glucose and insulin (Hirsch et al, 1991). This is uniquely important in the perioperative period when nutritional uptake is altered.

Glucagon

Glucagon is a catabolic hormone acting to mobilize glucose, fatty acids, and amino acids into the circulation (Fig. 52-8) (Berne and Levy, 1988). These responses are the reciprocal of the insulin effects, emphasizing that these two hormones are also reciprocally secreted (Table 52-9). Indeed, the principal stimulus for secretion of glucagon is hypoglycemia. Glucagon is able to abruptly increase the blood concentrations of glucose by stimulating glycogenolysis in the liver. This reflects activation of adenylate cyclase by glucagon and the subsequent formation of cyclic AMP. In this regard, the metabolic effects of glucagon at the liver mimic those produced by epinephrine. Indeed, the study of the mechanism by which glucagon and epinephrine act as hyperglycemics led to the discovery of cyclic AMP (Rall and Sutherland, 1958). Glucagon also causes hyperglycemia by stimulating gluconeogenesis in hepatocytes. Other effects of glucagon such as enhanced myocardial contractility and increased secretion of bile probably occur only when exogenous administration elevates plasma concentrations of this hormone far above those that occur normally (see Chapter 13). Amino acids enhance

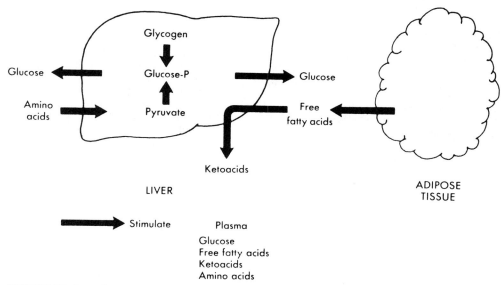

FIGURE 52–8. Glucagon stimulates tissue release of glucose, free fatty acids, and ketoacids and hepatic uptake of aminoacids. (From Berne RM, Levy MN. Physiology. 2nd ed. St. Louis: CV Mosby, 1988; with permission.)

Table 52–9
Regulation of Glucagon Secretion

Stimulation	Inhibition
Hypoglycemia	Hyperglycemia
Stress	Somatostatin
Sepsis	Insulin
Trauma	Free fatty acids
Beta-agonists	Alpha-agonists
Acetylcholine	
Cortisol	

the release of glucagon and thus prevent hypoglycemia that would occur from ingestion of a pure protein meal and associated stimulation of insulin secretion. Glucagon undergoes enzymatic degradation to inactive metabolites in the liver and kidneys and at receptor sites in cell membranes. The elimination half-time of glucagon is brief, being only 3 to 6 minutes.

REFERENCES

Babad AA, Eger EI II. The effects of hyperthyroidism and hypothyroidism on halothane and oxygen requirements in dogs. Anesthesiology 1968;29:1087–93.

Berne RM, Levy MN. Physiology. 2nd ed. St. Louis. CV Mosby. 1988.

Bovill JG, Sebel PS, Fiolet JW, Touber JL, Kok DM. The influence of sufentanil on endocrine and metabolic responses to cardiac surgery. Anesth Analg 1983; 62:391–7.

Faden AI. Opiate antagonists and thyrotropin-releasing hormone. I. Potential role in the treatment of shock. JAMA 1984;252:1177–80.

Ganong WF. Review of Medical Physiology. 13th ed. Norwalk CT. Appleton and Lange. 1987.

Gingerich R, Wright PH, Paradise PR. Inhibition by halothane or glucose-stimulated insulin secretion in isolated pieces of rat pancreas. Anesthesiology 1974;40:449–52.

Hirsch IB, McGill JB, Cryer PE, White PF. Perioperative management of surgical patients with diabetes mellitus. Anesthesiology 1991;74:346–59.

Hume DM, Bell CC, Bartter FC. Direct measurement of adrenal secretion during operative trauma and convalescence. Surgery 1962;52:174–87.

Mazze RI, Scwartz RD, Slocum HC, Barry KG. Renal function during anesthesia and surgery—The effects of halothane anesthesia. Anesthesiology 1963;24:279–84.

Palahniuk RJ, Shnider SM, Eger EI II. Pregnancy decreases the requirement for inhaled anesthetic agents. Anesthesiology 1974;41:82–3.

Philbin DM, Coggins CH. Plasma antidiuretic hormone levels in cardiac surgical patients during morphine and halothane anesthesia. Anesthesiology 1978;49:95–8.

Rall TW, Sutherland EW. Formation of a cyclic adenine ribonucleotide by tissue particles. J Biol Chem 1958;232:1065–76.

Sebel PS, Bovill JG, Schellekens APM, Hawker CD. Hormonal responses to high-dose fentanyl anesthesia. Br J Anaesth 1981;53:941–8.

Strout CD, Nahrwold ML. Halothane requirement during pregnancy and lactation in rats. Anesthesiology 1981;55:322–3.

Symreng T, Karlberg BE, Kagedal B, Schidt B. Physiological cortisol substitution of long-term steroid treated patients undergoing major surgery. Br J Anaesth 1981;53:949–53.

Taylor AL, Fishman LM. Corticotropin-releasing hormone. N Engl J Med 1988;319:213–21.

Walsh J, Puig MM, Lovitz MA, Turndorf H. Premedication abolishes the increase in plasma beta-endorphin observed in the immediate preoperative period. Anesthesiology 1987;66:402–5.

Williams LT, Lefkotwitz RJ, Watanabe AM. Thyroid hormone regulation of beta-adrenergic receptor number. J Biol Chem 1977;252:2878–91.

Chapter
53
Kidneys

The principal function of the kidneys is to stabilize the composition of the extracellular fluid as reflected by electrolyte and hydrogen ion (H^+) concentrations. End-products of protein metabolism such as urea are excreted, whereas essential body nutrients including amino acids and glucose are retained. The kidneys also secrete hormones for the regulation of blood pressure (angiotensin II, prostaglandins, kinins) and the production of erythrocytes (erythropoietin). Anatomically, the kidneys are paired organs weighing 115 to 160 g each and located retroperitoneally just beneath the diaphragm. Each kidney consists of a cortical (outer) and medullary (inner) portion with the center of each kidney corresponding to about the level of L2.

NEPHRON

The functional unit of the kidney is the nephron, which is composed of capillaries known as the *glomerulus* and a long tubule in which the fluid filtered through the glomerular capillaries is converted into urine on its way to the renal pelvis (Fig. 53-1) (Pitts, 1974). Each kidney contains approximately 1.2 million nephrons; this number does not change after birth.

Glomerulus

The glomerulus is formed only in the renal cortex by a tuft of capillaries that invaginate into the dilated blind end of the renal tubule known as *Bowman's capsule.* Capillaries that form the glomerulus are unique anatomically in being interposed between two sets of arterioles. Blood enters the glomerular capillaries through afferent arterioles and leaves through efferent arterioles. Pressure in glomerular capillaries can be altered by changing the vascular activity of either the afferent or efferent arterioles. It is the pressure in glomerular capillaries that causes water and low molecular weight substances to filter into Bowman's capsule, which is in direct continuity with the proximal renal tubule.

Renal Tubule

Components of the renal tubule are the proximal convoluted tubule, the loop of Henle, and the distal convoluted tubule. From the proximal renal tubule, glomerular filtrate passes into the loop of Henle. Those loops of Henle that extend into the renal medulla are termed juxtamedullary nephrons; those that lie close to the surface of the kidneys are designated as *cortical nephrons* (Fig. 53-1) (Pitts, 1974). From the loop of Henle, fluid flows back into the renal cortex by way of the distal renal tubule. Finally, the glomerular filtrate enters the collecting duct, which delivers fluid from several nephrons into the renal pelvis.

As the glomerular filtrate travels along the renal tubule, most of its water and varying amounts of solutes are reabsorbed from the renal tubular lumen into peritubular capillaries (Table 53-1) (Ganong, 1987). In addition, small amounts of other solutes are secreted by renal tubular epithelial cells into the lumen of the renal tubule. Unwanted metabolic waste products are filtered through glomerular capillaries but, unlike water and electrolytes, are not reabsorbed as the glomer-

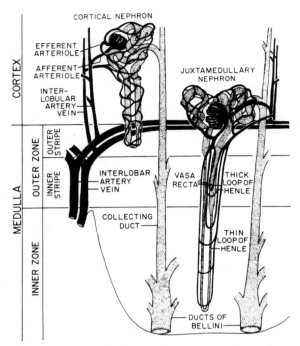

FIGURE 53–1. Schematic depiction of the nephron and accompanying blood supply. (From Pitts RF, Physiology of the Kidney and Body Fluids. 3rd ed. Chicago. Year Book Medical Publishers, 1974; with permission.)

ular filtrate progresses through the renal tubule (Table 53-1) (Ganong, 1987). Ultimately, the urine that is formed is composed mainly of substances filtered through the glomerular capillaries

in addition to small amounts of substances secreted by the renal tubular epithelial cells into the lumen of the renal tubule.

RENAL BLOOD FLOW

Renal blood flow is 1 to 1.2 L·min^{-1}, which represents 20% to 25% of the resting cardiac output. The pattern of renal vasculature parallels the structure of the nephron and has important functional implications. Anesthetics may reduce renal blood flow by decreasing the cardiac output, whereas sympathetic nervous system stimulation associated with surgical stimulation can increase renal vascular resistance to reduce renal blood flow.

Glomerular Capillaries

Blood enters the renal artery, which divides and ramifies, eventually providing the afferent arteriole of the glomerulus. This afferent arteriole is separated from the efferent arteriole by the glomerular capillaries (Fig. 53-1) (Pitts, 1974). The efferent arteriole offers significant resistance to blood flow, causing the glomerular capillaries to be a high-pressure system (Fig. 53-2) (Guyton, 1986). High pressure in the glomerular capillaries causes them to function in the same manner as arterial ends of tissue capillaries, with fluid filtering continuously out of the glomerular capillaries into Bowman's capsule.

Table 53-1
Magnitude and Site of Solute Reabsorption or Secretion in the Renal Tubules

	Filtered (24 h)	Reabsorbed (24 h)	Secreted (24 h)	Excreted (24 h)	Percent Reabsorbed	Location
Water (L)	180	179		1	99.4	P,L,D,C
Na$^+$ (mEq)	26,000	25,850		150	99.4	P,L,D,C
K$^+$ (mEq)	600	560	50	90	93.3	P,L,D,C
Cl$^-$ (mEq)	18,000	17,850		150	99.2	P,L,D,C
HCO$_3^-$ (mEq)	4900	4900		0	100	P,D
Urea (mM)	870	460		410	53	P,L,D,C
Uric acid (mM)	50	49	4	5	98	P
Glucose (mM)	800	800		0	100	P

P, proximal tubule; L, loop of Henle; D, distal tubule; C, convoluted tubule.

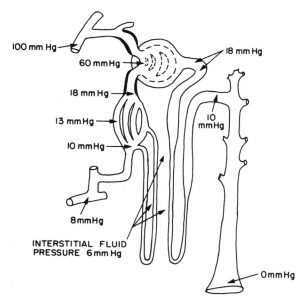

FIGURE 53-2. Intravascular pressures in the renal circulation. (From Guyton AC Textbook of Medical Physiology, 7th ed. Philadelphia: WB Saunders, 1986; with permission.)

Peritubular Capillaries

In the renal cortex, blood flows from the efferent arteriole into a second capillary network known as *peritubular capillaries*. In contrast to the high-pressure glomerular capillaries, the peritubular capillaries are a low-pressure system, which allows these capillaries to function in much the same way as the venous ends of tissue capillaries (Fig. 53-2) (Guyton, 1986). As a result, fluid from the renal tubules is absorbed continually into low-pressure peritubular capillaries. Indeed, of the 180 L of fluid filtered daily through the glomerular capillaries, all but approximately 1.5 L is reabsorbed from the renal tubules back into the peritubular capillaries, which eventually empty into the inferior vena cava.

Vasa Recta

The vascular pattern of the juxtamedullary nephrons is similar to that of the cortical nephrons except for a specialized portion of the peritubular capillaries known as the *vasa recta*. The vasa recta are capillaries that descend with the thin loops of Henle into the renal medulla before returning to the renal cortex to empty into the veins. Only 1% to 2% of renal blood flow passes through the vasa recta, emphasizing that blood flow through the medulla of the kidney is sluggish compared with the rapid blood flow that occurs in the renal cortex. Vasa recta capillaries are particularly important in the formation of concentrated urine because they control the rate of solute removal from the interstitium (countercurrent system).

Autoregulation of Renal Blood Flow

Changes in mean arterial pressure between approximately 60 and 160 mmHg autoregulate both renal blood flow and glomerular filtration rate (Fig. 53-3) (Guyton, 1986). Autoregulation of renal blood flow is due to an intrinsic mechanism that results in vasodilation or vasoconstriction of afferent renal arterioles. For example, reductions in mean arterial pressure and renal blood flow cause a decrease in glomerular capillary pressure and glomerular filtration rate. As a consequence, a negative feedback mechanism is activated, and signals from the macula densa cells cause vasodilation of the afferent renal arterioles (see the section entitled "Juxtaglomerular Apparatus"). This vasodilation allows renal blood flow to increase despite a persisting reduction in mean ar-

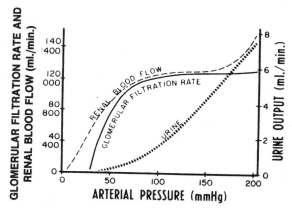

FIGURE 53-3. Renal blood flow and glomerular filtration rate, but not urine output, are autoregulated between a mean arterial pressure of approximately 60–160 mmHg. (From Guyton AC. Textbook of Medical Physiology, 7th ed. Philadelphia: WB Saunders, 1986; with permission.)

terial pressure. The same mechanism operates in the opposite direction, causing afferent arteriole vasoconstriction when mean arterial pressure becomes elevated. The fact that autoregulation occurs even in denervated kidneys confirms the intrinsic nature of the mechanism responsible for this response. The impact of anesthetic drugs on autoregulation of renal blood flow has not been extensively studied, although autoregulation has been demonstrated to be intact during administration of halothane to an animal model (Fig. 53-4) (Bastron et al, 1977).

Autoregulation of renal blood flow is not sustained in the presence of persistent changes in mean arterial pressure (approximately 10 minutes), which contrasts with sustained effects of autoregulation on glomerular filtration rate. This allows the glomerular filtration rate to remain near normal despite marked reductions in renal blood flow, which can be redistributed to other vital organs during prolonged periods of hypotension.

Juxtaglomerular Apparatus

Anatomically, the juxtaglomerular apparatus is the site where the distal renal tubule passes in the angle between renal afferent and efferent arterioles. Epithelial cells of the distal renal tubule that actually contact these arterioles are designated *macula densa cells,* whereas corresponding cells in the arterioles are known as *juxtaglomerular cells.* These juxtaglomerular cells release renin into the circulation during hypo-

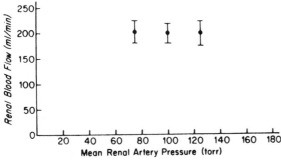

FIGURE 53–4. Autoregulation of renal blood flow seems to remain intact during halothane anesthesia. (From Bastron RD, Perkins FM, Pyne JL. Autoregulation of renal blood flow during halothane anesthesia. Anesthesiology 1977; 46: 142–4; with permission.)

tension, renal ischemia, or sympathetic nervous system stimulation in an effort by the kidney to maintain a normal renal blood flow and glomerular filtration rate. For example, formation of angiotensin II causes vasoconstriction of the efferent renal arterioles, which raises the glomerular capillary pressure so as to increase the glomerular filtration rate toward normal.

GLOMERULAR FILTRATE

Fluid that filters across glomerular capillaries into the renal tubule is designated *glomerular filtrate.* Permeability of glomerular capillaries is 100 to 1000 times as great as that of the usual tissue capillary. This increased capillary permeability reflects the presence of pores in the endothelial cells of the glomerular capillary membrane. These pores are of sufficient size to allow rapid filtration of fluid and small molecular weight substances with diameters less than 8 nm while excluding plasma proteins that have high molecular weights (albumin is the smallest protein, with a molecular weight of 69,000). For all practical purposes, glomerular filtrate is plasma without proteins.

Glomerular Filtration Rate

Glomerular filtration rate is the amount of glomerular filtrate formed each minute by all the nephrons. In normal persons, glomerular filtration rate averages 125 ml·min^{-1} or approximately 180 L each day. Reabsorption of approximately 99% of this 180 L of glomerular filtrate occurs during its passage through the renal tubule resulting in a daily urine output of 1 to 2 L. Urinary sodium ion (Na$^+$) excretion parallels glomerular filtration rate with approximately 1% of the filtered Na$^+$ being excreted in the urine (Table 53-1).

Mechanism of Glomerular Filtration

Glomerular filtration occurs by the same mechanism by which fluid filters out of any tissue capillary. Specifically, pressure inside glomerular capillaries causes filtration of fluid through the capillary membranes into the renal tubules. Normal filtration pressure is approximately 10 mmHg, which is calculated as glomerular capillary pressure (60 mmHg) minus colloid osmotic pressure (32 mmHg) and pressure in Bowman's capsule (18 mmHg). Normal glomerular filtration rate is 12.5 ml·min^{-1}·mmHg^{-1} of filtration pressure resulting in a glomerular filtration rate of 125 ml·min^{-1} when the net filtration pressure is 10 mmHg.

Filtration pressure responsible for glomerular filtration rate is influenced by mean arterial pressure, cardiac output, and sympathetic nervous system activity. Anesthetic-induced changes in these factors can exert profound effects on glomerular filtration rate and urine output. Indeed, virtually all anesthetic drugs and techniques are associated with decreases in glomerular filtration rate and urine output.

Mean Arterial Pressure

The impact of mean arterial pressure on glomerular filtration rate is blunted by autoregulation. Tubuloglomerular feedback, which probably occurs at the juxtaglomerular apparatus, is responsible for autoregulation of glomerular filtration rate. Specifically, signals from the macula densa cells in the distal renal tubules cause efferent or afferent renal arterioles to vasodilate or vasoconstrict and thus adjust the capillary pressure in the glomerulus to maintain an almost constant glomerular filtration rate, regardless of changes in the mean arterial pressure, between approximately 60 and 160 mmHg. Nevertheless, even a 5% change in glomerular filtration rate can result in substantial increases or decreases in urine output.

Cardiac Output

Because glomerular filtration rate parallels renal blood flow, it is clear that changes in cardiac output including those produced by anesthetics will have an important impact on glomerular filtration rate.

Sympathetic Nervous System

Innervation of the kidney is principally from T4 through T12. Sympathetic nervous system stimulation such as may occur in the perioperative period or exogenous administration of catecholamines results in preferential constriction of afferent renal arterioles, decreased pressure in glomerular capillaries, and a reduction in glomerular filtration rate. Excessive sympathetic nervous system stimulation can reduce glomerular capillary blood flow such that urine output decreases to almost zero.

RENAL TUBULAR FUNCTION

Glomerular filtrate flows through renal tubules and collecting ducts, during which time substances are selectively reabsorbed from tubules into peritubular capillaries or secreted into tubules by tubular epithelial cells. The resulting glomerular filtrate entering the renal pelvis is urine. The reabsorptive capabilities of various portions of renal tubules are different (Table 53-1) (Ganong, 1987). Reabsorption is more important than secretion in the overall formation of urine. Secretion, however, is particularly important in determining the amounts of K^+ and H^+ that appear in the urine. Secretion of H^+ by renal tubular cells is analogous to that which occurs in the stomach. Approximately two thirds of all reabsorptive and secretory processes in renal tubules take place in proximal renal tubules. As a result, only approximately one third of the original glomerular filtrate normally passes the entire distance through proximal renal tubules to reach the loops of Henle. The major physiologic determinants of the reabsorption of Na^+ and water are aldosterone, antidiuretic hormone (ADH), renal prostaglandins, and atrial natriuretic factor.

Active transport is responsible for the movement of Na^+ against a concentration gradient from the lumens of proximal renal tubules into the epithelial cells lining renal tubules and then into peritubular capillaries. Energy necessary for reabsorption of Na^+ is supplied by the Na^+–K^+ ATPase enzyme system. Glucose and amino acids share a common carrier (cotransport) with Na^+ to pass from renal tubules with epithelial cells. Inside the epithelial cells, glucose or amino acids split from the carrier and then diffuse through the cell membrane to enter peritubular capillaries. Aldosterone promotes reabsorption of Na^+ and secretion of H^+ and K^+ in the distal convoluted tubule.

More than 99% of the water in the glomerular filtrate is reabsorbed into peritubular capillaries as it passes through renal tubules. Nevertheless, lining epithelial cells in some portions of the renal tubule are more permeable to water, regardless of the concentration gradient for osmosis. For example, osmosis of water through proximal renal tubules is so rapid that the osmolar concentration of solutes on the peritubular capillary side of cell membranes is almost never more than a few mOsm greater than in the lumens of the tubules. Conversely, distal renal tubules are almost completely impermeable to water, which is important for controlling the specific gravity of urine. The permeability of the epithelial cells lining the collecting ducts is determined by ADH. ADH works by activating adenylate cyclase in the lining epithelial cells leading to formation of cyclic adenosine monophosphate and increased permeability of the cell membranes to water. As a result, when ADH levels are increased, most of the water is reabsorbed from the collecting ducts and returned to peritubular capillaries, resulting in excretion of minimal amounts of highly concentrated urine. In the absence of large amounts of ADH, little water is reabsorbed and large volumes of dilute urine are excreted. Painful stimulation as produced by surgery may evoke the release of ADH. Conversely, anesthetic drugs and opioids in the absence of surgical stimulation do not predictably cause the release of ADH. Likewise, positive end-expiratory pressure-induced antidiuresis is not associated with changes in the circulating plasma concentrations of ADH (Payen et al, 1987).

Countercurrent System

A *countercurrent system* is one in which blood inflow runs parallel and in the opposite direction to outflow. In the kidneys, the U-shaped anatomic arrangement of peritubular capillaries known as the vasa recta, to those loops of Henle that extend into the renal medulla make the countercurrent system possible. As a result, the kidneys are able to eliminate solutes with minimal excretion of water. The first step in the excretion of excess solutes in the urine is the formation of a high osmolarity renal medullary interstitial fluid. Indeed, osmolarity increases from approximately 300 mOsm·L^{-1} in the renal cortex to nearly 1200 mOsm·L^{-1} in the pelvic tip of the renal medulla. In addition, a sluggish medullary blood flow minimizes removal of solutes from the interstitial fluid of the renal medulla.

TUBULAR TRANSPORT MAXIMUM

Tubular transport maximum (Tm) is the maximal amount of a substance that can be actively reabsorbed from the lumens of renal tubules each minute. The Tm depends on the amounts of carrier substance and enzyme available to the specific active transport system in the lining epithelial cells of renal tubules.

The Tm for glucose is approximately 220 mg·min^{-1}. When the amount of glucose that filters through the glomerular capillary exceeds this amount, the excess glucose cannot be reabsorbed, but instead passes into the urine. The usual amount of glucose in the glomerular filtrate entering proximal renal tubules is 125 mg·min^{-1}, and there is no detectable loss into the urine. When the tubular load, however, exceeds approximately 220 mg·min^{-1} (threshold concentration), glucose first begins to appear in the urine. A blood glucose concentration of 180 mg·dl^{-1} in the presence of a normal glomerular filtration rate results in delivery of 220 mg·min^{-1} of glucose into the renal tubular fluid. Loss of glucose in the urine occurs at concentrations above the Tm for glucose. The presence of large amounts of unreabsorbed solutes in the urine such as glucose (or mannitol) produces osmotic diuresis.

REGULATION OF BODY FLUID CHARACTERISTICS

The kidneys are the most important organs for regulating the characteristics of body fluids. This regulation is apparent in the control of (1) blood volume; (2) extracellular fluid volume; (3) osmolarity of body fluids; and (4) plasma concentration of various ions, including H$^+$, and the resulting pH of body fluids. Thirst also plays a vital role in controlling some characteristics of body fluids.

Blood Volume

Blood volume is maintained over a narrow range despite marked daily variations in fluid and solute intake or loss. The basic mechanism for the control of blood volume is the same feedback loop that also influences blood pressure, cardiac output, and urine output. Specifically, an increase in blood volume increases cardiac output, which increases blood pressure. Increased blood pressure subsequently leads to renal changes (increased renal blood flow and glomerular filtration rate) that cause an increased urine output and a return of blood volume to normal. The reverse sequence occurs when the blood volume is decreased. The effect of changes in blood pressure on urine output seems to be sustained indefinitely.

The effects of blood volume on blood pressure, cardiac output, and urine output are slow to develop, requiring several hours to produce a full effect. This process, however, can be accelerated by (1) volume receptor reflexes, (2) ADH, (3) aldosterone, and (4) inherent vascular capacity of the circulation. For example, increased blood volume causes increased pressure in the atria, and the resultant stretch of the volume receptors initiates reflex responses that facilitate renal excretion of fluid and decelerate the return of blood volume toward normal. Increased circulating concentrations of ADH (water reabsorption is facilitated), aldosterone (Na^+ reabsorption leads to osmotic reabsorption of water), or both produce a decrease in urine volume and a tendency to restore blood volume. Persistent stimulation of the sympathetic nervous system and associated vasoconstriction as may occur in the presence of a pheochromocytoma leads to a reduction in blood volume, reflecting the inherent vascular capacity of the circulation. A similar decrease in blood volume may accompany chronic blood pressure elevations associated with essential hypertension. Conversely, blood volume may be increased by chronic drug-induced vasodilation or the effects of severe varicose veins.

Extracellular Fluid Volume

Control of extracellular fluid volume by the kidneys occurs by the same mechanisms and at the same time as control of blood volume. It is not possible to alter blood volume without also simultaneously changing extracellular fluid volume. Indeed, extracellular fluid becomes a reservoir for excess fluid that may be administered intravenously during the perioperative period.

Osmolarity of Body Fluids

Osmolarity of body fluids is determined almost entirely by the concentration of Na^+ in the extracellular fluid. Control of Na^+ concentration and, thus, osmolarity of body fluids is under the influence of the osmoreceptor–ADH mechanism and the thirst reflex. In contrast, the effect of aldosterone on plasma Na^+ concentration and the resulting plasma osmolarity are insignificant (Fig. 53-5) (Guyton, 1986). This is due to the fact that aldosterone-induced reabsorption of Na^+ is accompanied by a simultaneous reabsorption of water. Indeed, patients with primary aldosteronism often manifest an increased extracellular fluid volume but the plasma Na^+ concentration rarely increases more than 2 to 3 $mEq \cdot L^{-1}$.

Osmoreceptor–Antidiuretic Hormone

An increase in osmolarity of extracellular fluid owing to excess Na^+ causes osmoreceptors in the supraoptic nuclei of the hypothalamus to shrink and thereby increase the discharge rate of impulses through the pituitary stalk to the posterior pituitary where ADH is released. The resulting ADH-induced retention of water dilutes the plasma concentration of Na^+ and returns os-

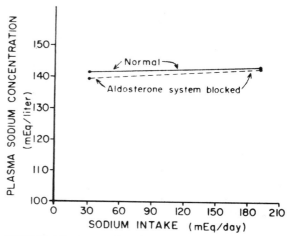

FIGURE 53-5. In the absence of aldosterone, the plasma concentration of sodium varies less than 2% over a sixfold range in sodium intake. (From Guyton AC. Textbook of Medical Physiology, 7th ed. Philadelphia: WB Saunders, 1986; with permission.)

molarity downward toward a normal value. Conversely, when extracellular fluid becomes too dilute, the osmoreceptors inhibit the release of ADH and more water than solute is excreted by the kidneys, thus concentrating Na^+ and returning osmolarity upward toward normal. Changes in osmolarity of 1% to 5% evoke substantial alterations in the circulating concentration of ADH. In contrast, changes in blood volume must usually exceed 10% to evoke changes in ADH release by the osmoreceptors. For all practical purposes, osmoreceptors may be considered as Na^+ concentration receptors.

Thirst Reflex

The most common cause for thirst is an increased Na^+ concentration in the extracellular fluid. Any change in circulation that leads to increased production of angiotensin II, such as acute hemorrhage or congestive heart failure, also leads to thirst. Although the sensation of a dry mouth is often associated with the thirst reflex, the blockade of salivary secretions, as by anticholinergic drugs, does not cause humans to drink excessively. The thirst reflex is activated when the plasma concentration of Na^+ increases approximately 2 $mEq \cdot L^{-1}$ above normal or when the plasma osmolarity rises approximately 4 $mOsm \cdot L^{-1}$. Humans typically drink the correct amount of water, allowing precise maintenance of the osmolarity of extracellular fluid. Indeed, relief from thirst occurs almost immediately after drinking water, even before this water has been absorbed from the gastrointestinal tract.

Plasma Concentration of Ions

Potassium

The role of the kidneys in controlling the plasma concentration of K^+ is mediated principally by the effects of aldosterone on the renal tubules. Indeed, small changes in the plasma concentration of K^+ evoke large changes in the plasma concentration of aldosterone (Fig. 53-6) (Guyton, 1986). In the presence of aldosterone, there is increased secretion of K^+ into renal tubules, leading to increased loss of this ion into the urine. Excessive amounts of aldosterone in patients with primary aldosteronism produce hypo-

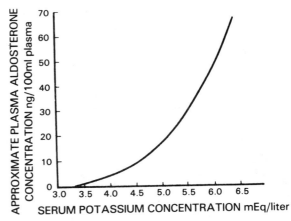

FIGURE 53–6.   Small changes in the plasma concentrations of potassium evoke large changes in the plasma concentrations of aldosterone. (From Guyton AC. Textbook of Medical Physiology, 7th ed. Philadelphia: WB Saunders, 1986; with permission.)

kalemia with associated skeletal muscle weakness owing to nerve transmission failure because of hyperpolarization of nerve membranes. When aldosterone activity is blocked, as by certain diuretics, the plasma K^+ concentration parallels intake of K^+, making hypokalemia or hyperkalemia possible (Fig. 53-7) (Guyton, 1986). Absence of aldosterone, such as is associated with Addison's disease, may result in hyperkalemia.

In addition to aldosterone, the plasma concentration of H^+ and Na^+ may exert modest effects on K^+ elimination in the urine. For example, H^+ competes with K^+ for secretion into the renal tubules. In the presence of acidosis, H^+ are preferentially secreted into the renal tubules and plasma K^+ concentrations may increase. Conversely, alkalosis is associated with hypokalemia. The level of Na^+ intake may influence plasma concentrations of K^+ because Na^+ is transported through renal tubular epithelial cells in exchange for K^+.

Sodium

The role of the kidneys in controlling the plasma concentration of Na^+ reflects active transport of Na^+ across renal tubular epithelial cells into peritubular capillaries. Approximately two thirds of Na^+ is reabsorbed from the proximal renal tubules and no more than 10% of Na^+ that initially

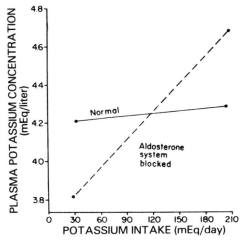

FIGURE 53-7. Plasma concentrations of potassium parallel intake when aldosterone activity is impaired. (From Guyton AC. Textbook of Medical Physiology, 7th ed. Philadelphia: WB Saunders, 1986; with permission.)

enters the glomerular filtrate is likely to reach the distal renal tubule. Aldosterone influences reabsorption of Na^+ from the distal renal tubules and collecting ducts. In the presence of large amounts of aldosterone, almost all the remaining Na^+ is reabsorbed and urinary excretion of Na^+ approaches zero. Aldosterone acts by entering the lining epithelial cells of the renal tubules where it combines with a receptor protein. This receptor protein activates DNA molecules to form messenger RNA, which subsequently causes the formation of the carrier proteins or protein enzymes necessary for the Na^+ and K^+ transport process. The formation of these substances requires approximately 45 minutes following the release of aldosterone.

Hydrogen

The kidneys secrete excess H^+ by exchanging a H^+ for a Na^+, thus acidifying the urine, and by the synthesis of ammonia, which combines with H^+ to form ammonium.

Calcium

Calcium ion (Ca^{2+}) concentration is controlled principally by the effect of parathyroid hormone on bone reabsorption. For example, a decrease in the plasma concentration of Ca^{2+} releases parathyroid hormone, which causes the release of Ca^{2+} from bone. When plasma Ca^{2+} concentrations are elevated, the secretion of parathyroid hormone is reduced to the point at which almost no release of Ca^{2+} from bone occurs. In addition to effects on bone, parathyroid hormone increases reabsorption of Ca^{2+} from the distal renal tubules, collecting ducts, and gastrointestinal tract.

Magnesium

Magnesium is reabsorbed by all portions of the renal tubules. Urinary excretion of magnesium parallels the plasma concentration of the ion.

Urea

Urea is the most abundant of the metabolic waste products that must be excreted in urine to prevent excess accumulation in body fluids. The major factors in determining the rate of urea excretion are the plasma concentration of urea (blood urea nitrogen or BUN), and glomerular filtration rate. Typically, approximately 50% of the urea that initially enters the renal tubules appears in the urine.

When the glomerular filtration rate is low, the glomerular filtrate remains in the renal tubules for prolonged periods before it becomes urine. The longer the period that the filtrate remains in the renal tubules, the greater is the reabsorption of urea. As a result, the amount of urea that reaches the urine is reduced and the BUN is increased. Conversely, when the glomerular filtration rate is increased, glomerular filtrate passes through renal tubules so rapidly that very little urea is reabsorbed into peritubular capillaries.

ATRIAL NATRIURETIC FACTOR

Cardiac atria synthesize, store, and secrete via the coronary sinus an amino acid hormone known as *atrial natriuretic factor* (ANF). This hormone produces a dose-dependent increase in urine volume and Na^+ excretion primarily by increasing glomerular filtration rate. As a potent vasodilator, ANF decreases blood pressure and elicits renal artery vasodilation. ANF antagonizes the release and end-organ effects of renin, aldosterone, and ADH.

Circulating plasma concentrations of ANF are linearly related to right and left atrial pressure and also proportional to atrial diameter. Inhibition of ANF release diminishes urine output and urinary Na^+ excretion while increasing plasma renin activity. Positive end-expiratory pressure-induced decreases in atrial distension result in reduced ANF release, which may mediate in part the antidiuretic and antinatriuretic effects of positive end-expiratory pressure (Kharasch et al, 1988). Hypothermic cardiopulmonary bypass is also associated with reductions in plasma concentrations of ANF (Kharasch et al, 1989).

ACUTE RENAL FAILURE

Acute renal failure is most often a result of acute glomerulonephritis or acute damage or obstruction to the renal tubules. Renal tubular injury, which may lead to acute renal failure, is likely due to an imbalance of the oxygen supply and demand of medullary ascending limb tubular cells (Byrick and Rose, 1990). High oxygen demand of these renal tubular cells is secondary to active reabsorption of solute, especially Na^+, which is increased in the presence of hypovolemia. In the presence of decreased renal blood flow, injury to ascending-limb tubular cells is exacerbated by arterial hypoxemia and endothelial cell swelling, which reduces further the perfusion of these metabolically active cells.

The normal kidney can autoregulate both its blood flow and its glomerular filtration rate in response to changes in cardiac output or perfusion pressure. This autoregulation is controlled by neural and humoral mechanisms that mediate intrarenal adjustment of vascular resistance and blood flow. When the limits of autoregulation are exceeded, ischemic renal injury can occur.

Acute Glomerulonephritis

In approximately 95% of patients, the abnormal immune reaction that causes acute glomerulonephritis occurs 1 to 3 weeks following an infection with group A beta streptococci at a site other than the kidneys. Antibodies that develop against the streptococcal antigen become entrapped in the basement membrane of the glomerular capillar-

ies. Once the immune complex has deposited in the glomerular capillaries, the cells begin to proliferate and large numbers of leukocytes become entrapped in the glomeruli. Many glomeruli become occluded because of this inflammatory reaction, and those that are not blocked often become excessively permeable, allowing both protein and erythrocytes to leak into the glomerular filtrate. In severe cases, acute renal failure may occur, but in most cases, the acute inflammation of the glomeruli subsides in 10 to 14 days and renal function recovers.

Acute Tubular Necrosis

Acute tubular necrosis reflects destruction of epithelial cells lining the renal tubules and is most often due to nephrotoxins (chloroform) or renal ischemia as produced by prolonged decreases in blood pressure and renal blood flow (shock). A transfusion reaction may cause acute tubular necrosis owing to hemolysis of erythrocytes and precipitation of free hemoglobin in the renal tubules, causing blockage of the nephron.

CHRONIC RENAL FAILURE

Despite different causes (chronic glomerulonephritis or pyelonephritis), the common denominator present in patients who develop chronic renal failure is progressive loss of nephron function and decline in glomerular filtration rate (Table 53-2). Renal reserve is decreased but patients remain asymptomatic when at least 40% of the nephrons continue to function. Renal insufficiency is present when only 10% to 40% of nephrons are functioning. These patients are compensated, but there is no renal reserve such that excess catabolic loads or toxic substances (aminoglycosides) can exacerbate renal insufficiency. Polyuria and nocturia in these patients most likely reflect decreased urine concentrating ability. Loss of more than 90% of functioning nephrons results in uremia (urine in the blood) and the need for dialytic treatment.

Chronic Glomerulonephritis

Chronic glomerulonephritis begins with the accumulation of precipitated antigen–antibody

Table 53-2
Stages of Chronic Renal Failure

	Estimated Number of Nephrons (Percent of Total)	Glomerular Filtration Rate (ml·min⁻¹)	Signs	Laboratory Changes
Normal		125	None	None
Decreased renal reserve	40	50–80	None	None
Renal insufficiency	10–40	12–50	Polyuria Nocturia	Increased blood urea nitrogen Increased creatinine
Uremia	10	12	See Table 53-3	See Table 53-3

complex in the glomerular capillary membrane, although this is rarely caused by streptococcal infection. Inflammation of the glomeruli results in progressive thickening of the glomerular membrane, which is eventually invaded by fibrous tissue. In the final stages of this disease, many of the glomerular capillaries are replaced by fibrous tissue, and the function of the nephron is lost.

Pyelonephritis

Pyelonephritis is an infectious and inflammatory process that usually begins in the renal pelvis but extends progressively into the renal parenchyma, destroying glomeruli and renal tubules. Infection can result from many different types of bacteria but is most often due to colon bacilli that originate from fecal contamination of the urinary tract. Infection usually affects the structures in the renal medulla of the kidney more than the cortex. As a result, the countercurrent system may be impaired, manifesting as an inability to excrete concentrated urine.

Manifestations of Chronic Renal Failure

Chronic renal failure is associated with multiple derangements affecting several organ systems (Table 53-3). A comprehensive preoperative evaluation must include assessment of these multiple derangements and review of renal function tests (Table 53-4).

Specific gravity of the urine approaches the glomerular filtrate (approximately 1.008) as progressively more nephrons are lost and the countercurrent system fails. Anemia is severe but usually well tolerated, reflecting its slow onset and compensatory increases in tissue blood flow and oxygen delivery made possible by reductions in blood viscosity and rightward shift of the oxyhemoglobin dissociation curve in response to acidosis and increased concentrations of 2,3-diphosphoglycerate. It is presumed that anemia associated with chronic renal failure reflects decreased renal secretion of the enzyme that splits erythropoietin from a plasma protein. Erythropoietin normally stimulates bone marrow to produce erythrocytes. Inability of the kidney to eliminate H^+ produced by metabolic processes of the body predictably results in metabolic acidosis. Hyperkalemia reflects inability of diseased

Table 53-3
Manifestations of Chronic Renal Failure

Accumulation of metabolic waste products in blood
Excretion of fixed–specific-gravity urine
Metabolic acidosis
Hyperkalemia
Anemia
Platelet dysfunction
Fluid overload and hypertension
Nervous system dysfunction
Osteomalacia

Table 53–4
Renal Function Tests

	Normal Value	Interpretation Influenced by
Blood urea nitrogen	8–20 mg·dl^{-1}	Dehydration Variable protein intake Gastrointestinal bleeding Catabolism
Creatinine	0.5–1.2 mg·dl^{-1}	Age Skeletal muscle mass Catabolism
Creatinine clearance	120 ml·min^{-1}	Accurate urine volume measurement

kidneys to eliminate K^+ and has important anesthetic implications especially with respect to cardiac rhythm and responses at the neuromuscular junction. Accumulation of metabolic waste products in the blood interferes with platelet aggregation while prothrombin time and plasma thromboplastin time usually remain normal. Retention of Na^+ and water results in fluid overload that may manifest as congestive heart failure and hypertension. Neurologic complications occur in the central nervous system (confusion or coma); peripheral nervous system (neuropathy); and autonomic nervous system. Uremic coma is most likely due to reductions in pH, whereas rapid and deep breathing during uremic coma is presumed to reflect an attempt to compensate for metabolic acidosis. Dialytic therapy is useful in correcting electrolyte, fluid, and platelet function. Alternatively, an analogue of vasopressin, DDAVP, is effective in shortening bleeding time within one hour following its intravenous infusion.

Dialytic Therapy

Chronic dialytic therapy is a complex technical challenge associated with multiple side effects (Table 53-5).

Hemodialysis

Hemodialysis is based on diffusive transport of solute down an osmotic gradient across a semipermeable membrane (cellophane). The dialysate should contain little or none of the substance to be removed from the patient's blood such that there will be a net transfer of solutes from the plasma into the dialyzing fluid. During hemodialysis, blood flows continually from an artery through the artificial kidney and back into a vein. Heparin is added to the blood as it enters the artificial kidney and protamine is added before the blood is returned to the patient. The need to maintain chronic vascular access via a surgically created arteriovenous fistula is a major cause of morbidity in patients with chronic renal failure.

Peritoneal Dialysis

The capillary network present in the peritoneal cavity provides a large surface area for contact of the patient's blood with the dialysate and is the basis for peritoneal dialysis. Surgical placement of an indwelling peritoneal catheter (Tenckhoff catheter) is necessary. Peritonitis is the major complication associated with peritoneal dialysis.

NEPHROTIC SYNDROME

Nephrotic syndrome is characterized by loss of large amounts of plasma proteins (up to 30 g daily) into the urine, reflecting increased permeability of the glomerular capillary membrane. The loss of protein causes a reduction in colloid osmotic pressure that manifests as edema, ascites, and accumulation of fluid in the pericardium, pleural cavity, and joints. Causes of the nephrotic syndrome include chronic glomerulonephritis, amyloidosis, and lipoid nephrosis. Glucocorticoids will usually cause complete remission of lipoid nephrosis but not the other causes of the nephrotic syndrome.

Table 53–5
Complications of Dialytic Therapy

Dementia

Hypotension

Hypoxemia

Skeletal muscle cramping

Protein depletion

Infection

Anticoagulation

Access failure

TRANSPORT OF URINE TO THE BLADDER

Urine is transported to the bladder through the ureters, which originate in the pelvis of each kidney. Each ureter is innervated by the sympathetic and parasympathetic nervous system. As urine collects in the renal pelvis, the pressure in the pelvis increases and initiates a peristaltic contraction that travels downward along the ureter to force urine toward the bladder. Parasympathetic nervous system stimulation increases the frequency of peristalsis, whereas sympathetic nervous system stimulation decreases peristalsis. At its distal end, the ureter penetrates the bladder obliquely such that pressure in the bladder compresses the ureter, thereby preventing reflux of urine into the ureter when bladder pressure increases during micturition.

Ureters are well supplied with nerve fibers such that obstruction of a ureter by a stone causes intense reflex constriction and pain. In addition, pain is likely to elicit a sympathetic nervous system reflex (ureterorenal reflex) that causes vasoconstriction of the renal arterioles and a concomitant reduction in urine formation in the kidney served by the blocked ureter.

As the bladder fills with urine, stretch receptors in the bladder wall initiate micturition contractions. Sensory signals are conducted to the sacral segments of the spinal cord through the pelvic nerves and then back again to the bladder through parasympathetic nervous system fibers.

The micturition reflex is a completely automatic spinal cord reflex that can be inhibited (tonic contraction of the exteral urinary sphincter) or facilitated by centers in the brain. Spinal cord damage above the sacral region leaves the micturition reflex intact, but it is no longer controlled by the brain.

REFERENCES

Bastron RD, Perkins FM, Pyne JL. Autoregulation of renal blood flow during halothane anesthesia. Anesthesiology 1977;46:142–4.

Byrick RJ, Rose DK. Pathophysiology and prevention of acute renal failure: The role of the anaesthetist. Can J Anaesth 1990;37:457–67.

Ganong WF. Review of Medical Physiology. 13th ed. Norwalk CT. Appleton and Lange. 1987.

Guyton AC. Textbook of Medical Physiology. 7th ed. Philadelphia. WB Saunders. 1986.

Kharasch ED, Yeo K-T, Kenny MA, Amory DW. Influence of hypothermic cardiopulmonary bypass on atrial natriuretic factor levels. Can J Anaesth 1989;36:545–53.

Kharasch ED, Yeo K-T, Kenny MA, Buffington CW. Atrial natriuretic factor may mediate the renal effects of PEEP ventilation. Anesthesiology 1988;69:862–9.

Payen DM, Farge D, Beloucif S, Leviel F, DeLaCaussaye JE, Carli P, Wirquin V. No involvement of antidiuretic hormone in acute antidiuresis during PEEP ventilation in humans. Anesthesiology 1987;66:17–23.

Pitts RF. Physiology of the Kidney and Body Fluids. 3rd ed. Chicago. Year Book Medical Publishers. 1974.

Chapter

54

Liver and Gastrointestinal Tract

LIVER

The liver lies in the right upper quadrant of the abdominal cavity and is attached to the diaphragm. It is the largest gland in the body, weighing approximately 1500 g and representing 2% of adult body weight. In the neonate, the liver accounts for approximately 5% of body weight. Hepatocytes represent approximately 80% of the cytoplasmic mass within the liver. These cells perform diverse and complex functions (Table 54-1).

Anatomy

The liver is divided into four lobes consisting of 50,000 to 100,000 individual hepatic lobules (Fig. 54-1) (Bloom and Fawcell, 1975). Blood flows past hepatocytes via sinusoids from branches of the portal vein and hepatic artery to a central vein. There is usually only one layer of hepatocytes between sinusoids so the total area of contact with plasma is great. Central veins join to form hepatic veins, which drain into the inferior vena cava. Each hepatocyte is also opposed to bile canaliculi, which coalesce to form the common hepatic duct. This duct and the cystic duct from the gallbladder join to form the common bile duct, which enters the duodenum at a site surrounded by the sphincter of Oddi (Fig. 54-2) (Bell et al, 1976). The main pancreatic duct also unites with the common bile duct just before it enters the duodenum.

Hepatic lobules are lined by Kupffer's cells, which phagocytize 99% or more of bacteria in the portal venous blood. This is crucial because the portal venous blood drains the gastrointestinal tract and almost always contains colon bacteria.

Endothelial cells that line the hepatic lobules contain large pores, permitting easy diffusion of large substances, including plasma proteins, into extravascular spaces of the liver that connect with terminal lymphatics. The extreme permeability of the lining endothelial cells allows large quantities of lymph to form, which contain protein concentrations that are only slightly less than the protein concentration of plasma. Indeed, approximately one third to one half of all the lymph is formed in the liver (see Chapter 45).

Hepatocyte plasma membranes contain adrenergic receptors (alpha-1, alpha-2, and beta-2) whose activity may be influenced by volatile anesthetics. Alpha-1 receptors predominate and their activation results in increased intracellular calcium ion (Ca^{2+}) concentrations. A similar response accompanies hypoxia. Excessive intracellular accumulation of intracellular Ca^{2+} is associated with toxicity and cell death.

Hepatic Blood Flow

The liver receives a dual afferent blood supply from the hepatic artery and portal vein (Fig. 54-3). Total hepatic blood flow is approximately 1450 ml·min^{-1} or approximately 29% of the car-

782

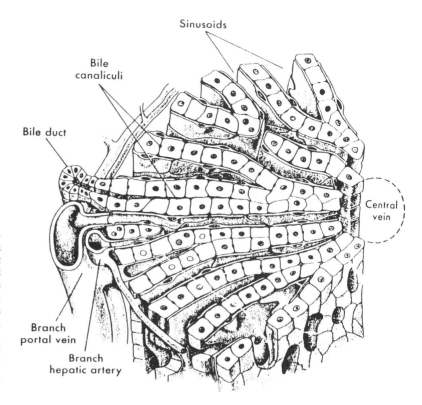

FIGURE 54–1. Schematic depiction of a hepatic lobule with a central vein and plates of hepatic cells extending radially. Blood from peripherally located branches of the hepatic artery and vein perfuses the sinusoids. Bile ducts drain the bile canaliculi that run between the hepatocytes. (From Bloom W, Fawcell DW. A Textbook of Histology. 10th ed. Philadelphia: WB Saunders. 1975; with permission.)

diac output. Of this amount, the portal vein provides 75% of the total flow but only 50% to 55% of the hepatic oxygen supply because this blood is partially deoxygenated in the preportal organs and tissues (gastrointestinal tract, spleen, and pancreas). The hepatic artery provides only 25% of total hepatic blood flow but provides 45% to 50% of the hepatic oxygen requirements. Hepatic artery blood flow maintains nutrition of connective tissues and walls of bile ducts. For this reason, loss of hepatic artery blood flow can be fatal

because of ensuing necrosis of vital liver structures.

Control of Hepatic Blood Flow

Portal vein blood flow is controlled primarily by the arterioles in the preportal splanchnic organs. This flow, combined with the resistance to portal vein blood flow within the liver, determines portal venous pressure (normally 7 to 10 mmHg) (see the section entitled "Portal Venous Pressure"). Sympathetic nervous system innervation is from T3 to T11 and is mediated via alpha receptors. This innervation is principally responsible for resistance and compliance of hepatic venules. Changes in hepatic venous compliance play an essential role in overall regulation of cardiac output and the reservoir function of the liver (see the section entitled "Reservoir Function").

Fibrotic constriction characteristic of hepatic cirrhosis can increase resistance to portal vein blood flow as evidenced by portal venous pressures of 20 to 30 mmHg. Conversely, congestive

Table 54–1
Functions of Hepatocytes

Absorb nutrients from portal venous blood

Store and release proteins, lipids, and carbohydrates

Excrete bile salts

Synthesize plasma proteins, glucose, cholesterol, and fatty acids

Metabolize exogenous and endogenous compounds

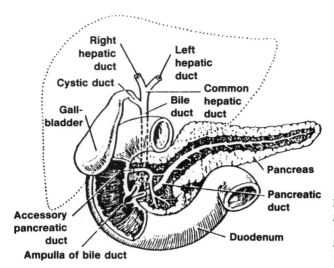

FIGURE 54–2. Connections of the ducts of the gallbladder, liver, and pancreas. (From Bell GH, Emslie-Smith D, Paterson CR. Textbook of Physiology and Biochemistry. 9th ed. New York: Churchill Livingston, 1976; with permission.)

heart failure and positive pressure ventilation of the lungs impairs outflow of blood from the liver because of increased central venous pressure, which is transmitted to hepatic veins. Ascites results when elevated portal venous pressures cause transudation of protein-rich fluid through the outer surface of the liver capsule and gastrointestinal tract into the abdominal cavity. Hepatic artery blood flow is influenced by arteriolar tone that reflects local and intrinsic mechanisms (autoregulation). For example, a decrease in portal vein blood flow is accompanied by an increase in hepatic artery blood flow. Presumably, a vasodilating substance such as adenosine accumulates in the liver when portal vein blood flow decreases, leading to subsequent hepatic arterial vasodilation and washout of the vasodilating material.

Halothane decreases hepatic oxygen supply to a greater extent than isoflurane or enflurane when administered in equal potent doses (Gelman et al, 1984) (see Fig. 2-24). Enflurane and particularly isoflurane preserve the ability of hepatic arterial blood flow to increase when portal vein blood flow decreases. Conversely, halothane preserves this autoregulation to a limited extent and only when used in doses that do not decrease blood pressure greater than approximately 20%. Surgical stimulation may further decrease hepatic blood flow independent of the anesthetic drug administered (Gelman, 1976). The greatest reductions in hepatic blood flow occur during intraabdominal operations presum-

ably owing to mechanical interference to blood flow produced by retraction in the operative area as well as the release of vasoconstricting substances such as catecholamines.

Reservoir Function

The liver normally contains approximately 500 ml of blood or approximately 10% of the total blood volume. Elevation of the right atrial pres-

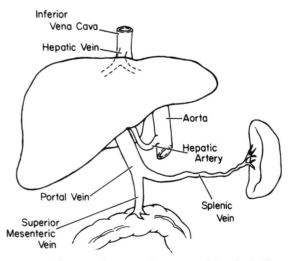

FIGURE 54–3. Schematic depiction of the dual afferent blood supply to the liver provided by the portal vein and hepatic artery.

sure causes back pressure, and the liver, being a distensible organ, may accommodate as much as 1 L of extra blood. As such, the liver acts as a storage site when blood volume is excessive, as in congestive heart failure, and is capable of supplying extra blood when hypovolemia occurs. Indeed, the large hepatic veins and sinuses are constricted by stimulation from the sympathetic nervous system, discharging up to 350 ml of blood into the circulation. Therefore, the liver is the single most important source of additional blood during strenuous exercise or acute hemorrhage.

Bile Secretion

Hepatocytes continually form bile (500 ml daily) and then secrete it into bile canaliculi, which empty into progressively larger ducts ultimately reaching the common bile duct (Fig. 54-2) (Bell et al, 1976). Between meals, the tone of the sphincter of Oddi, which guards the entrance of the common bile duct into the duodenum, is high. As a result, bile flow is diverted into the gallbladder, which has a capacity of 35 to 50 ml. The most potent stimulus for emptying the gallbladder is the presence of fat in the duodenum, which evokes the release of the hormone cholecystokinin by the duodenal mucosa. This hormone enters the circulation and passes to the gallbladder, where it causes selective contraction of the gallbladder smooth muscle. As a result, bile is forced from the gallbladder into the duodenum. When adequate amounts of fat are present, the gallbladder empties in approximately 1 hour.

The principal components of bile are bile salts, bilirubin, and cholesterol.

Bile Salts

Bile salts combine with lipids in the duodenum to form water soluble complexes (micelles) that facilitate gastrointestinal absorption of fats and accompany fat-soluble vitamins. In the absence of bile secretion, steatorrhea and a deficiency of vitamin K develop in a few days.

Bilirubin

After approximately 120 days, the cell membranes of erythrocytes rupture and the released

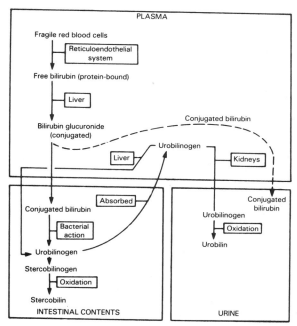

FIGURE 54-4. Schematic depiction of bilirubin formation and excretion. (From Guyton AC. Textbook of Medical Physiology. 7th ed. Philadelphia: WB Saunders, 1986; with permission.)

hemoglobin is converted to bilirubin in reticuloendothelial cells (Fig. 54-4) (Guyton, 1986). The resulting bilirubin is released into the circulation and transported in combination with albumin to the liver. In hepatocytes, bilirubin dissociates from bilirubin and conjugates principally with glucuronic acid. Unlike conjugated bilirubin, unconjugated bilirubin may be neurotoxic and may even cause a rapidly fatal encephalopathy. In the gastrointestinal tract, bilirubin is converted by bacterial action mainly into urobilinogen.

JAUNDICE. Jaundice is the yellowish tint of body tissues that accompanies accumulation of bilirubin in extracellular fluid. Skin color usually begins to change when the plasma concentration of bilirubin increases to approximately three times normal. The most common types of jaundice are hemolytic jaundice, owing to increased destruction of erythrocytes, and obstructive jaundice, owing to obstruction of bile ducts.

Cholesterol

Cholesterol in the bile may precipitate as gallstones if there is excess absorption of water in the gallbladder or the diet contains too much cholesterol. Gallstones occur in 10% to 20% of individuals; 85% are cholesterol stones. Daily oral administration of a naturally occurring bile salt, chenodeoxycholic acid, results in an increased volume of bile formation with a resulting dilution of cholesterol concentration. As a result, cholesterol becomes more soluble, and over a period of 1 to 2 years, cholesterol stones may be dissolved (Boucheir, 1980).

Metabolic Functions

Metabolism of carbohydrates, lipids, and proteins is dependent on normal hepatic function (see Chapter 58). Furthermore, the liver is an important storage site for vitamins and iron (see Chapter 34). Degradation of certain hormones (catecholamines and corticosteroids) as well as drugs is an important function of the liver. Formation of many of the coagulation factors occurs in the liver.

Carbohydrates

Regulation of the blood glucose concentration is an important metabolic function of the liver. When hyperglycemia is present, glycogen is deposited in the liver, and when hypoglycemia occurs, glycogenolysis provides glucose. Amino acids can be converted to glucose by gluconeogenesis when the blood glucose concentration is reduced.

Lipids

The liver is responsible for beta oxidation of fatty acids and formation of acetoacetic acid. Lipoproteins, cholesterol, and phospholipids, such as lecithin, are formed in the liver. Synthesis of fats from carbohydrates and proteins also occurs in the liver.

Proteins

The most important liver functions in protein metabolism are deamination of amino acids, formation of urea for removal of ammonia, formation of plasma proteins, and interconversions among different amino acids. Deamination of amino acids is required before these substances can be used for energy or converted into carbohydrates or fats. Reduction of portal vein blood flow as may occur with the surgical creation of portacaval shunt to treat esophageal varices can result in fatal hepatic coma owing to accumulation of ammonia.

GASTROINTESTINAL TRACT

The primary function of the gastrointestinal tract is to provide the body with a continual supply of water, electrolytes, and nutrients. To achieve this goal, the contents of the gastrointestinal tract must move through the entire system at an appropriate rate for digestive and absorptive functions to occur. Each part of the gastrointestinal tract is adapted for specific functions such as (1) passage of food in the esophagus, (2) storage of food in the stomach or fecal matter in the colon, (3) digestion of food in the stomach and small intestine, and (4) absorption of the digestive end-products and fluids in the small intestine and proximal parts of the colon. Overall, approximately 9 L of fluid and secretions enters the gastrointestinal tract daily and all but approximately 100 ml is absorbed by the small intestine and colon (Fig. 54-5) (Berne and Levy, 1988). The pH of gastrointestinal secretions varies widely (Table 54-2).

Anatomy

The smooth muscle of the gastrointestinal tract is a syncytium such that electrical signals originating in one smooth muscle fiber are easily propagated from fiber to fiber. Mechanical activity of the gastrointestinal tract is enhanced by stretch and parasympathetic nervous system stimulation, whereas sympathetic nervous system stimulation reduces mechanical activity to almost zero.

Tonic contraction of gastrointestinal smooth muscle at the pylorus, ileocecal valve, and anal sphincter helps regulate the rate at which materials move through the gastrointestinal tract. In other parts of the gastrointestinal tract, rhythmic movements (peristalsis) occur 3 to 12 times·min^{-1} to facilitate mixing and movement of food.

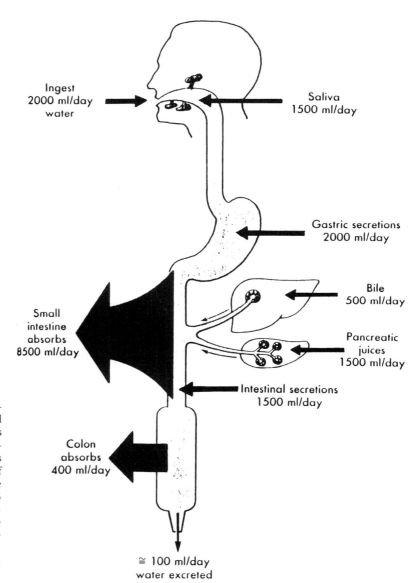

FIGURE 54–5. Overall fluid balance in the human gastrointestinal tract. Approximately 2 L of water is ingested each day and approximately 7 L of various secretions enters the gastrointestinal tract. Of this 9 L, 8.5 L is absorbed from the small intestine. Approximately 0.5 L passes to the colon, which normally absorbs 80% to 90% of the water presented to it. (From Berne RM, Levy MN. Physiology. 2nd ed. St. Louis: CV Mosby, 1988; with permission.)

Blood Flow

Most of the blood flow to the gastrointestinal tract is to the mucosa to supply energy needed for producing intestinal secretions and absorbing digested materials. Blood flow parallels digestive activity of the gastrointestinal tract. Approximately 80% of portal vein blood flow originates from the stomach and gastrointestinal tract with

the remainder coming from the spleen and pancreas.

Stimulation of the parasympathetic nervous system increases local blood flow at the same time it increases glandular secretions. Conversely, stimulation of the sympathetic nervous system causes vasoconstriction of the arterial supply to the gastrointestinal tract. The reduction in blood flow, however, is transient, because local

Table 54-2
pH of Gastrointestinal Secretions

Secretion	pH
Saliva	6–7
Gastric fluid	1–3.5
Bile	7–8
Pancreatic fluid	8–8.3
Small intestine	6.5–7.5
Colon	7.5–8

metabolic vasodilator mechanisms elicited by ischemia return blood flow to normal. The importance of this transient sympathetic nervous system-induced vasoconstriction is that it permits shunting of blood from the gastrointestinal tract for brief periods during exercise or when increased blood flow is needed by skeletal muscles and the heart.

Portal Venous Pressure

The liver offers modest resistance to blood flow from the portal venous system. As a result, the pressure in the portal vein averages 7 to 10 mmHg, which is considerably higher than the almost zero pressure in the inferior vena cava. Cirrhosis of the liver, most frequently caused by alcoholism, is characterized by increased resistance to portal vein blood flow owing to replacement of hepatic cells with fibrous tissue that contracts around the blood vessels. The gradual increase in resistance to portal vein blood flow produced by cirrhosis of the liver causes large collateral vessels to develop between the portal veins and the systemic veins. The most important of these collaterals are from the splenic veins to the esophageal veins. These collaterals may become so large that they protrude into the lumen of the esophagus, producing esophageal varicosities. The esophageal mucosa overlying these varicosities may become eroded, leading to life-threatening hemorrhage.

In the absence of the development of adequate collaterals, sustained elevations of portal vein pressure may cause protein-containing fluid to escape from the surface of the mesentery, gastrointestinal tract, and liver into the peritoneal cavity. This fluid, known as *ascites,* is similar to plasma, and the high protein content causes an elevated colloid osmotic pressure in the abdominal fluid. This high colloid osmotic pressure draws additional fluid from the surfaces of the gastrointestinal tract and mesentery into the peritoneal cavity.

Splenic Circulation

The splenic capsule in humans, in contrast to that in many lower animals, is nonmuscular, which limits the ability of the spleen to release stored blood in response to sympathetic nervous system stimulation. A small amount (150 to 200 ml) of blood is stored in the splenic venous sinuses and can be released by sympathetic nervous system-induced vasoconstriction of the splenic vessels. Release of this amount of blood into the systemic circulation is sufficient to increase the hematocrit 1% to 2%.

The spleen functions to remove erythrocytes from the circulation. This occurs when erythrocytes reenter the venous sinuses from the splenic pulp by passing through pores that may be smaller than the erythrocyte. Fragile cells do not withstand this trauma, and the released hemoglobin that results from their rupture is ingested by the reticuloendothelial cells of the spleen. These same reticuloendothelial cells also function, much like lymph nodes, to remove bacteria and parasites from the circulation. Indeed, asplenic patients may be more prone to bacterial infections.

During fetal life, the splenic pulp produces erythrocytes in the same manner as does the bone marrow in the adult. As the fetus reaches maturity, however, this function of the spleen is lost.

Innervation

The gastrointestinal tract receives innervation from both divisions of the autonomic nervous system as well as from an intrinsic nervous system consisting of the myenteric plexus, or Auerbach's plexus and the submucous plexus, or Meissner's plexus. In the absence of sympathetic nervous system or parasympathetic nervous system innervation, the motor and secretory activities of the gastrointestinal tract continue, reflecting the function of the intrinsic nervous system. Signals from the autonomic nervous system influence the activity of the intrinsic nervous system; for example, impulses from the parasympathetic nervous system increase intrinsic activity, whereas signals from the sympathetic nervous system decrease intrinsic activity. A large number of neuromodulatory substances act in the gastrointestinal tract.

The cranial component of parasympathetic nervous system innervation to the gastrointestinal tract (esophagus, stomach, pancreas, small intestine, and colon to the level of the transverse colon) is by way of the vagus nerves. The distal portion of the colon is richly supplied by the sacral parasympathetics via the pelvic nerves from the hypogastric plexus. Fibers of the sympathetic nervous system destined for the gastrointestinal tract pass through ganglia such as the celiac ganglia.

Motility

The two types of gastrointestinal motility are mixing contractions and propulsive movements characterized as peristalsis. The usual stimulus for peristalsis is distension. Peristalsis occurs only weakly in portions of the gastrointestinal tract that have congenital absence of the myenteric plexus. Peristalsis is also reduced by increased parasympathetic nervous system activity and anticholinergic drugs.

Ileus

Trauma to the intestine or irritation of the peritoneum as follows abdominal operations causes adynamic (paralytic) ileus. Peristalsis returns to the small intestine in 6 to 8 hours, but colonic activity may take 2 to 3 days. Adynamic ileus can be relieved by a tube placed into the small intestine and aspiration of fluid and gas until peristalsis returns.

Salivary Glands

The principal salivary glands (parotid and submaxillary glands) produce 0.5 to 1 ml·min^{-1} of saliva (pH 6 to 7) largely in response to parasympathetic nervous system stimulation. Saliva washes away pathogenic bacteria in the oral cavity as well as food particles that provide nutrition for bacteria. In the absence of saliva, oral tissues are likely to become ulcerated and infected. The bicarbonate ion (HCO_3^-) concentration in saliva is two to four times that in plasma, and the high potassium ion content of saliva can result in hypokalemia and skeletal muscle weakness if excess salivation persists.

Esophagus

The esophagus serves as a conduit for passage of food from the pharynx to the stomach. The swallowing or deglutition center located in the medulla and lower pons inhibits the medullary ventilatory center, halting breathing at any point to allow swallowing to proceed. The upper and lower ends of the esophagus function as sphincters to prevent entry of air and acidic gastric contents respectively into the esophagus. The sphincters are known as the upper esophageal (pharyngoesophageal) sphincter and lower esophageal (gastroesophageal) sphincter.

Lower Esophageal Sphincter

The lower esophageal sphincter is difficult to identify anatomically, but the lower 1 to 2 cm of the esophagus functions as a sphincter with a resting pressure of approximately 30 mmHg. A large portion of the resting tone of the lower esophageal sphincter is mediated by the vagus nerves as well as the intrinsic nervous system. Anticholinergic drugs and pregnancy decrease lower esophageal sphincter tone and gastrin, metoclopramide, and antacids increase tone. The influence, if any, of changes in lower esophageal sphincter tone and barrier pressure (lower esophageal sphincter pressure minus gastric pressure) and subsequent inhalation of gastric fluid during anesthesia remains undocumented (Hardy, 1988).

Failure of the lower esophageal sphincter to relax appropriately results in achalasia. Chronic incompetence of the lower esophageal sphincter permits reflux of acidic gastric contents into the esophagus with associated esophagitis (heartburn). This condition may be treated surgically by making a fold of gastric tissue (fundoplication).

Stomach

The stomach is a specialized organ of the digestive track that stores and processes food for ab-

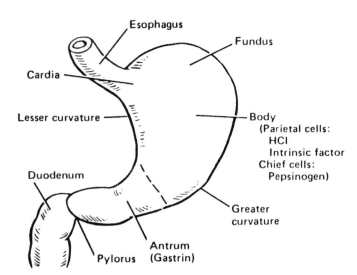

FIGURE 54-6. Anatomy of the stomach indicating site of production of secretions. Mucus is secreted in all parts of the stomach.

sorption by the gastrointestinal tract (Fig. 54-6). The ability to secrete hydrogen ions (H^+) in the form of hydrochloric acid is a hallmark of gastric function. The secretory unit of gastric mucosa is the oxyntic glandular mucosa. The stomach is richly innervated by the vagus nerves and celiac plexus.

Gastric Secretions

Total daily gastric secretion is approximately 2 L with a pH of 1 to 3.5. The stomach secretes only a few milliliters of gastric fluid each hour during the periods between digestion. Strong emotional stimulation, such as occurs preoperatively, can increase interdigestive secretion of highly acidic gastric fluid to 50 ml·h^{-1} or more. The major secretions are hydrochloric acid, pepsinogen, intrinsic factor, and mucus. Mucous secretion protects the gastric mucosa from mechanical and chemical destruction. Substances that disrupt the mucosal barrier and cause gastric irritation include ethanol and drugs that inhibit prostaglandin synthesis (aspirin or nonsteroidal antiinflammatory drugs).

PARIETAL CELLS. These cells secrete an H^+-containing solution with a pH of approximately 0.8. At this pH, the H^+ concentration is approximately 3 million times that present in the arterial blood. Hydrochloric acid kills bacteria, aids protein digestion, provides the necessary pH for pepsin to start protein digestion, and stimulates the flow of bile and pancreatic juice.

Secretion of hydrochloric acid depends on stimulation of receptors in the membrane of parietal cells by histamine; acetylcholine (vagal stimulation); and gastrin (Wolfe and Soll, 1988). All of these receptors increase the transport of H^+ into the gastric lumen by H^+–K^+ ATPase (Fig. 54-7) (Ganong, 1987). Activation of one receptor type potentiates the response of the other receptors to stimulation. Blockade of receptors with specific blocking drugs (see Chapter 21) produces effective reduction of acid responses because it removes the potentiating effect of stimulation of this receptor on the responses to other stimuli. Blockade of M-1 muscarinic receptors is produced by atropine or the more specific anticholinergic pirenzepine. Gastrin receptors can be inhibited by proglumide. Alternatively, the H^+–K^+ ATPase system can be inhibited by ameprazole. Pharmacologic manipulation of gastric fluid pH has special importance in management of patients considered at risk for pulmonary aspiration during the perioperative period.

Intrinsic factor, which is essential for absorption of vitamin B_{12} from the ileum, is secreted by parietal cells. For this reason, destruction of parietal cells as associated with chronic gastritis produces achlorhydria and often pernicious anemia.

CHIEF CELLS. Pepsinogens secreted by chief cells undergo cleavage to pepsins in the pres-

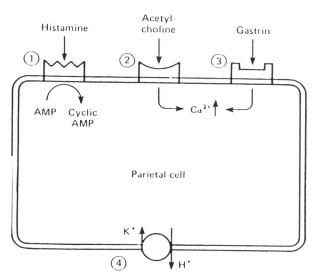

FIGURE 54–7. Gastric hydrogen ion (H^+) secretion by the parietal cells is stimulated by histamine acting on H-2 receptors (*1*), acetylcholine acting on muscarinic receptors (*2*), and gastrin acting on gastrin receptors (*3*). All receptors increase the transport of H^+ into the gastric lumen by H^+–K^+ ATPase (*4*). (From Ganong WF. Review of Medical Physiology. 13th ed. Norwalk, CT. Appleton and Lange, 1987; with permission.)

ence of hydrochloric acid. Pepsins are proteolytic enzymes important for the digestion of proteins.

G CELLS. Gastrin is excreted by G cells into the circulation, which carries this hormone to responsive receptors in parietal cells to stimulate gastric H^+ secretion. Gastrin also increases the tone of the lower esophageal sphincter and relaxes the pylorus.

Gastric Fluid Volume and Rate of Gastric Emptying

Neural and humoral mechanisms greatly influence gastric fluid volume and gastric emptying time. In general, parasympathetic nervous system stimulation enhances gastric fluid secretion and motility while sympathetic nervous system stimulation has an opposite effect.

Foods pass through the stomach at variable rates. For example, foods rich in carbohydrates leave the stomach in a few hours. Protein-rich foods leave more slowly, and emptying is slowest after a meal containing fat. More than 90% of a 750-ml bolus of saline leaves the stomach in 30 minutes. In fact, preoperative oral fluids (up to 150 ml 1 to 2 hours before induction of anesthesia) may stimulate peristalsis and expedite gastric emptying (Maltby et al, 1986; Sutherland et al, 1987). Clearly, a small amount of water to facili-

tate administration of oral medications shortly before induction of anesthesia does not produce sustained increases in gastric fluid volume and may even contribute to lower gastric fluid volumes. Events that predictably slow gastric emptying include enhanced sympathetic nervous system activity (fear or pain), active labor, and administration of opioids. There does not seem to be a difference in the rate of gastric emptying between parturients and nonpregnant patients (O'Sullivan et al, 1987). Prolonged fasting does not ensure an empty stomach.

Absorption from the Stomach

The stomach is a poor absorptive area of the gastrointestinal tract because it lacks the villus structure characteristic of absorptive membranes. As a result, only highly lipid-soluble liquids such as ethanol, and some drugs such as aspirin, can be significantly absorbed from the stomach.

Small Intestine

The small intestine consists of the duodenum (from the pylorus to the ligament of Treitz), the jejunum, and the ileum (ending at the ileocecal valve). There is no distinct anatomic boundary between the jejunum and ileum but the first 40% of small intestine after the ligament of Treitz is often considered to be the jejunum. The small intestine is presented with approximately 9 L of fluid daily (2 L from the diet and the rest representing gastrointestinal secretions) but only 1 to 2 L of chyme enters the colon. The small intestine is the site of most of the digestion and absorption of proteins, fats, and carbohydrates (Table 54-3).

Chyme moves through the 5 m of small intestine at an average rate of 1 cm·min^{-1}. As a result, it takes 3 to 5 hours for chyme to pass from the pylorus to the ileocecal valve. On reaching the ileocecal valve, chyme is sometimes blocked for several hours until the person eats another meal. An inflamed appendix can increase the tone of the ileocecal valve to the extent that emptying of the ileum ceases. Conversely, gastrin causes relaxation of the ileocecal valve. When more than 50% of the small intestine is resected, the absorption of nutrients and vitamins is so compromised that development of malnutrition is likely.

Secretions of the Small Intestine

Mucous glands (Brunner's glands) present in the first few centimeters of the duodenum secrete mucus to protect the duodenal wall from damage by acidic gastric fluid. Stimulation of the sympathetic nervous system inhibits the protective mucus-producing function of these glands, which may be one of the factors that cause this area of the gastrointestinal tract to be the most frequent site of peptic ulcer disease.

The crypts of Lieberkühn contain epithelial cells that produce up to 2 L daily of secretions that lack digestive enzymes and mimic extracellular fluid, having a pH of 6.5 to 7.5. This fluid provides a watery vehicle for absorption of substances from chyme as it passes through the small intestine. The most important mechanism for regulation of small intestine secretions is local neural reflexes, especially those initiated by distention produced by the presence of chyme.

The epithelial cells in the crypts of Lieberkühn continually undergo mitosis with an average life cycle of approximately 5 days. This rapid growth of new cells allows prompt repair of any excoriation that occurs in the mucosa. This rapid turnover of cells also explains the vulnerability of the gastrointestinal epithelium to chemotherapeutic drugs (see Chapter 29).

The epithelial cells in the mucosa of the small intestine contain digestive enzymes that most likely are responsible for digestion of food substances because they are absorbed across the gastrointestinal epithelium. These enzymes include peptidases for splitting peptides into amino acids, enzymes for splitting disaccharides into monosaccharides, and intestinal lipases.

Absorption from the Small Intestine

Mucosal folds (valvulae conniventes), microvilli (brush border), and epithelial cells provide an absorptive area of approximately 250 m^2 in the

Table 54-3
Site of Absorption

	Duodenum	Jejunum	Ileum	Colon
Glucose	++	+++	++	0
Amino acids	++	+++	++	0
Fatty acids	+++	++	+	0
Bile salts	0	+	+++	0
Water-soluble vitamins	+++	++	0	0
Vitamin B$_{12}$	0	+	+++	0
Na$^+$	+++	++	+++	+++
K$^+$	0	0	+	++
H$^+$	0	+	++	++
Cl$^-$	+++	++	+	0
Ca^{2+}	+++	++	+	?

small intestine for nearly all the nutrients and electrolytes as well as approximately 95% of all the water. Daily absorption of Na^+ is 25 to 35 g, emphasizing the rapidity with which total body Na^+ depletion can occur if excessive intestinal secretions are lost as occurs with extreme diarrhea. Active transport of Na^+ in the small intestine is important for the absorption of glucose, which is the physiologic basis for treating diarrhea by oral administration of saline solutions containing glucose. Bacterial toxins as from cholera and staphylococci can stimulate the chloride ion–HCO_3^- exchange mechanism, resulting in a life-threatening diarrhea consisting of a loss of Na^+, HCO_3^- and an isosmotic equivalent of water.

Colon

The functions of the colon are absorption of water and electrolytes from the chyme and storage of feces. A test meal reaches the cecum in approximately 4 hours and then passes slowly through the colon during the next 6 to 12 hours, during which time 1 to 2 L of chyme are converted to 200 to 250 ml of feces (Fig. 54-8). Circular muscle of the colon constricts and, at the same time, strips of longitudinal muscle (tineae coli) contract, causing the unstimulated portion of the colon to bulge outward into baglike sacs, or haustrations. Vagal stimulation causes segmental contractions of the proximal part of the colon and stimulation of the pelvic nerves causes expulsive movements. Activation of the sympathetic nervous system inhibits colonic activity. Bacteria are predictably present in the colon.

Secretions of the Colon

Epithelial cells lining the colon secrete almost exclusively mucus, which protects the intestinal mucosa against trauma. The alkalinity of the mucus owing to the presence of large amounts of HCO_3^- provides a barrier to keep acids that are formed in the feces from attacking the intestinal wall. Irritation of a segment of the colon as occurs with bacterial infection causes the mucosa to secrete large quantities of water and electrolytes in addition to mucus, diluting the irritating factors and causing rapid movement of feces toward the anus. The resulting diarrhea may result in dehydration and cardiovascular collapse.

Pancreas

The pancreas lies parallel to and beneath the stomach, serving as both an endocrine (insulin or glucagon) and exocrine gland. Exocrine secretions (approximately 1.5 L daily) are rich in HCO_3^- to neutralize duodenal contents and digestive enzymes to initiate breakdown of carbohydrates, proteins, and fats.

Regulation of Pancreatic Secretions

Pancreatic secretions are regulated more by hormonal than neural mechanisms. For example, secretin is released by the duodenal mucosa in response to hydrochloric acid. This hormone enters the circulation and causes the pancreas to produce large amounts of alkaline fluid necessary to neutralize the acidic pH of gastric fluid. In addition to the release of secretin, the presence of food in the duodenum causes the release of a second polypeptide hormone, cholecystokinin. Cholecystokinin also enters the circulation and causes the pancreas to secrete digestive enzymes (trypsins, amylase, or lipases). Trypsins are acti-

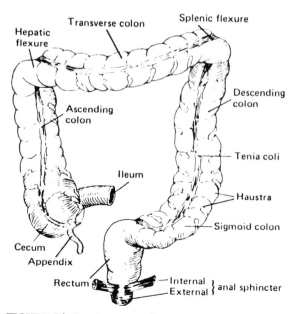

Hepatic flexure

Transverse colon

Splenic flexure

Descending colon

Ascending colon

Tenia coli

Ileum

Haustra

Sigmoid colon

Cecum

Appendix

Rectum

Internal
External } anal sphincter

FIGURE 54–8.   Anatomy of the colon.

vated in the gastrointestinal tract by the enzyme enterokinase, which is secreted by the gastrointestinal mucosa when chyme comes in contact with the mucosa. Damage to the pancreas or blockade of a pancreatic duct may cause pooling of proteolytic enzymes, resulting in acute pancreatitis owing to autodigestion by these enzymes. In general, pancreatic secretions are stimulated by the parasympathetic nervous system and inhibited by the sympathetic nervous system.

REFERENCES

Bell GH, Emslie-Smith D, Paterson CR. Textbook of Physiology and Biochemistry. 9th ed. New York. Churchill Livingston. 1976.

Berne RM, Levy MN. Physiology. 2nd ed. St. Louis. CV Mosby. 1988.

Bloom W, Fawcell DW. A textbook of histology. 10th ed. Philadelphia. WB Saunders. 1975.

Boucheir IAD, The medical treatment of gallstones. Annu Rev Med 1980;31:59–77.

Ganong WF, Review of Medical Physiology. 13th ed. Norwalk, CT. Appleton and Lange. 1987.

Gelman SI. Disturbances in hepatic blood flow during anesthesia and surgery. Arch Surg 1976;111:881–4.

Gelman SI, Fowler KC, Smith LR. Liver circulation and function during isoflurane and halothane anesthesia. Anesthesiology 1984;61:726–30.

Guyton AC. Textbook of Medical Physiology. 7th ed. Philadelphia. WB Saunders. 1986.

Hardy JF. Large volume gastroesophageal reflux: A rationale for risk reduction in the perioperative period. Can J Anaesth 1988;35:162–73.

Maltby JR, Sutherland AD, Sale JP, Shaffer EA. Preoperative oral fluids: Is a five-hour fast justified prior to elective surgery? Anesth Analg 1986;65:1112–6.

O'Sullivan GM, Sutton AJ, Thompson SA, Carrie LE, Bullingham RE. Noninvasive measurement of gastric emptying in obstetric patients. Anesth Analg 1987;66:505–11.

Sutherland AD, Maltby JR, Sale JP, Reid CRG. The effect of preoperative oral fluid and ranitidine on gastric fluid volume and pH. Can J Anaesth 1987;34:117–21.

Wolfe MM, Soll AH. The physiology of gastric acid secretion. N Engl J Med 1988;319:1707–15.

Chapter

55

Skeletal and Smooth Muscle

Muscle is generally classified as skeletal, smooth, and cardiac muscle. Skeletal muscle is responsible for voluntary actions, while smooth muscle and cardiac muscle subserve functions related to the cardiovascular, respiratory, gastrointestinal, and genitourinary systems. Muscle composes 45% to 50% of total body mass, with skeletal muscles accounting for approximately 40% of body mass. An estimated 250 million cells are present in the more than 400 skeletal muscles of humans. Inappropriate activity of smooth muscle is involved in many illnesses including hypertension, atherosclerosis, asthma, and disorders of the gastrointestinal tract.

SKELETAL MUSCLE

Skeletal muscle is made up of individual muscle fibers, each fiber being a single cell. There are no syncytial bridges between cells. Cross striations characteristic of skeletal muscles are due to differences in the refractive indexes of the various parts of the muscle fiber. Each skeletal muscle fiber comprises thousands of fibrils that consist of the contractile proteins myosin, actin, tropomyosin, and troponin. Myofibrils are suspended inside skeletal muscle fibers in a matrix known as *sarcoplasm*. The sarcoplasm contains mitochondria, enzymes, potassium ions (K^+), and an extensive endoplasmic reticulum known as the *sarcoplasmic reticulum*. The cell membrane of the muscle fiber is known as the *sarcolemma*. At the ends of skeletal muscle fibers, surfaces of the sarcolemma fuse with tendon fibers, which form tendons that insert into bones. *Hypertrophy* is synthesis of new myofibrils; *hyperplasia* is formation of more cells. Skeletal muscle has only limited capacity to form new cells.

Excitation-Contraction Coupling

The process by which depolarization of the sarcolemma and propagation of an action potential initiates skeletal muscle contraction is described as excitation–contraction coupling. An action potential occurs only in response to motor nerve activity and reflects opening of fast channels in the membrane, allowing rapid inward movement of sodium ions (Na^+) followed by outward K^+ movement and repolarization. The resting membrane potential of skeletal muscle is approximately −90 mV. The action potential lasts 2 to 4 ms and is conducted along the muscle fiber at approximately 5 m·sec^{-1}, which is slower than the velocity of conduction in large myelinated nerve fibers.

The action potential is transmitted deep into skeletal muscle to all myofibrils by way of transverse (T) tubules. The T tubule action potentials in turn cause the sarcoplasmic reticulum to release calcium ions (Ca^{2+}) in the immediate vicinity of all myofibrils. The Ca^{2+} binds to troponin, thus abolishing the inhibitory effect of troponin on the interaction between myosin and actin. As a result, the head of a myosin molecule links to an actin molecule (cross-bridging), producing movement of myosin on actin, which is repeated in serial fashion to produce contraction of the muscle fiber (Fig. 55-1) (Ganong, 1987). The immediate source of energy for contraction is provided by adenosine triphosphate (ATP). Hydrolysis of ATP to adenosine diphosphate (ADP) is provided by ATPase activity present in the heads of the myosin molecules where they are in contact with actin. Each interaction of myosin with actin results in hydrolysis of ATP. The amount of

ATP present in a skeletal muscle fiber is sufficient to maintain full contraction for less than 1 second. This emphasizes the importance of rephosphorylation of ADP to form ATP.

Shortly after releasing Ca^{2+}, the sarcoplasmic reticulum begins to reaccumulate this ion by an active transport process. This transport mechanism can concentrate Ca^{2+} up to 2000-fold inside the sarcoplasmic reticulum. ATP provides the energy for Ca^{2+} transport. Once the Ca^{2+} concentra-

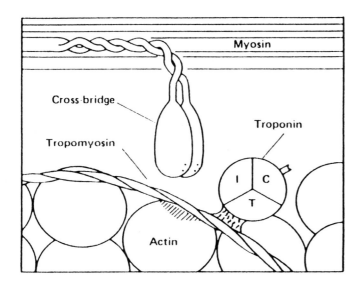

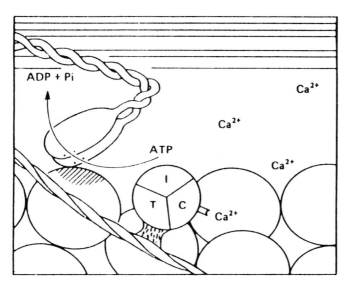

FIGURE 55–1. Contraction of skeletal muscle is initiated by attachment of calcium ions (Ca^{2+}) to troponin leading to hydrolysis of adenosine triphosphate (ATP) and cross-bridging between actin and myosin. (From Ganong WF. Review of Medical Physiology. 13th ed. Norwalk, CT. Appleton and Lange, 1987; with permission.)

tion in the sarcoplasm has been lowered sufficiently, cross-bridging between myosin and actin ceases and the skeletal muscle relaxes. Failure of the Ca^{2+} pump results in sustained skeletal muscle contraction and marked increases in heat production leading to malignant hyperthermia. The gene for this Ca^{2+} channel (ryanodine receptor) is on chromosome 19 (McCarthy et al, 1990). A mutation in this gene is speculated to be responsible for malignant hyperthermia susceptibility.

Rigor mortis reflects ATP depletion and failure of the Ca^{2+} transport mechanism, leading to permanent cross-bridging between myosin and actin. Skeletal muscles remain rigid until muscle proteins are destroyed. This occurs in 15 to 25 hours after death and is due to autolysis caused by enzymes released from lysosomes.

Neuromuscular Junction

The *neuromuscular junction* is the site at which presynaptic motor nerve endings meet the postsynptic membranes of skeletal muscles (motor end-plates) (see Fig. 8-2). The motor nerve ending branches to form a complex of nerve terminals that invaginate into the skeletal muscle fiber but lie outside the sarcolemma. The space between the nerve terminal and the sarcolemma is known as the *synaptic cleft* and is filled with extracellular fluid. Acetylcholine is synthesized in the cytoplasm of the nerve terminal and stored in synaptic vesicles. A nerve impulse arriving at the nerve ending causes the release of approximately 60 vesicles, each containing an estimated 10,000 molecules of acetylcholine (Ganong, 1987). In the absence of Ca^{2+} or in the presence of excess magnesium ions, the release of acetylcholine is greatly reduced. Acetylcholine diffuses across the synaptic cleft to excite skeletal muscles, but within 1 millisecond, the neurotransmitter is hydrolyzed by acetylcholinesterase enzyme (true cholinesterase) in the folds of the sarcolemma. This rapid inactivation of acetylcholine prevents reexcitation after skeletal muscle fibers have recovered from the first action potential.

Mechanism of Acetylcholine Effects

Nicotinic acetylcholine receptors comprise five subunits arranged in a nearly symmetric fashion that extend through the cell membrane (see Fig. 8-3). An average end-plate contains an estimated 50 million nicotinic acetylcholine receptors. Binding of two acetylcholine molecules (one molecule at each alpha subunit) causes a conformation change in the receptor such that Na^+ enters into the interior of the cell. As a result, the resting transmembrane potential rises in this local area of the motor end-plate, creating a local action potential known as the *end-plate potential*. This end-plate potential initiates an action potential that spreads in both directions along the skeletal muscle fiber. The threshold potential at which skeletal muscle fibers are stimulated to contract is approximately 50 mv.

Altered Responses to Acetylcholine

Nondepolarizing neuromuscular blocking drugs compete with acetylcholine at alpha subunits of the receptor and thus prevent changes in permeability of skeletal muscle membranes (see Chapter 8). As a result, an end-plate potential does not occur and neuromuscular transmission is effectively prevented. Anticholinesterase drugs inhibit acetylcholinesterase enzyme, allowing accumulation of acetylcholine at receptors and subsequent displacement of nondepolarizing neuromuscular blocking drugs from the alpha subunits (see Chapter 9). Myasthenia gravis is characterized by a reduction in the number of nicotinic acetylcholine receptors; the resulting end-plate potentials are too weak to initiate a propagated action potential.

Blood Flow

Skeletal muscle blood flow can increase more than 20 times (a greater increase than in any other tissue of the body) during strenuous exercise. At rest, only 20% to 25% of the capillaries are open, and skeletal muscle blood flow is 3 to 4 ml·100 g^{-1}·min^{-1}. During strenuous exercise, almost all skeletal muscle capillaries become patent. Opening of previously collapsed capillaries diminishes the distance that oxygen and other nutrients must diffuse from capillaries to skeletal muscle fibers and contributes an increased surface area through which nutrients can diffuse from blood. Presumably, exercise lowers the local concentration of oxygen, which in turn causes vasodilation because the vessel walls cannot maintain contraction in the absence of adequate amounts of oxygen. Alternatively, oxygen deficiency may cause release of vasodilator substances such as K^+ and adenosine. The increase in cardiac output that occurs during exercise results principally from local vasodilation in active skeletal muscles and subsequent increased venous return of blood to the heart. Among inhaled anesthetics, isoflurane is a potent vasodilator, producing marked increases in skeletal muscle blood flow.

Exercise is associated with a centrally mediated stimulation of the sympathetic nervous system manifesting as vasoconstriction in nonmuscular tissues and increases in blood pressure. Excessive increases in blood pressure, however, are prevented by vascular vasodilation that occurs in the large tissue mass represented by skeletal muscle. Exceptions to vasoconstriction induced by exercise are the coronary and cerebral circulations. This is teleologically understandable because the heart and brain are essential to the response to exercise, as are the skeletal muscles.

Innervation

Skeletal muscles are innervated by large myelinated nerve fibers that originate from the ventral (anterior) horn of the spinal cord (Fig. 55-2) (Berne and Levy, 1988). The nerve axon exits via the ventral root and reaches the muscle through a mixed peripheral nerve. Motor nerves branch in the skeletal muscle with each nerve terminal innervating a single muscle cell. A motor unit consists of the motor nerve and all of the muscle fibers innervated by that nerve. The motor unit is the functional contractile unit. Skeletal muscle tone is a residual degree of skeletal muscle contraction that persists even at rest. Presumably, skeletal muscle tone reflects nerve impulses that are emitted continuously from the spinal cord.

Denervation Hypersensitivity

Denervation of skeletal muscle causes atrophy of the involved muscle and development of abnormal excitability of the skeletal muscle to its

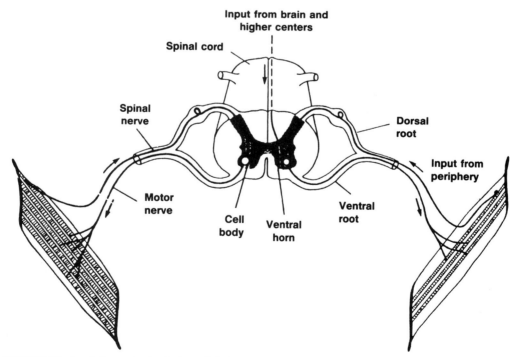

FIGURE 55–2.   Schematic depiction of skeletal muscle innervation. (From Berne RM, Levy MN. Physiology. 2nd ed. St. Louis: CV Mosby, 1988, p. ; with permission.)

neurotransmitter acetylcholine. Initially, after the motor nerve is interrupted, fasciculations occur owing to the release of acetylcholine from the terminals of the degenerating distal portion of the axon. Approximately 3 to 5 days after denervation, skeletal muscle fibrillation appears, reflecting spread of cholinergic receptors over the entire cell membrane and development of increased sensitivity (denervation hypersensitivity) to acetylcholine. After several weeks, atrophy of skeletal muscle fibers is so severe that fibrillation impulses cease. An *electromyogram* is the recording from skin electrodes of the electrical current that spreads from skeletal muscles to skin during simultaneous contraction of numerous skeletal muscle fibers.

SMOOTH MUSCLE

Smooth muscle is categorized as multiunit or visceral smooth muscle. Multiunit smooth muscle contraction is controlled almost exclusively by nerve signals and spontaneous contractions rarely occur. Examples of multiunit smooth muscles are the ciliary muscles of the eye, iris of the eye, and smooth muscles of many large blood vessels.

Visceral smooth muscle is characterized by cell membranes that contact adjacent cell membranes, forming a functional syncytium that often undergoes spontaneous contractions as a single unit in the absence of nerve stimulation. These spontaneous action potentials are particularly prominent in tubular structures, accounting for peristaltic motion in structures such as the bile ducts, ureters, and gastrointestinal tract, especially when they are distended. Plateaus in the action potentials of visceral smooth muscle lasting up to 30 seconds may occur in the ureters and uterus. The normal resting transmembrane potential is approximately −60 mv, which is approximately 30 mv less negative than in skeletal muscles.

In addition to stimulation in the absence of extrinsic innervation, smooth muscles are unique in their sensitivity to hormones or local tissue factors. For example, smooth muscle spasm may persist for hours in response to norepinephrine or antidiuretic hormone, whereas local factors such as lack of oxygen or accumulation of hydrogen ions cause vasodilation. It is believed that local factors and hormones cause smooth muscle contraction by activating the Ca^{2+} transport mechanism. Drugs relax smooth muscle by increasing the intracellular concentration of cyclic adenosine monophosphate or cyclic guanosine monophosphate.

Mechanism of Contraction

Smooth muscles contain both actin and myosin but, unlike skeletal muscles, lack troponin. In contrast to skeletal muscles, where Ca^{2+} binds to troponin to initiate cross-bridging, in smooth muscle the Ca^{2+}-calmodulin complex activates the enzyme necessary for phosphorylation of myosin. This myosin has ATPase activity, and actin then slides on myosin to produce contraction.

The source of Ca^{2+} in smooth muscle differs from that of skeletal muscle because the sarcoplasmic reticulum of smooth muscle is poorly developed. Most of the Ca^{2+} that causes contraction of smooth muscles enters from extracellular fluid at the time of the action potential. The time required for this diffusion is 200 to 300 msec, which is approximately 50 times longer than for skeletal muscles. Subsequent relaxation of smooth muscles is achieved by a Ca^{2+} transport process that pumps Ca^{2+} back into extracellular fluid or into the sarcoplasmic reticulum. This Ca^{2+} pump is slow compared with the sarcoplasmic reticulum pump in skeletal muscles. As a result, the duration of smooth muscle contraction is often seconds rather than milliseconds as is characteristic of skeletal muscles.

Smooth muscles, unlike skeletal muscles, do not atrophy when denervated but they do become hyperresponsive to the normal neurotransmitter. This denervation hypersensitivity is a general phenomenon that is largely due to synthesis or activation of more receptors.

Neuromuscular Junction

A neuromuscular junction similar to that of skeletal muscle does not occur in smooth muscles. Instead, nerve fibers branch diffusely on top of a sheet of smooth muscle fibers without making actual contact. These nerve fibers secrete their neurotransmitter into an interstitial fluid space a few microns from the smooth muscle cells. Two different neurotransmitters, acetylcholine and norepinephrine, are secreted by the autonomic nervous system nerves that innervate smooth muscles. Acetylcholine is an excitatory neuro-transmitter for smooth muscles at some sites and functions as an inhibitory neurotransmitter at other sites. Norepinephrine exerts the reverse effect of acetylcholine. It is believed that the presence of specific excitatory or inhibitory re-ceptors in the membranes of smooth muscle fi-bers determines the response to acetylcholine or norepinephrine. When the neurotransmitter interacts with an inhibitory receptor instead of an excitatory receptor, the membrane potential of the muscle fiber becomes more negative (hyperpolarized).

Uterine Smooth Muscle

Uterine smooth muscle is characterized by a high degree of spontaneous electrical and contractile activity. Unlike the heart, there is no pacemaker, and the contraction process spreads from one cell to another at a rate of 1 to 3 cm·sec^{-1}. Con-tractions of labor result in peak intrauterine pres-sures of 60 to 80 mmHg in the second stage. Resting uterine pressure during labor is approxi-mately 10 mmHg. Movement of Na^+ appears to be the primary determinant in depolarization, whereas Ca^{2+} is necessary for excitation–contrac-tion coupling. Availability of Ca^{2+} greatly influ-ences the response of uterine smooth muscle to physiologic and pharmacologic stimulation or in-hibition. Alpha excitatory and beta inhibitory re-ceptors are also present in the myometrium.

REFERENCES

Berne RM, Levy MN. Physiology. 2nd ed. St. Louis. CV Mosby. 1988.

Ganong WF, Review of Medical Physiology. 13th ed. Norwalk, CT. Appleton and Lange, 1987.

McCarthy TV, Healy JMS, Heffron JJA et al. Localization of the malignant hyperthermia susceptibility locus to human chromosome. Nature 1990;343:562–4.

Chapter

56

Erythrocytes and Leukocytes

ERYTHROCYTES

Erythrocytes (red blood cells or RBCs) are the most abundant of all cells in the body (25 trillion of the estimated total 75 trillion cells), emphasizing their irreplaceable role in delivery of oxygen to tissues. Indeed, the major function of RBCs is to transport hemoglobin, which, in turn, carries oxygen from the lungs to tissues. In addition to their function of transporting hemoglobin, RBCs contain large amounts of carbonic anhydrase. This enzyme speeds the reaction between carbon dioxide and water, making it possible to transport carbon dioxide from tissues to the lungs for elimination. Also, hemoglobin in RBCs is an excellent acid-base buffer, providing approximately 70% of the buffering power of whole blood.

Anatomy

RBCs are biconcave disks with a mean diameter of 8 μ. The shape of these cells can change, conforming to the capillaries through which RBCs must pass. The average number of RBCs in each milliliter of plasma, and thus the hemoglobin concentration and hematocrit, varies with the person, sex, and barometric pressure (Table 56-1). Each RBC contains approximately 29 pg of hemoglobin and each gram of hemoglobin is capable of combining with 1.34 ml of oxygen.

Bone Marrow

In the adult, RBCs, platelets, and many of the leukocytes are formed in the bone marrow. Normally, approximately 75% of the cells in the bone marrow belong to the leukocyte-producing myeloid series and only 25% are maturing RBCs, even though there are over 500 times as many RBCs in the circulation as there are leukocytes. This difference reflects the short half-time of leukocytes compared with RBCs. In the fetus, RBCs are also produced in the liver and spleen. The marrow of almost all bones produces RBCs until approximately 5 years of age. The marrow of long bones, except for the proximal portions of the humerus and tibia, becomes fatty and produces few or no RBCs after approximately 20 years of age. After 20 years, most RBCs are produced in the marrow of membranous bones, including the vertebrae, sternum, ribs, and pelvis. When the bone marrow produces RBCs at a rapid rate, many of the cells are released into the blood before they are mature. For example, during rapid RBC production, the number of circulating reticulocytes may increase from less than 1% to as great as 30% to 50%. Overall, the bone marrow is one of the largest organs of the body, approaching the size and weight of the liver.

Control of Production

The total mass of RBCs in the circulation is regu-

Table 56–1
Erythrocytes in the Plasma

	Content
Erythrocytes (ml)	
Male	4.3–5.9×10^6
Female	3.5–5.5×10^6
Hematocrit (percent)	
Male	39–55
Female	36–48
Hemoglobin (g·dl⁻¹)	
Male	13.9–16.3
Female	12.0–15.0

lated within narrow limits so that the number of cells is optimal to provide tissue oxygenation without an excessive number that would adversely increase viscosity of blood and reduce tissue blood flow (Fig. 56-1) (Ganong, 1987). It is not the concentration of RBCs in the blood that controls the rate of their production but rather the ability of cells to transport oxygen to tissues in relation to tissue demand for oxygen. Any event that causes the amount of oxygen transported to tissues to decrease, as in the presence of anemia, chronic pulmonary disease, or cardiac failure, will stimulate production of RBCs by the bone marrow. Destruction of bone marrow by radiation or drugs or inadequate amounts of iron predictably results in anemia (Fig. 56-1) (Ganong, 1987).

ERYTHROPOIETIN. Erythropoietin is a glycoprotein synthesized in response to arterial hypoxemia as produced by ascent to altitude or chronic pulmonary disease. It is speculated that hypoxemia evokes release of renal erythropoietic factor into the circulation from the kidneys. This enzyme acts on a globulin to split away the erythropoietin molecule. Erythropoietin stimulates RBC production in the bone marrow with the peak effect occurring in approximately 5 days. After this peak effect is reached, RBCs continue to be produced at an increased rate as long as hypoxemia persists. When hypoxemia is corrected, erythropoietin production decreases to zero almost immediately, followed in a few days by a similar decline in RBC production. Red blood cell production in the bone marrow remains at a low level until enough cells have lived out their life spans, thus reducing the number of circulating RBCs to a level consistent with normal tissue oxygenation (a negative feedback mechanism). The absence of kidneys removes the source of renal erythropoietic factor, which is consistent with the anemia that accompanies chronic renal failure.

Vitamins Necessary for Formation

Vitamin B_{12} (cyanocobalamin) is necessary for the synthesis of deoxyribonucleic acid (DNA). Lack of this vitamin results in failure of nuclear maturation and division, which is particularly evident in rapidly proliferating cells such as RBCs. In addition to failing to proliferate, maturation failure is reflected by formation of megaloblasts

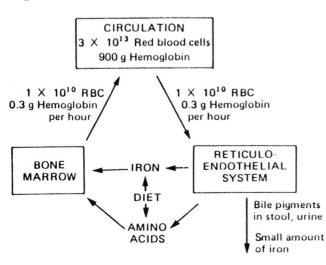

FIGURE 56–1. Erythrocyte formation and destruction. (From Ganong WF. Review of Medical Physiology. 13th ed. Norwalk, CT: Appleton and Lange, 1987; with permission.)

and macrocytes. The amount of vitamin B_{12} required each day to maintain normal RBC maturation is less than 1 μg and the normal store in the liver is approximately 1000 times this amount. As a result, many months of impaired vitamin B_{12} absorption are necessary before maturation failure macrocytic anemia manifests. Macrocytes have a weak cell membrane, causing them to exhibit a shorter life span than normal erythrocytes.

Folic acid, like vitamin B_{12}, is necessary for formation of DNA and maturation of RBCs. Deficiency of this vitamin predictably leads to a macrocytic anemia.

Destruction

Red blood cells normally circulate an average of 120 days after leaving the bone marrow. With increasing age, the metabolic system of RBCs declines (cytoplasmic enzymes capable of metabolizing glucose to form adenosine triphosphate) and cell membranes become fragile. Many fragile RBCs rupture in the spleen. Hemoglobin released from ruptured RBCs is rapidly phagocytized by reticuloendothelial cells (Fig. 56-1) (Ganong, 1987). Iron is released from hemoglobin back into the blood to be carried by transferring either to bone marrow for production of new RBCs or to the liver and other tissues for storage as ferritin. The heme portion of the hemoglobin molecule is converted by the reticuloendothelial cells into bilirubin.

BLOOD GROUPS

Genetically determined antigens (agglutinogens) are present on the cell membranes of RBCs. The most antigenic are the A, B, and Rh agglutinogens; other agglutinogens (Kell, Duffy, Lewis, M, N, and P) are less antigenic. A and B antigens are glycoproteins that differ in composition by only a single substitution. Blood is divided into different groups and types on the bases of the antigens present on RBC membranes.

ABO Antigen System

Blood is grouped for transfusion as A, B, AB, or O on the basis of the ABO antigen system (Table 56-2). A and B antigens can occur alone or in combination on RBC membranes, and in some individuals, both antigens are absent. There are six possible combinations of genes resulting in six different genotypes (Table 56-2). In addition to RBCs, A and B antigens are present in many other tissues and fluids including kidneys, liver, testes, salivary glands, saliva, semen, and amniotic fluid.

In the absence of the A or B antigen, the opposite antibody (agglutinin) is present in the circulation (Table 56-2). These antibodies are gamma globulins, most often being immunoglobulin M (IgM) or IgG molecules. It seems paradoxical that antibodies are produced in the absence of the respective antigen on RBC membranes. It is likely that small amounts of A and B antigens enter the body by way of food or bacteria, thus initiating the development of corresponding antibodies. Indeed, immediately after birth, the circulating level of antibodies to A or B antigens is almost zero. It is only at 2 to 8 months of age that a person begins to produce antibodies to the antigen not present on RBC membranes. A maximum titer of antibodies is usually reached by 8 to 10 years and then gradually declines with increasing age.

Table 56-2
ABO Antigen System

Blood Type	Incidence (percent)	Genotype	Antigens (Allutinogens)	Antibodies (Agglutinins)
O	47	OO		Anti-A, Anti-B
A	41	OA, AA	A	Anti-B
B	9	OB, BB	B	Anti-A
AB	3	AB	A, B	

Blood Typing

Blood typing is the *in vitro* mixing of a drop of the patient's blood with plasma containing antibodies against the A or B antigen. This mixture is observed under a microscope for the presence or absence of agglutination (Fig. 56-2) (Ganong, 1987). Using this procedure, blood can be typed as O, A, B, or AB. Cross-matching is the procedure that determines compatibility of the patient's blood with the donor's RBCs and plasma. Failure of agglutination when the RBCs from the donor and plasma from the recipient are mixed and when the RBCs of the recipient are mixed with plasma from the donor confirms compatibility. Typing of blood is also used to determine parentage, although it can only prove that a male is not the father.

Rh Blood Types

There are six common types of Rh antigens, designated C, D, E, c, d, and e, that are collectively known as the Rh factor. Only the C, D, and E antigens are sufficiently antigenic to cause development of anti-Rh antibodies that are capable of causing transfusion reactions. A person with C, D, or E antigens in RBC membranes is Rh-positive, and an individual with c, d, or e antigens is Rh-negative. Approximately 85% of Caucasian Americans are Rh-positive. Typing for Rh factors is performed in a manner similar to that for typing A and B antigens.

A person who is Rh-negative develops anti-Rh antibodies only when exposed to RBCs containing the C, D, or E antigens. This exposure may occur with transfusion of Rh-positive blood to an Rh-negative patient, or during pregnancy, when an Rh-negative mother is sensitized to the Rh-positive factor in her child. The development of anti-Rh antibodies is usually slow and these antibodies are less potent agglutinogens than are antibodies to the A and B antigens. Nevertheless, multiple exposures of an Rh-negative person to Rh-positive blood results in exaggerated responses.

If an Rh-negative individual is transfused with Rh-positive blood, there is often no immediate reaction. In some persons, however, anti-Rh antibodies develop in sufficient amounts after 2 to 4 weeks to cause agglutination of any transfused cells that are still circulating. These cells are then hemolyzed in the reticuloendothelial system, producing a delayed and usually mild transfusion reaction. On subsequent transfusion of Rh-positive blood to this same person, however, the severity of the transfusion reaction is greatly enhanced and can be similar to reactions resulting from ABO incompatibility.

An Rh-negative mother typically becomes sensitized to the Rh-positive factor in her child during the first few days following delivery, when degenerating products of the placenta release Rh-positive antigens into the maternal circulation. If these Rh antigens are destroyed at this time before an anti-Rh antibody response occurs, the mother will not become sensitized for subsequent pregnancies. This goal is achieved by injecting serum containing antibodies (Rh [D] immune globulin) against the antigen before it can evoke the formation of antibodies. If anti-Rh antibodies form, any subsequent pregnancy in which the fetus is Rh-positive may result in erythroblastosis fetalis.

Hemolytic Transfusion Reactions

Transfusion of ABO type blood that is different than that of the recipient results in agglutination

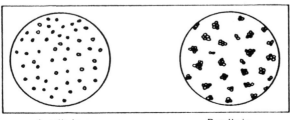

A cells in
A plasma

B cells in
A plasma

FIGURE 56–2. Erythrocyte agglutination in incompatible plasma. (From Ganong WF. Review of Medical Physiology. 13th ed. Norwalk, CT: Appleton and Lange, 1987; with permission.)

of the transfused RBCs by antibodies present in the plasma of the recipient. Agglutination of the recipient's RBCs is less likely because antibodies in the incompatible blood are rapidly diluted in the recipient's plasma. In addition to agglutination, this antigen–antibody interaction may result in immediate hemolysis of the transfused RBCs. Hemolysis reflects activation of the complement system, which releases proteolytic enzymes that cause lysis of RBCs. Indeed, blockage of blood vessels by agglutinated RBCs and concomitant intravascular hemolysis are well-recognized hazards of transfusion of incompatible blood. Nevertheless, immediate intravascular hemolysis is less common than agglutination, presumably reflecting the need for very high titers of antibody to evoke hemolysis. Ultimately, however, even agglutination leads to hemolysis of agglutinated RBCs. When the rate of hemolysis is rapid, the plasma concentration of hemoglobin may exceed the binding capacity of haptoglobin, and free hemoglobin continues to circulate. This free hemoglobin is converted to bilirubin, and jaundice may occur. Nevertheless, if liver function is normal, jaundice does not appear unless more than 300 to 500 ml of blood is hemolyzed in less than 24 hours. Acute renal failure often accompanies a severe transfusion reaction.

LEUKOCYTES

Leukocytes are classified as granulocytes (polymorphonuclear leukocytes), monocytes, and lymphocytes (Table 56-3). Granulocytes are further subdivided as neutrophils, eosinophils, and basophils based on the staining characteristics of granules contained in these cells. Acting together, leukocytes provide an important defense against invading organisms (bacterial, viral, or parasitic) and are necessary for immune responses. Normally, each milliliter of blood contains 4000 to 11,000 leukocytes, the most numerous being neutrophils. Granulocytes and monocytes are formed from stem cells in the bone marrow. After birth, some lymphocytes are formed in bone marrow but most are produced in the thymus, lymph nodes, and spleen from precursor cells that came originally from the bone marrow. Lymphocytes enter the circulation via the lymphatic system.

Neutrophils

Neutrophils are the most numerous leukocytes in the blood, representing approximately 60% of the circulating leukocytes. These cells seek out, ingest, and kill bacteria (phagocytosis) and thus represent the body's first line of defense against bacterial infection. Neutrophils contain lysosomes filled with proteolytic enzymes capable of digesting bacteria. Eventually, neutrophils are killed by toxic products released by lysosomes. Hydrogen peroxide produced by neutrophils also exerts an antibacterial effect. Neutrophils also release thromboxanes (vasoconstriction and platelet aggregation) and leukotrienes (increased vascular permeability).

Once neutrophils are released from bone marrow into the circulation, they have a life span of 6 to 8 hours. To maintain a normal circulating blood level of neutrophils it is necessary for the bone marrow to produce over 100 billion neutrophils daily. In the presence of infection, the need for neutrophils is even greater because these cells are destroyed in the process of phagocytosis. Indeed, a marked increase (up to fivefold) in the number of circulating neutrophils (leukocytosis) occurs within a few hours following bacterial infection or onset of inflammation. Leukocytosis is stimulated by release of a chemical substance from inflamed tissues known as leukocytosis-inducing factor. This factor is believed to dilate venous sinusoids of bone marrow, thus facilitating release of stored neutrophils. A similar increase in circulating neutrophils may accompany nonbacterial tissue injury such as myocardial infarction. Even intense exercise lasting only

Table 56–3
Classification of Leukocytes

	Cells in Each ml of Plasma (range)	Percent of Total (range)
Granulocytes		
Neutrophils	3000–6000	55–65
Eosinophils	0–300	1–3
Basophils	0–100	0–1
Monocytes (Macrophages)	300–500	3–6
Lymphocytes	1500–3500	25–35
Total Leukocytes	4000–11,000	

1 minute can cause the number of circulating neutrophils to increase threefold (physiologic neutrophilia).

Eosinophils

Eosinophils account for approximately 2% of circulating leukocytes. Following release from the bone marrow into the circulation, most eosinophils migrate within 30 minutes into extravascular tissues where they survive 8 to 12 days. These cells are weak phagocytes but enter the circulation in increased numbers following ingestion of foreign proteins. The most common chronic cause of increases in the circulating concentration of eosinophils is the presence of parasites in the blood, perhaps reflecting the role of eosinophils in detoxifying foreign proteins. Eosinophils show a special propensity to collect at sites of antigen–antibody reactions in tissues most likely in response to a chemotactic stimulus. The effect of this accumulation is to dampen the host's response by limiting antigen-induced release of chemical mediators from mast cells and basophils. The total number of circulating eosinophils increases during allergic reactions presumably because tissue reactions release products that selectively increase the production of eosinophils in the bone marrow.

Basophils

Basophils in the blood are similar to mast cells in tissues in that both types of cells contain histamine and heparin. Release of heparin into the blood inhibits coagulation and speeds removal of fat particles after a meal. Degranulation of these cells occurs when IgE selectively attaches to the membranes of previously sensitized basophils or mast cells. The subsequent release of histamine and perhaps other chemical mediators is responsible for the manifestations of allergic reactions.

Monocytes

Monocytes enter the circulation from the bone marrow, but after approximately 24 hours migrate into tissues to become macrophages. These macrophages, like neutrophils, contain peroxidase and lysosomal enzymes and are actively phagocytic. Macrophages constitute the reticuloendothelial system. In addition to bacteria, these cells phagocytize large particles including RBCs, necrotic tissue, and dead neutrophils. Monocytes also participate in the immune process by secreting interleukin, which promotes the proliferation and maturation of T lymphocytes.

Macrophages in different tissues are designated by different names; for example, macrophages in the liver are known as Kupffer's cells; in lymph nodes, spleen, and bone marrow, as reticulum cells; in alveoli of the lungs, as alveolar macrophages; in subcutaneous tissue, as histiocytes; and in the brain, as microglia.

Kupffer's Cells

Kupffer's cells line hepatic sinuses and serve as a filtration system to remove bacteria that have entered the portal blood from the gastrointestinal tract. Indeed, these tissue macrophages are capable of removing almost all bacteria from the portal blood.

Reticulum Cells

Reticulum cells line sinuses of lymph nodes. These macrophages effectively phagocytize foreign particles as they pass through lymph nodes. Invading organisms that manage to find their way into the general circulation are vulnerable to phagocytosis by reticulum cells in the bone marrow and spleen. The spleen is similar to lymph nodes except that blood rather than lymph flows through the substance of the spleen. The spleen is also important for the removal of abnormal platelets and erythrocytes.

Alveolar Macrophages

Alveolar macrophages are present in alveolar walls and can phagocytize invading organisms that are inhaled. If the phagocytized particles are digestible, the resulting products are released into the lymph. If the particles are not digestible (carbon), the macrophages often form a giant cell capsule around the particles.

Histiocytes

Histiocytes are tissue macrophages that are present in subcutaneous tissues. These cells phagocytize invading organisms that gain access when the skin is broken. When local inflammation occurs in the subcutaneous tissues, histiocytes are stimulated to divide and form additional macrophages.

Lymphocytes

Lymphocytes account for approximately 30% of circulating leukocytes. These cells play a prominent role in immunity (see the section entitled "Immunity")

AGRANULOCYTOSIS

Agranulocytosis is the acute cessation of leukocyte production by the bone marrow. Within 2 to 3 days, ulcers appear in the mouth and colon, reflecting the uninhibited growth of bacteria that normally populate these areas. Irradiation of the body by gamma rays associated with a nuclear explosion, or exposure to drugs or chemicals containing benzene or anthracene ring (sulfonamides, chloramphenicol, thiouracil), can cause acute bone marrow aplasia in which neither erythrocytes nor leukocytes are produced. Usually sufficient stem cells (hemocytoblasts) remain after injury to allow recovery of bone marrow function if fatal infection is prevented by appropriate antibiotic therapy. This regeneration, however, may require several months.

BACTERIAL DESTRUCTION

Leukocytes participate in destruction of bacteria by the processes of diapedesis, chemotaxis, and phagocytosis. Opsonization also makes bacteria susceptible to phagocytosis.

Diapedesis

Neutrophils and monocytes can squeeze through pores in blood vessels by diapedesis. Specifically, even though the pore is smaller than the leukocyte, a small portion of the cell slides through the pore at a time, the portion sliding through being momentarily constricted to the size of the pore.

Chemotaxis

Chemotaxis is the phenomenon by which different chemical substances in tissues cause neutrophils and monocytes to move either toward or away from the chemical. For example, inflamed tissue may contain substances (C5a, leukotrienes, bacterial toxins, or products of coagulation) that cause neutrophils and monocytes to move toward (chemotaxis) the inflamed area. Chemotaxis is effective up to 100 μ away from an inflamed tissue. Because almost no tissue is more than 30 to 50 μ away from a capillary, the chemotactic signal can rapidly attract large numbers of leukocytes to the inflamed area. Chemotaxis may be inhibited by inhaled anesthetics (see Chapter 2).

Opsonization

Opsonization is the coating of bacteria by IgG and complement proteins (opsonins), thus making the microorganisms susceptible to phagocytosis.

Phagocytosis

Neutrophils and monocytes are known as phagocytes. On approaching a particle to be phagocytized, the neutrophil projects pseudopodia around the particle. These pseudopodia fuse, creating a chamber containing the ingested particle. Phagocytosis is likely to occur when (1) the surface of the particle is rough, (2) the particle is electropositive, and (3) the particle is recognized as foreign. Most natural substances of the body, including neutrophils and monocytes, have electronegative surfaces. Conversely, necrotic tissues and foreign particles are often electropositive and, thus, are attracted to phagocytes.

INFLAMMATION

Inflammation is a series of sequential changes that occur in tissues in response to injury. Tissue injury, whether it is due to bacteria or trauma, causes the release of local substances (histamine, bradykinin, or serotonin) into the surrounding fluid. These substances, particularly histamine, increase local blood flow as well as the local permeability of capillaries, allowing fibrinogen to leak into tissues. Local extracellular edema results, and the extracellular fluid and lymphatic fluid coagulate because of the coagulating effects of fibrinogen present in extravasated fluid. As a result, brawny edema develops in the spaces surrounding damaged tissues.

Tissue spaces and lymphatics in the inflamed area are blocked by clots of fibrinogen; thus, blood flow through the area is minimal. This effectively isolates the injured area from normal tissues and minimizes the dissemination of bacteria or toxic products. Staphylococci liberate potent cellular toxins, causing the rapid onset of inflammation and isolation of the infected area. In contrast, streptococci cause less intense local destruction, such that the walling-off process develops slowly, allowing streptococci to spread extensively. As a result, streptococci have a greater tendency to produce disseminated and life-threatening infection than do staphylococci, even though staphylococci produce more intense local tissue damage.

Soon after inflammation begins, the inflamed area is invaded by neutrophils and macrophages. These cells immediately begin their function of phagocytosis. Products of inflamed tissues also stimulate movement of neutrophils into the inflamed area from the circulation. When neutrophils and macrophages engulf large numbers of bacteria and necrotic tissue, almost all the neutrophils and many of the macrophages die. The collection of dead leukocytes and necrotic tissue is known as pus. The pus cavity may digest its way to the exterior or into an internal cavity and thus discharge its contents. Alternatively, the pus cavity may remain closed, and eventually its contents will undergo autolysis and absorption into surrounding tissues.

IMMUNITY

Humoral immunity and cellular immunity represent the two types of immune defense systems designed to protect the body against organisms or toxins that cause tissue damage (Stevenson et al, 1990). The principal defense against bacterial infection is provided by humoral immunity owing to circulating antibodies in the gamma globulin fraction of plasma proteins. Cellular immunity is responsible for delayed allergic reactions, rejection of foreign tissue, and destruction of early cancer cells. Cellular immunity also serves as a major defense against infections owing to viruses, fungi, and bacteria such as myobacterium tuberculosis. Signals mediating interactions between immune system effector cells are termed *biologic response modifiers.* Substances responsible for these signals are polypeptides as represented by colony-stimulating factors, interferons, and interleukins.

Lymphocytes responsible for humoral immunity are designated B lymphocytes and those responsible for cellular immunity are T lymphocytes (Fig. 56-3). The designation as B lymphocytes reflects the original discovery in birds, in which the formation of these cells occurs in the bursa of Fabricius, while the T designation emphasizes the role of the thymus gland in the origin of these cells. Morphologically, B lymphocytes and T lymphocytes are indistinguishable.

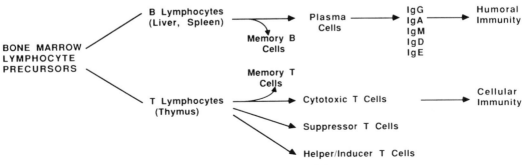

FIGURE 56–3. Schematic depiction of the development of the immune system.

B lymphocytes differentiate into memory B cells and plasma cells. Plasma cells are the source of gamma globulin antibodies responsible for humoral immunity. T lymphocytes are categorized as helper/inducer T cells, suppressor T cells, cytotoxic T cells, and memory T cells. Helper/inducer T cells and suppressor T cells are involved in the regulation of antibody production by B lymphocyte derivatives and cytotoxic T cells destroy foreign cells as represented by organ transplants. Helper/inducer T cells may be designated T4 cells because they often have on their surface a glycoprotein marker called T4; cytotoxic and suppressor T cells may be designated T8 cells for a similar reason.

Most of the preprocessing of B lymphocytes that prepares them to manufacture antibodies occurs before and shortly after birth. In humans, it is likely that this preprocessing occurs predominantly in the lymphoid tissue in the fetal liver and to a lesser extent in bone marrow and gastrointestinal mucosa. Most of the preprocessing of T lymphocytes occurs in the thymus shortly before birth and for a few months after birth. Removal of the thymus gland after this time usually will not interfere with cellular immunity. After formation of processed B and T lymphocytes, these cells are delivered by the circulation to lymphoid tissues where they are trapped. The location of lymphoid tissues (gastrointestinal tract, spleen, tonsils, and adenoids) is optimal for intercepting ingested or inhaled antigens as well as those that reach the circulation.

It is believed that during the processing of B and T lymphocytes, all those clones of lymphocytes capable of destroying the body's own tissues are self-destroyed because of their continued exposure to the body's antigens. This immune tolerance to the body's own tissues may diminish, resulting in autoimmune diseases such as thyroiditis, rheumatic fever, glomerulonephritis, myasthenia gravis, and lupus erythematosus. Likewise, selective suppression of T lymphocytes as with cyclosporine may interfere with early destruction of cancer cells manifesting as an increased incidence of cancer as in patients who are chronically immune-suppressed to improve acceptance of organ transplants. The human immunodeficiency virus specifically attacks help/inducer T lymphocytes (T4 cells) with eventual loss of immune function and death from infections due to normally nonpathogenic bacteria or cancer.

Antigens

Antigens are foreign proteins or chemicals that evoke the production of antibodies. Bacteria or toxins contain unique chemical structures that differ from normal body constituents, resulting in their role as antigens. For a substance to be antigenic, it typically must have a molecular weight more than 8000. Nevertheless, immunity against low–molecular-weight substances can occur if the material acts as a hapten and binds to a protein, the combination resulting in an antigenic response. Haptens that elicit such an immune response are usually drugs, chemical constituents in dust, or shed breakdown products of animal skin.

Antibodies

Prior to exposure to a specific antigen, clones of B lymphocytes remain dormant in lymphoid tissue. Entry of antigens into lymphoid tissues causes clones of B lymphocytes to form plasma cells capable of producing gamma globulin antibodies specific for activity against that antigen (primary response) (Fig. 56-4) (Guyton, 1986). Each antibody that is specific for a particular antigen has a different organization of amino acids that lends steric shape. This steric shape fits the antigen and results in a rapid and tight chemical or physical bond between the antibody and antigen. Some B lymphocytes, however, remain dor-

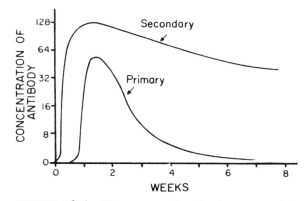

FIGURE 56–4. Time course of antibody response following primary and secondary injection of antigen. (From Guyton AC. Textbook of Medical Physiology. 7th ed. Philadelphia: WB Saunders, 1986; with permission.)

CLASSICAL PATHWAY   **ALTERNATIVE PATHWAY**

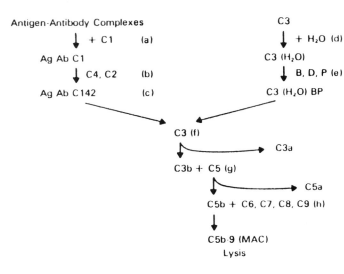

FIGURE 56–5. Diagram depicting the classical and alternative pathways of the complement system. (From Frank MM. Complement in the pathophysiology of human disease. N Engl J Med 1987; 316: 1525–30; with permission.)

mant in the lymphoid tissue, functioning as B memory cells. Subsequent exposure to the antigen causes these memory cells to participate in an exaggerated antibody response (secondary response) compared with the primary response (Fig. 56-5) (Frank, 1987). The increased intensity and duration of the secondary response is the reason why vaccination is often achieved by injection of the antigen in multiple small doses several weeks apart.

Structure

Plasma cells form gamma globulin antibodies that are grouped into five classes of immunoglobulins: IgG, IgA, IgM, IgD, and IgE (Table 56-4). IgG can cross the placenta to enter the fetal circulation and is the principal antibody that reacts with bacteria and probably viruses. IgA is elaborated by plasma cells localized to secretory tissues (tears, saliva, respiratory mucosa, gastrointestinal mucosa, or cervical mucosa), thus providing a topical and localized defense against infection. IgM is the most prominent immunoglobulin on the surface of lymphocytes and is the first type of antibody synthesized after initial exposure to an antigen. Natural antibodies against antigens on RBC membranes are IgM. IgD is important in antigen recognition by B cells. IgE antibodies are uniquely important in evoking degranulation of mast cells and basophils, result-

ing in release of chemical mediators, especially histamine, that are responsible for the symptoms of an allergic reaction.

Mechanism of Action

Antibodies act by (1) direct effects on the antigen, (2) activation of the complement system, or (3) initiation of an anaphylactic reaction. Examples of direct effects of antibodies that destroy antigens are (1) agglutination such as occurs with transfusion of incompatible blood, (2) precipitation, (3) neutralization, and (4) lysis. More important, however, than these direct effects are the amplifying effects of the complement system or the anaphylactic reaction.

COMPLEMENT SYSTEM. Complement is a system of enzyme precursors that are normally present in the plasma in an inactive form. These enzymes are designated as C1 through C9 for the classical pathway and B, D, H, I, and P (properdin) for the alternative pathway (Fig. 56-5) (Frank, 1987). Complement activation proceeds in a sequential fashion comparable with the clotting cascade. Classical pathway activation occurs when IgG or IgM binds to an antigen on the cell membrane of mast cells and basophils. This antigen–antibody complex initiates a sequential cascading process by initially activating the normally quiescent C1. Hereditary angioedema is periodic swelling

Table 56-4
Properties of Immunoglobulins

	IgG	*IgA*	*IgM*	*IgD*	*IgE*
Location	Plasma Amniotic Fluid	Plasma Saliva Tears	Plasma	Plasma	Plasma
Plasma concentration $(mg \cdot dl^{-1})$	600–1500	85–380	50–400	<15	0.01–0.03
Plasma half-time (days)	21–23	6	5	2–8	1–5
Function					
Complement activation	+	–	+	–	–
Degranulation of mast cells	–	–	–	–	+
Bacterial lysis	+	–	+	–	–
Opsonization	+	?	–	–	–
Agglutination	+	+	+	–	–
Virus inactivation	+	+	+	–	–

owing to decreased functional activity of the C1 esterase inhibitor. Activation of the alternative pathway occurs via nonimmunologic mechanisms (endotoxins, bubble oxygenator membranes, radiographic contrast media, or protamine) independent of antibodies. Activation of C3 and C5 occurs via either pathway, leading to the formation of active fragments known as anaphylatoxins (C3a, C5a). These active fragments evoke changes characterized by (1) lysis of bacterial cell membranes, (2) facilitation of phagocytosis by the phenomenon of opsonization, (3) attraction of leukocytes to the site of injury (chemotaxis), and (4) degranulation of mast cells and basophils manifesting as an allergic reaction. Activation of the complement system by endotoxin may be important in the development of renal failure and vasodilation in gram-negative sepsis. Generation of C5a may be responsible for the neutropenia and arterial hypoxemia that accompanies adult respiratory distress syndrome (Hammerschmidt et al, 1980). Protamine and heparin-protamine complexes can activate the complement cascade.

ANAPHYLACTIC REACTION. An anaphylactic reaction occurs when an antigen attaches to IgE antibodies on the cell membranes of circulating basophils or tissue mast cells. This antigen–antibody interaction changes the permeability of the cell membrane, leading to degranulation and release of chemical mediators (histamine, leukotrienes, or prostaglandins) into the circulation. These chemical mediators are responsible for the symptoms (hypotension, bronchoconstriction, or edema) of an anaphylactic reaction. Chemotactic factors are also released during degranulation serving to attract neutrophils, eosinophils, and platelets to the site of the antigen–antibody interaction. It is important to recognize that an anaphylactic reaction requires prior exposure to the antigen causing production of IgE antibodies that attach to cell membranes, rendering that cell sensitized should a repeat exposure to that antigen occur.

In some highly sensitized individuals, the degranulation resulting from the antigen–antibody interaction may be so explosive that life-threatening hypotension or bronchoconstriction occurs. Less explosive reactions are characterized by urticaria in which an antigen enters the skin and evokes the local release of histamine. Hay fever results when the antigen–antibody reaction occurs in the nose, in contrast to asthma, where the reaction occurs in the bronchioles of the lungs. Histamine seems to be primarily responsible for the symptoms of hay fever, whereas bronchospasm characteristic of asthma may be mainly due to leukotrienes. Indeed, antihistamines have beneficial effects in the treatment of hay fever; however, less effect is seen in their use for the prevention and treatment of asthma.

TISSUE TYPING

Tissue typing is possible in much the same way the blood is typed. For example, the most important antigens that cause rejection of transplanted tissue are the human leukocyte antigens (HLA). These HLA antigens are also present on cell membranes of leukocytes. As a result, tissue typing can be accomplished by determining the types of antigens on the recipient's lymphocyte membranes. Some HLA antigens are poorly antigenic, negating the need for precise tissue matching of all antigens.

REFERENCES

Frank MM. Complement in the pathophysiology of human disease. N Engl J Med 1987;316:1525–30.

Ganong WF. Review of Medical Physiology. 13th ed. Norwalk, CT. Appleton and Lange. 1987.

Guyton AC. Textbook of Medical Physiology. 7th ed. Philadelphia. WB Saunders. 1986.

Hammerschmidt DE, Weaver LJ, Hudson LD, Craddock PR, Jacob HS. Association of complement activation and elevated-C5a with adult respiratory distress syndrome. Lancet 1980;1:947–9.

Stevenson GW, Hall SC, Rudnick S, Seleny FL, Stevenson HC. The effect of anesthetic agents on the human immune response. Anesthesiology 1990;72:542–52.

Chapter

57

Hemostasis and Blood Coagulation

HEMOSTASIS

Hemostasis in the presence of loss of blood vessel integrity is achieved by several mechanisms, including (1) vascular spasm, (2) formation of a platelet plug, (3) clot formation, and (4) growth of fibrous tissue into the blood clot to seal the break in the blood vessel.

Vascular Spasm

The wall of a cut blood vessel immediately contracts, which serves to reduce blood flow from the damaged vessel. This contraction results from neural reflexes initiated by pain impulses from the traumatized vessel and release of vasoconstricting substances such as serotonin from platelets. Vascular spasm is most intense in severely traumatized or crushed blood vessels. The sharply cut or transected blood vessel, as occurs during surgery, undergoes less vascular spasm, and blood loss is reduced less. Vascular spasm lasts 20 to 30 minutes, providing time for additional mechanisms of hemostasis to become active.

Platelet Plug

The second event in hemostasis is an attempt by platelets to form a plug in the opening of the blood vessel. Within seconds after the endothelial lining of the blood vessel is disrupted, receptors on surfaces of platelets interact with exposed collagen and adhere to the site of injury. Factor VIII:vWF and thrombin are also important in platelet activation and adhesion. Contents of cytoplasmic granules of these platelets are extruded into the circulation (release reaction), providing the stimulus to attract other platelets (aggregation) to this site of vascular disruption and further enhance the platelet plug. Substances extruded from platelets include adenosine diphosphate (ADP) and thromboxane A_2. Aspirin inhibits the platelet release reaction and subsequent aggregation by irreversibly acetylating cyclooxygenase. Prostacyclin, presumed to come primarily from the vessel wall, allows clot to form in the wall of the vessel without extending into the vessel lumen.

The platelet plug mechanism is very important for closing minute breaks in small blood vessels that occur hundreds of times daily. When the number of platelets is reduced, small hemorrhagic areas appear under the skin and internally.

Megakaryocytes

Megakaryocytes are giant cells in the bone marrow from which cytoplasmic fragments are pinched off and extruded into the circulation as nuclear platelets. It is estimated that each megakaryocyte gives rise to 1000 to 1500 platelets. Thrombopoietin is a circulating substance that stimulates the formation of megakaryocytes and thus regulates the production of platelets. There are normally approximately 150,000 to 350,000 platelets in each milliliter of blood with an average life span of 8 to 12 days. Aged platelets are removed by the reticuloendothelial system and spleen.

Clot Formation

The fundamental reaction in blood clotting is conversion of fibrinogen to fibrin by the action of activated thrombin (Fig. 57-1). Activator substances from the traumatized vascular wall and platelets initiate this process within 15 to 20 seconds, and after 3 to 6 minutes the cut end of a blood vessel is filled with clot. If whole blood is allowed to clot and the clot is removed, the remaining fluid is serum. Serum is thus plasma with factors I, II, V, and VII removed.

Growth of Fibrous Tissue

Invasion of a blood clot by fibroblasts causes formation of connective tissue throughout the clot.

Conversion of the clot to fibrous tissue is complete in 7 to 10 days.

BLOOD COAGULATION

More than 30 different substances that promote (procoagulants) or inhibit (anticoagulants) coagulation have been identified in blood and tissues (Guyton, 1986). Normally, anticoagulants predominate, and blood does not coagulate. When a blood vessel is transected or damaged, activity of the procoagulants in the area of damage becomes predominant and clot formation occurs. Continued clot formation occurs only where blood is not flowing. This is true because the flow of blood dilutes thrombin and the other procoagulants released during the clotting process, thus preventing their concentration from rising high enough to sustain continued formation of clot.

Within a few minutes after the clot is formed, it begins to contract and typically expresses most of the fluid from itself after 30 to 60 minutes. Platelets are necessary for this clot retraction to occur. Indeed, failure of clot retraction is an indication that the number of circulating platelets is inadequate. Normally, as the blood clot retracts, the edges of the broken blood vessel are pulled together, restoring the integrity of the vascular lumen.

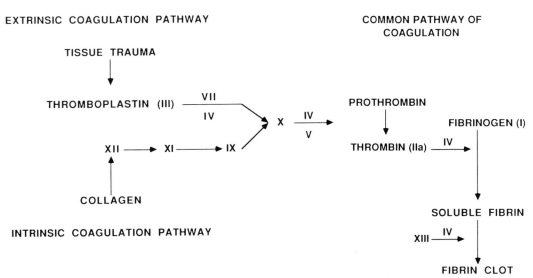

FIGURE 57–1. Schematic depiction of the extrinsic and intrinsic coagulation pathway culminating in the formation of a fibrin clot.

Initiation of Coagulation

Initiation of coagulation requires activation of prothrombin by mechanisms that are stimulated by trauma to tissues or to walls of blood vessels. Regardless of the mechanism, the result is formation of prothrombin activator, which then facilitates the conversion of prothrombin to thrombin.

The two pathways by which prothrombin activator is formed are known as the intrinsic coagulation pathway and extrinsic coagulation pathway (Fig. 57-1). In both pathways, a series of plasma proteins, often beta globulins, function as clotting factors (Table 57-1). Normally, those clotting factors exist as inactive forms of proteolytic enzymes, which, when activated, cause successive reactions of the clotting process. Blood coagulation culminates in the formation of fibrin, following the interaction of more than a dozen proteins in a cascading series of proteolytic reactions (Fig. 57-1).

Extrinsic Coagulation Pathway

The extrinsic coagulation pathway is stimulated to form prothrombin activator when blood comes into contact with traumatized vascular wall or extravascular tissues. Traumatized tissue releases a proteolytic enzyme, tissue thromboplastin (factor III), that initiates a succession of catalytic events (Fig. 57-1). Formation of prothrombin activator by the extrinsic pathway is rapid, often resulting in the appearance of clot within 15 seconds. The prothrombin time reflects the integrity of the extrinsic pathway.

Intrinsic Coagulation Pathway

The intrinsic coagulation pathway is stimulated to form prothrombin activator when there is trauma to the vascular wall that exposes collagen to circulating platelets and factor XII (Fig. 57-1). When blood is removed from the body and placed in a test tube, it is the intrinsic pathway alone that must initiate the coagulation process. The importance of calcium ions (Ca^{2+}) in the clotting process is emphasized by the ability of citrate or oxalate ions, which react with Ca^{2+}, to prevent clotting of blood when it is removed from the body. Clotting of blood is also greatly slowed if the surface of the container or tubing is smooth, such as the siliconized surfaces used

Table 57-1
Nomenclature of Blood Clotting Factors

Factor	Synonyms	Plasma Concentration ($\mu g \cdot ml^{-1}$)	Half-time (h)	Stability in Stored Whole Blood
I	Fibrinogen	2000–4000	95–120	No change
II	Prothrombin	150	65–90	No change
III	Thromboplastin			
IV	Calcium			
V	Proaccelerin	10	15–24	Half-time 7 days
VII	Proconvertin	0.5	4–6	No change
VIII	Antihemophilic factor	50–100	10–12	Half-time 7 days
	VIII:vWF	50–100		
	VIII:C	0.05–0.1		
IX	Christmas factor	3	18–30	No change
X	Stuart-Prower factor	15	40–60	No change
XI	Plasma thromboplastin factor	5	45–60	Half-time 7 days

during cardiopulmonary bypass. The intrinsic pathway proceeds slowly, usually requiring 2 to 6 minutes to cause clotting. A variety of inhibitors act at different sites in the intrinsic pathway. The partial thromboplastin time reflects the integrity of the intrinsic pathway.

Factor VIII

Factor VIII is a complex molecule that can be dissociated into two subcomponents. The larger subcomponent, designated von Willebrand factor (factor VIII:vWF) is synthesized in vascular endothelial cells and megakaryocytes. This factor is important for enhancing adhesion of platelets to vascular endothelial surfaces. The smaller subcomponent (factor VIII:C) is most likely synthesized in the liver and is important in the coagulation cascade. This factor is deficient or absent in patients with hemophilia A. The plasma concentration of factor VIII is precisely controlled with increases in the circulating level of this factor being evoked by epinephrine, vasopressin, and estrogens.

Conversion of Prothrombin to Thrombin

Prothrombin activator is responsible for the conversion of prothrombin to thrombin. Prothrombin as well as factors VII, IX, and X is synthesized in the liver. Vitamin K is required by the liver for formation of these factors. Indeed, lack of vitamin K resulting from absence of bile salts or the presence of severe liver disease may prevent normal prothrombin formation. Failure of the liver to synthesize prothrombin leads to a decline in the plasma concentration below acceptable levels within 24 hours.

Conversion of Fibrinogen to Fibrin

Fibrinogen is a high–molecular weight (340,000) protein present in the plasma in concentrations between 200 to 400 mg·dl^{-1}. This clotting factor is formed in the liver, and severe liver disease can lead to inadequate synthesis. Plasma concentrations of fibrinogen are often increased in the presence of pregnancy, tissue damage, inflammation, or cancer. An increased plasma concentration of fibrinogen accelerates the settling of erythrocytes (erythrocyte sedimentation rate) when the blood is allowed to stand. Because of its large molecular weight, little fibrinogen normally leaks into interstitial fluids, accounting for

the lack of coagulation that occurs in this fluid. When capillary permeability increases, however, as in the presence of inflammation, fibrinogen can enter interstitial fluids and initiate coagulation.

Thrombin is a proteolytic enzyme that acts on fibrinogen to remove two low–molecular weight peptides from each molecule of fibrinogen, resulting in a fibrin monomer that can polymerize with other fibrin monomers. A large number of fibrin monomers polymerize within seconds into long fibrin threads that form the reticulum of the clot. The strength of this fibrin clot is subsequently greatly enhanced by the action of fibrin-stabilizing factors, which are present in the plasma and are also released from adjacent platelets. Ultimately, the blood clot comprises a meshwork of cross-linked fibrin threads that adhere to the damaged surfaces of blood vessels, entrapping platelets, erythrocytes, and plasma.

Impact of Progressive Blood Loss

It is likely that stress, tissue trauma with release of tissue thromboplastin, and elevations in the plasma concentrations of catecholamines offset any hypocoagulable tendency resulting from hemodilution and loss of coagulation factors during progressive blood loss. These offsetting factors are probably responsible for the increase in coagulability seen in many surgical patients experiencing moderate to massive blood loss (Tuman et al, 1987).

Endogenous Control of Coagulation and Clot Formation

The two factors that normally prevent intrinsic initiation of the clotting process are the smoothness of the vascular endothelium, which prevents contact activation of the intrinsic clotting system, and a monomolecular layer of negatively charged protein on the inner layer of the vascular endothelium that repels clotting factors and platelets. In addition, plasma contains substances that inhibit activated clotting factors and facilitate lysis of intravascular clots.

Endogenous Anticoagulants

Antithrombin III is a circulating substance that binds to thrombin, thus preventing conversion to fibrin. This binding of antithrombin III to thrombin is greatly facilitated by heparin. Heparin is present in circulating basophils and mast cells located in tissues around capillaries. Mast cells are particularly abundant in tissues surrounding capillaries of the lungs and, to a lesser extent, those of the liver. This is important because capillaries of the lungs and liver receive many embolic clots formed in the slowly moving venous blood. Heparin may prevent further growth of these clots. Protein C is a circulating substance that inhibits the activity of factors VIII:C and V. Protein S enhances the effects of protein C. There is an increased incidence of thrombosis in patients with deficient amounts of antithrombin III, protein C, or protein S. Furthermore, heparin is not an effective anticoagulant when administered to patients with deficient antithrombin III levels.

Endogenous Lysis of Clots

Blood has the capacity to redissolve fibrin clots via a plasma proteolytic enzyme, plasmin (fibrinolysin), which is generated from its inactive precursor, plasminogen. Plasmin is formed in response to thrombin and tissue plasminogen activator, leading to the lysis of fibrin clots and production of fibrin split products. Urokinase, which is secreted by the kidneys, is capable of converting plasminogen to plasmin. Likewise, certain bacteria such as streptococci secrete substances (streptokinase) capable of converting plasminogen to plasmin. The therapeutic use of plasminogen activators is dissolution of intravascular clots by plasmin without a major effect on circulating fibrinogen. The principal importance of the endogenous fibrinolysin system is the removal of minute clots from small peripheral vessels that otherwise would become occluded. Conversely, opening of large blood vessels by this process rarely occurs. Excess activity of plasmin causes destruction of clotting factors such as factors I, II, V, VIII, and XII. As a result, lyses of clots may also be associated with hypocoagulability of the blood

Thromboembolism

Formation of clot inside a blood vessel is called thrombus to distinguish it from normal extravas-

cular clotting of blood. An embolus is a fragment of the thrombus that breaks off and travels in the blood until it lodges at a site of vascular narrowing. For this reason, an embolus originating in an artery usually occludes a more distal and smaller artery. Conversely, an embolus originating in a vein commonly lodges in the lungs, causing pulmonary vascular obstruction.

Thromboembolism is likely to occur in the presence of (1) any condition that causes a roughened endothelial vessel wall, such as arteriosclerosis, infection, or trauma; and (2) a slowing of blood flow. Slow or sluggish blood flow means activated clotting factors are not diluted and carried, away thus increasing the likelihood of localized clotting. Indeed, vascular stasis in leg veins associated with pregnancy or postoperative immobility is a common precipitating event for formation of a venous thrombus and subsequent pulmonary embolism.

Disseminated Intravascular Coagulation

Disseminated intravascular coagulation (DIC) reflects entrance of substances into the circulation that cause elaboration of thrombin leading to widespread thrombosis in small blood vessels. Hypofibrinogenemia occurs when fibrinogen is consumed in formation of these thrombi. Other clotting factors along with platelets may also be consumed. Spontaneous hemorrhage is likely while the presence of fibrin split products reflects activity of plasmin in dissolving (lysing) intravascular clots. Events that provoke DIC are complications of pregnancy and childbirth, sepsis, incompatible blood transfusions, and the presence of cancer.

REFERENCES

Guyton AC. Textbook of Medical Physiology. 7th ed. Philadelphia. WB Saunders. 1986.
Tuman KJ, Spiess BD, McCarthy RJ, Ivankovich AD. Effects of progressive blood loss on coagulation as measured by thrombelastography. Anesth Analg 1987;66:856–63.

58

Metabolism of Nutrients

Metabolism refers to all the chemical and energy transformations that occur in the body. Oxidation of nutrients (carbohydrates, fats, and proteins) results in production of carbon dioxide, water, and high energy phosphate bonds necessary for life processes. The most important high energy phosphate bond is adenosine triphosphate (ATP) (Fig. 58-1). This ubiquitous molecule is the energy storehouse for the body, providing the energy necessary for essentially all physiologic processes and chemical reactions. Probably, the most important intracellular process that requires energy from hydrolysis of ATP is formation of peptide linkages between amino acids during protein synthesis. Skeletal muscle contraction cannot occur without energy from ATP hydrolysis. ATP from metabolism of nutrients is necessary to provide energy for transport of ions across cell membranes and thus to maintain the distribution of these ions, which is necessary for propagation of nerve impulses. In renal tubules, as much as 80% of ATP is used for membrane transport of ions. In addition to its function in energy transfer, ATP is also the precursor of cyclic adenosine monophosphate.

For adults, total daily energy expenditure averages 39 kcal·kg^{-1} in males and 34 ml·kg^{-1} in females. Approximately 20 kcal·kg^{-1} is expended as basal metabolism necessary to maintain energy-requiring tasks essential for life. In the resting state, the necessary basal expenditure of calories is equivalent to approximately 1.1 kcal·min^{-1}, which requires use of 200 to 250 ml·min^{-1} of oxygen. Activities increase caloric requirements in proportion to the energy expenditure required

(Table 58-1). The caloric values of carbohydrates, fats, and proteins are approximately 4.1 kcal·g^{-1}, 9.3 kcal·g^{-1}, and 4.1 kcal·g^{-1} respectively. Fat forms the major energy storage depot because of its greater mass and high caloric value (Fig. 58-2) (Berne and Levy, 1988).

CARBOHYDRATE METABOLISM

At least 99% of all the energy derived from carbohydrates is used to form ATP in the cells. The final products of carbohydrate digestion in the gastrointestinal tract are glucose, fructose, and galactose. After absorption into the circulation, fructose and galactose are rapidly converted to glucose. As a result, glucose is the predominant molecule in carbohydrate metabolism. This glucose must be transported through cell membranes into cellular cytoplasm before it can be used by cells. This transport uses a protein carrier known as carrier-mediated diffusion, which is enhanced by insulin. Immediately, upon entering cells, glucose is converted to glucose-6-phosphate under the influence of the enzyme glucokinase. This phosphorylation of glucose prevents escape of glucose from cells back into the circulation.

The fetus derives almost all of its energy from glucose obtained by means of the maternal circulation. Immediately after birth, the infant stores of glycogen are sufficient to supply glucose for only a few hours. Furthermore, gluconeogenesis is limited in the neonate. As a result, the neonate be vulnerable to hypoglycemia.

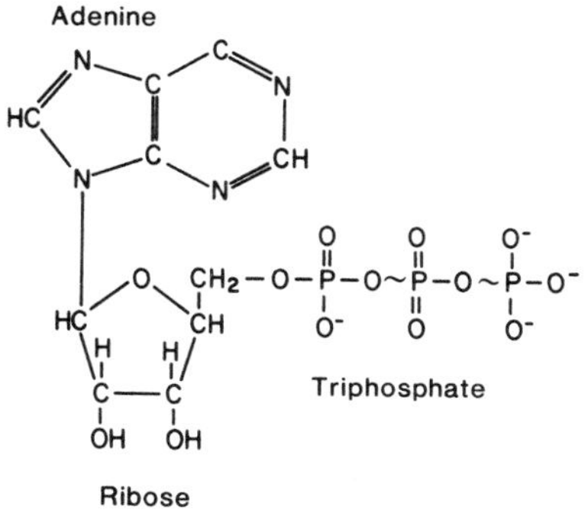

FIGURE 58–1. Metabolism of nutrients in cells is directed toward the ultimate synthesis of adenosine triphosphate (ATP). Energy necessary for physiologic processes and chemical reactions is derived from the high energy phosphate bonds of ATP.

Table 58–1
Estimates of Energy Expenditure in Adults

Activity	Calorie Expenditure $(kcal \cdot min^{-1})$
Basal	1.1
Sitting	1.8
Walking (2.5 miles·h⁻¹)	4.3
Walking (4 miles·h⁻¹)	8.2
Climbing stairs	9.0
Swimming	10.9
Bicycling (13 miles·h⁻¹)	11.1

Glycogen

After entering cells, glucose can be used immediately for release of energy to cells or it can be stored as a polymer of glucose known as *glycogen.* Although all cells can store at least some glucose as glycogen, the liver and skeletal muscles are particularly capable of storing large amounts of glycogen. The ability to form glycogen makes it possible to store substantial quantities of carbohydrates without significantly alter-

ing the osmotic pressure of intracellular fluids. Glycogen breakdown is catalyzed by activation of phosphorylase in liver and skeletal muscle by the action of epinephrine on beta receptors.

Gluconeogenesis

Gluconeogenesis is the formation of glucose from amino acids and the glycerol portion of fat. This process occurs when body stores of carbohydrates decrease below normal levels. An estimated 60% of the amino acids in the body's proteins can be converted easily to carbohy-

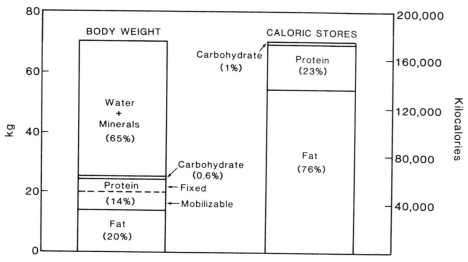

FIGURE 58–2. Comparison of the composition of body weight to caloric store. (From Berne RM, Levy MN. Physiology. 2nd ed. St. Louis: CV Mosby, 1988; with permission.)

drates, whereas the remaining 40% have chemical configurations that make this difficult.

Gluconeogenesis is stimulated by hypoglycemia. In addition, simultaneous release of cortisol mobilizes proteins, making these available in the form of amino acids for gluconeogenesis, especially in the liver. Thyroxine is also capable of increasing the rate of gluconeogenesis.

Energy Release from Glucose

Glucose is progressively broken down, and the resulting energy is used to form ATP. For each mole of glucose that is completely degraded to carbon dioxide and water, a total of 38 mol of ATP is ultimately formed. The most important means by which energy is released from the glucose molecule is by glycolysis and the subsequent oxidation of the end-products of glycolysis. Glycolysis is the splitting of the glucose molecule into

two molecules of pyruvate, which enter the mitochondria. In the mitochondria, pyruvate is converted to acetyl-coenzyme A (CoA), which enters the citric acid cycle (tricarboxylic acid cycle or Krebs cycle) and is converted to carbon dioxide and hydrogen ions (H^+) (Fig. 58-3). H^+ released during glycolysis, formation of acetyl-CoA, and in the citric acid cycle enters into oxidative chemical reactions to form large quantities of ATP (oxidative phosphorylation). Oxidative phosphorylation occurs only in the mitochondria and in the presence of adequate amounts of oxygen.

Anaerobic Glycolysis

In the absence of adequate amounts of oxygen, a small amount of energy can be released to cells by anaerobic glycolysis because conversion of glucose to pyruvate does not require oxygen. Indeed, carbohydrates are the only nutrient that can form ATP without oxygen. This release of

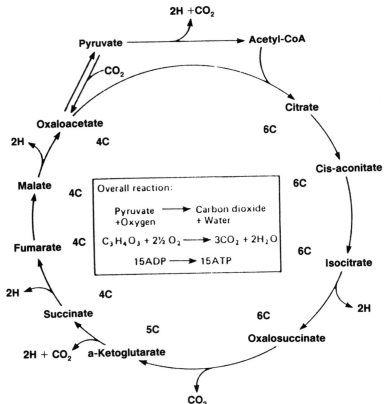

Overall reaction:

Pyruvate $\longrightarrow$ Carbon dioxide
+Oxygen $\qquad$ + Water

$C_3H_4O_3 + 2\frac{1}{2}O_2 \longrightarrow 3CO_2 + 2H_2O$

$15ADP \longrightarrow 15ATP$

FIGURE 58-3. Citric acid cycle resulting in production of 15 moles of adenosine triphosphate (ATP) by oxidative phosphorylation.

glycolytic energy to cells can be lifesaving for a few minutes when oxygen becomes unavailable.

During anaerobic glycolysis, most pyruvic acid is converted to lactic acid, which diffuses rapidly out of cells into extracellular fluid. When oxygen is again available, this lactic acid can be reconverted to glucose. This reconversion occurs predominantly in the liver. Indeed, severe liver disease may interfere with the ability of the liver to convert lactic acid to glucose, leading to metabolic acidosis.

LIPID METABOLISM

Lipids include phospholipids, triglycerides, and cholesterol. The basic lipid moiety of phospholipids and triglycerides is *fatty acids.* Fatty acids are long-chain hydrocarbon organic acids that, when bound to albumin, are known as *free fatty acids* (Fig. 58-4). An important role of free fatty acids is as precursors for prostaglandins. Phospholipids include lecithins, cephalins, and sphingomyelins, which are formed principally in the liver, and are important in the formation of myelin and cell membranes. The basic structure of the triglyceride molecule is three long-chain fatty acids bound with one molecule of glycerol (Fig. 58-5). Triglycerides, following absorption from the gastrointestinal tract, are transported in the lymph and then by way of the thoracic duct into the circulation in droplets known as *chylomicrons.* Chylomicrons are rapidly removed from the circulation and stored as they pass through capillaries of adipose tissue and skeletal muscles. Triglycerides are used in the body mainly to provide energy for metabolic processes similar to those fueled by carbohydrates. Cholesterol does not contain fatty acids, but its sterol nucleus is synthesized from degradation products of fatty acid molecules, thus giving it many of the physical and chemical properties characteristic of lipids (Fig. 58-6).

Lipoproteins are synthesized principally in the liver and are mixtures of phospholipids, triglycerides, cholesterol, and proteins (Table 58-2). The presumed function of lipoproteins is

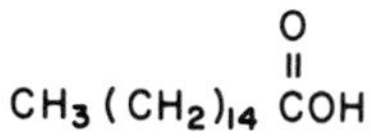

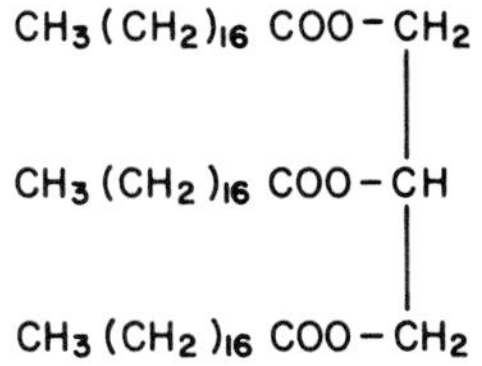

FIGURE 58–5. The basic structure of the triglyceride molecule is three long-chain fatty acids bound with one molecule of glycerol.

to provide a mechanism of transport for lipids throughout the body. Lipoproteins are classified according to their density, which is inversely proportional to their lipid content (Table 58-2) (see Chapter 32). All the cholesterol in plasma is in lipoprotein complexes with low-density lipoproteins (LDL) representing the major cholesterol component in plasma. These LDL provide cholesterol to tissues where it is an essential component of cell membranes and is used in the synthesis of corticosteroids and sex hormones. In the liver, LDL are taken up by receptor-mediated endocytosis. An intrinsic feedback control system increases the endogenous production of cholesterol when exogenous intake is decreased, explaining the relatively modest lowering effect on plasma cholesterol concentrations produced by low-cholesterol diets. If this endogenous increase in cholesterol synthesis is blocked by drugs that inhibit HMG–CoA reductase, then there is an appreciable decrease in the plasma cholesterol concentration.

The first step in the use of triglycerides for energy is hydrolysis into fatty acids and glycerol and subsequent transport of these products to tissues where they are oxidized. Almost all cells, except for brain cells, can use fatty acids interchangeably with glucose for energy. Degradation and oxidation of fatty acids occur only in mitochondria, resulting in progressive release of two

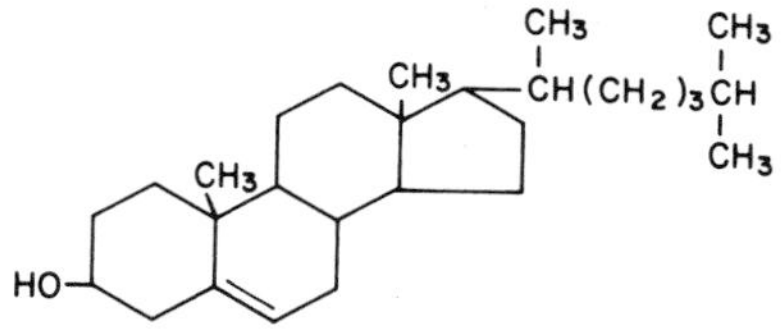

FIGURE 58–6. Cholesterol contains a sterol nucleus that is synthesized from degradation products of fatty acid molecules.

FIGURE 58–4. Palmitic acid.

Table 58–2
Composition of Lipids in the Plasma

	Phospholipid (percent)	Triglyceride (percent)	Free Cholesterol (percent)	Cholesterol Esters (percent)	Protein (percent)	Density
Chylomicrons	3	90	2	3	2	0.94
LDL	21	6	7	46	20	1.019–1.063
HDL	25	5	4	16	50	1.063–1.21
IDL	20	40	5	25	10	1.006–1.019
VLDL	17	55	4	16	8	0.94–1.006

HDL, high-density lipoprotein; IDL, intermediate-density lipoprotein; VLDL, very low-density lipoprotein.
LDL, low-density lipoprotein

carbon fragments (beta-oxidation) in the form of acetyl-CoA (Fig. 58-7). These acetyl-CoA molecules enter the citric acid cycle in the same manner as acetyl-CoA forme d from pyruvate during the metabolism of glucose, ultimately leading to formation of ATP. In the liver, two molecules of acetyl-CoA formed from the degradation of fatty acids can combine to form acetoacetic acid (Fig. 58-7). A substantial amount of acetoacetic acid is converted to beta-hydroxybutyric acid and small amounts of acetone. In the absence of adequate carbohydrate metabolism (starvation or uncontrolled diabetes mellitus), large quantities of acetoacetic acid, beta-hydroxybutyric acid, and acetone accumulate in the blood to produce ketosis because almost all the energy of the body must come from metabolism of lipids.

In contrast to glycogen, large amounts of lipids can be stored in adipose tissue and in the liver. A major function of adipose tissue is to store triglycerides until they are needed for energy. Epinephrine and norepinephrine activate triglyceride lipase in cells, leading to mobilization of fatty acids.

PROTEIN METABOLISM

Approximately 75% of the solid constituents of the body are proteins (Table 58-3). All proteins are composed of the same 20 amino acids, and several of these must be supplied in the diet because they cannot be formed endogenously (es-

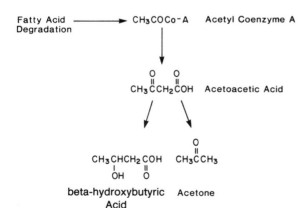

FIGURE 58–7. Fatty acid degradation in the liver leads to the formation of acetyl-CoA. Two molecules of acetyl-CoA combine to form acetoacetic acid, which, in large part, is converted to beta-hydroxybutyric acid, and in lesser amounts, to acetone.

Table 58–3
Types of Proteins

Globular	Fibrous	Conjugated
Albumin	Collagen	Mucoprotein
Globulin	Elastic fibers	Structural components of cells
Fibrinogen	Keratin	
Hemoglobin	Actin	
Enzymes	Myosin	
Nucleoproteins		

Table 58-4
Amino Acids

Essential	Nonessential
Arginine	Alanine
Histidine	Asparagine
Isoleucine	Aspartic acid
Leucine	Cysteine
Lysine	Glutamic acid
Methionine	Glutamine
Phenylalanine	Glycine
Threonine	Proline
Tryptophan	Serine
Valine	Tyrosine

sential amino acids) (Table 58-4). Endogenous synthesis of amino acids depends first on the formation of appropriate alpha-keto acids. For example, pyruvate formed during the glycolytic breakdown of glucose is the keto acid precursor of alanine. Each amino acid has an acidic group (COOH) and a nitrogen radical usually represented by an amino group (Fig. 58-8). In proteins, amino acids are connected into long chains by peptide linkages. Even the smallest proteins characteristically contain more than 20 amino acids combined by peptide linkages, whereas complex proteins have as many as 100,000 amino acids. In addition, more than one amino acid chain in a protein may be bound together by hydrogen bonds, hydrophobic bonds, and electrostatic forces. The type of protein formed by the cell is genetically determined.

Amino acids are relatively strong acids and exist in the blood principally in the ionized form. Even after a meal, the blood amino acid concentration increases only a few milligrams, reflecting a rapid tissue uptake, especially by the liver. Passage of amino acids into cells requires active transport mechanisms, because these substances are too large to pass through channels in cell membranes. In proximal renal tubules, amino acids that have entered the glomerular filtrate are actively transported back into the blood. These transport mechanisms have maximums above which amino acids appear in the urine. In the normal person, however, loss of amino acids in the urine each day is negligible.

Storage of Amino Acids

Immediately after entry into cells, amino acids are conjugated under the influence of intracellular enzymes into cellular proteins. As a result, concentrations of amino acids inside cells remain low. Indeed, storage of large amounts of amino acids does not occur, but rather these substances are stored as actual proteins in the liver, kidneys, and gastrointestinal mucosa. Nevertheless, these proteins can be rapidly decomposed again into amino acids under the influence of intracellular liposomal digestive enzymes. The resulting amino acids can then be transported out of cells into blood to maintain optimal plasma amino acid concentrations. Tissues can synthesize new proteins from amino acids in blood. This response is especially apparent in relation to protein synthesis in cancer cells. Cancer cells are prolific users of amino acids, and, simultaneously, the proteins of other tissues become markedly depleted.

Plasma Proteins

Plasma proteins are represented by (1) albumin, which provides colloid osmotic pressure; (2) globulins necessary for natural and acquired immunity; and (3) fibrinogen, which polymerizes into long fibrin threads during coagulation of blood. Essentially, all plasma albumin and fibrinogen and 60% to 80% of the globulins are formed in the liver. The remainder of the globulins are formed in lymphoid tissues and other cells of the reticuloendothelial system. The rate of plasma protein formation by the liver can be greatly increased in situations, such as severe burns, where there is loss of large amounts of fluid and protein through denuded tissues. The synthesis rate of plasma proteins by the liver depends on the blood concentration of amino acids. Even during starvation or severe debilitating diseases, the

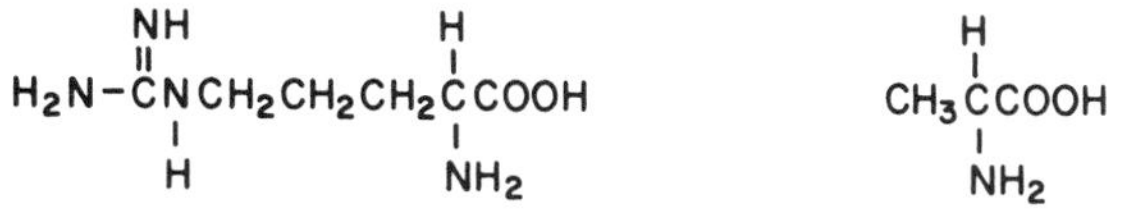

FIGURE 58–8. Examples of amino acids containing an acidic group (COOH) and an amino group (NH_2).

ratio of total tissue proteins to total plasma proteins in the body remains relatively constant at approximately 33:1. Because of the reversible equilibrium between plasma proteins and other proteins of the body, one of the most effective of all therapies for acute protein deficiency is the intravenous administration of plasma proteins. Within hours, amino acids of the administered protein become distributed throughout cells of the body to form proteins where they are needed.

Use of Proteins for Energy

After cells contain a maximal amount of protein, any additional amino acids are either deaminated to keto acids that can enter the citric acid cycle to become energy or are stored as fat. Certain deaminated amino acids are similar to the breakdown products that result from glucose and fatty acid metabolism. For example, deaminated alanine is pyruvic acid, which can be converted to glucose or glycogen, or it can become acetyl-CoA, which is polymerized to fatty acids. The conversion of amino acids to glucose or glycogen is gluconeogenesis, and the conversion of amino acids into fatty acids is *ketogenesis*. In the absence of protein intake, approximately 20 to 30 g of endogenous protein are degraded into amino acids daily. In severe starvation, cellular functions deteriorate because of protein depletion. Carbohydrates and lipids spare protein stores because they are used in preference to proteins for energy.

Growth hormone and insulin promote the synthesis rate of cellular proteins, possibly by facilitating the transfer of amino acids into cells. Glucocorticoids increase the breakdown rate of extrahepatic proteins, thereby making increased amino acids available to the liver. This allows the liver to synthesize increased amounts of cellular proteins and plasma proteins. Testosterone increases protein deposition in tissues, particularly the contractile proteins of skeletal muscles.

REFERENCE

Berne RM, Levy MN. Physiology. 2nd ed. St. Louis. CV Mosby. 1988.

Drug Index

Drugs are listed by generic name followed by trade name(s) in parentheses.

Subject Index

Numbers followed by an *f* indicate a figure; *t* following a page number indicates tabular material. For listing of trade names corresponding to generic drug names, see Drug Index.

properties of, 35, 35t
structure of, 34f
Isoniazid
excretion of, 497
interaction with inhaled
anesthetics, 498, 498f
side effects of, 497-498
structure of, 497, 497f
Isophane insulin, 438t, 440
Isoproterenol, 274-275
add original entries
Isoproterenol, 266f
pharmacology of, 265t, 274
Isosorbide dinitrate, 335, 451

J

Jaundice, 785
cholestatic, erhythromycin-
induced, 492
hemolytic, 785
obstructive
in phenothiazine-treated
patient, 368
in thioxanthene-treated
patient, 368
Juxtaglomerular apparatus,
772

K

Kallikrein, 411
Kanamycin, 485, 487
Kappa receptor, 72-73, 72t,
92
Kent's bundle, 713
Ketamine
action of, 134
allergic reaction to, 139
effects of
on airway, 139
cardiovascular, 138-139,
138t
on central nervous system,
137-138
on hepatic function, 139
on renal function, 139
ventilatory, 139
emergence delirium with,
140-141
interaction of, 139-140,
140f
with neuromuscular
blockers, 146

mechanism of action of,
134-135
metabolism of, 135-136, 136f
pharmacokinetics of, 135-136,
135t
receptor theories of, 134-135
structure activity relationships
of, 134
structure of, 134f
tolerance to, 136, 140
uses of, 136-137
Ketogenesis, 824
Ketoprofen, 258f
Ketorolac, 259-260
Kidney, 769-781. See also
Nephron; under Renal
anatomy of, 769f, 769-770
in blood pressure control, 407,
408f
clearance via
of anticholinesterase drugs,
231
of barbiturates, 105
of drug, 12-13
of local anesthetics, 155
drug effect on
of aminoglycosides, 485
of barbiturates, 113
of inhaled anesthetics, 57, 58f
of prostaglandins, 388,
389-390, 389f
of salicylates, 255
dysfunction of
neuromuscular blockers, 212
salicylate effect on, 255
effect on, of cardiac failure
regulation by
of acid—base balance,
747-748, 748f
of blood volume, 774-775
of extracellular fluid, 775
of osmolality of body fluids,
775, 775f
of plasma ion concentration,
776-777, 777f
Kinetics
first-order, 13
zero-order, 13
Kininogenase, 410
Kupffer's cells, 782, 806

L

Labetalol, 308-309, 308f

Larynx
edema of, corticosteroid
treatment of, 427
innervation of, 720
Laudanosine, plasma concentration of, 206, 207f
Lecithin, 593, 821
Left atrial pressure, 687
Lens of eye, 632-633, 632f
Lente insulin, 438t, 440
Leucovorin calcium, 511, 554
Leukemia, treatment with
corticosteroids, 428
Leukocytes, 805-807
bacterial destruction by, 807
characteristics of, 805
classification of, 805t, 805-807
formation of, 801, 807
Levodopa, 530-533
drug interactions of, 532-533
metabolism of, 531
side effects of
on anesthetic requirement,
532
behavioral disturbances, 531
cardiovascular, 532
endocrine, 532
gastrointestinal, 531
involuntary movements,
531-532
structure of, 531f
Levorphanol, 70t, 96
Levothyroxine, 416
LH. See Luteinizing hormone
Lidocaine
effect of
on anesthetic requirement,
167, 167f
cardiovascular, 160-161, 161t
on central nervous system,
159-160
in grand mal seizure
suppression, 168
on ventilatory response to
hypoxia, 161
efficacy of, 343t
history of, 148
interactions of
with cimetidine, 402
with neuromuscular
blockers, 198
mechanism of action of,
345-346
metabolism of, 153-154, 154f

ISBN 0-397-51129-9